FAMILY MEDICAL GUIDE

Edited by A. M. Cooke, DM FRCP

Designed by Arthur Lockwood

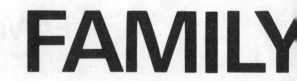

The Royal Society of Medicine

MEDICAL GUIDE

PEERAGE BOOKS

First published in Great Britain in 1980 by
Longman Group Limited

This edition published in 1988 by
Peerage Books
Michelin House
81 Fulham Road
London SW3 6RB

ISBN 1 85052 118 2

Printed in Hungary

Dr. A. M. Cooke is an Honorary Consulting Physician to
the Radcliffe Infirmary and United Oxford Hospitals.
Formerly May Reader in Medicine at Oxford, he is an
Emeritus Fellow of Merton College. He has served as Senior
Censor of the Royal College of Physicians of London,
President of the Section of Medicine of the Royal Society of
Medicine, and as a member of the General Medical
Council. He is an Honorary Fellow of the Royal Society of
Medicine, an Honorary Member of the Association of
Physicians of Great Britain and Ireland, and an Honorary
Member of the Royal College of Radiologists. He was
editor of the *Quarterly Journal of Medicine* for 28 years, and is
the author of two books and a number of papers on
medicine and the history of medicine.

Donald G. Cooley, the editor of the Better Homes and
Gardens Family Medical Guide, has had a distinguished
career spanning four decades as an editor and writer of
medical subjects. Formerly science and medicine editor of
The Literary Digest, he was the editor of *Your Health and Your
Life* from 1938–60 and has written and edited more than
twelve medical books, including the Better Homes and
Gardens best-selling *Eat and Stay Slim*, the *Diet Book*, and
Nutrition For Your Family.

Foreword

This book derives from the original American version of the *Family Medical Guide*, first published in 1964 by the Meredith Corporation in their Better Homes and Gardens Series, with various reprintings and a revision since. Its 30 original contributors included many of the most distinguished names in American medicine, to whom we gladly offer our thanks and admiration for their work. The book at once appealed to the American public, and has rightly enjoyed phenomenal sales in the U.S.A.

Adaptation of the American book for the United Kingdom seemed at first sight a simple task, but it soon became apparent that there were many problems to be solved. To be expected were the minor differences in spelling and phraseology; less expected were more serious differences. Some diseases occur in the U.S.A. but not in Britain, while others are more important in Britain than in the U.S.A. Some aspects of medical practice differ surprisingly between the two countries. Public interest in various aspects of medicine is different on the two sides of the Atlantic. Progress in medical knowledge proceeds not in a steady stream, but in a series of starts and stops, first in one branch of the art and then in another. As a result of these and other factors, after only a few years some chapters have been thought to require considerable emendation, while others have been little changed.

Whatever alterations we have felt it necessary to make, our immense debt to the learning and labours of the original American authors remains, and is warmly acknowledged.

Contents

When should I call my doctor?

This is a complicated question but some general principles can be stated. A basic fact is that the family doctor exists to serve his patients. Just as there is an art in how he handles them, there is an art in how to handle your doctor. You will receive the best from him if you use him wisely and with consideration.

If you move to a new district or for some other reason change your doctor, it is wise to call on the new one. It will help him to know something about your past medical history, and any current problems. What is also important, he will know what you look like when you are well.

Doctors have been heard to say that patients should not bother them with trivial complaints. This may be so, but how is the patient to know whether his symptom is trivial or is the beginning of something serious? It is certainly true that there are more minor illnesses than major ones.

For complaints that do not seem urgent or serious you would go to see your doctor rather than summon him to you. By doing so you would save his time because visiting patients in their homes takes longer than seeing them in the surgery. As many doctors operate an appointment system, it is wise to telephone for an appointment at a time convenient to yourself and to the doctor.

Most complaints can safely be left for 24 hours or until the next morning. In fact, many diseases can be difficult to diagnose in the earliest stages, so some hours delay may simplify diagnosis. You should consult your doctor without delay for any

Going into hospital

If your illness requires you to be admitted to hospital, you may find it a strange and bewildering world, but you may be sure that the unusual features are all there for good reasons. Some hospitals provide an explanatory booklet for patients, some have special booklets for the parents of children about to be admitted, and some even notes for visitors. Each booklet will naturally apply in detail to a particular hospital, but some general advice common to all can be given.

You will require pyjamas or a nightdress and at least one spare set, face flannels, toothbrush and toothpaste, hairbrush and comb, handkerchiefs (preferably disposable), a small mirror, dressing gown and slippers, writing materials, and something to read. Ladies will require make-up and a bedjacket, gentlemen shaving materials. Hospitals do not like aerosol containers (such as hair spray, deodorants, shaving cream). Many hospitals ask patients to bring their own towels and soap. It is wise to have your property marked with your name. For light sleepers, earplugs are a boon.

Do not take valuables or much money; you will need only a small amount of money to buy newspapers. If you do have to take valuables, the hospital will not be responsible for them unless they are given to the Ward Sister for safe keeping; she will give you a receipt.

Many hospitals do not have storage space for day clothes, so your relatives may be asked to take them home until you are ready to leave hospital. Also, most hospitals require personal laundry to be taken home for washing.

The doctor must know about any medicines that you are already taking, so hand any drugs over to the Sister. Tell the doctor or Sister if you are allergic to any drug or other medical preparation (for example, sticking plaster).

Visitors provide an enjoyable break in ward routine, but they can be very tiring. Two at a time is enough, and they should not stay too long. Ask them both to sit on the same side of the bed, otherwise you will have to keep turning your head, and that too is tiring. Relatives or friends should keep away if they have a cough, cold, or other infection, both for your sake and that of the other patients in the ward. Visitors should ask the Ward Sister what foods or drinks (if any) are suitable for the patient. Many hospitals have special rules for visiting by children.

Smoking in wards is discouraged, on health grounds and for the comfort of non-smokers.

sort of lump or swelling, whether painful or not, and for the passage of blood, even small amounts, from any orifice of the body.

There are of course occasions, fortunately not common, when the doctor must be summoned to the patient, even in the middle of the night. Doctors, like other people, appreciate an undisturbed night's rest, and they do better work when not tired, but it is part of their job to turn out in the night when necessary. Situations where it would be reasonable to summon the doctor urgently include the following, but no list can be complete:

loss of consciousness (other than the transient loss from an ordinary faint)
sudden paralysis of a limb or limbs
a fit
a large loss of blood from any orifice of the body

obvious difficulty in breathing
an obvious fractured bone
a burn of any severity
pain which makes the victim grey or sweating
the development of persistent extreme pallor
severe vomiting and/or diarrhoea
very severe and persistent headache
poisoning, especially in children
a high temperature, 40°C (104°F) or over.

If there is any doubt in your mind, it is wise to communicate with the doctor. He may be able to reassure you or suggest immediate action, or he may decide to come and see the patient.

If no doctor can be found, and the condition is obviously *serious*, dial 999 for an ambulance to take the patient to hospital.

Most hospitals provide amenities such as wireless, television, telephone trolley, shop or newspaper and sweet trolley, library, hairdressing facilities for ladies and barbering for men. If you take in your own radio, it must of course be fitted with earphones.

You should remember to take your National Health Service medical card and your National Insurance number. If in receipt of a Retirement Pension, National Insurance Benefit, Sickness or Invalidity Benefit, Attendance Allowance or any other Social Security Benefit, you should look at your payment book to see if the Social Security Office should be notified of your admission to hospital. The hospital's Social Service Department is there to help you with these sorts of problems. The Ward Sister can provide you with sickness certificates, but remember to ask straight away because delay may result in loss of entitlement to Sickness Benefit. If you should develop a disability likely to affect your ability to drive a car, you are required to notify the Licensing Authority.

Your illness is a personal matter. If relatives or friends enquire about you they will be told of your progress, but no information about the diagnosis, treatment, or outlook will be given without your permission. Strictly speaking, this rule applies to everybody, but in practice such information is usually given to husband or wife, parents, or someone directly responsible for the patient.

Although the prime function of a hospital is the care of patients, some have another important function, the training of doctors and nurses. If you are in a Teaching Hospital you may have a medical student allotted to you, who will study and take a special interest in your case. You may be asked to be the subject of a ward round or lecture. These occasions are in fact quite interesting, and they mean that your illness will be gone into in great detail. By taking part you will be making an important contribution to the teaching. If you do not like the idea, you only have to say so.

When you leave the hospital, take care to remove all your belongings. Leave your address with the Sister, in case there is mail to be forwarded.

If you wish to complain about something, tell the Sister. Most hospitals have special machinery for investigating complaints. Do not just bottle it up or complain to your relatives and friends. If you have a complaint the hospital would like to know all about it, so that steps can be taken to put it right and prevent it happening again.

Lastly, do not be afraid to ask questions of the doctors and nursing staff.

Prevention is better than cure

No human being can go through life without facing hazards, such as illness or accident. Fate deals out health to some and illness to others as randomly as good and bad luck. It is plainly a help to be descended from a healthy and long-lived family – unfortunately no one can choose his or her parents. On the whole, therefore, we have to accept what happens, but some illnesses and accidents are preventable and it is worth considering factors that can cause or prevent bad health.

Everyone knows that adequate housing, a congenial job, good food, plenty of sleep, fresh air, exercise, rest, recreation, and cleanliness are aids to health. Avoidable hazards to health include smoking, alcohol, obesity, and accidents at home.

Smoking is an important hazard, especially cigarette smoking. It has been proved beyond doubt by many surveys in different countries, carried out with properly matched controls and strict statistical methods, that cigarette smoking increases the risk not only of cancer of the lung, mouth, and throat, but of coronary artery disease, bronchitis, emphysema, and gastric ulcers. Pregnant women who smoke have smaller babies than nonsmokers and are more liable to have stillborn babies. These are incontrovertible facts.

Cigars and pipes do less harm, but are still a health risk. The argument that one has to die of something is also true, but it is not wise to choose a particularly unpleasant mode of death years before the normal time. Experience shows that it is less difficult to give up smoking altogether than it is merely to cut it down. As well as the cost of the tobacco, smokers pay about £1,300 million annually in tax. They could enjoy many pleasures and indeed luxuries if they spent this money in some other way.

Alcohol is scientifically speaking "a general protoplasmic poison" and as such should obviously be avoided. Actually, if used sensibly and in moderation it is not a serious danger to health. All forms of alcohol are fattening, especially beer. Most alcoholics who die with hobnail liver and other unpleasant complications have drunk large amounts of spirits – whisky, gin, or brandy. Alcohol is a good servant, but a bad master, and the answer in short is moderation. For those who cannot control their addiction there exists *Alcoholics Anonymous*, 11 Redcliffe Gardens, London, SW10 9BG (Telephone 01–351–3344).

Obesity is a serious danger to health in developed countries. Primitive man had to hunt for his food or grow it by laborious agriculture. Modern man has shops or a supermarket in the next street, crammed with the produce of the world, displayed in an attractive manner. This is a great temptation. In the young, obesity is mainly a matter of appearance. In the middle-aged and elderly it is a major matter of health. It was pointed out by the famous Greek physician Hippocrates over two thousand years ago that fat people do not live as long as the thin. The obese are more liable to high blood pressure, arteriosclerosis, diabetes, gallstones, and arthritis of the hips and knees. They are bad subjects for surgery, and stand up to serious illness, such as pneumonia, less well than those who have stayed slim.

Dietary advice on weight reduction is to be found in countless newspapers and magazine articles, which it may be noticed often give conflicting advice. The simple truth is that the recipe for weight reduction can be summed up in two short words – eat less. This is admittedly difficult and requires great determination, but it can be done, and the rewards of success are great. Advice on dieting will be found in chapter 15.

Accidents in the home   After the roads, the home is the most common site for accidents. The most dangerous room in the house is the kitchen, followed by the bathroom, both being especially hazardous for children. A government committee that studied accidents in the home found that 28 per cent could be traced to defective design or maintenance of stairs, hand rails, or lighting. These are not difficult things to put right.

Fire is a hazard to be reckoned with. Metal waste-paper containers, fine-mesh fireguards, and not leaving bedding to air in front of an open fire are all sensible precautions. A fire extinguisher on each floor of the home is a good investment. Oil stoves should be self-extinguishing if knocked over, and alternative fire escapes to the staircase should be considered. Never let children play with matches. Never leave a frying-pan in use unattended – it may catch fire. If it does, cover it with a metal lid or damp towel (which should be kept handy). If you cannot extinguish the flames, carry the pan outside, walking backwards to avoid being burnt.

Electrical equipment can be dangerous. Do not allow any bare wires, do not have wires trailing across the floor, and do not use adaptors to attach more appliances to a socket than it was intended to carry. Children are apt to poke their fingers or metal objects into electrical sockets and may be electrocuted. Child-proof sockets are obtainable. Never use any electrical appliance that can be reached or touched by anyone in the bath.

Medicines and pills Most houses have a cabinet in the bathroom in which medicines or pills are kept. This is a potential source of danger to young children. Such a cabinet should be kept locked, if possible, and every attempt made to keep medicines out of reach of children. When a medicine prescribed by the doctor is no longer needed, dispose of any that is left by throwing it in a dustbin or flushing down the lavatory. Then dispose of the container.

Household cleaners, sprays, and liquids should also be kept well away from children. Never use unlabelled or wrongly-labelled containers. For example, lavatory cleanser in a lemonade bottle has caused tragic and unnecessary deaths.

Pets are a source of great pleasure and instruction to children, but can carry hazards. The younger the child, the closer contact it enjoys with its pets, which may bite or scratch, or transmit parasites or diseases. For example, dogs can transmit leptospirosis, toxocariasis, or hydatid disease. Some kinds of bird can cause psittacosis. All the above conditions are extremely unpleasant and dangerous. If a pet becomes ill, it should at once be removed from contact with the children, and be seen by a vet. Children should be taught never to let a pet lick the face. It is difficult or impossible to prevent contamination of the hands, and this is another very good reason for ensuring that the hands are washed before meals. Pets should have their own food receptacles and never be allowed to feed off or lick family crockery.

Teeth Decayed teeth are ugly and inefficient, and should be repaired, but they have little effect on general health. From the health point of view the teeth that we chew with are more important than those that we smile with. Inadequate chewing is liable to cause various stomach troubles. Some people dread the prospect of false teeth quite unnecessarily. When first worn, dentures seem uncomfortably large, but with perseverance become part of their owner, who eventually feels uncomfortable without them.

Coughing and sneezing Much respiratory disease, coughs, colds, bronchitis, and even pneumonia, could be prevented if people learned how to cough and sneeze correctly into a handkerchief. An unchecked cough projects droplets of infected material ten feet and an uninhibited sneeze travels fifteen feet.

Cleanliness Personal washing needs no recommendation. To wash the hands after using the lavatory is a social and hygienic duty. The possible germs on door handles and money are an unpleasant thought, so it is a commonsense precaution, especially for children, to wash the hands before a meal. Contrary to claims in advertisements, the germs in the water of a lavatory pan do no harm to anyone. It is impossible to eradicate them completely, and if it were possible, they would be there again the next time the lavatory was used.

Recreations Wise men and women have two recreations, a physical one for out-of-doors, and a mental one for indoors. It is important for wives and mothers to have some activity that will for a time keep them away from the kitchen and nursery.

Worry We all become worried at times, and may even fear for our mental health. Some worries have an obvious cause, such as money troubles, family affairs, or bereavement. These are distressing but often fade, and time is a healer, although a slow one. Other worries are sometimes unnecessary or even irrational. A talk with an understanding relative or friend, or your doctor, should help. It is better to share worries, rather than bottle them up inside.

Lastly, adequate insurance against fire, accident, injury, disability, and death will help the peace of mind. Further advice on prevention of accidents will be found in chapters 12 and 29.

Chapter 1

Home care of the patient

Revised by John Fry, OBE MD FRCGP

To every family there comes a time when someone who is ill or injured or convalescent must be, or could be, taken care of at home. An illness may be so trivial and fleeting that no special nursing skill is needed, other than soothing an irritable and grumpy patient. Other illnesses may be prolonged, require rearrangement of a room of the house, perhaps some special equipment, and continuous care of a bedridden patient. For some illnesses, of course, hospital care is essential, at least in the acute stages.

The decision to undertake home care of a patient for any extended time is not to be made lightly. Yet home care is often possible and in the best interests of the patient, if there is someone who cares and can give care. There is increasing emphasis on long-term medical care in the home, for patients who do not need full-time medical attention in hospital. This is also made necessary by earlier discharge from the hospital of both surgical and medical patients, and by shortages of hospital beds in some areas. This chapter describes some common nursing procedures, sickroom equipment, and know-how, which make care both easier to give and more comforting to the patient. Of course, not every measure will apply to every patient. A patient with an ordinary minor upset can be kept in his ordinary bedroom in an ordinary way. But fever, vomiting, weakness, or pain may indicate that the illness is not ordinary at all and that the doctor should be called.

Illnesses that can be nursed at home Most of those who are ill are cared for at home. Only one in a hundred is sent to hospital. It is children and the elderly who are most liable to illness and most likely to be nursed at home. It is normal for children to pass through a period of repeated coughs and colds and stomach upsets between the ages of three and seven. They will also pick up the common infections such as chicken pox, measles, and mumps at this time.

Everyone who lives long enough will be likely to experience the effects of ageing. They will be liable to rheumatism, heart strain, degeneration of arteries (for example of the brain), and eventually to some terminal illness. About one in every three persons still dies in his own home. In their last illness they are usually nursed there by relatives and friends supported by doctors and nurses.

In addition there are those who suffer, unfortunately, from chronic incapacitating illnesses such as strokes, mental illness, disabling arthritis, and other serious troubles that may affect any age group and require long-term care at home. Recently hospitals have been tending to discharge their patients earlier and earlier, and patients convalescent after surgical operations and certain medical conditions such as heart attacks will now often need to be nursed at home. The home care team of nurses and doctors is organized to help with all these problems. Access to it is through the family doctor. Not only is this team able to give regular medical and nursing care, but its members are available to help in times of personal stress and sorrow such as bereavement and other human disasters.

Organization and assistance Home care has always been customary in Britain, and since the introduction of the National Health Service (NHS) it has been more soundly based, with much more support and assistance available. Everyone is entitled to the care of a general practitioner, supported when required by nurses, health visitors, midwives, home helps, and social workers. Usually home care is arranged through the family doctor, who works closely with the hospital services.

All the services provided by these health workers are part of the NHS and do not carry any costs. Through the district nurse or midwife a wide range of equipment is available for home care, such as plastic aprons, syringes and needles, towels, dressings, thermometers, and surgical equipment. Bedpans or commodes may be borrowed and so may walking frames and other aids. Wheelchairs (suitable for indoor and outdoor use) can be ordered by the family doctor. There are services available for the collection and disposal of infectious or soiled material, and there is a special laundry service available for incontinent and similar patients. Special beds and mattresses (such as ripple beds which are needed for patients who must be still) can be borrowed, and local authorities are also able to make structural alterations in the house to help in long-term care.

Home helps will give assistance with household tasks on a regular basis, and meals-on-wheels are available for those who cannot easily cook or shop for themselves. There are special grants for those in the family who care for the chronic sick, as well as social security payments for other needs. Physiotherapy and rehabilitation services are available in the home in some districts for those who require their help.

Good nursing habits   Regardless of the nature of the patient's illness, certain nursing practices should be applied as a matter of routine. Measures which apply to specific situations will be discussed later.

Handwashing   Hands should be washed thoroughly – preferably under running water – before and after attending to the patient. Rub the hands together vigorously and work soap between the fingers and around the nails. Nurses keep their fingernails trimmed closely. Wash around the wrists. Rinse well. If running water is not available, pour clean water from a jug over the hands. Repeat the lathering and rinsing. Rinse the bar of soap after each use. Dry hands well with a clean towel. A combination of moisture and cold predisposes to chapping. Hand cream or lotion can be applied to help keep the skin supple.

Some sort of gown for the home nurse looks professional and protects the clothing. If the patient has a minor upset, an apron or washable cotton dress may be the most practical. If he has an infectious disease (see page 30) the doctor may recommend a gown to be worn and kept in the sickroom.

Waste disposal   Dispose of the patient's bowel and bladder discharges immediately. Provide a container for soiled tissues and bandages. Line it with a paper bag which can be closed without touching the contents. Place it where the patient can reach it. Pick up soiled materials through a fold of newspaper, or use tongs. Provide paper tissues for nasal and throat discharges. The district nurse can arrange for disposal of waste from incontinent and surgical cases.

Dishes   It is a good idea for the patient to have separate dishes and eating utensils. However, washing with hot water and soap, followed by rinsing with hot water and drying, will remove or destroy most germs. Usual dishwashing methods will be adequate unless the patient's illness requires special precautions. Mechanical dishwashers which use water at a temperature higher than human hands can stand are excellent. Dirty dishes, of course, should be washed promptly. Scrape the patient's food scraps onto a newspaper, wrap them up, and put them into the dustbin.

Linen   Collect soiled sickroom linen in a bag or newspaper and wash it in the usual way. After washing, the linen may be dried and ironed together with the rest of the family laundry, unless other advice has been given. A special laundry service is available for the chronic sick.

The sickroom

The ideal sickroom should be cheerful, light, quiet, uncluttered, and well-ventilated, with an adjoining bathroom. A room on the ground floor, at a level with the kitchen, saves stair climbing. Also, a ground floor room is usually closer to household activities and easier to get to when an unattended patient calls for attention. However, a compromise may be required if an upstairs room is quieter and easier to isolate. If there is a choice, select a room that is close to a bathroom. Place the bed to avoid dazzling light or glaring reflections.

Equipment   The needs of patients vary, and different kinds of necessary or desirable equipment will be described later. The main thing is that pieces of equipment should be kept tidily in a cupboard of the sickroom, or the bathroom, or neatly arranged on a table or shelves, so that they are at hand when the nurse needs them.

A few things are essential. The patient should have some means of attracting attention – a bell or a buzzer. There should be a bedside table within the

Chapter 1 Home care of the patient

patient's reach, for a glass of water, paper tissues, perhaps a book or magazine or clock. The doctor will usually allow a radio. An ordinary night table may be too small to accommodate the desired items. A tea trolley on castors, with a shelf, is quite practical and can be rolled aside while the bed is being made.

There should be a wastepaper basket, lined with newspapers or a paper bag into which used tissues and dressings may be dropped. A paper bag, rolled at the top to make a rim that keeps it open, can be pinned to the side of the mattress within easy reach of the patient.

Furnishings No sickroom should be cleared to a state of bareness. Leave some of the amenities that soften harshness and cheer the patient. His emotional attitudes are important to his getting well.

A rug or carpet that covers most of the floor may be left where it is, but remove small rugs that could be tripped over or may slide when the patient steps on them.

Leave everything that is easily laundered – curtains that soften glare, dressing table covers, table mats. Get rid of excesses that give a cluttered look or impair nursing efficiency. A table will be needed – a sturdy card table or something comparable – for washbasins, jugs, trays, and the like, so that articles are within reach when needed.

A comfortable chair for the patient, if he can sit up, is essential. Add a plain chair for the nurse, and another chair if visitors are permitted and the room is large enough. Removal of a large upholstered chair may leave room for one or two plain ones, and give the room a more airy look. A footstool which helps the patient to get out of bed can also serve as a rest for his legs when he is sitting in a chair.

Check the position of room lamps so they do not cause glare to the patient. A sick person should not look at a lamp that has part of a bare bulb visible – and neither should a well person. A switch for turning on a lamp at night should be within reach of the patient in bed.

Dust the room with a damp cloth or mop. Keep the carpets clean and avoid stirring up dust. The woodwork and exposed floors can be washed down occasionally with water and soap or detergent.

Room ventilation In cool weather the room temperature should be kept evenly at about 18° to 21°C (65° to 70°F) in the daytime and a few degrees lower at night. Fresh air is not necessarily cold air. A cold sleeping room is not ideal for everybody, and certainly not for people who are ill. Babies put

carefully to bed in a warm room with a wide open window may kick off the bedcovers and suffer severe chilling when cold blasts of air make the temperature drop sharply.

Keep the sickroom free of draughts. To ventilate a room when it is cold and windy outside, open opposite windows a little way at the top to create a gentle crossflow of fresh air. If draughts are inevitable, the patient can be protected by placing a screen or a couple of chairs draped with a blanket on the draughty side of his bed.

People fall ill in hot weather as well as in winter. Excessive heat is uncomfortable, particularly if the patient has a fever, and is a physical burden on the heart. Fans do not cool the air, but move it. Air moving over the skin, however, assists the evaporation of perspiration, causing cooling. A properly placed fan can draw cool night air into the house, or into a single room. For instance, a good-sized fan can be placed directly in front of an open window of the sickroom, to expel air from the room. Close the sickroom door and open another window. Cool night air can then enter and replace hot room air that is being blown out.

Cooling part of the body cools the whole of it. A good body cooler is a basin of tepid water in which the patient can submerge his hand and wrist or entire forearm. This is practical for a patient in bed. A cool sponge bath is also comforting, and particularly valuable in reducing body temperature in a feverish child.

The patient's bed For a brief illness, the patient's own bed is quite satisfactory. For more extended home care, choice of a bed that saves the nurse's energy is more important. A single or twin bed is easier to make, and walk around, than a double bed, and the patient is more accessible. If the patient is completely bedridden and requires care for a long time, equipment may be loaned by community agencies. The doctor or nurse should be able to answer queries.

The mattress should be firm and resilient. Foam rubber mattresses are good. The patient should not sink into a too-soft mattress. If the bedsprings sag, a piece of plywood across the frame between mattress and springs will add stiffness.

Ordinary beds are lower than hospital beds. This makes little difference if the patient is in and out of bed frequently, and sits in a chair. But if the bed is made slightly higher, this saves much wear and tear on the home nurse, is kinder to the back, and reduces bending and reaching, particularly if the patient

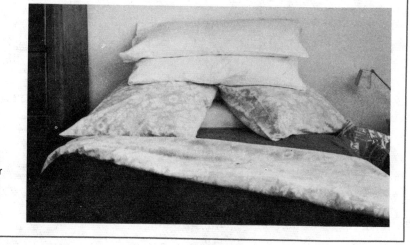

Arrangement of pillows
Pillows may be arranged as shown to give good support for a patient who is partially sitting up. Support should be given to the shoulders and small of the back.

needs constant care for a considerable time. Some height can be added by putting a second mattress on top of the first or by pieces of wood under the legs. Place the bed so that neither the sides nor foot are against a wall.

Comfort with pillows There is considerable comfort for the bedridden patient in the careful positioning of pillows. The human body has joints, bony ridges, and curves that are ill-designed for lying in flat planes on a flat surface. The home nurse should make sure that pillows give support to body parts that are in a state of tension or pressure and help to keep each part as relaxed as possible. A patient in bed needs frequent changes of position not only for comfort, but to help sustain good muscle tone and spread the labour fairly among different structures.

In addition to pillows of conventional size, there should be one or two smaller ones. Pillows for support need not necessarily be ordinary pillows. A small cushion can be put into a pillowcase or a blanket rolled to make a long bolster, or cloth pads may be folded to any shape and thickness. There are no hard-and-fast rules about positioning pillows. You will know that you have done it properly if, when you have tucked a pillow in place, the patient says that he feels comfortable.

Foot supports Footrests serve two purposes. They keep the bedclothes from pressing heavily on upturned toes, and they give the patient something to brace his feet against. It is very uncomfortable for a patient who lies on his back to have his feet pulled down by a tight top sheet that leaves no room for

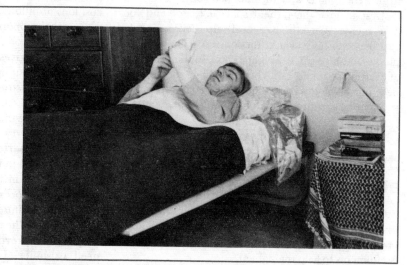

Resting a slipped disc in bed
A slipped disc will often respond to a period of strict bed rest, during which the patient is not allowed to sit up. A board must be placed under the mattress to give support. Note the bag for refuse, which is pegged to the bedclothes.

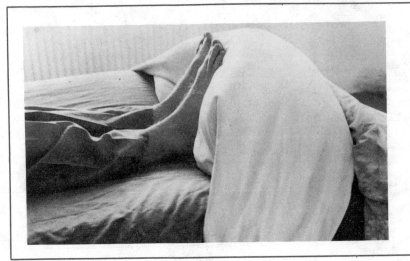

A footrest prevents footdrop
and gives the patient
something to push against.

movement. In time this may cause a condition known as footdrop.

It is quite simple to give footroom to a bedridden patient. All that is necessary is to support the bedding an inch or two above the patient's upturned feet. This can be done in a variety of ways. A fat roll of blanket or one or two pillows can be placed under the top sheet at the foot of the bed. A piece of plywood, a fold of thick foam rubber, or cushions from upholstered furniture can be placed between the end of the mattress and the footboard of the bed. A "bumper" of proper size can be made by cutting and taping a corrugated cardboard box. If the bed has no footboard, a piece of wood can be nailed and braced at right angles to a piece of plywood which fits between mattress and springs. The plywood can be tied to the bedrails if mattress pressure does not hold it firmly enough. Drape the top bedclothes over the footrest to give the patient space for foot and toe movements. When the patient sits up there may be a gap between his feet and the footrest. Close it with pillows, cushions, or a weighted box, so that the soles of his feet are comfortably braced. When making the bed, pinch the top bedclothes together in a pleat or two so they can give and afford room to move.

Common nursing procedures and equipment

Some items of sickroom equipment make it easier to give care to the patient, or make him more comfortable and contented, or both. Here are some useful items to help the patient:

Bed table This should be a flat surface on which the patient's meals are served and which he can use for writing and reading when he sits up or is propped up in bed. Simple U-shaped tables with long feet that slide under the bed and a top that projects above the bedclothes can be bought, and are useful pieces of furniture for many purposes. The tops can be tilted and adjusted for height. Or else a folding ironing board or padded board can be supported by the backs of chairs pushed against the sides of the bed. With a little cutting, taping, and ingenuity, a stout cardboard box can be made into a functional bed table. Cut holes in opposite sides of the box, to accommodate the patient's legs.

A bed cradle is a means of keeping the weight of bedclothing off the patient's body. Here, too, a cardboard box cut with holes that arch over the patient's outstretched body is serviceable. Often, firm cushions or pillows placed strategically alongside the patient will support the weight of sheets and blankets and keep him comfortable.

A bed rope gives the patient something to pull on, to help him to sit up or turn in bed, if he is permitted to. Tie a rope, strap, or nylon clothesline securely to the foot of the bed, with the loose end in reach of the patient. Be sure the rope is strong.

Moving the patient in bed The less time that is spent lying still in bed the better, to avoid weakness, blood clotting in the leg veins, and soreness of the back and buttocks. Always let the patient move or help to move himself if possible. If he is in bed for any length of time the patient must be moved and turned frequently to prevent bedsores. If he is helpless he will need assistance. Tell him what you are going to do before you do it. Remove or pull down top bedding to allow freedom of movement. Roll and slide the patient gently; do not lift unnecessarily. Think of the hips and shoulders as pivots of the body. The patient should be fairly close to the edge of the bed so that the nurse does not have to bend awkwardly.

Turning from back to side Put the patient's ankles together and straighten his legs. Keep your knees against the edge of the bed. Reach across and put one hand around and partly under his far shoulder near the arm joint. Put your other hand similarly around and under his hip. Roll him towards you with an upward pulling motion until he is on his side. Arrange his arms comfortably. You can also put your hands under his near shoulder and hip and roll him away from you. But it is usually easier to pull than to push.

If there is a drawsheet under the patient, loosen it, grasp its far edge and pull upwards and towards you to roll the patient on his side. A drawsheet may also be used to pull the patient towards the foot or head of the bed, or to roll him from a face-down position onto his side or back.

Turning from side onto back Reverse the above procedure. Standing at the patient's back, put your hands on his near hip and shoulder and roll him downwards and towards you.

Helping the patient to sit up Curl one arm under and round the patient's shoulder so that your hand has a good grasp round the shoulder joint. Let your other forearm lie along the patient's chest so he can place his arm under your armpit and grasp the top of your shoulder. At the ready signal, lift upwards and forwards. The patient can use his free arm as a brace

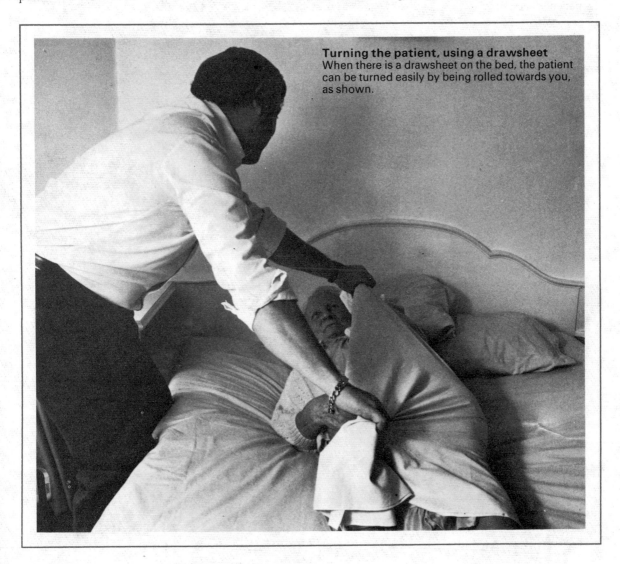

Turning the patient, using a drawsheet
When there is a drawsheet on the bed, the patient can be turned easily by being rolled towards you, as shown.

Chapter 1 Home care of the patient

Making a bed with the patient in it

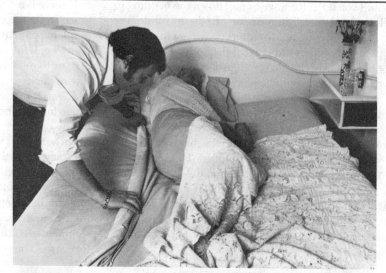

1 Turn the patient onto one side, having crossed one leg over the other to facilitate turning. Untuck the dirty sheet and roll it up against the patient's back.

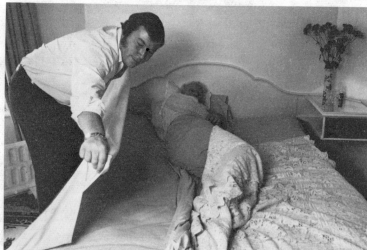

2 Tuck in the clean sheet.

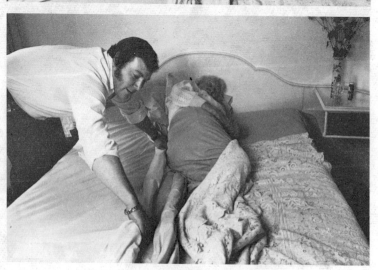

3 Roll the clean sheet up against the dirty sheet.

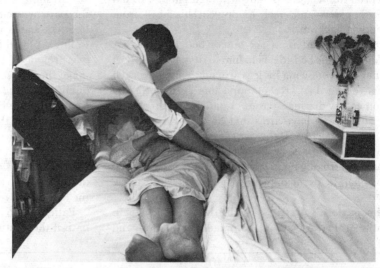

4 Roll the patient across onto the clean sheet. The patient's head should be supported by a pillow.

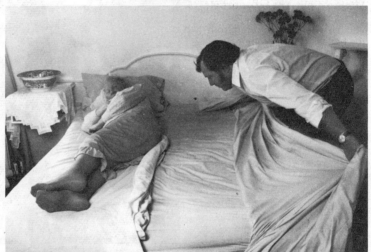

5 Remove the dirty sheet.

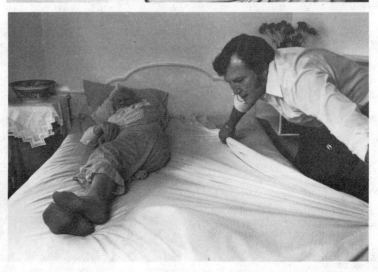

6 Tuck in the clean sheet.

to prop himself. Keep your arm high enough round his shoulders and neck to prevent his head from flopping backwards.

If the patient is to get out of bed into a chair brought to the bedside, help him to sit up and support him while you swing his legs around to hang over the edge of the bed. Keep supporting him until any momentary dizziness passes. A patient's chair should be sturdy and have arms that he can grasp to help himself out of bed. If the patient cannot help himself you may need assistance to get him safely into the chair. An ironing board used as a bridge between bed and chair helps the patient to slide over.

The patient's bath The district nurse can help with bathing. A bed bath stimulates circulation, and is refreshing as well as cleansing. A daily bath for the patient is customary. But use judgement. More frequent baths may be necessary if there is much soiling. On the other hand, overfrequent and overprolonged baths can be tiring and may even make the skin sodden. The skin of elderly patients is often dry, and too much soap and water too frequently applied may cause itching and other discomforts. If the patient has a skin rash, eruptions, or sores, ask the doctor about bath precautions.

You may want to change the sheets when you give the bath. The sickroom should be warm and free of draughts. Keep the patient covered except for parts of the body that are being washed.

Patients who are not too ill may take an ordinary bath if the doctor permits. The mild activity can be

Lifting a patient by yourself
Always be careful to protect you own back by bending from the knees. If the patient is partially mobile and able to help:

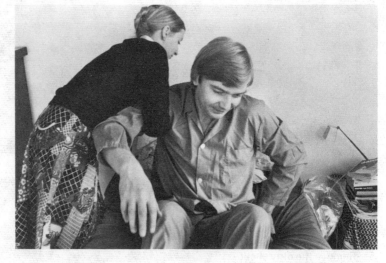

Place your arm under one side of the patient. Ask him to help by pushing down with his heels.

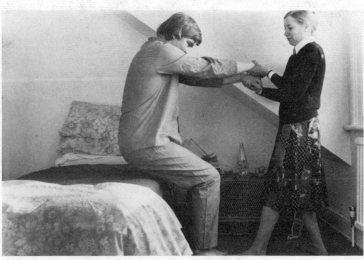

Steady yourself and the patient by placing your foot over his. Grasp both his hands firmly and pull him up by leaning backwards.

helpful. Fill the bath to the desired level with water a little warmer than body temperature 38° to 40°C (100° to 105°F). Have all the essentials – soap, towels, fresh nightclothes – handy. Do not leave the patient alone in the bathroom with the door locked. Keep within earshot outside and speak to him occasionally. Never leave a small child alone in a bath.

Bed baths   The art of bathing a patient in bed is not very complicated if you keep some simple general principles in mind. The photographs on the next page show how to wash a child – the technique applies equally well to an adult patient.

Protect bedding with towels or blankets. Wash each part quickly, rinse off the soap, dry thoroughly, cover, and proceed to the next area. Let the patient help to wash himself if he is able to, even if it is only his face and hands. Collect everything you need: a bowl, towels, flannels, and soap. If the sickroom is not near a bathroom, provide an extra bowl for clean rinsing water, a jug of warm water, and a bucket for dirty water.

It is a good idea to have two lightweight cotton bath blankets. Put one of them on top of the bed blankets, ask the patient to hold it, and strip the bed blanket and top sheet from underneath. Move the covered patient to one side of the bed. Spread the second bath blanket over the bottom sheet with the loose edge folded along the patient's back. Move the patient back onto the bottom blanket and smooth it out on the other side of the bed. Remove the pyjamas or nightdress.

Two people lifting a patient

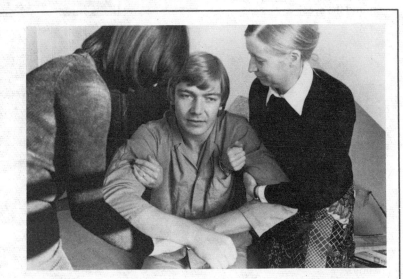

A gentle but safe way to help the patient get out of bed.

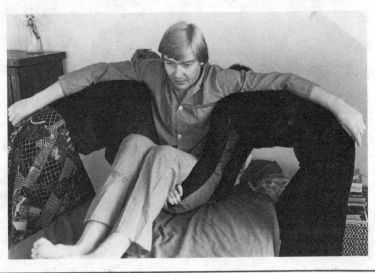

If the patient is immobile and unable to help, two people will usually be needed to lift him. Put one arm under the patient's thigh and grasp your helper's arm. Place the shoulder under the patient's armpit with your other arm supporting his lower back. Bend from the knees when lifting.

Chapter 1 Home care of the patient

Washing a patient in bed
The technique described here can be used for patients of all ages who are confined to bed, for example by a wound or fracture.

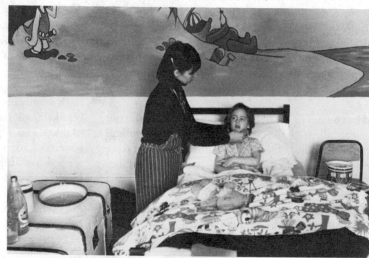

1   Place a towel over the patient's lap. Wash the face, neck, and ears. Do not use soap around the eyes.

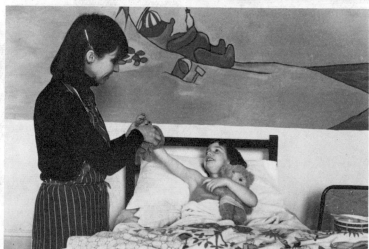

2   Remove the pyjamas or nightdress. Wash arms and hands.

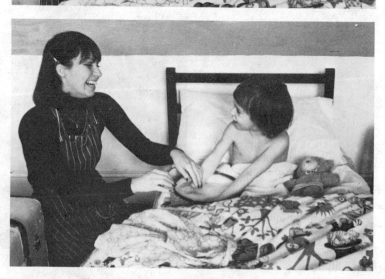

3   The patient may prefer to wash his own hands.

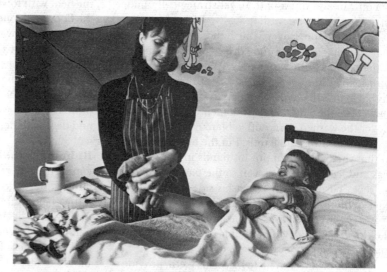

4   Wash the legs and feet. Limbs are easier to wash if they can be straightened. Put a towel under each limb as it is being washed. Work quickly and cover washed parts.

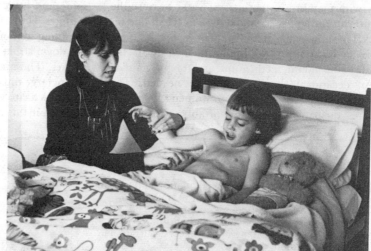

5   Wash the chest and abdomen.

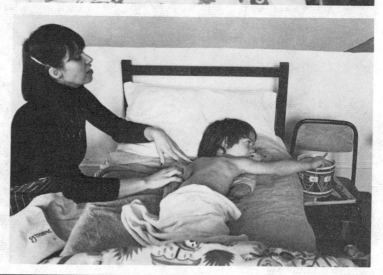

6   Turn the patient on his side – wash the back of his neck, back, and buttocks.

You can also put a bath towel strategically under an arm or leg as you wash it.

Fold the flannel over your hand like a mitten so that dangling ends cannot drip. Wash around the patient's eyes with water only. Wash face and ears with soapy water, rinse and dry. With the patient on his back, pull the bath blanket part of the way down, and wash the chest and abdomen. Work quickly. Cover the washed parts with a blanket or bath towel.

Wash the arms and hands. Put the bowl on the bed so that the patient can put his hands in it. Wash the legs and feet. Place the basin so the patient can soak his feet. Turn the patient on his side and wash the back of his neck, back, and buttocks.

Leave the genital area to the last. Here the patient should wash and dry himself if he can, but assistance may be needed.

If the patient can sit up to brush his teeth, provide a tray with toothbrush, toothpaste, water to rinse the mouth, and an empty basin. Drape a towel around his neck for protection. If the patient is helpless, use moistened cotton-tipped applicators to swab the inside of the mouth, teeth, gums, and tongue gently.

An occasional shampoo may be needed. The easiest technique, especially with women's long hair, is to rest the patient's head comfortably on an edge of the bed, with towels underneath. Put a large basin on the floor, with one end of a tray resting in it, the other end slanted upwards to rest under the patient's head. Wet the patient's hair with water from a jug, work up a lather with the shampoo, rinse and dry. Let the hair stream down the tray so that dirty water collects in the basin on the floor. It is very good for a woman patient's morale if a professional hairdresser can come and deal with her hair.

Rubbing of the back   A good backrub can be very comforting in relieving numbness and stimulating circulation. A good time for this is during or after the bath, before fresh nightclothes are put on. The patient may lie on his side or face down if that is more comfortable. Wet the hands with warm surgical spirit and place them flat on the patient's back. Move the hands to the neck, around and down to the lower spine and buttocks, up and down again for several minutes. Use firm, long, gentle strokes with a kneading motion, a little stronger on the up than on the down stroke. Do not remove the hands between strokes. The area at the sides and back of the neck where large muscles connect with the upper shoulder region is a site where muscular tensions often begin. Massage in this area will be appreciated by the patient.

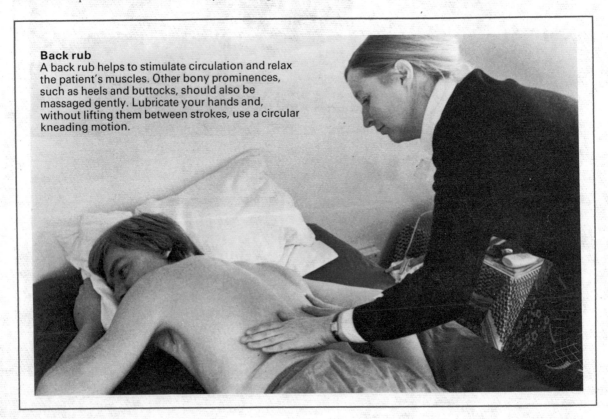

Back rub
A back rub helps to stimulate circulation and relax the patient's muscles. Other bony prominences, such as heels and buttocks, should also be massaged gently. Lubricate your hands and, without lifting them between strokes, use a circular kneading motion.

Pressure care
Pressure sores are easier to prevent than to cure. Frequent turning is required for patients who are unable to move themselves – they should be turned about every two hours.

Right, a simple device to keep bedclothes off the toes.

Below, correct side-lying position; a pillow or pad should be placed between the patient's knees to prevent rubbing.

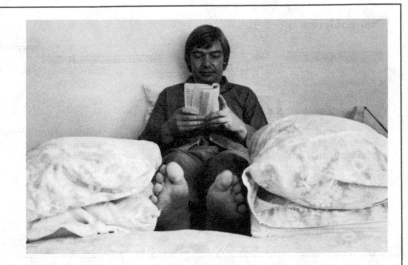

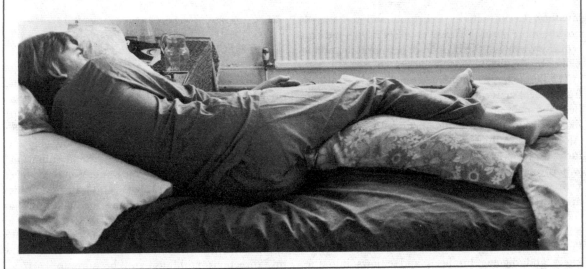

Pressure sores Pressure sores result from continued pressure by the weight of the body resting on bony ridges where the overlying skin is poorly padded. Vulnerable areas are the hips, elbows, sacrum, knees, shoulder blades, heels, and ankles. The earliest sign of pressure sores is tender, warm, slightly reddened skin. Watch for such signs when caring for a patient, and call them to the doctor's attention. In later stages the skin is purplish and may be raw, circulation is impaired, and treatment is difficult. The best treatment of pressure sores is prevention. Here the home nurse is very important. When bathing the patient, inspect the skin for any unusual redness, breaks, or discoloration.

Moisture from discharge is likely to cause the skin to break down. Keep the patient's skin dry. Be prompt in attending to incontinent patients.

Change the position of the patient frequently. Ease pressures on reddened tender skin areas. A pad of foam rubber under the pressure area is comforting. Pads of cotton or resilient layers of soft cloth may be bound or taped over a reddened area. Do not use inflated air cushions unless the doctor approves. Do not rub reddened tender skin areas too vigorously. Wash the area with warm soapy water, rinse, and pat dry, sponge with baby lotion or surgical spirit – unless the skin is broken – and cover with large cotton pads unless the doctor advises other measures. Keep sheets dry, free of wrinkles and crumbs. Be careful to avoid skin friction when lifting the patient onto a bedpan or moving him in bed.

The bedpan Whenever it is at all possible, patients should be encouraged or aided to get up and go to the

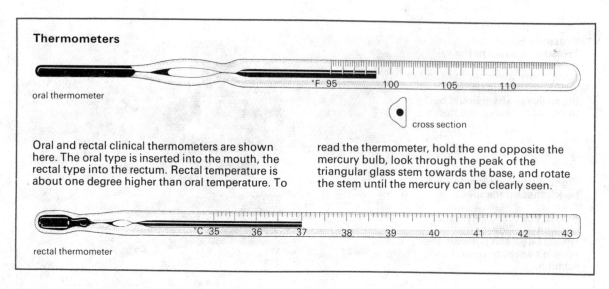

Thermometers

oral thermometer

Oral and rectal clinical thermometers are shown here. The oral type is inserted into the mouth, the rectal type into the rectum. Rectal temperature is about one degree higher than oral temperature. To

cross section

read the thermometer, hold the end opposite the mercury bulb, look through the peak of the triangular glass stem towards the base, and rotate the stem until the mercury can be clearly seen.

rectal thermometer

lavatory. Useful activity is helpful and the seated posture more natural. However, a bedridden patient requires the use of the bedpan or a commode, and a bell or buzzer to let his wants be known.

It is best to buy a commercial model, or borrow one from a local source through the nurse. A cover for the bedpan can be made by folding newspapers around it like a sleeve and fastening them with safety pins. Alternatively a thick towel may be used. It is a good idea to place a large sheet of plastic or other waterproof material under the patient. When the bedpan is needed, remove the cover and put a towel around the opening, or warm it. A bedpan kept at room temperature may feel warm enough to the hands, but not when sat upon. Unless he is totally helpless, the patient can assist matters by flexing the knees and digging his heels and elbows into the mattress. Put your hands under the small of his back, and help to raise the hips while with the other hand you slide the pan under and adjust it with the open end towards the feet. Cover the patient, leave toilet paper at hand, and leave him in private.

Provide a basin of warm water, soap, flannel, and towel. Patients want to clean themselves if they can. Give help if necessary. Empty the bedpan into the lavatory unless the doctor instructs otherwise or there is something unusual about the contents. Rinse the pan with cold water, then brush with hot soapy water. Rinse again, dry, cover the pan, and put it away. If the rim of the pan is chipped, padding is advisable to avoid skin scratches. Be careful to raise the patient so that the skin is not injured by friction when the pan is given and removed. If the patient can sit up, but no lavatory is nearby, a commode is helpful. Protect the floor with newspapers. Male patients may need a urinal.

How to take the temperature

Body temperature varies slightly through the day and in different parts of the body. The skin is cooler than the internal organs. The average normal temperature taken by mouth is around $36 \cdot 5°C$ ($97°$ to $98 \cdot 4°F$). But fever – excessively high temperature – over $37 \cdot 8°C$ ($100°F$) usually signifies illness, and a subnormal temperature may also have meaning. Whether a fever fluctuates, increases, disappears and returns, subsides or does not subside after taking medicines, or has other characteristics, may be important for a doctor to know. The doctor may ask you to take the patient's temperature at certain times or intervals. If so, follow his directions faithfully and be sure to keep an accurate written record of the time and reading.

The clinical thermometer is the familiar instrument for taking temperatures. There are two common types, one for insertion into the mouth, the other into the rectum (oral and rectal). The latter has a somewhat fatter bulb (the part that holds the mercury). The narrow glass tube of the thermometer is about three and a half inches long with short and long lines that look like markings on a ruler on one side of the triangle, and figures beginning with $34°$ and ending with $43°C$ ($94°$ to $110°F$) on the opposite side.

Read the thermometer by holding the end opposite the mercury bulb in your fingers, in good light, and looking through the peak of the triangular glass toward the flat base. There is a little bubble where the clear glass joins the bulb. Rotate the thermometer slowly; the bubble appears to widen. Above it you

26

should see a flat silver ribbon of mercury. If you do not, turn the thermometer one way or the other until the ribbon appears. It disappears completely if the viewing angle is slightly changed.

The end of the silver ribbon marks the temperature reading. The long lines of the ruler-like markings correspond to degrees of temperature on the other side of the triangle. The short lines are usually fifths (two tenths) of a degree. An arrow points to the 98·4° mark (37° C).

Temperatures are most commonly and conveniently taken by mouth. Be sure the mercury is shaken down to about the 35°C (95°F) mark. To shake it down, hold the thermometer firmly between thumb and fingers by the end opposite the bulb and give two or three sharp downward flicks of the wrist. Read the thermometer to be sure that the mercury is actually shaken down.

Place the thermometer bulb well under the patient's tongue, and keep it there for at least three minutes. He must keep his lips closed and not talk or bite on the stem. Do not take the temperature immediately after a hot bath, smoking, or eating hot or cold foods.

Rectal temperature is about one degree higher than mouth temperature. For various reasons, such as dry or inflamed mouth, or nasal congestion with mouth breathing, it may be necessary to take the temperature rectally. The thermometer bulb should be lubricated with cold cream or oil and inserted about one inch into the rectum, preferably by the patient himself. It should be kept in place three minutes or more. In babies and small children it is often easier to take the temperature in the rectum than in the mouth. Place the child face down across your knees, separate the buttocks, and insert the thermometer bulb about one inch. Hold it in place by keeping the buttocks together.

Sometimes the temperature is taken by placing the thermometer in the armpit, with the arm well pressed against the body for five minutes or more. Normal armpit temperature is one degree lower than mouth temperature.

After use, clean the thermometer with cool or tepid water and soap. Hold the thermometer by the top, wipe it with cotton wool and put it in its container. It is not necessary to use powerful antiseptics. Do not hold the thermometer under hot tap water, or in a basin of hot water. The mercury might expand enough to break the instrument. If you cannot read the thermometer, put it away until someone else can. The silver ribbon will stay where it is until it is shaken down. What happens if a clinical thermometer breaks

in the mouth? Spit out the glass. If some mercury is swallowed, it does not matter. Metallic mercury is inert and non-poisonous.

Pulse and respiration

The doctor may ask you to take the patient's pulse and respiratory rate. If so, keep a written record of the reading, the date, and the hour. You will need a watch or clock with a second hand. The pulse is usually taken at the wrist. A little below the base of the thumb, just inside the point where a projection of the wristbone can be felt on the thumb side, an artery runs under the skin of the patient's wrist. Place three finger tips on the artery with the thumb behind. Press just hard enough for pulsation to be felt. Count for 30 seconds and multiply by two to get the pulse rate. Take the pulse when the patient is quiet. For extra accuracy, count the pulse for two 30-second intervals, a little time apart, and add the two figures to get the rate per minute. The average adult has a pulse rate of 72 per minute when sitting, but this can vary a little in either direction and still be normal. Activity and excitement as well as illness can cause changes in the pulse rate. The pulse can also be taken in other areas where an artery crosses bone near the skin surface –

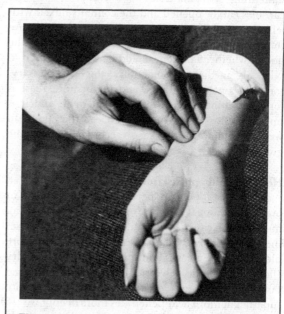

The usual pulse to be felt is at the radial artery. Lightly place the examining fingers (not the thumb) on the bone on the thumb side of the wrist and gently advance them until the bone can no longer be felt and is replaced by the pulsating artery.

Chapter 1 Home care of the patient

for instance, at the temples, or between the anklebone and heel on the inner side of the foot.

Respiration, or breathing rate, is best counted when the patient is not aware of what you are doing. The rate of breathing is affected by apprehension, exertion, and other factors. The resting respiratory rate of adults ranges between fourteen and eighteen per minute, is faster in children, and faster still in infants.

Nursing treatments

The important thing in giving treatment to patients is to be sure that you know what you are doing. A hot-water bottle to warm a bed is safe enough, but a hot-water bottle on the abdomen of a patient whose pains are caused by appendicitis can be dangerous. If you have any uncertainty about doing the right thing, ask the doctor for advice. It is very easy to burn patients with a hot-water bottle.

Giving medicines Check the label and directions each time you give a medicine. You might be mistaken about similar-looking bottles. Measure the amount exactly. Ask the doctor whether tablets should be crushed and given in orange juice (or something else palatable) to a child; or whether capsules can be opened and the contents mixed with jelly for a small child. Set an alarm clock to be sure that medicines are given at specified times. Ask the doctor whether a patient should be woken at night to take his medicine. Sometimes this is necessary, sometimes not. Medicines, and the doctor's reasons for prescribing them, differ a great deal, and it is important for the nurse to get clear directions, to write them down, and to keep a record of the doses she gives.

Hot and cold applications

Heat applications can be of considerable help in many conditions. Heat is soothing, helps to relax muscles, and eases tensions and pains. Heat increases the flow of blood, dilates vessels, and brings more blood to local areas. Heat applications may be dry (hot-water bottle, electric heating pad, infrared lamp) or moist (hot compresses). Dry heat is more superficial, moist heat penetrates more deeply.

Too much heat can, of course, burn. Do not apply anything to the patient's body that it too hot to hold in your own hands, or which feels too warm to the skin of your inner forearm. Check electrical devices for broken wires and be sure to follow the manufacturer's directions. Check a hot-water bottle for leaks. Fill it about half full with hot but not boiling water. Screw in the stopper a little way and squeeze out the air so the bottle is floppy, not inflated like a tyre. Tighten the stopper and hold the bottle upside down to be sure there is no leakage. Wrap in a warm towel and apply. Refill with warm water when the bottle cools and reapply as necessary.

Remember that a comatose or disorientated patient or a baby cannot tell you that a hot-water bottle is so hot that it is inflicting a burn. Be very careful in applying a hot-water bottle to an infant or a patient who is sedated or semiconscious, or who cannot move. In fact, it is best not to do so.

A hot compress furnishes moist heat. Use folded gauze, flannel, or soft woollen fabrics. Hold with tongs and dip into boiling water. Shake off excess water. Or you can lay a towel over the bottom and sides of the basin, place the compress in it, and pour hot water over it. Lift the towel by its ends and twist to squeeze out excessive moisture. Test the compress on your own skin. Apply loosely to the affected part. A strip of plastic sheeting can be laid over the compress. Cover with a towel or soft cloth, or else use a hot-water bottle to maintain heat and hold the compress in place. Replace the compress with a warm one when the first begins to cool. Continue for as long, and repeat as often, as the doctor orders.

Cold applications Cold compresses may be ordered for comfort, to reduce swellings or bruises, and for other purposes. Cold reduces local circulation, the opposite of heat applications. Check with the doctor that cold treatment is appropriate.

Soak some folded gauze, flannel, or a soft cloth in a basin of iced water. Wring thoroughly so that there are no drips and apply to the affected part. Replace with a freshly wrung compress when the first becomes warm. Stop if there are signs of chilling.

Sponge baths to reduce fevers are sometimes ordered. Rubbing surgical spirit mixed with water is an efficient cooler because of the evaporative qualities of the spirit. However, alcohol may be inadvisable if the skin is broken, dry, or weeping from eruptions, and fumes may be inhaled if rubbing spirit is used lavishly and frequently in poorly ventilated rooms. Cool but not freezing water is always safe (except in emergency treatment of heatstroke). Dip cloths in cool water, squeeze out excess moisture, and bathe the entire body. Apply moist cool cloths to the armpits and groin. Watch for signs of chilling and stop at once if the patient begins to shiver.

Inhalation Steam inhalation is very soothing to congested breathing passages. Inhaled steam helps to soften thick secretions, to ease coughing, hoarseness, and a sore throat, and to make breathing easier. Technically, what the patient inhales is not live steam but water vapour. But this vapour may be hot enough to burn, or a container of scalding water may be tipped over, so take safety precautions. An electric vaporizer is a worthwhile investment. Follow the manufacturer's directions. Quite satisfactory steam inhalation can be obtained from simple household equipment. Pour steaming water into a wide-mouthed jug or container and set it in a pan or basin on a table low enough for the seated patient to lean over it. Drape a blanket over the patient's head and shoulders and above the jug, so that the steamy vapour is concentrated for inhalation. Alternatively a paper bag can be slipped upside down over the jug, with a hole cut under a top edge to deliver vapour to the patient. A rolled newspaper can be used in a similar way.

A croup tent is simply a means of concentrating warm water vapour for inhalation by an infant. Put a steaming kettle or other vapour source at the side of the baby's crib. Be sure it is secure and, of course, out of the baby's reach. Roll newspapers into a funnel which directs vapour into the crib. Any tent-like arrangement which is secure and which confines vapours within the crib space will serve. The top of the crib can be covered with a card table or umbrella and the top and sides with a blanket, except for the side through which the warm water vapour enters the crib.

Enemas Enemas are most commonly given to flush waste from the lower bowel, but there are other medical purposes, and sometimes medications are included. Soap enemas are irritating to membranes. Unless the doctor specifies some other liquid, use plain water. The nurse will usually give the enema, but it is useful to know what she needs and what she does.

Prudent considerations – waterproof sheeting, nearness of a bedpan, commode, napkins, or the lavatory – can be left to common sense. Have everything ready: enema bag or container, nozzle, rubber tubing with stopcock (if necessary tubing can be pinched with the fingers to control the flow), and something from which to hang the enema bag about 50 cm (18 in) above the bed. Unless otherwise ordered, about 600 ml (1 pt) of solution is standard for adults – and it must be warmed. Fill the enema bag, hang it up, and allow the solution to fill the tube. Preferably, the patient should lie on his side with knees partly drawn up. Lubricate the nozzle and insert it gently about 5 cm (2 in) into the rectum. The patient will prefer to hold it in place, but give assistance if necessary. Let the solution flow in slowly; stop if the patient complains of pressure or pain. The patient should retain the solution for a few minutes, if he can. In case he cannot, the bedpan should be placed before giving the enema.

Disposable enemas containing bowel-cleansing solutions can be bought. These contain about 300 ml ($\frac{1}{2}$ pt) of solution which can be expelled by squeezing a plastic bag. The entire unit is discarded after use.

Children and infants Give smaller amounts of enema fluid to children – 300 ml ($\frac{1}{2}$ pt) for children, 100 ml (3 fl oz) for a baby. Use a smaller rectal tube. To give an enema to a baby, lay him on his back and remove the nappy. Protect your lap or the table with waterproof material. The baby probably will not retain the solution so it is best to have him on a bedpan. A tube and funnel or a bag is preferable to an enema syringe, which, if the bulb is squeezed forcefully, can be dangerous. A small soft rubber catheter or baby enema equipment can be bought from a chemist's shop. Fill the enema bag or funnel. Lift the baby's legs by the ankles. Insert the lubricated nozzle about 2·5 cm (1 in) into the rectum, gently. Let the solution flow in slowly. Press the baby's buttocks with a folded nappy to help hold the solution. Have a basin or nappy ready to receive the expelled enema and bowel movement.

Special diets

Sometimes when a child has a minor illness or a patient is convalescing at home the doctor advises a light diet or a bland diet and the home nurse may not be sure exactly what foods are suitable. Doctors also prescribe special purpose diets as part of the treatment of certain conditions. No one should ever go on a very restricted diet without the orders and advice of a doctor. However, some understanding of the properties of various common foods is helpful in carrying out a doctor's suggestions for the feeding of a patient who is not seriously or chronically ill.

Light or convalescent diet A light, soft, or convalescent diet should provide appetizing, easily digested, plainly cooked foods with a limited amount of coarse roughage. To tempt the appetite, serve meals attractively. Do not overload trays. The following are recommended:

Beverages: The usual hot or cold drinks. Nutritious liquid snacks.

Bread, cereal products: Biscuits, fine white or brown bread, or rolls. Cooked cereals, such as rice pudding, cornflour, sago. Cereal with sugar and milk. Rice, macaroni, spaghetti.

Meat, eggs, cheese: Bacon, tender beef, poultry, liver, lamb chops, fresh fish. Tinned salmon or tuna. Soft-boiled eggs. Cream or cottage cheese, cheddar cheese used in cooking.

Fats: Butter, margarine, cream.

Vegetables: Strain if necessary to remove coarse fibres (or use strained vegetables or fruit for infant feeding). Vegetables can be rubbed through a sieve and served as purees or used in cream soups. Or fold sieved vegetables into egg white and bake as soufflés.

Fruit: Juices, purees, strained fruit, ripe bananas, cooked or tinned apples, apricots, pears, peaches (no skins or seeds should be left).

Soups: Broths, clear soups. If cream soups are served, the vegetables should be puréed.

Puddings and sweets: Sugar and jam. Plain cakes. Jelly and custards. Ice cream, mousse, fools. Rice, tapioca, semolina.

AVOID: Fried foods, batter, rich pastries, fat-rich foods and sauces, nuts, pickles, coarse and raw vegetables.

Bulk-forming (high-residue) diets A certain amount of bulky material and plentiful fluids are necessary for normal bowel regularity. Foods that help to correct chronic constipation are those containing extra bulk, water, lubricants, sugars, and organic acids that have laxative effects. Some foods wrongly believed to be constipating are merely foods that are well assimilated and consequently leave very little residue.

High-residue foods: Whole-grain breakfast cereals or those containing bran. Raw fruit. Leafy green vegetables. Vegetable pulps that are high in fibre content.

Low-residue foods: Finely ground, polished, refined cereals; fruit juices, puréed vegetables, milk, cheese, meat, fish, poultry, eggs.

Bland diets The list below gives some common foods that are soft, smooth, free of rough fibres and seeds, and unlikely to cause irritation or any increased secretion of acid juices in the stomach.

Fruits: Remove the skin and strain to remove any coarse fibres and seeds. Raw ripe banana or pear;

cooked or tinned apples, apricots, cherries, peaches, pears.

Fruit juices: Strain and dilute drinks by mixing with equal parts of water.

Cereals: Breakfast cereals, cooked cereals, macaroni, spaghetti.

Breads: White, toast, rolls, water biscuits.

Milk and milk products: Whole or skim milk, butter, cream.

Meat and fish: Lean meat, chicken, turkey, liver, fresh fish, tinned tuna or salmon.

Eggs: Soft-boiled, poached, soufflé, or omelette.

Vegetables: Potatoes (baked, boiled, mashed), beetroot, carrots, peas, spinach, green beans.

Soups: Creamed soups of allowed vegetables.

Desserts: Jelly, custards, ice cream, tapioca, rice pudding, sponge cake, plain sweet biscuits.

Beverages: Weak tea, milk.

AVOID: Coarse breakfast cereals, bran-based cereal, wholemeal bread, fizzy drinks, coffee, pork, veal, broth, bouillon, meat extracts, chili, highly spiced foods, fried foods, gravy, raw fruits and vegetables, nuts, and pickles.

Salt-poor (low-sodium) diets A rigid low-sodium diet requires medical supervision. The doctor will be able to give advice. See chapter 15.

If the patient has an infectious disease

Infectious diseases require extra nursing precautions. If at all possible, the sickroom should be isolated and removed from the flow of family traffic. While it is true that members of the family may have been exposed to the patient's germs during the incubation stage of his disease, it is best to have a separate sickroom and to keep family members, pets, and visitors out of it. Transmission of infection works both ways. A visitor may pick up the patient's germs, but the patient may also acquire some of the visitor's germs, which, on top of those he already has, may complicate his illness.

A gown for the nurse is essential. This can be any suitable light garment which covers the clothing and arms – a housecoat, full apron, long smock. Preferably, it should fasten at the back. Hang it up inside the sickroom. Put it on when you go in and take it off when you go out.

Think of the inside of the gown, next to your clothing, as the clean side, the outside as the contaminated side. Wash your hands before you put it on. Grasp the inside of the gown and work your arms into the sleeves without touching the outside. Fasten. Wash your hands before removing the gown, slip your arms out of the sleeves, and put it on its hanger with the inside in. Wash your hands again. Remember that the inside of the gown is clean, the outside contaminated.

Dishes should be kept separate from the family's. Soak them in boiling water for about ten minutes, immediately after use, then wash with soap or detergent. Paper dishes are convenient; they can be wrapped in a newspaper, with the food scraps, for immediate disposal.

Linen may need boiling for ten minutes before laundering. Some diseases may require special management of bowel discharges. The doctor will give any special directions that may be necessary. He can also advise on what is required by health regulations, and whether or not it is necessary to keep family members away from school or work. There are local facilities for disposal and laundering of infectious and soiled linen.

Cleaning of the sickroom

The final cleaning of the sickroom after the patient has recovered is, in essence, little more than good housekeeping. Fumigation is hardly ever practised now except in special circumstances, such as ridding premises of ticks and mites. Sunlight and dryness destroy most germs in a short time.

Launder everything washable in the usual way. Nonwashable things such as the mattress, thick rugs, pillows, and stuffed toys should be given an all-day outdoor airing in bright sunlight if possible. Rubber equipment which cannot be boiled should be washed in soap and water, dried, and aired in the sun. Wash down the bathroom, the floors, woodwork, doorknobs, and unupholstered furniture with soap and water. Air the room for several hours on a dry, sunny day. Help in these matters is often available from local health services through the district nurse.

Staphylococci

Staphylococcus germs are common inhabitants of the skin and nasal passages. Some strains of these germs cause little trouble, and if they do, are controllable by common antibiotic drugs. The worst strains are called "resistant staphs" because antibiotics have little if any effect on them. Sometimes they are called "hospital staphs" because the resistant varieties tend to proliferate under hospital conditions. Strenuous aseptic techniques and housekeeping measures have done a great deal to reduce epidemics of the hospital staph, but resistant strains are sometimes unknowingly carried into the home. What happens then may not be recognized as due to staph germs. A baby may have impetigo; an older brother a nasty crop of styes. Father may have boils, mother a severe fingernail infection, sister a bad sore throat. There may be minor troubles that clear up without medical attention. The illnesses may come weeks or months apart, and probably will not be attributed to a common cause – a bad strain of staph germs in the house. Suspicion may be aroused by a repeated infection, revealing itself in different ways, which seems to run through the family.

Hygienic measures, some of them quite simple, others calling for a little more effort or alertness than usual, can do a great deal to interrupt chains of staph transmission. Here are some recommended precautions if the doctor confirms that bad staph germs are present in the house.

Take showers instead of baths.

Give everybody an individual towel and flannel. No common towel.

Do not share brushes, combs, or toilet articles.

Keep washbasins, toilet seats, bathrooms, and fixtures scrupulously clean.

Use disposable tissues instead of handkerchiefs. Put paper towel dispensers in the kitchen and elsewhere. Drop these soiled disposable articles into a paper bag, close the top, and burn or discard promptly.

Wash the hands before eating, and after handling the dressings, bandages, or contaminated clothing of an infected person. There are germicidal soaps and liquid germicidal detergents that have longer-lasting germ-suppressing action than ordinary soap.

After laundering towels and linens, press with a dry iron.

Chapter 2
Infectious diseases

Revised by A. B. Christie, MA MD FRCP FFCM

The study of infectious disease is really the study of man and his environment, a study of the struggle for survival. The main difference between man and microbe is size. Man is much larger, but in other respects the two are very similar. Each must adapt to the environment. Each requires food, warmth, air, or some part of it, each must excrete waste products, and each must reproduce. Many microbes find the conditions they need on or inside man's body. They become parasites on him. Sometimes this parasitism causes man no trouble at all. On his skin there are always microbes of which he is completely unaware, and those inhabiting his intestines perform vital functions for him, such as the manufacture of certain vitamins or the breaking-down of substances into simpler forms, but there are many microbes which cause man inconvenience or serious disease. These are termed pathogenic or disease-producing. They may cause a simple skin infection such as a sore or boil, or a severe ulcer such as anthrax; a mild respiratory infection such as the common cold, or a life-threatening attack of pneumonia; a short sharp bout of diarrhoea, or a severe prolonged illness such as typhoid fever. These examples indicate the various ways in which microbes attack the body. Skin contact is enough to cause anthrax; a punctured wound can cause tetanus; a bite from an insect can inject the microbes of plague or malaria into the body; the air we breathe can carry the agents responsible for influenza, whooping cough, smallpox, psittacosis, and many other infections into or through the respiratory tract; if we swallow contaminated food or water, the germs of dysentery, typhoid fever, hepatitis, or cholera can enter the intestinal tract and cause disease there, or they may pierce the lining of the bowel and cause disease in distant parts of the body. So the air we breathe, the food and water we eat and drink, the insects flying around us, and even the earth we walk upon can all harbour dangerous agents of disease, the pathogenic microorganisms. In fact, man and microbe are engaged in a struggle for survival. If man survives his illness he does so by killing the invading microbes, but while he is ill, they are multiplying in or on his body and they can pass from him to other people by droplets from the mouth, in the excreta, or by direct contact; or they may be carried from him in an insect which proceeds to bite someone else. In all these instances the multiplying microbes are enabled to get around. In other words, the patient is in an infectious condition. The disease he suffers from is an infectious disease.

The word microbe used here covers all the microscopic or submicroscopic agents of disease such as bacteria, viruses, and protozoa. These are all different forms of life, differentiated by their size, their ability to lead an independent existence, and many other biological, chemical, and physical factors. Viruses are the smallest, and they can survive only by penetrating the cells of a larger animal, man for example, and by using some of the vital chemical elements in those cells to make new substances essential to their own multiplication. The new viruses then leave the cell in which they have multiplied and pass to neighbouring cells to begin the process all over again, leaving behind them damaged or dead cells. Bacteria are larger than viruses; protozoa are larger still, and both can exist and multiply outside animal cells. Typhoid germs can multiply in warm food, and typhoid fever is often spread by contaminated food. Microbes causing anthrax or tetanus can, in certain conditions of temperature and moisture, multiply in soil. All these organisms are very small and can be seen only under the microscope. There are other agents of infectious disease which are much larger. The mite which causes the itch, or scabies, is just visible as a black speck under the skin. Higher up the scale are the helminths or worms; they may be several feet long. The characteristic which all these agents share is that for at least part of their life they must parasitize another living organism, and for our purpose this means man.

So far we have spoken about infection and illness as if they were the same thing, but this is not always true. Man has protective devices in his body which enable him to tackle and often defeat the invading agents. If it were not so he could hardly have survived in the midst of so many competitors for a place in his environment. One of these defence mechanisms is the ability to produce substances in his blood and tissues which neutralize any foreign, invading substance. Certain germs produce poisonous toxins which circulate through man's body and cause damage in some of his organs or tissues. The diphtheria germ behaves in this way. The germ itself causes some inflammation in the patient's throat, but in addition it produces a toxin there which gets into the bloodstream and can damage the heart, or cause paralysis by invading the nervous system. Tetanus also acts in this way; the germ itself remains in the wound but its toxin spreads to the nervous system and causes the convulsions which characterize the disease. Man's body can produce protective chemicals called antitoxins which, when they meet toxins, rapidly neutralize them. In any one infection the outcome is a mathematical one, depending on speed and quantities. If the dose of toxin is large, it may get round the body and cause damage before the body has time to produce enough antitoxin to deal with it; the patient becomes ill. If the dose is small and the body quick to react, all the toxin is neutralized before any damage is done; the patient does not become ill but suffers from what is called a subclinical infection. In some cases this symptomless infection may render the patient immune against the germ for the rest of his life. This was often the case when diphtheria was common in Britain. Many older children and adults were immune to the disease though they had never suffered from it. They had had one or more subclinical attacks in the past. Antitoxins are specific for the toxins which provoke them. The diphtheria antitoxin protects only against diphtheria toxin; it is useless against tetanus toxin, and vice versa. These antitoxins are part of the humoral, or fluid defences of the body; they are

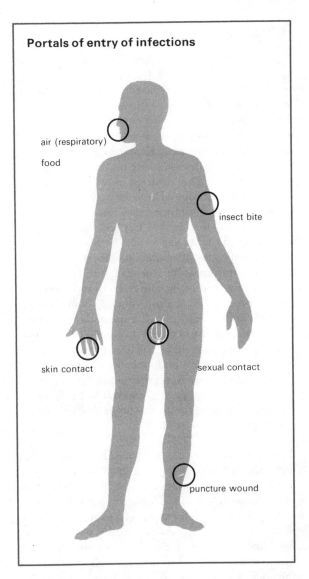

Portals of entry of infections

air (respiratory)
food
insect bite
skin contact
sexual contact
puncture wound

carried in the blood or tissue fluids. The body can produce different varieties of antibodies, which attack and neutralize germs, even those which do not produce toxins. There is a large number of them, able to attack different parts of invading germs, each specific for one germ, and each a part of the humoral defences of the body. There is a second method of defence in which some cells of the human body change their character in response to infection, and this change can protect against infection if it is quick enough and if the dose of infection is small enough. The ability of the human body to react to small doses of infection without causing disease is the basis of immunization programmes. The body is made to react to small doses of injected material just as it does to small doses of natural infection.

33

Chapter 2 Infectious diseases

Immunization

Vaccine is a word derived from the Latin word vacca meaning a cow. Edward Jenner's original vaccine against smallpox was prepared from material taken from the sores of cowpox, a disease of cows, very like the smallpox of man. Jenner noticed that milkmaids who had had cowpox did not catch smallpox, and that set his mind working. He would give his patients a dose of the mild disease and so prevent them getting the severe one. That concept is still the basis of modern immunization. The word vaccine has come to mean any substance used in immunization programmes though it now has nothing to do with cows, and the term vaccination is used loosely to mean any process of immunization. Inoculation is another word meaning the same thing; it is a horticultural term really, and refers to the grafting of a bud or eye (Latin oculus) from one plant into the stock of another. Someone with imagination realized that the implanting of a microbe, a living thing, into man, another living thing, was a very similar process. So we have vaccines and inocula, vaccination and inoculation. Immunology, the science of immunization, is one of the most complicated branches of modern medicine. Our interest here is limited to some of its practical applications.

Toxoids We have already considered toxins and antitoxins. Clearly, it could be highly dangerous to inject a toxin into man in order to stimulate the production of antitoxin in his body; it might kill him instead. So the germ is encouraged to grow in a broth in the laboratory, and produce its toxin which diffuses into the broth. The broth is then centrifuged. That means it is spun round in tubes at high speed so that the bodies of the germs are flung to the bottom of the tubes but the toxin remains in the fluid. This fluid, which contains the toxin, but not the germs, is then separated and treated with chemicals; formalin is often used. The chemicals destroy the harmfulness of the toxin, which is now called a toxoid. The toxoid is harmless, but when injected into the human body it still stimulates the production of antitoxin; if repeated, this process eventually renders the body immune, or resistant, to subsequent doses of toxin. The first dose of toxoid alerts the antitoxin-producing mechanism of the body, but very little antitoxin is produced. After a second dose, given several weeks later, a great deal of antitoxin is produced, and after a third dose still more. The immunity so produced is long-lasting, possibly lifelong in some cases, but a booster dose is usually given some years later to make

sure. The two commonest toxoids are those against diphtheria and tetanus. These are usually given together to infants, two doses separated by six weeks, a third after six months, and a booster when the child goes to school; a final dose of tetanus toxoid may be given when the pupil leaves school. A child given this preventive treatment will escape diphtheria and tetanus, both deadly but completely avoidable diseases.

Bacterial vaccines Some germs produce their damage by invading the human body and attacking different organs directly. Immunization is not then a question of destroying a toxin; we have to try to attack the germ itself. This is done by growing the germ in the laboratory, killing it by heat or some chemical, and then making a suspension of the dead germs called a vaccine. Injected into a patient, the vaccine is harmless but stimulates the production of antibodies against the bodies of the germs, and if the immunized person is later attacked by living germs, these antibodies destroy the invaders before they have time to do any damage. There can in fact be many different antibodies against one germ, each aimed at a different part or property of it; these parts or properties are called antigens. Anything which can stimulate the production of an antibody is an antigen, and one of the aims of the immunologist is to find out which antigen of a germ is the one which stimulates the production of the protective antibody in the patient, for not all antibodies are protective. If the immunologist can separate the protective antigen he may then be able to produce a vaccine containing just that antigen, excluding all the unnecessary antigens and so making a vaccine less likely to cause unpleasant reactions in the recipient. This work is continuing but some vaccines still contain the whole germ and all its antigens. Such a vaccine is TAB, which contains the dead germs of typhoid and paratyphoid A and B. Two injections are usually given and these provide protection which lasts for about three years. The protection is not absolute; nothing in medicine is. If the vaccinated person swallows a large enough dose of typhoid germs, for example in highly contaminated food, he will probably contract typhoid fever, quite possibly a bad attack. If the dose is small, for example in water, he will probably escape. There is no doubt that in military campaigns TAB has greatly reduced the incidence of the disease in soldiers. The ideal way to combat typhoid fever is not by injections, but by good sanitation and pure water supplies. These are often not available in underdeveloped countries, and the

Defences against infection

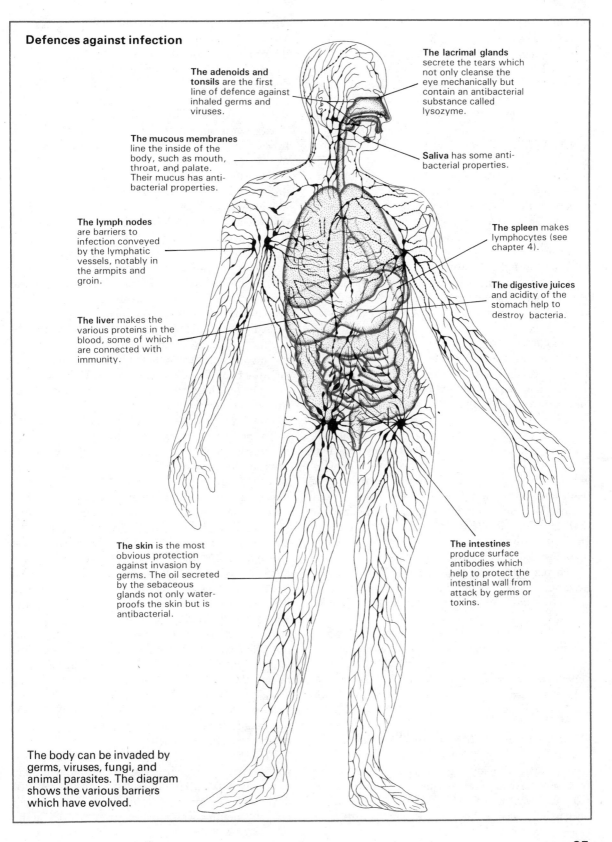

The adenoids and tonsils are the first line of defence against inhaled germs and viruses.

The lacrimal glands secrete the tears which not only cleanse the eye mechanically but contain an antibacterial substance called lysozyme.

The mucous membranes line the inside of the body, such as mouth, throat, and palate. Their mucus has antibacterial properties.

Saliva has some antibacterial properties.

The lymph nodes are barriers to infection conveyed by the lymphatic vessels, notably in the armpits and groin.

The spleen makes lymphocytes (see chapter 4).

The digestive juices and acidity of the stomach help to destroy bacteria.

The liver makes the various proteins in the blood, some of which are connected with immunity.

The skin is the most obvious protection against invasion by germs. The oil secreted by the sebaceous glands not only waterproofs the skin but is antibacterial.

The intestines produce surface antibodies which help to protect the intestinal wall from attack by germs or toxins.

The body can be invaded by germs, viruses, fungi, and animal parasites. The diagram shows the various barriers which have evolved.

Chapter 2 Infectious diseases

traveller intending to go to such places should therefore have a course of TAB.

Whooping cough, cholera, and anthrax vaccines are all killed vaccines. Whooping cough vaccine gives good protection, though very rarely it may cause severe reactions. Cholera vaccine protects for six months only; it may prevent the illness but it does not save a person from becoming a carrier of the germ, and so does little, if anything, to prevent or control epidemics. It is no longer officially required for travellers, except for those coming from infected areas. Anthrax vaccine is effective, but in Britain the disease is rare, and the only people who require vaccination are workers in certain trades who have to handle animals or animal products from abroad. In countries where anthrax is common, animals and their herdsmen should be given vaccine.

Sometimes a vaccine is prepared from germs that are still alive though in a weakened state. This weakening, or attenuation, is brought about by growing the germ under unfavourable conditions in the laboratory. The germ continues to reproduce but loses its ability to cause disease, though retaining its ability to produce antibodies, rather like the toxoids already mentioned. BCG vaccine is one of the most important examples. BCG means Bacillus Calmette Guérin, called after the two doctors who developed it. It is composed of attenuated tuberculosis germs and protects against that disease. In some countries where the incidence of tuberculosis is still very high, BCG is given to newborn babies to protect them against being infected by adult sufferers, and it protects them against tuberculous meningitis, a particular hazard at that age, and fatal unless diagnosed and treated early. In countries where the disease has become uncommon the usual policy is to test children at about eleven years old. Only those shown to be susceptible need be vaccinated. The skin test should also be used for nurses and doctors who are going to look after patients with tuberculosis.

Another live attenuated bacterial vaccine is plague vaccine. Two injections give protection for about a year, and in plague areas doctors and others who may come in contact with the disease should be revaccinated every year. Plague occurred during the Vietnam war, but troops given the vaccine were protected.

Viral vaccines Antibiotics and other drugs are effective against many bacterial diseases, but so far we have no drug with any real effect against viruses. In that respect, then, viral vaccines are more essential than bacterial vaccines. Many viral vaccines are live, attenuated vaccines. Smallpox vaccine is grown on one of the membranes inside the shell of a hen's egg. When scratched or injected into the skin of the patient this causes a sore or pustule to develop at the site. The patient may have a mild feverish illness as the sore develops. He is really suffering from an active infection caused by the live attenuated virus. We call the condition vaccinia, and this is an infectious disease, for it can spread to the skin of another person by careless contact. Although in itself a very mild disease, vaccinia stimulates antibodies in man which are indistinguishable from smallpox antibodies, so it protects against smallpox. In most viral diseases live attenuated vaccines have proved more effective than killed vaccines. With a live vaccine one injection is often enough; with a killed vaccine, as we have seen, at least two are usually required. Measles vaccine is live and attenuated; it is given to children after their first birthday. It may cause a mild febrile illness, usually trivial, but it gives protection, probably for life. Rubella (German measles) vaccine is also live. It should be given to all girls before the age of puberty, because the great danger from rubella is to the unborn baby of a mother unlucky enough to suffer an attack of the disease in the early months of pregnancy. The virus can get through the bloodstream from the mother to the baby in her womb and can cause very severe damage to it in the early months when the baby's organs are taking shape, especially the heart, the eyes, and the ears. Rubella vaccine must not be given to pregnant women because the vaccine virus may get through to the baby too, though it seems doubtful that this attenuated virus could cause damage to the developing baby. If any woman of childbearing age is given the vaccine she must be warned not to become pregnant for at least two months, because of the theoretical danger to the baby. Rubella often causes subclinical infections and by the time they become pregnant most women in Britain fortunately have developed their own resistance to the disease. A blood test can decide if this has occurred and is now routine in antenatal examinations. There are both live and killed vaccines against mumps, but neither has been used to any extent in Britain, because the disease is not thought serious enough to justify its addition to the already crowded vaccination programme. The vaccine has been used successfully in military units in which mumps can be a troublesome disease in new recruits.

There are two vaccines against poliomyelitis, a live and a killed one, the former called the Sabin and the latter the Salk vaccine after the names of the two doctors who did most to develop them. The live one is given by mouth on a lump of sugar or as drops on the tongue, the killed one must be given by injection. There are three separate polio viruses, types 1, 2, and 3, and three doses of the mixed viruses must be given to make sure that the child forms antibodies to all three types. So there must be three injections or three sugar lumps, and obviously most authorities, and most children, prefer the sugar lumps. Theoretically, the live vaccine is probably to be preferred in that, as well as stimulating antibodies in the recipient, it also makes the intestinal canal resistant to any future invasion by wild (that is, nonattenuated) virus, so that the vaccinated child cannot become a carrier of wild virus. The killed vaccine virus, on the other hand, produces only antibodies, without this intestinal immunity. There is some controversy on this point, and it is true that in at least one country, Norway, polio has been abolished by the use of killed vaccine. The live vaccine virus is excreted in the faeces of the vaccinated child for a week or two after he gets the sugar lump, and it is thought that very rarely this virus may regain some of its virulence and cause poliomyelitis in a contact. This is a serious hazard of very rare occurrence; in Britain probably not more than once in four million doses. No process in medicine is entirely safe, and risk has to be balanced against benefit.

There are several vaccines against influenza, most of them killed, though live vaccines are being tried. So far all have been disappointing. The protection is short-lived, not more than a few months, but the main difficulty with influenza is that there are many different strains of virus, and these strains keep changing. Making a vaccine takes time, and by the time one has been developed against a virus currently causing influenza in the population, that virus may have disappeared and a new strain taken its place against which the vaccine may give little, if any protection. It seems likely that the total number of strains of flu virus is limited; a "new" strain may not be a new strain at all, but an old strain which has not been around for many years. Thus, when the "new" Hong Kong virus appeared in 1968 it was found that people born around 1900 already had antibodies in their blood against it. Virologists are now trying to manipulate the influenza virus in their laboratories in an effort to make it produce all its possible changes or mutations in the hope that a vaccine against them all might be prepared. That would be a great achievement, but meanwhile we must make do with the vaccines we have. Mass vaccination with these is not worthwhile. They should be used only for more vulnerable people—the elderly and those with chronic chest or heart disease.

Hepatitis is a common infectious disease and we have no vaccine against it. Two viruses are concerned, the A and the B viruses. Both have been seen under the electron microscope, but until we are able to grow them in the laboratory making a vaccine is difficult. Meanwhile we can do something by giving antiserum and this will be discussed shortly.

Rabies is at present not seen in Britain except in patients infected abroad. There have been several vaccines against it, but until recently most have had very severe side effects, including brain damage. This was due to nonhuman or foreign material in the vaccine. The virus can now be grown on tissue cultures of human cells in the laboratory, and the resultant vaccine has no harmful side effects and is much more effective. One or two injections are enough, whereas with the earlier vaccines large numbers of injections had to be given. Rabies vaccination may be given to people who have to handle potentially dangerous animals, for example in quarantine stations, or to anyone bitten by an infected animal. In the latter case, antiserum is given as well (see below).

There are many more vaccines, those against botulism, Q fever, and brucellosis, for example. These are used mainly for people at special risk.

Antisera The human body takes time to produce antibodies in response to vaccines. Sometimes time presses. One cannot wait for a child infected with the diphtheria germ to produce its own antibodies; the toxin may get round too quickly. An antiserum is serum separated from blood which already contains antibody. Diphtheria antiserum comes from a horse which has previously been immunized against diphtheria toxin. It contains a great deal of antitoxin and can be given to a patient either as a prevention after exposure, or to treat the disease in its early stage before the patient has time to manufacture his own antibody. Horse antiserum is a foreign substance; the human body does not like it, and there may be unpleasant reactions. These have to be accepted when a life is at stake. Rabies is another disease where time is short and antiserum is always given along with the vaccine; it is again a horse serum, with its resulting disadvantages. Antiserum from the blood of people immunized against rabies has been used and, not being a foreign substance, does not cause reactions, but obviously human rabies antiserum will always be in short supply. Hepatitis is a very common disease in Britain and indeed all over the world. Very often it causes a subclinical infection; this means that many adults have antibody in their blood without ever having suffered from the disease. Antiserum

37

prepared from pools of such blood is called human immunoglobulin and can be given to people likely to be heavily exposed to infection – nurses, doctors, and others who deal with hepatitis patients. It is also useful in residential institutions, especially for the subnormal where personal hygiene may be poor. Also, it may be recommended for people going to areas of high incidence and poor hygiene. One can count on antiserum protection against hepatitis A for six months. What often happens in this period is that one gets only a subclinical infection, even after a heavy dose of the virus. This, however, gives permanent active immunity. Active immunity occurs when a person produces his own antibody in response to infection or to a vaccine. Active immunity tends to be long-lasting in most diseases. Passive immunity occurs when a person is injected with antibody from another source, animal or human; such immunity lasts for only a short time, usually only a few weeks or months. Human antiserum against hepatitis B is available but is in rather short supply; antibody must be present in high concentration against hepatitis B to be effective.

Human antisera against measles and mumps are available and may be useful in certain circumstances. A child exposed to measles from a brother or sister has no time to respond to a vaccine; a dose of antiserum, prepared from the blood of someone who has had measles, may protect him, but he should be given vaccine later. Human antiserum against mumps has been used in outbreaks occurring in military units. Antiserum against tetanus (ATS) prepared from horses has long been used to prevent tetanus after wounds. It sometimes causes troublesome reactions. Human antiserum from the blood of people immunized against tetanus is now available though in short supply. It has no unpleasant side effects and is used in selected cases, but active immunization in childhood is a much better way of avoiding tetanus.

Before we leave immunization, why, it may be asked, is there no vaccine against the common cold? The answer is simple. At least 100 different viruses can cause the common cold. So consider the problem of giving 100 different injections to 50 million people. It is not really feasible. The hope may lie instead with antiviral drugs, though there is no sign of a good one at the moment; or perhaps it may become possible to induce specific antiviral protective substances, such as interferon, in the body. This substance is produced in human cells infected by viruses and helps to bring infection to an end. Virologists are studying the possibility of stimulating it artificially, but there is no quick answer to the problem of the common cold.

Prevention has been discussed before describing the diseases themselves for a purpose. Prevention is undoubtedly better than cure in the field of infectious disease.

We can best look at these diseases by grouping them according to their route of entry into the body, respiratory infections, gastrointestinal infections, and so on.

Respiratory infections

A respiratory infection is one in which the germ enters the body in the breath. The germ may attack the upper part of the respiratory tract – the nose or the throat, in the common cold or tonsillitis, or the lower parts of the tract, as in bronchitis or influenza. Alternatively, it may pass through the cells of the respiratory tract without damaging it to reach other parts of the body, as in chickenpox, measles, smallpox, and many others. The most frequent respiratory infection is the common cold.

The common cold Over 100 viruses can cause the common cold. Most of these are rhinoviruses (rhinos is from the Greek, meaning of the nose). The virus enters the nose in a droplet which has, of course, come from someone else's nose or throat. The virus settles on the cells lining the airway and immediately penetrates them because a virus must get into a living cell in order to survive and multiply, thus forming new virus particles. These new viruses escape from the first cell and pass to new ones, where they again use cell materials to form more new viruses. So the process goes on. The invaded cells produce a substance called interferon which has been mentioned already; this tends to stop the multiplication of viruses inside the cells, and meanwhile antibody is being produced elsewhere in the body. Antibody cannot enter cells; it attacks the virus as it passes from one cell to another. So man produces two main weapons in his battle against the invading virus. Interferon tries to stop the viral process inside the cell, and antibody to stop the virus spreading to other cells. It is a question of timing. Whether the person gets a cold or not depends on how quickly his cells form interferon and whether he already has his antibody mechanism stimulated by a previous infection. If the virus gains a foothold, other weapons against it are brought into play, for the virus irritates the lining cells of the nose, and these pour out a watery fluid to try to wash it out: the patient now has a streaming cold. Sensory organs in the nose are irritated; this causes sneezing, and if the virus gets lower down in the respiratory tract the irritated

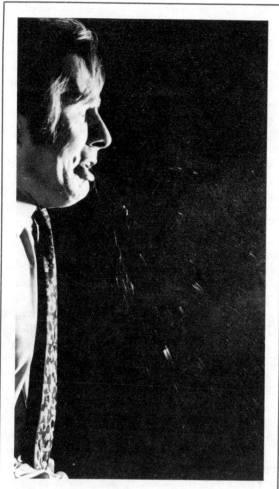

An uncontrolled sneeze. The infected droplets can be propelled for several metres.

It should be added that a cold temperature has nothing to do with the common cold. Experiments have been carried out in which volunteers have been soaked with cold water and left sitting in cold rooms without getting colds. Other volunteers, given every comfort but also a dose of virus into their nose, go down with the common cold. It is true that one often feels cold or has noticed a draught just before the onset of a cold, but this is because one has already caught the cold and is more sensitive to outside temperatures. We get more colds in winter than in summer, but this is much more likely to be due to our change of habits in winter. We stay indoors more and crowd together at parties so that rhinoviruses can rapidly spread from one person to another. Scientists wintering in the Arctic or Antarctic do not get colds in the winter, but they get them in the early summer when relief ships arrive with viruses carried by the crew, or even when they return home to warmer climates and catch viruses from their friends and relations.

Tonsillitis In this condition the germs attack the tonsils and the throat. They cause inflammation in the cells there and this results in pain. The tonsils and throat look redder than normal and there may be a white coating or exudate over the tonsils. Many germs can cause tonsillitis. Streptococci, a type of bacteria, are among the commonest but many viruses cause exactly similar appearances. The doctor must try to distinguish between them, and he can do this by taking a swab of the tonsils. If streptococci are present the antibiotic drug called penicillin is usually the correct treatment, but antibiotics are useless against viruses and should not be given. It is important to make a correct diagnosis, for streptococci can sometimes cause serious complications. The germs may get through to the glands of the neck and cause an abscess, or may, by some process which is not fully understood, cause serious damage to the heart, rheumatic heart disease, or damage to the kidney, nephritis. So it is wise to get rid of the streptococci quickly with a course of penicillin. All these serious complications have become much less common in Britain in the last 30 years, but doctors cannot claim the credit; the decline has been due to a change in the virulence or striking power of the germ itself. If one studies the history of infectious disease over long periods, one finds evidence of waxing, waning, and waxing again in some diseases. The change in virulence of streptococci has not occurred all over the world. In Libya, for example, rheumatic heart disease is still a common disease. Libya is a hot

cells there cause coughing. The secretions, the sneezing, and the cough are all ways by which the body tries to get rid of the virus. It is a question of balance, virus versus man's defences. If the defences win, the cold is over in a day or two with little trouble to the victim. If the virus wins, the victim gets a heavy cold; the thin fluid from his nose changes to a thick, sticky fluid which is full of debris from dead cells killed by the virus, and the coughing brings up thick phlegm from the dead cells deeper down in the breathing tubes. A cold is a fairly simple example of a battle between a virus and the body's defences. It occurs in a restricted field, the cells of the nose and the upper respiratory tract, but it does illustrate what happens in every such encounter in other parts of the body between virus and man. The outcome is not always so simple.

Chapter 2 Infectious diseases

country, so the idea that rheumatic disease is caused by cold and damp is not true. Respiratory infections, so often thought to be due to our cold damp climate are, in fact, just as common in hot tropical climates. Respiratory germs are adaptable and if they can flourish in the hot moist atmosphere of our lungs and breathing tubes, they can be quite as much at home in the hot moist tropics.

Exudate on the tonsils is also seen in other diseases, diphtheria and infectious mononucleosis (glandular fever) in particular. In these the respiratory aspect of the infection is only a minor feature.

Croup This is a condition where a germ attacks the voice box or larynx, the upper part of the breathing tube in the neck (the trachea), and sometimes the higher part of the bronchi in the chest; the medical name for one form of the disease is laryngotracheo-bronchitis, but croup is simpler. The lining cells of the tract are swollen and inflamed. This causes loss or hoarseness of voice and some obstruction to the entry of air. The latter feature depends on the size of the trachea. In an adult it is quite wide and there is usually little obstruction, but in a baby or young child the tube is very narrow and even slight swelling of the lining cells can cause alarming obstruction. Rarely, an urgent operation called tracheostomy is required, in which an incision is made into the trachea and a metal or plastic tube inserted. In less urgent cases, moistening the air breathed by the child may tide it over the worst, and sometimes drugs are useful. Croup may be caused by several different bacteria or viruses, or it may occur in the early stages of more general infections. It is fairly common in the first day or two of measles, sometimes in whooping cough; in both these conditions simple measures are usually enough. The most dangerous type of croup is caused by the diphtheria bacillus, where the larynx is swollen and sometimes covered with exudate. Most of these patients require tracheostomy or some other form of mechanical help. Fortunately, diphtheria is now a rare disease in Britain due to immunization.

Bronchitis When a virus or bacterium attacks the lining cells of the lower part of the breathing tract, the bronchi, the resulting inflammation is called bronchitis. The main symptom is a cough. This is caused by the irritating effect of the inflammation but it fulfils a purpose when there is excess fluid in the bronchi in response to the inflammation. In the later stages of the infection the fluid is thick and sticky because of cell debris, and until this is coughed up the bronchitis will not settle. Some unfortunate people suffer repeated attacks of bronchitis and eventually this leads to a condition where the lining cells are destroyed and are replaced by tissue which lacks the defensive properties of normal lining cells. Germs getting on to this tissue can often pass through it and cause further damage to the lungs. This is the condition of chronic bronchitis and it can lead to extensive loss of lung cells. The patient may suffer from repeated attacks of acute bronchitis which make the condition worse and worse, and he may become a respiratory cripple. This is not an infectious disease in the strict sense in that it does not pass from person to person, but it is the result of germs attacking the cells of the respiratory tract and eventually destroying many of them.

Influenza We have already seen that there are several strains of influenza virus. Influenza A virus tends to cause the large epidemics, the B virus causes outbreaks in between the epidemics. The C virus seems not to be important. The viruses keep changing in type; the virus of one winter may be quite different from that of the next winter. The virus attacks the lining cells of the respiratory tract. In the upper part of the tract it can cause symptoms of the common cold, and a sore throat is common. Lower down it causes the symptoms of bronchitis with cough, some pain behind the breastbone, and sometimes pain on deep breathing. Always there is some feeling of chill and general malaise. In most people the illness lasts only a few days though there is general tiredness for a few more days. In some the illness is more severe and keeps the patient in bed for a week or more. Influenza is often more severe in the elderly, and it is especially dangerous in patients who already have some other illness such as chronic bronchitis or heart disease. That is why vaccine is recommended for such patients every autumn, just before the most likely time for an outbreak. Rarely the virus invades the whole body causing viraemia, or virus in the blood. When this happens there may be no respiratory symptoms, but severe general illness and extreme weakness – this is seldom fatal. The commonest cause of severe illness from influenza is damage to the lining cells of the lower respiratory tract by the virus, for this lets other germs in and allows them to pass through into the lung beyond. These germs may have been present in the patient's body for a long time, never doing any harm, or they may be breathed in from outside. When they reach the lung they set up severe inflammation, which is called pneumonia. As in the other inflammations of the respiratory tract, fluid is poured out in response to the infection, but this now enters into the tiny spaces of the lung where the air meets the fine blood vessels and the interchange of gases takes place, oxygen from the air into the blood, and carbon dioxide from the blood to the air. The affected parts of the lungs become solid and airless.

The patient has fever and rapid respiration, and is often blue. These features are due partly to the areas of the lungs that are out of action, but more so to the toxic effects of the germs. Death in pneumonia is usually due to heart failure, but antibiotics have greatly reduced the risks.

Pleurisy and pneumonia often go together. Several types of bacteria can cause this complication of influenza – streptococci, pneumococci, *Haemophilus influenzae*, and staphylococci. The names do not matter much except to the doctor who has to choose the correct treatment. Penicillin is nearly always the best for streptococci and pneumococci, but not for *Haemophilus influenzae* and sometimes not for staphylococci. The doctor must make a choice of the best antibiotic based on past experience and published data, and on the known history of his patient's reaction to drugs given in previous infections. He cannot wait for laboratory information on the sensitivity of the germ in his patient's sputum to various antibiotics, but he must be ready to alter the treatment if necessary when that information becomes available in 24 to 48 hours. Usually he finds that his guess was near the mark and his patient is already improving when the sensitivity tests come through. Antibiotics have certainly changed the outlook in influenzal pneumonia, but it is still a killing disease, especially in the elderly, the frail, and in those with other illnesses or those who come too late for treatment. Most patients who are properly treated recover nowadays. The germ *Haemophilus influenzae* has nothing to do with the cause of influenza. It is a common organism, often found in the throat or sputum of healthy people. It can become dangerous, as shown above, and it was so often found in influenzal pneumonia, before the influenza virus was discovered, that it was thought to be the cause of the disease. The name has stuck, but the disease it most commonly causes is a form of meningitis, not influenza.

Pneumonia Pneumonia can occur without being a complication of influenza. The same germs and some others may be involved. The changes in the lungs and the symptoms are the same as in influenzal pneumonia though the onset may be less sudden and severe. Pneumonia of this type used to be a long illness of several weeks and it caused many deaths, but now

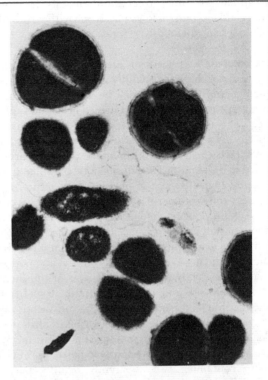

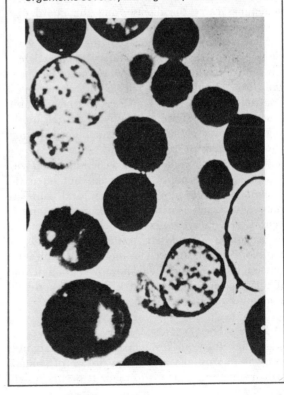

Above, a greatly enlarged photograph of normal staphylococci. Lower photograph shows these organisms severely damaged by an antibiotic.

41

Chapter 2 Infectious diseases

treatment with the correct antibiotic cuts the illness short and mortality is low. This is one of the triumphs of modern medicine.

Psittacosis Psittacosis is a disease spread to man by birds of the parrot family. At least 70 different members of this family may be infected, including budgerigars and similar birds which are often kept as pets. The disease is caused by a germ (chlamydia), a species of bacteria, and it passes from infected birds in their faeces and in beak discharges. It can survive dried in dust and this fine dust can be breathed in by people. It is a disease of bird fanciers, of pet shop owners and customers. It can spread in unexpected ways. One lady, a budgerigar fan herself, visited another lady who had recently installed cages of parakeets in her music room. The visitor noticed that the birds did not look too healthy but she also noticed that there was some dust on the rims of the sherry glasses that she and her father drank from before leaving. She and her father both got psittacosis and they learned later that some of her friend's birds were dead, and her helper was in hospital with psittacosis. On another occasion 26 people who passed through a room containing two apparently healthy parrots caught psittacosis, and in a third incident twelve actors on a stage caught the illness from the thirteenth member of the cast, a parrot. Racing pigeons sometimes carry the disease, and the guard of a railway train carrying crates of pigeons once caught the infection. The way to avoid the spread of the disease is to rear birds in sanitary aviaries where preventive treatment can be given, and to buy birds only from such sources. The import of parrots is controlled by law. Pigeons do carry the infection, but it seems that the strain of chlamydia carried by the pigeons in our public squares is less virulent than those carried by the parrot family.

The disease takes the form of a chest infection with symptoms and signs of pneumonia, but often the general symptoms of malaise, aches, and pains are more severe and sometimes there are symptoms of central nervous system disease such as delirium and even coma. Fortunately psittacosis responds to antibiotic treatment, but it is a thoroughly unpleasant disease. Bird fanciers should know more about it, and if they become ill and need a doctor they should remember to tell him they keep birds.

Q fever The Q stands for query because its cause was at first unknown. It was first described in abattoir workers in Australia and it is a disease of animals which sometimes spreads to man. It occurs widely among animals, notably cattle and sheep, and whole herds may be infected though the animals are not usually ill in any way. The germs are shed in vast quantities in the urine, faeces, vaginal discharges, placentae, and milk, and pastures and sheds can be widely contaminated. Yet somehow the infection does not readily spread to man. It tends to occur in little outbursts. All the people on one farm suddenly go down with the disease though on neighbouring farms, just as heavily contaminated, no one gets the disease. Q fever has been caught from sculpture packed in straw, and it has been spread by drinking infected milk. If blood samples are taken from farmers and others exposed to infected animals antibodies are sometimes found in the blood showing that subclinical infection has occurred, but in other areas where infection in animals seems just as high, no antibodies are found in man. So it is an odd disease, particularly when one learns that the micro-organism is a highly dangerous germ to handle in the laboratory, and bacteriologists prefer to test for antibodies in blood for diagnostic purposes rather than to attempt to grow the germ and risk catching the infection.

The symptoms of the disease are general malaise, aches and pains, and fever, and usually there are some respiratory symptoms such as cough, but the X-ray often shows far more damage to the lungs than the cough suggests. It can be a very unpleasant illness but it responds to antibiotics.

Legionnaires' disease This disease first came into prominence in 1976 in Philadelphia when there was an outbreak among legionnaires attending a conference. There were 183 known cases and 29 patients died. The disease resembles pneumonia in its symptoms. The unusual thing was the very high incidence among one group of people in one place. The disease was related to residence in one hotel only, even to the time spent in the lobby of the hotel or in the street just outside. The other puzzling thing was that at first no germ could be found in the sputum of the patients or in tissues after death. Usually in pneumonia there is no difficulty in finding the responsible germ. Only after six months laboratory work was a germ found – it is a small bacillus, but has not yet been fully classified. The disease is probably not a new one at all. There was a similar outbreak in Michigan in 1968. Blood from some of the patients had been kept in the laboratory and when it was tested against this "new" germ it was found to be positive for antibody against it. There was also an outbreak among holidaymakers who returned from

Spain to Scotland in 1973: again the blood had been saved and was positive. There is still some doubt about the source of the disease, and more outbreaks may occur.

Whooping cough This can be a distressing disease which affects mainly babies and young children, interfering with their nutrition and growth. It lasts for weeks or months, and can throw a great strain not only on the child but also on the mother who has to look after him. A baby in a whooping cough spasm is an alarming sight, and the mother can become very distressed and frightened. After a month both she and her baby can be exhausted. In hospital the child in spasm is dealt with by an experienced nurse who knows what to expect; at home it is very different. Whooping cough is not always a mild disease.

It is caused by a germ called *Bordetella pertussis*. Jules Bordet was a doctor and pertussis is the Latin for bad cough. The germ attacks the lining cells of the bronchi and penetrates into lung tissue where inflammation develops which squeezes the air spaces and produces areas of airless lung; in the bronchi themselves there is thick sticky fluid so that breathing is made very difficult for the child. He tries to overcome this by spasms of violent expiratory coughs, often twenty or more in rapid succession with no intake of air at all. At the end of the spasm there is often a long pause and the mother wonders if the child is going to breathe again; finally he does take a deep breath and as the air rushes into the chest through the narrow larynx it makes a high, hollow whooping noise from which the disease gets its name. The spasm is often followed by vomiting. Some children have 20 or 30 such spasms in a day, others may have only two or three. Older children usually have milder attacks than young babies, though in babies there is often no distinct whoop.

The commonest complication of the disease is pneumonia caused by other germs, such as streptococci and pneumococci, which invade the damaged lung, and this pneumonia used to be the cause of many deaths. Antibiotics usually cure the pneumonia but they unfortunately have no effect on the disease itself, except perhaps in the very early stages when the disease is usually undiagnosable. Treatment consists mainly of patient but firm nursing. A certain amount of firmness is required, because oversympathetic care tends to prolong the coughing. Sometimes whooping cough causes convulsions, probably due to lack of oxygen in the brain during long spasms. Very occasionally it causes coma or death from brain damage.

Tuberculosis Tuberculosis has been partially conquered in most developed countries, but it remains a great scourge in underdeveloped countries and is not uncommon in immigrants in Britain. It can cause damage in the lungs, and the germ can spread through the body; there is no organ which cannot be affected, bones, joints, kidneys, brain, skin, and so on. The disease is discussed in chapter 6.

Other respiratory infections

We are using the term respiratory to indicate the mode of entry, but not all such infections cause respiratory symptoms, as will now be seen.

Smallpox and chickenpox The viruses of these two diseases enter by the respiratory tract but they pass right through the air spaces and into the bloodstream. This carries them to distant parts of the body where for a time they multiply without causing symptoms. This time is called the incubation period. Every infectious disease has a characteristic incubation period. At the end of this time the viruses have multiplied and now they spill back into the bloodstream and spread through the body. In smallpox this causes severe general illness; in the worst cases the patient may die before the rash has time to develop, but in most cases after two or three days of illness the rash appears. In chickenpox the initial illness is usually absent or very mild and the rash is the first thing noticed. The two rashes are similar in many ways but they differ in the pattern of their distribution over the body. In chickenpox the rash is centripetal, that is, it seeks the centre of the body and is more profuse on the trunk than on the limbs. In smallpox the rash is centrifugal, it flees from the centre and is more profuse on the limbs than on the trunk. It sounds easy to diagnose and usually it is easy to tell one from the other, but sometimes diagnosis is difficult, and can be the most critical in medicine; critical, because if one misses a case of smallpox the disease will most certainly spread to someone else. Smallpox is one of the great killing diseases of human history, but in recent years it has been almost eliminated. The virtual abolition of smallpox has been the greatest triumph of modern preventive medicine. It has been achieved by almost unbelievably hard work in remote areas of the world by workers who have searched out every case and vaccinated every contact. In many countries, including Britain, routine vaccination against smallpox has been stopped for several years now, for there has been so little danger of the disease coming into Britain and such sound methods of preventing its spread if it did, that the risks of vaccination are greater than the risks of smallpox. There are risks in vaccination, but while smallpox was rampant these risks were acceptable, serious as they sometimes were. Perhaps in the near future there will be no need for vaccination in any part of the world.

Chickenpox is still with us. Usually a trivial disease, it can be serious, for example in the newborn, or in patients with other diseases such as leukaemia who may be on powerful drugs which reduce resistance to infection. At present human immune serum, from the blood of adults who have recovered from chickenpox, can be used to protect such children. A vaccine has been prepared, for the virus can be grown in the laboratory, but it would not be worthwhile adding it to the already crowded vaccine programme. It can be used in special cases.

Measles and rubella Rubella is often called German measles but it has nothing to do with measles at all, or with Germany. The diseases are often considered together because they cause similar rashes on the body. They both enter by the respiratory tract and, like smallpox and chickenpox, they multiply during their incubation period in some other part of the body. When it spills over into the bloodstream the measles virus causes quite a sharp general feverish illness, with cough, croup, head cold, and conjunctivitis. Spots in the mouth are present for several days before the rash comes out, and are diagnostic of measles. The patient is often very ill, the

Rashes caused by infectious diseases

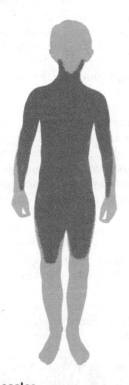

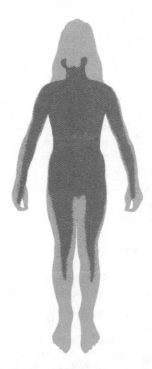

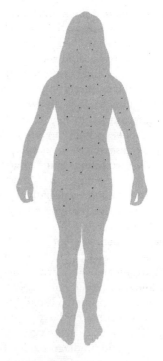

Measles
The rash consists of regular flat pink spots a few millimetres in diameter, which first appear behind the ears and across the forehead, and spread to the trunk and limbs.

Rubella (German measles)
The rash is similar to measles, but less severe, and is usually accompanied by enlargement of lymph nodes, particularly those at the back of the head.

Chickenpox
The rash consists of small pink pimples which become clear blisters and are followed by scabs. The distribution is mainly on the trunk with very few spots on the face or limbs.

disease affecting adults more seriously than children. The rash of measles consists of pink-brownish blotches spread all over the body. It begins to fade after a few days but staining of the skin may persist for a week or two. The temperature also falls after a few days and by the end of a week the patient feels well again. There are unfortunately several complications. Bronchopneumonia is the commonest and, like the pneumonia of whooping cough, used to cause many deaths, but it responds to treatment with antibiotics. The other serious complication is encephalitis (inflammation of the brain), which develops usually as the rash is fading and the child appears to be getting better. It may lead to coma, severe brain damage, or death. It occurs in probably 1 in a 1000 cases. Measles can be a serious disease. In some countries, notably Nigeria, it is still a killing disease.

Measles vaccine is effective in prevention. The only difficulty is that it is easily destroyed by high temperatures or sunlight. Unless good refrigeration facilities are available, vaccine may be rendered useless before it is given to the patient. In the very countries where measles can be serious these facilities are often lacking, so this kind of prevention cannot be carried out. The difficulties in health programmes are not always medical.

Rubella is a much milder disease. There is usually very little general illness, the rash is faint and quickly disappears, there are no important complications and no need at all for any treatment, certainly no antibiotics. Were it not for its serious effects on the unborn child (described earlier in this chapter), we could dismiss rubella as a trivial disease. As it is, it is one of the most worrying; but vaccination with rubella vaccine can prevent the disease.

Mumps This disease is caused by a virus, which gets right through the body and can cause symptoms in several organs. The commonest site of trouble is in the salivary glands, especially in the parotid gland. Parotid means beside the ear, and that is where the typical swelling of mumps takes place, from the front of the ear down into the neck. The swelling is very painful and makes opening of the mouth and chewing most uncomfortable; both parotid glands are usually inflamed, occasionally only one: Mumps virus sometimes causes pain and swelling in the testicle (orchitis) and in the epididymis, the small tubes behind the testicle. This complication is fairly common when young men get mumps and may occur without any parotid swelling. The young man is always worried about possible effects on his virility. He can be reassured that sterility is a rare sequel. Meningitis

may also occur as a complication of mumps, often without parotitis, but fortunately it is a mild self-limiting condition. Mumps cannot be dismissed as trivial. It can be unpleasant, but in at least half the infections with mumps virus the illness is subclinical. There is no drug or antibiotic treatment for mumps; bed and careful nursing are required for complicated cases.

Diphtheria The word (from Greek, diphthera) literally means a hide or membrane and refers to the membrane which forms in the throat in this disease. The germ multiplies on the tonsils and other parts of the throat and forms its toxin there. This toxin passes into the bloodstream and so reaches the heart and the nervous system where it causes its main damage. It is a treacherous disease, because it often begins quietly with very little pain in the throat and a few vital days can pass before one realizes that the child is seriously ill; vital, because early treatment with antitoxin is lifesaving. It is also treacherous because the child often appears to have made a good recovery from the early illness only to develop severe paralyses many weeks later. In the first two weeks, poisoning of the heart muscle by the toxin is the great danger, and many of the most severely ill patients die at this stage. Even if they recover from the heart damage, they may develop paralysis of the throat, eye, swallowing muscles, larynx, heart nerves, breathing muscles, or the limbs from three to seven weeks later and children sometimes die from these late complications. Early treatment with antiserum certainly saves lives and antibiotics may help too, but there is no doubt that the proper way to deal with this disease is to prevent it. Fortunately, diphtheria is now rare in Britain because diphtheria vaccine is one of the best and safest vaccines, which should be given to every child. In many poor countries diphtheria is still a common cause of death.

Infectious mononucleosis This is also called glandular fever, a bad name, for many of the patients do not have swollen glands. The disease is caused by a virus, and one of the striking features is an increase in one type of the white cells of the blood – the mononuclear cells. A patient, of course, is not aware of this. He usually gets an exudate on the tonsils and a sore throat; his neck glands may enlarge and he is feverish. Sometimes he gets a fever and nothing more, and his illness can be puzzling until the doctor carries out some special blood tests. The patient usually recovers within a week or at most two, but somehow this illness has become a fashionable one and the patient often expects a long convalescence. There is rarely any need for this, and there is certainly no need for repeated blood examinations. Some patients have a second attack, but this is never so severe or prolonged as the original attack. Blood tests and other tests in this and many other diseases often take a long time to return to normal – months perhaps, or years. When the patient feels better he usually *is* better and should get back to work or studies. Studies are mentioned because this is often a disease of students: in America it has been called college disease. The virus is called the Epstein-Barr or EB virus. This is very common and is spread all over the world. Most people get infected with it in childhood but suffer no symptoms; the infection is entirely subclinical. If, however, the first infection is in adolescence, then there are symptoms, the symptoms of infectious mononucleosis. Tests have been carried out on university students before entry. Most have evidence of past infection. They do not get infectious mononucleosis, but those who are negative to the test become positive after they enter the university and, in doing so, most get the symptoms too. In several diseases adults suffer more from the infection than do children. This is true, for example, of measles and chickenpox. It is best to get your EB virus before you grow up.

Meningitis Meningitis means inflammation of the meninges, the membranes which cover the brain and spinal cord. It can be caused by many different viruses and bacteria, the former being the more common in this country. The meningococcus is the cause of meningococcal meningitis, sometimes called cerebrospinal fever, which is the commonest type of bacterial meningitis in Britain, except in newborn babies in whom a large variety of different germs can cause meningitis, many of them derived from the bowel. *Haemophilus influenzae* and the pneumococcus are also common causes after the neonatal period, but any germ which can invade the cerebrospinal fluid which bathes the brain and spinal cord can cause meningitis. Not all these germs enter the body by the respiratory route. It is difficult to find a classification which fits all cases. Pneumococci may be present as resident, harmless, and symptomless germs in the throat of a person for years, but reach the brain when something affects part of the skull bones, or if there is a tiny fracture of the bone between the roof of the mouth or the orbit of the eye and the base of the brain. When there is an outbreak of meningitis, however, the cause is usually the meningococcus and this spreads from patient to patient by the respiratory route. Most infected people do not get meningitis; they become temporary carriers of the germ and this can be discovered only by routine swabbing of the throat. Why one person gets meningitis and another remains perfectly well is not known, but it is a characteristic of many infectious diseases. In those who do get meningitis, the germ enters the bloodstream and then passes into the cerebrospinal fluid to set up inflammation of the meninges. In some unfortunate people the germs multiply very rapidly in the blood and the patient may die from a severe septicaemia (blood infection) before the germ has time to cause signs of meningitis. Oddly enough, the onset of meningitis can be a hopeful sign, for meningitis is a curable disease whereas the sudden and severe form of septicaemia is nearly always fatal.

Headache, stiff neck, and vomiting are the leading signs of meningitis. When the infecting organism is a bacterium, these signs increase rapidly and soon signs of brain upset appear – delirium, clouding of consciousness, and in the worst cases coma. Untreated, most cases of viral meningitis are self-limiting, but untreated bacterial meningitis is often fatal, or the patient may survive after a long illness but with signs of permanent brain damage such as paralysis or mental deficiency. Nowadays, provided treatment is not too late in starting, the outlook is good; even patients in coma make good recoveries, but this is not true in neonatal meningitis. Early diagnosis is essential in all cases. This depends on an examination of the cerebrospinal fluid, which is obtained by passing a needle into the spinal canal low down in the back. The procedure is called lumbar puncture. The causal germ can be detected in the fluid, sometimes very quickly, by looking at a smear of the fluid on a microscope slide, but often only after growing it in the laboratory over 24 to 48 hours. The doctor gets exact information about the type of germ and can adapt his treatment to it, but usually he will make a guess at the best drugs to use and be ready to alter this if necessary when results come through. What he usually does is to give a combination of the antibiotics likely to be effective against the severest germs of meningitis and to drop unnecessary ones according to the tests.

Gastrointestinal infections

Gastrointestinal means relating to the stomach and intestines. If a germ enters by the mouth the infection is regarded as a gastrointestinal one. There are many such infections and most of them, but not all, cause gastrointestinal disease. Common symptoms are diarrhoea and vomiting, and when these are mild, viruses are usually the cause. Dysentery and enteritis are gastrointestinal infections which cause typical gastrointestinal illnesses. Poliomyelitis and hepatitis also enter by the mouth but the illnesses they cause are very different.

The route of infection in both groups is through the mouth, mainly by bowel organisms. It is best to be clear about this unpleasant fact. Germs are passed in the faeces of a patient or carrier and they find their way into the mouth of another person in food or drink. Sometimes the germ is passed from the faeces of an animal to the mouth of man, as in salmonellosis. In a few cases the germ is derived from the environment and gets into food, as in some types of food poisoning and botulism. Quite clearly these unpleasant things can happen only where there are faults in hygiene or sanitation. The prevention of these infections requires extensive precautions which are constantly being carried out. Waterworks, sewage works, factory and catering hygiene are all devised to prevent these infections. In developed countries they can be controlled, but in poorer countries control is a daunting matter.

Typhoid fever Typhoid fever is a disease of man only. This at once makes control easier. In a developed country steps can be taken to deal with infected excreta from a patient. The treatment of sewage can reduce the level of infection that passes into rivers and other sources of water supply, and at the waterworks any germs that still remain are destroyed. So water from such a source cannot cause typhoid fever unless there is a breakdown somewhere in the final stages. The germ may get into milk or cream, usually from the hands of a carrier, but pasteurization will destroy it. The germ can pass from a carrier to cold prepared foods and multiply on them, and this remains a danger. Typhoid fever is rare in a country like Britain but this is only because preventive measures are going on all the time. In underdeveloped countries typhoid remains a very common disease. Sanitation can be nonexistent, drinking water comes straight from a polluted river, and there is no pasteurization and very little hygiene.

The typhoid germ enters by the mouth and passes very quickly from the intestine into the bloodstream. It settles down in some internal organ, usually the liver or spleen, and multiplies there. After a period of about fourteen days the germs spread into the blood and the illness begins. The main symptoms are general ones such as fever, headache, and malaise, but there are no obvious diagnostic signs or symptoms like the measles rash. There are many causes of such a fever — the doctor must sort them out by careful examination of his patient and by doing various tests. In typhoid there are often a few small rose spots on the abdomen. These give a clue to an experienced doctor though the inexperienced are likely to miss them. Examination of the blood may show the presence of antibodies to the typhoid germ or the germ may be grown from blood, faeces, or urine. These tests may have to be repeated several times before the diagnosis is made, but meanwhile the doctor has to guess and put the patient on a likely drug. For typhoid fever the best is probably chloramphenicol. During the illness the typhoid germ attacks the lining cells of the bowel wall. This sometimes causes diarrhoea though typhoid is not characteristically a diarrhoeal illness. It does cause ulceration of the bowel wall, and dangerous complications may follow. Each patient must be carefully watched and nursed. Nevertheless, modern treatment with antibiotics has changed the disease pattern. The period of fever is much reduced, but this depends on early diagnosis and early treatment. Both are often unavailable in poorer countries and it is still common there to see patients who are untreated and seriously ill.

Drug resistance in infections All is not straightforward in the treatment of typhoid fever and other infections. We have powerful drugs, but germs do not readily give up their place in nature. Many of them develop resistance to one or more drugs, including antibiotics. This resistance can pass from one microbe to another by a process known as conjugation. One type of germ can infect a different type with its resistance pattern. The common and usually harmless bowel germ, *E. coli*, may become resistant to several antibiotics. This may not matter much, but if *E. coli* comes in contact with the typhoid germ and passes on its resistance, then this can matter a great deal. This has happened, and on quite a large scale, so that there are now many typhoid germs that have acquired resistance to chloramphenicol in this way – a serious matter. This has come about largely through the indiscriminate use of antibiotics, when they are prescribed for trivial infections or for viral and other infections when they cannot possibly do any good. Doctors are sometimes to blame, but in this enlightened age some patients think that they know all about antibiotics and expect to get them for their colds and their aches and pains. It is not only typhoid germs that are affected and not only chloramphenicol. Many other germs acquire resistance in this way and other antibiotics are rendered useless. The solution, at best partial, lies in more intelligent use of these drugs, by doctors and public alike.

Dysentery There are two main forms of dysentery, amoebic, which is mainly a tropical disease, and bacillary, which is common all over the world. Amoebic dysentery is caused by a tiny one-celled organism, similar in appearance to the amoeba we are taught about at school. It is often a lingering disease with no marked diarrhoeal phase, but with late and serious complications, notably amoebic abscess of the liver. It does not occur in Britain except in patients who have been infected abroad. Bacillary dysentery is an acute diarrhoeal disease caused by bacteria. The germ lodges in the wall of the bowel and fluid is poured out into the gut. Watery, sometimes bloodstained diarrhoea results. There are several different types of dysentery bacilli and they cause different grades of illness. The Sonne bacillus is common in Britain and causes mainly mild attacks, which are over in a day or two. Flexner and Shiga bacilli (called after Drs Simon Flexner and Kiyoshi Shiga) are not so common in Britain, but they may cause more severe illness. In tropical countries the diarrhoea may last for many days and lead to exhaustion and dehydration and severe loss of blood from the bowel. If untreated, it may be fatal. Most of the mild dysentery seen in Britain needs no special treatment, though in babies and in frail, elderly patients it may be necessary to set up an intravenous drip to counteract loss of fluid. In the severe Flexner and Shiga infections antibiotics may do some good, but the essence of treatment is to replace water lost from the body.

Like typhoid, dysentery is a disease of man only and infection therefore passes only from man to man. Defective sanitation and polluted water supplies are the main cause of spread, but a carrier can contaminate food and, especially with the Sonne strain, infection can be spread on the hands directly from one person to another. This is often the case in outbreaks in nursery classes and play schools. Control in such outbreaks can be difficult; it consists of careful toilet hygiene, which is not easy with young children.

Salmonellosis Salmonellae are among the most widespread of germs. They infect man and a host of other animals as well. Nearly all domestic animals can be infected, such as cows, pigs, and poultry, and, to a lesser degree, sheep. Even elephants, snakes, seals, pet tortoises, rats, and shellfish may suffer, but the main problem is with cattle, pigs, and poultry. Often infection causes no illness in these animals, though calves can suffer severely. The animals are frequently healthy carriers, and, of course, carry their infection with them to the abattoirs and poultry processing plants and from there into food factories, shops, and homes. The illness caused by salmonella infection is usually inflammation of the intestines (enteritis) with diarrhoea, some abdominal pains, and sometimes vomiting. Most attacks are fairly mild, lasting for only a few days, but some are severe and exhausting. Occasionally the salmonellae penetrate the bowel and invade the bloodstream and then the condition is one of salmonella septicaemia, a condition like typhoid fever. Except for these cases, the treatment of salmonellosis is simple and no antibiotics are required. In fact these can do harm by interfering with the normal bowel germs and allowing the salmonellae more room to multiply. If the salmonellae are grown in the laboratory it can be shown that some antibiotics destroy them. It does not follow at all that in the very different conditions inside the bowel the antibiotic will still work and, in fact, it does not. But, of course, if the laboratory reports the germ as sensitive to an antibiotic it is very tempting to prescribe that antibiotic. Salmonellosis is a common disease in Britain, and if antibiotics are used in this unintelligent way drug resistance, sometimes serious, can result. When the germs get into the bloodstream causing septicaemia, the situation is different and antibiotics must be tried, though results are often not as good as laboratory results might lead one to hope for. The laboratory is, after all, a very artificial environment for germs, and laboratory reports can tell us only what has happened in the test tube. Patients and doctors sometimes regard the laboratory as the place with all the answers, but it is at the bedside that decisions, with laboratory help, have to be made.

Food poisoning Food and poison might be regarded as contradictory terms, yet food poisoning is a common condition in Britain and all over the world. The trouble is that microbes like the same kind of food as human beings and if they can get into it they flourish and multiply. We have already seen that salmonellae can be present on our raw animal food as it comes from the farms. Chickens are probably the commonest source of salmonella food poisoning. Other germs can get on our food from various sources and at various stages in the production and preparation of food. Staphylococci are common skin germs;

Gastrointestinal infections

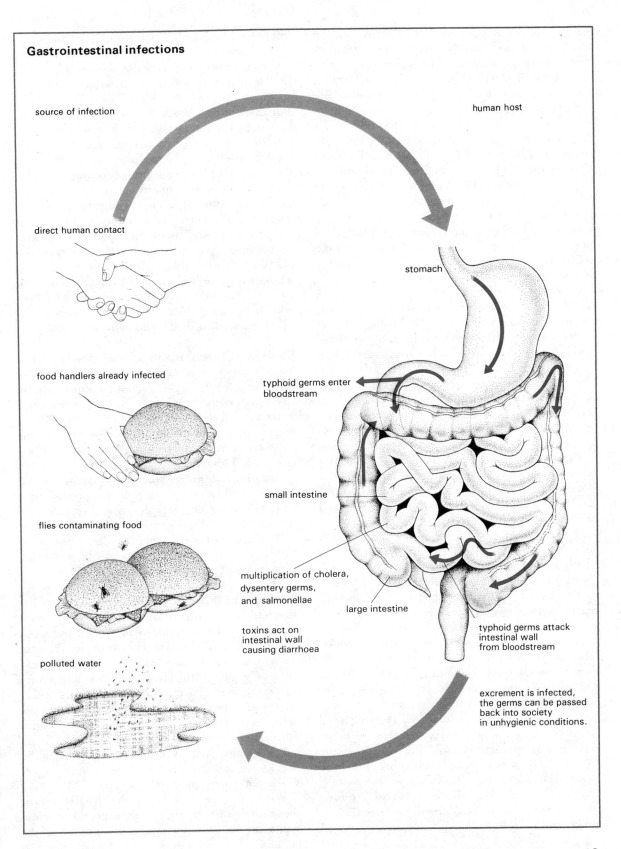

source of infection

human host

direct human contact

food handlers already infected

flies contaminating food

polluted water

stomach

typhoid germs enter bloodstream

small intestine

multiplication of cholera, dysentery germs, and salmonellae

large intestine

toxins act on intestinal wall causing diarrhoea

typhoid germs attack intestinal wall from bloodstream

excrement is infected, the germs can be passed back into society in unhygienic conditions.

49

Chapter 2 Infectious diseases

most are harmless, but some form a toxin which, if swallowed in food, rapidly causes intense vomiting and sometimes diarrhoea. The staphylococci may come from a food handler who carries the germ in his nose, or on his hands, or he may have a sore somewhere on his hands or arms. If the staphylococcus gets into the kind of food that is right for staphylococci, and that food is kept at the right temperature, then it will produce its toxin. The germ likes moisture and a moderate room temperature, it likes creamy foods, and cold meats and pies. If the food is later heated thoroughly, the germs are destroyed, but the toxin remains; it is unaffected by heat and will still cause food poisoning. The moral is not to leave food in the warm; put it in the refrigerator till it is required, and if any food handler has skin sores he should be taken off duty.

Another food poisoning germ is *Clostridium welchii*. The first part of the name refers to the shape of the germ, the second comes from Dr William Welch. This is a soil germ that gets into dust and onto shoes, and is sometimes found in human and animal faeces. It produces a toxin which resists heat, and it likes conditions where there is not much oxygen but some warmth. So it is at home in a stew that has been kept warm. The germ is killed by heat but the toxin survives. Stew should be served hot; any leftovers should be cooled quickly and kept in the refrigerator.

Bacillus cereus is another food poisoning germ. It is present in soil and so is found on green vegetables and potatoes. It can easily get into kitchens, and has caused food poisoning mainly in connection with rice served in Chinese restaurants. The danger is that boiled rice may be left overnight in a warm room, and time is important for multiplication. Next day the rice is gently fried when required for customers, and the frying may not be enough to kill the masses of bacilli.

The causal factors are obvious – germs will multiply in moist warm food. If food is not to be eaten as soon as it is cooked, it should be kept very hot or very cold; food should not be kept warm for hours. Thorough cooking is required to kill salmonellae in poultry, for the germs are often deep in the carcase. On beef the germs are on the surface and are easily killed in the oven. Two things are important with poultry, which is so often sold frozen. Thawing must be thorough, and a large turkey requires 36 to 48 hours in a warm room, not a cold garage, to thaw out. When fully thawed, thorough cooking to ensure heat penetration is essential. In poultry food poisoning outbreaks, one or other, often both, of these requirements are found to have been neglected. The prevention of food poisoning is, of course, a major public health measure ranging from good husbandry on the farm, through first class abattoir management and on to inspection of factories, shops, and kitchens, but the good housewife has a part to play too.

Botulism This is a rare kind of food poisoning, caused by *Clostridium botulinum*. The germ is a strict anaerobe, that is, it lives only in areas of restricted oxygen, so it is never caused by fresh food but only by foods that have had some form of cooking leading to low oxygen content. Inadequately preserved foods may cause botulism. Commercial canneries are all geared to the killing of botulism germs by high temperatures, and botulism from commercially canned food is very rare. Up to 1978, there have been only three outbreaks in Britain in the present century. The last was due to a contaminated tin of salmon. It has been commoner in other countries and it has been said that a study of botulism in various countries becomes a study of food habits in those countries.

Cholera Cholera is one of the great epidemic diseases which at times sweep over the world. The germ is passed in the faeces and gets into water in rivers and wells. People who drink this untreated water are infected with the cholera germ. Most of them do not suffer from the disease but become temporary carriers and they excrete the germ in their faeces too. This in part explains how the disease can spread over wide areas of the world where sanitation is absent or poor. Where there is efficient sanitation and a safe water supply, cholera cannot spread. So in spite of alarms when a single imported case is reported in Britain, there is no danger of the disease spreading within the country on anything other than a minor, local scale and even that is highly improbable.

The symptoms of cholera are severe watery diarrhoea and dehydration. It is the dehydration that kills, and in a severe case the loss of fluid from almost constant diarrhoea can cause dangerous dehydration within the first day of illness. The treatment of cholera is essentially the treatment of dehydration. The fluid must be replaced quickly. Antibiotics play a very minor part in treatment. They may help to get rid of the germ but that is not important in the acute stage of the illness. On the other hand efficient emergency rehydration stations save lives, and cholera is no longer a highly fatal disease. The treatment must be taken to the patient. Cholera patients do not travel well in hot, humid climates.

We now come to some of the diseases which, though they enter by the mouth, cause no intestinal symptoms but cause damage in distant parts of the body. There are many of these but we will consider only a few important examples such as poliomyelitis, brucellosis, and hepatitis.

Poliomyelitis Poliovirus is one of the enteroviruses, a group which enters the body by the mouth and digestive tract. After entry, poliovirus multiplies in the glandular tissue of the throat, in the intestine, and in the lymph nodes which drain it. In most infected people there are no symptoms. For every one patient who develops symptoms there are a hundred or perhaps a thousand others infected. So poliomyelitis is a highly infectious disease but most attacks are subclinical. Polio to most people means paralysis, but paralysis is in reality an uncommon effect of infection. It is not clear how the virus spreads. An infected person harbours the virus in his throat for about two weeks and he might spread it by droplets which another could then breathe in, thus it becomes a respiratory infection. He passes the virus in his faeces for at least three weeks and may do so for up to three months, and during epidemics the virus can be grown with ease from city sewage. Spread by the mouth is always higher in young children where hygiene is poor; thus it fits the pattern of the poorer countries, but not that of the more developed countries. In temperate countries polio was a disease of the summer months and this is not characteristic of respiratory infections. So there is some mystery about exactly how the disease spreads. A very important aspect is that in underdeveloped countries severe paralysis is uncommon while in developed countries the worst forms of paralysis, including the often fatal paralysis of breathing, were common. It was in older patients that the severe paralyses were seen. This seems to mean that the nervous tissue of the youngest children is more resistant to the virus than that of older children and adults. This need not surprise us, for there is considerable difference in the histology (fine structure) of nervous tissue at the two ages.

One uses the word "was" for developed countries and "is" for poorer countries. In the former, polio has been almost abolished by the vaccine, while in the other countries vaccination programmes are still incomplete and polio is still a common disease. It is easy to get children vaccinated in modern towns, with a health clinic just round the corner, but in underdeveloped countries the nearest clinic may be hundreds of miles away. The danger in the developed countries is that with the disappearance of the disease people will get careless about vaccination. The virus has *not* disappeared.

In most infected children the virus multiplies in the gastrointestinal tract but then dies out. In a few the virus invades the bloodstream and causes a mild feverish illness; we call it the minor illness of polio. In many of these the virus dies out and there is no further trouble, but in the unfortunate the virus passes into the central nervous system and the major illness develops. The child has severe headache and stiff neck, the signs of meningitis in fact. Even now the disease may go no further, and we call this nonparalytic poliomyelitis, but in some the nerve cells are attacked and destroyed and these patients become paralysed. The paralysis may be mild, affecting only a few muscles, perhaps one of the leg muscles only, a crippling condition indeed, but not life threatening; this is the kind of disease most often seen in tropical countries. Sometimes the paralysis is widespread; both arms and both legs are paralysed and in the worst cases the breathing muscles or the swallowing muscles are paralysed. These are the patients who require a tracheostomy and some form of artificial respiration. There were many such cases twenty years ago in Britain, and in some countries there are still patients, usually adults, who have been in iron lungs for up to twenty years. Polio can be a tragic disease, but it can also be prevented.

There is no real treatment for the paralysis. Some nerve cells may be poisoned but not permanently damaged; and as these recover, so does the paralysis. When the cells are actually destroyed there can be no true recovery of muscle power. The patient can be taught to make the best use of the power that remains, and for this physiotherapy is rewarding work. Residual weakness or deformity can sometimes be helped by orthopaedic appliances or operation. Polio units are not unhappy places. There is always a spirit of endeavour and determination, and paralysed patients can lead useful, happy lives within their physical limitations. But it is much better to prevent this disease. There is some evidence that physical exercise in the pre-paralytic phase increases the amount of paralysis. Therefore young patients with fever, especially in a polio epidemic, should be put to bed as a precaution.

Brucellosis Brucellae (the germ is named after Sir David Bruce) are common germs in goats, sheep, cows, and pigs; different strains attack different animals. In the Mediterranean the disease is common in sheep and goats and the germ is *Brucella melitensis*: in Britain the disease is found mainly in cattle and the germ is *Brucella abortus* (it causes abortion sometimes in cattle). It spreads to man in two ways: by excretion in the milk and in the vaginal discharges of the animals. Man can get the disease by drinking infected milk, or occupationally by contact with the uterine and vaginal discharges in animal obstetrics. There are two ways of stopping the spread. Pasteurization of milk kills the germs and the milk is safe to drink. The other way is to try to stamp out the disease in animals. The best way to do this is to remove infected animals from the herd and to build up brucellosis-free herds. A brucellosis eradication programme is now under way in Britain, though other developed countries have long since got rid of the disease.

The disease in man takes two forms, acute and chronic. The acute form is sometimes called undulant fever because the temperature swings up and down like waves of the sea; it is a bad name, for often the temperature does not behave like that at all. But it is a feverish illness with much sweating and general aches and pains, especially in the joints. Tiredness is a prominent feature. The acute form of the disease usually responds to antibiotics. The chronic type may follow an untreated acute attack or it may come on slowly on its own. It may take several forms. Arthritis and bone disease are common, but often the commonest symptoms are sheer tiredness and, with it, depression. Mistakes can easily be made. The patient may be diagnosed as suffering from psychological depression before the correct diagnosis of chronic brucellosis is made. Treatment of this chronic form is much more difficult, and may require repeated courses of antibiotics.

Hepatitis   This is one of the commonest infectious diseases throughout the world. There are two main forms, hepatitis A and hepatitis B. They cause a similar disease but the viruses are different. Hepatitis A is spread by the faecal contamination of water and food. Hepatitis B is spread mainly by the transfer of blood from one person to another, by blood transfusion, for example, but also by the sharing of syringes – it is a common disease in drug addicts. It is highly infectious, the merest trace of blood being enough to carry the infection, and can be a dangerous disease in kidney and other dialysis units where blood is handled during treatment. The disease can also be transmitted by more usual routes in families.

The leading symptom is jaundice, due to liver damage. Along with this go fever, abdominal discomfort, and malaise. It is a very weakening disease and the patient may take months to get back fully to normal. Chronic liver disease with much ill health may finally result. Rarely the whole liver is destroyed and the patient dies in liver coma.

In hepatitis B tiny particles in the blood can be seen under the electron microscope. These form the Australia antigen (so called because it was first seen in the blood of Australian aborigines); the particles are parts of the virus of the disease, but so far it has not been possible to grow the virus in the laboratory, which is unfortunate. Hepatitis A virus has been seen, under the electron microscope, in the faeces of patients in the early stages of the disease, but again the virus has not been grown. Blood containing antibody can be used for the preparation of antiserum and this is used with some success in prevention, but it obviously cannot be used on a wide scale, and it does nothing to eradicate the disease.

Skin infections

This is not an exact classification, for in some of the diseases, rabies for example, the virus cannot enter through unbroken skin. Moreover, most of the diseases are not diseases of the skin itself, but of some distant part of the body. But we are concerned with mode of entry, and the term skin infection will serve for that purpose. The diseases we will consider are boils, herpes, anthrax, tetanus, leptospirosis, rabies, Lassa fever, and Marburg disease.

Boils   These are true infections of the skin and underlying tissues. The germ probably enters the skin by a hair follicle or the opening of a sweat gland or sebaceous gland. It sets up inflammation under the skin and pus forms. Eventually the pus bursts through and forms a discharging boil. The commonest germ is a staphylococcus, which is a germ often found on the skin. Just why the germ sometimes lies quietly on the skin and at other times breaks through it and causes a boil is not clear. Many people carry staphylococci in their noses and the same staphylococcus may be found in a boil on their skin, so it may be carried on the fingers and scratched into the skin. On the other hand, many people scratch and many people pick their noses, but not many get boils. In some people boils can be a recurring nuisance, especially in moist areas like the armpits. All sorts of antiseptic preparations are tried without much·success. Sometimes a vaccine prepared from the patient's staphylococcus helps, and sometimes antibiotics do, but it is wrong to treat such patients with one antibiotic after another.

Cold sore or herpes   This is a common infection. A cold sore is caused by the herpes simplex virus. This infects most people in early childhood, usually without causing symptoms, but sometimes an infant gets a severe inflammation of the gums and lips with the first or primary infection. Thereafter, possibly not till adult life, he gets recurring sores on the lips or mouth. The virus can be found in these sores. The odd thing is that patients develop antibodies to the virus after the primary infection and theoretically there should be no recurrences, though the relationship between antibody and antigen is not quite so exact as this. It seems that the virus lies dormant in the tissues for years and emerges in response to some stimulus. What the stimulus is is not clear. Strong sunlight seems to provoke it in some people, minor injuries in others; some diseases, especially meningitis and pneumonia, seem to stimulate it, for herpes on the lips is a common sign in these diseases. Sometimes the virus affects the eye and this may damage the cornea. Occasionally it invades the bloodstream in primary infections in older children and causes a severe illness. Very rarely, in primary infection in adults, the virus invades the brain and causes a severe, even fatal form of encephalitis.

One hopeful point is that antiviral drugs are available for treatment. One is iododeoxyuridine or IDU. This can be applied to a cold sore of the lips and seems to stop it in its early stages. The drug and other antiviral drugs, the cytosines, have been used in encephalitis. The results are not always successful, sometimes there is complete failure, but the importance lies in their being among the first of several drugs to have any antiviral effect at all. Others may follow.

Anthrax   This is mainly a disease of animals, such as cattle, sheep, and goats. It can be highly fatal. In some hot humid countries it can kill hundreds of thousands of animals in a season. The germ is one which forms spores. These are microbial bodies which can remain alive for years in unfavourable conditions but germinate and produce the ordinary forms when conditions improve. These ordinary or vegetative forms multiply in soil, but they are usually killed off by soil bacteria. This is what happens in temperate climates. In hot countries in summer the herbage dries and animals have to graze close to the soil; they may then take in spores lying in the dry pasture and these spores can germinate in the animal and cause death from anthrax. Hot humid climates favour the development of spores. The carcase of an animal dead of anthrax, and any discharges from the body, are heavily infected with anthrax germs. This includes the hide or wool, and the bones. Hides, wool, hair, and bones are exported in huge quantities to other countries and if these are infected, anthrax can be caused in workers who handle them, often thousands of miles away. Anthrax can occur in dockers, in workers in glue factories (glue comes from bones), in upholsterers who handle hair, and in gardeners who sprinkle bone meal on their gardens. Most bone meal is now sold after sterilization, but hides and wool can be damaged by sterilization processes. The best protection for exposed workers is anthrax vaccine, and this is now routine. Man is, however, highly resistant to anthrax, and when exposed to infected material may not contact the disease.

There are two main types of this disease in man, cutaneous and pulmonary. The pulmonary form is called woolsorters' disease, a form of acute lung infection which is frequently fatal. Early diagnosis and treatment with penicillin may save some lives, but the best protection comes from antidust measures in the factory and vaccination of the workers. Cutaneous or skin anthrax is commoner. This causes a sore on the skin, often called a malignant pustule, a bad name, for the sore is neither malignant nor is it a pustule. If there is pus in a sore it is not anthrax. The patient suffers chills and general malaise. Very rarely he develops anthrax septicaemia or severe internal haemorrhage. Penicillin is effective in treatment, but the sore takes a long time to disappear.

Tetanus   This is another disease caused by a sporing germ. *Clostridium tetani* is a soil germ and it gets into the human body in wounds contaminated with soil. The wound may be tiny and unnoticed; a thorn prick may be enough. The germ is found in animal faeces, so soil which has been manured is more likely to contain tetanus germs. The spore germinates only in conditions of low oxygen; hence deep dirty punctured wounds are more likely to be followed by tetanus than surface wounds. However, tetanus can follow trivial wounds. The spore germinates in the tissues of the body and in doing so produces tetanus toxin. The toxin passes to the central nervous system and there attacks the nerve cells. The cells are thrown into a highly excitable state and send impulses down the nerve into the muscles; this causes the muscles to contract strongly, thus producing the spasms and convulsions of tetanus.

The first muscles to contract are those of the mouth and jaws. This causes tightening of the jaws which gives the name of lockjaw to the disease. In bad cases convulsions come on every few minutes and lead to complete exhaustion and death unless treated. Sometimes spasm of the swallowing, larynx, and breathing muscles causes death. The essence of

Chapter 2 Infectious diseases

treatment is to stop the spasms. This can sometimes be done by sedative drugs in large doses, but it is usually safer to perform a tracheostomy (putting a tube in the airpipe) early in the disease. This gives control of breathing if spasm of the throat or breathing muscles does occur. Treatment of severe cases consists of giving a drug called curare intravenously. This drug has the property of paralysing all the muscles of the body, including the breathing and swallowing muscles. The patient must be connected through his tracheostomy tube to a breathing machine and all feeding is done by a tube passing into the stomach through the mouth. Tetanus is a self-limiting condition. If the patient can be kept alive long enough, which usually means about three weeks, the chances are that he will survive. But it is hard going for the patient and all his attendants. With modern prevention, nobody should ever get tetanus, and it is now rare in Britain.

Leptospirosis The term leptospirosis covers a wide class of diseases all caused by one or other of the leptospirae, fine spiral-shaped germs. Typically the germ infects an animal, which sheds the germ in its urine, and the germ then finds its way, usually by water, to the skin of man, which it penetrates. One disease called Weil's disease is caused by *Leptospira icterohaemorrhagica*; ictero means yellow, and the disease is characterized by jaundice and haemorrhage. The animal host is the common rat. The disease in man is found in connection with certain occupations – miners, fish curers, and farmers for example, all of whom may come in contact with rat's urine in water. The germ dies rapidly in acid waters, and a small difference in environment can have a great effect on the incidence of the disease. Another disease is swineherds' disease caused by *Leptospira pomona*; it is carried in pigs and the highest incidence in man is in summer in Switzerland. Canicola fever is caught from dogs carrying *Leptospira canicola*; the dogs suffer from excessive passing of urine, and the germ is excreted in it. Canefield leptospirosis in Australia is carried by *Rattus conatus*, a native rat which becomes infected with *Leptospira australis*. The rat urinates against the low stems of the canes and the workers scratch their legs on the sharp canes and get the disease. There are many more types of leptospirae and of leptospirosis but the only two usual in Britain are Weil's disease and canicola fever, and both are uncommon, thanks to preventive measures.

Weil's disease is usually a fairly mild feverish illness. Occasionally it is severe and the patient develops pronounced jaundice, haemorrhages of the skin and often of the eye, violent muscular pains, and, in the worst cases, kidney failure which may be fatal. Canicola fever is quite different. The illness begins with fever and malaise, and after a few days signs of meningitis develop. This is fortunately self-limiting in most cases, but penicillin hastens recovery.

Rabies Rabies is normally a disease of animals only. Its spread to man is an epidemiological accident. The man dies and the virus dies with him. This is of no advantage to the virus in its struggle for survival. Rabies is a disease of small animals: polecats, mongooses, martens, ferrets, skunks, weasels, and probably many others. Foxes and wolves prey on these, and when the infection builds up, it spills over into these larger animals which then become rabid. Rabies is the Latin for madness. A rabid animal will bite anything that comes in its way. A fox or a wolf can bite man and give him rabies, but more often the victim is a stray dog, and the dog, becoming rabid, bites man. Rabies could reach Britain from the Continent through a smuggled dog or cat. Once in, the virus could spread to our native wild life and it would then be almost impossible to stamp it out. Even in countries in which the disease is endemic, however, human rabies is a rare infection.

An infected dog often first becomes more friendly than usual and tends to lick anyone around. The lick can be dangerous if it touches a broken piece of skin. After a day or two the dog leaves its home and wanders off on its own. It may have paralysis of its vocal cords so does not bark, but it will attack and bite anyone in its way. The dog's saliva is full of rabies virus. After a few more days the dog returns and now slinks into a corner and dies very soon. From start to finish its illness does not last more than ten days. If a dog is alive ten days after biting someone, it was not rabid at the time of the bite. Cats are less often infected than dogs. They tend to hide away during the whole illness but can spring out and attack man unexpectedly. The bite is just as infectious as the dog's.

The disease in man begins quietly, with malaise, headache, possible tingling in the bitten limb, and fever. Soon the stage of excitement comes on with the characteristic frightening reactions to the sight of water or to the idea of drinking. This is called hydrophobia or fear of water. From then on the course is steadily downwards. The patient may develop paralysis of various muscles but he dies soon from heart failure, conscious almost to the end. The whole illness lasts only about a week, one of the most unpleasant deaths known to man. Once symptoms have appeared there is no specific treatment. All the methods of intensive care, including artificial respiration, have been used and in only three cases did this appear to be effective, but in others, even in the most skilled hands, it has only prolonged the dying.

In rabies, more than in almost any other disease, prevention must be the aim. For Britain, an island, the first aim must be to keep it out by rigid quarantine laws. Those exposed to risk by their occupation should be actively immunized at regular intervals. Anyone bitten by a dog or cat which might be rabid should be treated at once with antiserum and vaccine, and the new human diploid vaccine promises well. The dog or cat must, if caught, be kept under observation. If it proves not to be rabid, the treatment on the man can be stopped. If the dog cannot be found or if the bite is by a fox or wolf then full prevention must be given.

Lassa fever   This disease first came into the news in 1969. It has occurred mainly in Nigeria, Liberia, and Sierra Leone. It is caused by a virus and seems to behave in two distinct ways. It may smoulder in villages, affecting many of the inhabitants without making them noticeably ill. Some have a fairly mild illness. Moreover it seems not to be highly infectious. At other times it flares up, perhaps in a hospital environment, is highly infectious, and causes a severe, sometimes fatal disease. Why there should be this difference is not known. There seems no doubt that the virus can be carried by a small rodent which gets into the village houses. Whether these animals are the source of the human disease and how it spreads from one to the other is not known, but it seems likely that this is a zoonosis, a disease spread from animal to man. The symptoms are fever, sore throat, and malaise. In severe cases the patient develops symptoms of shock. In its severest form Lassa fever seems to be a very rare disease, quite out of proportion to the alarm it causes in Britain where there have been only one or two cases in travellers and these have never spread to anyone else. If a patient from Africa has a high fever he is much more likely to be suffering from malaria than from Lassa fever. Malaria has killed millions, Lassa fever very few.

Marburg disease   This disease was first diagnosed in Marburg, West Germany, in 1967 when there was an outbreak among laboratory workers handling blood and other materials from imported African green monkeys. There were cases in Belgrade at about the same time. The infection obviously came first from the monkeys but it was able to spread from one patient to another. The symptoms include high fever, headache, backache, and a dull red rash. The patient tends to bleed from body openings and there is a fall in the cells which help blood to clot (thrombocytes). The disease is thought to be uncommon.

Insect-borne infections

Most insects are beneficial to man in various unseen ways in nature. A few cause some of the worst epidemic diseases. In Britain none of these are now important and occur only in people infected abroad. The one exception is scabies, which is described in chapter 5.

Malaria   Malaria has been, and still is, one of the great scourges of mankind. The disease is caused by a protozoon somewhat larger than most germs, called a plasmodium. There are several varieties, *Plasmodium falciparum* and *Plasmodium vivax* being the most important. They have a complicated life-cycle. Part of their life must be lived inside man, and part inside a mosquito, and during these two lives the plasmodium undergoes a series of changes. In one series, in man, the plasmodium multiplies mainly in the liver and in red blood cells. The multiplication consists of the splitting of one swollen plasmodial body into a host of new small bodies and each time such a host is released into the bloodstream the patient gets a rigor, or shivering attack. The other series of changes can take place only in the body of a mosquito, and multiplication now is a sexual process, the male plasmodium mating with the female. The sexual forms do develop in man but mating cannot take place there. So the mosquito must bite man to take in the gametocytes or sexual forms. The sexual process produces hosts of new forms of the plasmodium in the mosquito and these reach its mouth parts. When next it bites, it injects these into its victim and the nonsexual splitting process starts all over again. Clearly the survival and the spread of the plasmodia, and so the spread of malaria, depends on close and frequent contact between man and mosquito. This association still exists in many parts of the world and it is a difficult one to break. Mosquitoes breed in standing water and they can fly a long way from the water to bite man. There are two ways of preventing malaria. The first is to try to get rid of the malaria mosquito near inhabited areas. Swamps need to be cleared, but small pools of water near human habitation must be cleared too. All this can involve major civil engineering. The second method of attack

The malaria cycle

Prevention of malaria can be achieved by either destroying mosquitoes, protecting man from their bites, or by preventive drugs.

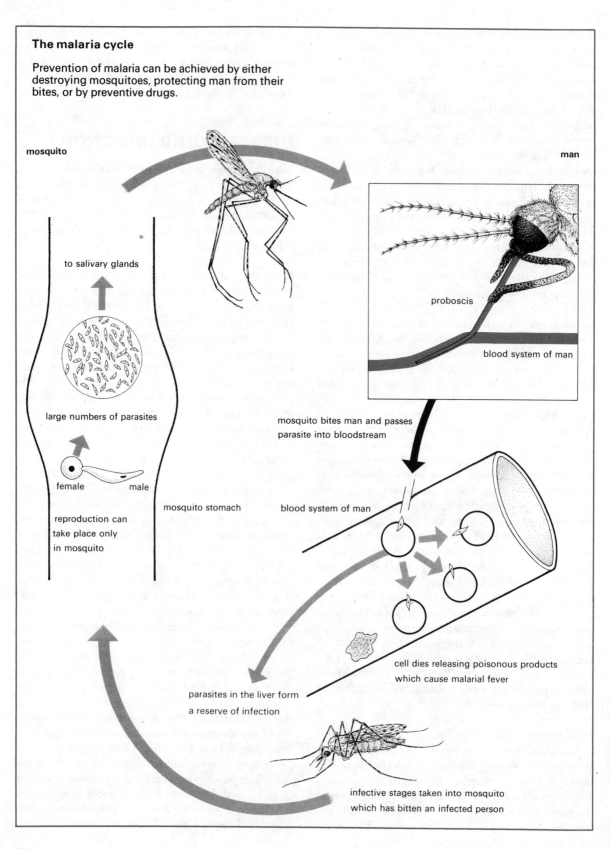

mosquito

man

to salivary glands

large numbers of parasites

female   male

reproduction can take place only in mosquito

mosquito stomach

proboscis

blood system of man

mosquito bites man and passes parasite into bloodstream

blood system of man

cell dies releasing poisonous products which cause malarial fever

parasites in the liver form a reserve of infection

infective stages taken into mosquito which has bitten an infected person

is to try to destroy mosquitoes by poisoning them with chemicals. This can mean spraying stretches of water from a plane and also spraying the inside of huts and houses, an enormous task, and one of the difficulties is that the mosquito can become resistant to the drug. On a simpler scale man can prevent contact by sleeping inside mosquito nets, as the mosquito bites mainly at night. A totally different approach is for man to take antimalarial drugs in a malarious area. This does not prevent the spread of malaria but it does prevent the onset of disease and it is vitally important for travellers to take these drugs if they enter a malarious area, even for a stopover of an hour or two.

The symptoms of the disease are caused by the splitting of the plasmodia in man's body, and the typical symptom is the rigor. There is first a cold shivering stage as the temperature rises, then a hot stage and sweating as it falls. Blood cells are destroyed by the parasites, and anaemia is a common feature of malaria. The liver is invaded and jaundice follows. Sometimes there is vast destruction of blood cells and the pigment of the dead cells discolours the urine; this is the blackwater fever of malaria. The worst complication is cerebral malaria, caused by severe attacks of *Plasmodium falciparum*, which can be rapidly fatal if not diagnosed and treated early. Treatment of malaria by drugs is successful if begun early. The main difficulty is in thinking of the disease in a country such as Britain where the disease no longer occurs except in those infected abroad, for malaria can mimic other less serious diseases. Any patient who has been abroad and is taken ill at any time on return home must tell his doctor where he has been, and when.

Typhus fever   This is still a serious epidemic fever in some parts of the world. It is caused by a germ called a rickettsia (after Dr Howard Ricketts, who himself died from this disease) and the germ is carried in the common body louse, which bites man and injects the rickettsia. There are several forms of typhus but the important one is epidemic typhus. The symptoms are high fever, a rash, cerebral symptoms such as delirium, and often signs of bronchitis. The disease fortunately responds to the antibiotic chloramphenicol, but without it patients often die in the second week of the disease. Prevention of typhus means getting rid of lice. Patients' bodies must be dusted with an antilouse powder, usually DDT.

Plague   This is another of the great epidemic scourges of mankind. There have been vast outbreaks in the past. The Black Death that swept across the world in the Middle Ages was plague, and plague is still around today, though no longer in Britain, fortunately.

Plague is caused by a germ called *Yersinia pestis*. The germ is carried in rats and many other animals. It is transferred to man by the bite of a flea which sucks the infected blood of the rat and then, when the rat dies, jumps on to man and injects the germ into him. That is a highly simplified account of what is a most complicated and fascinating story. All sorts of factors come into it, such as temperature, humidity, rainfall, aridity, the different digestive processes in different fleas, and the different breeding habits of different rodents.

There are two main forms of plague, bubonic and pneumonic. In bubonic plague, swellings or buboes form in the lymph nodes near the bite, often in the groin, the armpits, and the neck. They are painful and full of pus. The germ can leak into the bloodstream and cause plague septicaemia, and this is often fatal. Bubonic plague is not infectious from man to man unless the patient lives long enough to develop plague pneumonia. When he does so, his sputum is full of plague germs and these spread rapidly to contacts who breathe the plague-ridden air, and develop not bubonic, but pneumonic plague, a highly infectious condition. Both pneumonic and septicaemic plague are highly fatal diseases. If the disease is immediately recognized and treated with the correct antibiotics, streptomycin and tetracycline, the outlook is good.

The prevention of plague consists of breaking contact between man, rat, and flea. The worldwide spread of plague has been checked by keeping rats out of ships, but containers may not be so safe. Warehouses are kept as free of rats as possible.

Venereal infections

The two great venereal diseases are gonorrhoea and syphilis. There are others, but we will deal only with these two. There is little need to dwell on the mode of infection. They are both transferred in sexual intercourse. Sexual deviations can lead to unusual presentations in the throat or in the rectum. In one stage of early syphilis the tonsils are infected and the disease can pass in kissing. Children can be affected, with syphilis congenitally, with gonorrhoea by contact with an infected mother, and these will be discussed shortly. Stories of infection from lavatory seats and the like are not true.

Chapter 2 Infectious diseases

Syphilis Syphilis is a disease of the whole body. It is caused by a germ called *Treponema pallidum* and this enters the body through the genital mucous membranes during intercourse. There is an incubation period of about one month and then the sore or chancre appears. In males this chancre is usually seen on the penis and there is enlargement of the associated lymph nodes in the groin. In women the chancre may be in the vagina or on the neck of the womb and so is not seen. This is primary syphilis. If treated now with penicillin the disease can be eradicated, but in women this stage may be missed. After about six months the second stage begins. By now the germ is all through the body but the commonest symptoms are sore throat, hoarseness, headache, and a rash on the body. This stage is still fully treatable. The third stage in an untreated case may come on at any time after the second, but often it is many years later. In the interval the disease has been damaging many organs of the body. It can cause liver, heart, or brain disease. At this stage the disease can be stopped by treatment but the damage done to the internal organs is beyond repair. Liver disease can undermine general health, heart damage can lead to heart failure, and brain and spinal cord damage can lead to paralysis and insanity. General paralysis of the insane is a rather frightening title of a disease caused by syphilis. Fortunately the third stage of syphilis is not now often encountered in Britain. The disease is curable in the early stages before permanent damage is done. It is therefore essential to examine carefully any patient who has been exposed to possible infection, and to continue to carry out blood tests until the doctor is satisfied that infection has not occurred. The final test may be

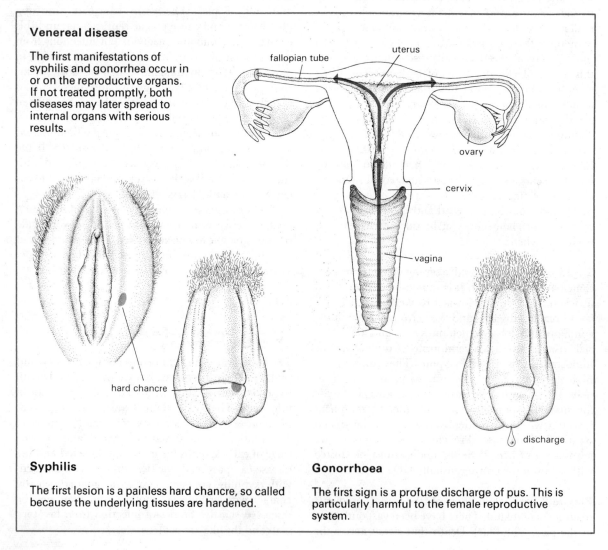

Venereal disease

The first manifestations of syphilis and gonorrhea occur in or on the reproductive organs. If not treated promptly, both diseases may later spread to internal organs with serious results.

fallopian tube

uterus

ovary

cervix

vagina

hard chancre

discharge

Syphilis

The first lesion is a painless hard chancre, so called because the underlying tissues are hardened.

Gonorrhoea

The first sign is a profuse discharge of pus. This is particularly harmful to the female reproductive system.

required six months after the exposure. Such tests must also be done on patients with gonorrhoea, for it is quite possible to contract both diseases from one exposure. The gonorrhoea may be cured rapidly in a day or two, but the syphilis may be overlooked.

A syphilitic mother may transmit the disease to the fetus. The baby may be affected in various ways, some serious. The condition can be treated, but is best prevented.

Gonorrhoea Gonorrhoea means a flow from the genitals, and a discharge from the penis or the vagina is the characteristic sign. Along with discharge there is usually pain or difficulty in passing urine. A man always knows if he has the symptoms of gonorrhoea. In a woman the signs may be slight or absent and she may not know she is infected. This is one of the main causes of the wide spread of gonorrhoea – an apparently healthy woman with gonococci in her genital passages. Untreated gonorrhoea may spread up the genital tract. In man this spread can cause inflammation of the testis and the tubes behind them, epididymo-orchitis. It can cause inflammation of the prostate gland at the base of the bladder, and narrowing or stricture of the urethra through which the urine passes from the bladder to the outside. All these are serious and unpleasant local complications. The germ can enter the bloodstream and cause inflammation in the joints, the skin, and the heart, all rather uncommon but serious when they occur. In women the great danger is inflammation of the womb and of the tubes leading from the ovaries to the uterus; this is known as salpingitis. Blockage of the tubes may then cause sterility. During birth, the baby may be infected, possibly with serious damage to the eyes, even causing blindness. The treatment of gonorrhoea with sulphonamides and penicillin is very successful, so long as the gonococcus remains sensitive. Many strains have long been resistant to sulphonamides and some are now resistant to penicillin, so new drugs are being tried. When the gonococcus is sensitive the disease is cured very quickly indeed. This has its own danger, for the patient comes to regard the infection as a minor incident, easily curable if he gets it again. So it is possible that the successful drug has increased the incidence of infection. Contraception has probably played its part too by removing the fear of conception following intercourse. Young persons should remember that although "the pill" is effective against pregnancy, it does *not* protect against venereal diseases. The prevention or reduction of venereal infection encounters social, moral, and educational problems.

Meanwhile venereal disease forms one of the great epidemics of modern life.

Miscellaneous infections

Travellers' diarrhoea One could write a book under this heading for there are many infections, tropical and temperate, to which man is exposed. One of the commonest these days is travellers' diarrhoea. This has all sorts of other names, gyppy tummy, turista, and many others, but there is little doubt that it is an infection of the bowel caused by the ingestion of contaminated food: in fact, just a type of food poisoning. Natives of a place probably become immune to the local germs in food, but strangers go down with diarrhoea within a day or two. They in turn become immune, but if they move on elsewhere they may get another attack from different local germs. This kind of occurrence is sometimes seen at international conferences; the local delegates remain well but the foreigners become ill. The best way of avoiding this is to be careful about eating raw food, especially salads, cold meats, or any buffet foods, and not to drink local water unless one can be assured it is safe. See also chapter 30.

Intestinal worms There are many worms which afflict man. The round worm, or ascaris, is a common one all over the world. The eggs are passed in the faeces of an infected person and are resistant to heat, cold, and drying. They are carried in dust and can be swallowed in food or drink. They mature in the intestine and grow to several inches in length. One or two worms in the intestine cause little trouble; the idea that they steal the patient's food is mistaken. They may migrate to other parts of the body occasionally, to the lungs, for example, where they certainly cause symptoms, or into the stomach where they may be vomited up. They may even creep up the oesophagus and come down the nose. If there are large numbers in the intestine they can cause abdominal swelling and discomfort and in extreme cases a bunch of worms can cause obstruction of the bowel, which requires operation. The worms can be driven out of the body by drugs given by mouth. There are many other kinds of worm; threadworms are very common in children, but are often symptomless and can be eradicated. Tapeworms are rare in Britain.

Pets and infection

Are pets the cause of infections in man? We have seen that they can carry the germs of some forms of leptospirosis. A rabid dog or cat can cause rabies in man, although rabies has not yet come to Britain. Dogs and cats sometimes suffer from salmonella infections and can infect people with the disease, but they are not important causes and may, in fact, be infected by man and his food just as much as the other way round. Tortoises and terrapins do convey salmonellosis, even paratyphoid fever, but again they are not common causes. Pet birds are a different matter: they are the commonest cause of psittacosis. The way to avoid trouble is to be careful where one buys these pets. An infection whose importance has recently been realized is toxocariasis. This is caused by *Toxocara canis* or *Toxocara cati*, tiny worms passed in the faeces of dogs and cats; the eggs can be found quite easily in soil fouled by them. The worms get into the body and can cause symptoms, usually mild, in children. These include fever, bronchitis, and malaise, but sometimes the eyes are damaged. A skin test can show if a child has been infected. It is important to be aware constantly of the dangers from pets.

Diagnosis, treatment, and prevention

This account is not meant to teach anyone to diagnose, treat, or prevent infectious diseases. But perhaps one can have an intelligent interest in the problems. As regards diagnosis one scarcely needs to be a doctor to recognize a florid measles rash. The diagnosis of other infections, or indeed of measles if it is unusual, can be extremely difficult. Body fluids and tissues may be tested, blood, urine, sputum, cerebro-spinal fluid, or saliva; faeces, vomit, snips of skin, or pieces of liver and other organs obtained by needle puncture or biopsy. They may be examined for cellular changes, or the presence of antibodies, or cultured for the growth of germs. Some of the tests are easy, and results are available in minutes or hours. Others are complicated and may take days, weeks, or months. One test may tell nothing of importance; a repeat test may show a diagnostic change. Tests may put a diagnosis beyond dispute, or they may just give a vague clue. They may be negative, yet still helpful in excluding some disease. The history of the onset and the previous contacts may be more important than the most elaborate tests.

In some diseases specific treatment is available. Chloramphenicol will cure most cases of typhoid fever, if the organism has not become resistant, but there is no specific treatment for measles or mumps or many others. The essence of specific treatment is to be sure that the drug does kill or inhibit the germ and that it does so in the human body. Antibiotics are good drugs but they have their limitations.

Prevention is an enormous subject. It will be clear that simple rules of cleanliness and hygiene will prevent some infections, but it must be equally clear that the prevention of others would involve the reversal of some areas of natural history, for man is not alone in the struggle for survival. Germs and other animals also strive for their place in the natural world. Man has provided one form of protection for himself and some of his animals, and that is immunization. This can be highly successful as in smallpox and poliomyelitis. But it is an artificial process and it must be kept going. Infectious diseases can be controlled, but they are unlikely to disappear.

AIDS is an acronym for Acquired Immune Deficiency Syndrome. This means that the body of the person affected loses the ability to fight infections and other diseases.

It is a new condition, unknown before 1981.

AIDS is caused by a minute organism, the HIV virus (human immunodeficiency virus). Once inside the body the HIV virus attacks certain white blood cells which make antibodies that act as natural defenders against infections, cancers and other conditions.

AIDS is caught and spread through *sex* with an infected person or through infected blood. The virus can enter the body through the vagina (front passage), anus (back passage) or penis. Small amounts of blood and other fluids pass from person to person during sex and allow the virus into the blood stream. Most of those infected so far have been male homosexuals or bisexuals.

AIDS can also be passed on through the *blood* by sharing of infected needles by drug users; by some haemophiliacs, who need certain blood products to help clotting, when the blood has been infected by HIV virus (all bloods are now specially heat treated to destroy the virus). Very rarely nurses, doctors and dentists may become infected from needlepricks or through cuts after contact with infected patients.

During *pregnancy* a woman with the HIV virus can pass it on to her unborn child who will be born infected.

AIDS is *not* caught through normal social contacts, such as kissing, shaking hands, coughs or sneezes, or from toilet seats, bed linen, cups and other crockery, or from sharing a house, contact at work or at school. Nor can it be caught through being a blood donor.

A person infected with the HIV organism does not always suffer from AIDS. It is believed that some persons infected with HIV suffer no apparent illness, but nevertheless are infectious to others. Between one-third and one-half develop an illness termed AIDS-related-complex (ARC) with persistent enlargement of glands.

Persons with ARC will become excessively tired; lose appetite and weight; have swollen glands in neck, groin and armpits, have night sweats and fever, persistent diarrhoea, and skin rashes; will cough and have mouth ulcers.

AIDS itself is the most serious result of HIV infection, and one in three develop it. Serious diseases take hold, such as pneumonia, infections of intestines and meningitis. Cancers of skin and other parts may develop and mental deterioration can result.

Almost all persons with full-blown AIDS will die.

The only way of diagnosing AIDS is by a test on a small amount of blood taken from an arm vein. The test checks the blood for antibodies against HIV. These may take three or more months to develop from the time of infection. A *positive result* indicates that infection with HIV has occurred and the person is infected. A *negative result* means that there is no evidence of infection but it may need to be repeated a few weeks later to be certain. The test in itself does not predict whether or not a person will develop AIDS.

At present there is no cure for AIDS. Once infected, the virus stays in the body for life. There is much that can be done to relieve and comfort a person with AIDS.

The only hopes at present are *prevention* and in plain words this means "safe sex". There is no vaccine against AIDS yet. Safe sex means avoidance of unprotected sex with unknown partners who may have the HIV. Using a condom gives protection, but not complete protection. Sharing of needles for injecting drugs is dangerous and should be avoided.

A person with a positive blood test should seek expert advice and must avoid unprotected sex and shared needles, and must not be a blood donor; infected women must not have a baby. Doctors and dentists should be informed so that they may take protective measures.

Although AIDS is a terrifying prospect and little can be done to save those who have it now, if the causes are understood and steps taken to avoid them, then it should be controllable until a cure and/or a protective vaccine is developed.

Chapter 3
The heart and circulatory system

Revised by A. M. Cooke, DM FRCP

The human heart is a remarkably tough hollow muscle about the size of its owner's fist. In principle, it is an electrically-fired pump which squeezes and relaxes at one point in a closed system of flexible pipes, to keep the fluids within the pipes in constant circulation. All tissues depend on this circulation for their nutrition and disposal of wastes. Perhaps because we can feel our hearts beat, and thump and

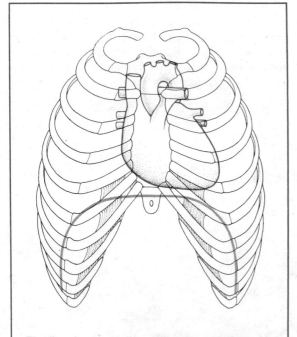

The fist-sized heart lies well protected within the rib cage, above the diaphragm. Its apex (where the beat is felt) tapers downwards to the left, but the mass of the heart lies centrally in the chest, rather than on the left side of the body.

pound sometimes in our ears when we exert ourselves, and know that when the heart stops, we stop, some people feel that the heart is a delicate organ that needs coddling. On the contrary, it is about the sturdiest organ we possess, designed to do its vital work with a minimum of fuss or complaint.

The amount of work done by the heart – even when its owner merely lies in bed – is awe-inspiring. The heart beats about 70 times a minute, which is 38 million times a year. Less than one month after conception, the heart of a fetus begins to beat and continues for a lifetime. An adult heart pumps about a quarter of a pint of blood at each stroke, or 3,000 gallons a day, which weigh thirteen tons. All this unceasing labour is accomplished without conscious effort on our part. Yet the heart rests between beats, and is resting a little more than half the time. In a lifetime of 70 years, the heart rests for about 40 years. It rests even when it is working its hardest, and gives an excellent lesson in the value of pacing exertion.

Externally, the heart is roughly pear-shaped, with the apex or tapered part at the bottom. It lies almost centrally in the chest behind the breastbone in a diagonal position, its broad part pointed up and to the right, and its apex downwards to the left. The apex is where the beat is felt, which is no doubt the reason for the belief that the heart is in the left side of the body. The heart is well protected by the rib cage, and other defences. It is almost impossible to injure a healthy heart by short periods of extreme physical exertion, partly because other muscles become exhausted before the heart muscle. And the heart has considerable resilience so that it can rebound from fairly severe blunt blows. It more or less hangs from blood vessels that give flexible support and allow a certain amount of mobility.

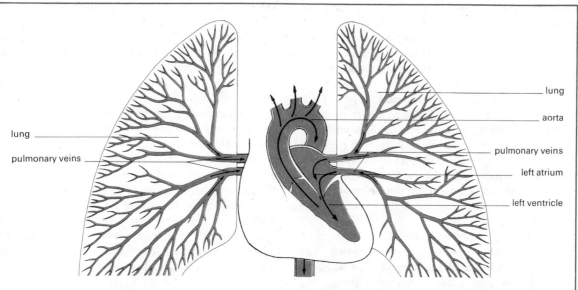

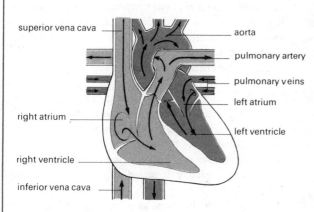

The two sides of the heart are normally separated from each other – the left heart pumps freshly oxygenated blood to the body, the right heart pumps "used" venous blood to the lungs for purification.

Top. Oxygenated blood from the lungs enters the left atrium by the pulmonary veins, flows into the left ventricle, and is pumped to the body through the aorta.

Bottom. "Used" blood from the body enters the right atrium from the superior and inferior vena cavae, then flows into the right ventricle, and is pumped to the lungs through the pulmonary artery.

Centre. The different circulations of the two sides of the heart.

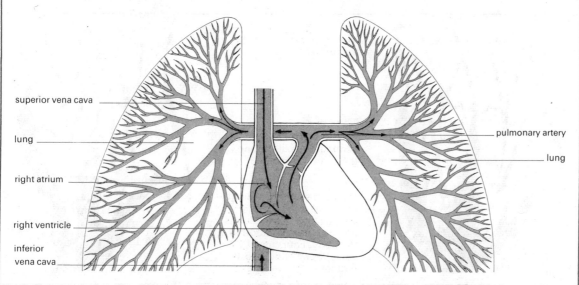

Chapter 3 The heart and circulatory system

Chambers and valves Functionally, we have two hearts which sustain separate circulations and beat as one. The complete heart is divided into a right and a left heart by a solid muscular wall, the septum, which runs down the centre and prevents blood in the two sides of the heart from mixing.

The right side of the heart receives "used" blood, returned from the veins of the body, and pumps it to the lungs where it gets rid of carbon dioxide and picks up oxygen from inhaled air. The left side of the heart receives freshly oxygenated bright red blood from the lungs and pumps it to the body through a vast network of vessels. This is quite simple in principle, although a cross section of the heart makes matters look rather complicated.

Each side of the heart has two hollow chambers, an atrium (also called an auricle) and a ventricle. The atrium is mainly a receiving room and its walls are relatively thin since it does not have to pump very hard. The atrium opens into the ventricle below it. Ventricles do most of the pumping work and have thick muscular walls. The left ventricle which gives fresh blood its initial propulsion to all parts of the body is more muscular than the right which has only to pump spent blood under a lower pressure to the nearby lungs.

As in a car engine which has no power without compression, valves in the heart are necessary to seal pressure chambers tightly, so that the contracting muscles have something to work against. This is accomplished by four sets of heart valves which open and shut in precisely timed sequences, prevent the backflow of blood, and so keep it moving in one direction.

In the right heart, blood moves from atrium to ventricle through the tricuspid valve, which has three triangular-shaped flaps. Contraction of the ventricle moves blood through a semilunar valve (which has three cusps shaped like half moons) into an artery that leads to the lungs. The semilunar valve opens at the same time that the tricuspid valve closes.

Simultaneously, the left side of the heart goes through the same cycle. Blood in the atrium goes to the ventricle through the mitral valve, so called because its two leaflet flaps resemble a bishop's mitre. The valve closes and the contracting ventricle moves the blood through another set of semilunar valves into the main artery, the aorta, for distribution to the body. Under resting conditions these cycles are repeated about 72 times a minute – the rate of one's pulse. The rate of the heartbeat varies with age, size, bodily activity, rest, or excitement.

Heartbeat regulators Both sides of the heart beat in unison. The atria beat first and then the ventricles. The part of the beat during which the heart relaxes and the ventricles are filling is called diastole. The period of contraction is called systole. Thus, as well as a two-sided heart, we have two levels of blood pressure – systolic and diastolic.

Diastolic pressure is the lower of two figures (such as 120/90) with which doctors express blood pressure readings. Here, 90 is the low pressure level in the arteries during the period when the heart is resting. The figures record the number of millimetres a column of mercury is raised by the force of blood pressure.

The fine mechanisms and forces that trigger the

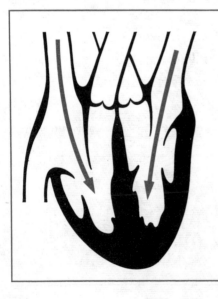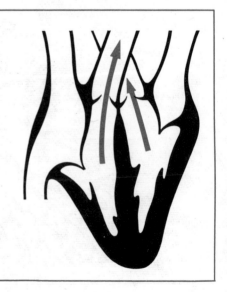

Mechanical pumping action of the heart

Left. In diastole the ventricles are filling and the heart is relaxed or resting.

Right. In systole the heart contracts and forces venous blood to the lungs and oxygenated blood to the body. Four sets of valves open and close as required.

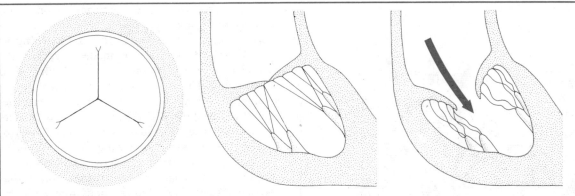

The tricuspid valve
This valve controls the flow of blood between the right atrium and ventricle. The diagram on the left shows the valve when shut. The central diagram shows the valve's position during systole, when the heart is pumping blood out. The valve prevents backflow of blood from ventricle to atrium. On the right, the valve relaxes to allow blood to flow from atrium to ventricle during diastole.

heartbeat are not known completely. A small knot of tissue known as the pacemaker or sinus node is a vital "spark plug". It is located in the upper part of the heart near where great veins enter the right atrium. It consists of specialized nerve and muscle cells which start a wave of muscle contraction in the heart. The wave spreads over the atrial muscle and is transmitted by a special band of tissue (the atrio-ventricular node) from the atria to the ventricles. In some cases of disease or injury which interrupt communications between the sinus and A–V nodes, the ventricles may continue to beat independently.

The electrical nature of impulses that start the heartbeat is shown by the success of artificial pacemakers in triggering normal rhythms in some forms of heart disease. Artificial pacemakers are battery-powered devices, worn over the shoulder like a camera or implanted under the skin, which are connected to electrodes in heart tissue. The devices feed tiny shocks of electric current to the heart, to keep it running rhythmically. Various abnormalities of the heartbeat are called arrhythmias.

Anatomy   A little knowledge of anatomy helps one to understand terms such as "myocardial infarction" and "endocarditis" that doctors use when discussing heart functions and disorders.

The heart is enclosed in a tough bag of tissue called the pericardium. Lubricating fluid permits the heart to glide freely within it. Occasionally, the pericardium becomes inflamed, or the two layers may stick together, from causes such as rheumatic fever or extension of infections from neighbouring parts.

The heart muscle is called the myocardium. It is a specialized and very powerful form of muscle, laid down in crisscross layers. The myocardium may become inflamed, or weakened, or even starved to death by impairment of its blood supply.

The internal lining of the heart which includes the valves is the endocardium. Bacteria may sometimes cause serious inflammation of the endocardium, especially of the valves.

The broad upper part of the heart is entered by great vessels which branch in quite confusing ways. Perhaps the easiest way to clarify the tangle is to think of these as input and output vessels. Two great outward vessels emerge side by side from the top central part of the heart. One is the pulmonary artery which carries blood from the right heart to the lungs. It branches almost immediately into two divisions, one of which leads to the left, and the other to the right lung. The other output vessel is a great artery, the aorta, which arches over the pulmonary artery. The aorta carries freshly oxygenated blood from the left side of the heart and distributes it through smaller and smaller vessels to all parts of the body.

Four vessels, two on each side, bring the blood to the heart. These enter at the top and sides of the broadest part of the upper heart and discharge into their respective atria. Two large veins, the superior (upper) and inferior (lower) vena cavae open into the right atrium and bring blood that is returned to the heart for pumping to the lungs. The upper vena cava brings blood from the head and arms, and the lower from the legs and lower parts of the body. Two similar pulmonary veins opening into the left atrium bring oxygenated blood from the right and left lungs.

Blood inside the heart cannot nourish the heart

65

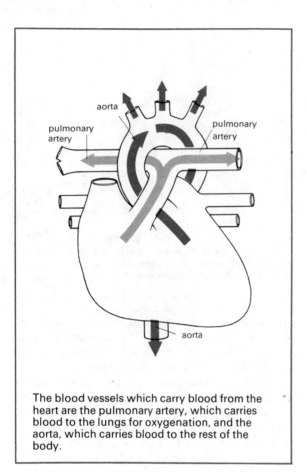

The blood vessels which carry blood from the heart are the pulmonary artery, which carries blood to the lungs for oxygenation, and the aorta, which carries blood to the rest of the body.

muscle. Like other tissues, the heart muscle must obtain its blood through circulatory channels. It gets its blood through coronary arteries and the blood is returned by a collecting system of veins that drain into the right atrium. The two coronary arteries are easily seen on the surface of the heart, arising separately from the root of the aorta just above its semilunar valves. The vessels follow a tortuous course and branch into finer and finer subdivisions. The name coronary was bestowed by early anatomists who fancied that the vessels resembled a crown encircling the heart.

Diagnosis A careful history of the patient, his complaints and symptoms and physical examination are essential in diagnosing heart troubles. The doctor's judgment is aided by tests and instruments which give important information about the heart's behaviour. All tests require expert interpretation and their results sometimes may be inconclusive. For instance, a patient may be asked to do a measured amount of exercise, such as stepping up and down a short flight of stairs. The time needed for his pulse rate

to return to normal gives some indication of his heart's reserve capacity.

Sounds and murmurs Heart sounds are better heard than described. Words are inadequate, but the typical heart sound is commonly approximated as "lubb-dup". The dull low lubb is caused by the closing of the valves between the atria and ventricles and is partly the sound of the ventricular muscles contracting. The dup sound, shorter, higher pitched, almost clicking, is caused by closing of the semilunar valves in the exit arteries. There is a fraction of a second pause between a dup and the next lubb. At that moment the heart rests. Other sounds from particular hearts are distinguishable by a trained ear. A rather soft swishing or hissing sound – a murmur – may indicate that blood is leaking back through an imperfectly closed valve but there are other types of murmur that are of no significance. They can occur in normal persons.

Electrocardiograms A minute electrical impulse is set up whenever a muscle contracts. These impulses can be magnified by instruments, and their strength and character can be recorded on paper. An instrument called the electrocardiograph detects these electrical changes in contracting heart muscles; its record is an electrocardiogram. Several leads from the surfaces above different parts of the heart transmit impulses to the instrument for amplification. Normal hearts produce characteristic tracings. Disordered

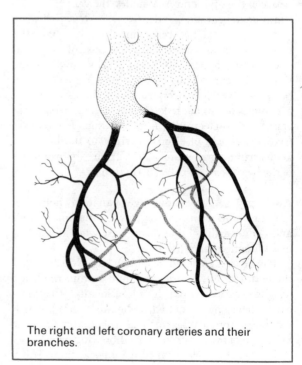

The right and left coronary arteries and their branches.

hearts may produce tracings which differ in some particular way and give clues to the nature of the trouble. The ECG can reveal a lot about disorders of heart rhythm and obstruction of the coronary arteries, but some heart disorders cause little or no change in the ECG. Its interpretation requires much experience.

X-rays The heart imprints its shadow on an X-ray photo of the chest. Comparison with healthy hearts gives information about enlargement, distortions, and abnormalities of the heart and its four chambers.

With a fluoroscope (see Encyclopedia of medical terms), the doctor may watch the living heart in action.

Some more complex procedures which must be carried out in hospitals using special equipment are not used routinely and are seldom necessary. However, they are of value in assisting diagnosis of rare, puzzling, and complicated heart disorders, and some of them are useful tools in heart research.

By a technique called angiocardiography the course of radiopaque dyes through the heart valves and circulation can be followed, and defects seen by taking X-ray pictures at split second intervals.

The heart has a kick which jolts the body imperceptibly. The kick, not unlike the recoil of a gun, is the recoil of the heart when it contracts and pumps blood into the aorta. This slight nudge can be picked up by apparatus called the ballistocardio-graph, which consists essentially of a delicately suspended cot on which the patient lies, and instruments which amplify the minute heart-impelled quiverings of his body. The device gives information about the heart's energy output.

By another procedure, cardiac catheterization, blood can be withdrawn from the right and left heart through a tube inserted through a vessel of the arm. Measurement of pressures and analysis of the blood samples give information that in some circumstances is of great value.

The nature of heart disease It may seem inconsistent to discuss diseases of the heart as if these were detached from the blood vessels, that is, the arteries and veins through which the heart pumps the blood. The heart and the arteries are interdependent – the whole system is the circulation.

In another sense, however, heart disease in its major forms is really artery disease. The common types of heart disease are congenital, rheumatic, hypertensive, and coronary. Other ailments also cause heart damage, such as infections, notably syphilis and virus diseases. These disorders of the heart are chiefly vascular (that is, of blood vessel origin).

Congenital heart disease originates before birth. It results from failure of the necessary twisting, joining, and division of two primitive arteries to take place in proper sequence, and with necessary completeness, as the heart is forming its four chambers, valves, and major inlets and outlets. For example, in one irregularity, patent ductus arteriosus, the artery which bypasses the lungs in the unborn child fails to close after birth and blood continues to flow through it. This can be corrected by surgery.

In *rheumatic heart disease* the inflammation in the heart muscle is often perivascular, that is, around the arteries in the heart muscle. Other blood vessels in the body may also become inflamed in rheumatic fever. Its most important effects are damage to the heart valves, obstructing the flow of blood or causing leakage of the valves with loss of compression.

In *hypertensive heart disease* the heart muscle becomes overworked because of contraction of the fine branches of the arterial system throughout the body, producing an increase in resistance which prevents easy flow of blood into the organs. Thus the pressure in the arteries is raised and the heart is forced to pump blood against a high resistance.

In *coronary heart disease* we see the most obvious example of the role of the narrowing arteries in producing heart failure. Coronary heart disease is

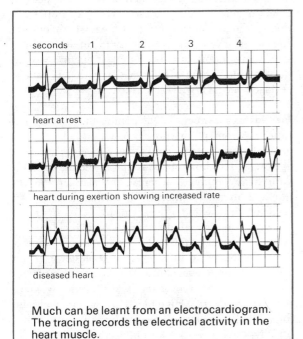

seconds   1   2   3   4

heart at rest

heart during exertion showing increased rate

diseased heart

Much can be learnt from an electrocardiogram. The tracing records the electrical activity in the heart muscle.

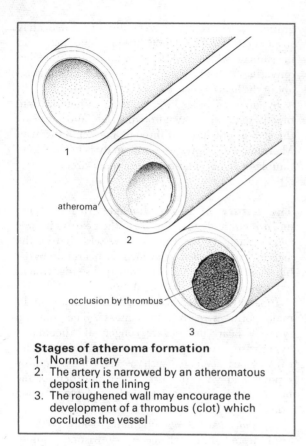

Stages of atheroma formation
1. Normal artery
2. The artery is narrowed by an atheromatous deposit in the lining
3. The roughened wall may encourage the development of a thrombus (clot) which occludes the vessel

Heart failure The heart can fail in three main ways: by inability to pump out the blood adequately (congestive heart failure); by sending painful sensations to the chest (anginal failure); or by losing its normal beating and becoming irregular, or extremely slow or fast, or by having periods of complete stopping of the beat. The last is called heart block and this refers to blocking of the electrical impulse which passes from atria to ventricles with each heartbeat. It should not be confused with blocking of a coronary artery by a clot.

Coronary artery disease

Different doctors use different terms for the commonest type of arterial degeneration, such as arteriosclerosis, atherosclerosis, and atheroma. All these words indicate impairment of elasticity, thickening of the wall, and narrowing of the vessel by fatty and fibrous plaques in the lining layer.

Arteriosclerosis of the coronary arteries is the most common form of heart disease. Arteries undergo thickening of their walls as they grow older. This occurs earlier and more severely in some people than others, probably because of differences in heredity. This is in fact a common way for a person to age and die.

Atheroma (athere is Greek for porridge) is a fatty cholesterol deposit appearing in the lining and walls of affected arteries. Later there may be a deposit of calcium salts in these diseased areas. An important question in the control of this disease is whether or not the tendency to it is hereditary or sufficiently dependent upon environmental influences to be preventable. There is little evidence that it can be reversed once it is well established.

Hereditary aspects One point is that young men suffering from premature coronary attacks are, in general, muscular and tend to put on weight after the age of 25. This body shape is that of the mesomorph with heavy muscles, whereas the slender, poorly muscled man (ectomorph) is almost immune to coronary disease under the age of 40.

There are also families with a high incidence of coronary attacks and early death, and in some a family tendency to high levels of cholesterol in the blood, or a high level of uric acid. Diabetes increases the susceptibility to coronary disease, even in women, to a striking degree. High blood pressure may also be found with coronary disease, especially in women, and hypertension adds an important burden to the heart.

really coronary artery disease, because the heart muscle itself is normal except where the circulation to it has been reduced or cut off by narrowing or blocking of branches of the coronary arteries. It is also called ischaemic heart disease, which is a good term, because it describes the real damage to the heart from local reduction of blood supply to a portion of the muscular wall. So in coronary heart disease we should always think of the constantly changing pattern of the circulation in the complex branching distribution of the coronary arteries. Some have become thickened and narrowed, or blocked with clots or fatty deposits. In some a clot in the artery has become partially dissolved. New channels then open to replace those which have blocked, but this takes time.

Of course, the arteries in other organs are also subject to degeneration by arteriosclerosis, when the arteries are obstructed to a point where the increased demand for blood flow cannot be satisfied. We recognize cramping pain in the calves of the legs when walking as evidence of ischaemia or restricted blood supply. In general, however, people with ageing changes in their arteries continue much as normal unless the arteries predominantly affected are in the brain, the heart, or the kidney.

Another outstanding fact is that in the early age period, especially under the age of 40, coronary sclerosis is almost entirely a male disease. Only after the menopause or after early removal of the ovaries does its occurrence become equal in male and female subjects. Women's hormonal arrangements before the menopause seem to provide a considerable degree of protection against coronary disease.

Incidence   There is a great deal of interest in heart attacks and in what seems to be an increase in heart disease as a cause of death. Sudden death is almost always a heart death. Coronary artery disease is by far the most common type of heart disease responsible for these events. However, there are factors, apart from a true increase in the occurrence of coronary disease that account for what has been called an epidemic of heart diseases. These are; the increase in the average age of our population, the conquest of many infectious diseases which were previously fatal, the general improvement in the health of the population, and the greater accuracy in the diagnosis of coronary disease. There is also a tendency to label some deaths as coronary when other fatal diseases are present.

It is a popular belief that coronary disease is something new, and indeed the recognition of acute coronary thrombosis is only about 60 years old. Heart deaths did not appear in the mortality figures of 150 years ago, but they must have existed.

In any event, this epidemic seems to have reached its peak and to be tapering off to some degree. But so long as more years are added to our life expectancy we may expect a high incidence of both coronary disease and cancer.

Environmental factors   The chemical and anatomical features that each man carries for his life are predetermined by his heredity. What are the things he may do or that are done to him that will bring on a coronary attack? We actually know relatively little about what these influences may be in an individual case. We have some knowledge of differences in the prevalence of coronary disease in different countries, but if these countries are medically primitive the information is highly inaccurate.

In general, two factors seem to be involved – one is the effect of arteriosclerosis and narrowing of the coronary vessels; the other is the tendency to thrombosis or clotting in these vessels. Not only are these two different things, but there is doubt as to which comes first.

Whatever may be the genesis of this disease, it seems certain that prosperous nations have more sclerosis and a greater tendency to abnormal clotting than do the less wealthy ones. The usual explanations for these differences are that the men in prosperous countries tend to be overweight, less physically active, consume richer diets, smoke more cigarettes, and live more competitive lives.

Exercise and diet   Thin, active men living in the country and doing hard physical work each day are likely to be long-lived. It makes little difference what a man eats so long as he uses up calories and does not gain weight. Men who do not exceed their top weight at the age of 25 have a good life expectancy.

A great deal of work has been done on the influence of the polyunsaturated fats (vegetable oils) as compared to animal fats and hardened fats (some of the margarines). It seems reasonable to reduce the total fat calories of our diets.

Cholesterol   Much of the apprehension concerning diet centres on cholesterol, which has become a popular scare word, and the usual assumption is that fat or cholesterol in the food causes fat or cholesterol in the arteries. This is too simple an explanation. It is not really known whether the cholesterol in the lining of the arteries comes from the diet or is a product of the degenerative changes. Furthermore, a certain amount of fat and cholesterol is necessary in our food. Fat has virtues ranging from vitamin supply to energy production and lubrication. Cholesterol is needed in almost every tissue of the human body and, if not supplied in the diet, it will be produced by the liver. It is also essential to sex hormone production.

So active has been the investigation of dietary factors that almost everything has been incriminated, either from excess or deficiency in the diet – fats, proteins, carbohydrates, trace elements, vitamins, and soft water. It is better not to be dogmatic, but to realize that man has changed from an essentially protein and fat-eating savage to a civilized creature enjoying palatable, calorie-rich carbohydrates and sugars in the past 10,000 years – which is too short a time for him to make a satisfactory adjustment. This dietary shift may well be a primary factor in the increase of obesity, dental caries, myocardial infarction, peptic ulcer, diabetes, and other diseases.

Susceptibility prediction   The prediction of who is likely to suffer from coronary disease is best made by family history, weight gain after the age of 25 (from eating too much), presence or absence of high blood pressure, and roughly the level of cholesterol in the blood. We must use caution against too much emphasis on cholesterol levels. The level fluctuates greatly in the same person and is influenced by emotion and other factors.

Chapter 3 The heart and circulatory system

Tobacco and stress   Of the many other factors in a man's life that have been blamed for his developing coronary artery disease, two deserve mention – tobacco and emotional stress.

There is no heart condition which is helped by tobacco, and men with angina are always better if they do not smoke.

Coronary disease is ubiquitous in civilized society because of the age of the population, and it is found at all economic levels and with all degrees of nervous stress. Studies show that regardless of occupational stress, the incidence of coronary disease is inversely related to the degree of physical effort of the job – that is, the physically active are less affected regardless of whether they have jobs with much or little nervous tension.

Professor Arnott has stated this well: "Psychological stress and strain has for long been popularly believed to play an important part in a wide variety of disease, including ischaemic heart disease and essential hypertension. So far as I can see, this hypothesis has no scientifically credible basis whatsoever – in fact, most of the evidence adduced in its support is dubious and much of it absurd. . . . The ready acceptance of this stress and strain concept is very understandable. It nourishes the amour propre of the believer and it is readily acceptable to the unfortunate victim and his relatives. It places ischaemic heart disease in being in the position of the unjust reward of virtue. How much nicer it is when stricken with a coronary thrombosis to be told that it is all due to hard work, laudable ambition, and selfless devotion to duty than to be told it is due to gluttony and physical indolence."

This is not to say that an emotional stimulus may not start an attack of angina; there is evidence to show that it may. But nervous tension does not cause the deposit of fatty substances in coronary arteries other than in a secondary sense, that is, that it encourages compensatory excessive smoking and eating, without enough exercise.

The pattern of coronary artery disease   It may seem a pessimistic statement, but physicians today possess no method, test, or instrument for the early detection of coronary artery disease and are no more capable of making the diagnosis of its clinical manifestations than they were in 1768 when the English physician, William Heberden, first described it.

The earliest sign of coronary insufficiency is the sensation of pressure or strangling in the chest, or angina pectoris, and the diagnosis is made by the skilled assessment of what the patient tells the doctor and by whether or not a nitroglycerine tablet under the tongue relieves the patient of his distress.

Nitroglycerine was first given for this disease in 1867 and is still in use. The character of the distress and its relationship to causative factors must be studied by the doctor. It is not a good idea for the patient to diagnose his own ailment. A great many chest pains are harmless and related to organs other than the heart.

It is true that in some instances an electrocardiogram will reveal abnormal electrical waves in the heart to support a diagnosis of coronary disease, but when these are present the disease is well advanced. Indeed, by the time angina develops, one or more branches of the coronary system have already been blocked by gradual narrowing of the particular vessels that are involved.

Angina

By and large, angina shows itself by chest discomfort or pain and a sense of constriction, brought on by situations which demand more work by the heart and greater blood flow through the coronary arteries. These may be physical effort, emotional stress, the increased circulation required by the digestion of a meal, and, particularly, exertion in cold windy weather. Combinations of these factors are especially bad.

Living with angina   Development of angina pectoris does not mean an invalid's life. Often, simple alterations in daily living will reduce the symptoms considerably. Weight reduction, cutting out smoking, taking more holidays, rearranging work commitments, and more suitable exercise will help.

A man with angina should realize that, while he has progressive narrowing in his coronary arteries, so do other men over the age of 45. Furthermore, the body is always attempting to compensate for this by widening other arteries in the coronary system to produce a new circulation. The patient's course depends upon the balance of the state of the arteries and the collateral circulation in his heart.

One must face the fact that coronary artery disease is a common cause of sudden death. On the other hand, the average length of life after the diagnosis is made is well over ten years and many live much longer. Indeed, men who recover from the more severe forms of coronary thrombosis, to the degree that they can return to work, die at a rate only about fifteen per cent greater than unaffected persons with normal life expectancy.

Coronary thrombosis

The term heart attack is commonly given to the condition that kills its victim within a few minutes or causes a collapse which is survived long enough for him to be put to bed at home or in the hospital. Usually the patient has a history of previous angina, but this new attack often comes when he is at rest or asleep and not involved in any exertion such as he has learned to avoid in the past. On the other hand, he may have had no earlier chest distress but is awakened by a severe crushing chest pain with sweating, nausea, and collapse. Nitroglycerine fails to relieve him and may make him worse. Morphine and other sedatives, oxygen, and heart-supporting drugs may be needed.

Usually a fresh clot is found in a narrow coronary artery and in those surviving a few hours or days an area of heart muscle supplied by the blocked artery will be found to have died from loss of blood supply; that is, the structure of the muscle and its function of contraction will be lost (myocardial infarction), and in those who recover this area will be replaced by scar tissue. The extent of the muscle damage determines the events of the next few days and weeks. Unfortunately, some patients with coronary thrombosis die within a few hours. But, although it sounds obvious, every day that the patient survives steadily increases the outlook of a good recovery.

The state of the heart rate and rhythm, the recovery of blood pressure, the disappearance of pain, and the subsidence of fever are all signs to be evaluated. There are more delicate indications also, certain blood enzyme tests, sedimentation rate, and so on, to guide the doctor. For this condition, the electrocardiograph can not only make the diagnosis, but tell the area of involvement of the heart muscle, and something about the severity and extent of the damage and the likely speed of recovery.

Treatment   The treatment of each patient must be individual but is always greatly aided by good nursing. Where conditions for home nursing are good, and particularly in elderly patients, there seems to be no advantage in hospital admission in cases without disorders of heart rhythm. Though complications are more easily dealt with in hospital, they occur less often in cases nursed at home. The use of oxygen, heart drugs, blood pressure stimulants, and anticoagulant medicines is the province of the physician. The question of anticoagulants is still a vexed one throughout the world, and different statistical studies support either the use or omission of them. They are

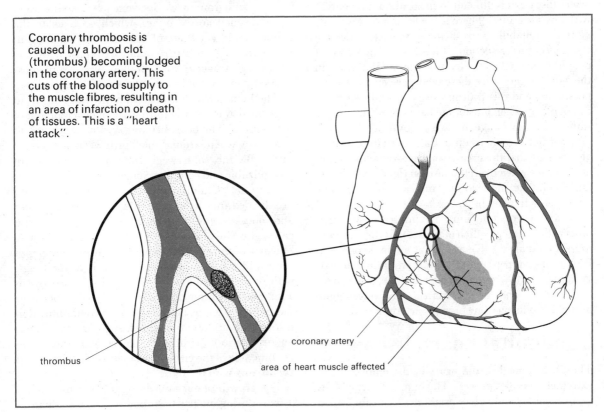

Coronary thrombosis is caused by a blood clot (thrombus) becoming lodged in the coronary artery. This cuts off the blood supply to the muscle fibres, resulting in an area of infarction or death of tissues. This is a "heart attack".

thrombus

coronary artery

area of heart muscle affected

difficult and dangerous to use but prevent some secondary thrombosis in the veins of very ill patients with sluggish blood flow in the legs. Early mobilization from bed has greatly reduced the number of deaths from this common complication. Recent experience in industry shows that most men with good recovery and no subsequent heart muscle failure may return to their usual jobs even with moderately heavy labour. The exception is the operation of public transport, even though the risk may be slight.

After recovery As in the case of angina, coronary thrombosis need not lead to invalidism. Most men go through a period of anxiety and depression after a coronary thrombosis, but as the years go on they realize that recovery usually means a return to a comfortable effective life. Patients should be advised to resume as normal a life as possible, and sexual activity is not prohibited. Obviously, they should avoid situations beyond their control – do not get caught in snow storms, do not swim out to a raft when you have to swim back, do not drink so much that you lose your judgment, do not smoke, do not gain weight, and exercise regularly. Losing one's temper is a luxury.

Prevention In view of the fact that many influences appear to be involved in the development of coronary artery disease, it is difficult to speak about prevention with any assurance. There is the feeling that it is one of the inevitabilities of civilized society, indeed a result of natural selection. It has been suggested that people who survived the terrible famines in Europe in the Middle Ages were those who were efficient body fat storers, and this trait has been transmitted to an age of plenty when fat storage has become dangerous rather than advantageous. We are putting in calories and not burning them up in daily activities. It may also be true that the greatest harm is done to men in adolescence when overemphasis on rapid growth and large fat intakes in the form of milk are common. The adolescent girl takes in far less.

In any event, one must be impressed by such observations as that which indicates that the only way to make a male rat live as long as a female one is to feed it only 70 per cent of what it would like to eat. Weight control, regular physical exercise, reduced fat and sweets, and no cigarettes may have some protective influence on coronary arteries.

Congenital heart disease

The development of the heart in the embryo is an extremely complex process. The human heart with its four chambers and valves originates as a tube which divides and twists in a fashion that permits a great variety of errors of construction. Disturbances in oxygen supply to the mother, infections – chiefly viral – and deficiencies in nutrition, seem to be of major importance. Recently, we have seen the effect of certain drugs, notably thalidomide, in producing congenital defects of the limbs, and similar defects may appear in the heart.

The possibilities of combinations of cardiac defects are almost limitless, hundreds are known but most of these are so severe that they lead to death of the infant before, or shortly after, birth. The errors of assembly consist chiefly of failures in the development of the valves; or of septal defects, that is, failure of holes in the partitions between heart chambers to close properly; or of persistence of the artery that bypasses the lungs (ductus arteriosus) which fails to close and cease its fetal function after birth.

Many others occur, such as the emptying of veins from the lungs into the wrong atrium; origin of coronary arteries from the pulmonary artery, instead of the aorta, so that the heart muscle is being fed blue unoxygenated blood, instead of red blood; lack of proper division of the heart into four chambers so that it may have only three, or even only two chambers; incomplete rotation of the heart so that its main arteries arise from the wrong ventricle; persistence of the unneeded aortic arches, which go back to the primitive gill slit stage of the embryo, resulting in rings of blood vessels surrounding and constricting the breathing (trachea) and swallowing (oesophagus) tubes; and narrowing (coarctation) of the aorta.

The human heart, at first a simple tube, begins to be formed at about the third week of development of the embryo. The heart begins to twitch, and then to beat, somewhere around the fourth week of development. By the sixth week the four chambers are recognizable and complex changes are under way.

Diagnosis Children with congenital heart disease are divided into two main groups – cyanotic (blue) and noncyanotic (with normal colour). In some cases, the child may become blue in attacks. The blueness of the cyanotic type is due to the mixing of venous blood, that has not gone through the lungs, with oxygenated blood. This may be caused by an abnormal communication or septal defect between the right and left heart chambers, or communication through an abnormal channel, such as a persistent ductus arteriosus, if there is a high enough pressure on the blue side of the circulation to force the blue blood over to mix with the red.

The growth of our knowledge of congenital heart defects during life has been built upon two advances

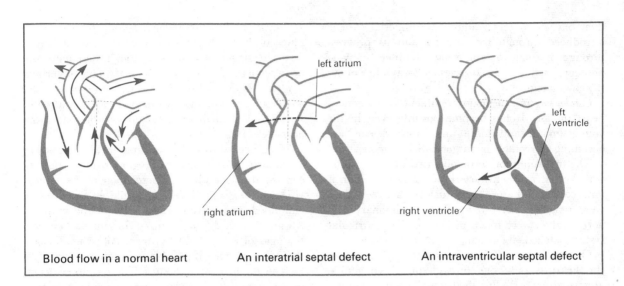

| Blood flow in a normal heart | An interatrial septal defect | An intraventricular septal defect |

of recent years – the cardiac catheter, and the development of cardiac surgery, with and without the heart pump. The latter permits stopping of the patient's own heart and the carrying on of an effective circulation by a mechanical pump beside the operating table. The cardiac catheter is a thin tube filled with saline, which can be threaded into an arm vein and pushed into the heart – most readily into the right atrium, right ventricle, and lung vessels; special techniques are necessary for left heart catheter study. The tube may be seen on the fluoroscopic screen of the X-ray and guided into the heart, it can be photographed by X-ray, it can be used to measure pressures in the heart and lungs and passed through septal defects. Through it can be drawn samples of blood from various areas in the heart for measurement of

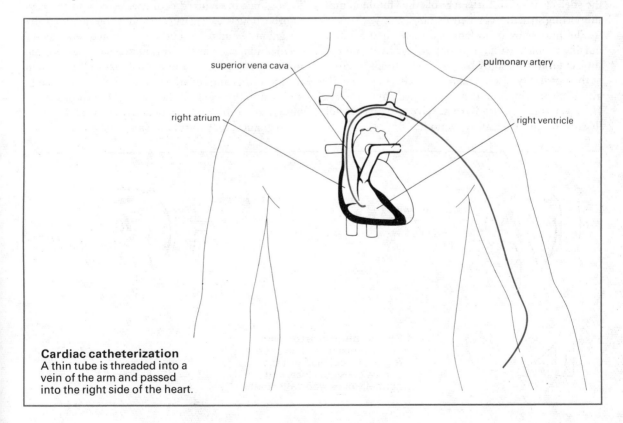

Cardiac catheterization
A thin tube is threaded into a vein of the arm and passed into the right side of the heart.

their oxygen content; radiopaque material can be introduced through the catheter and its progress through normal or abnormal channels can be photographed by a rapid series of X-ray films or X-ray cinematography.

Cardiac surgery is the major treatment for congenital heart disease. It has become possible even in the young infant, and more and more defects are becoming correctable by surgery. (See chapter 23.)

The first condition to be operated on successfully was the patent ductus arteriosus. This operation is now common. Later, septal defects between atria were repaired, narrowed stenotic pulmonary and aortic valves were freed, defects in the ventricular system patched, abnormal pulmonary veins resited.

Of course there are instances where the defect in the heart is only one of widespread congenital abnormalities including the brain. This may be true in Down's syndrome where surgery of the heart will not correct the fundamental inherited genetic defect. Another combined congenital anomaly is Marfan's syndrome. These patients have a typical association of cardiac defect and dislocation of the lenses of the eyes. They are tall and slender with very long spider-like fingers and toes (arachnodactyly). They are not usually suitable for cardiac surgery since the defect is a disturbance of the fundamental supporting structures of their tissues.

The blue baby is no longer a mere medical and nursing problem with only a hope of survival, but is a subject for intense study by modern methods because of the possibility of surgical relief. Still, by no means all of these children can be helped by surgery. However, blue babies have survived to live useful lives even when constantly cyanotic.

Prevention Present evidence favours the view that illness of the mother in early pregnancy is the major factor in congenital defects, although there may also be a genetic or family tendency. This inherited tendency is exceedingly small, and does not justify advice to a woman against having other children if she has given birth to an infant with a congenital heart defect.

It has been shown that German measles (rubella) in the first three months of pregnancy may result in cardiac abnormalities in a percentage of the babies. It is best for girls to have their children's diseases in childhood, especially German measles and mumps. All girls should be ummunized for rubella between the ages of eleven and fourteen. All virus diseases should be avoided if possible in pregnancy, particularly in the first three months. There is no evidence that colds or influenza can cause congenital defects.

Similarly, it is believed by some embryologists that any exposure to anoxia (low oxygen) can be dangerous to the fetus at this time – even trips in aircraft and high altitude travel. The latter view is supported by the high incidence of congenital heart disease in babies born in races living at high altitudes, as in the Andes Mountains of South America.

Errors in nutrition are not likely to be of great importance in civilized countries, except in the very poorly nourished. Drugs should be avoided by pregnant women except for accepted emergency medication, such as the antibiotics, but these should not be given for every minor ailment. Only certain tranquillizers and sedatives should be used. Smoking and consumption of alcohol by pregnant women are most undesirable and, particularly in the early weeks of pregnancy, may harm the baby.

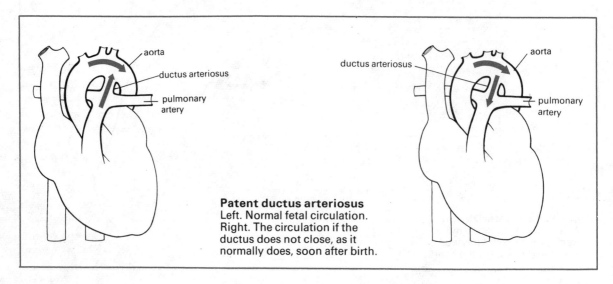

Patent ductus arteriosus
Left. Normal fetal circulation.
Right. The circulation if the ductus does not close, as it normally does, soon after birth.

Congestive failure

Like other organs in the body, the heart often does not announce the early stages of its diseases. It is only when it has used up its reserve of muscular power, or of blood supply in its coronary arteries, that it begins to produce a warning signal. In coronary disease this is usually the distress on exertion called angina pectoris.

In situations where the trouble is in the heart muscle or valves, the symptom is breathlessness (dyspnoea). This is a particular kind of shortness of breath, with an increased rate of breathing, coming on with exertion or sometimes waking the patient from sleep with oppression in the chest, desire to sit up in order to breathe better (orthopnoea), wheezing, and cough.

This disturbance is sometimes known as cardiac asthma, but this is an undesirable term, because it has nothing to do with bronchial asthma.

All these breathing difficulties are a prominent part of what is known as congestive failure. It should not be confused with the shortness of breath which is intermittent, not regularly associated with exertion, and characterized by a sensation which is usually referred to as being an inability to take a deep breath. This leads to deep sighing breathing and finally one of these breaths is effective. Then the symptom subsides, only to start again later. This is an uncomfortable, but never serious sensation and is found in all sorts of fatigue and anxiety conditions. It is usually worse when the person is resting or working quietly rather than when he is asking the heart to do extra work.

True congestive failure occurs only with damaged hearts, but is often reversible with treatment and it may be kept under control for years with careful diet and medicine. It is of two kinds – right and left heart failure – but there is usually a combination of these. The reason for differentiating the two types is partly to help in deciding the underlying cause of the heart disease.

In right heart failure, the right ventricle has difficulty in delivering to the lungs the venous blood, which banks up in the right atrium and then in the veins in both upper and lower parts of the body and in the liver. This venous stasis (slowing of normal flow in the veins) with increased pressure results in leakage of fluid through the small vessel walls and collection of the fluid (oedema) in the ankles, later the legs, or even most of the body in bedridden patients. Fortunately, this is not seen so often since the treatment has been better understood. The old term for oedema was dropsy; both mean "too much water in the tissues",

and one may speak of a waterlogged patient. Actually, in pure right heart failure the congestion is in the outer or peripheral parts of the body and the lungs are spared, but this is very rarely seen, since both sides of the heart generally weaken together, especially if there is heart muscle disease, but the thinner right ventricle tends to fail first.

In left heart failure, the difficulty lies in the ineffective discharge of the left ventricle. This can arise from hypertension, obstruction of the aortic valve (stenosis), leakage of the aortic valve (regurgitation), leakage of the mitral valve, and other less common conditions. Mitral stenosis, on the other hand, spares the left ventricle and causes back pressure in the circulation behind it, that is, in the left atrium, and the blood vessels in the lungs. There is then hypertension in the lesser circulation, namely, high blood pressure in the lung arteries and veins. The right ventricle, in trying to pump against this, will fail first. In fact, when the left ventricle weakens and has trouble in emptying, this will result in much the same increase in pressure in the lung vessels, so that secondary failure of the right ventricle will occur. It is clear that either mitral stenosis or left heart failure will reveal itself by causing the sufferer to become breathless on exertion because the effort calls for an increase in the amount of blood pumped by the heart which in turn will bank up in the lungs.

Treatment The most important advance in the treatment of congestive heart failure was made by a British doctor, William Withering, in 1785. He discovered, after investigating various herbs used by an old woman to treat dropsy, that the foxglove, whose leaves produce the drug digitalis, was the active agent. He therefore used a decoction of the leaves and published a little book describing the effects. Digitalis is particularly effective when atrial fibrillation is associated with the failure since it causes a blocking of many of the irregular useless signals from the atrium and slows the ventricles, as well as strengthening the heart muscle. The proper use of this drug was forgotten after Withering's day and only in the present century have the dosage and methods of administration in the individual patient become well established.

Another important step was the introduction of effective diuretics, that is, drugs stimulating kidney activity to eliminate the retained water.

In recent years, one more valuable drug has been added and that is the diuretic compound that does not contain mercury and may be taken by mouth. The basic drug is chlorothiazide, of which several modifications are available.

A third advance was the re-emphasis of the importance of sodium in the diet of people subject to congestive failure. The body's congestion by water is encouraged by the retention of sodium in the tissues and, indeed, the action of most diuretics seems to be the elimination of sodium through the kidneys and this takes the water with it. Careful attention to the amount of sodium in the diet may make the use of diuretics unnecessary or, at least, permit smaller or less frequent doses. (See low sodium diets, page 372.)

The most common source of sodium in our food is table salt, sodium chloride, and this is readily controlled, but a person with a need for sodium restriction should be under careful medical control; firstly, to receive instructions about the sodium content of foods which are not obviously salty, and, secondly, to be sure that the sodium and other necessary salts, such as potassium, are not unduly depleted to a point where the chemistry of the body is so disturbed as to produce further complications. The level of restriction is an individual prescription for each patient. It should be remembered that in certain areas of the country drinking water is so rich in sodium as to be a factor in the total sodium intake.

The next step in treatment was the technical ability to operate on the mitral valve and relieve stenosis. When this is the cause of heart failure, direct attack on the mechanical obstruction is the most valuable treatment, but secondary treatment is usually also necessary.

As well as these treatments, one must not disregard the common-sense measures advisable for anyone with heart disease. These include a routine of life within the limits of the patient's physical ability, and one which does not produce symptoms; weight control; omission of tobacco (often a most important step in controlling a cough); and the correction of any complicating disease. For example, anaemia from the bleeding of a stomach ulcer, infections of various sorts, diabetes, hypertension, and other ailments may precipitate or perpetuate congestive failure.

Congestive failure is not necessarily a final stage of heart disease; it may be a temporary situation responding to treatment, and after recovery the patient may lead a reasonably active, productive, comfortable life for years. The cardiac patient must learn to live with his disability and to cooperate fully with his doctor.

Rheumatic heart disease

The most common cause of heart disease in children and young adults is rheumatic fever. This disease is a streptococcal infection which may appear also as scarlet fever or acute streptococcal nephritis (kidney inflammation). It has been decreasing in prevalence in Britain for over 30 years, but tends to occur in epidemic form wherever large groups of young men are brought together, as in military training camps. It is more common in the colder months, especially the spring, and in temperate climates, but rheumatic heart disease is also found in the tropics, although the premonitory symptoms of sore throat and joint pains may be less obvious.

Symptoms The characteristic stage of onset of rheumatic fever is a respiratory infection with sore throat. Culture of the bacteria from the throat shows a particular variety of streptococci. Two or three weeks after this sore throat the patient will have joint pains with swelling and redness of the larger joints of arms and legs, possibly nosebleeds, skin eruptions, a form of pneumonia, inflammation of the sac around the heart (pericarditis), heart murmurs, and changes in the electrocardiogram. Another sign may be chorea (St. Vitus dance) and, in severe cases, small fibrous nodules may appear over bony prominences like knuckles, elbows, knees, ankles, and spine.

At the present time, the disease seems to be less severe than it was 40 years ago. The patient may have only mild joint pains, yet the heart valves and muscles may be affected. The earliest sign of heart muscle inflammation may be the electrocardiographic evidence of a delay in the passage of the electrical impulse from atrium to ventricle. In rare cases this may lead to a degree of blocking of the impulse by inflammatory reaction, so that heartbeats are dropped, that is, the heart pauses momentarily. The patient has fever and an increased heart rate. The white blood cell count is elevated, and other indicators, such as the sedimentation rate, show signs of disturbance.

Valve damage Murmurs and changes in the heart sounds occur. Some of these decrease and disappear with recovery, but loud murmurs produced at the mitral valve and those from the aortic valve mean true inflammation of the valve leaflets. While the heart has four valves – tricuspid, pulmonary, mitral, and aortic – the last two are commonly affected by rheumatic fever, the tricuspid rarely, and the pulmonary never.

With recovery from the acute stage, the inflamed valve becomes scarred and does not close properly, resulting in a leak (regurgitation), or it becomes narrowed by adhesion of the valve leaflets (stenosis). The effects of these mechanical disturbances in the valves are greatly influenced by the degree of injury to the heart muscle (myocarditis) which accompanies the valvular inflammation.

The heart enlarges by thickening of the muscle because of the greater work demanded by the leaking or obstructed valves, and stretches out by weakness brought on by the inflammation of the heart muscle. Later it may develop irregularities of rhythm and finally atrial fibrillation with total and continuous irregularity.

We think of rheumatic heart disease as a malady of childhood and early life, but many patients with rheumatic hearts live into the late adult years and even old age. It is believed that some cases of calcified aortic valve stenosis have their origins in childhood rheumatic infection, but this is notoriously an elderly person's type of heart disease and may be seen in the 70's and 80's.

Rheumatic infection is unlike most other diseases of childhood in that it does not characteristically run an acute course and then subside with complete recovery that makes the child immune to other attacks. Quite the reverse, it may lead to a low grade smouldering infection lasting for months or years. The tendency to recurrence is ever present, especially after colds and sore throats. This moderately acute state may be shown by vague joint pains (sometimes wrongly called growing pains), skin rashes, the nervous twitching of chorea, nosebleeds, poor appetite, weight loss, abdominal pain (sometimes mistaken for appendicitis), and the picture of a child who is ill and out of sorts. Recurrent acute attacks may appear at intervals of a few months or, more often, ten to twelve months apart.

Rheumatic infection occurs most commonly in cities and in poor economic conditions. There seems also to be some family tendency. It has been thought that improved economic conditions are largely responsible for its decline. Patients with acute rheumatic fever do occur, however, in families of a high economic level.

Wherever the streptococcus is prevalent, rheumatic fever is found. It may well occur throughout the world and its present decrease is probably only a phase in which it is waiting to appear, like many diseases that re-emerge in times of war, overcrowding, and poor nutrition.

Clinical course The common cold with running nose and no fever is not the precursor of an attack of rheumatic fever. The sore throat is the potential danger signal, if accompanied by fever, and if a throat culture shows the typical streptococcus. This is the infection that should be treated early, and if this is done the incidence of rheumatic fever following it is strikingly reduced. Prompt treatment with penicillin is essential. If such treatment is not given, rheumatic infection may appear two or three weeks later, but it should be remembered that the number of children or young adults who develop this after a sore throat is really very small. Since, however, it is unpredictable, treatment should be given early and after a throat culture has been taken. If the beta haemolytic streptococcus (group A streptococcus) is not found in this culture, no harm is done; but if it is, the full course of ten days of penicillin is advisable.

It may be very easy or very difficult to be sure of the diagnosis of rheumatic fever or even of the early stages of rheumatic heart disease. Some signs are unmistakable, such as pericardial inflammation or characteristic murmurs and electrocardiograms. Often a period of several weeks of bed rest may be necessary before the child can be judged free from active rheumatic infection. This is also the reason why a child should be seen by his doctor at intervals of a few months for at least three years after a bout of rheumatic fever, even if the heart appears to have escaped damage.

Generally, it is best for a rheumatic child to have daily preventive penicillin by mouth for several years after an attack, though how long for is not really known. Some say for life, but after a child grows up the treatment can be stopped if valvular disease is not clearly present and if he is alert to the knowledge that he should always have penicillin when he has a sore throat or other severe respiratory disease. An attack of active rheumatism may subside in two or three weeks but usually we think of this as a disease lasting for six weeks, or longer. Return to normal life may be permitted by the end of three months. Complications and daily symptomatic treatment in the acute phase should be in the doctor's hands. Penicillin, aspirin, and the newer steroid hormones (cortisone derivatives) are the usual drugs for this disease.

Chronic rheumatic heart disease When the heart is permanently damaged by rheumatic fever, the course of the disease may be rapid and fatal in children in a matter of a few weeks or months, but the usual progression is slow and the most striking fact is that adults in their thirties to fifties, or even later, who can remember no episode of acute rheumatism in their earlier life, may be found to have valvular deformities due to rheumatic infection. There may be only a history of vague pains or frequent sore throats.

Patients of this sort may be unaware of their heart disease until some severe strain is put upon the heart, such as infection, pregnancy, or competitive athletics; or on routine examination for life insurance or military service. Sometimes the arrival of sudden total irregularity of the heart at a rapid rate (atrial fibrillation), will lead to heart failure and reveal underlying mitral stenosis.

The two valves commonly affected are the mitral and the aortic. Either one may develop a leak (regurgitation) or a narrowing from thickening and scarring (stenosis). The mitral valve is particularly liable to stenosis and the aortic to regurgitation. Furthermore, the stenosis of the mitral valve, which puts a back pressure on the left atrium, is commonly associated with atrial fibrillation. Aortic regurgitation is a more serious condition, but there are gradations of stenosis and regurgitation as well as combined damage to either or both valves, that is, a valve may have some degree of both obstruction and leakage.

Surgery It is in this area of rheumatic valvular disease that cardiac surgery has played one of its most successful roles. The technique of cardiac catheterization permits study of the actual amount of blocking or leaking of the valves and a good estimate of the actual size of the valve opening.

It is now possible to relieve the stenosis of the mitral valve; it is somewhat more difficult to remove the aortic valve obstruction; and it is still more difficult to repair leaking valves. Progress, however, is being made in fashioning artificial valves of human tissue or plastic materials. The ability to perform open heart surgery is aiding these advances, since the heart can be stopped while an artificial pump takes over the circulation during the operation.

Men and women with rheumatic heart disease usually live moderately active, useful lives under medical care, and now after cardiac surgery their life expectancy and work ability have been greatly improved. A certain number, perhaps fifteen per cent, have to undergo second operations because of the return of valve deformity from scarring. It is hoped that this percentage will decrease with improved surgical techniques.

Irregularities of the heartbeat (the arrhythmias)

Among the early discoveries concerned with the action of the heart and circulation, the observation of the pulse beat and its disturbances was very important. In ancient days the wrist pulse bore many names from which the physician was supposed to make the diagnosis of different diseases. It was described as slow or fast, hard or soft, full or weak, bounding, paradoxical (when it rose and fell in

volume in an abnormal fashion during breathing), and so on. The relationship between what went on in the heart and what could be felt by the finger on the artery at the wrist was not understood, but it is still true that careful observation of the character of the pulse can give a great deal of information about the heart and blood pressure.

Although much was learned in the last century by simple mechanical recording of the pulse with levers moving writing pens, the invention of the electrocardiograph by Willem Einthoven in Holland in 1903 provided us with an instrument of extreme delicacy, capable of recording every kind of disorder of heart rate and rhythm. Indeed, the electrocardiograph was first used chiefly to study these disturbances. It was not until about 40 years ago that its value in diagnosing heart muscle injury, as in coronary thrombosis and infarction, became recognized.

Rapid heart When exercise, emotion, or any other stimuli ask the heart to provide more blood for the tissues, it will accelerate. It retains its normal sequential beating, that is atrium and then ventricle, but just goes faster. This is sinus tachycardia, or rapid heartbeat under control of the sino-auricular node, or pacemaker. The rate may be quite fast, up to 160.

Normal heart rate is variable throughout the day. It may average 72, but normal men can have daily resting rates of 50 to over 80. The rate is usually slower in the morning; it rises after exercise and emotion, a meal, or with smoking.

There are great differences at different ages. An infant before birth may have a heart rate of 120, and when he is 80 it may be 60. The difference in animals is striking. The heart rate of an elephant is 46 per minute and that of an ostrich is 60, while that of a small bird may be 900. The canary's heart beats 1000 times a minute.

A rapid heart from excitement or exertion is a normal response and is one of nature's reflexes to prepare the individual to fight or run away. The reason we have this tachycardia when we are anxious is often because we cannot decide which to do.

Normal irregular heart Another normal alteration of the heartbeat is called sinus arrhythmia. The heart speeds up when we breathe in, and slows down when we breathe out. This is more noticeable in children and young people and if any characteristic is to be applied to it, it should be considered a sign of a normal heart.

Other disturbances The most common disorder of heart rhythm is the extrasystole or premature beat. This is a hesitation of the heart which, when felt in the pulse at the wrist, seems to be a skipping or dropping out of a heartbeat. Actually what happens is that a small area in the atrium, or ventricle, or even in the electrical network of heart nerves, becomes irritable and sends out a message before the next normal signal from the sinus node is due. This triggers off an early or premature beat and the expected normal one does not occur because, having just responded, the heart is not ready. What we usually feel is a temporary flutter in the chest or neck and a heavy thump when the next beat comes. This thump is caused by a larger ejection of blood because the heart has paused and therefore has had more time to fill.

Few, if any, of us go through life without occasional or many premature beats. Often the subject does not even feel them at a time when we are actually recording them in the electrocardiogram. They are more common at rest and sometimes make it difficult to get to sleep, especially for someone who is apprehensive about them. They are never serious and probably occur in normal hearts more often than in those with disease. They may come singly or in groups, irregularly with periods of freedom, or be present for weeks, months, or years. Most of us learn to live with premature beats and disregard them as merely a nuisance, but they may mean that fatigue, coffee, tea, (or other drinks containing caffeine), cigarettes, alcohol, late hours, or anxiety are affecting us.

When a series of premature beats gets strung together at a rapid rate it is called paroxysmal tachycardia. Such attacks may show heart rates over 300, but mainly from 120 to 180. They start or stop abruptly and run from a few seconds up to several hours. Occasionally the attack may last for days or weeks.

Paroxysmal tachycardia may originate in the atrium or ventricle. The latter type is usually more serious and harder to treat. Drugs are available that are generally helpful in preventing paroxysmal tachycardia. The most commonly used is some form of quinidine, a relative of quinine. Various measures to stop an attack should of course be under the control of a doctor.

The rapid, totally irregular rhythm of atrial fibrillation is found most often with rheumatic valvular disease (chiefly mitral stenosis), thyroid overactivity, or coronary disease with congestive failure. However, it can also occur at intervals as short attacks for as long as 60 years in apparently normal hearts. Its occurrence should always lead to a careful medical survey because all organic causes should be ruled out before it can be considered harmless or

functional. Digitalis is the drug chosen for treatment of acute attacks.

A far more serious and often fatal disturbance of rhythm is *ventricular fibrillation*. Since the ventricle is not pumping in this condition, it is rapidly fatal unless the heart can be defibrillated by the new electrical machines that shock the heart out of its dangerous standstill. Ventricular fibrillation occurs more often in acute coronary attacks and during cardiac surgery, although it may unexpectedly occur during other forms of surgery. The ability to terminate such attacks by defibrillating has been of dramatic service on many occasions. The onset of this form of fibrillation probably accounts for many sudden and unexpected deaths in people going about their daily tasks, as well as in those in the serious stages of obvious acute coronary disease.

There is one other form of rhythm disorder of varying degrees of seriousness. This is *heart block*. In its mildest form there is a delay between the beat of the atrium and that of the ventricle which exceeds the normal interval. This is called first stage block or prolonged P-R interval in the electrocardiogram. It is seen in a few apparently normal people with slow hearts, but may be a sign of early rheumatic disease of the heart muscle, especially in children.

The second stage is dropped beats when the block is sufficient to prevent the electrical impulse from passing from the atrium to the ventricle at certain intervals of time. If this block becomes established in a proportional form, namely blocking at regular intervals, the atrium may beat twice as often as the ventricle (2:1 block) or three times to the ventricle's twice (3:2 block) or in some other relationship (3:1, 4:1, and so on).

Finally, in serious disease the impulse may be entirely blocked and we speak of complete heart block. This is a somewhat confusing term because it sounds as if the heart is jammed up. It refers, however, only to the electrical message being blocked. Inflammation or degeneration of tissue near the A-V node is responsible, chiefly in coronary artery disease. If this complete blocking is intermittent, the heart stops and the patient will be dizzy for a moment, or faint, go into convulsions, or die depending on how long the ventricle stops beating. Actually, however, another pacemaker below the A-V node may take over and it is possible to live for years with a heart in which the ventricles are beating slowly and independently, paying no attention to the atria which are also beating regularly at a faster normal rate.

It is in these conditions of high grade or complete block that the new electrical pacemakers are useful.

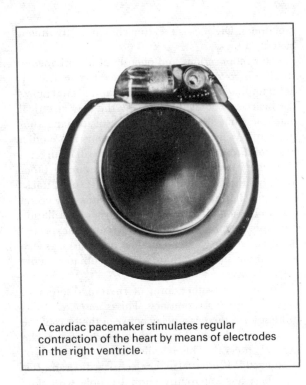

A cardiac pacemaker stimulates regular contraction of the heart by means of electrodes in the right ventricle.

One can be applied to the chest in an emergency, and later a small one can be implanted under the skin, with a wire going to the heart. These devices send a stimulating current to electrodes in contact with the heart muscle, thus triggering the beat and producing contractions at near the normal rate when the heart itself cannot do so reliably. Cardiac pacemakers have increased greatly in sophistication and reliability since the first ones, which were carried in an awkward and bulky package at the waist, with wires connected with electrodes in the heart.

Many patients need the permanent protection of a pacemaker implanted under the large muscle on the left side of the chest. The original installation of course requires surgery. Replacement of the battery every five or more years requires surgery but this is a relatively minor procedure. It is possible that battery replacement may become unnecessary in improved pacemakers if tiny nuclear power plants, currently under development, that run on and on for many years prove practicable.

Obliterative arterial disease

As long as arteries function as tubes conveying blood, they can be said to be adequate. A major occurrence that can render an artery inadequate to convey blood

is obstruction. The most common cause of obstruction to an artery is arteriosclerosis – closure of the arterial tube brought about by degenerative disease. Reduction in size of the lumen (the internal tubelike channel) of an artery often occurs, but sufficient reduction of blood flow to cause malfunction of tissues supplied by the artery does not occur unless the reduction is severe. It is obvious that considerable disease of the arterial wall must exist before tissue malfunction can occur.

Blockage within an artery develops from an atheromatous plaque or deposit of fatty material within the lining of the artery. Thrombosis of an artery is the usual factor which precipitates the patient's symptoms. A thrombus is a blood clot which remains at the point of its formation; an artery in which this occurs is said to be thrombosed. The artery, which at first was partially blocked, becomes completely occluded or thrombosed over a length varying from a half inch to six to twelve inches. Any artery in the body is susceptible to being blocked in this manner.

Arteriosclerosis is a rather broad category which includes diseases of the major arteries such as the aorta, iliac, and femoral arteries. Loss of elasticity and changes in the appearance and structure of lining coats of the arteries are brought about mainly by degenerative changes which increase in frequency with age and which affect the arterial system of such vital organs as the heart, brain, kidneys, and major blood vessels to the extremities. Arteriosclerosis may be prevalent throughout the arterial system, but it is rarely generalized to the extent that all arteries of the body are affected equally or similarly.

Processes of thrombosis When an artery thromboses due to sclerotic disease, a sequence of changes occurs. The thrombus, or clot, sets up severe inflammatory reaction which spreads to the covering (adventitia) of the artery and then into surrounding tissues. Frequently, collateral circulation (a new network of blood vessels) develops around the blockage. This may be sufficient to keep the tissues alive, but not sufficient to supply adequate blood to muscles during exercise.

Once an artery has thrombosed and caused symptoms, there is danger that other arteries in the body will become blocked in a similar fashion. Arteriosclerosis is a progressive disease. Fortunately its course is not steadily downhill, but rather, after each thrombosis, there may be a period of improvement as collateral circulation develops. Intervals of improvement vary in different patients from a few weeks to twenty years or more between episodes.

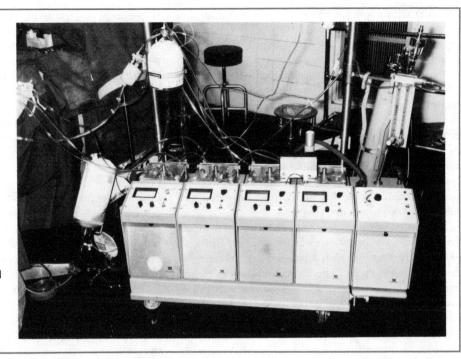

A heart lung machine, used for bypassing the blood from the patient's heart and lungs during certain operations on the heart.

This tendency to spontaneous improvement between episodes of thrombosis makes it difficult to assess the disease process accurately. While patients with symptoms of arteriosclerotic thrombosis have decreased life expectancy, it is important to stress that the course of the disease is highly variable. Some patients are markedly affected, but others lead long, active and useful lives with an interval of years between thrombotic episodes.

Absence of arteriosclerosis is very rare in middle-aged and elderly persons. The disease is much more prevalent among men than women. Atheroma formation is uncommon in women before the menopause. However, in patients with diabetes the sex incidence of arteriosclerotic symptoms is about equal, perhaps because diabetes is more prevalent in women.

Symptoms Arteriosclerotic disease rarely causes symptoms until an artery becomes completely or partially blocked. Thrombosis of the lower portion of the aorta and major vessels of the legs (a common area for arteriosclerosis) causes three main types of symptoms.

Intermittent claudication, which means intermittent limping, is the most common symptom. The patient, after walking a certain distance, develops pain in the calf muscles, due to inadequate flow of blood through these muscles. The blood flow is adequate when the patient rests, but inadequate to meet the greater demands of increased physical activity. Patients with this symptom usually state that pain comes on after they have walked a specific distance. The pain may of course come sooner if the patient walks at a faster rate or walks uphill.

Another symptom is pain at rest. This is ominous evidence of severe blockage of arterial blood flow to the affected area. As a rule, these pains are worse at night, and may be eased by letting the leg hang down or aggravated by elevating the leg.

Another distressing symptom may be anaesthesia, or loss of sensation in the entire extremity or a portion of it. This frequently occurs after a major blockage of blood flow involving the entire foot.

Arteriosclerosis of major vessels of the lower limbs rarely causes a patient to complain of symptoms other than intermittent claudication or rest pain. However, a frequent complaint is that the feet and toes are unduly sensitive to cold. Some patients may complain of numbness of the feet and toes without a feeling of coldness. These symptoms may manifest themselves before major symptoms of advanced arteriosclerosis of the major vessels of the lower limbs occur.

Treatment Perhaps the best advice that can be given to a patient with obliterative arterial disease is to recommend some form of physical exercise every day, such as a walk. In this manner a compensating circulation may be built up to improve blood flow to the affected limb.

A diet with a low content of fat which contains a predominance of unsaturated fatty acids is advisable. It is essential that tobacco be eliminated, as its blood vessel constricting tendencies contribute to the development of symptoms associated with the disease.

Alcohol is a vasodilator (that is, an agent which dilates small blood vessels, so that more blood flows through) and it can be useful in the treatment of this disease when taken in moderate amounts, not only for its vasodilating role, but also for its mild sedative action, particularly in patients who have some pain associated with the thrombosis. Some doctors think that anticoagulant therapy should be instituted after thrombosis of a major artery.

Prevention of infections of the extremities is most important. An infection may often precipitate gangrene in a patient with advanced arteriosclerotic disease of an extremity. The feet should be kept clean and dry, the toenails carefully cut, and corns or bunions treated by a chiropodist. Shoes should be comfortable and well-fitting, neither too tight or too loose. At the slightest suspicion of infection, inform your doctor immediately.

Posture in bed is of great importance for patients with thrombosis of a major vessel of the leg. The ideal position for the affected limb is slightly below the level of the heart. Raising the head of the bed about six inches achieves a satisfactory sleeping posture. On no account should an affected limb be raised above the level of the heart.

Exposure to cold should be assiduously avoided. Patients with advanced disease whose occupation exposes them to cold weather may have to change occupations. The feet should not be allowed to become wet and the patient should avoid chilling, since it will constrict blood vessels. No hot objects should ever be placed in contact with the skin. Hot-water bottles and electric heating pads should never be used to warm the feet, however cold.

Anything which may produce cuts in the skin, bruises, or crushing injury should be avoided. This means avoidance of crowded places where the patient's feet may be stepped on. Should a minor injury occur, the patient should go to bed and call his doctor. The importance of proper care of the feet in all cases of arteriosclerosis cannot be overstressed. Prevention of any mechanical, chemical, or heat injury to the skin of the feet and toes is very important. Many cases of gangrene which occur in patients with this disease can be traced to some supposedly minor and usually preventable injury to the feet.

Patients with occlusive arterial disease may benefit by surgical reconstruction of the affected artery after thrombosis, if the arterial vessels beyond the thrombosis are open and adequate. In the patient who meets these requirements there is a good chance of restoring adequate circulation with the relief of disabling symptoms. The involved artery may be opened and the thrombus removed. Another operation is a bypass procedure, using an artificial artery of synthetic fabric to convey blood around the obstruction.

The outcome of arterial reconstructive procedures depends on many factors, such as the amount of collateral circulation, the degree of blood insufficiency, and the age and general condition of the patient. However, in patients who meet the necessary criteria for surgery, results are gratifying in about 90 per cent. In these successful cases, restoration of adequate flow to the blood-starved limb will be manifested by relief of symptoms.

Another form of surgery sometimes used is sympathectomy, in which an attempt to overcome arterial contraction accompanying the disease is made by cutting certain of the sympathetic nerves to the involved arteries. At present it is the only procedure that can be offered to patients with extensive and irreparable arterial disease. Though many drugs are prescribed for this condition, none have been proved effective.

Arterial aneurysms

An aneurysm or ballooned-out weak spot of a major artery such as the aorta may occur at any point along its course. The portions of the aorta in the chest and in the abdomen are common sites.

The essential factor in aneurysm formation is damage to the middle layer of the artery wall. When only the thin lining and outer fibrous tissue layers remain to withstand repeated pulsing forces of blood flow, the artery begins to dilate or balloon out. Progressive dilatation ensues in the weakened area, and as the aneurysm develops, pressure is exerted upon tissues that surround it.

Syphilis is a major cause of aneurysms of the thoracic aorta, which lies within the chest. Arteriosclerosis may also lead to aneurysms in this region, but as a rule it is more likely to produce diffuse dilatation of the aorta than the characteristic sac-like aneurysm seen in syphilis. In its early stages the aneurysm may cause no symptoms, or may be associated with only slight discomfort. Usually, symptoms result from pressure upon adjacent organs and tissues. Thus, the symptoms produced depend largely upon the location and size of the aneurysm.

Aneurysm of the abdominal aorta

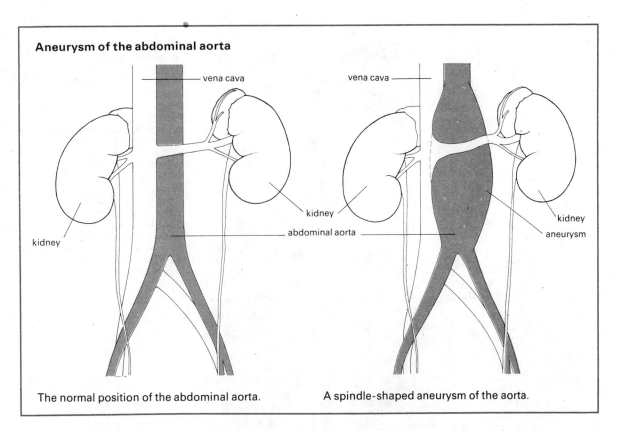

The normal position of the abdominal aorta.

A spindle-shaped aneurysm of the aorta.

Most aneurysms of the abdominal aorta occur just below the area where the renal arteries branch off to serve the kidneys, and the dilatation usually extends downward to involve the common iliac arteries which lead to the legs. These aneurysms result not from syphilis, but from arteriosclerotic disease. The major symptom is generally pain in the upper abdomen or lower back, which may extend to the lower extremities. Presence of pain is an important symptom, for it often indicates a rapid and progressive enlargement of the aneurysm. The outlook in this disease, if untreated, is grave. The majority of patients may develop actual rupture of the aneurysm, with intense pain and death due to blood loss. The average period of survival after occurrence of symptoms from an aneurysm is from one to two years, with rupture of the aneurysm being the most common cause of death.

Recent advances in vascular surgery have greatly improved the outlook for patients with arterial aneurysms. The involved segment of the artery, including the aneurysm, is removed, and replaced with a synthetic artery which restores normal blood flow within the arterial system. Results of operative treatment for aneurysms have been increasingly gratifying and surgery has been a major factor in reducing the extremely high death toll of the past.

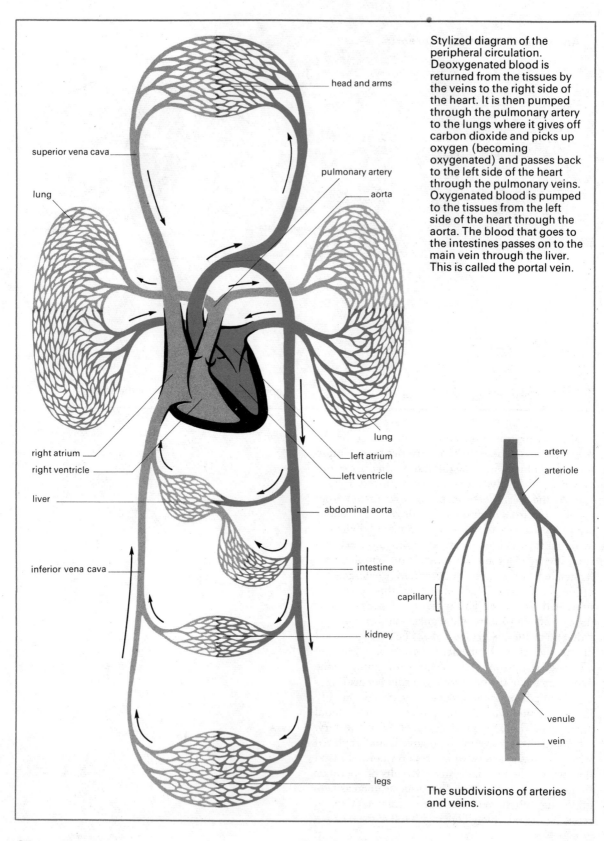

head and arms

superior vena cava

lung

pulmonary artery

aorta

right atrium

right ventricle

lung

left atrium

left ventricle

liver

abdominal aorta

inferior vena cava

intestine

kidney

legs

Stylized diagram of the peripheral circulation. Deoxygenated blood is returned from the tissues by the veins to the right side of the heart. It is then pumped through the pulmonary artery to the lungs where it gives off carbon dioxide and picks up oxygen (becoming oxygenated) and passes back to the left side of the heart through the pulmonary veins. Oxygenated blood is pumped to the tissues from the left side of the heart through the aorta. The blood that goes to the intestines passes on to the main vein through the liver. This is called the portal vein.

artery

arteriole

capillary

venule

vein

The subdivisions of arteries and veins.

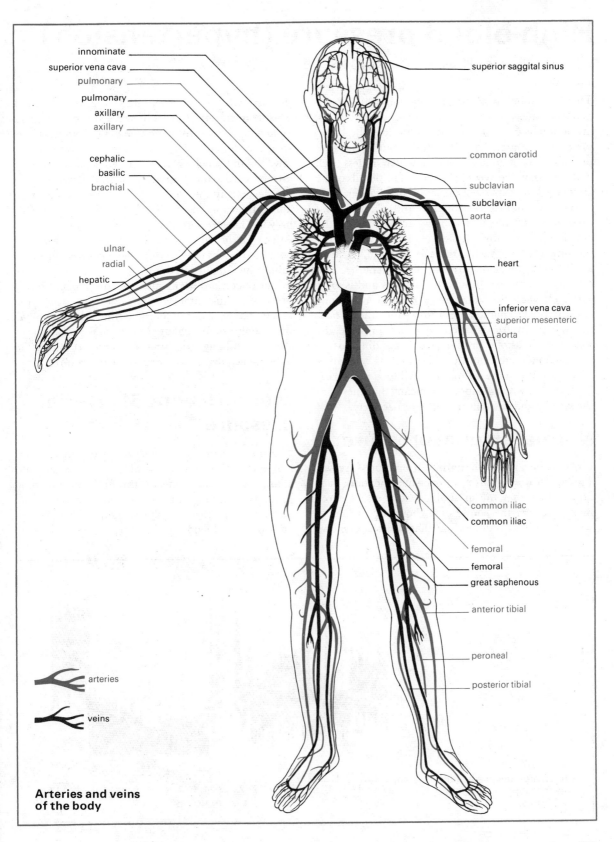

innominate

superior vena cava

pulmonary

pulmonary

axillary

axillary

cephalic

basilic

brachial

ulnar

radial

hepatic

superior saggital sinus

common carotid

subclavian

subclavian

aorta

heart

inferior vena cava

superior mesenteric

aorta

common iliac

common iliac

femoral

femoral

great saphenous

anterior tibial

peroneal

posterior tibial

arteries

veins

**Arteries and veins
of the body**

High blood pressure (hypertension)

Revised by Sir George Pickering, MD FRCP FRS

There is probably no bodily function which commands greater attention, or has graver connotations, in the minds of the lay public, than does the blood pressure reading. On the other hand, there is probably no common function which is less well understood by the average layman. The details of the circulation are explained earlier in this chapter.

When we talk of arterial pressure and of high arterial pressure or high blood pressure we are referring to the circulation from the left side of the heart and the pressure in arteries such as those to the brain, the arm, and the leg. The blood leaves the heart in pulses. The pulse is transmitted through the arteries and is most easily felt where the radial artery passes over the bone at the wrist. The highest pressure to which the blood is raised in the arteries is called the systolic pressure, the lowest the diastolic pressure, corresponding to the contraction (systole) of the heart and its relaxation (diastole). When the doctor says the blood pressure is 120 over 90, written 120/90, he means that these are the systolic and diastolic pressures respectively.

Normal arterial pressure

It used to be said that the normal arterial pressure was 120/70. However, this is an oversimplification. It is now known that the arterial pressure varies enormously during the course of 24 hours according to what the subject is doing. The diagram below shows

the arterial pressure measured continuously in a healthy doctor of 31 years of age. Between 1400 and 1600 hours he was listening to me discussing patients with the students. The arterial pressure was rather low, around 90/65, perhaps because he was nearly asleep. At 1600 the head nurse, on instruction, stuck a needle sharply into his buttocks. The pressure rose abruptly to 150/70. At 2400 he had intercourse with his wife. The pressure again rose abruptly to 160/100. Afterwards he fell asleep and the pressure fell as low as 60/30. This sort of variation has occurred in every subject investigated in this way.

The doctor ordinarily measures his patient's blood pressure in his surgery, clinic, or ward when the patient has been at rest for some time. Measurements show only small changes from one occasion to another, although the pressure tends to fall as the patient becomes accustomed to the procedure.

Measurement of arterial pressure

The most accurate way of measuring arterial pressure is to insert a tube containing salt solution (saline) into a large artery and connect it through a flexible tube containing saline to a tube containing mercury (the mercury manometer). The height to which the pressure of the blood raises the mercury then gives the

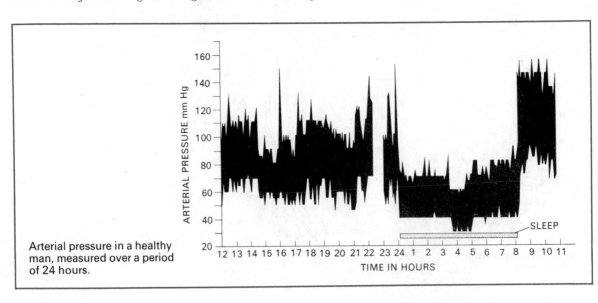

Arterial pressure in a healthy man, measured over a period of 24 hours.

pressure in millimetres of mercury, which is the unit used throughout the world. It is now possible through a device developed in Oxford to use this method to measure arterial pressure in men who are going about their ordinary business. A long thin nylon tube containing saline is introduced into the arm artery at the elbow. The other end of the tube is connected with a pressure recorder, which records on moving photographic paper. The pressure recorder is carried by a harness on the chest and the photographic recorder in the pocket. Surprising information has been obtained in this way.

In routine medical examinations a simpler method is used. A rubber cuff covered by nonstretching fabric is wrapped round the upper arm. The cuff is connected to a hand pump and a mercury manometer. The physician listens through a stethoscope to the artery at the elbow below the cuff. As the cuff is inflated he hears a sound with each pulse beat which stops when the pressure is raised above systolic. As the pressure is reduced the sound reappears, becomes louder and then abruptly decreases and finally disappears. The point at which the sounds first appear on reducing the pressure in the cuff is the systolic pressure. The point at which they disappear gives the diastolic pressure.

The delivery of blood to the organs of the body is regulated by the size of the smaller arteries, whose walls are largely composed of muscle and elastic tissue. The degree of contraction of the arterial muscle is regulated by the sympathetic nerves, see page 162, and also by the composition of the blood, particularly its content of adrenalin and noradrenalin secreted by the adrenal glands which powerfully constrict arterial muscle. When a person is frightened or angry the sympathetic nerves are excited and adrenalin is poured out into the blood; the arteries contract and the arterial pressure rises. When the subject exercises, the arteries to the muscles dilate and the output of the heart increases enormously, up to five times in trained athletes.

The flow of blood through the blood vessels comprising the circulation obeys the ordinary laws of hydrodynamics. The arterial pressure depends on the output of the heart, which determines the rate of flow through the arterial system, and the resistance offered by the arteries, which depends on their diameter and the viscosity of the blood. The viscosity is to all intents and purposes constant. Alterations in arterial pressure are thus due to alterations in the output of the heart and the calibre of the arteries.

High arterial pressure (hypertension)

As the diagram below illustrates, normal arterial pressure tends to rise with age. Age in years plus 100 is the average systolic pressure in the population at large. So far as we know systolic pressures of 150 and less and diastolic pressures of 95 and less do no harm. Above that they may, and the harm is proportional to the height of the pressure. The harmful effects are chiefly on the heart and arteries.

Varieties of hypertension In systolic hypertension the systolic pressure alone is raised. It occurs in maladies in which the output of the heart is

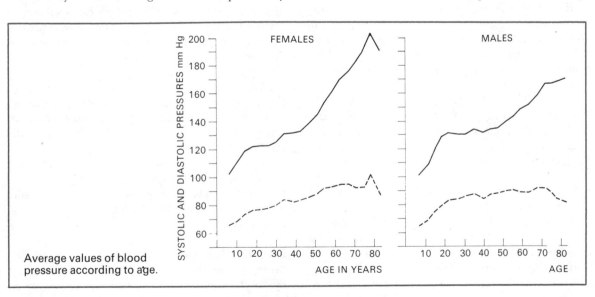

Average values of blood pressure according to age.

increased, such as anaemia and oversecretion of thyroid hormones, but its commonest cause is the rigidity of arteries that occurs with advancing age. In itself it requires no treatment. In diastolic hypertension both systolic and diastolic pressures are raised. This is what is ordinarily meant by hypertension. When the diastolic is over 110 mm it always requires treatment. When it is persistently over 100, it may require treatment.

The heart has more work to do. It therefore tends to grow bigger to compensate for this, but the process can be reversed by reducing the arterial pressure.

The arteries are most seriously affected with the following results.

The accelerated or malignant phase of hypertension is a complication of the very highest pressures. It may show itself in loss of eyesight, by heart failure, or kidney failure. Fortunately the doctor can now reduce the arterial pressure quickly and keep it down. This cures the malignant phase and prevents its recurrence.

Coronary artery disease is usually part of a generalized disease (atheroma or arteriosclerosis) of large arteries. Small patches form on the lining of arteries and on these a thrombus (a special kind of blood clot) may form. When this happens in a coronary artery the blood supply to that part of the heart stops. If the area affected is extensive enough the result is fatal. If it is smaller the patient suffers severe pain and may develop heart failure. This is myocardial infarction. Severe narrowing produces pain in the chest on walking (angina pectoris). Both conditions are described earlier in this chapter on page 68. Coronary artery disease is due to many factors, in addition to high arterial pressure. The main ones are age, smoking cigarettes, lack of exercise, and a high cholesterol value in the blood. All of these are quantitatively related to the disease.

Stroke The commonest cause of a stroke is the stopping of blood supply to a part of the brain following the formation of a clot on an arteriosclerotic plaque in a neck or brain artery. High blood pressure is again an important factor; for a reason not understood, reducing the arterial pressure is more effective in preventing strokes than preventing coronary artery disease.

Cerebral haemorrhage is the other (and less common) form of stroke. It is a consequence of the rupture of a small expansion (aneurysm) on a small artery of the brain. These aneurysms may develop in people with high arterial pressure (diastolic persistently over 110)

as they get older. They are prevented by reducing arterial pressure.

Renal artery disease is complex because it can be a result of hypertension and it can be a cause. In young people congenital narrowing of a renal artery may produce hypertension which is cured if the diseased segment of the artery is cut out and replaced by a graft. In older people surgical treatment is often less successful and medical treatment is usual.

Causes of hypertension The common specific diseases accompanying hypertension are:

Renal disease In addition to renal artery disease already mentioned, nephritis (inflammation of the kidney, Bright's disease) and pyelonephritis (infection of the kidney) may cause hypertension. The treatment of the hypertension is just the same as when these diseases are absent.

Diseases of the adrenal gland These are relatively well understood. The medulla of the adrenal gland produces adrenalin and its close relative noradrenalin which raise arterial pressure. Tumours of the medulla and similar tissue occur rarely and produce paroxysmal hypertension because they suddenly pour out their secretions into the bloodstream. The tumours usually occur in the abdomen along the aorta or in the adrenal itself. Surgical removal of the tumour cures the hypertension.

Conn's syndrome, in which a tumour of the cortex of the adrenal produces an excess of salt retaining hormone. Sodium is retained and potassium lost. Hypertension, thirst, polyuria, and muscular weakness are common symptoms.

Cushing's syndrome may be due to an adrenal or to a pituitary tumour, resulting in an oversecretion of cortisol by the adrenal cortex. The development or accentuation of male secondary sex characteristics, diabetes, and hypertension are manifestations. It usually requires surgery.

Hypertension of pregnancy The blood pressure may rise excessively in the last three months of pregnancy. If it rises very high the patient may have fits (eclampsia). It may be necessary to reduce the arterial pressure by drugs. The blood pressure nearly always returns to normal levels after the baby is born.

Contraceptive pills Occasionally the taking of contraceptive pills produces a rise of blood pressure which may be severe. Stopping the pills will cure the hypertension.

Essential hypertension means that no specific cause has been found for the high blood pressure. It is by far the commonest condition and represents an exaggeration of the normal rise with age. Two factors are known to be concerned, inheritance and environment. Inheritance helps to determine the arterial pressure at any age. As in the case of stature it is a graded inheritance due to the influence of many genes derived from both parents. But the resemblance is less for blood pressure than for stature. Environmental factors determine the rate of rise with age. We do not know exactly what they are. In tribal societies blood pressure does not rise with age, but it does if members leave their tribes for another kind of life. Despite the popular notion to the contrary, there is no special psychological type associated with hypertension. There is no association between the amount of salt eaten and arterial pressure. Nor is there any definite association with smoking, though there is with obesity.

Treatment   The higher the blood pressure, the less the expectation of life. It is now known that if very high pressures are reduced and kept down, expectation of life is increased and complications prevented. The level of diastolic arterial pressure above which the benefit to the patient exceeds the nuisance value of treatment is somewhere between 95 and 110 mm Hg. The case for treatment is greater the higher the pressure. If the pressure is very high (over 130 mm Hg diastolic) it must be reduced at once since complications are likely.

Thirty years ago blood pressure reduction entailed a diet of boiled rice supplemented by some fruit but excluding everything else. The diet was almost salt free and had to be adhered to strictly as any indulgence sent the blood pressure up again. A surgical operation to remove the sympathetic nerves was sometimes successful and sometimes not. Nowadays drug treatment is successful in lowering blood pressure. Surgery is restricted to repair of coarctation of the aorta, removing tumours of the adrenal glands, and to some cases of renal vascular disease.

The drugs of choice belong to the thiazide diuretics and the beta ganglionic blockers. The former increase the excretion of water and salt by the kidney but whether this is the mechanism by which they reduce blood pressure is uncertain. The beta blockers block conduction through the beta fibres of the sympathetic nerves. With these drugs, given either singly or in combination, it is usually possible to keep the diastolic arterial pressure below 95 without undesirable side effects. Sometimes it is necessary to use other drugs to increase the effect. Today it is usually possible to avoid producing depression, fatigue, diarrhoea, and

sexual impotence which used to be side effects with drugs used previously.

Because of the risk of coronary disease it is sensible for patients with hypertension to pay particular attention to the known risk factors in that disease. Thus they should not smoke cigarettes, should avoid putting on weight, and should take exercise. Many doctors would also advise them to avoid eating animal fats.

Those whose work involves hard physical labour tend to have rather lower blood pressure. Regular exercise and moderation in the use of alcohol are perhaps even more important in those with elevated pressures than in the population at large. The popular picture of the patient with hypertension as the hard driving business executive with a red face and a large belly who smokes too much and who drinks too much corresponds rather to the patient with coronary artery disease, to which of course hypertension may contribute.

Low blood pressure

When arterial pressure and its variations were less well understood it was common for arterial pressures below 90 mm Hg to be classified by doctors as low pressure and the patient so informed. A variety of symptoms was attributed to it. However, insurance statistics show that such patients tend to have an unusually long expectation of life. It is therefore not diagnosed as a disease.

Low pressure used to occur in pulmonary tuberculosis when this was a common disease. It is an important manifestation of Addison's disease; see chapter 9.

Varicose veins

Revised by Stanley Rivlin

When a doctor speaks of varicose veins, he is thinking only of enlarged and inefficient veins in the leg, between the toes and groin. He is not referring to swollen veins in the anal canal (piles) which are entirely different in every way and are discussed in chapter 14.

How the vein circulation works

It is often assumed that the pumping action of the heart, which forces the blood down the arteries into the legs, is sufficiently strong to send the blood back up the legs again into the general circulation. This is not so, for all the heart's effort is used in persuading the blood to flow through thousands of smaller and smaller arteries and arterioles into the capillaries, where it delivers its nutrients to the tissues and collects up waste products, to be recycled. The blood from the capillaries then passes into the venules (the smallest veins) whence it returns to the heart by larger veins, served by a totally different pumping action, which is located in the muscles of the calf.

If the legs are crossed so that the left leg is resting on top of the right, and the foot is moved up and down, pivoting at the ankle, it is possible both to see and feel the calf muscles contracting (see diagram below). These muscles, which are called the calf muscle pump or peripheral venous heart, pump the blood back up normal legs to the heart and it is the proper use of these muscles which is the key to successful treatment of the various complications of varicose veins such as ulcers, eczema, phlebitis, and thrombosis.

The diagram opposite illustrates the two types of vein in the leg. Firstly, the deep veins, so called because they lie deeply between the muscles, and secondly, the superficial veins, which lie just under the skin. The superficial veins are connected to the deep veins at a number of points by veins called communicating veins. Each communicating vein contains a one-way valve which is constructed so as to ensure that the blood must pass from the surface veins into the deep veins. The deep veins in their turn have one-way valves which direct the blood up towards the heart. Every time the calf muscles contract, blood is propelled up the deep veins towards the heart and, as the muscles relax, blood flows in from the surface veins to refill the empty deep veins, ready for the next muscular contraction to speed the blood on its way. It is this contraction and relaxation of the calf muscles in normal legs which is primarily responsible for the venous return from the lower limbs. It follows that a decrease in active leg movements, particularly ankle movements (which control the calf muscles), leads to a reduced venous return which in turn causes back pressure in the veins leading to swollen legs, ulcers, phlebitis, and thrombosis.

How varicose veins develop

Contrary to popular belief, chefs, dentists, hairdressers, and others with standing occupations are no more liable to varicose veins that anyone else. But should they be unlucky enough to be one of the ten per cent of the population who have varicose veins then trouble will appear much earlier, owing to their occupational lack of leg movement which leads to stagnation of blood in the veins, producing the symptoms of aching, heavy, and tired legs, swollen ankles, skin irritation, and sudden cramp of the calf in bed.

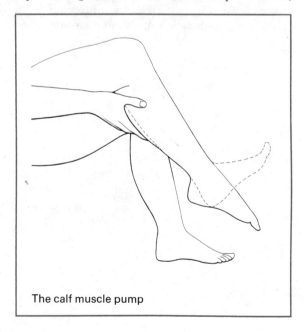

The calf muscle pump

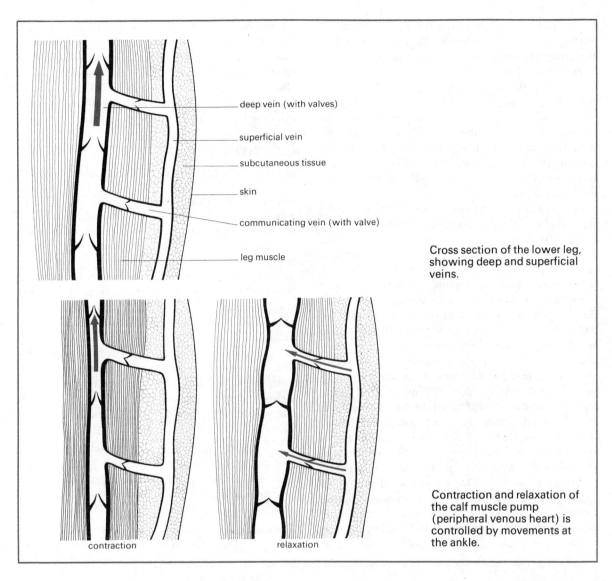

deep vein (with valves)

superficial vein

subcutaneous tissue

skin

communicating vein (with valve)

leg muscle

Cross section of the lower leg, showing deep and superficial veins.

contraction

relaxation

Contraction and relaxation of the calf muscle pump (peripheral venous heart) is controlled by movements at the ankle.

Whether or not you are one of the ten per cent who actually have varicose veins is purely a matter of chance. There is possibly a hereditary factor but this is not proven, and is certainly absent in many cases. The fact is that the development of veins and their valves in the human embryo is, unlike most of the body's systems, extremely inefficient. No two people ever have exactly the same venous system – in fact even the two legs in the same person often have a different pattern of veins – and, most significant of all, this strange state of affairs even applies to the all-important valves within the veins. In short, one out of every ten people is born with a faulty valve, or a valve which at some time or other will cease to function efficiently, allowing some of the blood to fall back down the veins, upsetting the pressures in the venous system and giving rise to the swollen veins which we call varicose (from Latin, varix – a dilated vein).

Fortunately, it is usually only one or two valves which are faulty and when these valves are isolated and removed from the system the patient is cured. In other words varicose veins is not a general disease which, despite treatment, gets worse as the years go by. It is a localized congenital fault (like a harelip or prominent ears) which can be cured surgically.

Varicose veins in pregnancy

Varicose veins in pregnancy are brought about by the damming back of the blood in the leg veins, produced by the increase in venous blood returning from the enlarged uterus. This causes an obstruction as it joins the stream of blood from the leg veins on the way back to the heart. It occurs only in those people who are liable to varicose veins by reason of having a potentially faulty valve which is given the final push by the temporary increase in back pressure. Indeed, in many women the valve goes back to near normal after the child is born, and the veins disappear. A second pregnancy may render the valve permanently faulty – in which case the veins will remain varicose after the pregnancy.

It is very rare for a patient to require active surgical treatment for varicose veins in pregnancy. If the legs ache, then it is worth wearing support tights. If they do not ache, there is no point, for elastic support does not prevent the onset of varicose veins, and in hot weather the preventive wearing of support hose is just one more extra (and in this case unnecessary) burden for the pregnant woman. However, there are two simple procedures worth carrying out. The first is to wear lace-up shoes during the working day (never slippers, and never wooden exercise sandals). This will ensure that the calf muscles are used to their fullest extent and that blood is pumped back up the legs and prevented from stagnating. Not only will this prevent heavy aching legs but it will greatly lessen the chances of phlebitis (inflammation and clotting of the surface veins during pregnancy). The second procedure is to sleep with the foot of the bed raised by 23 cm (nine inches). This works only if the bed is tipped as in the diagram below. It is a waste of time putting anything under the mattress, for the whole objective is not so much to raise the legs but to lower the heart in relation to the rest of the body. This ensures that when the patient is asleep and unable to move the ankles, the blood in the legs runs back of its own accord into the general circulation instead of stagnating in the veins. Raising the foot of the bed is also a cure for calf cramp which affects so many pregnant women and is due to blood collecting in the calf muscle veins during the night.

Complication of untreated varicose veins

Varicose eczema Varicose eczema is a chronic, rough, sometimes weeping area which usually commences in the skin overlying varicose veins and is brought about by the patient who (one cannot blame her or him) scratches the skin, often while half-asleep in a warm bed, owing to the intense irritation produced by the veins. The eczema is itself irritating and promotes further scratching and rubbing. This produces a vicious circle of irritation – scratching – irritation. In a number of cases both legs, the arms, and the trunk also become eczematous, all stemming from one leg with varicose veins. No matter for how many weeks or months the eczema has been present there is a simple rapid way to bring it to a halt, which the doctor will probably suggest and which is as follows.

Take a deep plastic bin which is wide enough to accommodate your foot when placed flat on the bottom, and fill it up with lukewarm water so that when your leg is inside it, water does not overflow on to the floor.

Measure the amount of water in the bin, and for every gallon add half a teaspoon of crystals of

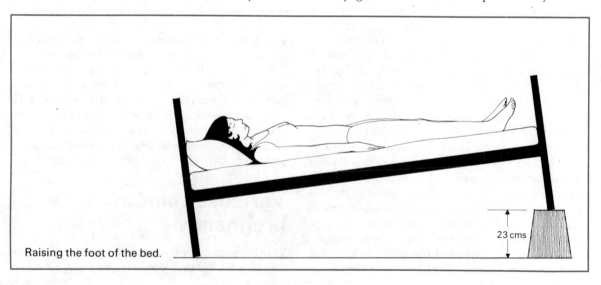

Raising the foot of the bed.

23 cms

potassium permanganate, obtainable from the chemist. (Keep these crystals out of reach of children.)

Stir the crystals until they are all dissolved and put your leg in so that all the eczema is covered. Soak your leg for ten to fifteen minutes, twice a day for three to four days and then once a day for a further three to four days (if the level of the fluid in the bin is not high enough, a mop or sponge can be used to splash it up and down your leg).

After each soaking, take your leg out and let it dry in the air. DO NOT dry it with a towel. In between soakings a bandage may be worn if desired, but there is no harm in allowing the air to reach your leg.

After the first two or three soakings the leg will cease to itch, and after the course is finished the leg can be washed, and the skin will look reasonable again. Any irritation on the body will stop of its own accord – there is no need to bathe it.

The permanganate mixture is very strong and will stain your hands and leg brown. Rubber gloves should be worn and the bin should stand on a sheet of plastic.

Once the eczema is controlled it is essential to have the varicose veins dealt with, otherwise the eczema will recur.

Varicose ulcer There are a number of different causes of ulcerated legs. When the less common causes such as diabetes, and arteriosclerosis are excluded, no less than 75 per cent of leg ulcers are directly due to varicose veins. Of the remainder, two thirds are due to deep vein thrombosis and one third to a varied group of conditions, including rheumatoid arthritis, osteoarthritis of the hip, and damaged knee and hip joints following accidents.

It may seem strange to learn that all these conditions, varicose ulcers, post-thrombotic ulcers and "damaged joint" ulcers all have one common factor. This is fortunate, for it means that they all respond to the same basic treatment.

The common factor in all these ulcerated legs is oedema and by this term is meant a collection of fluid in the legs which is sufficiently noticeable to cause a dent in the skin when it is pressed firmly with the finger. This oedema effectively prevents the normal healing processes from operating. Thus a simple graze or cut, instead of healing, becomes a chronic ulcer.

In varicose veins and deep vein thrombosis the oedema results from faulty valves which prevent efficient pumping away of the blood during normal use of the leg. In the case of damaged or diseased hip, knee, or ankle joints, the resultant difficulty in walking reduces the use of the calf muscles and hence brings to a halt the venous pump (see page 90) which normally returns the blood to the heart. In every case the result is the same, a reduction in venous return, leading to an increase in venous back pressure which prevents the watery part of the blood from leaving the tissues, which in turn become waterlogged, or in medical terms, oedematous.

The doctor will do everything possible to banish oedema so that an ulcer has the opportunity to heal. The simplest way is to put the patient to bed for 24 hours, lying flat on the back with one pillow for the head and with the foot of the bed raised 23 cm (nine inches).

While the patient is awake, simple pumping exercises may be carried out (a cradle in the bed to keep the bedclothes off helps here), but while the patient is asleep, the fluid will drain away because the heart is lower than the legs.

At the end of 24 hours the swelling will have disappeared and the doctor or nurse will apply a comfortably firm (not tight) bandage which will remain on until it is changed every week or two. During this time further oedema can be prevented from developing by keeping to the following simple list of rules, which are designed to increase the pumping action of the calf muscles in order to overcome the problem of the faulty valves or damaged joints. (In the case of damaged ankle joints, for example rheumatoid arthritis, the treatment can be carried out in bed – probably without the need for bandaging.)

Rules for ulcer patients

1 Use your leg normally while under bandage treatment.

2 Avoid standing still. Take a few steps whenever possible.

3 Wear leather *lace-up* shoes with low heels, *never* slippers, in the house. If the feet feel hot and tired at the end of the day, change into another pair of lace-up shoes, *not* slippers.

4 Do not sit with the legs crossed.

5 Do *not* sit with the legs up.

6 Sit normally but move the ankles up and down (as if beating time to music) every now and again.

7 Do not go to sleep in an armchair.

8 Walk as much as you please.

9 Do not sit close to the fire.

10 Never bath in the morning – only at night before bed.

11 Raise the foot of the bed on 23 cm blocks.

With this regime, the most difficult and obstinate ulcer will be well on the way to healing in twelve weeks while the easy ones will be soundly healed at the end of ten weeks.

After healing there is the problem of permanent cure. With varicose ulcers, that is, ulcers due to varicose veins, there is little difficulty provided the veins are adequately treated with surgery. Post-thrombotic ulcers and "damaged joint" ulcers can be kept at bay provided the patients keep to the rules (which are not very onerous) for the rest of their lives. But it must be emphasized that this includes sleeping with the foot of the bed raised nine inches.

Superficial phlebitis   This is a clotting of blood in the surface veins arising from the fact that the larger the vein becomes, the slower the blood moves within it. Eventually it moves so slowly, particularly where there is a large varicose bulge, that the blood clots, and the clot spreads up and down the vein. When this happens the surface vein becomes hard, red, and very tender, so that walking is painful.

The danger of superficial phlebitis is that the clot can spread into the deep veins where a piece could come loose and travel to the lung. This is called a pulmonary embolus and gives rise to pain in the chest and sometimes more serious symptoms.

It must be obvious that the danger of this happening is multiplied a hundredfold if the patient rests the leg, for the less the leg is used, the slower the venous return and it is the more likely that the clot will spread. On the other hand, if the leg is *used* so as to speed up the blood flow in the deep veins, the clot in the surface veins is sealed off and cannot spread.

But how, it may be asked, can one use the leg if it is acutely painful, with red, tender, and hard veins? Fortunately the answer is simple. The doctor, or nurse, will bandage the leg firmly with an elastic adhesive bandage from the toes to the knee or to the groin, depending on the extent of the phlebitis and you will help both the doctor and yourself by adhering to the above rules. The bandage may need to be changed after a week or two and usually one or two bandages will suffice.

Once the veins have settled down and returned to their previous state, which may take three to six months, it is wise to have them dealt with to prevent further attacks of phlebitis.

Deep vein thrombosis   This is a more serious condition than superficial phlebitis, for the clot must be prevented from moving to the lung. The symptoms in this case are usually a cramp-like pain in the calf often accompanied by a pain in the groin and almost invariably by a very swollen leg from ankle to knee or ankle to groin. This condition often demands hospital treatment for a few days so that the appropriate dose of anticoagulant drugs (which prevent further clotting) can be determined for each individual case.

When the patient returns home from hospital the doctor will advise a supporting bandage whilst the swelling slowly improves and you can help him greatly by keeping to the rules.

Treatment of varicose veins

The successful treatment of varicose veins has defied the medical profession throughout the world since time immemorial. This is not because it is impossible to cure varicose veins, indeed with the appropriate treatment well over 90 per cent of cases can be permanently cured. It is the sheer weight of numbers which defeats the system. Estimates are that there are five million people in the United Kingdom with varicose veins. Assuming one half of these people to have varicose veins in one leg and the other half to have varicose veins in both legs, this means seven and a half million legs. It is agreed by all those surgeons who are specially interested in varicose veins that successful surgery may take at least one and a half hours per leg. This brings us to a staggering eleven million hours of surgical operating time. To use up all this time for varicose veins would effectively prevent the treatment of hernias, piles, stomach ulcers, cancer, and many other conditions. It is true that there are a number of specialist centres where such treatment can be given, but places are naturally limited, and waiting lists are long.

Surgery   Should you be fortunate enough to be admitted to a centre specializing in the surgical cure of varicose veins, you will find that the surgeon will first examine your leg in detail to establish the site of the faulty valve(s). He will then carry out an operation designed firstly to seal off the faulty valve and thus allow a normal venous return, and secondly to remove the ugly dilated veins.

If you have normally healing skin, any scars should almost disappear, leaving you with no signs of ever having had varicose veins. For this operation you would need to be in the hospital for only four to five days, and you should be able to walk (with bandaged legs) without a limp within 24 hours of the operation.

Injections   As surgery is not easily available to all, other methods of treatment have to be considered and the chief of these is of course injections. With this method a substance known as a sclerosing agent is injected into the vein. The effect of this is to damage physically the vein wall so as to produce a chemical superficial phlebitis which is controlled by immediate bandaging, walking, and adherence to the rules. This phlebitis narrows the vein walls, sometimes permanently, but in many cases will need to be repeated a number of times.

Chapter 4

Blood and blood-forming organs

Revised by E. C. Gordon-Smith, MA BM MSc FRCP

Blood is a fluid which has two main constituents, the plasma which is a clear yellow fluid containing many different substances in solution, and the blood cells which are suspended in the plasma. The blood circulates round the body in the blood vessels. In the tissues, the larger blood vessels divide into smaller ones until they are finer than hairs, and surrounded only by a single cell layer. This allows diffusion of substances into the tissues and the re-collection of waste products back into the circulation, the blood being pumped along constantly by the heart and muscles in the limbs. This thorough distribution is essential for the normal working of all organs in the body.

Blood has four functions. Firstly it must carry oxygen, without which most body cells will not survive, from the lungs to the tissues by means of the red cells. Carbon dioxide produced by the tissues is transported to the lungs in the plasma. Secondly, it must present a line of defence against the constant threat of invasion by bacteria, parasites, and other hostile organisms which inhabit our environment. Thirdly, it must carry the energy-giving substances produced by food to the tissues and carry the waste products to the kidneys and liver for removal and chemical neutralizing respectively. Fourthly, it distributes heat, mostly from the centre to the periphery.

This chapter deals with the first two of these functions. The special property of the blood to remain liquid in blood vessels, but to clot when damage to these vessels occurs is also discussed. The study of the production, function, and destruction of these cells in health and disease is called haematology.

The cells of the blood

Blood cells were the first ever to be seen with a microscope, by the Dutch scientist Jan Swammerdam in 1658. Three main groups of cells were eventually recognized, red cells (erythrocytes), white cells (leucocytes), and platelets. These cells are important in the transport of oxygen, the defence against infection, and the coagulation of the blood respectively.

Red blood cells The normal red blood cell is a flat disc-shaped cell, concave on both surfaces. This description is accurate for cells which are examined in a stationary environment, but in the circulation the red blood cell has to be flexible enough to pass through channels, such as capillaries, which are narrower than the cell itself. The shape of red cells may be altered by disease, and the examination of blood films is an important part of the investigation of many illnesses.

The colour of the red blood cells is caused by the presence of an iron-containing compound, haemoglobin. This complex substance has the special property of being able to combine with molecules of oxygen when the concentration is high, as in the lungs, and to give up these molecules when the oxygen concentration in the surrounding tissues is low. It has a lesser ability to combine with carbon dioxide, though in this case it picks up molecules in the tissues and gives them up in the lungs. The physical structure of haemoglobin is now known, as well as the way in which it combines with and releases oxygen. This affords hope for the treatment of many

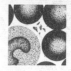

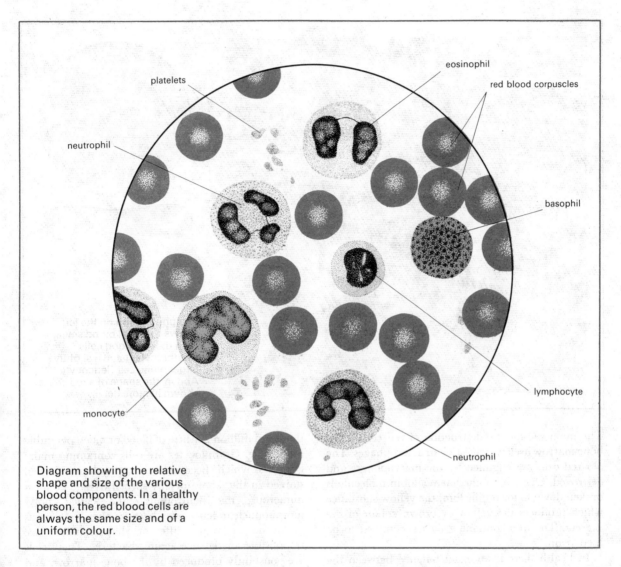

Diagram showing the relative shape and size of the various blood components. In a healthy person, the red blood cells are always the same size and of a uniform colour.

disorders of the red cell which afflict hundreds of thousands of people in different parts of the world.

When haemoglobin is combined with oxygen it is bright red. When the oxygen is released the haemoglobin becomes darker and appears blue when seen through the skin. This is why in heart and lung diseases, or asphyxiation, which prevent the blood being offered sufficient oxygen, the lips and extremities look blue. This blue colour (cyanosis) may also be produced by a wide variety of disorders where there is an increase in the amount of de-oxygenated blood in the superficial circulation.

Red cells are formed in the bone marrow, found in the interior of bones. Marrow cells are similar to most other cells of the body, having a nucleus, which contains genetic information. They divide and produce substances for the proper function of the cell,

including in this case haemoglobin, using oxygen as a source of energy. Two or three days before the mature red cell leaves the marrow, the nucleus is extruded together with many other cellular structures so that the mature cell which finally enters the circulation contains no nucleus. It is a simple receptacle for carrying oxygen, and never divides again until it is broken up about four months later.

The destruction of the red cells is accomplished by certain types of white cell which have left the circulation and taken up residence in particular tissues. The many different names given to these cells reflects the difficulty which earlier workers had in identifying their origin but it now seems certain that the cells are derived from monocytes about which more will be said later. In the tissues these cells are called macrophages, histiocytes, or reticulum cells.

Blood and blood-forming organs

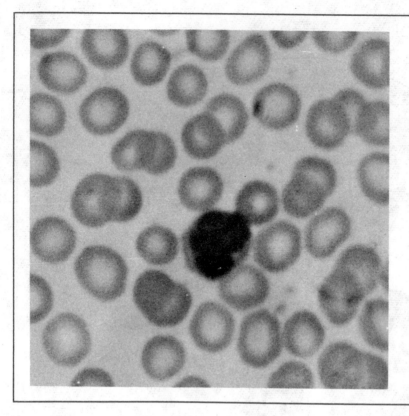

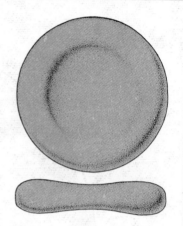

The photograph on the left shows a normal blood smear with the red blood cells (erythrocytes) and a slightly larger white cell (leucocyte). Above, the shape of a red cell is shown in more detail.

The main site for the destruction of red cells is the bone marrow itself which is rich in macrophages. The old red cells are engulfed by the macrophages and destroyed. One part of the haemoglobin molecule is broken down to form bilirubin, the yellow substance which produces the yellow or brown colour of the excreta. The iron-containing part is retained to be used again.

In health there is an exact balance between the number of red cells destroyed each day and the number produced. The total number of red cells in a healthy adult man is about 25 million million or five million per cubic millimetre of blood. The total blood volume of an adult is about five litres. Each day about one per cent of the cells die so that the marrow produces about 250 thousand million cells a day. Apart from the number of red cells the amount of haemoglobin that the cells contain is important for life.

White blood cells (leucocytes) These are less numerous than red cells and are made up of several different types of cell which can be recognized by their appearance, when stained, under the microscope. Generally, white cells are larger than red cells and the normal numbers present are about five thousand million per litre of blood or 5,000 per cubic millimetre. Granulocytes are cells containing many granules which become brightly coloured when stained in the laboratory by special dyes. The most numerous, the neutrophils (also called polymorphonuclear leucocytes because their nucleus is made up of many different shaped lobes) are responsible for defence against bacteria. These cells are constantly produced by the bone marrow, and enter the blood. They have the ability to penetrate the capillary wall to enter the tissues and scavenge for bacteria. When bacteria do break through the outer defences of the skin or lining of the intestine, neutrophils are chemically drawn to the site of infection. Here the neutrophils will devour the bacteria if the organisms have been properly prepared for digestion by other cells. Pus is formed by the casualties in the fight against infection, and is made up of dead bacteria and white cells. The bone marrow stem cells are activated by cells returning from the infected area to produce an increase in young neutrophils to meet the requirements of the situation.

Eosinophils, whose granules stain red, and basophils, whose granules stain blue, are other types of granulocytes which have important functions that are

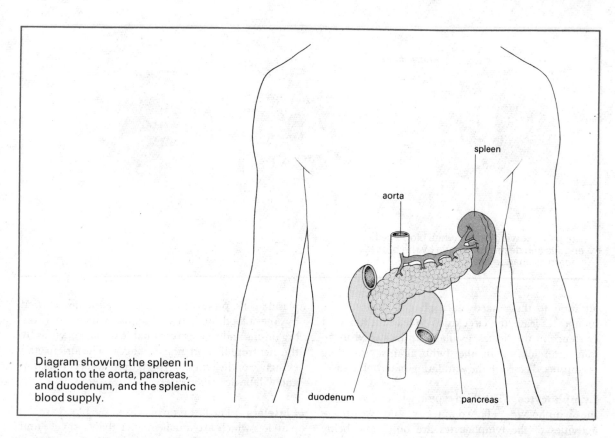

Diagram showing the spleen in relation to the aorta, pancreas, and duodenum, and the splenic blood supply.

aorta

spleen

duodenum

pancreas

not fully understood. In certain allergies the number of eosinophils in the blood may be greatly increased.

Mention has already been made of macrophages and their role in the destruction of red cells. These cells are derived from monocytes which are produced in the bone marrow, enter the circulation and leave, like granulocytes, through the vessel walls. Unlike granulocytes these cells do not die in fighting infection, but settle down in special sites of the body where they form the fixed macrophage system. These special sites include the liver and spleen. Here the macrophages line specially designed blood vessels where they can screen the blood for damaged red cells, foreign organisms, and other abnormal substances which they engulf. The process of cells eating particles or organisms is called phagocytosis. In

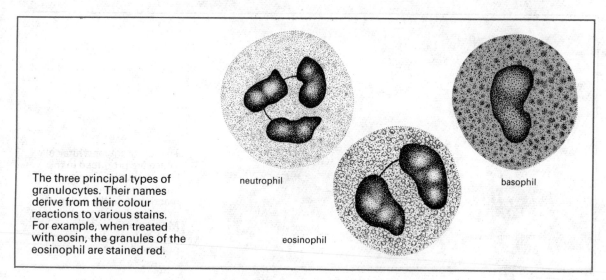

The three principal types of granulocytes. Their names derive from their colour reactions to various stains. For example, when treated with eosin, the granules of the eosinophil are stained red.

neutrophil

basophil

eosinophil

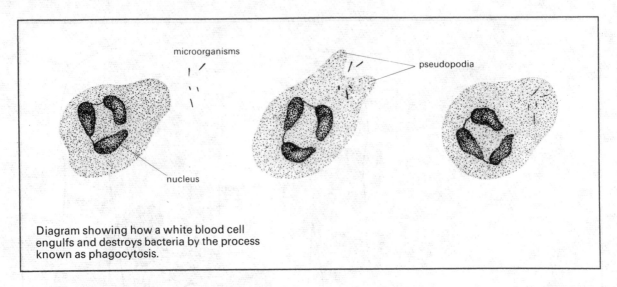

Diagram showing how a white blood cell engulfs and destroys bacteria by the process known as phagocytosis.

addition to these fixed macrophages, some of the monocytes leave the circulation to lead an itinerant existence in the tissues, available to be called up to join granulocytes in the fight against invading organisms. These are the wandering macrophages.

Lymphocytes The third type of white blood cell is the lymphocyte. The complexity and wealth of activities of the lymphocytes are only now being appreciated. These cells provide the mechanism by which foreign substances or organisms are recognized as being different from the body's own cells. They are the basis of the immune system. Some types of lymphocyte are the "memory" where knowledge of previous assaults by organisms is stored, and which "recognize" subsequent invasions by the same organisms. The descendants of these cells, called plasma cells, produce substances, antibodies, carried by the blood and tissue fluids, which coat the organisms and render them liable to phagocytosis by the neutrophils and macrophages. The origin and existence of the lymphocytes require a special section and will be described later.

Platelets The last type of cells in the blood are the platelets which are much smaller than red cells and are important in the coagulation of the blood. They are more numerous than white cells, the normal range being 150,000 to 400,000 per cubic millimetre. Platelets have the property of sticking together when vessel injury occurs, forming platelet plugs which stop the flow of blood in the damaged blood vessel. The relationship of platelets to other substances in the clotting system is discussed under bleeding disorders.

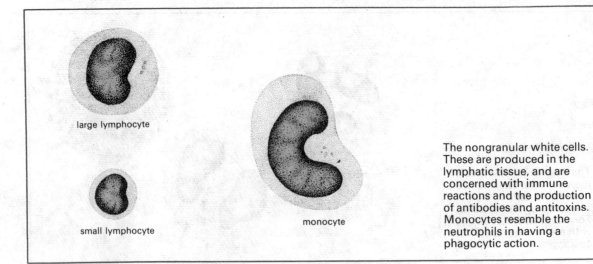

The nongranular white cells. These are produced in the lymphatic tissue, and are concerned with immune reactions and the production of antibodies and antitoxins. Monocytes resemble the neutrophils in having a phagocytic action.

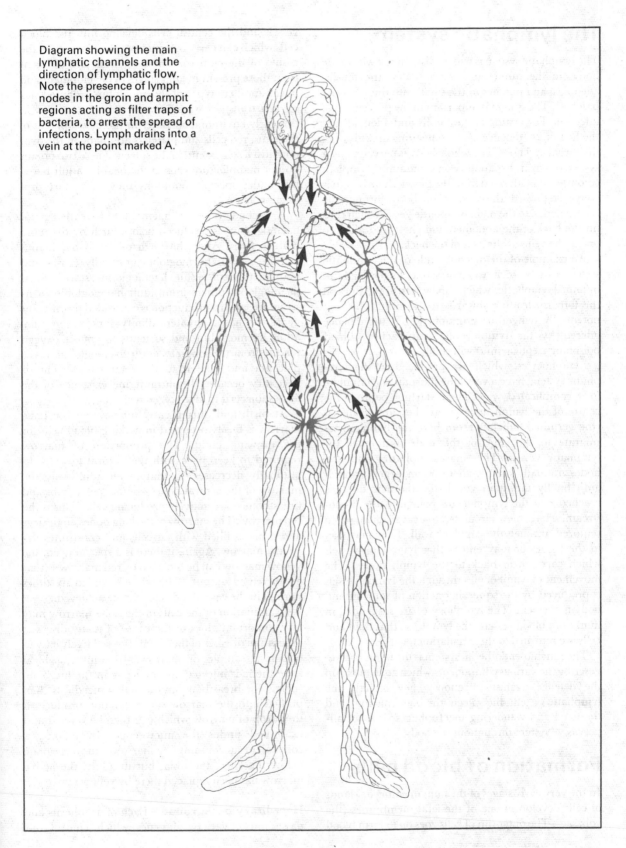

Diagram showing the main
lymphatic channels and the
direction of lymphatic flow.
Note the presence of lymph
nodes in the groin and armpit
regions acting as filter traps of
bacteria, to arrest the spread of
infections. Lymph drains into a
vein at the point marked A.

The lymphatic system

The lymphatic system is widely distributed within the body, in the numerous lymph nodes, the tonsils, adenoids, and patches in the small intestine (Peyer's patches). The system is important in the prevention of infection. For example, the tonsils and adenoids are the first line of defence against invading organisms in the throat and nose. The whole body is pervaded by a system of tiny transparent vessels containing lymph (a colourless fluid derived from the blood). The lymph is conveyed towards the centre of the body, through the lymph nodes, to the main lymphatic vessel which runs up the back of the abdomen and chest to drain into one of the veins at the root of the neck.

An example of the defensive role of the lymphatic system can be seen when a septic finger leads to inflamed lymphatics which can be seen as red lines on the forearm leading towards the armpit. This is a potentially dangerous situation, for, if the defence offered by the lymph node is breached, blood poisoning (septicaemia) will result.

Lymphocytes, which are produced in the lymphatic system, have a very long life span and circulate in a complicated way. Their starting point is the centre of the lymph node where they are produced (the germinal follicle). From here the lymphocytes migrate to the edge of the node and enter the lymphatic vessels. The small lymphatics from the nodes gradually join together to form larger channels until finally the main vessel, the thoracic duct, is reached and the lymphocytes pour into the blood-stream. Here they circulate, to leave again when required, through the capillary wall. They may stay in the tissues or may enter other lymphatic vessels which carry them back to the lymph nodes. The movement of lymphocytes through the lymph vessels is produced by the squeezing action of muscles and body movement. The lymphocytes are suspended in fluid from blood vessels (the lymph) so that fluid and cells are returned to the circulation together.

The reticulo-endothelial system is the name used to describe the various components which go to make up the defence against infection. They include the lymphatic system, the spleen, the bone marrow, and the fixed and wandering macrophages. It is an all-pervasive system throughout the body.

Formation of blood cells

In the very early stages of the human embryo, islands of cells develop in one of the fetal membranes (the yolk sac). The outer rim of cells goes on to form blood vessels and the central cells develop into red blood cells which can carry oxygen from the placenta to the tissues of the embryo. These red cells are different from those present in later stages of development and have another type of haemoglobin adapted for oxygen transport where oxygen tensions are low in this early environment. Later in the development of the fetus, red cells and platelets are made in the liver and, to a lesser extent, in the spleen. These two organs do not manufacture cells in the healthy adult body, but under special conditions they may start production again.

A second type of haemoglobin (called fetal haemoglobin) is produced before birth by the more mature fetus. After the birth of the baby, manufacture of fetal haemoglobin gradually ceases and manufacture of adult haemoglobin starts. Fetal haemoglobin differs from adult haemoglobin in its structure, and its production is controlled by different genes. It has a greater affinity for oxygen than adult haemoglobin and so tends to collect oxygen readily from the mother's adult haemoglobin at the placenta and take it to the fetal tissues. This is necessary because the intrauterine existence of the fetus subjects it to low oxygen tension.

At birth and during early infancy, all the bone marrow is busily occupied in making blood cells for the growing child. The proportion of marrow required to keep pace with the natural loss of cells gradually decreases, so that in an adult only the marrow of the central bones – spine, pelvis, ribs and breastbone – are actively producing cells. This is the red marrow. The marrow of the long bones, in the legs and arms, is filled with fat cells and constitutes the yellow marrow. Again, if there is a special need, the yellow marrow can be replaced by red marrow so that an increased output of blood cells, up to six times normal in the case of red cells, can be achieved.

Examination of the cells in the bone marrow may give important clues to the cause of many diseases, other than diseases of the blood. It is relatively easy to obtain a sample of marrow. In adults, a local anaesthetic is injected around a site in the hip bone (pelvis) or breastbone and a hollow needle is then pushed into the marrow space. Suction produces a tiny drop of marrow which can then be stained and examined under the microscope. In infants, a convenient site for sampling marrow is the large bone below the knee, the tibia, but in adults the active marrow has been replaced there by yellow marrow.

Hereditary background   Each of us inherits and passes on a variety of genes which control our

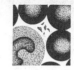

individual characteristics such as appearance, hair, eyes, skin colour, and so on. Some of the inherited characteristics, such as height, and weight, may be modified by factors in our environment, like nutrition or illness.

In some cases a single gene controls a very important function, whereas in other cases a whole group of genes together produce a particular end result. An example of the first situation is the production of haemoglobin. The molecule of haemoglobin is made up of two types of protein chain called alpha and beta chains. Each of these two chains is under the control of one gene. A very slight change in the gene may cause a marked change in the structure and function of the haemoglobin produced, and lead to severe anaemia. An example of the second situation is the inheritance of a tendency to certain disorders of the whole reticulo-endothelial system. It has already been mentioned that the lymphocytes are responsible for the recognition of foreign substances as opposed to those that are part of the body, ("self"). In some patients disorders arise because the lymphocytes fail to recognize "self" and start to order the production of antibodies to the body's own tissues. This produces a variety of disorders called autoimmune diseases, and the tendency to acquire these diseases may run in families.

In assessing diseases of the blood and reticulo-endothelial system the doctor has to be aware of the genetic and environmental background of the patient and will enquire into the family history of the patient as well as dietary habits and work environment, each of which may modify the course or features of a disease.

Blood groups and blood transfusion

The recognition of "self" and "foreign" by lymphocytes depends upon differences on the surface of cells from other persons or species. These differences are caused by the presence of complicated molecules, usually proteins combined with fats or sugars, which, if foreign, have the property of stimulating lymphocytes to produce antibodies. The substances are collectively known as antigens. They are determined by the genes which a person inherits. Identical twins inherit exactly the same genes, so that lymphocytes of one twin recognize as "self" all the tissues of the other. It is thus possible to transfer or transplant any organ or tissue from one identical twin to the other without fear of rejection. The more distant the relationship between donor and recipient, the less likely it is that transfer of tissues or organs will be successful unless the antigens on the surface of the donor's cells can be matched with those of the recipient. Fortunately there are only a few important antigens in red blood cells and their identification is relatively easy.

Blood transfusions have been attempted for centuries. Often transfer of blood was used in an attempt to convey special characteristics from one person to another. Thus blood from a docile man, or even from a lamb, would be given to an aggressive patient. Of course, these experiments failed and the recipients were probably saved from death only because the amount of blood used was very small.

In 1898, Dr Karl Landsteiner observed that when blood from one person was mixed with the blood of another person the cells sometimes clumped together (agglutinated) whereas with others no clumping occurred. He divided the people into three groups, those with factor A, B, or both A and B (AB) in their blood. Later, a fourth group of people who lacked both A and B were identified and called O. These factors are determined by antigens on the red cell surface and this system, the ABO system, divides blood cells into four groups: A, B, AB, and O. The proportion of a population which has each of these groups varies throughout the world since they are determined by inheritance. In the United Kingdom Group O is the commonest, but even in these islands there is variation, group A being more common in the south of England and group O more common in Scotland. In addition to the blood group antigens on the red cells, some people have antibodies in their plasma against the A or B substances which are not their own. Thus people with blood group AB have no antibodies, people with A have anti-B and those with blood group O have both anti-A and anti-B. In practice there are no anti-O antibodies.

There are many other blood group systems apart from the simple ABO system. The next most important in practical terms is the Rhesus blood group system, so called because it was first identified using rhesus monkeys. Three closely connected genes determine this system and a person either has Rhesus antigen on the surface of the red cells (Rhesus positive), or it is lacking (Rhesus negative). People who are Rhesus negative will make antibodies if given Rhesus positive blood. These antibodies will cause clumping together and then destruction (lysis) of the Rhesus positive red cells. The importance of this system lies in the fact that mothers who are Rhesus negative may have Rhesus positive babies. A small

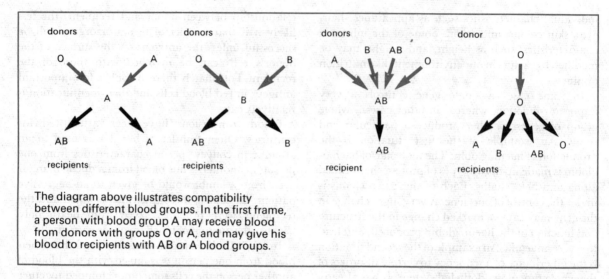

The diagram above illustrates compatibility between different blood groups. In the first frame, a person with blood group A may receive blood from donors with groups O or A, and may give his blood to recipients with AB or A blood groups.

amount of an earlier baby's blood may have entered the mother's circulation during labour, causing the production of antibodies. In a subsequent pregnancy these antibodies are hostile to the baby's blood, causing neonatal jaundice, severe anaemia, or even death of the baby before birth. The prevention of this condition – haemolytic disease of the newborn – by giving appropriate antisera after the birth of each child of a Rhesus negative mother is one of the recent triumphs of medicine.

Blood transfusion is now a standard practice and saves thousands of lives each year but is made possible only by the generosity of thousands of voluntary blood donors. It will be appreciated that the large reserve capacity of the bone marrow for making blood compensates rapidly for the loss of one pint (568 ml) of blood, about one tenth of the total blood volume.

The general health of a blood donor is also assessed before blood is collected. For the donor's protection the haemoglobin is measured and any donor who appears to be anaemic is not bled, but is advised to consult his doctor. Certain diseases can be transmitted by blood transfusion, the most dangerous being one form of hepatitis. Fortunately modern tests are available to detect the presence of hepatitis virus in a potential donor and these people, who are otherwise entirely healthy, are rejected as donors. Syphilis and malaria are other disorders which may be transmitted but there are screening tests for the former, and the latter is rare in the United Kingdom.

The matching of blood groups and identification of antibodies require sophisticated techniques, and despite careful cross-matching of blood, reactions by a patient to transfusion may occur. These reactions commonly take the form of fever and even shivering

(rigors). Although most unpleasant for the patient, these reactions do no lasting harm. They are caused by incompatibility of the white cells in the transfusion. On the whole this can be prevented by giving anti-allergic drugs or by removing the white cells from the blood before the transfusion is given.

Serious reactions to blood transfusion are extremely rare. The usual cause is the giving of the wrong blood to a patient, the mistake occurring because of human error in labelling tubes or reading names on packs of blood. If the blood given contains red cells against whose antigens the patient already has antibodies, so that the blood is incompatible, the blood will be destroyed and damage to the kidneys may occur. Fortunately, the damage is reversible and modern artificial kidney techniques will keep the patient alive long enough for these organs to recover.

Disorders of the blood

Anaemia Anaemia literally means "want of blood". In medical terms it means that a person has less haemoglobin than is usually found in healthy people of the same age group. Nearly everyone has mild anaemia at some time of their life and it is important for doctors to sort out which of the many causes of anaemia are present, and which are potentially serious. Anaemia may develop because the bone marrow is unable to make sufficient blood to keep pace with normal losses or because there is an increased loss of blood with which the normal marrow cannot cope.

Iron deficiency anaemia The most common anaemia in the world is iron deficiency anaemia. The body is very efficient at conserving iron to make haemo-

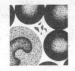

globin, but in two situations the iron stores may be lost and anaemia results. Insufficient iron in the diet is probably the commonest reason for iron deficiency, but in most affluent societies small, continuous, or intermittent blood loss is the more serious cause. Nutritional iron deficiency is most often found in the premature infant, the growing child, and the pregnant woman. At these times there is an increased demand for the production of haemoglobin and the iron reserves may not be sufficient to provide all the iron necessary.

WARNING: No child should ever be given iron tablets unless prescribed by a doctor since iron in this form is extremely poisonous to children. A not uncommon tragedy is the accidental taking of iron tablets prescribed for a pregnant mother, but mistaken for sweets by a young child.

In children such iron deficiency is usually temporary and will get better without treatment. Oral doses of medicinal iron of almost any type will promptly correct iron deficiency anaemia.

Chronic blood loss may be quite unsuspected. A symptomless peptic ulcer, piles which bleed only intermittently, excessive menstrual flow, and other conditions may cause chronic blood loss and iron deficiency anaemia. More sinister causes are cancers of the bowel. It is essential to detect and correct the cause of the blood loss, preferably before providing iron supplements.

During the early years of life the normal haemoglobin values are identical for both sexes. With the onset of menstruation in girls and until the menopause, the haemoglobin levels of women average one to two grams lower than in men of the same age (women 11·5 to 16·5 gm; men 13·5 to 18 gm). After the menopause there should be no significant difference. In a man any iron deficiency anaemia is likely to be due to chronic blood loss and the site of bleeding must be sought.

Sometimes a patient cannot tolerate any form of oral iron because of intestinal upsets. There are forms of iron that a doctor may inject intravenously or intramuscularly to bypass the digestive tract.

Any kind of anaemia may be virtually symptomless, or symptoms may be severe to the point of incapacitating the patient. So gradual is the onset of anaemia in many instances that the person may not be conscious of any significant change in strength or endurance; in others, noticeable symptoms appear early and increase. The widespread use of cosmetics masks the developing pallor to the casual observer who ordinarily does not inspect the conjunctivae, gums, and mucous membranes of the mouth as the doctor does. Even this may be misleading except in extreme cases. The only real test is to take blood and examine it. Many women adjust to a lowered haemoglobin level by sheer force of will and attribute their tiredness to the excessive demands of home, job, or age. They do not realize how much more they could do and how much better they would feel with more normal haemoglobin levels.

Indirectly, many vague aches and pains may derive from anaemia. The heart muscle may protest with attacks of angina pectoris due to anaemia rather than to disease of the blood vessels of the heart.

Only a doctor can distinguish between simple iron deficiency anaemia and the more serious and complicated anaemias. A simple blood test may give the lead, and when indicated, a bone marrow examination and suitable laboratory tests to rule out other possible complicating factors will confirm the diagnosis. It pays to be sure. Do not accept a therapeutic test for iron deficiency anaemia – that is, to try the effect of an iron-containing prescription or proprietary brand – before proof that all that is needed is iron. Precious days or weeks may be lost on self-medication by guesswork if anaemia is due to one of the causes other than iron deficiency.

Pernicious anaemia This is a disease of middle and later life. Giant red cells (macrocytes) are found in the blood in certain anaemias. Each red cell appears to be overloaded with haemoglobin while the total red cell count is decreased. This is one of the characteristics of pernicious anaemia – a name that once was all too apt, but now is retained only out of respect for tradition. As recently as 1925 this disease was invariably fatal; today the life expectancy of the properly treated pernicious anaemic patient is the same as that of the general population. However, it is simpler to continue to call the disease pernicious anaemia than a macrocytic hyperchromic megaloblastic anaemia.

In sharp contrast to the small pale haemoglobin-deficient red blood cells of simple iron deficiency anaemia, the fewer large cells in pernicious anaemia are fully filled with haemoglobin and appear to be more highly coloured than normal. Many misshapen red blood cells appear as the anaemia becomes more severe and there is an accompanying decrease in blood platelets and white cells.

The life span of the abnormal red cells in pernicious anaemia is quite short. They are easily disintegrated and give up their haemoglobin more readily (haemolysis). This breakdown results in an increase of pigments, which frequently give a lemon yellow colour to the skin. The urine also takes on a deeper colour because of excreted red cell breakdown products.

Pernicious anaemia may first be suspected because of three quite different sets of symptoms.

1 Most frequently there is a gradual increase of fatigue and weakness, with pallor which progresses to the typical lemon yellow colour of the skin and mucous membranes. The tongue becomes smooth, red, and sore.

2 The onset may be heralded by gastrointestinal symptoms, more particularly indigestion, which reflects the destruction of certain glands in the stomach wall.

3 Even before external signs of anaemia appear, there may be evidence of spinal cord degeneration though this is rare. Deterioration of parts of the nervous system is made apparent by unbalanced gait and the gradual onset of numbness and tingling in the toes and fingers, spreading to the feet, hands, legs, and arms. Impaired sensitivity to pinprick, light touch, heat, and cold often develops in a "glove and stocking" distribution. In men impotence occurs early and disturbances of bladder control are common.

The neurological features are the most serious manifestation of pernicious anaemia. If the condition is recognized early and treated adequately, the nervous system symptoms may be reversed.

One of the triumphs of modern medicine is the discovery of the chemical factors involved in blood cell production and of the treatment which has changed pernicious anaemia from an invariably fatal disease to one that can be controlled with practically complete success.

An incredibly small amount of vitamin B_{12} – one microgram, or about 1/28,000 of an ounce a day – is often sufficient to keep a pernicious anaemia patient in good health. In the average patient, injection of a maintenance dose of vitamin B_{12} every month is sufficient to maintain normal red cell production. Treatment must, of course be continued for the rest of the patient's life, since vitamin B_{12} does not cure the basic biochemical defect but is needed to replace the deficiency.

Folic acid, another vitamin essential for normal blood cell production, has the same ability as vitamin B_{12} to overcome the purely anaemic symptoms of pernicious anaemia. Folic acid, however, is powerless to protect against the potentially serious effects of the disease on the central nervous system. So there is a danger that if multiple vitamins including folic acid are taken as self-medication without a doctor's advice, the characteristic anaemia may be masked and go unrecognized while the neurological degeneration progresses beyond the point of no return. Whenever the previously described neurological symptoms appear, whether or not there are typical symptoms of anaemia, it is very likely that pernicious anaemia is in the background, and immediate medical diagnosis is imperative.

There is a slightly higher incidence of stomach cancer in patients with pernicious anaemia than in normal persons.

Other macrocytic anaemias These are mostly caused by a deficiency in folic acid which may arise in two ways. First there may be a lack of the vitamin in the diet. Folic acid is present in green vegetables but is inactivated by excessive cooking. People who live on tea and toast, mainly old age pensioners, are liable to develop anaemia due to folic acid deficiency. Another common cause is alcoholism, where poor diet combined with damage to the liver and to the intestinal tract leads to a complicated pattern of vitamin deficiencies. Pregnant women may have a deficiency of folic acid, and supplements of the vitamin are often given as a routine precaution. The second cause of folic acid deficiency is a failure to absorb the vitamin normally from the intestinal tract. Malabsorption syndromes include diseases such as coeliac disease, tropical sprue, and the results of extensive surgery to the small intestine.

There remains a small group of patients who have macrocytic anaemia which is not due to vitamin B_{12} or folic acid deficiency. These patients usually have a fundamental disorder of red cell production. The only treatment for them may be repeated transfusion or a reliance on the adaptation of the body to chronic anaemia.

Polycythaemia Polycythaemia, or erythrocytosis, is the condition of too many red cells in the blood. A relative polycythaemia occurs when there is loss of plasma without comparable loss of blood cells, with a corresponding concentration of red cells. Restricted fluid intake alone may lead in a few days to a decrease in plasma volume, or loss of water and salts due to vomiting, diarrhoea, excessive sweating, extensive burns, or traumatic shock can lead to excessive plasma loss. Restoration of fluid balance with proper amounts of water and salts promptly abolishes the relative polycythaemia.

The red blood cell forming mechanism in the bone marrow is very sensitive in its response to increased oxygen needs by the body. People who live at high

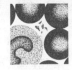

altitudes have higher red cell counts to compensate for the lowered oxygen pressure. There are also certain diseases of the lung which prevent the proper oxygenation of the blood and result in compensatory increases in red cells.

Primary polycythaemia, or polycythaemia rubra vera, is a chronic disease which involves an increase in all the cellular elements of the bone marrow – red cells, granulocytes, and blood platelets. The diagnosis is usually made just by looking at the patient, who characteristically shows marked redness of the skin, especially of the face and cheeks, with purplish lips (cyanosis), bluish nail beds, and purple colouring of the fingers. The whites of the eyes are pink. Symptoms develop gradually, mainly as a result of the increased thickness or viscosity of the blood. The patient feels generally unwell, is easily tired, has difficulty in thinking clearly and a headache or heaviness in the head. Itching may be a troublesome symptom, particularly following a hot bath. A patient with well-developed polycythaemia rubra vera may suffer from a venous thrombosis and, at the same time, have a bleeding tendency. The thrombosis is understandable since many of these patients have a great increase in blood platelets, but the function of these platelets may be abnormal so that they fail to form the platelet plugs in response to injury.

Treatment consists basically of decreasing the number of circulating cells and slowing down their overproduction, if possible. The blood volume in polycythaemia is often increased to seven or eight litres and as much as 75 per cent of the blood volume is comprised of cells, whereas the normal level is around 45 per cent. The obvious remedy is to remove the surplus red cells, and this can be done by bloodletting (venesection), but this has no influence on the increased number of blood platelets and white cells.

Treatment is either by repeated bloodletting or by radioactive phosphorus (32P). Both methods alleviate the condition, but neither is a complete cure.

The haemolytic anaemias The term haemolysis means a shortening of the normal red cell life span. Haemolytic anaemia occurs when the bone marrow cannot compensate for the increased destruction of red cells. Haemolysis occurs when there is a genetic defect in the metabolism or structure of the red cell or an abnormality in the structure of the haemoglobin. These are the inherited haemolytic anaemias. The red cell life span may also be shortened by changes in the plasma – the acquired haemolytic anaemias. In all haemolytic anaemias there is an increased production of bilirubin, the yellow breakdown product of haemoglobin, and an increase in the numbers of immature red cells (reticulocytes).

Hereditary spherocytosis (also called familial acholuric jaundice) is one of the common inherited haemolytic disorders in white-skinned people. It is a condition which results in the production of small globular fragile red blood cells (microspherocytosis) by the bone marrow. Spherical red cells are less resistant to normal wear and tear than normal red cells. This susceptibility to destruction with the resultant escape of haemoglobin gives rise to the most prominent signs of the disease – jaundice and anaemia.

From birth, the inherited trait results in a precarious balance of red cell production and destruction. The balance may be tipped towards destruction by the ordinary events of life, or by stress such as a mild infection or a fracture, which may precipitate a haemolytic crisis with an increase in jaundice and pallor. In such circumstances, there is always a sharp increase in the percentage of young red cells recently delivered into the circulation. The disease may be inactive and symptomless, or produce chronic ill health. An acute crisis may threaten life itself. Such crises are a constant threat to a person who has inherited the trait. For that reason, when the diagnosis is certain, it is advisable to consider removal of the spleen as a preventive measure during a time of inactivity rather than to undertake surgery during an acute crisis. The spleen is the principal site of red blood cell destruction in this disease and its surgical removal (splenectomy) should alleviate the disorder. Splenectomy is the treatment of choice for hereditary spherocytosis at any age when any degree of symptomatic activity has been demonstrated. Smaller accessory spleens are often found in these patients and all splenic tissue must be discovered and removed by the surgeon if a relapse is to be avoided. Splenectomy carries an increased risk of infection in very young children so it is desirable, though not always possible, to wait until the child is in its teens before carrying out the operation.

Chronic haemolytic anaemia over a prolonged period will almost certainly result in formation of stones in the gallbladder which are derived from blood pigments. Splenectomy not only controls the anaemia but when performed early prevents the formation of this type of gallstone.

Acquired haemolytic anaemia is closely associated with immunological mechanisms. In many such cases, specific antibodies to the patient's red blood cells can be found in the blood.

Adrenal corticosteroids (cortisone) and similar

Chapter 4 Blood and blood-forming organs

drugs are the usual treatment for these patients. Drugs which suppress the body's natural immune reactions, such as azathioprin, may be used in addition if the dose of steroid is unacceptably high. In this disease, also, the spleen is sometimes the main site of destruction of the red cells and splenectomy may prove helpful.

Molecular diseases of blood (haemoglobino-pathies) Haemoglobin is a complex molecule containing iron. Its iron-containing part (haem) is smaller than the globin portion, which is a protein. Relatively simple chemical units known as amino acids are linked together in precise sequences to form proteins. As an analogy we can imagine a word spelt with a large number of letters. If a couple of letters are transposed, or a wrong letter used, the word is obviously misspelt. A similar seemingly trifling error in a sequence of hundreds of amino acids creates a unique molecule. It may closely resemble another molecule, but it will be subtly different. If the molecule is important to some body function, the apparently trifling difference gives rise to some form of disease. This is the reason for the term molecular disease – because it is caused by a change in the structure of a molecule.

Such hereditary "misspellings" of haemoglobin do occur in some people. Linus Pauling, the Nobel prize-winning chemist was the first to demonstrate that such an error is responsible for a disease, namely sickle-cell anaemia. Many similar chemical errors, called haemoglobinopathies, have been identified. More than a hundred different abnormal haemo-globins have been recognized. Initially they were designated by a letter of the alphabet but recent practice utilizes the name of the place from which the patient came, for example "Hb Shepherd's Bush". Only the usual adult and fetal haemoglobins are considered normal. Abnormal haemoglobins do not always cause disease. Sometimes they do, however, and the application of this modern knowledge has greatly enhanced our understanding of once mys-terious blood disorders.

Sickle-cell anaemia occurs predominantly in the Negro race, although a few instances in white people have been reported. The name of the disease reflects the tendency of these abnormal red blood cells to take sickle- or oat-shaped forms when the level of oxygen in the blood falls, because of the distorting effect of the abnormal haemoglobin molecule. As the sickling increases, the blood becomes more viscous and the red cells more fragile, leading to haemolytic anaemia and impairment of blood supply to many organs, including the lungs, central nervous system, and long bones. The course of the disease is punctuated by crises with fever and attacks of pain felt in the arms and legs, heart, or abdomen. Treatment of such crises is to relieve the symptoms, with or without oxygen administration or blood transfusions. In children there is often enlargement of the spleen which may be associated with abnormal blood destruction, for which splenectomy may be needed. If the patient survives to adult life the spleen shrinks greatly in size with repeated thromboses and fibrosis but crises nevertheless occur. Patients should avoid going to high altitudes because crises are precipitated by a reduction in available oxygen.

Research efforts are under way to improve the treatment and recognition of sickle-cell disease – a disease that is perfectly well understood but is not at present curable because the inherited defect is hidden in the structure of haemoglobin molecules. Of those who carry the sickle-cell trait and can transmit it to offspring, only about one in four hundred has evident sickle-cell anaemia.

Sickle-cell disease is inherited recessively (see chapter 26). If only one parent has the trait, there is an even chance that each child born to them will or will not have the trait, but none will have anaemia. If

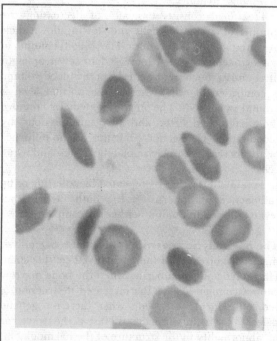

A photograph showing the distortion of red cells due to an inherited abnormality of the haemoglobin molecule, called sickle cell anaemia.

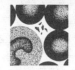

both parents carry the trait, for each child born to them, there is a 50 per cent chance that it will inherit only the trait, a 25 per cent chance that it will have evident sickle-cell anaemia, and a 25 per cent chance that it will be normal, with neither the trait nor the anaemia. The gene originated in West Africa and it is believed that inheritance of only one gene protects against the ravages of malaria – perhaps the reason why the abnormal gene survives.

Experimental treatments of painful sickle crises, not without potential hazards, give hope that better methods will become available. Since crises generally abate when the symptoms are treated, the benefits of medication are hard to evaluate, and there is some doubt that medicines can actually reach the blocked sites. No known treatment can change the basic defect in the haemoglobin molecule.

The most important factors in avoiding crises and preventing the cumulative damage which may occur are good nutrition, avoidance of dehydration, and prompt management of infections. The higher the standard of living and general medical care, the less is the eventual harm.

Thalassaemia or Mediterranean anaemia derives its name from the fact that it occurs predominantly in the peoples bordering on the Mediterranean sea and their descendants elsewhere in the world. Like sickle-cell anaemia, it may occur either as a relatively symptomless trait, thalassaemia minor, or as a severe anaemia, thalassaemia major. The disorder arises because there is a failure in the manufacture of one or other of the globin chains of haemoglobin.

In the major disorder, which is frequently fatal during childhood, the red cells are small and very low in haemoglobin concentration. Usually both the spleen and liver are enlarged. If the spleen begins to destroy too many red blood cells the patient may benefit from splenectomy. The only effective treatment is transfusion, which eventually leads to problems of iron overload and it is to be hoped that knowledge gained from molecular biology will eventually help these patients. In general it may be said that splenectomy is beneficial, in theory and usually in practice, in all of the haemoglobinopathies whenever increased haemolytic action of the spleen is shown to exist.

Haemoglobinuria (haemoglobin in the urine)

Paroxysmal nocturnal haemoglobinuria is a rare form of chronic haemolytic anaemia. The patient's morning urine has a dark red appearance. The characteristic feature of the disorder is iron from the blood in the urine. The defect is in the red blood cell which is abnormally sensitive to attack by complement, one of the immune defence substances. The reason for increased haemolysis during sleep is not known. Onset of the disorder is gradual and the course chronic. Splenectomy has not proved to be of any value.

Paroxysmal cold haemoglobinuria The patient passes dark-coloured urine after exposure to cold during the winter months, or more rarely after strenuous exercise. The dark red or almost black urine contains haemoglobin, other substances, and sometimes intact red blood cells. The paroxysmal attack comes on at any time from a few minutes to six or eight hours after the patient is chilled. The chilling may be surprisingly slight. There is headache, pain in the back and legs or abdomen, chills followed by fever of 40° C (104° F) or higher, blueness of the skin, and a transient rise in blood pressure. A test shows that haemoglobin separates from the patient's blood when a sample is chilled in a test tube and subsequently warmed. Congenital syphilis used to be the commonest cause of this disorder, but various virus infections are now the usual causative agents.

Red cell enzymes The red cell carries a number of enzymes. These are protein molecules which speed up chemical processes of the body. Sometimes the red cell does not inherit normal enzymes and a deficiency of one particular enzyme leads to a type of hereditary haemolytic anaemia which is associated with haemoglobinuria. It was noticed that some black soldiers in the United States army who were given the antimalarial drug primaquine, developed haemolytic anaemia. They were said to be primaquine sensitive. The cause of this unusual reaction is now known to be due to a deficiency of a specific red cell enzyme. No harm results unless primaquine or something else triggers a haemolytic anaemia. Various other drugs – sulphonamides, some common pain relievers, and even some kinds of bean, an ordinarily harmless food – have been shown to cause haemolytic reactions in persons who lack a protective enzyme because of their inherited make-up. In addition, infective hepatitis, infectious mononucleosis, and certain bacterial pneumonias and viral infections of the upper respiratory tract seem to take advantage of the enzyme deficiency to produce a haemolytic anaemia. Treatment is not usually required for this disorder except to warn the patient about the possible dangers of certain drugs.

Other relationships of specific enzyme deficiencies to various disorders are now being shown, and further developments are expected in this relatively new area of research.

Chapter 4 Blood and blood-forming organs

Bleeding disorders

Purpura (purple patches in skin and mucous membrane) Blood platelets (thrombocytes) are essential for the normal coagulation of blood, assisting in the formation of clots when we cut ourselves. Platelets are small fragments of mother cells (megakaryocytes) in the bone marrow. If for any reason there is a reduction in the number of platelets, evidence of bleeding from tiny blood vessels may appear in the skin and mucous membranes. A general term for such bleeding is purpura.

Small haemorrhages may occur spontaneously as well as after mild injury. Tiny pinpoint haemorrhages (petechiae) often occur in healthy people and are of no significance, but larger purplish patches in and beneath the skin or black and blue spots are warnings to seek the cause of bleeding. If these painless signs are ignored, bleeding gums, prolonged nosebleeds, or severe urinary or gastrointestinal haemorrhages or prolonged menstrual periods may follow. At the first appearance of these signs a doctor should be consulted. If investigation shows that normal blood platelets are present in normal quantity, then other mechanisms of abnormal bleeding such as vitamin C or K deficiency or infections may be identified and treated. When bleeding is due to a great reduction in the numbers of circulating blood platelets the next step is a careful study of the bone marrow to determine whether the megakaryocytes in the marrow are capable of producing normal populations of platelets.

One of the most dangerous crises is uncontrolled and uncontrollable bleeding. Transfusions of fresh whole blood or platelet suspensions can be only temporarily effective. The precise mechanism underlying such bleeding must be established at the earliest possible moment, in case a specific remedy is available.

Immune thrombocytopenic purpura (ITP) means bleeding occurring with deficiency of platelets due to their destruction by antibody reaction. The antibody may arise in response to known or unknown causes. The bone marrow shows an increase in numbers and activity of platelet-producing cells without a parallel increase of platelets in the blood, indeed a severe deficit results. The spleen is the major site of destruction of the antibody coated cells in most, though not all, patients with ITP.

ITP in childhood is often acute and self-limiting. Bleeding from the mouth is common. A recent viral infection, particularly in children, may diminish the number of marrow cells, which can be confirmed by microscopic observation. This demands whole blood transfusions while efforts to demonstrate an auto-immune basis – reaction of the body's own cells to foreign substances – are made. Corticosteroid drugs should also be started immediately and if it is a true immune reaction spontaneous recovery may be expected, beginning within a few hours to a few days. Should stopping of the drugs be followed by a relapse with a dangerous decrease in platelets, and the marrow still shows an increase of megakaryocytes, splenectomy is indicated and is successful in about two thirds of patients. Expert bone marrow interpretation is the key to diagnosis and treatment of both chronic and acute thrombocytopenic purpuric crises.

The term hypersplenism means an excessive increase in the destructive processes of the spleen. If the spleen is enlarged in a case otherwise suggestive of ITP, the possibility of hypersplenism must be considered. If confirmed, splenectomy is desirable in such patients. Not infrequently, when the spleen is removed for an apparent hypersplenic ITP, an unsuspected disease, for example, splenic tuberculosis, sarcoidosis, or Hodgkin's disease, is uncovered, and specific treatment can be begun for the underlying disease.

The spleen is not essential to life, and in most cases can be removed without detrimental effect. Lord Dawson of Penn made long-term studies of patients who had had their spleen removed for congenital haemolytic anaemia and who later fought in the First World War. They were not weaker or more liable to infection than their comrades. Patients whose normal spleens have been removed after rupture from injury or for ITP and other hypersplenic states have been studied since 1930, without finding any evidence of heightened susceptibility to infections or interference with normal health and longevity, or of any handicap to normal growth and development in children. Nevertheless, some doctors have indicated an increased risk from certain types of infection after splenectomy in small children. Penicillin is often given preventively to such children.

Other bleeding diseases

Haemophilia is the best known of the hereditary bleeding disorders. It is no longer so hopeless a disease as it once was, although the defect in clotting ability of the blood is permanent, and the patient must learn to live with it and adapt his activities to his inborn handicap. Classic haemophilia is the result of varying degrees of a deficiency of a substance in the blood plasma which has an essential role in the very complicated processes of blood coagulation. The substance is called antihaemophilic globulin or AHG.

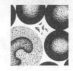

In the numbering system of blood-clotting factors, it is Factor VIII. Inability to produce this factor, or not enough of it, is passed on by female carriers who do not themselves have symptoms but transmit the disease to male descendants. There is remarkable variation in the bleeding tendencies of haemophiliacs. In some patients the condition is troublesome only when a tooth must be extracted or some fairly severe wound is suffered. Other patients are so sensitive that even ordinary activities may produce haemorrhage into joints. They may thus develop crippling joint deformities.

Treatment is important and should be given however minor the cut or accident, since recurrent delayed bleeding is common and may be difficult to control. Appropriate coagulation tests evaluate the activity of AHG, which not only varies from person to person but in the same person from time to time. Treatment has been revolutionized by the introduction of concentrated preparations of AHG, either as a precipitate prepared from blood at National Blood Transfusion Centres or more concentrated material available commercially. The AHG is given by injection into a vein and many haemophiliacs learn how to do this for themselves at home so they do not have to attend hospital.

Care of haemophiliac infants and children taxes the emotional and financial resources of parents. Babies who inherit the trait gradually learn to avoid bumps and bruises as they grow up. A session or two in a hospital teaches the important lesson – prevention!

Parents should do all within reason to safeguard their small haemophiliac boy. The sides of the child's bed, playpen, or high chair should be padded. Toys should be soft, without sharp edges. Finger and toenails should be trimmed regularly. Be careful to keep cutlery and other objects that the child might pull onto himself out of his reach. Early treatment of even minor bleeding is very important despite the natural reluctance of parents to subject their child to injections.

Christmas disease is named not after the season, but after the family in which it was first discovered. It is also called haemophilia B. Symptoms are indistinguishable from classic haemophilia, but are caused by hereditary deficiency of a different blood clotting element, Factor IX. It is unlike haemophilia in two important respects: some of the female carriers may themselves have a mild bleeding tendency, and Factor IX, unlike Factor VIII, is relatively stable in stored blood which therefore may be used effectively in treating bleeding episodes.

Other bleeding disorders There are twelve numbered coagulation factors and inherited deficiencies of each of them have been described. Compared with haemophilia they are rare and most are not so severe. Treatment depends upon replacement of the missing factor by transfusion.

White cell disorders A lack of circulating granular white cells (granulocytes) leads to an increased risk of bacterial infection. Such a deficiency may occur only in white cells (neutropenia) or in association with reduced numbers of all blood cells (pancytopenia). The deficiency may arise because of a production failure or because of increased destruction.

Production failure occurs in various diseases of the bone marrow. Sometimes patients react in an abnormal way to certain drugs, and shortage of neutrophils (neutropenia) occurs. Excess destruction may occur when the spleen is enlarged and destroys the neutrophils. This may occur in association with rheumatoid arthritis (Felty's syndrome), tropical disorders, especially malaria (tropical hypersplenism) and some disorders of the liver circulation (Banti's syndrome).

Careful study of the interreactions of spleen and bone marrow is vital in understanding the group of diseases involving either or both organs. Also, autoimmune reactions may initiate hypersplenism and must be distinguished. The spleen lies in the abdominal cavity high up under the diaphragm on the left side behind the ribs. The normal spleen can not be felt, but if it enlarges to twice or more its normal size (200 to 280 gm – 7 to 10 oz), the doctor can feel it on abdominal examination. In some diseases the spleen may become enormously enlarged, filling the entire abdomen and weighing as much as 4·5 kg (10 pounds) or more. Tests using radioactive chemicals can provide much evidence about the role of the spleen in destruction, pooling, or even production of blood cells in various disease states. The idea that radioactive substances may be injected often alarms patients but the amount of radioactivity which the patient receives is rigidly controlled and very rarely exceeds the amount present in a conventional X-ray.

In myelofibrosis the bone marrow is gradually replaced by fibrous tissue. In most instances the spleen enlarges, and it is important to know whether the spleen itself is involved in this process or whether it is resuming its embryonic function of blood cell production. In this disease needle aspiration often fails, and it is necessary to obtain a bone marrow sample by a surgical procedure. This helps the haematologist to decide the relative role of the spleen in any given patient and whether splenectomy would be beneficial. In selected patients, removal of the spleen will relieve increasing discomfort and increase the blood cell survival time, thus prolonging life more comfortably without weekly blood transfusions which otherwise might be required for many months and even years. Radioactive isotopes are particularly useful in this disorder in helping the doctor to decide whether the spleen should be removed or not.

The leukaemic states

The word leukaemia creates alarm in the minds of many people. It is true that leukaemia, like many other disease states, may be fatal sooner or later. But, as is also true of many other diseases now, there are increasing numbers of patients with this disturbance in the white cell equilibrium who live normally and die of unrelated diseases.

It has been customary to divide the leukaemic states into the acute and chronic leukaemias. The terms were originally descriptive of the clinical course of the disease. The acute disease, frequently having an onset similar to an acute infection, is the kind most frequently seen in children and has a fatal outcome in four to eight weeks if untreated. On the other hand, chronic leukaemia characteristically has a gradual onset, occurs in middle and later life, and may remain inactive or progress very slowly over a period of months and years before symptoms develop which interfere with the normal life of the patient.

While it is true that we do not yet know the basic causes of the leukaemias, research is leading closer to those factors which either cause these changes or lower a person's resistance to them. Considerable progress has been made in the variety and specificity of drugs and other agents which may be used to alter, and in many cases, stop the progress of this group of diseases. Thus the term leukaemia does not necessarily carry the same fatal connotation as it used to, any more than pernicious anaemia any longer denotes an invariably progressive and fatal red blood cell disease.

Chronic leukaemias Any kind of white blood and connective tissue cells may occur in excess without involving any of the others.

Chronic lymphocytic leukaemia, relatively benign, is the most common form in patients in the late fifties and extending through the sixth and seventh decades of life. Fortunately, this is the easiest of all the leukaemias to control for long periods of time. In the absence of symptoms and without any serious disturbance of bone marrow function or any vital organ, no treatment may be necessary for months or years.

The doctor who finds a mild elevation in the lymphocytes in circulating blood will know that sooner or later they may increase. Watchfulness and periodic blood and physical examinations of the patient are needed, to determine if specific therapy is needed. When the bone marrow is invaded, early or late enlargement of the regional lymph nodes, or spleen, or both, may develop in addition to slowly worsening anaemia and a decrease in blood platelets. Increase in lymphocyte production with swelling of lymph nodes may also occur without any change in the circulating blood cells.

More frequently, however, when a patient notices any lymph node swelling or discovers a solid mass in the upper left quadrant of his abdomen, a look at the blood will reveal an increase in the lymphocytes but they will still be small, qualitatively normal, mature lymphocytes. A bone marrow study will reveal the degree, if any, of lymphocyte infiltration of the marrow with displacement of red cell and platelet formation.

Whenever chronic lymphocytic leukaemia is recognized, many doctors prefer the patient to be seen by a haematologist who, from the fairly broad choice of agents now available, will decide the treatment programme best fitted for the individual patient. Generally, the choice is between corticosteroids or relatively mild cytotoxic drugs.

There are several complications to be kept in mind in chronic lymphatic leukaemia:

About fifty per cent of such patients show a lowering of the antibody globulins, and if, as sometimes happens, the granulocytes are also reduced in number, there may be increased susceptibility to infections. When acute bacterial infections develop they must be treated promptly with the appropriate antibiotic. If the antibody globulins are very low, replacement injections may also be given.

Herpes zoster (shingles), a painful virus disease of the sensory nerves, has a close association with chronic lymphatic leukaemia patients. Shingles is a self-limiting disease, but requires great patience on the part of both the patient and the doctor, although better treatments are becoming available.

If the spleen becomes involved, hypersplenism may cause haemolytic anaemia and reduction in the number of platelets, so splenectomy is advised. When such a situation develops there need be no hesitancy in proceeding with surgery. The specific deficiency of cells can be corrected, and there seldom follows any exacerbation of the leukaemia or any later complication which might have been a result of the splenectomy.

Haemolytic anaemia or a low platelet count may develop as a consequence of abnormal antibody production. Treatment with corticosteroids is usually effective.

Chronic lymphocytic leukaemia, then, is the least dangerous type of leukaemia and there is better than a fifty-fifty chance of continuing to live a useful life with this disease.

Chronic granulocytic leukaemia   The various types of cells in the bone marrow – neutrophils, basophils, and eosinophils – may be involved either singly or jointly along with the megakaryocytes in this disease. The lymph nodes are not usually involved, but the spleen becomes enlarged early – in some patients it fills the entire left side of the abdomen – and may be the first sign. Characteristically in chronic granulocytic leukaemia, the cells are relatively mature, with only a small percentage of immature cells in blood and bone marrow. The spleen, being a reservoir for bone marrow elements, tends to become engorged with excess white cells resulting from overproduction.

There is an increasing number of therapeutic agents which are helpful. X-ray irradiation is the time-honoured method of reducing the enlarged spleen and in most cases is still the best initial treatment, though it is possible that early removal of the spleen may be helpful. Along with reduction in the size of the spleen there is a diminution in the production of cells from the bone marrow. At times, a remission which will last months, and even as long as three years may be induced by direct irradiation over the spleen.

New chemotherapeutic agents are finding a place in the treatment of this disease as in the other leukaemic states. Some are more effective in one type of leukaemia than in another, and at different times in the same patient. Duration of control with the usual agents ranges from two to seven years, rarely longer. It is, however, the continuing medical advice of the haematologist which must be followed if maximum benefit is to be obtained for the patient during the prolonged course of this chronic disease. Unlike chronic lymphocytic leukaemia, which seldom, if ever, changes to more acute forms, chronic granulocytic leukaemia characteristically evolves sooner or later into the subacute or acute myeloblastic phase (proliferation of cells from which the myelocytes develop). It is not certain why this change in the maturation of the cells occurs, but when it does occur in the blood, reflecting a sudden bone marrow predominance of myeloblasts, there is usually a change for the worse in the condition of the patient. A reversal of the previously high platelet level causes spontaneous bleeding, secondary infections reflect the marked immaturity of the granulocytes, fever and malaise develop, and the patient for the first time feels ill. This phase usually ends fatally. Its treatment requires a prompt change in medication. Combinations of four or more cytotoxic drugs is the standard treatment at present. Transplantation of normal bone marrow from a brother or sister after whole body irradiation of the patient has been tried, but this form of treatment is still experimental and its value has yet to be proved.

This field of therapy is changing so rapidly that no published volume can keep up with the speed of development of new and better agents. The family doctor will seek the best current advice in centres of haematological specialization. This will give assurance that every possible therapeutic measure will be made available to the patient as soon as it is approved for clinical use. Approximately 85 per cent of patients developing this disturbance begin with chronic cellular changes, and therefore may be assured months and years of normal activity. Some types of leukaemia are particularly susceptible to infection and require nursing with particular care, usually in specialized units.

Other varieties of chronic leukaemia include the rare chronic monocytic leukaemia and the so-called erythroleukaemia. In the latter the abnormality appears to be in the red cell precursors during the chronic phase but often the disease finishes with an acute leukaemia. Treatment of these rarer types of leukaemia and of the preleukaemia states is mainly supportive – that is correction of anaemia and bleeding by transfusion and early treatment of infections with antibiotics.

Acute leukaemias   The acute leukaemias were so called because of their rapidly fatal course in the untreated state. There are two main types, acute lymphoblastic leukaemia which affects mainly children, and acute myeloblastic leukaemia which affects older children and adults. There are other varieties of acute leukaemia and as more work is carried out to identify the cell type involved, so the classification of acute leukaemia becomes more complex. The manifestations of all types of acute leukaemia tend to be similar and the symptoms are due to lack of red cells, white cells, and platelets. Fatigue, infections,

Chapter 4 Blood and blood-forming organs

and haemorrhage may be the first signs of the disease, either singly or in combination. It will be appreciated from what has already been said that these factors are not specific for leukaemia but may occur in a variety of blood diseases. In the blood of patients with leukaemia are found the telltale primitive cells. From their appearance it may be possible to identify the cell type involved but frequently other tests are needed. It is important to identify the type of leukaemia because treatment of each type is different.

The treatment of acute lymphoblastic leukaemia in childhood has been revolutionized in the past ten years so that some doctors now speak guardedly of cure. Untreated children with acute leukaemia die in four to eight weeks. The main basis of treatment of all types of acute leukaemia is the destruction of the malignant cells by drugs given in intermittent doses so that normal bone marrow cells have the chance to recover between courses. With acute lymphoblastic leukaemia, the drugs used are vincristine and prednisone. With this combination of drugs about 90 per cent of the children enter what is called remission, that is disappearance of the abnormal cells from the blood and the bone marrow, and a return to normal health. Formerly leukaemia was likely to relapse, partly because leukaemic cells remained in the central nervous system where they were protected from the effects of the drugs by the so-called blood-brain barrier. Modern treatment overcomes this barrier by the use of radiotherapy to the brain and spinal cord which destroys the dividing leukaemic cells but spares the brain cells. The treatment with cytotoxic drugs is continued for two years and during this time the child is subjected to repeated bone marrow examinations and lumbar punctures to examine the fluid which bathes the nervous system. Even with the greatest care and understanding it is a harrowing time for children and parents. Nevertheless, the ordeal is well worthwhile, for now some 50 per cent of the children enter a remission which lasts five years or more without relapse.

The treatment of acute myeloblastic leukaemia is less satisfactory. The drugs used to produce remission are more toxic and have more unpleasant side effects than those used in the acute lymphoblastic type. About three quarters of the patients obtain a remission, often short-lived. Some new hope is offered by the use of bone marrow transplantation, but this is still in the development phase and no one yet knows whether it will be of lasting use in this disease.

The lymphomas The lymphomas are a group of malignant diseases which affect the lymphatic system – the lymphocytes, the lymph nodes, and the patches of lymphoid tissue throughout the body. Twenty years ago the treatment of these malignancies was very unsatisfactory though some relief of symptoms could be achieved with radiotherapy. Since then, the introduction of more powerful and diverse chemotherapeutic agents together with improved radiotherapy has greatly increased the success of treatment. These improved therapeutic measures have in turn led to a greater understanding of the different types of lymphoma, since accurate diagnosis is now important rather than just interesting. The classifications of the lymphomata are many and varied, and tend to produce confusion rather than clarity. From the viewpoint of treatment there are two groups – one is Hodgkin's disease, the other comprises the rest. The reason for this is that the treatment of Hodgkin's disease, once an almost invariably fatal disorder, is now established in principle and successful in practice whereas the treatment of the other lymphomas is uncertain.

Hodgkin's disease This disease, named after the English doctor Thomas Hodgkin who described it in 1832, is a disorder about which many facts are now known but the origin of which is unknown. It is only recently that it has been universally accepted that Hodgkin's disease is malignant but it is still not clear which are the malignant cells. The disease, as Hodgkin recognized, starts in a group of lymph nodes, often in the neck, and then spreads to involve other nodes, the spleen, and eventually organs other than those of the lymphatic system. The lymph nodes are replaced by abnormal tissue which consists basically of two types of cell, lymphocytes and large cells, called Reed-Sternberg cells after the two people who first described them in detail. Possibly the latter cells are the malignant cells and the lymphocytes represent the body's reaction to them. Certainly there is considerable variation between cases in the number of lymphocytes in proportion to the Reed-Sternberg cells and in the amount of scar tissue present. The microscopic appearances bear some relationship to the degree of malignancy of the disease.

Doctors divide Hodgkin's disease into four stages. In stage one a single group of nodes is involved. In stage two adjacent groups are involved but the disease is present above or below the waist only, and not on both sides. In stage three there is universal involvement of lymphoid tissue, but only in stage four are organs other than the lymphoid system involved. In addition, the various stages of the disease are classified A or B depending on whether generalized symptoms, such as fever, sweating, or pain are present – (B), or not, (A). The stage is important since the treatment is different. This usually means that patients with Hodgkin's disease are subjected to an operation to remove the spleen and a small piece of liver for microscopic examination. In addition, X-rays are carried out following injection of a dye into the lymphatic vessels in the foot. The dye is then carried up the lymphatic vessels, through the lymph nodes and eventually into the thoracic duct in the chest. It outlines the lymph glands as it goes so that their size and texture can be evaluated.

The treatment is, on the whole, successful. Over 95 per cent of stage one disease is curable, and even in stage four over half the patients are alive and apparently well five years after diagnosis.

The many other types of lymphoma vary considerably in their malignancy and their distribution in the body. The characterization of each type depends upon differences in the cell type involved, its surface and functional properties, the speed with which the cells are dividing and the pattern of the malignant cells within the blood, lymphoid tissue, and other organs. With this information, which may be obtained only by careful investigation, it may be possible to offer a diagnosis and prognosis, that is, the outlook, in an individual case. Treatment will depend upon these findings, varying from no treatment, only observation in those types known to be very benign, to vigorous treatment with multiple drugs, or radiotherapy, or both in the more malignant varieties. The advances made in the therapy of these disorders are not as great as those in Hodgkin's disease but are none the less important.

Diseases of abnormal proteins (paraproteinaemias)

In certain diseases, the multiplication of lymphocytes and the production of antibodies become deranged and a variety of disorders, from malignant to relatively benign, result. The hallmark of these diseases is the presence of an abnormal amount of a single type of protein in the blood – the paraprotein – which may be relatively simply identified.

Multiple myeloma (or myelomatosis) is the most common and most malignant of these disorders though even here the course of the disease is long. The symptoms and signs develop because of the proliferation and infiltration of the plasma cells themselves and because of the presence of an abnormal protein. The proliferation of plasma cells occurs mainly in the bone marrow with erosion of surrounding bone. This produces pain and weakness with spontaneous fractures. The calcium released from the bone is excreted by the kidneys but the excessive load may seriously damage these organs and produce kidney failure. Thirst and frequency of urination occur before this phase. Infiltration of the marrow space leads to anaemia, a low platelet count, and low white cell count with the attendant risks of bleeding and infection. Other organs may be infiltrated, or large masses of plasma cells (plasmacytomas) may develop. The excessive protein may damage the kidneys, alter the function of platelets and cause bleeding, increase the viscosity of the blood so that a feeling of heaviness and fatigue develop, or may be associated with the deposition of a curious substance, amyloid, in many organs. The diagnosis is made on the basis of bone marrow examination, the detection of the abnormal protein in the blood and its product, Bence Jones protein, in the urine. This protein is named after its discoverer Dr Henry Bence Jones (1847). It is now clear that this disease is a slowly progressive disorder and that the production of abnormal protein may have been present for many years before symptoms develop. Only the symptoms of the disease need be treated, not the protein itself. Once symptoms develop, treatment depends upon the nature and distribution of the lesions. Localized lesions which produce pain may be treated with radiotherapy. The proliferation of the plasma cells is arrested by the use of cytotoxic drugs. These drugs are derivatives of the First World War chemical weapon, mustard gas. The original gas, sulphur mustard, caused blistering of the skin and red eyes but severe overexposure caused bone marrow and lymphoid failure. These observations led doctors during the Second World War to look at the effect of derivatives of this gas, which were again being developed for military purposes, on malignant lymphomas. This was the birth of modern cytotoxic therapy.

Treatment of myeloma is moderately effective in controlling the disease for a while but almost inevitably after a period of months or years symptoms return and lead inevitably to death.

Waldenström's macroglobulinaemia is a more benign condition affecting older people. It is named after its discoverer, a Swedish physician and biochemist, who described the presence of a large protein molecule in the plasma of patients who complained of headache, heaviness, fatigue, and other symptoms of increased blood viscosity. In the bone marrow is found a mixed proliferation of lymphocytes and plasma cells but symptoms arise only from the effects of the protein, not from the proliferation of cells. The condition is very slowly progressive. Treatment used to be with cytotoxic drugs but the results were disappointing. Now it is possible to remove large quantities of plasma from patients and replace it with normal plasma – virtually to cleanse the blood. This may be achieved by centrifuging the blood so that plasma and cells separate, removing the plasma and replacing it with normal plasma, and then reinfusing it back to the patient. Modern machines allow this to be done as a continuous procedure so that patients with macro-globulinaemia can be treated rapidly and efficiently.

Bone marrow failure

Bone marrow failure is a general term given to a variety of disorders in which there is a failure by the bone marrow to produce mature cells for the circulation. The most extreme example of these disorders is aplastic anaemia. In this disease there appears to be a destruction or functional abnormality of the stem cells so that they fail to produce any mature cells. The condition may follow exposure of susceptible persons to drugs which normally have no harmful effects, it may follow exposure to industrial poisons, virus infections, particularly hepatitis, and is the inevitable consequence of an overdose of radiation or cytotoxic drugs. The symptoms produced are those caused by the lack of cells – a great increase in infection, bleeding, and anaemia. Nearly all patients with severe aplastic anaemia die despite modern treatment.

Bone marrow transplantation Many attempts were made to replace the destroyed bone marrow by normal bone marrow but none was successful before the work of Donnall Thomas and his associates in Seattle in 1969 showed that bone marrow transplantation could be made to work. The reasons for the failure of earlier attempts were many. It was not possible to match the marrow between donor and recipient accurately, and control of rejection was poor. The support procedures, antibiotics, trans-fusions, and so on were not all available. The Seattle doctors appreciated these difficulties and contri-buted, through experimental work, to their solution. The technique of marrow transplantation is relatively simple. Marrow is aspirated from the hip bone and other sites rich in marrow of the donor, processed so that there are no clumps of cells present and then infused into a vein of the recipient. The marrow cells lodge in various organs, including the bone marrow, and those in a suitable environment will grow. The main difficulties lie in keeping the patient alive long

enough for this to happen and preparing the recipient to accept the graft. Large doses of cytotoxic or immunosuppressive drugs have to be used to achieve the latter end and these have severe toxic effects on the patient. Strict isolation facilities, the facility to give white cell transfusions as well as red cells and platelets must all be provided. Even when the marrow has repopulated the blood with mature cells, troubles are not over. It is inevitable that cells concerned with immunity are transferred from the donor to the recipient and that these cells may react in an attempt to reject the recipient. This produces a reaction called "graft versus host disease" which itself may destroy the graft and lead to death of the patient. Despite all these troubles it is possible to establish successful grafts in about half the patients with severe aplastic anaemia – an enormous advance on a previously hopeless situation.

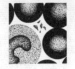

Chapter 5

The skin

Revised by H. R. Vickers, MA MSc MD FRCP

The skin is one of the most important organs of the body. It consists of two layers, the epidermis and dermis. The outermost, the epidermis, consists of living and dead cells, those in its deepest layer are constantly dividing and these new cells are pushed towards the surface. On this journey they gradually alter in nature and, at the surface, die, giving the outer protective layer of the skin, which is composed of keratin. This layer of dead cells varies greatly in thickness on different parts of the body, being thickest on the palms and soles where protection from pressure is of paramount importance, and thinnest on the areas where rapid fine movement is necessary, such as the eyelids and lips. The dead cells on the surface are constantly being shed and the process of keratin formation from the deepest layer takes about twenty-eight days.

Dipping down into the dermis are the specialized appendages of the skin, the sweat glands and the hair follicles into which open the sebaceous glands secreting grease. In the dermis are the blood vessels supplying nourishment to the keratin factory of the epidermis and these also, by regulation of the flow of blood through the skin, play an important role in the regulation of the body temperature. The nerve endings by which we receive all different types of sensation are present in the dermis, and the whole is filled with the supporting structures of collagen and elastin. The colour of the white-skinned races is influenced by the redness of the blood vessels shining through the epidermis. In dark-skinned races the colour is due to melanin pumped out by melanocytes situated among the cells in the deepest layer of the epidermis. The number of melanocytes is roughly the same in all races, but those in the dark-skinned are much more efficient producers of melanin.

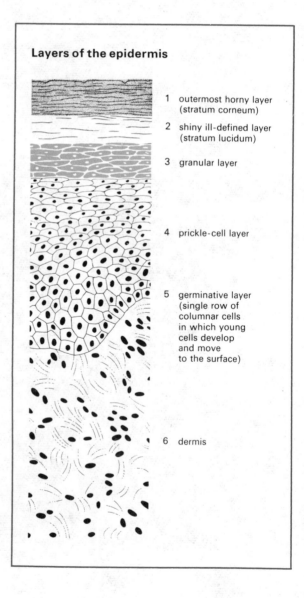

Layers of the epidermis

1 outermost horny layer (stratum corneum)

2 shiny ill-defined layer (stratum lucidum)

3 granular layer

4 prickle-cell layer

5 germinative layer (single row of columnar cells in which young cells develop and move to the surface)

6 dermis

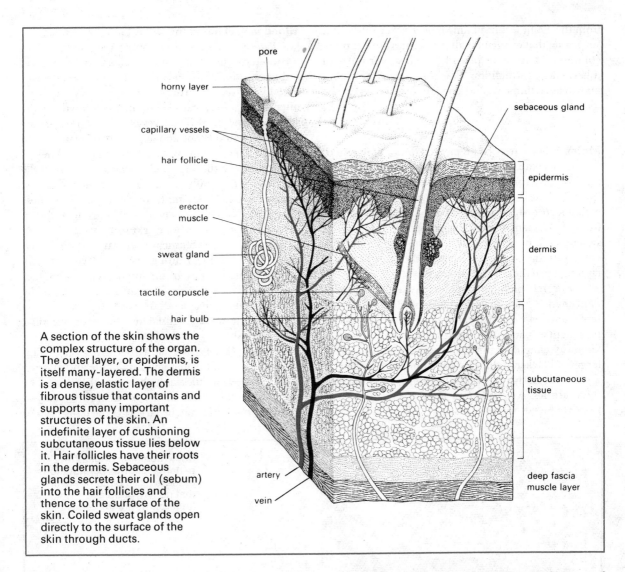

pore

horny layer

capillary vessels

hair follicle

erector muscle

sweat gland

tactile corpuscle

hair bulb

sebaceous gland

epidermis

dermis

subcutaneous tissue

artery

vein

deep fascia muscle layer

A section of the skin shows the complex structure of the organ. The outer layer, or epidermis, is itself many-layered. The dermis is a dense, elastic layer of fibrous tissue that contains and supports many important structures of the skin. An indefinite layer of cushioning subcutaneous tissue lies below it. Hair follicles have their roots in the dermis. Sebaceous glands secrete their oil (sebum) into the hair follicles and thence to the surface of the skin. Coiled sweat glands open directly to the surface of the skin through ducts.

Functions

The three main functions of the skin are protection, temperature control, and sexual attraction.

Protection The methods by which this is achieved are pain, so that we withdraw rapidly from destructive agents such as heat; the protective layer of keratin; the grease film on the surface of the skin helping to keep us waterproof; protection from noxious bacteria; and pigment which protects us from the harmful effects of sunlight.

Body temperature This is controlled largely by regulation of the blood flow through the skin, by constriction or dilatation of the blood vessels. If the body is getting overheated sweat is poured onto the surface and the evaporation of this cools the skin.

Sexual attraction The skin plays a great part in all sexual attraction, and it is on this that the fortunes of the cosmetic industry are founded.

Disorders of the skin

These can be considered in distinct groups: congenital malformations, abnormal function, the reaction of the skin to noxious agents, diseases peculiar to the skin whose cause is at present unknown, neoplasms (new growths) benign and malignant, the involvement of the skin in internal disease, emotion and the skin, and the hair and nails.

Congenital malformations

When one considers the extraordinarily complex processes taking place in the development of a baby

119

from the ovum fertilized nine months previously, it is surprising that congenital abnormalities are not more common. The skin provides many varieties of inherited abnormalities. The commonest are often known as birthmarks, and small or large moles can be found in most people.

Moles   These may be pigmented or nonpigmented, may be accompanied by a growth of coarse hair, and may be very small or cover large areas of the body surface. They arise from the cells forming the melanocytes which migrate early in embryonic life from the region of the developing central nervous system to disperse eventually at the junction of the epidermis and dermis. If some of these cells remain clumped together, the result is a mole.

Very rarely pigmented moles may undergo malignant change. Such change is particularly rare in hairy moles and before puberty, but medical advice should be sought for any pigmented nonhairy mole which alters its character in any way, such as becoming larger or blacker, itching, or becoming surrounded by a red halo. Early removal is life-saving and although there are less serious causes for these changes, it is better to be safe than sorry.

Blood vessel naevi (naevus is Latin for "mole")

Capillary haemangioma (port-wine stain)   Unfortunately this type often occurs on the face, although other parts of the body may be affected. The livid reddish purple patch is present at or soon after birth and is caused by an overgrowth of the smallest superficial blood vessels (capillaries) in the skin. The cause is not known, but it is certainly not due to maternal injury during pregnancy. A few – particularly on the nape of the neck and centre of the forehead – gradually fade, but the majority persist throughout life. Attempts made to destroy these superficial blood vessels usually result only in destroying the overlying skin as well, leaving unsightly scarring. Surgical removal of the affected area, followed by grafting, is again cosmetically unacceptable because of the impossibility of matching facial skin with skin from any other part of the body. Fortunately, modern cosmetic camouflage techniques now offer satisfactory methods of hiding these blemishes.

Cavernous haemangioma (strawberry naevus)   This is usually seen in the first few days of life and appears as raised red nodules anywhere on the skin. The majority are not more than two inches (five cm) in diameter but some may be larger. If the baby cries or

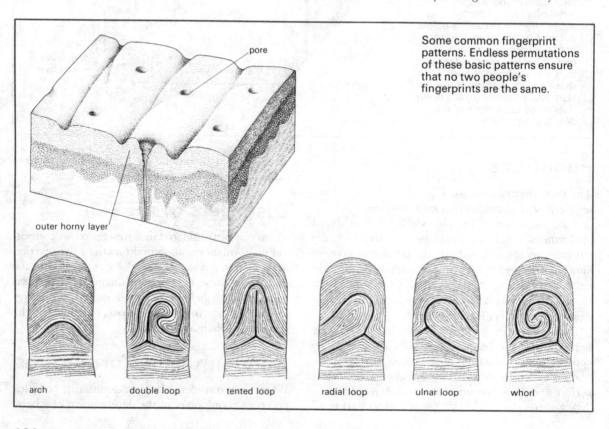

pore

outer horny layer

Some common fingerprint patterns. Endless permutations of these basic patterns ensure that no two people's fingerprints are the same.

arch   double loop   tented loop   radial loop   ulnar loop   whorl

strains, the mark increases in size, and if squeezed, the blood can be emptied out only to fill when the pressure is released. This type of birthmark consists of blood-filled spaces which are probably due to a delay in the normal formation of the blood vessels. The naevus often increases in size for the first twelve months of life and then slowly clears up over the course of the next few years. Treatment, which may result in scarring, is therefore unnecessary unless the naevus is situated on the eyelids or interferes with sucking.

Spider naevi   These little abnormalities of the blood vessels are not true naevi and can appear at any age. They appear as small red spots – the body of the spider – from which small capillaries may be seen to radiate. They may be numerous in pregnancy and are also associated with liver disease. They never disappear spontaneously, but are easily cured by cauterization of the central blood vessel. Since these are small arterioles, damage can result in brisk bleeding which can be easily controlled by pressure.

Atopic eczema (infantile eczema: the asthma-eczema syndrome)   In most books this distressing condition is usually considered in the section on dermatitis, but these two conditions are quite

different. The tendency to atopic eczema is inherited and it is now known that these patients have abnormalities in immunological reactions. The eczema usually occurs between the third and sixth month of life. The face is first affected, as a rule, and the rash then spreads to most of the body. This is accompanied by intense irritation, and the consequent rubbing and scratching damages the skin reddened by the eczema, often resulting in bleeding and secondary infection. The babies are restless, often thin, and do not sleep well. The natural course of the condition is to persist up to the age of two or three years when it may completely subside, although some cases show thickened irritable areas of skin around the neck, behind the knees, and in front of the elbows. A proportion of these patients also suffer from asthma.

It was formerly thought that the cause of the condition was allergy to a particular food, and this supposition was based on skin testing. Unfortunately, withholding the supposedly provocative food did not result in cure, and a much more reasonable explanation is that these patients inherit a very reactive skin which breaks down when exposed to irritants. Because of this hyperreactive skin, false positive reactions to skin testing are produced.

Modern treatment consists of control of any

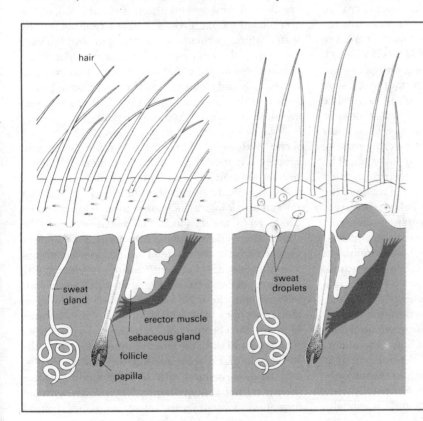

Each hair has a very small muscle attached near its root. Cold and fear make the muscles contract, the hairs stand on end, and the skin surrounding them rise in small bumps (gooseflesh).

infection of the skin by cleanliness and antibiotics, the control of the inflammatory reaction by corticosteroid preparations, the avoidance of irritants in the surroundings, and the use of such well-tried preparations as tar products on the skin, together with sedation when necessary. These measures have made a great difference to control of the condition. Parents are understandably anxious about their baby's affliction, and the problem of management must be explained carefully. Even though the rash should clear in the first few years of life it must be remembered that these patients will always have an overreactive skin and so should avoid entering any occupation where they are likely to come into contact with skin irritants, such as nursing, hairdressing, engineering, building, and medicine. This is one of the conditions in which vaccination against smallpox is contraindicated since the skin has no inborn immunity to the vaccine.

Psoriasis This common condition is not usually included under the heading of congenital abnormalities, but all the evidence points towards the view that the tendency to psoriasis is inherited and that the disease process can be started by many stimuli. Once the condition has been established by such a trigger, it persists even when the provoking stimulus has ceased. Psoriasis occurs in about two per cent of the population in the United Kingdom. There are marked racial differences in its incidence. Although children can be affected, the disease is unusual before puberty. After puberty it may appear for the first time at any age – even in advanced old age. The characteristic lesions are well-defined reddened scaling plaques, which may vary in size from a few millimetres in diameter to patches covering most of the body surface. They usually do not itch. The principal sites are the knees and elbows. Scaling plaques may occur on the scalp, but fortunately the face is usually spared. The nails may also be involved.

The problem with psoriasis is very largely cosmetic. The condition itself is not associated with any internal disease although chronic arthritis is more common in psoriasis sufferers. In spite of a great deal of research, the cause is not known. What is known is that the rate of turnover of the epidermal cells is greatly increased, the time taken for cells to pass from the basal layer to the surface being as little as six days, compared with twenty-eight days in normal skin. Since the abnormality in psoriasis is genetically determined, it is impossible to promise cure, although in the majority of patients the condition can be successfully controlled by various local applications and occasionally by internal treatment in severe cases. This may have serious side effects and so is given only under strict medical supervision. The recent introduction of so-called black light, ultraviolet light of a particular wavelength, is still under evaluation but the results seem to be favourable and if easily accessible treatment centres can be established to treat patients without interfering with their work this would be of enormous benefit to many unfortunate sufferers. The condition is not infectious.

Abnormal function

This group of diseases arises from some alteration in the functioning of parts of the skin.

Ichthyosis This is a common condition in which the skin is abnormally dry. The usual variety is inherited as a dominant trait, and the dryness is most marked on the legs, diminishing progressively towards the head. In severe cases the skin is thickened, looks dirty, and gives the appearance of crocodile or fish skin, from which the disease derives its name. The skin on the front of the elbows and back of the knees (the flexures) is often unaffected, which distinguishes ichthyosis from atopic eczema. The condition is due essentially to a diminution of the secretion of sebum (grease), and as a result of this the water which normally keeps the skin supple evaporates from the surface cells. Treatment is designed to conserve what little natural grease there is, and various oils and creams help. The condition improves in hot weather, possibly from the beneficial action of sweat, which helps to hydrate the skin.

Acne vulgaris This very common condition arouses an enormous amount of mental anguish because it occurs at puberty just when the sufferer is becoming aware of the opposite sex. It is due to a normal physiological increase in the amount of sebum produced by the sebaceous glands responding to the stimulation of the hormones responsible for establishing the mature adult state. This increased sebaceous secretion occurs in every normally developing teenager. The sebaceous glands open into hair follicles, and where the follicles are very small – as on the face, upper back, and chest – they may become blocked. Each blocked follicle appears as a blackhead (comedo) and since the sebum cannot escape onto the surface, the gland becomes distended ("whitehead"), and then may burst into the surrounding tissues producing an irritant inflammatory reaction with pus formation. Sometimes the sebaceous glands, instead of bursting, become very distended and appear as unsightly swellings. Whether or not a boy or girl develops acne in adolescence therefore depends on the reactivity of the sebaceous gland to normal hormone secretion, and the size of the openings on the skin. Both these factors tend to be inherited characteristics. When full maturity is established the stimulus to the sebaceous gland diminishes, and so the often-stated comfort that the condition will eventually subside is true.

However, this is of very little solace to the sufferer, who may bear ugly scars later. Treatment is designed to remove the blockage from the mouth of the glandular opening and to diminish sebaceous activity.

The first is achieved by hot soaking, washing with soap and water, the use of degreasing lotions and the applications of different lotions and ointments, all of which have a drying, desquamating (descaling) action. In addition, small doses of the tetracycline group of drugs taken by mouth on an empty stomach

blackhead

Occasionally the opening of a sebaceous gland becomes blocked by a plug of hard sebum. This often becomes black on contact with air – a blackhead.

over a long period of time have a beneficial action, the mechanism of which is not fully understood. It is probably a biochemical as opposed to an antibiotic action. The small doses used have been shown to be harmless, even though taken for many months. The only contraindication is in early pregnancy when the drug may cause yellow discoloration of the developing baby's teeth. Fresh air and sunshine undoubtedly help, and it was shown in vitamin C deprivation experiments during the Second World War that shortage of vitamin C aggravates the acne tendency. Chocolate seems to contain a factor which stimulates sebaceous activity and should be avoided, but other foods seem to have little activity in this respect. Severe residual scarring can be greatly relieved by surgical treatment, but only when all activity has ceased.

Chilblains are red, swollen, itching, or painful swellings, usually on the hands and feet. In severe cases the skin may become ulcerated. This common and annoying complaint is caused by the action of cold on the skin. Prevention is to keep warm by means of adequate clothing and a warm house. Calcium is of no value and any drugs given to increase blood flow, if given in effective doses, have undesirable side effects produced by depriving other organs of blood.

Varicose eczema and ulceration This unpleasant condition is caused by a breakdown in the function of the veins in the leg. Venous blood, which has delivered its oxygen content and nutrient factors to nourish the lower extremity, is pumped back to the heart and so to the lungs, largely by the compression action of the muscles surrounding the veins. Valves in the veins prevent the blood from flowing back, but if these are inefficient and the veins dilate, used blood accumulates in the tissues. The skin is then not adequately nourished and breaks down to give red weeping areas of varicose eczema. Any small injury produces breaks in the skin surface, resulting in ulceration. Cure depends on restoring the circulation. This can be achieved by firm supporting bandages preventing dilatation of the veins and, in severe cases, by surgical treatment of the inefficient veins. See page 94.

Reaction to noxious agents

Under this heading are considered the reactions of the skin to harmful agents encountered in the environment, including irritants, infection, and insects.

123

Chapter 5 The skin

Dermatitis This is the word used to describe a very well-defined reaction in the skin produced by external agents. The stages seen are redness, often accompanied by irritation, vesicle (small blister) formation, weeping of the surface, then healing.

There are two main varieties of dermatitis. Firstly, contact irritant dermatitis which will occur whenever the normal skin comes into contact with an irritant. The commonest example of this is seen on the hands of women who come into contact with strong cleansing agents; secondly, contact sensitization dermatitis which occurs only in a patient who has become specifically sensitized (allergic) to a particular substance which nonsensitized people can handle with impunity. The establishment of this state of sensitivity is governed by several factors, the most important of which is previous contact with the sensitizing substance. Thus a keen gardener may handle the *Primula obconica* for years and then suddenly develop severe dermatitis every time he comes into contact with the plant. This sudden change is often difficult for the patient to understand.

Many substances are potential sensitizers, but all have the power of combining with the proteins in the skin. Trying to find the cause requires the skills of a detective. The area of the skin affected often provides the first clue, for example, lips affected by lipstick, earlobes by earrings, and so on. The range is very wide – cosmetics, chemicals used in the rubber industry, dyes, metals such as nickel and chrome, ointments, plants, including weeds, adhesives, cement, match heads. Once sensitivity is established, the whole of the skin is reactive, not only that part originally in contact with the sensitizer, and this fact is utilized in patch testing. The substance under suspicion is applied to the apparently unaffected skin in concentrations which would not affect a normal person, and left on for 48 hours. If the patient is sensitized to this substance, the skin in contact with the patch test will develop dermatitis. Cure of the patient depends on avoiding the causative agent in his environment because unfortunately, with the great majority of sensitizing substances, desensitization is impossible. Treatment includes: avoiding contact with the cause, soothing lotion applied frequently during the acute phase, steroid-containing preparations to reduce inflammatory reaction, and bland cream to hasten the return of the skin to normal.

Infection The skin is normally covered with harmless organisms, but comes into contact with germs of many types. The natural powers of self-sterilization are well-developed in normal healthy skin. Invasion takes place when the skin surface is damaged or when the general resistance of the patient is lowered.

Erysipelas This is caused by the invasion of the skin by a particular type of streptococcus. The organism usually gains access by way of a crack in the skin such as can occur around the nose, the corners of the mouth, or the ears. The patient feels ill, has a high temperature, and often has a shivering attack (rigor). The affected skin is reddened and raised with a well-defined edge. The condition responds quickly to antibiotics.

Folliculitis, boils, and carbuncles Staphylococci normally invade the skin through a hair follicle. If the infection is superficial, a little septic spot – a pustule – is seen, often with the hair sticking up through the middle of the pus. If the infection is deeper there is much more inflammation and the result is a boil. If several adjacent hair follicles are affected, this produces a carbuncle, a large boil with several discharging openings.

Staphylococci gain access only when the natural resistance of the skin to infection is lowered, and cure of recurrent boils depends not only on eliminating the infection, but also on restoring the natural resistance of the skin. This lowering may be caused by internal diseases such as diabetes or leukaemia, but in the majority of cases patients harbour reservoirs of staphylococcal infection, sometimes in the nose and also in cracks in the perianal region. These patients, when asked, will often admit to chronic irritation in that area (pruritus ani).

The staphylococcal infection is treated with the appropriate antibiotic and, at the same time, application of a local antiseptic to the affected area. The organisms which are present on the whole of the skin surface should be dealt with by antiseptic baths or generalized ultraviolet light. In very resistant cases it is possible that a member of the family may be a staphylococcal carrier.

Impetigo This common condition is one of the few contagious skin diseases. It is usually seen in children and appears as well-defined crusts which look as though they are stuck onto the skin. The earliest change seen in the skin is slight redness, followed by small blisters which burst in a matter of hours giving a discharge which coagulates on the skin, forming a golden crust. Staphylococci can usually be grown from these lesions which respond quickly to the local application of an appropriate antibiotic. Unfortunately many skin conditions are now treated with powerful corticosteroid ointments which reduce the inflammatory reaction of the skin. This interference with the natural defence mechanism controlling the infection allows the lesion to spread. As a result, impetigo has now assumed many weird and wonderful patterns. Impetigo may also occur as a secondary infection on any irritating skin condition such as scabies, lice infestation, and atopic eczma. Such conditions, when present, must also be treated.

Lupus vulgaris As the name implies, this used to be very common, but with the increasing control of tuberculosis, this manifestation of infection of the skin with the tubercle bacillus is becoming less common; in the United Kingdom it is seen in Asian immigrants.

Lupus vulgaris usually attacks the exposed skin and appears as a very slowly growing nonitching coppery red patch. If left untreated, over the course of years it slowly extends, causing scarring of the skin. It is cured quickly by antituberculosis drugs, but when diagnosed it is important that all members of the family and close contacts should be examined for evidence of internal tuberculosis which might have been the source of infection in the patient.

Leprosy This disease is still common in certain parts of the world, but no new cases have been reported for decades in people born and living in the United Kingdom. However, there are people who have lived in countries where leprosy is common in whom the disease appears for the first time in this country. The manifestations often occur in the skin and the clinical picture is determined by the degree of immunity of the patient to the disease. If immunity is low, the disease appears as lepromatous leprosy, in which nodules laden with bacilli appear in the skin. If immunity is high, the variety of leprosy is tuberculoid, and in this presentation it is difficult to find any bacilli except in the nerve trunks. These patients are found to have areas of skin in which there is loss of sensation, although involvement of the nerves occurs in all varieties of leprosy since the bacilli have a predilection for nerve trunks. This gives rise to muscle weakness, contractures, and skin damage as a result of loss of sensation.

Modern treatment controls the disease well and there is no need to segregate these patients on the grounds of infectivity.

Virus diseases Most people become only too aware of the impact of virus infection on their skin in childhood, when they are suffering from measles and chickenpox (see chapter 2).

Warts (verrucae) are probably the commonest of the virus diseases affecting the skin, and can be most annoying. The wart virus, although visible in the lesions when examined by the electron microscope, has not yet been grown in a culture.

The areas commonly affected are the hands (verruca vulgaris), the soles of the feet (verruca plantaris), the cleft of the buttocks and genitals (condyloma accuminata), and the face (verruca plana). It is probable that the same virus is responsible for each of these, the appearance of the lesions depending on the site involved. On the sole of the foot and palm of the hand, the wart is pushed into the surrounding skin by pressure and this is largely responsible for the pain. Warts around the fingernails are particularly prone to occur in nail biters.

Warts have been known for hundreds of years, and folklore is full of infallible cures. All of these have two features in common, the performance of some unusual act – such as burying meat in the garden – and a time interval of about three weeks. Many warts disappear after charming although it is difficult to understand the mechanism of such cures. Whether it is psychological or merely coincidental is not clear. More resistant cases are treated either with destructive preparations, such as salicylic and lactic acids, or destroyed by freezing or electric cautery, or removed by curetting under local anaesthesia.

The infectivity of warts is difficult to assess. Not all children suffer from warts, and there is no point in stopping children with plantar warts (verrucas) from using public swimming baths if children with warts on the hands are not also excluded. Many more people die from drowning than from warts and children who happen to have plantar warts should also be taught to swim. Treatment may work quickly or the warts may be very resistant.

Herpes simplex (cold sores) This common malady can be extremely unpleasant. The lips are usually affected, although recurrent attacks may occur on other parts of the body, particularly the cheeks and genital area. The attack starts with a feeling of discomfort, in a few hours the area becomes red, and small blisters appear which burst to form a crust, sometimes difficult to distinguish clinically from impetigo. This crust lasts for about a week then separates, leaving slight redness which quickly fades. Recurrent attacks at the same site are the rule, so it is thought that the virus remains dormant after each attack, ready to be reactivated by such stimuli as rise of body temperature and bright sunlight. It is not easy to kill the virus, but local application of some of the newer antiviral agents will probably control each attack and may reduce the frequency of recurrence.

Herpes zoster (shingles) It is unfortunate that the word herpes occurs in the name of two different diseases since herpes simplex and herpes zoster are caused by two different viruses. Herpes simplex gives recurrent attacks throughout life, whereas it is extremely uncommon to have more than one attack of herpes zoster. Herpes simplex heals without any residual scar, but herpes zoster may leave deep scars and gives rise to a great deal of pain which may persist for months after the attack. Herpes zoster virus is the same as that causing chickenpox. It attacks one or more sensory nerves on one side of the body and this accounts for the unilateral distribution. Not infrequently the patient experiences quite severe pain in the affected area many hours before the eruption appears. This consists of small deeply situated blisters which then burst and dry into crusts which separate in ten to fourteen days. The most serious area to be involved is the eye since blisters occurring on the cornea may result in scarring and interference with vision. Very occasionally, if the general resistance of the body is lowered by serious internal disease, the herpes zoster may become widespread and this is probably the foundation of the old wives' tale that if the shingles meets in the middle the patient will die. Frequent local application of an antiviral agent in the early stages probably has a beneficial action on the course of the disease.

Fungus infections   Of the many fungi, only a few affect the skin. The most simple, *Candida albicans* (monilia), gives rise to thrush, and the others cause various varieties of ringworm. This descriptive name dates from very early times. The typical lesion on the skin appears as a well-defined ring which slowly expands like a "fairy ring" in a field as the fungus invades new areas of keratin in its search for food.

Thrush   The effects of this infection with *Candida albicans* are probably most easily recognized in the mouths of babies where it produces well-defined white plaques, but it also affects the nappy area of infants. The increased incidence in this age group may be due to the modern habit of enclosing nappies in plastic pants. The organism may invade at any age and the most common site of infection is the genital area in women. The patient experiences intense irritation and may be conscious of a creamy vaginal discharge. Skin folds in the groin, the cleft of the buttocks, and the area under the breasts are also frequently attacked, and diabetics are particularly vulnerable to such infection. The organism may also invade the nail folds.

Except in rare congenital deficiencies favouring the growth of the organism, thrush is of no dire significance and can usually be quickly brought under control by ointments or pessaries containing nystatin.

Pityriasis (tinea) versicolor   This low-grade fungus infection is commonly seen on the chest and back of young adults. In white-skinned races it causes slightly scaling non-itching yellowish brown plaques with an irregular margin which may cover large areas or consist of many isolated irregular patches. If the patient has been exposed to the sun, affected areas are paler than the surrounding normal sunburnt skin, and this is not entirely due to the screening action of the fungus because in pigmented races the disease appears as paler slightly scaling patches. The fungus is killed by fungicidal ointments, but probably the easiest way to clear up the condition is to paint the area once a week with selenium sulphide and wash it off after twelve hours. The scalp should also be shampooed with the substance. Four applications are usually sufficient, but reinfection is common – probably from contaminated clothing worn next to the skin, or possibly from organisms lurking in the hair follicles. Even after cure it takes time for the depigmented areas to attain the same colour as the surrounding normal skin.

Tinea pedis (athlete's foot)   This infection is very common and is easily acquired from infected scales of skin dropped on the floor of changing rooms and shower baths. The fungus lives in the damp softened skin between the toes, particularly in the space between the fourth and little toes. From there it may spread both onto the sole, causing small blisters, and onto the upper surface of the foot. It usually causes little trouble, but occasionally may give rise to blisters on the palms and between the fingers, particularly in hot weather. It may also damage the skin to enable invasion by more potentially harmful organisms. Cure is not easy and reinfection is common. The toes should always be dried carefully, communal bath mats and duckboards should be avoided whenever possible. Most patients are helped by the application of fungicidal ointments twice daily and these should be continued for at least a month after the condition has apparently healed. See later for Griseofulvin.

Tinea cruris (dhobi itch)   This is much more common in men and is often associated with infection of the feet. There is an itching reddened scaling patch on the inner aspect of the thigh, especially where it is in contact with the scrotum. This again responds quickly to a fungicidal ointment. If the condition is treated with corticosteroid preparations which suppress the inflammation only in order to ease the irritation, the organism is not eradicated but allowed to spread. When the ointment is stopped the irritation recurs, so it is reapplied, and if used repeatedly over a long period of time will damage the skin, causing degeneration of the collagen in the dermis and resulting in unsightly red streaks.

Tinea corporis (ringworm of the smooth skin) The round slightly scaling lesions with a well-defined spreading edge are the usual manifestations of ringworm, but it must be remembered that not all round scaling patches on the skin are ringworm, and again the pattern may be modified by inappropriate treatment. The usual sources of infection are animals, in the home or on the farm.

Tinea capitis (ringworm of the scalp) Several fungi invade the keratin of the hair, and ringworm of the scalp used to be common in children. The affected hairs are brittle and break off close to the scalp giving a round area of apparent baldness, but when the scalp is examined closely the presence of the short hairs distinguishes this from true baldness. This type of ringworm is caused by a particular variety of fungi of the microspora, or small-spored type, and these will not grow in the presence of adult sebum, so this disease occurs only in children. Diagnosis is made either by examining the affected hair microscopically or by making use of the fact that the affected hair, when examined in a darkened room by a specially filtered ultraviolet light (Wood's light), fluoresces with a brilliant green glow. This is a quick way of tracing contacts, isolating infected domestic pets, and also finding out when the patient is free from the disease.

The scalp may also be attacked at any age by other fungi, particularly those carried by cattle, giving rise to carbuncle-like lesions which are sometimes known as kerion. These may heal with a certain amount of scarring which is made worse if an unsuspecting surgeon incises the inflamed mass.

Tinea unguium (ringworm of the nails) The keratin of the nails may be attacked by fungi. The infection usually enters the nail at the free edge and spreads along the under surface of the nail, which becomes discoloured and brittle. One or more nails may be involved and are made unsightly. The condition has to be differentiated from other diseases of the nail, and one difficulty is that fungus may invade a nail previously damaged by some other condition, and cure of the fungus will then not necessarily restore the nail to normal.

Treatment of ringworm infection Although local fungicides should be applied to the skin, the whole outlook for patients suffering from this type of infection has been altered since the discovery of the drug Griseofulvin. The drug is taken by mouth and is eventually taken up by the skin. Many fungi are unable to invade keratin impregnated with Griseofulvin and although the drug does not kill the

fungus, as the keratin grows out, the fungus is shed. The time needed for cure is therefore dependent on the rate of keratin turnover. On the skin this is about 28 days, the fingernails six months, the toenails perhaps eighteen months to two years, and the hair several months, depending on how short it is cut. Griseofulvin has very few side effects. It is absorbed better if taken with a meal containing fat, but will not work in patients taking barbiturates. Although effective in the great majority of fungal diseases which affect the skin, it is of no value in the treatment of thrush or pityriasis versicolor.

Insects and mites Those causing most trouble are the acarus, lice, fleas, cheyletiella, and mosquitoes.

Scabies This common disease is caused by a minute mite which is just visible to the naked eye, acarus or *Sarcoptes scabiei*. The sufferer complains of severe irritation, which is usually worse at night. The typical signs are small superficial wavy lines sometimes up to one cm ($\frac{1}{2}$ in) in length, which mark the site of the burrows made by the fertilized female in the superficial layer of the skin as she pushes along laying

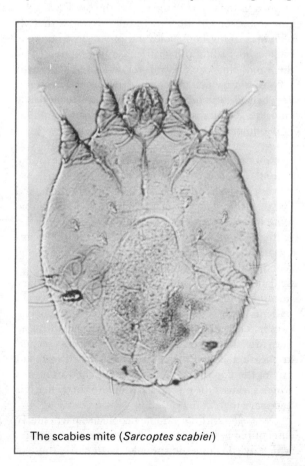

The scabies mite (*Sarcoptes scabiei*)

her eggs. She burrows in selected sites and these are, in descending order of preference, the skin between the fingers, the outer side of the hand, the inner surface of the wrist, the external genitals in men, the elbows, around the navel, the nipples, the front of the armpits, the buttocks, and in babies the feet. The face is never involved except in suckling infants. With skill and the aid of a lens, the doctor can remove the mite from the end of its burrow and give a demonstration to the patient of an active mite, which should ensure that the treatment is carried out thoroughly. Although the mites are present only at the sites mentioned above, the patient's body may be covered with irritating papules. These result from an allergic response provoked by the presence of the mites in the skin.

The eggs hatch into larvae which mature into active adults and the fertilized female again burrows into the skin, either of the patient or a close contact. Spreading is almost entirely the result of personal contact.

Cure is easy provided that two rules are observed. These are that the application prescribed must be applied to the whole of the skin of the body from the chin to the soles of the feet, and the second is that all members of the household and other close contacts such as boyfriends and girlfriends must be treated at the same time to prevent reinfestation. The two preparations which are effective when used properly are benzyl benzoate and gamma benzene hexachloride. Scabies is rarely contracted from clothing or bedding.

Lice There are three varieties which live in separate sites – the head, the body, and the pubic region. The last is sometimes called the crab louse because of its shape. Each can be seen with the naked eye, but the diagnosis of the head louse and pubic louse is usually made by finding the eggs (nits) on the hairs in the affected region. Body lice and their eggs live in the seams of undergarments. All lice live on the blood of their host and their activities cause a great deal of itching. Scratching gives rise to secondary infection, and lice must always be sought for in patients with severely crusted infected scalps. The eggs hatch in about eight days. Head lice and pubic lice are treated with malathion, and a second application should be used in seven to nine days to kill any of the lice which might have hatched from nits which survived the first application. For body lice it is necessary to treat the clothing.

Fleas and cheyletiella Some people are particularly susceptible to flea bites and bites from various mites which live on domestic animals, particularly those of the cheyletiella group. The patients have grouped itching papules, which may be made raw by scratching. Cure depends on getting rid of the infestation from the household pets by a good anti-flea powder and for complete effectiveness, this can also be sprinkled in bedding. This is one of the commonest causes of heat spots (papular urticaria) in children. It is not understood why some members of the family are affected whereas others escape.

Mosquitoes Some people react very severely to mosquitoes. In girls and young women, bites on the legs may result in large tight blisters which take several days to subside.

Diseases peculiar to the skin

There are several diseases, the cause of which is not known, which predominantly affect the skin. The commonest of these are lichen planus, pityriasis rosea, nettle rash, vitiligo, and granuloma annulare.

Lichen planus This is a fairly common condition which is worrying to the patient because it itches and often lasts for months. The characteristic rash consists of small flat-topped shiny pimples usually found on the front of the forearms and on the lower legs, although any part of the body, including the genital area, may be affected. Lichen planus is uncommon on the face, but in 50 per cent of patients, the inside of the mouth is involved, although the patient may be unaware of this. Occasionally, the condition is first noticed by the dentist.

The cause is unknown, although a period of stress may precede the eruption. The condition is not infectious and usually fades within a few months, although recurrence is not unknown.

Pityriasis rosea This is a harmless condition usually seen in young adults who are alarmed to find their trunk covered with a rash which may, or may not, itch. The individual lesions consist of well-defined oval macules, 1 to $2\frac{1}{2}$ cm ($\frac{1}{2}$ to 1 in) in diameter. Characteristically, the long axis of the lesion is situated along the line of the ribs. The generalized eruption may be preceded by a single larger lesion which is known as the herald patch. The condition usually occurs in spring and autumn and lasts about six weeks. The cause is unknown, although it behaves like a virus infection, second attacks being very uncommon. It does not affect a developing baby even though the mother may be affected in the early days of pregnancy. There is no treatment apart from soothing lotions such as calamine to ease any irritation, and the condition fades in six to eight weeks.

Nettle rash (urticaria) Most people have an attack of nettle rash during their lives, and the itching red weals of many different sizes and shapes are well-known. The lesions fluctuate in shape in the course of hours and may occasionally be accompanied by quite alarming swelling of the soft tissues (angioneurotic oedema). This is one of the commonest manifestations of so-called food poisoning. Usually the attack lasts only for a few days, but it may persist for months or years. Familiar causes are foods such as shellfish and strawberries, but often the cause is elusive and unfortunately skin testing is of no help. Investigation demands a careful and detailed history of the patient's condition, and clinical examination to eliminate external causes such as scabies and similar agents. Some patients produce an urticarial reaction when the skin is stroked (dermographism) or when exposed to heat or cold. In addition to foods, drugs sometimes produce nettle rash, the commonest being penicillin, aspirin, and tartrazine, the yellow colouring agent used in the covering of many tablets.

Several factors have been implicated, such as lingering infection, emotional upset, and hormonal change, and the management of nettle rash can be difficult. Most patients respond satisfactorily to antihistamine drugs given in adequate dosage. Different patients seem to be helped by different drugs, and all these must be given under medical supervision.

Vitiligo (leukoderma) This condition is characterized by well-defined, often bizarrely shaped areas of skin in which, for quite unknown reasons, the melanin cells stop producing pigment. In white-skinned races this may not be noticed until the skin is exposed to sun and the normal skin becomes sunburnt, making a striking contrast with the white areas. In pigmented races the piebald effect is very noticeable. The depigmented areas may become larger and more numerous with time, but occasionally they may diminish and finally disappear. There is no certain cure but some, particularly the pigmented races, respond to a combination of light to the skin and a drug, psoralene, by mouth. In the great majority cosmetic camouflage is the only treatment available.

Granuloma annulare These striking ringed lesions which usually arise on the back of the hands of children and young adults are often mistaken for warts, but the well-defined edge of the ring, sometimes up to two cm ($\frac{3}{4}$ in) in diameter, with a slight central depression, is very characteristic. The cause is unknown and is not associated with any internal disease. Lesions may occur on other areas of the body, particularly the feet, and may last for years. For some unknown reason, they may disappear if a small wedge is taken out of the edge for microscopical examination, and may respond to injection with a cortisone preparation. Apart from their appearance they are of no serious significance.

Neoplasms (growths)

Neoplasms of the skin are of two varieties, benign and malignant (cancerous).

Benign neoplasms There are many forms of benign growths which affect the skin but only the common ones will be considered here. All cause a certain amount of worry to patients, not only because of their appearance, but also because of the fear of malignancy, and reassurance is important.

Seborrhoeic warts These are the very common brown to black, slightly raised plaques often two to three cm ($\frac{3}{4}$ to 1 in) in diameter which usually occur on the trunk or scalp, first appearing in middle age and increasing in number until there may be scores of them. They are more common in some families, and are of no significance, but they may itch slightly and sometimes become infected. It is relatively easy to remove them by scraping under local anaesthesia or by freezing with liquid nitrogen, but there is no way to stop new ones from appearing. They are not infectious, are quite distinct from virus warts, and never undergo malignant change.

Campbell de Morgan spots This is the name given to the bright red, often slightly raised spots which occur on the trunk in middle age. They are of no significance.

Skin tags These are often thought to be warts by the patient and commonly occur on the neck and in the armpits, especially in plump women. They are small superficial tags of skin; an effective home remedy is to tie a piece of cotton tightly round the base. They can also be cut off with scissors or destroyed by electric cautery.

Kerato-acanthoma Nodules arise on the face in middle age and grow in the course of a few days or weeks to the size of a large pea. The edge is rounded and may contain small dilated blood vessels. The

129

Chapter 5 **The skin**

whole is surmounted by a layer of keratin. In the past these were often mistaken for cancers of the skin, but it is now known that if they are left untreated, they will spontaneously drop off in about six months. However, they can be removed easily and safely by curetting under local anaesthesia without leaving any appreciable scar.

Malignant neoplasms   There are several varieties of cancer occurring primarily in the skin, and the skin may be involved secondarily from internal malignant disease. There are also a number of conditions which themselves are not malignant but which, if left untreated, would give rise to cancerous changes after several years. The commonest of these, solar keratosis, is produced by sunshine.

Solar keratoses   These occur as the result of long exposure of unprotected white skin to sunlight, and are common in white-skinned people. Although seen in any country, they are much more common in those living in hot dry climates such as Australia, South Africa, India, and Mexico. It is particularly the fair-skinned who are at risk, since their melanin-producing mechanism is not so active. The areas of exposed skin become freckled, and later scaly crusted wartlike lesions occur and the skin becomes dry and thin. These heaped-up areas may, in the course of years, develop the true invasive characters of skin cancer. Treatment of them is therefore important. Destruction by various methods is satisfactory, but probably the best way of dealing with them is by the application of a recently introduced ointment which contains the drug, 5-fluorouracil. This acts selectively on rapidly dividing cells without damaging the surrounding normal skin.

Rodent ulcer (basal cell carcinoma)   This is by far the commonest variety of malignant disease of the skin. The name is derived from the fact that if untreated, it slowly erodes into the adjacent tissues, including muscle and bone. Although classified as a cancer because the cells proliferate beyond their normal site, the growth invades only locally and never spreads to distant parts of the body. Growth is extremely slow.

Rodent ulcers occur usually on the face of white-skinned people in or after middle age. They occasionally arise on skin previously damaged by injury, but sunlight is probably the commonest cause. The early lesion is a small raised papule which slowly enlarges over the course of months. As the cells increase in number, the centre may break down giving a superficial ulcer with a characteristic raised pearly edge.

Treatment is very satisfactory but the smaller the nodule, the easier it is to treat, and it is important for patients to seek advice on any peculiar nodules which are noticed, particularly on the face, and which persist for several weeks.

Bowen's disease (intra-epithelial epithelioma)   This is a condition which usually arises on the trunk or legs in or after middle age. It appears as a well-defined slightly scaling reddened flat patch on the skin. The proliferating cells in the epidermis spread outwards at first within the epidermal layer and may remain confined to the skin for years, later changing into true invasive cancers. Bowen's disease is common in people who in earlier life have been exposed to inorganic arsenic, either in the course of their work, for example horticulture, or sheep-dipping, or who have taken arsenic in various medicines and tonics. The condition can be easily cured by cutting out or destroying the proliferating cells.

Squamous epithelioma   This is a true cancer arising in the cells of the epidermis. Again sunshine on white skin is the commonest cause, but it can also be caused by exposure to tars and certain mineral oils, and on skin damaged by X-ray burns.

The tumour grows rapidly and owing to its rapid growth may degenerate and bleed. As it is a true cancer, it may spread to involve the lymphatic glands draining the area. Fortunately, since the growth is visible, medical advice is sought early and it is usually successfully treated either by surgery or radiotherapy, or a combination of the two.

In addition to the skin, epitheliomata occur occasionally inside the mouth and used to be found on the lips because of burns produced by clay pipe smoking.

Melanoma (malignant moles)   These are quite deservedly the most feared of malignant diseases in the skin, but fortunately are not very common. They can occur on any part of the body and at any age, but are very rare before puberty. They may arise on already existing pigmented moles, particularly the small flat nonhairy type. The factors producing such changes are not known. In any case, the chance of such a change taking place is very small because almost everybody has a few pigmented moles, but the incidence of malignant moles is very low. However, it is rising with the increasing tendency of the white-skinned races to expose a great deal of their unprotected skin to strong sunshine on every possible occasion. Moles are also influenced by hormonal change and may alter in size during pregnancy. The changes which give rise to suspicion that malignant transformation is taking place can be summed up briefly in that anything which brings the attention to a mole must be taken seriously. If the mole itches, becomes blacker, increases in size either along or above the surface of the skin, is surrounded by a red halo, or if it ulcerates and discharges dark serum, medical advice should be sought without delay. Some of these changes may prove to have an innocent cause, but it is better to be safe than sorry, and successful treatment depends on early complete removal. Even when it has not been possible to eradicate the disease completely, the course is variable and apparently depends on little-understood factors associated with the patient's immunological mechanisms.

The skin and internal disease

The skin is involved in many disease processes, either directly or in an unspecific way, and one only has to consider that when a patient suffering from some internal disease looks ill, this is because of the effect of the disease on his skin, the only part visible to the visitor. It is impossible to deal here with all these conditions but it is appropriate to discuss pruritus.

Pruritus (itching) This very common symptom can be the most difficult of all dermatological problems. As discussed earlier, many skin diseases cause irritation, and scabies must always be remembered. The diagnosis may be difficult in clean patients and the acarus mite is no respecter of rank or title. However, the skin may itch for no apparent reason and the irritation may be generalized or affect only small areas of skin.

Generalized irritation This may be caused by internal diseases. Sufferers from diseases of the liver and kidneys may itch, internal malignant disease may cause irritation, as may some disorders of the blood. In many patients, the symptom is not due to any such cause and in older patients, quite severe irritation may be caused by the gradual diminution of the natural grease in the skin which occurs with increasing age. Relief can be obtained by conserving this as much as possible by cutting down the frequency of hot baths, by using as little soap as possible, and by the application of bland oils either directly onto the skin or by using these in the bath.

Localized irritation Areas of skin may itch for no apparent reason, and the almost uncontrollable desire to scratch will itself damage the skin, producing a vicious circle of irritation – scratching – skin damage – irritation – which may be difficult to break. Common sites of such localized irritation are the palms, outer aspect of the forearms, the elbows, nape of the neck, perianal and genital area, inner thighs, and outer sides of the lower legs. In many of these patients, the onset is associated with some emotional or domestic upset and a cure often depends on these difficulties either being resolved or understood. The old expression about things getting under one's skin is, perhaps, a relevant observation.

Irritation of the ano-genital region This localized form of irritation can be a source of great annoyance. It is important to eliminate and treat local causes. This type of itching may be a symptom in diabetes; in women vaginal discharge may cause intense irritation. Piles, skin tags, and threadworms all produce anal irritation, as do persistent dirt and faecal contamination. Unfortunately, some of the proprietary ointments sold to control the condition may themselves produce sensitization dermatitis after prolonged use. However, in many cases no cause can be found and there is often an emotional background to the problem which must be resolved. Since these are often social and domestic difficulties, the help of a sympathetic medical social worker can be invaluable.

Diseases largely associated with emotional upset

In addition to some cases of pruritus mentioned above, there are several diseases in which emotional disturbance seems to play a major role. The commonest two are dermatitis artefacta and rosacea.

Dermatitis artefacta This difficult problem usually arises in adolescent girls, but may occur at any age in either sex. The patients consciously or subconsciously damage their own skin. The underlying motives may be very complex. The usual method is to produce long scratches with the fingernails or a sharp instrument, but many bizarre methods of damaging the skin have been recorded. A girl who persistently burnt her upper chest with an ultraviolet lamp puzzled many experienced dermatologists for several years. Often there is an underlying emotional problem, perhaps associated with the current boyfriend or lack of boyfriend, and the patient may feel compelled to "take it out on herself". A protective dressing to the damaged area results in rapid cure of the skin, but this will not remove the underlying cause. The motive is much more obvious in patients who deliberately aggravate what may have been a relatively trivial injury sustained at work.

Rosacea (acne rosacea) This common condition usually occurs in women in their forties and fifties. It is characterized by a vivid flushing of the central part of the face, and in these areas small papules and pustules may appear. The patients are acutely conscious of their red face. It is more common in patients who blushed easily in younger life and also in those who take their meals and beverages very hot. The fundamental cause is a persistent dilatation of the blood vessels in the blush area, and many of these patients admit to difficulty in relaxing in their ordinary household duties. Rosacea may also be associated with the well-recognized instability of vasomotor control at the time of the menopause, which is manifested as hot flushes. Coming to terms with life is important as well as taking food and drinks as cool as possible, but the most effective form of therapy is to take a small daily dose of one of the tetracycline group of antibiotics (as used in acne vulgaris) over a period of time. The condition occurs less frequently in men and then may produce enlarging and reddening of the nose (rhinophyma) which is best reshaped by plastic surgery.

Emotion and skin disease Many skin diseases are very worrying to patients, and the doctor will, of course, bear this in mind in his treatment.

Diseases of the hair

The pattern of hair growth in man is very largely governed by racial and genetic factors, but loss of hair can cause a great deal of mental anguish which is aggravated by the commercial pressure exerted by wig makers and transplantation experts. In no other animal does the growth of hair behave as in man, and this has made research and understanding of hair growth difficult. Deductions can be made from observing changes in hair seen in different disease processes, and at adolescence there are obvious striking changes with the increased growth of hair on certain specific areas of the body in men and women.

Alopecia This is the name given to hair loss. It may be localized, diffuse, or complete, and may be brought about by conditions which attack the hair-growing mechanism, or diseases of the scalp.

The commonest variety of baldness is that seen in many men, male pattern alopecia. The hair stops growing first of all on the temples and on the top of the head. The areas affected gradually extend, and in severe cases the whole of the scalp from the forehead to the back of the scalp may be completely bald. The hair on the sides and back of the scalp is not affected. There is undoubtedly a familial factor and the process seems to be triggered off by the normal changes of puberty. Eunuchs castrated before puberty never go bald. At present there is no way of stopping this process although many attempts have been made. The much publicized and expensive treatment by transplantation makes use of the fact that the hair at the sides never falls, so hair-containing follicles are transplanted from the sides into the balding areas.

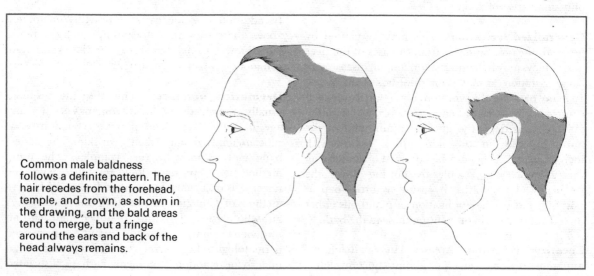

Common male baldness follows a definite pattern. The hair recedes from the forehead, temple, and crown, as shown in the drawing, and the bald areas tend to merge, but a fringe around the ears and back of the head always remains.

These follicles undoubtedly grow and produce hair in their new environment but since it is not possible to transplant individual hairs, the treated patient is left with rows of tufts of hairs on his previously bald areas which become more noticeable as the hair normally situated on the crown is shed.

A similar but usually less marked loss of hair may occur in women and although this is occasionally associated with hormonal abnormality, it is unusual. Fortunately, female wigs are very much less obvious than male wigs, largely on account of the difference in styles of hairdressing.

Hair loss in both men and women may occur with severe dandruff (seborrhoea capitis), and when this is controlled by antiseptic creams, lotions, and shampoos, the hair will regrow.

Diffuse hair loss in young women is occasionally associated with lowering of the amount of iron in the blood serum, and in these cases regrowth will occur when the deficiency is remedied.

Postfebrile and postpuerperal alopecia Diffuse hair loss may occur after both severe febrile illness and pregnancy, and since the loss may not be noticed for up to three months after these events, the patient may not associate these with the hair loss. In these cases the outlook is good, regrowth usually occurring in a few months.

Alopecia areata This is a common variety of hair loss producing well-defined round areas of complete baldness, usually on the scalp, but possibly in other areas such as the beard, eyebrows, and body. The round areas may coalesce giving bizarre shapes of baldness and may become extensive. The whole scalp may be affected (alopecia totalis) or indeed the whole of the body (alopecia universalis). The cause is unknown but some families are more prone to it than others. Regrowth in the milder varieties usually occurs within six months but recurrences are not uncommon and the prognosis both in these and in the very extensive cases is poor. Unfortunately there is no effective treatment.

Traumatic alopecia and trichotillomania Hair loss can be produced by mechanical removal of the hair which may occur without the knowledge of the patient. Very vigorous brushing, particularly in those having tightly curled hair of the African negro variety, when used in conjunction with chemicals for straightening the hair, will both pull out the hair and cause it to break. Hair styling in which the hair is pulled tightly will give areas of thinning. This was often seen when "ponytails" were fashionable and it occurs with the regular use of tightly wound rollers for curling the hair.

There is one particular form of hair loss seen usually in children and adolescents known as trichotillomania in which the hair is broken by the conscious or subconscious habit of twisting or pulling the hair. This habit in children is like thumb sucking or nail biting and may be difficult to stop, but wearing a glove on the unoccupied hand when writing, or a closefitting cap in bed may be effective. The habit usually subsides with increasing age.

Alopecia from underlying disease Some conditions, such as thyroid disease, or the actual treatment of some diseases may also cause hair loss.

Increased hair growth (hirsutes) Just as loss of hair is a great source of worry to some people, so does the increased growth of hair on normally smooth areas cause great distress to others, especially women. Hair is present on all parts of the body except the palms and soles but the density and type varies both in different races and in different members of the same race. Increased hair growth may be seen on the body in some children without any underlying disease and this is marked in those from the Indian subcontinent. However, it is after puberty that most of the problems occur and although hair on the face and chest is normal in men, it is when it appears on the face and chest in women that it causes trouble.

Increased hair on the face in women may be a genetic characteristic and is regarded as normal in many races. In Anglo-Saxons it tends to be the exception rather than the rule and the presence of such hair may produce great emotional disturbance. It is sometimes regarded as evidence of some hormonal abnormality and although such changes will result in abnormal hair growth, they are rare, and in the vast majority of cases intensive investigation reveals no abnormality.

Removal of excessive hair, particularly from the face, is difficult because it is the normal physiological pattern in that individual. Hormone therapy is not effective in the absence of hormonal abnormality, and although exposure to X-rays will destroy the hair follicles, the dose required inevitably destroys the skin overlying the hair follicles, giving rise eventually to unsightly scarring and even skin cancer. Preparations which dissolve the keratin of the hair are effective but may also adversely affect the keratin of the skin. Mechanical removal with tweezers or waxes is effective and is used by many. Shaving is thought by many women to emphasize loss of femininity, and the short shaved hairs are stubbly because they do not bend. Electrolysis is thought by many to be the answer to their problem and this is certainly effective for relatively isolated hairs but is difficult to carry out if there are many hairs. Passing a fine electrode down beside each hair to destroy the active part of the hair follicle with a small electric current is very time-consuming, and if not done carefully, scarring can result.

Many patients have been helped by friction, rubbing the affected areas gently but frequently (four to six times a day) with fine sandpaper or smooth pumice stone and this, together with bleaching for brunettes, is often effective.

Ingrowing hair If hair penetrates into the skin away from the hair follicle it produces a brisk foreign body reaction and this is a real problem in negroes with tightly curled hair. After shaving, the corkscrew-like short hair bores into the surrounding skin. These ingrowing hairs can be picked out easily with a needle but the only effective way to prevent the recurrent inflammation of the beard area is to grow a beard. When this is not desired, brushing the face against the direction of hair growth with a stiff nailbrush after shaving may help to prevent a certain amount of ingrowing.

Diseases of the nails

Nails are modified keratin and are affected by conditions in which there is abnormal keratinization. There are a number of rare congenital diseases characterized by abnormal formation of nails, hair, skin, and sometimes teeth.

If keratin formation has been affected as a result of a serious illness, grooves may be seen across each nail and since the fingernails take about six months to grow out, it is sometimes possible to tell when the patient had such an illness – one of the signs used by a clever palmist. Fungus infections, psoriasis, and lichen planus may all involve the nails and are discussed elsewhere.

Spoon-shaped nails (koilonychia)   These are seen in some varieties of anaemia.

Paronychia This condition was previously mentioned with thrush, which, together with other low-grade infections, may invade the potential space between the nail and the overlying nail fold. The space is normally sealed by the cuticle but if this is damaged, organisms may enter and give rise to a painful red swelling at the base of the nail. The nail itself may be damaged and growth is impaired. The condition is much commoner in women and is aggravated by frequent contact with water.

Cure depends on preventing water getting into the nail space, treating the infection, and encouraging regrowth of the cuticle. This can be achieved by working nystatin cream (both as an anticandida agent and as a barrier cream) into the affected nail fold whenever the hand is being put into water. For a busy housewife, it may mean applying the cream twenty to thirty times a day but this is much easier than to have the nail removed. Permanent cure usually takes about six weeks. Wearing rubber gloves, even lined household gloves, does not help because the inevitable sweating inside the glove encourages the growth of the organism.

Splitting nails This annoying condition is due to weakening of the cement substance at the free edge of the nail and may be the result of various solvents in household cleansers as well as the solvents of nail varnish remover.

Misshapen nails The commonest cause is previous injury to the nail bed and this is almost impossible to remedy. If it gives rise to great deformity of the toenails, the best form of treatment is to remove the nail bed, thereby preventing further nail growth.

Care of the skin

Although it is obvious that the colour of the skin is an inherited characteristic, it is not generally realized that many of the other properties of the skin and hair are determined by ancestry. Some white people inherit a translucent facial epidermis through which the colour of the underlying blood vessels shows as a desirable "pink and white" complexion. The degree of oiliness, the dryness and thickness of the skin all tend to be inherited. The amount of natural grease varies throughout life in each individual and this is influenced by changes in the secretions of the various endocrine glands at different ages.

A healthy body and contented mind are the first essentials for a healthy skin. Internal disease adversely affects the skin, and stresses and strains result in unbecoming expressions of tension.

The skin must be protected from harmful outside agents – excessive sunlight, cold, heat, and chemicals, particularly those which remove greases and keratin.

Oily skin should not be exposed to greases or local applications such as highly emulsified creams which block the openings of the grease glands.

Dry skin must be protected from degreasing agents, strong soaps, and household cleansers.

In industry, mechanical handling of potentially harmful substances must be, and usually is, installed whenever possible. If contact with potential sensitizing agents is inevitable, this must be for as short a time as possible and the contaminated skin cleaned immediately after contact ceases. Barrier creams are no substitute for personal hygiene and avoidance of contact with irritants.

Care of the hair

The keratin of the hair is a complex chemical compound which can be damaged by many agents, particularly those designed to alter the configuration of the chemical molecules. This is achieved often by destroying the bonds linking the molecular chains together and the hair is inevitably weakened. Occasionally it actually breaks. All curling and straightening agents must be used with great caution. It is a peculiar fact of the human make-up that those with naturally straight hair wish it to be curly and those with curly hair wish it to be straight. Hair dyes which combine with the keratin, such as the paraphenylene diamine group, probably do not weaken hair, but on the other hand they are potent skin sensitizers and may give rise to severe dermatitis even after previous satisfactory use.

Vigorous brushing and combing is also liable to break the hair, and excessive massage of the scalp has the same result. Greasiness of the hair is caused by secretion from the sebaceous glands in the scalp; the amount varies with each individual and at different ages. The hair should be washed either with soap and water or a mild shampoo as frequently as necessary.

The colour and natural shape of the hair are genetically determined as is the pattern of hair growth throughout life. Wise men and women make the best of the skin and hair with which they have been endowed and do not waste money on remedies and cosmetic preparations that claim miraculous powers.

Chapter 6
The lungs and chest

Revised by J. E. Cotes, MA DM FRCP and Peter Elmes, MD FRCP

An average adult breathes more than 12,000 litres (2,600 gallons) of air a day. This is not only the body's largest intake of any substance, but the most immediately important to life. We can go without food for many days and water for many hours without fatal results. But life cannot continue without air for more than a few minutes.

The life-giving component of air is oxygen, which constitutes approximately one fifth of its volume. Almost all the rest of air is nitrogen, with minute amounts of several other inert gases. Ordinary combustion is a rather violent combination of oxygen with fuels such as coal, wood, or petrol, producing flames and heat. A similar but marvellously controlled process called respiration goes on incessantly in every one of our millions of body cells.

The word respiration in ordinary usage means the breathing in and out that we all do, to take in oxygen and get rid of carbon dioxide. To the doctor or physiologist, the term also has a further meaning – the interchange of these gases that goes on in the body cells themselves. The former process is called "external respiration", and the latter "internal respiration".

Many small organisms obtain oxygen by absorbing it directly through the cell walls from their environment. In man and higher animals the problem is more complicated since their billions of internal cells do not have direct contact with the oxygen rich atmosphere. An efficient means of bringing oxygen from the outside world to every cell, and of removing the waste carbon dioxide is essential. This transport system is provided by the blood in conjunction with specialized organs, the lungs.

The lungs

The two lungs lie side by side in the chest cavity. In general appearance they are cone-shaped and greyish in colour. A baby's lungs are pink, and those of a coalminer are virtually black. The base of each lung rests on a dome-shaped muscle, the diaphragm, and the top part (apex) is in the root of the neck. The lungs normally have only one attachment, where the bronchi join the windpipe, and are freely movable.

A deep fissure divides each lung into a lower and an upper lobe. The left lung, slightly smaller than the right, has two lobes. In the right lung a horizontal fissure just below the middle produces a third or middle lobe. Each lobe is divided into segments, which can be readily separated from the others. Before this was known, surgical removal of a small area of diseased lung tissue required removal of an entire lobe (lobectomy) or even a whole lung (pneumonectomy). Today, if a condition is limited to one lung segment, only the involved segment is removed, leaving the remainder of the lobe for normal function.

Each lung is completely surrounded and encased by a thin glistening membrane, the pleura. The inner surface of the chest wall has the same pleural lining. Normally, there is no space between the lung and chest wall membranes, although the area of sliding contact is called the pleural cavity. In certain circumstances of disease or accident the pleural cavity may be occupied by air, blood, or other fluid.

The opposed fluid-lubricated surfaces of the pleura slide easily over each other as the lung expands and contracts during respiration. The lung pleura

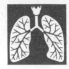

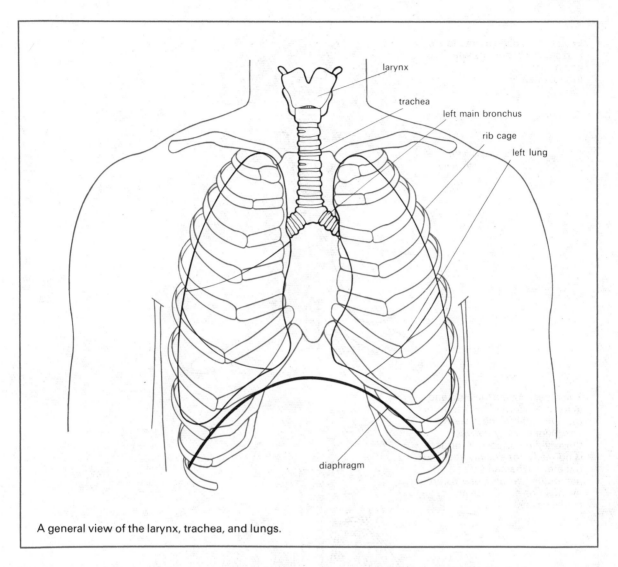

A general view of the larynx, trachea, and lungs.

Diagram labels: larynx, trachea, left main bronchus, rib cage, left lung, diaphragm

contains no pain-transmitting nerves. In this way abnormalities may arise in the lung or its pleura without causing pain. However, the pleural lining of the chest wall is richly supplied with sensory nerves, so that when it is involved in disease, pain may be experienced. It is often caused by inflammation following an infection of the lung. Pneumonia or tuberculosis may sometimes be responsible.

At birth the lungs are solid and contain no air. The baby's first breaths rapidly expand the lung to at least three times its former size. The expansion is assisted by a chemical substance (surfactant) which forms a lining layer in the lung. The surfactant reduces the suction which must be applied to open up the small air spaces (alveoli). Once the alveoli are open the surfactant prevents them from closing down entirely during breathing out. The substance is normally present in the lungs well before birth. Sometimes it is deficient; the baby then experiences respiratory distress and needs assistance from a respirator. Production of surfactant then rises to normal.

The shape of the lungs   When in the body, the lungs are in close relation to the chest wall, and in fact completely fill the chest cavity. If they are removed after death, their elasticity causes them to shrink immediately to about one third of their original size. Similarly, if one side of the chest is opened at operation that lung will collapse in the same way. In the body the shape of the lungs is maintained by a slight negative pressure (that is, a pressure slightly below that of the atmosphere) in the pleural cavity. This, as it were, sucks the lungs outwards and maintains them in contact with the chest wall.

137

Chapter 6 The lungs and chest

Each lung is divided into lobes
and smaller segments which
can be separated
independently.

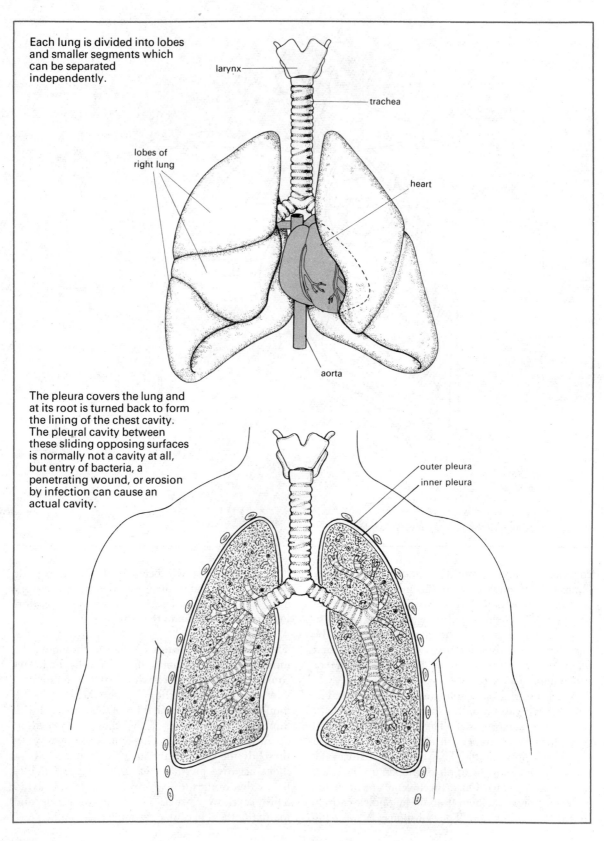

larynx

trachea

lobes of
right lung

heart

aorta

The pleura covers the lung and
at its root is turned back to form
the lining of the chest cavity.
The pleural cavity between
these sliding opposing surfaces
is normally not a cavity at all,
but entry of bacteria, a
penetrating wound, or erosion
by infection can cause an
actual cavity.

outer pleura

inner pleura

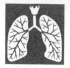

Controlled collapse of a lung may be performed by a doctor by introducing measured amounts of air through a needle into the pleural cavity. This procedure, known as artificial pneumothorax, was formerly used to rest a lung, as part of the treatment of tuberculosis. The therapeutic pneumothorax has now largely been replaced by drugs.

Fortunately, the pleural cavity of each lung is independent of the other. Collapse of one lung does not much affect the functions of the opposite lung.

Inside the lungs   Air that is drawn in through the nose or mouth is warmed and moistened on its journey to the lungs. In the upper part of the throat the air follows the same passageway as food on its way to the stomach. Then at about the level of the Adam's apple the passage divides to form the gullet at the back, and the voice box (larynx) at the front. The larynx is a tubular air passage about five cm (two in) long in women, somewhat longer in men. Its upper opening is guarded by an ingenious trapdoor, the epiglottis, which keeps the passage open for the passage of air, but closes it when food or liquids are swallowed. A mistaken attempt to swallow and inhale at the same time demonstrates that it cannot be done. Occasionally, if the opening is closed imperfectly or not in time, we experience a spasmodic choking reaction commonly called "swallowing the wrong way".

The lower part of the larynx is continuous with the trachea or windpipe, an air tube between ten and $12\frac{1}{2}$ cm (four and five in) long. The trachea is kept from collapsing by numerous C-shaped rings of cartilage, which can be felt by running a finger up and down over the lowest part of the front of the neck, just above where the breastbone begins. Here the trachea is very close to the skin surface and can be easily reached by a surgeon who can make an artificial opening (tracheotomy) to permit air to enter the trachea and bypass any suffocating obstruction of the larynx above it.

Approximately at a level with the top of the heart, which lies behind it, the trachea divides into two bronchi, one going to the right and the other to the left lung. The right bronchus is a wider and more direct continuation of the trachea than that on the left side, and therefore a more common site for lodgment of inhaled foreign material. The main trunk of a bronchus passes towards the base of the lung, but divides and subdivides into ever smaller air tubes. The so-called bronchial tree does resemble the branches of an inverted tree, branching into smaller

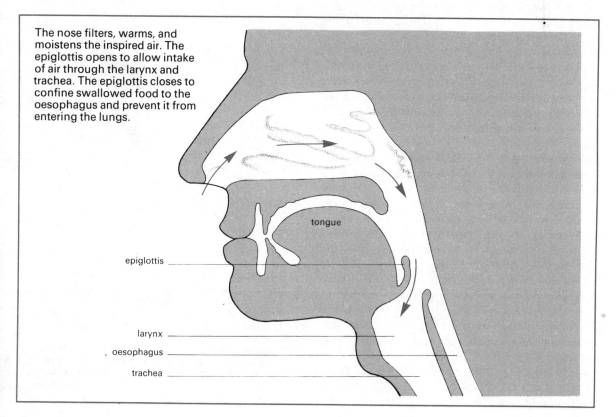

The nose filters, warms, and moistens the inspired air. The epiglottis opens to allow intake of air through the larynx and trachea. The epiglottis closes to confine swallowed food to the oesophagus and prevent it from entering the lungs.

tongue

epiglottis

larynx

oesophagus

trachea

Chapter 6 The lungs and chest

and smaller tubules. The tinest lung tubes, the bronchioles, terminate after many divisions in blind globular air sacs. These pouches, called alveoli, resemble microscopic clusters of grapes. We have some 400 million alveoli, each of which is an infinitesimal respiratory chamber. It is here that the exchange of gases takes place.

Exchange of gases The inner surfaces of the alveoli, continuous with the bronchioles, bronchi, and trachea, are technically outside the body, in contact with the atmosphere. If the walls of all the air cells were spread out as one continuous area they would cover a surface the size of a tennis court, but this immense surface is compacted into the small space of two lungs. The membrane is, however, extremely thin and delicate, to allow the absorption of oxygen from air and dispersal of carbon dioxide (the waste gas from the cells).

A single alveolus is a globular chamber open at one end. Oxygen-containing air is in contact with the inner wall. The blood supply of the alveolus is very rich. The capillary wall is only one cell thick, and so is the air sac wall. Gas molecules can move rapidly through these very thin layers. This process, in effect exposes a vast, thin, moving sheet of blood to the external world. After the exchange of gases in the lungs, bright red blood is pumped by the heart to the body. Deoxygenated dark blood is pumped by the heart to the lungs.

Haemoglobin in the red blood cells is the substance which picks up oxygen in the lungs and transports it to the tissue cells. Similarly, the carbon dioxide given off by the tissue cells is conveyed to the lungs and passes out in the breath.

How we breathe The smaller air tubes within the lungs have muscle fibres, but the alveoli have no muscle. They are passive organs, expanded and contracted by movements of ribs and diaphragm which force air to flow in and out, much like a bellows.

The lungs are enclosed in a flexible box, the thoracic cavity. Its top is the base of the neck; its sides are the ribs which are linked in front to the breastbone (sternum) and at the back to the backbone (vertebrae). At the bottom of the thoracic cavity is the diaphragm which separates the chest from the abdomen. Contraction of the diaphragm causes it to pull downward and expand the chest cavity, assisted by muscles which elevate the ribs. The lung surfaces, clinging to the sides of the box through the vacuum-like pull of the pleural cavity, necessarily expand with

the box and air flows in. Relaxation of the diaphragm and intercostal muscles allows the lung to shrink, and air is exhaled. The mechanical action is comparable to that of a bellows containing a very elastic sponge with its surfaces securely attached to the sides of the bellows.

Nerve centres The sequences of breathing – about eighteen respirations per minute, or some 26,000 diaphragm contractions a day – are under nervous control. The breathing centre is in the lower part of the brain (medulla) at the top of the spinal cord. This centre coordinates the movements of all the muscles of respiration. If it is damaged, as in some polio patients, the breathing muscles are paralysed from lack of nervous impulses. Respirators ("iron lungs") expand and relax the chest mechanically.

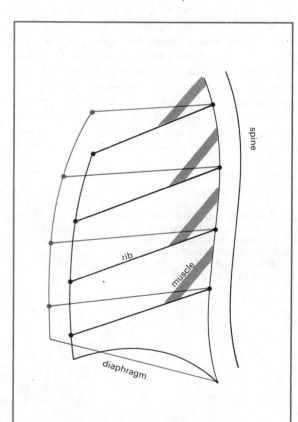

In expiration (black), the ribs slop downwards and the diaphragm is domed upwards. In inspiration (red), the ribs become more horizontal and the diaphragm is flattened. This results in an increase in the capacity of the chest, which then sucks in air. In quiet breathing, respiration is mostly performed by the diaphragm. With exercise, the muscles between the ribs (intercostal muscles) elevate the rib cage.

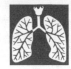

The structure of the lungs

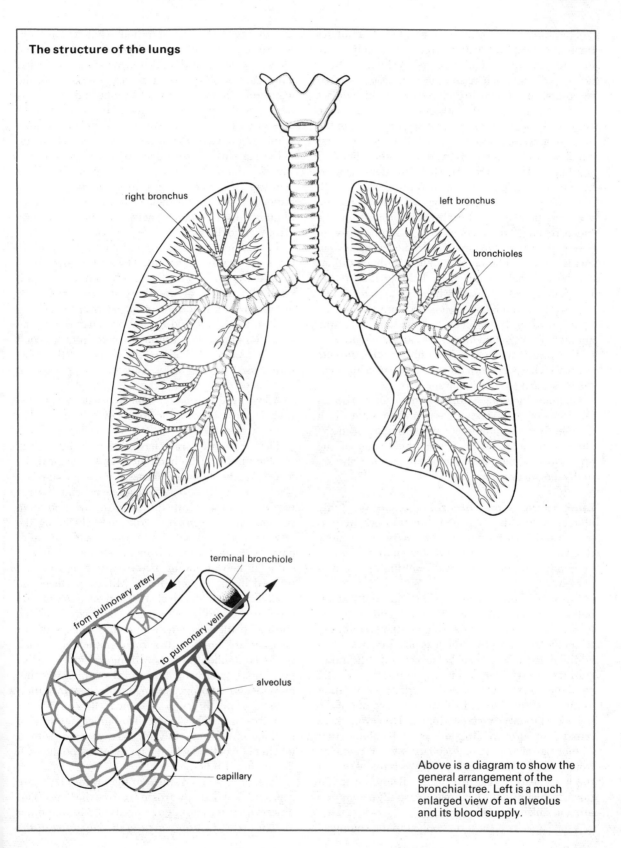

right bronchus

left bronchus

bronchioles

terminal bronchiole

from pulmonary artery

to pulmonary vein

alveolus

capillary

Above is a diagram to show the general arrangement of the bronchial tree. Left is a much enlarged view of an alveolus and its blood supply.

Chapter 6 The lungs and chest

The breathing centre alternately stimulates breathing in and breathing out. It is helped by information from several sources – in the lungs from nerve endings which record the expansion (stretch receptors) and also the irritant receptors which detect any small particles on the inside of the airways; in the chest wall from receptors in muscles and joints; in the arterial blood from specialized cells (chemoreceptors) which sense the amount of oxygen and other chemical substances. The amount of carbon dioxide is detected both by these cells and by the breathing centre itself. The information from the lungs and thorax mainly regulates the pattern of each breath; that from the blood regulates the amount – most importantly an excess of carbon dioxide or a deficiency of oxygen increase the ventilation of the lung. Both conditions can be artificially induced by holding the breath. Before long there is an overwhelming urge to inhale, so powerful that it is not possible to commit suicide by breath-holding. Intake of air into the lungs raises the amount of oxygen and dilutes the carbon dioxide.

The principal nerve of breathing is the phrenic nerve which passes down the sides of the neck through the chest cavity to the diaphragm.

Complex nervous pathways may give rise to sensations of pain in body areas remote from the site of trouble. It is not unusual for pain originating in the chest wall pleura to be felt in the region of the appendix, and pain from the diaphragm may be felt in the shoulder region.

Lung volumes and breathing capacity Only about one twelfth of our total breathing capacity is exercised in breathing at rest. The body's respiratory reserve is tremendous. An entire lung may collapse or be removed surgically without resulting in shortness of breath.

With each quiet breath-cycle of an adult, about half a litre (one pint) of air flows into and out of the lungs. This is known as tidal volume. If one continues to inhale at the end of quiet inspiration, about an additional two litres can be sucked into the lungs (inspiratory reserve volume). Similarly, if one continues to exhale at the end of ordinary expiration as much as a litre and a half can be forced out of the lungs (expiratory reserve volume). However, there remains about two litres of residual volume that cannot be exhaled. A lung collapses when removed from the body, but enough air always remains so that the lung floats if placed in water. Before an infant takes its first breath, the lungs are solid, contain no air, and sink if placed in water.

Vital capacity is the term applied to the volume of air displaced from full inspiration to full expiration. It is measured by inhaling as deeply as possible and blowing as much as possible into a measuring device. The quantity of expelled air varies with body size and age. A medium-sized man of European descent may have a vital capacity of 4.0 to 4.5 litres between the ages of 20 to 40 years; women and people of other ethnic groups have somewhat lower values. However, as the elasticity of tissues decreases with age, the vital capacity diminishes and may be as much as 20 per cent less at 60, and 40 per cent less at 75 years. It is important to allow for these factors since otherwise a diminished vital lung capacity may be erroneously attributed to disease.

Ventilatory capacity is the ability of the lungs to move air rapidly in and out. The average over a few breaths is about 120 to 180 litres per minute but falls off if the period of breathing is prolonged. The measurement is made either during forced breathing or from a single forced expiration starting with the lungs full of air. The volume expired in one second (forced expiratory volume, FEV 1·0) is the most widely used index, it is normally about 75 per cent of the vital capacity.

A low FEV is usually associated with breathlessness. It may also be due to overweight and other causes.

The respiratory tract has efficient self-cleansing mechanisms, and both physical and biological defences. Firstly physical defences. The air passages are bent and the air is deflected at each bend. Larger particles of dust breathed in with the air tend to go straight on. They mostly strike the cells lining the airways and stick in the mucous layer. Smaller particles float downwards in the stream of air and settle on the walls of the airways where they too are trapped in the mucous layer. Minute particles too small to sediment mostly float in and out and cause no problem. Secondly the biological defences. From the entrance of the larynx to the tinest bronchioles, the air passages are lined with special epithelium, which consists of millions of cells with microscopic hairlike projections (cilia) which beat in rhythmic, sweeping movements that propel a thin film of mucus over their surfaces. The direction of mucus flow is always outwards from the lungs. The inner surfaces of millions of air sacs (alveoli) are covered with a moving film of fluid which joins uninterruptedly with that of the air tubes.

Foreign particles trapped in the mucous layer are constantly carried upwards away from the lungs. This process prevents about 99 per cent of dust and other foreign materials from entering or remaining in the

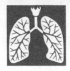

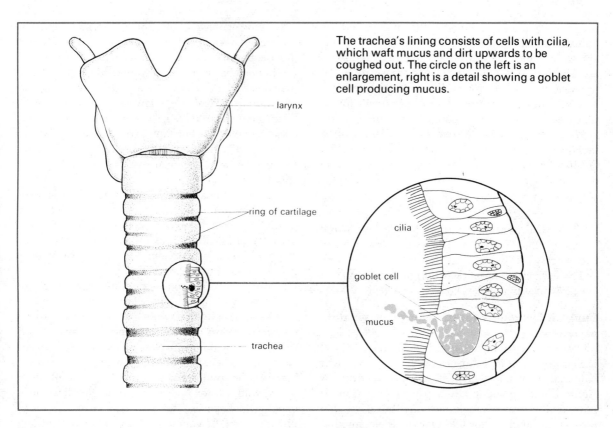

The trachea's lining consists of cells with cilia, which waft mucus and dirt upwards to be coughed out. The circle on the left is an enlargement, right is a detail showing a goblet cell producing mucus.

larynx

ring of cartilage

trachea

cilia

goblet cell

mucus

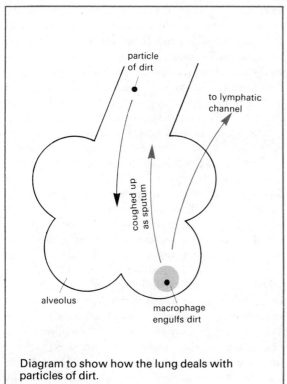

particle of dirt

to lymphatic channel

coughed up as sputum

alveolus

macrophage engulfs dirt

Diagram to show how the lung deals with particles of dirt.

lungs. The one per cent that is not eliminated is engulfed by scavenging cells and deposited in the lungs and their lymph nodes.

Lung diseases

Lung diseases are usually caused by agents carried by the air we breathe. If we were as careful to prevent the contamination of the air we breathe as we are with the water we drink, there would be very little lung disease. The diseases will be described under the following headings:

Infections (diseases due to microbes)
Asthma
Organic dust diseases
Toxic chemicals and dusts
Primary lung cancer
Benign pneumoconiosis (nuisance dust diseases)
Ageing

Infections

We breathe in microbes with every breath we take. Fortunately these are mostly prevented from invading the tissues and causing illness by protective

Chapter 6 The lungs and chest

proteins in the mucous lining of the airways and the lining material of the alveoli. Some of these proteins are agents which act against any microbes and some are specific antibodies developed as a result of previous exposure to a particular bacterium or virus. The protein defences are backed up by cells in the lung tissue and from the blood, whose main function is to destroy invaders and remove the debris (killed invading organisms as well as damaged human cells).

Microbes able to penetrate these defences can be divided into three groups:

Those which attack normal people and cause serious illness.

Those which attack normal people but cause serious illness only in people who have weak defences.

Those which are harmless to normal people but can cause illness in people who have no defences.

Lung infections caused by very virulent organisms

Influenza (a virus infection)   See chapter 2.

Pneumonic plague is an example of a virulent bacterial infection which is spread by droplets (spitting and coughing) from person to person. If untreated, it carries a high mortality, but those who recover are immune for life. Once an epidemic has spread through a population the disease disappears because there are no susceptible persons for the organism to live on. Throughout the Middle Ages there was an animal reservoir where the infection could lie dormant and cause outbreaks every fifteen to 40 years. Sporadic cases in young people gave warning of an epidemic. Fortunately modern sanitary conditions and active measures against rats have led to the disappearance of this illness as a serious world problem, but it could arise again in conditions of war.

Tuberculosis is an infection due to a virulent organism which takes a long time to establish itself in the lung (six weeks to three months). The primary infection of the alveolar part of the lung is usually insufficient to cause any symptoms or to interfere with lung function. Then two things happen, firstly the organisms start to spread to the rest of the body by the lymph channels and the blood, and secondly the body mobilizes its immune system which starts destroying the tubercle bacilli and causing an inflammation. The patient suffers a feverish illness sometimes associated with a collection of fluid round the lung called a pleural effusion. If the immune response is adequate the tuberculous infection dies down. If not the infection may spread and prove fatal.

In some people the infection lies dormant and can relapse as a result of malnutrition or some other disease. But in most the tubercle bacilli have died and the patient has a degree of protection from further infection which is shown by a positive skin reaction (Mantoux or Heaf test). This partial protection is lifelong but can be reduced as a result of malnutrition, disease, or old age. The same sort of protection lasting for ten to twenty years can be produced by vaccination with a special strain of tubercle bacilli (BCG).

The second phase of tuberculosis occurs in spite of the protection provided by the primary infection or by BCG vaccination. It probably requires a large quantity of bacilli such as results from repeated or intimate contact with someone with serious lung disease who coughs frequently. Again there is an interval of weeks or months after infection before the patient is aware of any illness. Then there is a gradual increase of symptoms including cough, breathlessness on exertion, loss of weight, sweating at night, and tiredness. Coughing up blood seldom occurs at an early stage. People should not wait until they see blood in the sputum but should always consult their doctor and ask for a chest X-ray if they develop a cough which persists for ten days or more. Early disease is usually confined to the upper part of one lung and only spreads first to the upper part of the other lung and later to the lower parts of the lungs after months or years. It is now possible to cure tuberculosis at almost any stage with antibiotics. Early treatment returns the patient to normal. But the treatment has to be prolonged in advanced cases and there may be permanent scarring of parts of the lungs with corresponding breathlessness and cough.

The treatment of early tuberculosis need take only nine months to a year on antibiotics with careful supervision. Bed rest is not necessary but the patient must be isolated from susceptible contacts for the first few weeks until the sputum no longer contains tubercle bacilli. Patients can return to light work as soon as they feel well and can regard themselves as cured by the end of six months. The difficulty lies in making the correct choice of drugs for the individual patient and in making absolutely sure that they are taken correctly for the full length of time. Although there are six or seven drugs which are effective against tuberculosis, they have to be used correctly.

Patients must always take two and sometimes three drugs simultaneously and must keep to the treatment for the full course without any breaks. The tubercle bacillus can continue its growth in spite of the presence of a single drug, but cannot do so in the

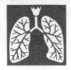

presence of two drugs at once unless the dose is too low. This interesting and important phenomenon is known as antibiotic resistance and is passed on to the offspring of the tubercle bacillus. It can prevent treatment working in the individual patient who can pass the resistant bacilli on to other patients who will also fail to respond to treatment.

Some patients become allergic or develop other toxic reactions to drugs. This means changing to another drug without delay if treatment is to be effective and to prevent resistance.

The choice of drug and the supervision of patients with tuberculosis is a complicated matter which needs to be done by experts with adequate assistance from social workers and laboratories. There are two essential aspects of the control of tuberculosis which require expert attention.

Firstly, ensuring the completion of adequate treatment. Patients with tuberculosis are infectious and should in theory live in some form of isolation hospital until their condition is no longer infectious. The doctors treating tuberculosis must have isolation facilities available for admission of patients who cannot be isolated sufficiently at home or who cannot be relied upon to take their treatment regularly. This applies especially to patients who relapse with infections resistant to antibiotics. It is sometimes necessary to resort to the surgical removal of the infected part of the lung if it proves impossible to achieve a curative course of antibiotic treatment.

Secondly, the tracing and treatment of contacts. These fall into two groups. 1 People found to have active infection including the person from whom the patient may have caught the disease. These contacts are treated as any other new case of tuberculosis and their contacts must be investigated too. 2 People who show no evidence of active tuberculosis infection but who may be incubating the disease. Those who are skin test negative need to be kept under observation to see whether the skin test becomes positive within three months. They then require treatment. Those who are skin test positive when first examined may need treatment if there is reason to believe that the test has become positive recently. (They may have been tested at some routine health examination at school or at work.)

BCG vaccination of school children and special populations such as nurses and medical students makes the detection of recent infection amongst contacts very difficult. For this reason the routine BCG vaccination of population groups is usually abandoned when the incidence of tuberculosis falls below a certain level. Contacts who have recently become skin test positive, or show other evidence of early primary (adult) type of tuberculosis need treatment. But because at this early stage there may be only relatively small numbers of tubercle bacilli in their bodies it may be possible to deal with the infections with a shorter course of antibiotic treatment and using only one drug for part of the period of treatment.

For nearly 30 years we have had the drugs with which to cure tuberculosis. It is now evident that all the complex treatments used before the modern treatment were of little or no value except that the isolation of patients in a sanatorium did help, together with the general improvement in the sanitation, to reduce the level of tuberculosis within the community. If for nearly 30 years we have had the opportunity to cure tuberculosis we have also had the opportunity to eradicate it. Why has progress been so slow? There were 8,102 new cases of respiratory tuberculosis in Great Britain in 1974 and 1,074 deaths in England and Wales in 1974. The majority of these deaths (830) occurred in people over the age of 60 and another 110 of those occurring below the age of 60 are described as "late results of tuberculosis". In other words, patients in whom the infection was cured but treatment was started late, and who died later because of scarring of the lungs. Effective treatment was possible from 1950 onwards, but there are many people who developed tuberculosis before then and in whom the infection has lain dormant. With the onset of old age and other diseases lowering their resistance the disease becomes reactivated. Such people act as a reservoir of infection in the community, a danger to their grandchildren. Their symptoms may be mistaken for chronic bronchitis (which they may also have). They respond poorly to treatment and the tuberculosis may be a contributory factor rather than the main cause of death. Young people who catch the disease from these old people, if diagnosed early and treated correctly, should not in their turn form a reservoir of continued infection. Immigrant populations living in overcrowded conditions have been particularly prone to infection after they have arrived in this country. The arrival of immigrants with active infection has not played an important part in maintaining tuberculosis.

Provided there is no serious influx of people with tuberculosis acquired overseas and provided the health service continues at its present level of efficiency, tuberculosis should become rapidly less important as the generation who developed their infections before 1950 die off in the normal way. There are parts of the world where for political or economic reasons tuberculosis eradication has not been nearly as successful.

Lung infections due to less virulent organisms
There are many agents which usually cause minor illnesses such as measles, mumps, whooping cough, the various viruses causing the common cold, and so on. They cause a fever accompanied by a varying degree of swelling of the lining of the airways and sometimes blockage. They may sometimes invade the alveolar part of the lung and cause pneumonia. This happens more often in chicken pox but antibodies arrive quickly enough to prevent serious damage. In people with an inherited defect the antibody response may be too slow and these childhood infections give rise to a serious illness and sooner or later death. It may soon be possible to identify the individuals with this defect in early childhood and give them replacement treatment. But up to the present this kind of immune deficiency has remained rare because few sufferers live long enough to have children.

Fibrocystic disease (cystic fibrosis) is an inherited condition in which the mechanical cleansing of the mucous lining of the airways is defective. Dirt, containing microbes, breathed into the lungs in the normal way gets caught and patches of inflammation

result. Owing to the delayed clearance these patches of inflammation heal slowly with scarring and destruction of the alveolar part of the lung. This scarring makes the lung less able to withstand future infections, and progressive lung damage occurs. The condition affects other parts of the body, particularly the pancreas, and can cause death in childhood. Careful management with a special diet and help with chest infections now means that sufferers live into adulthood but may still be unable to have children.

Chronic bronchitis Regular cigarette smoking also produces a disturbance of mucus clearance from the bronchi very like fibrocystic disease. Irritants which are present in all forms of smoke (smoke from domestic chimneys, motor vehicles, and factories as well as from cigarettes) cause an extra outpouring of mucus from the cells in the lining of the airway. At first this is brought up by the cilia and swallowed. But after a time the patient has to cough it up to clear it, especially in the mornings in order to clear the night's accumulation. Coughing is inefficient and at this stage blockage of small airways with excess of mucus occurs from time to time. Inhaled dirt and microbes are eventually caught behind such a block and a patch of inflammation develops. This is particularly

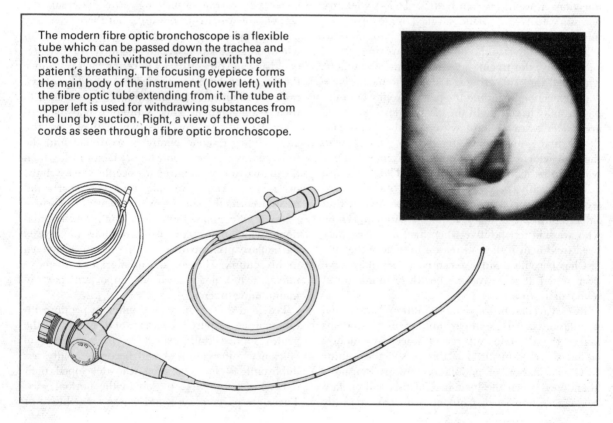

The modern fibre optic bronchoscope is a flexible tube which can be passed down the trachea and into the bronchi without interfering with the patient's breathing. The focusing eyepiece forms the main body of the instrument (lower left) with the fibre optic tube extending from it. The tube at upper left is used for withdrawing substances from the lung by suction. Right, a view of the vocal cords as seen through a fibre optic bronchoscope.

liable to occur as a result of an otherwise trivial chest infection or during a period of cold weather with high atmospheric pollution. Certain bacteria take advantage of the damage to the lung-clearing mechanism and become invaders. The body builds up an immunity to these organisms so that there is not an active inflammation all the time, but only when an extra load is put on the defence system. This condition of reduced defence against infection with narrowed swollen air passages is called chronic bronchitis. It comes on gradually over the years and is often referred to quite rightly as smoker's cough. Eventually the sufferer notices a cough with sputum and breathlessness on exertion, and an increasing tendency to have trouble with chest illnesses each winter. Even without the intervention of other diseases such as lung cancer, bronchitis caused 28.2 million days off work and 23,000 deaths in England in 1975. Dust and chemicals inhaled at work are relatively trivial contributors to the disease. As atmospheric pollution and cigarette smoking are the main causes of chronic bronchitis, sickness and death from this disease are largely preventable.

Pneumonia means inflammation of the lung. There are several varieties, see chapter 2.

Pleurisy When exposed to infection the pleura may become inflamed. In dry pleurisy the inflamed membranes rub together causing a sharp chest pain aggravated by breathing, and the doctor may hear with his stethoscope a rough scraping sound. In pleurisy with effusion, the two layers are separated by liquid so there is no pain, but there are likely to be other features such as fever or shortness of breath. Pleurisy is a common accompaniment of pneumonia and is sometimes caused by tuberculosis.

Infections in patients with weakened defences
Patients undergoing major surgical operations or who spend a long period of unconsciousness as a result of illness or injury are particularly liable to develop pneumonia. This is because the reflex mechanism which prevents food, drink, saliva, and so on from getting into the lung ("going down the wrong way") is out of action. The defences of the lungs are incapable of dealing with repeated inhalation of infected material from the mouth and throat even with the help of antibiotics. Therefore patients in this condition have to be barrier nursed, by which every possible precaution is taken to prevent virulent microbes reaching the patient.

The same situation arises in patients who have lost the ability to make the antibodies and the cells to cope with infections. Patients with leukaemia, aplastic anaemia, or who are receiving large doses of cortisone or other drugs which interfere with the immune system are at risk. Because of the failure of the immune system any microbe, even yeasts and fungi which are normally harmless, can invade the tissues and cause a fatal infection. Again antibiotics are of only temporary value. Treatment with drugs that may affect the immunity mechanisms is kept as short as possible and when the patients are most at risk they are kept in hospital in special isolation cubicles and allowed no visitors. After organ transplant, treatment with this sort of isolation may be needed for several weeks. When the treatment has stopped or the dosage of drugs has been reduced, the patient gradually recovers the ability to deal with infections, but the recovery may never be complete.

Lung abscess Sometimes a localized area of lung (a segment) becomes damaged and then infected. This can happen if the airway gets blocked, for instance by choking over a peanut, or a broken tooth, or other foreign material which drops down the trachea and lodges in one of the branches of the bronchial tree. It can also happen when the blood supply to part of the lung gets blocked by a clot (an embolus) or when cancer interferes with both the airway and the blood supply. Such a localized area of damage leads to complete destruction of a piece of lung and the formation of a hole (an abscess cavity) full of foul debris. This condition used to happen quite often before antibiotics were available and when medicines to suppress cough and pain were more widely used than they are now. In those days it was sometimes necessary to perform an operation to drain the contents of the abscess through the chest wall. With the correct treatment lung abscesses now usually drain into the airways and the contents are coughed up. The abscess heals leaving a scar, but the patient has permanently lost a piece of lung.

Allergies

See chapter 21 for a detailed account of allergy.

Asthma

If protein-containing dust gets into the lung the inflammation produced by the antibody-allergen reaction occurring amongst the cells lining the airways causes:

swelling of the lining
contraction of the special (smooth) muscle in the

wall of the airway

an outpouring of extra mucus

These combine to narrow the airway. The airflow becomes turbulent and noisy (wheezy) and breathing is hard work. It is especially bad during breathing out which normally requires no muscular effort but becomes a conscious hard squeeze in severe asthma.

Children and young adults, especially those who develop eczema and allergy to cow's milk in the first few months of life, may develop seasonal asthma. This coincides with the pollen hay fever season or the kind of dusty activity which causes hay fever. Although these children seem well between acute attacks they may have some trouble all the time and an acute attack may be brought on by exposure to a specific dust (from a horse or a cat) or just by violent exercise when the extra deep breathing brings more dust into contact with the airway lining.

It is relatively easy to determine which dusts are causing the asthma in young people and therefore they can reduce their difficulty either by avoiding the dust or by being desensitized as for hay fever. By contrast when asthma develops in adults (it often comes on in middle age) the relationship between a specific dust and the onset of symptoms is less clear. The trouble may start after an attack of "flu" or just a bad cold. Further attacks may be brought on by minor respiratory infections (colds), by cold foggy weather, or by sudden exertion or excitement. Wheeziness tends to become permanent in people who have had attacks of late onset asthma for some years. Luckier people have one or two spells during the course of a year and are never troubled by it again.

Doctors have tended to regard the asthma of childhood and that of the middle-aged and elderly as two separate diseases. They have called the childhood disease "extrinsic" asthma and have concentrated on looking for specific allergens in the inhaled dusts and treated the patients accordingly. Skin testing and desensitization was widely practised. They regarded the late onset disease as "intrinsic" that is to say some error in the patient making him or her react to all kinds of dusts and therefore not responding to the same treatment as children.

However, in recent years two things have conspired to alter the picture.

Symptomatic or palliative treatment has become much more effective in both groups of patients.

More detailed studies of children and adults reveal that an abnormality of the antibody response is present in all cases so that even in children there is a progressive tendency to react to a wider range of dusts. In adults with late onset disease there is also an element of specific allergy, often to the house dust mite (dermatophagoides – which lives in our bedding) and sometimes to foods and drinks as well.

Although more detailed knowledge of the allergic aspects of asthma has led to the development of more effective and safer vaccines for desensitization, they are still unpredictable in their usefulness in the individual patient and can cause uncomfortable and dangerous reactions. On the other hand the symptomatic or palliative treatments are very effective and although they do not all work in all patients they can be tried out quickly and safely.

Dilator drugs Many different preparations are available as tablets, injections, sprays, powders, or pressurized aerosols. They are drugs which reduce the swelling of the airway lining, relax the smooth muscle in the airway wall, and reduce the outpouring of mucus. Where possible these drugs are applied direct to the lining of the airways (by aerosol). Just enough should be administered leaving as little as possible to upset the workings of other parts of the body.

There are three kinds of dilator groups of drug used for this purpose. All are related to herbal remedies discovered in the Middle Ages. One group is related to belladonna (deadly nightshade), another group is related to ephedrine (which was first extracted from a herb by the Chinese), and the third group is related to the caffeine in coffee. Needless to say the new drugs are far more potent than the old herbal remedies but they have the same mode of action. The most modern derivatives have been selected for their relatively specific action in asthma and their relative lack of effect on other organs. As the drugs in one group have the same general effect it does not help to take two at the same time. But if a drug from one group does not produce adequate relief of symptoms adding one from another group may be helpful.

Sodium cromoglycate and similar compounds Intal was the first of these drugs to be widely used but other compounds are becoming available. Intal is taken as a powder sucked into the airways through a special device. The powder has no untoward effects (except that it makes some people cough). If used regularly and correctly it makes the lining cells unable to react and cause asthma. The drug prevents both constant symptoms and acute attacks in a proportion of asthmatics. It is of no value once an acute attack has started because the airways are too narrow to allow the powder to reach the relevant cells.

Cortisone and related compounds The body controls its response to infections and injuries by varying the

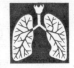

level of cortisol (the natural cortisone) in the blood. The cortisol is produced and stored in the adrenal glands and is released in response to chemical signals from the pituitary gland. If the body seems to be endangering its survival by too dramatic a response to a crisis (as happens in severe attacks of asthma called status asthmaticus) then the extra cortisol produced from the adrenal blocks the chain of reactions in the tissues which cause inflammation, swelling, narrowing of the airways, and fever. By administering cortisone or similar synthetic compounds it is possible to supplement the damping effect of the body's cortisol in asthma. But as in the case of the dilator drugs these cortisone derivatives have effects on all parts of the body which are not appropriate and can be harmful. Therefore, the dose of the drug must be kept to a minimum if possible by inhaling it. As in the case of the dilator drugs inhalation may be impossible during a severe attack. It is then necessary to give the cortisone by mouth or by intravenous injection to get it to the airway lining cells in the emergency.

Cortisone derivatives are used both for the treatment of acute attacks and in the control of continued asthma when the other drugs (the dilators and cromoglycate) are insufficient.

Unless the long-term use is carefully supervised and the dose kept to a minimum serious changes may occur in other parts of the body.

The dose of cortisone or its derivatives must be increased to cope with any operation, accident, or illness because the body loses its ability to respond to an emergency.

In the year 1974 there were 1,086 deaths due to asthma. These deaths were more frequent in women than men and the peak incidence is between the age of 60 and 74. Only 68 deaths occurred in the under 20's age group.

Organic dust diseases

In addition to hay fever and asthma there are a number of illnesses due to inhalation of particular dusts. Apart from byssinosis in flax workers most of these diseases have been recognized only recently and they are usually named after the occupation which causes the dust (farmer's lung, pigeon fancier's lung) or the material from which the dust arises (bagassosis, from handling bagasse which is the fibrous pulp left after molasses has been squeezed out of sugar cane). Truly allergic persons cannot work in these dusty environments because of the immediate symptoms of hay fever or asthma. Those who are able to work may

cough at the beginning of each working day, but have no other symptoms until they have been at the job for many years. Then on a Monday or the first day back after a holiday they notice gradually increasing weakness, sweating, tightness in the chest and then breathlessness. They may have to go home early but feel all right next day and can work without trouble for the rest of the week. The symptoms return with increasing severity on subsequent Mondays, extending to other days until some years later they occur every working day and retirement is necessary.

In farmers similar symptoms occur when they open bales of hay that have become mouldy. If this is not an everyday procedure the farmer may develop an acute severe illness requiring admission to hospital. Pigeon fanciers may notice minor symptoms for years especially when handling birds in the loft as they return from a long race. Then for no obvious reason they develop progressive breathlessness and (like the farmers) have abnormal shadows in their lungs on X-ray.

It is characteristic of this group of illnesses that there is a delay, usually of many years, during which repeated exposure causes trivial or no symptoms. Then when serious symptoms develop there is a delay of several hours between the exposure to the dust and the onset of symptoms. For instance workers exposed to a certain cedar wood dust during the day get the breathlessness in the night, just as exposure to certain isocyanate paints during the day may cause breathlessness in the night. Although the symptoms may resemble asthma serious lung damage is likely. The problem arises deep down in the lung in the small airways and alveoli. Here the cells react and their swelling fills the air space and prevents the oxygen reaching the blood. If no further exposure to dust is allowed inflammation will subside and the lung will return to normal. But if exposure continues or is repeated the inflammation will gradually increase and give way to scarring which either fills up the air spaces or renders the affected part of the lung so stiff that it cannot be ventilated. The inflammation can be reduced by giving cortisone or one of its derivatives, but this will not prevent scarring from occurring. It is very important that patients with this kind of illness should keep away from further exposure to avoid permanent damage with commensurate shortening of life. This is particularly true for the illness due to keeping pigeons.

Sarcoidosis There are a number of diseases causing inflammation of the lung which sometimes persist for long enough to leave scars. Bacterial or virus infection can be the cause but there are also those illnesses which have some of the features of an infection and some of the features of an allergy. The exact cause is not known, the severity of the illness varies very much from individual to individual and cortisone or its derivatives produce a temporary improvement. Sarcoidosis affects other parts of the body (the skin, the lymph nodes, liver, spleen, eyes) as well as the lung. The patient may notice painless red lumps on the legs and a little tiredness and may be unaware of any other trouble. X-rays show little nodules of inflammation in the lungs and enlargement of the lymph nodes in the centre of the chest. Damage to other organs may be revealed by blood tests or by taking a small piece of tissue for examination under the microscope. In most people the inflammation subsides leaving no detectable scarring after a few months. If the trouble is slow in clearing or seems to be spreading to interfere with the working of the lungs or other organs then treatment is needed.

Similar but more diffuse inflammation and scarring of the lower part of the lungs can occur in people with rheumatoid arthritis or cirrhosis of the liver. But the diffuse damage can also be cryptogenic (this means that the cause has not yet been found). This cryptogenic disease tends to produce permanent damage to the lungs in spite of treatment, and the outlook is poor.

Toxic chemicals and dusts

Some of the earliest illnesses recognized as related to occupation (miner's phthisis, potter's asthma) were due to dust and vapours inhaled into the lungs. Mercury poisoning suffered by those who gilded silver using amalgam was, for instance, due to inhalation of the mercury vapour. However, there were other occupational diseases due to the conditions of work which encouraged the spread of infections like tuberculosis, either because of overcrowding or the communal use of blow pipes as in glass blowers. Improved conditions at work which have occurred in the last hundred years have matched better housing and sanitation and have removed most of the infections related to occupation. Vapours and gases have also ceased to be an important problem. Those which cause coughing, sneezing, and running of the eyes and nose are socially unacceptable at a level which might have led to lung disease with prolonged exposure. Those which do not cause this local irritation are usually absorbed through the lungs into the blood. They tend to cause damage to the nervous system or other organs rather than the lung.

Dusts which are filtered off by the nose and by the mucous lining of the airways are usually rendered harmless. The dusts of animal and vegetable origin may cause allergic illnesses.

There remain the chemical and mineral dusts which are so fine that they pass through the filter system of the airways and reach the alveoli. Here if they are not too small they will settle on the walls of the alveoli. There is a range of particle sizes which can cause disease in this way, between 0.1 μ and 3 μ in diameter (1/10,000 of a millimetre and 3/1,000 of a millimetre) for rounded particles and a slightly wider range for fragments of fibres. The particles which are retained in the lungs are very small, too small to be seen by the naked eye and many are too small for the ordinary microscope. An electron microscope is needed to get a clear view of these particles. Particles even smaller than 0.1 μ in diameter may be present in the air we breathe in but cause no harm because they remain suspended in the air and do not have time to fall onto the walls of the alveoli before they are carried out when we breath out again.

Silica and asbestos The two most important toxic dusts are silica and asbestos. They are toxic because they damage the cells whose job it is to remove dust from the alveoli. These cells are called macrophages which normally collect the dust, move up into the airways, are carried up to the larynx, and are then swallowed with the dust particles still in them.

Silica dust damages these macrophages so that they move into the tissue of the lung and die. This releases the silica particles which are thought to be taken up by a succession of macrophages which die in turn releasing substances which lead to inflammation and a scar. The disease silicosis is due to the presence in the lungs of large numbers of little collections of silica dust surrounded by hard lumps of scar tissue. At first, although these scars can be seen on the X-ray the affected person notices no ill effect, but as the scars grow and join together the lungs become stiff, and breathing becomes harder work and less efficient. Once in, silica dust cannot be removed and as the scarring tends to be progressive it is not safe to allow people to work with silica so long that they develop X-ray changes. Any job which involves cutting, drilling, grinding, or milling rock carries with it the production of fine particles of silica which are potentially harmful to the lungs. It is now the practice to prevent the dust getting into the air as far as possible by doing these jobs wet, or by keeping the dust from the worker by good ventilation. Filter masks are too uncomfortable to wear except as a temporary measure. The air that workers breathe where there is a risk of silicosis is normally analysed regularly to ensure that the amount of fine (respirable) silica in the dust is below the safety limit. Other dusts present with silica (as in coal workers dealing with the rock above and below the coal seams, and slate and kaolin workers) may modify the effect of the silica dust so that different safety standards may have to be applied in each situation. Silica dust does not cause cancer but it may modify the course of other lung diseases such as tuberculosis. Pure coal dust causes much less harm than silica and may even reduce the effect of silica inhaled with it. But coal workers exposed to high levels of respirable dust used to get scattered and then coalescent scarring (progressive massive fibrosis) which led to breathlessness and eventually death. Miners in this country are not now permitted such high exposure so that if the periodic chest X-rays do show any changes they can be moved out of the pits and will suffer no serious harm.

Asbestos dust differs from silica in that it is made up of little rods, short fragments of fibres. The thickness, length, and straightness of these rods depend on the kind of asbestos and where it was mined. For many years it was thought to be a safe material and was handled like cotton and flax. However, under those conditions all kinds of asbestos gave rise to enough respirable dust to cause scarring of the lungs, which was sometimes fatal after only fifteen or twenty years working exposure. The mechanism of scarring is similar to silicosis in that the macrophages attempting to remove the rods become damaged and die. The body attempts to make the rods harmless by coating them with a brown crust, but if there is a lot of dust coating is incomplete and scarring occurs. This kind of illness is due to relatively large fibres which can be seen under the ordinary microscope. Reducing the number of these fibres to two fibres per cubic centimetre in the air breathed by workers has greatly reduced the liability to develop asbestosis.

Exposure to asbestos can also cause two forms of cancer. The dust from radioactive ores (radium, uranium) can also cause cancer and so can nickel. But because it has been so widely used and regarded as safe the problem of asbestos cancer has caused a great deal of alarm. Approximately 300 lung cancers and the same number of mesotheliomas (cancers of the pleural membrane) are occurring each year in the British Isles due to exposure to asbestos. The lung cancers result from a combination of cigarette smoking and asbestos dust. Although they occur in workers with insufficient asbestos exposure to cause serious lung scarring, these lung cancers are not expected to continue to be a serious problem for people exposed only to the dust levels now permitted in the industry. They have not been reported in people whose exposure to asbestos has occurred outside their place of work. They would disappear if people exposed to asbestos did not smoke. It is very important for all people with past exposure to asbestos to stop smoking to reduce their risk of lung cancer.

The lung cancers caused by asbestos usually develop in late middle age, even if exposure was started soon after leaving school. These cancers are essentially similar to those induced by cigarette smoke. Mesotheliomas are different, they are not related to cigarette smoke and are extremely rare except in people who have had some exposure to asbestos. The exposure needed can be quite brief (a few months) to dust levels well below that which causes scarring. More prolonged exposure due to living downwind from an asbestos factory where dust suppression was not practised has also caused mesothelioma. Very small fibre particles seem to be the most dangerous. The interval between first exposure and the development of the tumour averages over 40 years in adults. As the exposure has often been brief it is difficult to obtain the details of the kind of asbestos causing the tumour and the level of exposure. A great deal of work is being done at the present time to make it possible to use asbestos commerically without causing this tumour. Usual commercial practice within the official regulations in Britain at the present is thought not to create a risk to the general public. The chief danger remains in the handling and disposal of old insulation material containing amphibole asbestos (crocidolite and amosite). Mesotheliomas are cancers arising not in the lung itself but in the pleura, the space between the lung and the ribs or diaphragm. They can also arise in the space around the intestines (the peritoneum). They are fatal and treatment is aimed at relieving pain and perhaps a little prolongation of life. Mesotheliomas due to exposure to asbestos before the current regulations came into force will continue to occur for the next 30 to 40 years. They will increase in number at first, perhaps for the next fifteen to twenty years and then gradually decline. It is hoped that long before then a satisfactory treatment or, better still, a method of prevention in people already exposed to asbestos will have been discovered. In the meantime, it is essential that workers who may come into contact with this dust are thoroughly protected.

Primary lung cancer

A combination of prolonged heavy exposure to asbestos dust and lifelong cigarette smoking is one of the most likely ways of producing lung cancer. Such cancers develop in well over half of people who have spent their working life in this way. But such heavy asbestos dust exposure no longer occurs. By far the most important factor leading to the 33,000 deaths which occurred in England and Wales in 1974 is cigarette smoking. Reduction in atmospheric pollution in towns and cities, and the removal of occupational causes might reduce this by about a fifth, to 26,000. Removal of cigarette smoking (provided it was not replaced by some other damaging practice) would reduce these deaths to between one tenth and one twentieth, in other words to less than 3,000 per year. This change would occur quite rapidly and be complete within ten years. Although the total consumption of tobacco and of cigarettes has fallen in the last five years unfortunately the fall has been slight. Its effect may be increased by a change to filtered cigarettes with a relatively low tar content. But the greatest reduction in cigarette smoking has been in elderly men, members of the professions. Manual workers of all ages have not reduced their smoking, and young men and women of all ages are still increasing their cigarette consumption. The risks of dying of lung cancer have levelled off, falling a little in men, but still rising in women.

Cancer of the lung is usually fatal. Although the cancer starts in the lung and could be removed by operation or suppressed by X-ray treatment, it has usually spread to other parts of the body before the patient consults the doctor or even realizes that he or she is ill. Less than one in five reach the hospital at a stage when the disease seems curable and of these less than a quarter are apparently cured by treatment and live more than five years. Very few survive ten years.

The patient may first complain of a cough, especially a cough with streaks of blood in the sputum, and breathlessness or pain on breathing. These are the symptoms caused by the growth in the lung. However, it is equally likely that the patient's complaint arises from the spread of the growth to other parts of the body. Muscular weakness, tiredness, loss of weight, painful swelling of the joints, swelling of the fingertips, bone pain, or even the symptoms of a stroke – each of these can be the first thing that a patient with lung cancer may notice. All these may also develop during the course of the illness.

Some can be helped by surgery, some by X-ray therapy, and some by anticancer (cytotoxic) drugs. But usually the improvement is temporary and sometimes the treatment makes the patient feel worse. Ultimately all the doctor can do is keep the patient as comfortable and painfree as possible with drugs. With such an ugly prospect it is surprising why anyone continues to smoke.

Benign pneumoconiosis

Most of the fine dust that we breathe in and that gets caught in our alveoli is harmless. It is gathered up by the phagocytes and removed completely by the airways and swallowed. However continued exposure to high levels of nontoxic dust can cause problems. The continued heavy use of the dust removal system stimulates the cells concerned to grow, just as hard work makes muscles grow. This leads to an increased production of mucus and of cells coming up the airways which may be more than the cilia can cope with. Secretions may collect and have to be brought up by coughing. In other words excessive prolonged exposure to any dust can cause the changes of chronic bronchitis. Although this is normally reversible when exposure ceases, it can nevertheless cause permanent difficulties in people who have asthma and in people who smoke.

Overloading the system can also cause the dust to accumulate in the lung. As in the toxic dust diseases the phagocytes loaded with dust fail to reach the airways. They either lodge in the tissues around the openings of the airways or get carried from there along the lymphatics to the pleura or to the nodes near the centre of the chest. Here they remain for life, occupying space but causing no active harm. They may show up on X-rays and lead to a mistaken diagnosis of more serious chest disease. Heavy nontoxic dust exposure may overload the system and interfere with the clearance of what might otherwise be trivial levels of toxic dust, as well as increasing the effects of cigarette smoking and other types of atmospheric pollution on the lung.

Ageing

The main effect of ageing on the lung is the loss of its elasticity. The cells forming the alveoli and the airways are supported on a framework of elastic fibres which are capable of stretching nearly half as much again as their resting length. When we breathe in, we use the muscles in the chest and diaphragm to stretch the elastic fibres and make room for the air to rush in.

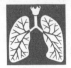

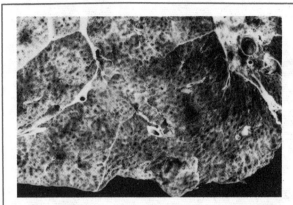 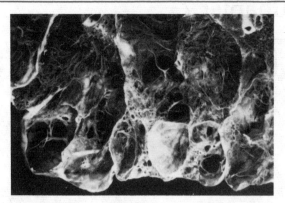

Left, a section of normal lung. The air-containing cavities (alveoli) are very small and very numerous. Right, a section taken from the lung of a patient with severe emphysema, showing fewer, but much larger cavities. In this condition, although the lungs contain more air, the surfaces for exchange of oxygen and carbon dioxide are much diminished.

When breathing out we simply allow the fibres to contract and blow the air out. The fibres do this while still supporting the airways and keeping them open. Elastic fibres are used all over the body and are formed while we are still growing. Few, if any, useful elastic fibres seem to be produced after about the age of twenty, by which time the ones present at birth are beginning to wear out. They continue to wear out and break as the years pass and lead to a loss of elasticity in the lungs as well as in the skin, giving rise gradually to the appearances of old age. This process seems to occur at a constant rate which varies from individual to individual (it is part of the pattern we inherit) and seems to be unaffected by illnesses. Within the lung this ageing process has two serious effects on function so that the maximum capacity of the lung to take in oxygen and remove carbon dioxide is reduced year by year.

The effects are firstly the breakage of alveolar walls leading to the formation of larger spaces, fewer partitions and therefore a smaller area of contact between the air and the blood. Secondly there is loss of the elastic recoil. Although this makes the work of breathing in less, the older subject has to do more of the work of breathing out. The lungs themselves no longer contract, the muscles of the chest wall and diaphragm must work to squeeze the air out. During this process, the airways which are no longer held open by the elastic framework of the lung tend to collapse and make it even more difficult to push the air out. This condition is called emphysema.

Viewed against this background of age change, lung diseases take on a more complex pattern. For instance in childhood before the lung is fully grown the airways are narrow and block easily. Inflammation of the airways whether due to infection or allergy (asthma) can produce illnesses of dramatic severity with equally dramatic recovery compared with the same illness in the adult. The elderly person with emphysema is also more vulnerable than the younger adult. He not only has airways which become blocked easily on breathing out but he is short of spare alveolar capacity. His filter system is defective so that infections of the airways are more likely to spread down into the alveolar part of the lung causing pneumonia (bronchopneumonia).

Chronic bronchitics and asthmatics already have narrowing of their airways due to swelling and scarring of the lining and the contraction of the muscle coat. This narrowing adds to that due to ageing and increases the speed of loss of function with age. The rate of loss of function in cigarette smokers is two to four times as rapid as in nonsmokers because of this effect on the airways. The point at which the lungs will no longer permit physical exertion and the point of no return are achieved at a younger age. Any illness which leaves a scar, whether it is a severe episode of pneumonia which does not resolve completely, the loss of a piece of lung because of blocking of the airway with a foreign body, delay in the treatment of tuberculosis or the result of exposure to dust, will reduce the reserves of useful lung tissue. Although they may not affect the rate at which the remaining lung tissue ages, nevertheless loss of useful lung continues relentlessly in the normal areas and the point at which there is not enough left to live on is reached that much sooner.

153

Chapter 7
The nervous system

Revised by C. J. Earl, MD FRCP

All that we know and remember about the world around us is brought to our consciousness by body cells that specialize in communication. These cells are collectively known as the nervous system. They carry messages which move muscles or give meaning to the printed page. They also regulate many automatic activities, such as the heartbeat and intestines, mechanisms of which we are not conscious. These cells, organized to form the nervous system, make up an elaborate mechanism similar to a computer, but much more complex than the largest electronic computer. The white cordlike structure which the anatomist calls a nerve consists of bundles of hundreds or thousands of individual nerve fibres. Sometimes the word nerves has been applied to emotional states (a nervous man) but this has nothing to do with what is being discussed here.

The nerve unit

The nerve cell consists of a cell body from which slender projections reach out. One of these is often longer than the others and may be many feet long. It is known as the axon and usually conducts impulses away from the cell body. The shorter projections are called dendrites and accept impulses from other nerve cells which are transmitted by means of special points of contact known as synapses. Some dendrites may be very long, for example, the long dendrite in a sensory nerve may start several feet from the spinal cord. The complete unit of cell body, axon, and dendrites is called a neuron.

Most nerve fibres are covered by a sheath of white fatty material called myelin. The white matter of nerve tissue largely consists of myelin-covered fibres, and the grey matter is composed of cell bodies and dendrites. Myelin acts partly as an insulator to prevent impulses jumping from one nerve fibre to another, but it is also essential for normal conduction, and in fact the thicker the myelin sheath, the more rapidly are the impulses able to travel along the nerve fibre. When the myelin sheath is defective, nerve fibre function is partially or completely lost. In some diseases the primary disturbance is loss of the normal myelin sheath (see demyelinating disorders).

We have billions of neurons – some 12,000 million in the brain alone. This is fortunate, for we cannot grow new nerve cells. The number we now have is the most we will ever have. Some are bound to be lost by the wear and tear of living. An elderly person has many fewer neurons than in youth, but the original supply was so generous that thousands can be lost without great impairment of function, provided that the losses are scattered and not concentrated into a particular nerve centre or tract. A limited amount of nerve repair is possible.

All the metabolic processes of a neuron are controlled by the cell body. If a nerve fibre is cut or injured, the part attached to the cell body remains alive, but the part beyond the injury gradually withers away. Sometimes the live part can extend itself through the withered component to reach its original destination and restore function. In favourable situations severed nerves can be rejoined by surgery. This can be done only with nerve tracts that can be reached by the surgeon. Many unfortunately can not, and in the central nervous system (brain and spinal cord) regeneration does not occur.

A midline section through the brain

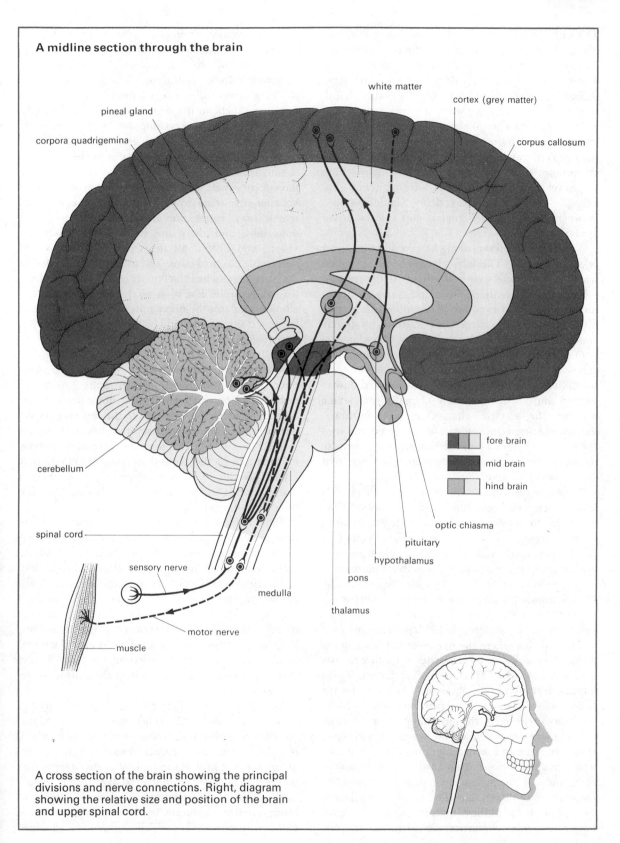

white matter

cortex (grey matter)

pineal gland

corpus callosum

corpora quadrigemina

fore brain

mid brain

hind brain

cerebellum

optic chiasma

pituitary

hypothalamus

spinal cord

pons

sensory nerve

thalamus

medulla

motor nerve

muscle

A cross section of the brain showing the principal
divisions and nerve connections. Right, diagram
showing the relative size and position of the brain
and upper spinal cord.

Chapter 7 The nervous system

The nerve impulse A nerve is not like a wire and what travels over it is not ordinary electricity. Neurons do not make direct contact with each other. There are countless breaks along pathways that nerve messages travel. Electricity, on the other hand, travels over a continuous wire, at a speed of 186,000 miles a second. The greatest speed at which nerve impulses travel in the human body is somewhat more than 200 miles an hour. This is quite fast, but far from instantaneous. It means that our nervous reactions are never immediate, even in an emergency. For example, there is a short delay (latent period) between seeing a traffic signal at stop and the driver applying the brakes.

Nerve impulses travel along a nerve fibre by a sort of chain reaction. This is an electrochemical process which is now quite well understood. It depends on movements of ions backwards and forwards across membranes of a nerve fibre. The inside of a resting fibre is negatively charged, the outside, positively charged. This is caused by the relative abundance of potassium ions in the interior and sodium ions in the exterior. Activity of a neuron changes the permeability of the membranes, with an inward flow of sodium and an outward flow of potassium, which reverses the electric charge. Almost instantly, sodium-potassium movements are reversed and so is the electric charge. These alternating movements of molecules across membranes produce currents that cause a nerve impulse.

Thus a nerve impulse is a series of tiny electrical leaks which travel over fibres and are boosted from one point to the next by chains of electrochemical relay stations which give local reinforcement of power. A stimulus either causes a single neuron to discharge or fire, or it does not. Possible communications between individual neurons are virtually infinite in number, since the cells are not physically attached to each other. These loose connections permit millions of different switching arrangements.

The junction where the fine terminal branches of an axon come close to the dendrites of another neuron is called a synapse. There is no direct contact. An impulse is transmitted from axon to dendrite by the action of a chemical intermediary (transmitter substance) released at the terminal part of the axon. One of these is the chemical known as acetylcholine. However, excessive accumulation of acetylcholine would make it impossible for further transmission to occur and so the acetylcholine is quickly destroyed by the enzyme cholinesterase. The paralyzing effect of nerve gases is due to their property of preventing the normal action of cholinesterase. At some synapses, other chemical substances act as transmitters. One of these is dopamine, lack of which is important in the production of the neurological symptoms of Parkinson's disease (paralysis agitans).

There is no difference whatever between nerve impulses except in frequencies per second. There is not a special kind of nerve impulse for seeing, another for hearing, or another for smelling or tasting. If some incredibly mischievous rerouting of nerve pathways should occur, we would perhaps be able to hear a flavour or smell a sunset. Something of this sort occasionally arises from lesions in nervous tissues which may cause unreal but vividly perceived sensations, and there are hallucinations of taste, vision, and indeed all the senses, which have no detectable physical basis. The pins and needles felt in the little finger when the "funny bone" is knocked are a good example. The blow on the ulnar nerve at the elbow stimulates the nerve fibres but the sensation is felt not at the site of the blow but far away where the fibres originate.

Input and output pathways Different neurons have certain differences in structure. A major distinction is between sensory and motor nerve tracts. Sensory nerves carry impulses to the central nervous system, and motor nerves carry impulses away from it to effect action. Thus a sensory nerve tract carries the information to the central nervous system that a finger is resting on a hot stove and the motor nerves cause muscles to contract which will withdraw the hand from danger.

Some nerve tracts are composed entirely of motor or sensory fibres, but others contain both kinds. Cell bodies of sensory nerves lie just outside the spinal cord, and those of motor nerves within it. From these cell bodies fibres run out to connect with distant body tissues, muscles, organs, glands, blood vessels, skin, eyes, ears, and so on. The finely branched end of a motor neuron fibre which connects with muscle fibre is called an end plate. Outlying endings of sensory neurons connect with a variety of receptor organs, such as pain receivers in the skin or the light sensitive cells in the eye.

Communications between sensory and motor nerve fibres and cell bodies may involve many complex links within the spinal cord and the brain. A red light at a street corner does not produce an automatic and inbuilt mechanism of the body to put on the brakes. The fact that a red light means "stop" has been learnt. A visual impression of colour must be interpreted by the brain before impulses are channelled to motor nerves which activate leg and foot

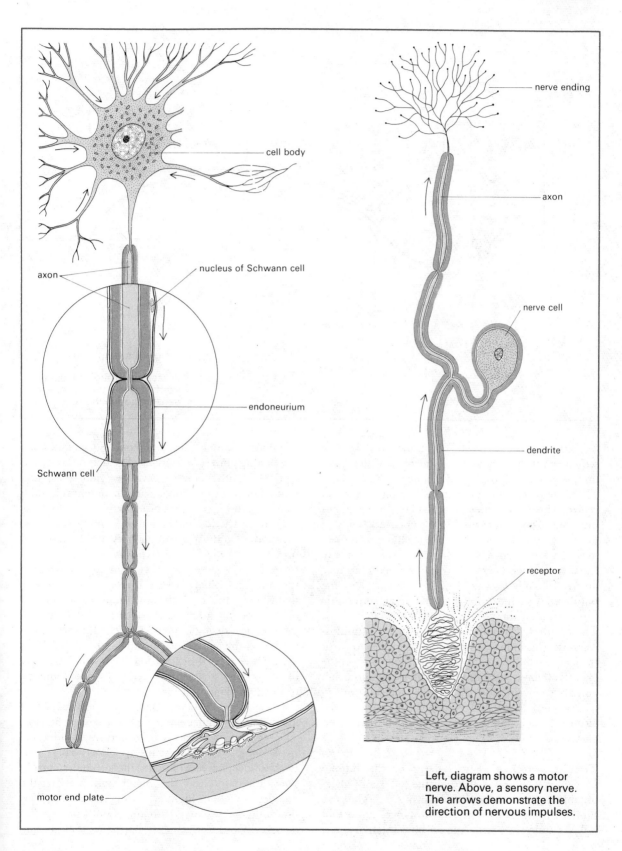

cell body

axon

nucleus of Schwann cell

endoneurium

Schwann cell

motor end plate

nerve ending

axon

nerve cell

dendrite

receptor

Left, diagram shows a motor nerve. Above, a sensory nerve. The arrows demonstrate the direction of nervous impulses.

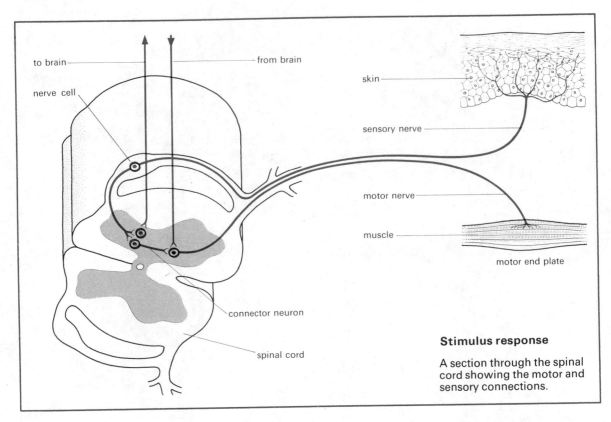

to brain

from brain

nerve cell

skin

sensory nerve

motor nerve

muscle

motor end plate

connector neuron

spinal cord

Stimulus response

A section through the spinal cord showing the motor and sensory connections.

muscles that push down the brake pedal. The sequence involves thousands of neurons which steer impulses in the appropriate directions.

The simplest "stimulus-response" circuit is a spinal reflex. This is an action in which the brain is not involved. A familiar example is the knee jerk reflex. A tap just below the kneecap of one leg hanging loosely over the other sends a stimulus over sensory nerve tracts to the spinal cord where motor nerves produce an irresistible jerk of the leg. In the same way the pupil reflex of the eye brings about an automatic constriction of the pupil when a light shines on it. There are also more complicated "stimulus-response" reactions, as when an object flies towards the face and the arm automatically rises to protect the eyes. Examining various reflexes gives the physician valuable information about the localization of neurological disorders. To use the terminology of the electrical engineer, they are used to test different circuits.

Traffic switches Few reflexes of the human nervous system are as simple as the reflexes of lower organisms which do a great deal of the organism's thinking for it. There are, for instance, important reflexes concerned with human bowel activity, but

emotions, training, social taboos, and conditioning can modify pure reflex actions. The nervous system is equipped with countless switches, junctions, and evaluation centres which, with incomparable skill, channel constant streams of nerve impulses towards the proper decision and action. It should be obvious, therefore, that drawings of the nervous system which present a schema of the pathways of major nerve tracts are, in a sense, deceptively simple. Drawings of the brain and spinal cord and their nerve connections to the body can show little more than a master plan of nervous organization. It must be remembered that infinite networks of finely branched nerve fibres permeate the entire body and control actions as minutely exact as the expansion or constriction of tiny blood vessels, so fine that red cells must squeeze through them in single file.

It would be a mistake to think of the nervous system as an entirely independent electrical switchboard. The central nervous system and the endocrine (hormone-producing) systems are closely associated. For instance, nerves stimulate the adrenal glands to pour adrenalin into the blood and prepare the muscles for fight or flight according to an order from the brain when danger threatens. But some special nerve cells also secrete neuro-hormones that in some respects act like adrenalin. We may think of the nervous system as a rapidly acting electrical system, and hormones as a more deliberately acting chemical system, not independent but complementary, working in intricate coordination for our welfare.

The central nervous system

The brain and the spinal cord are together known as the central nervous system. The spinal cord is a soft column of nerve tissue continuous with the lower part of the brain and enclosed in the bony vertebral column. Except for the twelve pairs of cranial nerves which connect directly with the brain, all the nerves of the body (spinal nerves) enter or leave the spinal cord through openings between the vertebrae. The cord is a slightly flattened cylinder, a little wider from side to side than front to back, about 2 cm ($\frac{3}{4}$ in) thick and 43 cm (17 in) long. All the functions of the body depend upon the integrity of this intricate mass of cord tissue which weighs only 42·5 gm ($1\frac{1}{2}$ oz). A cross section of the spinal cord reveals white tissue on the outside and a grey H-shaped mass in the centre. The tips of the H, which is composed of nerve cell bodies, are called the anterior and posterior horns. Paralysis and wasting (atrophy) of muscles result if nerve cells of the anterior horns are attacked or destroyed by disease, such as poliomyelitis. Sensory impulses enter the cord on its posterior aspect and travel up in the white fibre tracts to the brain, or enter the grey matter of the cord to trigger a reflex response at the same level.

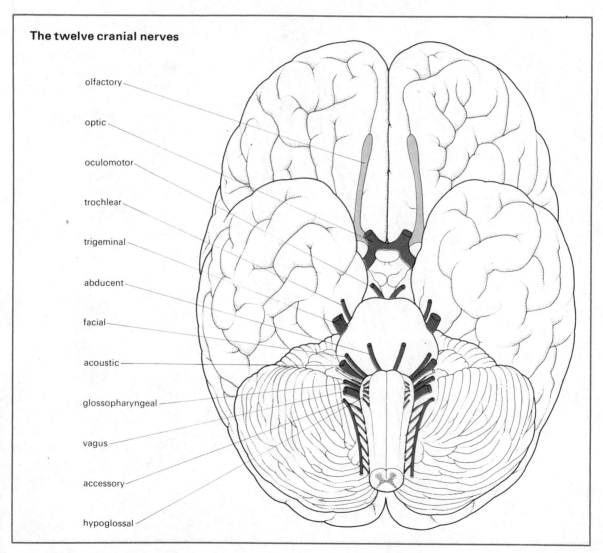

The twelve cranial nerves

olfactory
optic
oculomotor
trochlear
trigeminal
abducent
facial
acoustic
glossopharyngeal
vagus
accessory
hypoglossal

The central and peripheral nervous systems

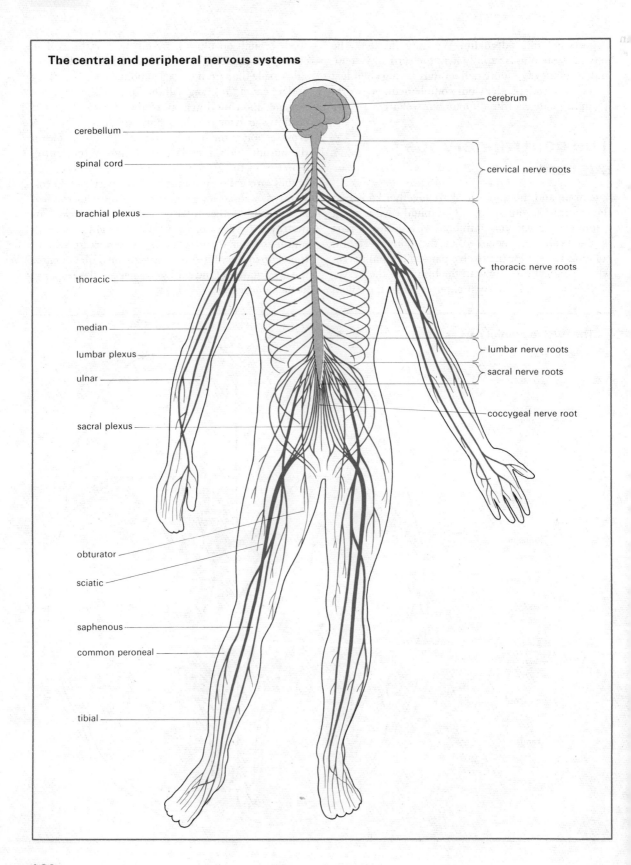

cerebellum

spinal cord

brachial plexus

thoracic

median

lumbar plexus

ulnar

sacral plexus

obturator

sciatic

saphenous

common peroneal

tibial

cerebrum

cervical nerve roots

thoracic nerve roots

lumbar nerve roots

sacral nerve roots

coccygeal nerve root

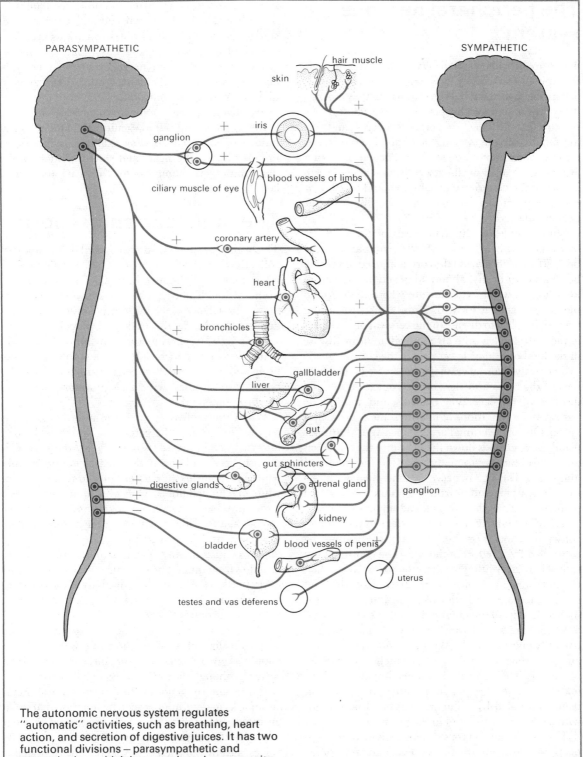

The autonomic nervous system regulates "automatic" activities, such as breathing, heart action, and secretion of digestive juices. It has two functional divisions — parasympathetic and sympathetic — which in general produce opposite and counterbalancing effects as the needs of the body demand.

Chapter 7 The nervous system

The peripheral nervous system

There are 31 pairs of spinal nerves which emerge from the spinal cord. They are named and numbered according to the vertebral level at which they emerge. They are a part of the peripheral nervous system which also includes the cranial nerves and the autonomic nervous system. Each spinal nerve divides into two roots, motor and sensory. The sensory root is attached to a small swelling, a collection of nerve cells known as the posterior root ganglion, and here lie the cell bodies of the primary sensory fibres in the peripheral nerve.

Spinal nerves at different levels of the cord are concerned with activities of different parts of the body. If a specific part of the cord is injured, there will be characteristically abnormal reactions to neurological tests, which will indicate where the diseased part of the cord is located. If an arm is weak and wasted, it points to disease in the cervical or neck part of the cord. If a leg is involved, it will indicate disease in the lumbosacral or lower part of the cord.

The twelve pairs of cranial nerves arise in the lower part of the brain and they branch out to supply the muscles of the face and eyeballs and to provide pathways for sensations of hearing, smell, taste, and vision. One of the cranial nerves, the vagus (Latin for wandering) extends down the neck into the abdomen and sends branches to many organs in the chest and abdomen. The vagus nerve is concerned with the rate of breathing and heartbeat, and the motility and gland secretion of the stomach and small intestine.

The heart muscle does not contract in response to conscious effort nor can its rate of beating be controlled by an effort of the will. The control of the rate of cardiac beating is carried out by what is called the autonomic nervous system. It controls this and other automatic activities of some internal organs such as activity of the intestinal canal or sweat glands. Some organs, such as the urinary bladder, though basically under control of the autonomic system, have an overriding control system which is normally voluntary. The control of another important automatic function, breathing, is different yet again, being controlled by ordinary peripheral nerves but with a central control unit in the brain stem.

The autonomic nervous system is divided into two parts – the sympathetic system and the parasympathetic. The two systems work in opposite senses (for example, stimulation of the sympathetic increases heart rate and stimulation of the parasympathetic slows it). Sympathetic nerve trunks lie on either side of the spinal column, connect with spinal nerves, and extend fibres to various organs of the chest and abdomen. Parasympathetic nerves (which include the vagus nerve) originate in the brain and the lower part of the spinal cord. In general, both divisions reach and control the same organs – lungs, heart, liver, spleen, stomach, pancreas, adrenals, kidneys, colon, intestines, genitalia, bladder – but induce opposite effects. For example, sympathetic impulses speed the heart and slow digestion, while parasympathetic impulses slow the heart and stimulate digestion.

The brain and spinal cord

The brain and spinal cord are covered by membranes collectively called meninges (hence, meningitis, inflammation of the membranes). The outer membrane of tough fibrous tissue is known as the dura mater, or often simply the dura. Under this lies a delicate membrane, the arachnoid (Greek for "like a spider's web"). The innermost membrane, the pia mater (or pia), closely follows the contours of the brain and spinal cord. Between the arachnoid and the pia is a space filled with a clear watery fluid, the cerebrospinal fluid.

When the skull is opened, the most conspicuous part of the brain is the cerebrum, which is divided into two hemispheres. Its outer layer, the cortex, is pinkish grey and the underlying structure mainly white in colour because it contains large numbers of white myelinated fibres, while grey matter contains a larger number of nerve cell bodies and short fibres. Deeper again inside the white matter lie more masses of grey matter known as the basal ganglia. White matter consists mainly of conducting tissue, carrying impulses from the cerebrum to the spinal cord and the lower parts of the brain, from one part of the cortex to another and from one cerebral hemisphere to its fellow on the opposite side.

The fissures, infoldings, and convolutions of the cerebrum slightly resemble those of a walnut. These infoldings greatly increase the surface area of the cortex. Although the folds may seem haphazard, they are quite uniform in normal brains and serve as useful landmarks in determining specific functional areas of the brain, such as those for speech, vision, and hearing. A deep vertical fissure divides the cerebrum into two halves, a right and a left hemisphere. The right hemisphere controls the left side of the body, and vice versa.

A great deal is known about the function of specific parts of the cerebral cortex, and although there is much overlapping of various functional areas, some areas are specially concerned with certain activities. The visual centre is located in the back part of the brain called the occipital lobe. Areas for hearing and smell are located in the temporal lobe at the side of the head. The sensory and motor centres are separated by a well-defined fissure. These centres were often first recognized through symptoms of disorders which affect them, and this special knowledge is helpful in diagnosing obscure neurological complaints and

affords landmarks to the neurosurgeon in locating and removing a brain tumour, an abscess, a bullet, or a clot in the brain. Several other centres of organization lie deep in the cerebral hemisphere. From the evolutionary point of view they are often older than the cerebral cortex although some have developed with it. Some of these are described below.

Thalamus and basal ganglia These are the masses of grey matter which lie deep in the cerebral

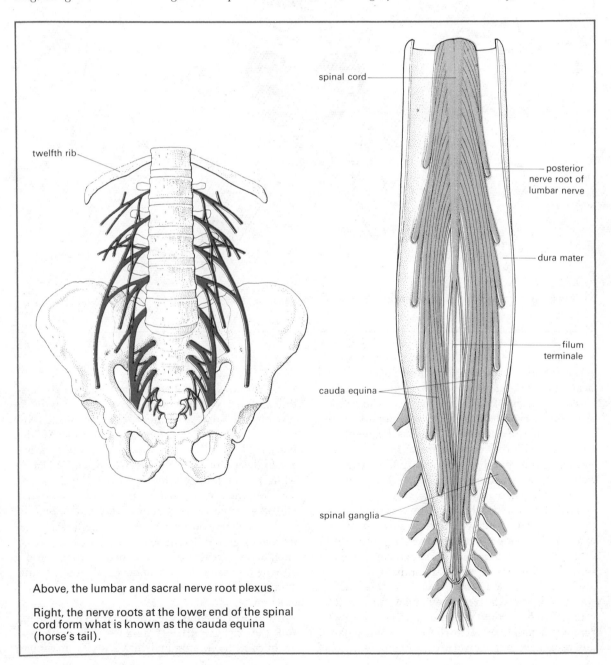

Above, the lumbar and sacral nerve root plexus.

Right, the nerve roots at the lower end of the spinal cord form what is known as the cauda equina (horse's tail).

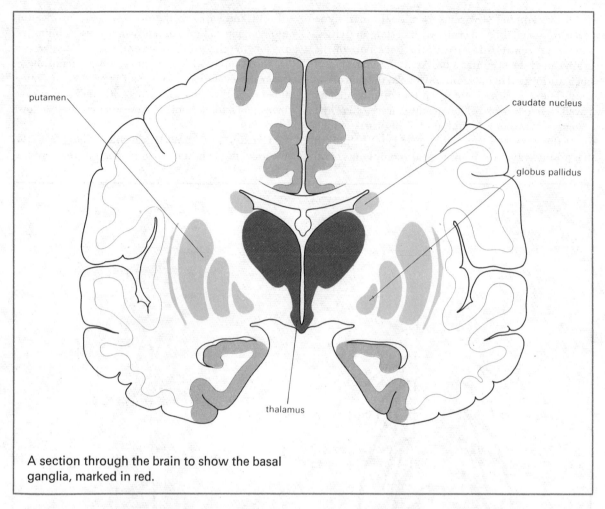

putamen

caudate nucleus

globus pallidus

thalamus

A section through the brain to show the basal ganglia, marked in red.

hemispheres. The thalamus is predominantly a main relay station on the sensory pathways of the body – head and neck, trunk and limbs, on the way to the cerebral cortex. Lesions of the thalamus might therefore be expected to cause loss of sensation on the opposite side of the body. The basal ganglia are concerned with the control of motor function. Their physiology is poorly understood and with the exception of Parkinson's disease (paralysis agitans), disease arising in them is rare.

The white fibre tracts which connect the brain to the spinal cord pass down the brain stem which also contains areas of grey matter. These are the cells of origin of the motor cranial nerves and correspond to the anterior horn cells of the spinal cord. There are also nuclei (that is, collections of cell bodies) concerned with the sensory cranial nerves. The cerebellum lies behind the brain stem and below the cerebral hemispheres. It is concerned with balance and coordination of muscular movement.

Sites of disorder

From knowledge of the structure and function of different parts of the nervous system, it is often possible to judge accurately what is affected by disease. Thus, weakness of the whole of one side of the body is likely to be due to a lesion in the opposite cerebral hemisphere. It may even be possible to know which part of the hemisphere is particularly involved. An abnormal reflex points to trouble along the pathways of nerves that activate the reflex. Spastic (stiff) paralysis and flaccid (flabby) paralysis result from damage at different points of nervous pathways. Inability to speak, or to recognize written words, although spoken words are understood, may indicate damage to those parts of the brain with a specific function.

All spaces around the central nervous system, and the four ventricles (cavities) of the brain, are filled with cerebrospinal fluid. This is very similar to other tissue fluids, but some diseases may cause certain chemical changes in its composition. In the lower back there is room for a needle to be inserted between the vertebrae to withdraw a sample of fluid. Chemical examination of the fluid is often helpful in the diagnosis of disease.

Diagnosis of disorders

The diagnosis of nervous disorders is based firstly upon a comprehensive history of the patient's family, past illnesses, and present symptoms, followed by a neurological examination. This consists of examination of motor power, all forms of sensation, and coordination, supplemented by examination of the eyes and blood pressure. Various investigations may be necessary, such as lumbar puncture, electroencephalogram, and X-rays.

Lumbar puncture is performed by withdrawing a sample of the fluid (cerebrospinal fluid) that surrounds the brain and cord through a needle inserted between the lumbar vertebrae. In disease it may be abnormal in various ways which provide valuable information.

The electroencephalograph is a machine which magnifies and records the minute electric currents given out by the brain cells. Abnormalities of the encephalogram are of diagnostic value, especially in epilepsy.

X-rays of the head will reveal abnormalities of the skull or its contents. Sometimes a dye is injected into the arteries that supply the brain (an angiogram), or air is introduced into the cavities of the brain through a lumbar puncture needle. These tests, which can be very unpleasant for the patient, have been largely superseded by computerized axial tomography. This is an outstanding invention by a British scientist, Godfrey Hounsfield. The pencil-like beams of X-rays rapidly scan the head at a series of angles, the X-ray energy which emerges being measured. The energy varies according to the density of the structures through which the beams have passed. A computer coordinates the results and produces a picture of the tissues within the skull. This test is rapid and harmless.

Brain injuries

Mild brain injuries that cause momentary unconsciousness (concussion) leave no lasting damage to the brain as a rule, although some patients may experience dizziness, nervousness, restlessness, and headache as an aftermath for weeks or months. Loss of consciousness that lasts several minutes or more following a head injury requires medical care. Some injuries, whether the skull is fractured or not, can cause lasting damage to brain tissue and leave persistent defects of neurological function. More severe injuries with haemorrhage and severe brain swelling may be fatal. The majority, however, leave no serious defects.

Intracranial tumours

Because the brain closely fills the compartment of the rigid skull, any added substance inside the skull cavity, whether it is a haemorrhage, inflammation of the brain (encephalitis), swelling of the brain due to injury, or a new growth within the skull, will cause an increase in intracranial pressure. The presence of raised intracranial pressure is always a serious matter, since if it is left untreated it will lead to progressive deterioration of cerebral function and vision, and even death.

There are many types of intracranial tumour. Some arise in particular structures, such as the pituitary gland. Others arise from the meninges which cover the brain. These are benign tumours and provided they are accessible to surgery, they can be completely removed. Other tumours, unfortunately often malignant, arise within the brain substance and can only rarely be completely removed. However their rate of growth is very variable and sometimes even partial removal is followed by years of freedom from symptoms. Radiotherapy is sometimes helpful. Chemotherapy has so far met with little success. Although these tumours arise within the brain substance their origin is not in nerve cells but in the glial cells, which are the supporting tissue for the neurons. Similar tumours may very rarely affect the spinal cord. Both spinal cord and brain may be affected by metastatic tumours, that is, tumours which have spread from a primary tumour at some other site. Tumours of the lung and breast in particular are liable to spread to the brain.

Demyelinating diseases

In this group of diseases, whose cause is usually unknown, the primary disturbance in the nervous system is a loss of the myelin sheaths of nerve fibres. This loss of myelin is often patchy, different parts of the nervous system being affected simultaneously or in succession. Demyelinated nerve fibres lose the power to conduct messages or impulses from the brain to the muscles, as well as messages of touch, pain, vision, and hearing to the brain. As a result there may be paralysis or numbness in an arm or leg, or unsteady gait, blindness, and loss of bladder and bowel control.

Multiple sclerosis is the commonest of this group of diseases. It may involve any part of the brain, spinal cord or the optic nerves, with patchy demyelination, and is characterized by varying paralysis, numbness, blindness, unsteady gait, impairment of speech, and mental changes. It usually begins during the early years of life, most often between 20 and 30 years of age. The first sign of illness may be the sudden paralysis of a leg, or half of the body, or the sudden loss of vision in one eye. This may persist and slowly progress to other symptoms, but usually the first symptoms disappear within weeks or months, only to recur over the course of some years with a succession of the same or other symptoms in various parts of the body. The disappearance of symptoms is referred to as a remission and the reappearance as a relapse. These remissions and relapses may spread over a period of five, ten, or more years, after which there is a tendency towards steady progression of the disease, until partial or total invalidism ensues, although occasionally the condition may be very mild. There is as yet no specific treatment nor any means of prevention, although at the present time there is a great deal of research going on into the disease.

Amyotrophic lateral sclerosis This illness differs from multiple sclerosis in that the nerve degeneration is not diffusely spread out through the entire nervous system, but involves only the cell bodies of the motor nerves, with subsequent degeneration in the motor tracts of the spinal cord and the motor roots of the peripheral nerves. This in turn causes a slowly progressive paralysis and wasting (atrophy) of muscles on both sides of the body, sometimes more on one side than on the other. The hands often show the first signs of wasting and weakness, and later the legs are affected. There is no loss of sensation. The disease is progressive and untreatable.

Infections of the nervous system

Infection may involve the brain, the spinal cord, or the peripheral nerves. Infection of the brain is called encephalitis, while infection of the meninges or covers of the brain is called meningitis. Infection or inflammation of the roots that stem from the spinal cord and brain is called radiculitis, and of the nerves, neuritis. Inflammation of the spinal cord is known as myelitis.

Inflammation of the brain may cause headache, fever, nausea, vomiting, drowsiness, or coma, together with paralysis and numbness in various parts of the body, blindness, or deafness. Encephalitis is usually due to a virus infection of the brain and has a variable outcome. In some cases full recovery is the rule, others can be fatal, or recovery may be incomplete, leaving some degree of disability.

Meningitis produces severe headache, vomiting, nausea, stiffness of the neck and back, with fever and other signs which can be easily recognized by the physician. Antibiotics have proved to be of great help in combatting the various bacterial infections that cause meningitis. A well-known type of meningitis which may occur in epidemics is due to an organism known as the meningococcus. There are also varieties of meningitis due to viruses, which are painful for the patient, but seldom fatal.

Myelitis Among infections of the spinal cord, probably the very worst and most crippling form was that caused by the virus of poliomyelitis. The virus specifically attacks the motor cells in the spinal cord. This disease which used to occur in large and frightening epidemics has been effectively prevented by the use of vaccines.

Neuritis The vague term neuritis describes a wide group of disturbances affecting the peripheral nerves and their roots after they leave the brain or spinal cord. Some are due to inflammation, others to compression of the nerves as they pass through narrow canals in the vertebrae and skull. Biochemical abnormalities which may occur as manifestations of diabetes and certain vitamin deficiencies are common causes of neuritis.

Bell's palsy (facial paralysis) is a neuritis of the facial nerve. It is caused by inflammation and compression of the swollen nerve as it passes through a tiny opening in the skull behind the ear in its course to the muscles of the face. As the weakness develops, the eye will not close fully, there is a droop of the lower part of the face, difficulty in drinking (because of weakness of the lips on one side), and a tendency to dribble from the corner of the mouth. The paralysis may be partial or complete. In most cases the condition clears up over several months. The sudden appearance of paralysis of the face may prove alarming and embarrassing. During the time when the eyelid cannot be closed, a patch must be worn to prevent dust or rough particles from injuring the delicate cornea of the eye which is normally moistened and cleaned by blinking. In patients with severe injury to the facial nerve, there may be only partial recovery or no recovery at all.

Neuralgias Neuralgia is a word used to describe a pain arising in a nerve. It is sometimes possible to discover the cause. Trigeminal neuralgia (tic douloureux) is a common form of neuralgia and is characterized by repeated attacks of excruciating pain in one side of the face, usually involving the lips and nose and sometimes the gums and tongue. The attack is often brought on by merely touching a trigger zone in the upper or lower lip, or the gum or nose, on the affected side. Speech is difficult, because as the lip moves the trigger zone can set off an attack of pain. Eating is also interfered with, because any contact of food with the sensitive zone of the lip or tongue may cause pain, leading the face to be sharply drawn up as a reaction. Similarly, washing the face becomes painful. The cause is not known, but it is believed that operations and procedures about the teeth and gums may have something to do with setting up the trigger area that leads to reflex irritation of some branch of the trigeminal nerve. A bout of attacks may last weeks or months, with each attack lasting seconds to half a minute and recurring countless times in a day. Bouts may occur at intervals over many years. A drug called carbamazepine (Tegretol) often relieves the pain, or permanent relief may be achieved by cutting the trigeminal nerve, which causes loss of sensation in the face.

Shingles (herpes zoster) is due to an infection by a virus of a ganglion, or group of nerve cells on a sensory nerve root. It leads to irritation and pain, followed by a rash of small blisters in the area of skin supplied by the nerve. The pain may be very severe. It tends to subside and disappear in weeks, but the discomfort in the area may remain for months. (See page 125.)

Sciatica This is due to pressure on the nerve roots in the lumbar region and causes pain in the back and down the leg. The cause is often pressure from a protrusion by an intervertebral disc (a plate of fibrous tissue lying between the vertebrae). The condition usually cures itself with rest but occasionally needs surgical treatment.

Polyneuritis is a disease of the peripheral nerves on both sides of the body at one time, sometimes of both arms and legs. It may affect the cranial nerves supplying the face, jaws, tongue, and eye muscles. Motor as well as sensory nerves are involved, so that there is weakness, loss of muscle tissue (atrophy), numbness, and loss of reflexes. It may be caused by infection, by alcohol, or by chemical abnormalities, as in uncontrolled diabetes, or by lack of vitamins of the B-group. It tends to subside with treatment, but may leave permanent minor abnormalities. Lead polyneuritis in painters was common in the past, but is now seldom seen.

Pressure neuropathies are fairly common. They may be due to external pressure on a peripheral nerve, for example, at the elbow or behind the knee. Mild pressure causes a transient paralysis (palsy) and often occurs during normal sleep. Prolonged unconsciousness may lead to more severe pressure

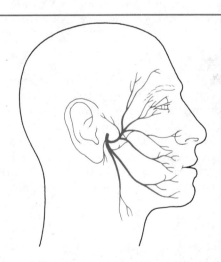

The facial nerve (seventh cranial nerve) emerges from a small opening in the skull. The nerve supplies the muscles of the face which are paralysed in a patient with Bell's palsy.

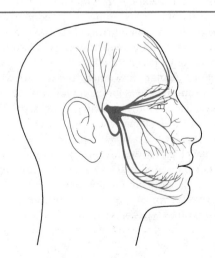

The trigeminal nerve, fifth of the twelve pairs of cranial nerves, transmits sensations from the facial area. Repeated attacks of excruciating facial pain are characteristic of trigeminal neuralgia.

which takes many weeks to recover. A common variety of palsy due to pressure occurs at the wrist where the median nerve (one of the important nerves in the hand) passes through a narrow tunnel where it may be compressed by the swelling of other structures lying in the same confined space. It may need surgical treatment for its relief. (See page 460.)

Headache

Headache is a common symptom. It is well to be clear what is meant by the term. To most people it means an aching or stabbing pain which always feels as if it is right inside the head. It may be continuous or rhythmical; it may be affected by exertion or posture. It is to be distinguished from other tension symptoms in the head, such as a sense of pressure or a weight on top, or the feeling that there is a tight band round the head. True headache does not extend to the neck.

Causes range from tiredness, worry, or too much tobacco and alcohol, to sinus pain from upper respiratory infections, certain eye diseases, migraine, the sequel to a head injury, occasionally to a raised blood pressure, and rarely to serious disease of the brain or its membranes. Fortunately, most headaches are not serious and will respond to aspirin or paracetamol and rest. The small proportion which are persistent or extremely severe will of course require the attention of the doctor.

A migraine headache may be of the classic type, on one side of the head, associated with nausea, vomiting, and weakness and sometimes preceded by an aura of flashing lights, shimmering geometrical patterns before the eyes, or blurring of vision. The liability to attacks of migraine frequently runs in families but attacks are often precipitated by special factors, such as hormone changes in women (the menstrual cycle and oral contraceptives for example), and by dietary factors such as cheese, chocolate, oranges, or alcohol. Treatment of migraine when the condition is mild may just involve the taking of a pain reliever when the attack develops or the use of ergotamine preparations. The pain itself is due to abnormal dilatation of blood vessels, and ergotamine acts directly on the blood vessels. Sometimes regular preventive treatment with other types of medication is used to reduce the frequency and severity of attacks.

Dizziness and vertigo

Dizziness or giddiness are words which have no exact meaning but are often used to describe various forms of nonpainful sensation in the head. Often, however, they refer to a symptom whose medical name is vertigo – a false sense of movement (often rotation) of the patient himself or his surroundings. This symptom is due to a disturbance of the vestibular system, a mechanism including the organs of balance of the inner ear and the nerve cells in the brain stem to which they are connected. Vertigo may be produced in normal persons by overstimulation of the organs of balance by rapid turning of the body in a rotating chair. Where the vestibular system is not working normally, even a quick turn of the head to one side or a sudden change of position may have the same effect. While the vertigo is present the patient's balance may be affected so that he is unable to stand or walk without support.

Vertigo is due to periodic disturbance of function of the semicircular canals (the organs of balance which are a part of the inner ear). In most instances it is not due to any serious cause. For example, it may follow a head injury or a virus infection involving the organs of balance. Sometimes, however, it may be a symptom of an impairment of the flow of blood to the brain stem from narrowing of the arteries supplying that part of the brain. Vertigo is often associated with noises in the ear and hearing loss. The attacks recur over many years and may be very severe. They lead over a long period of time to progressive hearing loss. The condition is probably due to changes in pressure in the fluid which lies in the semicircular canals and in the cochlea in the inner ear. On the assumption that raised pressure is the cause, surgical procedures to reduce the pressure have been used to arrest the hearing loss and prevent the attacks of vertigo.

Cramp

This is a painful, often violent, muscular contraction which may appear during exercise or relaxation – even during sleep. It is normally of no serious significance although it may occur more readily in muscles whose motor nerve supply has been damaged, for example, in sciatica, polyneuritis, and amyotrophic lateral sclerosis. If it is frequent it may be prevented by a small regular dose of quinine.

Spasms

Spontaneous muscle spasms of other sorts may occur in neurological disease. Some may be drug-induced (tranquillizers in common use may have this effect). Some are due to spinal cord disease in which the lower limbs may be drawn up involuntarily into a position of flexion (flexor spasms). A rare form of muscular spasm whose cause remains unknown is spasmodic torticollis, in which a spontaneous contraction of the muscles of the neck produces an involuntary twisting of the head to one side or the other. This is a very difficult condition to treat.

Tics are abnormal movements of a different sort. The movement is not truly involuntary but occurs as the result of a feeling of compulsion to move which the patient experiences. Resistance to this urge to move leads to a build-up of emotional tension which is relieved when the patient carries out the movement. Mild forms of tic (also known as habit spasm) are extremely common and rarely disabling. Occasionally, however, tics are so violent and involve such bizarre activities that they need medical treatment. Some respond to tranquillizing drugs.

Cerebral palsy

This term is applied to a variety of neurological defects from abnormalities in the brain arising before birth as the result of congenital abnormality, or in early infancy. The conditions do not normally progress but are often associated with poor intellectual development. The cause is uncertain; injuries to the brain at birth are often thought to be important and prematurity is frequently a factor. Infections in infancy may also be responsible. The commonest type of cerebral palsy is that in which there is a hemiplegia, that is, a weakness of one side of the body from damage to the opposite cerebral hemisphere. This may be associated with epilepsy. Spontaneous abnormal movements of the face and limbs may occur. These are slow sinuous movements to which the name athetosis is given. The condition was often due to damage to the fetal brain by antibodies in Rhesus factor incompatibility. Nowadays it is fortunately possible to prevent this where it is detected early in pregnancy. Stiffness and weakness of the legs may also occur (Little's disease, spastic diplegia). Some of these patients have low intelligence, but not all, and relatively normal intelligence may be masked by physical difficulties in communication. The incidence of cerebral palsy is reduced by proper antenatal care and skilled obstetrics.

Muscular dystrophy

Muscular dystrophy is not a disease of the nervous system, but an intrinsic disease of the muscles due to an unknown cause. The fact that it affects several members in a family would make it seem that some abnormal chemistry is inherited, which progressively destroys the muscle tissue so that in the course of several years there may be loss of muscle tissue with very severe paralysis. Although in many families the illness makes its appearance when the children are young, there are different forms of the disease that occur sporadically in only one member of a family during adolescence or adulthood. The most severe form is the so-called pseudohypertrophic dystrophy which affects young boys and is transmitted through the mother, whose own brothers will have suffered from the condition. The weak muscles become swollen before they waste, hence the term pseudo-hypertrophic (see also chapter 19).

Parkinson's disease (paralysis agitans)

This is one of the commoner neurological disorders and is named after James Parkinson who described it in 1817. In most cases the cause is obscure, although it is well known that the disease used to occur as a sequel to encephalitis lethargica (sleepy sickness) which attacks the basal ganglia, cerebrum, and brain stem, but which has not occurred in Britain in epidemic form since the 1920's.

The important symptoms are shaking of the limbs (tremor), slowness of movement, and impairment of balance. Shaking may be the first symptom to appear. It frequently begins in one hand and spreads to the other limbs over a period of some months or a year or so. The slowness of movement may show itself in walking, which becomes slow and shuffling. When similar slowness affects the upper limbs the arms fail to swing and there are difficulties with fine movements – fastening buttons for example. Handwriting becomes small and cramped and may be difficult to read. In some patients, other movements are affected, particularly those involving rapid alternation, such as brushing the teeth. Facial expression tends to be impassive due to lack of spontaneous movement and a reduction in blinking results in a staring look.

Once the disease has appeared, it tends to be progressive, but the rate at which the symptoms worsen is very variable and some sufferers remain with only the mildest disabilities for many years.

It is now generally agreed that the cause is a degenerative change in the pigmented cells of two masses of grey matter in the brain stem known, on account of their colour, as the substantia nigra. Treatment of the condition has been revolutionized in recent years. For a long period the only effective drugs were compounds related to atropine (the active principle of belladonna, a drug derived from the plant deadly nightshade). These drugs were effective in reducing rigidity and improving the speed of movement but had little effect on tremor or severe slowness of movement. About 25 years ago the first effective surgical treatment was introduced which has the great advantage of relieving tremor as well as rigidity. Many patients were treated by surgical means which involved making small lesions deep in the brain substance with a special apparatus. Recently it was observed that there was a deficiency of a substance known as dopamine in certain parts of the brain in Parkinsonism and a direct attempt was made to increase the dopamine levels by administering dopa (the precursor of dopamine in the body). This proved to be remarkably successful and has transformed the lives of many sufferers with the disease. Unfortunately the effect of dopa is to relieve the symptoms only and the progressive nature of the disease is unaltered.

Many elderly people become unnecessarily worried when they find themselves affected by a tremor, in case it is a symptom of Parkinson's disease. This is rarely the case and they can be reassured that although it is a nuisance, and sometimes causes a mild disability, there is no risk of severe disability in the future.

Congenital malformations

There is a wide variety of malformations of the brain and nervous system, but the most common of these, hydrocephalus and spina bifida, are of most concern because many sufferers of the former and most of the latter survive to a full life, whereas infants with severe malformations where a large part of the brain is missing do not survive birth.

Hydrocephalus is a term that expresses the true state of the problem (hydro meaning water and cephalus, brain) that is, "a brain filled with water". It is usually due to some malformation or infection of the brain while the child is still in the womb. At birth the head may not appear abnormal, but it rapidly expands with each month, and death usually occurs by the end of the second year of life. The problem is that the liquid usually present in the cavities of the brain is prevented from escaping, due to an abnormal blockage of the exit, so that the fluid accumulates, expands the head to extreme size and destroys the brain substance, causing paralysis, blindness, and convulsions. Sometimes there is only a partial block of fluid escape and such patients may survive for many

years or even to full life. It may be possible by surgical means to provide an escape route for the trapped fluid and the condition may be halted. There have been considerable advances in treatment in recent years.

Spina bifida is a spinal malformation in which some of the vertebrae fail to fuse, so that a sac containing the meninges, the cerebrospinal fluid, and even the spinal cord itself may protrude between the split vertebrae and appear under the skin. When present it indicates that the malformation occurred before the fetus in the uterus was three months old, since after that the vertebrae normally close and seal in the cord and its membranes. The abnormality usually appears in the lumbar or low part of the back; it is often associated with hydrocephalus. The sac-protruding type occurs rarely. The more common type is called occult, because there is no sac on the surface of the spine, but there is a slight separation in the lumbar vertebrae that shows up on X-ray examination. In such malformations there may be a tuft of hair on the surface, and because of some underlying defect in the spinal cord there may be slight unsteadiness in gait, some abnormalities in the reflexes of the legs, and sometimes inability to control the bladder and bowel. The sac type requires surgery, but for the occult type no specific treatment is usually needed.

Spina bifida may sometimes be detected by screening in early pregnancy for alpha-fetoprotein (AFP).

Epilepsy

Epilepsy has been known from antiquity, but our understanding of it has developed only in the past century. When it appears, the family may not only be perplexed by the illness, but confused by contradictory information about it. An understanding of what it is, what its problems are, and what can and should be done about it will provide the best basis for intelligent cooperation in medical care. Answers to some of the more common questions about epilepsy are presented here, but only the patient's own doctor can solve individual problems.

Epilepsy is a tendency to have fits or seizures. (Seizure is the word commonly used in the United States of America to describe attacks of epilepsy. In this country the word fit is more common. Seizure conveys better the meaning of the word epilepsy and has been used in this chapter.) Technically, it is a tendency to recurrent episodes of alteration of consciousness or control, associated with abnormal overactivity of at least some part of the brain at the time of an attack.

The brain is a complex organ, and is delicately balanced to control or modify everything a person does. Even the simplest sensations are registered in the brain and this information is used as the basis for actions ranging from the simplest of responses to highly complex activities, such as using a typewriter or playing a musical instrument. The whole brain appears to be used for abstract thinking and planning, but various parts of the brain specialize in particular activities such as speaking, or moving particular muscles. Normally, all these parts work in harmony, but if a small group of cells becomes abnormally active, this may result in a seizure. If the overactivity remains in one area, the result is a localized or special kind of seizure. If it spreads throughout the brain, a more generalized seizure may result. After the attack is over, the brain cells return to their normal activity. Thus, except for the brief time of a seizure, a person with epilepsy is usually able to live as normally as anyone else.

Seizures

Other terms for seizures include convulsions, spells, blackouts, fits, paroxysmal cerebral dysrhythmia, fainting spells. The old name for the disease was the falling sickness. Not everything called by one of these names is an epileptic fit. For example, a person may lose consciousness, or faint, from inadequate blood supply to the brain as a result of a temporary heart irregularity or from lowering of the blood pressure because of an emotional shock. Consciousness returns when the blood flow is restored. There are several kinds of epileptic seizure, depending partly upon the group of brain cells that become overactive and partly upon the person's age and other factors.

Convulsions or grand mal seizures are the most common form and may occur at any age. The attack may begin with a warning feeling or aura, after which a brief unnatural cry may be uttered. The person loses consciousness, his body stiffens and jerks, and his colour becomes darker because the muscles used in breathing are involved in the muscular spasms. This change in colour is not serious, because breathing is restored when the muscles relax again within a few minutes.

Grand mal seizures are not ordinarily harmful unless the person injures himself in falling, though he may sometimes bite his tongue or lips. If the bladder is full when the attack begins, the convulsive seizure may cause it to empty; or occasionally he may soil himself by a bowel action, which may add greatly to the embarrassment of an epileptic attack.

Very little need be done by a person witnessing the beginning of an attack as the seizure will come to an end by itself. The person having an attack should be eased to the ground and protected from injuring himself, but it is no longer thought necessary to attempt to insert anything between the jaws. Turning the person on his side towards the end of the seizure will help get rid of any saliva, and eliminate the risk of choking if there should be vomiting after the attack. A report of careful observation of the attack may greatly help the doctor in his diagnosis. Many persons can resume their usual activities almost immediately after a seizure, but others will need a short period of rest and reassurance. Since the person can not remember what happened during the seizure, he will be helped if the person who is with him is able to remain calm and explain to him that nothing very serious has happened.

A series of attacks in close succession is called status epilepticus and is a medical emergency. A doctor should be notified immediately and his instructions followed. Hospital treatment will usually be necessary for a patient in status epilepticus.

Petit mal epilepsy is seen mainly in children, and usually disappears after adolescence. Petit mal seizures consist of brief, sudden losses of consciousness, lasting for only a few seconds. In these spells, the child seems to daydream or stare briefly, and there is usually no falling and only a slight movement of mouth, face, or arms.

Psychomotor seizures may be highly variable, but there is always loss of memory for the attack. There is a clouding of consciousness accompanied by automatic performance of movements that often seem quite purposeful and have a varying degree of complexity. There may be restless, repetitive movements, automatic movements such as walking, chewing, or moving about the room, so that at first glance it is possible to confuse these episodes with emotionally disturbed behaviour.

Partial or localized seizures are so-called because the disturbance underlying the attack seems to remain limited to a focus in the brain, and so the manifestations are limited to one area of the body, as in the jerking of an arm or a leg. A peculiar feeling in one of the limbs may also represent a focal seizure. Any of these manifestations, as well as some of those applying to the special senses such as vision, hearing, taste, or smell may be followed by spread of abnormal activity to other areas of the brain and hence more widespread seizure manifestations. If such a peculiar disturbed feeling or warning comes on before a more general attack, it is called an aura, and often permits the person to take some kind of action to protect himself, such as lying down on a bed before the seizure starts.

There are other less common kinds of seizure which include muscle jerking, alteration of function of some of the internal organs, or peculiar feelings, and some of these require special study to determine their exact nature.

Causes of seizures

There are two categories of causes of seizures. One, the response of the brain cells to specific and discoverable injury or disturbance by an outside factor; the other, the intrinsic susceptibility of the person to seizures.

Many things can happen to the brain to make it susceptible to seizures. A direct injury to the brain, in a road accident or injury at birth, may cause some of the brain cells to become intermittently overactive and set off a chain of events that produces a seizure.

An infection of the brain, such as encephalitis, may cause irritation at the time of the infection and convulsions may occur during the acute illness, or long after the acute infection has passed.

Anything that seriously interferes with the blood flow to an area of the brain may cause a seizure, and this is the reason why epileptic attacks are sometimes a complication in persons who have had strokes. In a few cases, a brain tumour may produce interference with brain cell function.

The use of alcohol, particularly in excess, may provoke seizures. Inborn defects of brain structure or brain metabolism, and any change in the metabolism of the body, such as disturbance of the blood sugar supply to the brain, may also produce seizures of a similar type.

It is because of this variety of possible causes that the doctor may need to perform an extensive diagnostic investigation. Since some of these causes can be corrected by direct action, their elimination naturally represents the best means of treatment. A specific correctable cause may not be found and reliance must then be put on preventing seizures by the use of drugs and other measures.

If no definite cause of the seizures can be found, there are two possible conclusions. Firstly, the specific cause may have been relatively minor or obscure. For example, the occurrence of a head injury may not have been remembered, or the neurological changes may be too obscure to appear as part of the findings in the examination. Secondly, there may be a varying susceptibility to seizures in different people, especially in the case of petit mal spells in childhood.

Diagnosis of epilepsy

In the case of typical grand mal convulsions, the diagnosis may be readily apparent to the most casual observer, but the observation of this symptom would still leave uncertainty as to the cause of the attack. With the other types of seizure, a diagnosis may be made only after a careful investigation, as it is possible for other conditions to resemble seizures enough to produce some degree of uncertainty.

A careful review of the history given by the patient, as well as by observers who have witnessed an attack, is the basis for establishing the diagnosis. Since the patient may not be able to report anything except warning feelings or after effects, it is extremely important that someone who has seen an attack should give the doctor an accurate description of what took place during the period of unconsciousness. The history will also reveal clues to other kinds of illnesses that may contribute to an understanding of the cause of the attacks.

Physical and neurological examinations may lead to an understanding of the cause of a seizure. For example, evidence of abnormality of heart function may show that the seizures are in reality being triggered by changes in the blood supply to the brain. The finding of localized weakness or changes in the reflexes may point to some localized disturbance of the brain as the cause of the seizures. Many epileptics will require some or all of the investigations described on page 165.

Other tests include examination of the blood, urine, and chemical constituents of the blood, such as the level of blood sugar.

Since some cases of epilepsy are the result of serious injury to the brain, it is not unusual for psychological testing to take place as a means of assessing the patient's ability to cope with day-to-day challenges.

Control of seizures

Medication is the backbone of the management of epilepsy, but other general health and psychological considerations are also important. With appropriate regular treatment, control of seizures can be satisfactorily achieved for 85 per cent of patients, more than half of whom can be made completely free of attacks.

To be effective, drugs must be taken with regularity. The doctor will usually prescribe a regular drug dosage to be taken once or twice a day or, on occasion, several times a day. It may be that the initial dosage will be inadequate for control, and subsequently increased amounts of the same drug or other types of medication will be required. A growing child often requires some adjustment to dosage of the drug to keep pace with growth.

It is possible that some of the side effects of the treatment will be so troublesome that a particular drug will have to be replaced by another, but with perseverance and cooperation between the patient and his doctor, a satisfactory balance of preparations can usually be worked out.

Absolute regularity of taking a medicine is important for two reasons. Firstly, since control of the seizures depends on having an adequate level in the body tissues of the proper drug, a seizure may recur if this level is allowed to drop. Secondly, it has been observed that abrupt reduction of medication will accentuate the likelihood of seizures. It is of extreme importance that the patient and his family understand that regularity of medication is essential to successful treatment. Various means have been used to help ensure that no dose is missed, including marking a calendar, taking the drug in association with some other fixed function each day, such as with meals, or by counting out the tablets each time. Many families have been helped by the device of securing seven small containers from their chemist, labelling each one with a day of the week, and then at the beginning of the week putting the proper dosage for each day into a separate container. This permits the patient who should use the drug to check personally that the container is empty at the end of each day, or some other member of his family can unobtrusively check the container. If a dose is inadvertently missed, the doctor will usually give instructions for making up the missed medication. If a particular schedule is difficult to maintain, the doctor will often help by trying to simplify the dosage schedule so as to avoid having to take medicines at school or at work.

There should be no serious complications in connection with medication to control seizures, though it may take some time to find the most appropriate drug for an individual patient.

It used to be thought that drugs for epilepsy produced some mental dulling, but with modern drugs this is no longer true, except perhaps for a temporary effect if larger than optimal doses are being used, with the effect clearing when the medication is reduced. Some drugs will produce unsteadiness in walking, blurring of vision, or nausea, but these are temporary and disappear when the dosage is adjusted. A few can produce skin reactions or disturbances of blood, kidney, or liver function, so when these are used the doctor may request periodic laboratory tests. However, the patient should be alert to report any apparent side effects.

Treatment should be continued for one or more years after the last observed attack. For major epilepsy (grand mal), this is usually at least two or three years, but it may be longer, depending upon the appearance of the patient's EEG and other considerations. The treatment should never be discontinued except on the doctor's advice.

Brain surgery may occasionally be suggested if investigation reveals that the cause of the seizure is a blood clot, or tumour, or similar condition that can be helped by surgery. In other cases that have been found not to respond adequately to drug treatment, an attempt may be made to remove by surgery the limited area of cells causing the seizure discharges. This is not always possible, so surgery is approached only after very careful study of the problem.

Social and psychological factors

Although most persons with epilepsy are basically stable, emotionally healthy, and productive, there are social and psychological problems which may make life more difficult for them. Ancient superstitions about the illness may occasionally result in exclusion from social groups. The attitude of parents or teachers may alternate between overprotection and outright rejection of the child, and either of these may bring symptoms of emotional maladjustment to the surface. This illness is unusual because the attitudes of the people around the patient may create more of a handicap than the actual illness itself. Continuing public information and education are doing much to eliminate the unfortunate attitudes that may add to the patient's burden.

The person with epilepsy often has problems to deal with, including the uncertainty he feels about the possibility of recurring attacks, the uneasiness he may feel from isolation, uncertainty about himself because of appearing to be entirely well and yet having to take drugs and finally, by a lack of adequate understanding of his own illness. Many patients with epilepsy have been able to avoid the pitfalls of self-pity, anxiety, and feelings of rejection by seeking a clearer understanding of the illness from the doctor and others who are in a position to give advice. Many people find support through belonging to local Action for Epilepsy groups.

Persons with epilepsy may have emotional problems as other people do, and epilepsy itself is not considered a form of mental illness. In general, the intelligence of persons with epilepsy parallels that of the general population, with about as many having above normal as below normal intelligence. Famous people who are believed to have had epilepsy include Lord Byron, Dostoevski, Julius Caesar, Napoleon, Handel, Alexander the Great, and William Pitt.

Education In the limited number of patients whose seizures are the result of extensive damage to or disturbance of the brain, their capabilities will be limited by this underlying impairment, so that special schooling and other care may sometimes be necessary, even though the seizures themselves may be readily controlled by effective medication.

Since most patients with epilepsy have normal intelligence and the seizures can be reasonably well controlled, children can, and should, go to school normally. There are a few children with serious damage to the brain, or other causes of mental deficiency, who also have seizures, who should be placed in special classes because of the mental deficiency rather than because of the seizures. If seizures are too frequent to be tolerated in the classroom, special arrangements should be made temporarily until satisfactory control can be established.

Employment A person with even moderately well controlled attacks can perform well in an extremely wide range of employment so long as he is not required to operate high-speed or dangerous equipment such as motor vehicles, aeroplanes, hoists, or other things by which he or others might be injured in the event of an unexpected seizure. With proper placement and adequate training, a person with epilepsy can prove to be an excellent worker, and many highly skilled professional people are found among the ranks of persons with epilepsy. In Britain, the Employment Service Agency has produced a leaflet entitled "Employing someone with epilepsy" which "aims to reassure employers that they need have few apprehensions about employing people with epilepsy, and to tell them about the help and advice which the Employment Service Agency can give".

The Agency itself "can give expert advice to actual or intending employers of people with epilepsy through its Disablement Resettlement Officers (DROs). These officers have been specially selected and trained for the work of helping disabled people with various handicaps to get and keep suitable jobs and, collectively, they have considerable experience of the sort of problems likely to be encountered and the best solutions".

For employees, The British Epilepsy Association has published a leaflet on "Epilepsy and getting a job", which offers practical advice on how best to look for employment.

Marriage An increased susceptibility to seizures may occur in some families, although this familial tendency is not great enough in most cases to cause any real concern about a person with epilepsy having children. However, if two persons having epilepsy marry, the chance of their children having seizures is naturally greater than if only one of the parents is affected. In general, it is believed that there is no valid reason for persons with epilepsy not to marry and have children, but the individual circumstances should be thoroughly reviewed by the person's own doctor or sources of special help that may be suggested by him.

The Law   The law concerning driving varies from country to country. In Great Britain, a patient must declare that he has suffered from epilepsy in his driving licence application. If he has been free from attacks for three years, even though still taking anti-epileptic drugs, he may be given a licence.

In Great Britain further information and help may be obtained from the British Epilepsy Association, Crowthorne House, Bigshotte, New Wokingham Road, Wokingham, Berkshire RG11 3AY.

Strokes

Revised by John Marshall, MD FRCP

The patient who has suffered a stroke constitutes one of the major problems in medicine. The popular term stroke, or sometimes paralytic stroke, has about the same meaning as the medical word apoplexy – to cripple by a stroke. All these terms express the blow-like suddenness of symptoms. However, there is a great range of severity, from so-called little strokes which may cause a few minutes of confusion, passing dizziness, or slurring of speech, to major strokes which may quickly be fatal. A medical term that better describes the mechanism of strokes is cerebrovascular disease, since the underlying cause is disease of the cerebral blood vessels, which leads to impairment of blood supply to the brain.

Although the stroke victim is usually middle-aged or older, most often over 60 years of age, younger men and women are by no means immune. Until recent years there was no preventive or curative treatment for strokes. All that could be done was to apply general measures such as preventing obstruction of breathing in the acute stage and, once the acute stage was passed, mobilizing the patient as soon as possible. Accurate pinpointing of the cause of the trouble was relatively unimportant, since there was no definitive treatment.

In the past decade great advances in diagnosis and treatment of cerebrovascular disease have been made. A major advance has been the introduction of angiography, a method by which the cerebral arteries which cannot be seen on a plain X-ray film are made visible. A dye is injected through a needle or catheter introduced into an artery in the neck or groin while X-ray films are taken, so outlining the cerebral arteries and revealing obstructions and narrowed segments.

Causes

A stroke may manifest itself in a variety of ways and produce many widely varying effects or symptoms, even though the underlying cause of the stroke is the same in most cases. When a block occurs within one of the major arteries supplying the brain, the blood supply to that portion of the brain is halted and the affected brain area stops functioning. If this situation is prolonged for more than a few minutes, the brain cells in the affected area die. The agents that cause the block are a clot in an artery or a constriction of sufficient extent to interrupt the flow of blood. A clot forming in the cerebral artery itself is the most common cause of a stroke. If a clot forms elsewhere in the body and a piece becomes detached to be carried along the bloodstream to the brain, where it obstructs an artery, the term cerebral embolism is used. Another cause of the death of brain cells leading to a stroke is cerebral haemorrhage. This occurs particularly in people with high blood pressure; an artery ruptures because of the high pressure and the blood which escapes destroys the brain cells in the neighbourhood. Haemorrhage may also occur from an aneurysm, which is a blood-filled sac formed by local stretching of the arterial wall, or from an angioma, which is a mass of abnormal blood vessels. The effect of this disruption of the brain cells is prompt and in many instances far-reaching because of the role of the brain in maintaining normal body processes. For example, small areas on one side of the brain largely govern the control of the opposite arm and leg. Should one of these areas become damaged, the patient's control of that arm or leg is lost. The limb then becomes weak or paralyzed. If the affected area is big enough, the paralysis affects one whole side of the body and hemiplegia (one-sided paralysis) is the result.

Various other areas of the brain control speech, sight, and other complex activities. A stroke affecting one of these brain areas will be reflected in disturbance of the function that area controls. Persons who have suffered strokes often have difficulties with vision, speech, hearing, and gait.

Treatment

Despite major advances in many aspects, treatment of the stroke patient continues to offer many problems. As recently as ten years ago there was no treatment worthy of consideration to offer. Today, therapy is available under broad classifications such as surgery, anticoagulants, the cortisone drugs, and agents designed to dissolve clots. One form of therapy is the use of anticoagulants to reduce the clotting tendency of the blood. The intention is that, with the reduction in the clotting tendency, further clot formation in a narrowed and diseased artery may be prevented.

However, the administration of anticoagulants is never free from risk because of the danger of haemorrhage. The tendency of the blood to clot is normal and to some degree desirable as this prevents serious bleeding occurring in minor injuries. Without this every person would be in the situation of patients with haemophilia. In attempting to combat the undesirable clotting of cerebral thrombosis it is possible to swing to the other extreme so that cerebral haemorrhage occurs. For this reason anticoagulants are rarely used in strokes with a sudden onset.

Surgery Of all the forms of available treatment, surgery in suitable cases presents the most hopeful approach to the crisis caused by a stroke. In many instances, the obstruction of the blood flow to a portion of the brain does not occur in the brain itself, but in a major artery of the neck, the carotid artery. As it is situated close to the surface at the side of the neck, the carotid artery is readily accessible to the surgeon, and when a clot is present its surgical removal may bring about a dramatic reversal of the patient's symptoms.

Obstruction of a major blood vessel outside the brain is an important factor in the incidence of strokes, and as many as fifteen to twenty per cent of strokes are caused by a block in the carotid artery leading to the brain. A thrombus commonly forms at the site of an arteriosclerotic plaque. The origin of the plaque is complex, but the effect is that fat (and other material) is deposited at certain sites in the walls of arteries. The material builds up to form a mass which projects into the artery and thus narrows the channel. This in itself may be sufficiently severe to reduce the blood flow to a critical level but even when this is not the case, thrombosis often occurs and so the blood supply is obstructed.

In cases of partial obstruction of the carotid artery, symptoms may be temporary loss of vision or intermittent impairment of function (for example, impaired control of movements, or numbness) of a hand or foot, sometimes associated with a transient defect of speech or vision. These intermittent effects are known as transient ischaemic episodes and are very important as they give warning that a major stroke may develop soon. Appropriate treatment of transient ischaemic attacks may prevent this happening.

When a stroke has occurred due to a block of the internal carotid artery, the surgical procedure most frequently used is called thrombo-endarterectomy or thrombectomy of the artery. In this operation the artery is exposed, opened, and the clot removed.

Complications and fatalities are rare and in most instances the patient is up and about the day after the operation, is home within a week, and can return to work within a month.

Operations designed to diminish the occurrence of transient ischaemic attacks have a high percentage of good results. If the obstruction in the carotid artery is extensive, the site may be bypassed with one of the vascular prostheses now available. These are artificial blood vessels made of synthetic materials. Rapid advances in treatment of arterial obstruction outside the brain itself have shown the importance of early diagnosis and early recognition of an impending stroke. Prompt surgery may prevent a major stroke.

Cerebral haemorrhage

This is due to rupture of a small blood vessel, usually in a patient with a long history of high blood pressure. This type of stroke is uncommon in anyone with normal blood pressure. Usually the haemorrhage occurs deep within the brain, but in some instances it may occur in more superficial areas. Distinguishing between a haemorrhage within the brain and a stroke due to blockage of one of the blood vessels may often be difficult but the invention of computerized axial tomography has been an important breakthrough in this field. (See page 548.)

Cerebral haemorrhages are not necessarily fatal as was once commonly believed. Occasionally it may be possible to remove the blood by surgical operation. More important, however, is the prevention of cerebral haemorrhage by proper treatment of a raised blood pressure. It has now been shown that bringing the blood pressure down to a normal level and keeping it there reduces the risk of the patient having a stroke. This can be done by drugs which must be taken regularly under medical supervision.

Aneurysms, which are frequently congenital, are dilatations of an artery wall, which may pouch out from the artery like a thin-walled balloon, or like an inflated weak spot of a tyre inner tube. This weakened, overstretched area of a cerebral artery is filled with blood, and if it bursts, blood seeps out, accumulates, presses upon delicate brain tissue, and produces a stroke or strokelike symptoms with unconsciousness and one-sided paralysis. Not infrequently, as a consequence of the aneurysm, spasm narrows the arteries around the aneurysmal sac, further impeding the blood supply to the brain. Surgical treatment is generally direct, that is, a small clip is placed on the neck of the aneurysmal sac. If there is no neck, the sac may be wrapped with gauze or with a plastic material which hardens and supports the area from the outside. The clot resulting from the haemorrhage is of course removed at the same time.

An uncommon cause of stroke is angioma formation in a blood vessel of the brain. These areas tend to bleed at a relatively early age, the peak incidence being at about 25 years. As a rule, haemorrhage from this cause occurs at lower levels of blood pressure and so less damage is done, and the mortality rate in this form of stroke is lower.

Restoration of function

In restoration of function after a stroke, physiotherapy and occupational therapy play an important part. Certain deformities may occur after a stroke, which, if allowed to develop and progress, not only delay recovery but also impede the restoration of voluntary movements of affected parts. The most common deformities arise from adhesions of a joint, and contractures or shortening of a muscle or muscles of the paralyzed limb. These deformities occur most commonly in the patient who is paralyzed on one side of the body and who, either because of prolonged unconsciousness, the threat of further complications, or further brain haemorrhage, must remain in bed for a prolonged period.

One of the most important deformities that can be prevented is called foot-drop, with associated shortening of the Achilles tendon – the tough cord of tissue that runs up the back of the heel. In this condition the paralyzed foot drops so that the toes point downwards. Prevention or partial prevention can be achieved by using a bed-cradle to keep the weight of the bedclothes off the foot and a foot rest support (see chapter 1) to maintain the foot at an angle of 90 degrees to the leg, and by daily stretching of the calf muscles when they begin to become tight and shorten. Another measure is the placing of sandbags along the outside of the paralyzed leg to prevent outward rolling of the leg and foot. Equally important is the care of the upper limb. The fingers and wrist should be maintained in the normal position and not allowed to become bent. Splints are not advisable for this purpose as, although position is maintained, the joints tend to become fixed. Positioning on a pillow or sandbag, the patient being encouraged to move the paralyzed limb regularly by means of the good limb, is preferable.

Perhaps the most troublesome disability is so-called frozen shoulder, resulting from adhesions which form in and about the shoulder joint of the paralyzed limb. This condition generally occurs from immobilization of the joint. Every effort should be made by those who are caring for the patient to prevent frozen shoulder by moving the joint regularly. Alternatively the patient may be provided with a sling and pulley by which he can move the affected joint himself. The newer cortisone drugs are often used in treatment of frozen shoulder. These compounds are injected into the joint and may give early relief of pain. However, their effects in improving the range of motion in the joint are not so consistent, and restoration of joint function can take up to two years or more despite the injection of steroids and diligent physiotherapy, hence the importance of prevention.

Physiotherapy is aimed at restoring voluntary power and is based on repetitive use of various forms of active rather than passive exercise. Exercises are started at the earliest possible stage of the illness and are based on simple principles. The most important of these is that from the beginning it must be understood that it is the patient who has to make the major effort in moving the limb. Leg function is started first in an effort to make the patient walk. Knee and hip exercises should be introduced as soon as the patient's general condition allows. As soon as these exercises are accomplished, more complicated exercises are introduced and these again emphasize restoration of function. Examples are: moving up and down the bed, rolling from side to side in bed, and then sitting on the edge of the bed. At this stage an attempt is made to restore balance when sitting, and the patient is taught to resist attempts to unbalance him. It is important to re-establish balance awareness as early as possible. Once the patient has attained balance in sitting on the edge of the bed, he should be moved into a high-backed chair. With a stable foot and ankle he now requires only minimal power above the knee to stand or walk.

If the hemiplegic patient can raise his paralyzed leg only a few inches off the bed while lying on his back, there is sufficient muscle power in the thigh to permit walking. Once he has assumed the standing position, exercises are first based on weight-bearing, then marking time, and finally walking. A set of parallel bars is of great help when early attempts at walking are being made. This may be followed by use of a walking frame. When functional activity of the lower limb is achieved, mastery of the upper limb or restoration of its function may be more easily attained. Here the principle is simply a progression from passive movements to active assisted movements and then to unassisted voluntary movements.

Occupational therapy emphasizes the active exercises and incorporates them into the activities of daily living. For example, a functional pattern of rehabilitation can use those movements necessary for such activities as conveying food to the mouth, combing the hair, and other personal functions. The shoulder pulley can be used to assist shoulder movement. It is important to concentrate on outward rotation of the shoulder, this being the most difficult movement for a hemiplegic to regain. Bending and straightening of the forearm, and rotation of the arm inwards and outwards, are also difficult and must be practised through all stages from passive movement to active movement and then to unassisted voluntary activity. Quite often, however, the fingers cannot be re-educated to any return of the normal function the patient had before his stroke, except in mild cases. The fingers are often held tightly bent and full straightening is rarely possible.

Rehabilitation at home The advantages of starting physiotherapy and occupational therapy early in the management of residual paralysis after a stroke, and the realization that neither requires elaborate or complicated apparatus, lead the way to early therapy given in the home. Home physiotherapy has a great many advantages, not the least of which is that it can be given frequently throughout the day. The principal disadvantage of home physiotherapy is that the recovering stroke patient is deprived of association with others who are similarly affected, and thus does not have encouraging demonstrations of the heartening progress that can be made in overcoming disabilities.

There is no particular drug of value in helping the physiotherapy programme to produce relaxation of contracted muscles. Best results are achieved when the patient's efforts are encouraged by a firm, but sympathetic family or physiotherapist, who can understand the anxieties, lessened power of concentration, loss of memory, and difficulties of communication the patient may be experiencing. It should be remembered that in some cases of stroke the patient may not be able to speak clearly or at all, but may understand what is said to him.

The long-term outlook The best time to assess the patient's recovery of function, and of remaining disabilities, is about three months after the time of the stroke. However, continuing improvement in the level of independence of stroke victims can be expected up to one or even two years after onset. Of

particular relevance is evaluation of the patient's range of movement, his abilities to feed himself and manage his toilet, and capacities to perform household duties or undertake forms of employment. This assessment can be made by an occupational therapist. At about this stage a retraining programme may also be necessary. For example, the left hand may be retrained to take over some of the functions of a paralyzed right hand. Aids in retraining, such as alterations to clothing, perhaps replacement of buttons by zips, may be suggested. Modifications to the home may be desirable, such as handrails in the bathroom and elimination of stair climbing, where possible.

The most important factor in rehabilitation of stroke patients is to begin physiotherapy and occupational therapy as soon as this becomes feasible. Every patient is studied individually in an effort to apply the best possible treatment.

Chapter 8

Kidneys and genito-urinary tract

Revised by Alec Badenoch, MA MD ChM FRCS

The heart and circulatory system move blood to and from all parts of the body. The kidneys continuously filter various substances from the blood, reabsorb some of them, but concentrate waste products created by the chemical processes of the body, and pass them out as urine. In this way, they regulate the volume and composition of body fluids. The heart is a powerful organ which pumps blood, the kidneys monitor the quality of this blood, so that the body is not poisoned by an accumulation of harmful end products of its own metabolism, and at the same time allow it to retain essential fluids and salts for the tissues.

The labours of the kidneys are prodigious, but silent, and far less dramatic than the constant throbbing of the heart. About one quarter of the

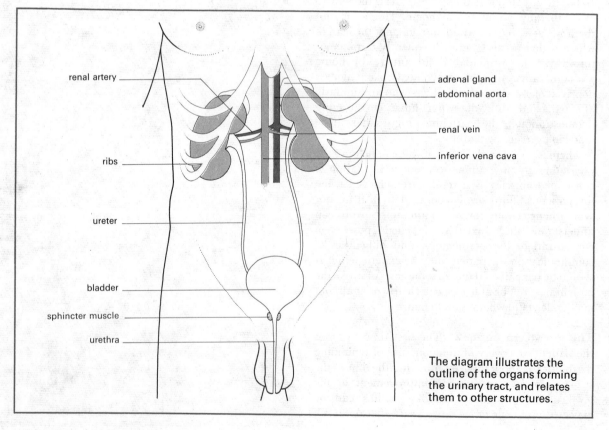

The diagram illustrates the outline of the organs forming the urinary tract, and relates them to other structures.

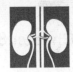

The kidney

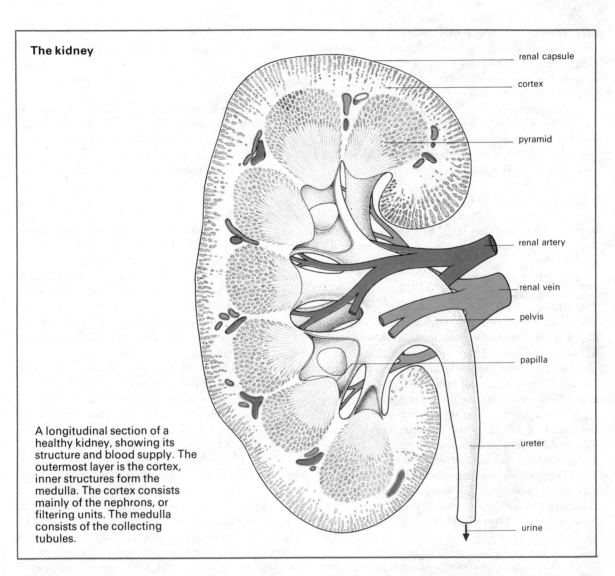

renal capsule

cortex

pyramid

renal artery

renal vein

pelvis

papilla

ureter

urine

A longitudinal section of a healthy kidney, showing its structure and blood supply. The outermost layer is the cortex, inner structures form the medulla. The cortex consists mainly of the nephrons, or filtering units. The medulla consists of the collecting tubules.

blood pumped by each stroke of the heart passes through the kidneys, and the total body fluid passes through the kidneys about fifteen times a day. This amounts to approximately 1,930 litres (1,700 quarts) of blood every day, of which only about one thousandth is converted into urine. The kidneys and urinary tract function as a unit, with a certain division of labour. The primary function of the kidneys is to form urine, that of the urinary passages is to dispose of it. Physicians who specialize in disorders of the kidney are called nephrologists, and surgeons who specialize in disorders of the urinary tract are called urologists.

The kidney

Most people have seen animal kidneys and are familiar with their shape and deep maroon colour.

The human kidney is not dissimilar, is bean-shaped and weighs about 150 gm (five oz). We have two kidneys, one on each side, lying behind the abdominal cavity (not in it) and protected at the rear by the spinal column and large muscles of the back. The kidneys are situated just underneath the lowest ribs. The right, which lies just below the liver, is usually a little lower than the left. They are surrounded by fat which cushions and supports them, allowing some range of movement and minor variations in position, which are not necessarily abnormal nor a threat to health.

A section of the kidney, cut vertically, shows a mass of tissue curved around the pelvis and hilum (see diagram above). The kidney receives its blood supply from the renal artery which is usually a single large artery although there may be two or more moderate-sized vessels. The artery divides into progressively smaller branches which make their way through the kidney tissue and filtering units. The blood is then collected by an intricate system of small veins which join to form larger vessels emptying into the renal vein, thus returning blood to the general circulation. The primary urine-forming function of the kidney is accomplished during the passage of blood through the tiny filtering units. Kidney cells have certain other functions. They manufacture pressor (pressure-elevating) substances which help to control the blood pressure, and when the blood supply to the kidney is diminished these substances are manufactured in larger amounts and may cause raised blood pressure in an attempt to increase the blood flow through the kidney. They also have other metabolic functions that are not clearly understood.

The filtering unit The urine-forming unit of the kidney is called a nephron. It is a complicated and highly efficient filtration plant and consists of several intricate structures. These units are packed tightly into the outer solid part of the kidney, and the naked eye cannot distinguish an individual nephron, only vague lines converging on the central cavity. At the top of the nephron is a cup-shaped structure known as Bowman's capsule. Projecting into the capsule is the glomerulus (Latin for little ball), a tufted network of intricately laced small blood vessels called capillaries. Practically all the constituents of the blood except cells and proteins can pass from the capillaries into the space between the double walls of the capsule. This fluid, or filtrate, contains many dissolved materials, some of which are indispensable for the body's welfare, and some of which are harmful.

The filtering process of the glomeruli is physical, not chemical. Blood in the capillaries is under much higher pressure than the tissue fluids around them and the filtrate is forced through the walls. If the blood pressure drops below a certain level, filtration is reduced or ceases. The filtering area of a kidney is astonishingly great. That of the total glomeruli of a single kidney is as large as the surface of the entire body, and the glomerular capillaries of both kidneys, if laid end to end, would stretch more than 56 km (35 miles).

The filtrate is very dilute, and out of some 200 litres (180 quarts) of filtrate a day, the average adult concentrates about 1.7 litres (three pints) of urine. If all the filtrate were lost from the body, we would be in a perpetual state of unbearable thirst, and the loss of fluid and the essential dissolved materials would quickly prove to be fatal. Obviously, most of the

filtrate and many of its dissolved materials must be reabsorbed, whilst harmful materials are not. This is a function of the kidney tubules, the lower part of the nephron, in which residues are gradually concentrated into urine.

The capsule forms the head of a tubule, into which the filtrate flows freely. The tubule descends, bends upon itself in a hairpin turn (Henle's loop), and takes an ascending course. This convoluted course, full of twists and turns, increases the length of the tubule which can fit into a small space. Most of the water and selected dissolved materials are reabsorbed and returned to the circulation as the fluid moves through the tubules. The concentrate at the lower end of the tubules is urine and is ultimately discharged.

There are more than a million nephrons in each kidney carrying out this system of filtration, selective reabsorption, and excretion. The nephrons of both kidneys if unwound and placed end to end would stretch well over 80 km (50 miles). If one kidney is removed, there is a temporary impairment of the excretory functions, but in a few months' time the remaining kidney will enlarge to do the extra work.

The kidneys regulate fluid and electrolyte balances and vital acid-base levels, which must be kept within extremely narrow limits to be compatible with life. In the biological sense, electrolytes are dissolved salts or ions which participate in the countless chemical processes of the body. Perhaps the most familiar electrolyte is sodium, an element of common salt. About 1·1 kg ($2\frac{1}{2}$ lb) of salt pass through the tubules daily, but rather less than nine gm ($\frac{1}{3}$ oz) is excreted in the urine. If salt intake is excessive, or the ability of the kidneys to excrete it is impaired, a condition of oedema – fluid retention and waterlogged tissues – results. On the other hand, salt depletion may cause dehydration and severe symptoms, such as the painful muscle cramps which occur in normally healthy persons who sweat profusely from continuous strenuous exertion in hot surroundings, when they drink large amounts of water, and lose excessive quantities of salt in perspiration. The kidneys safeguard the balance of many other electrolytes which are of profound importance to normal health. The kidneys can also excrete larger particles, such as germs.

Some kidney disorders primarily affect the glomerular filtration units and others the tubular reabsorption units. Many self-diagnosed complaints of kidney trouble such as pain in the loin or excessive or uncomfortable urination may have little or nothing to do with the kidneys, and only a doctor, after proper examination, can determine the true nature of the condition.

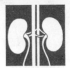

The filtering action of the kidneys

Blood flows into the kidney through the renal artery, which divides into smaller and smaller branches within the kidney tissue. The diagram on the right shows one of the filtering units, called a nephron. Below, the structure of a Bowman's capsule is illustrated in more detail. As blood passes through the glomerulus, it is filtered of impurities. This dilute filtrate enters the glomerular capsule and passes into the proximal tubule. Substances needed by the body (including water) are reabsorbed, and the impurities concentrated to be excreted as urine.

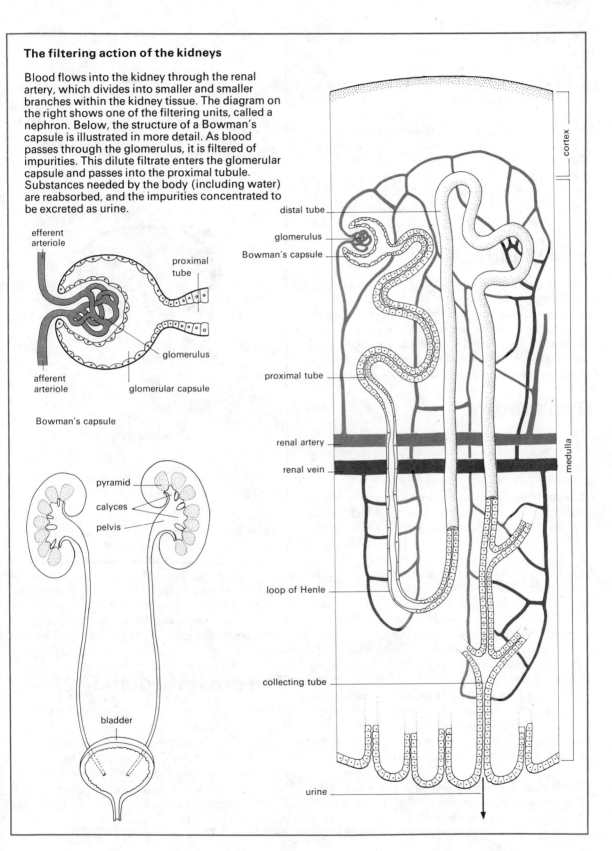

efferent arteriole

proximal tube

glomerulus

afferent arteriole

glomerular capsule

Bowman's capsule

pyramid

calyces

pelvis

bladder

distal tube

glomerulus

Bowman's capsule

proximal tube

renal artery

renal vein

loop of Henle

collecting tube

urine

cortex

medulla

The collecting system The collection and disposal of urine is a function of the urinary passages, as distinct from the manufacturing functions of the kidneys. Urine from the lower ends of the tubules flows into several small cuplike chambers called calyces (Latin for cups) which merge into two or three major calyces opening into a single cavity, the kidney pelvis. This is a funnel-shaped sac which extends partly outside the kidney. Its lower end becomes the ureter, a narrow tube through which urine from the kidney passes into the bladder. Urine passes steadily, drop by drop, out of each kidney along the ureter to the bladder.

The bladder

The bladder is a storage organ which retains urine until disposal is convenient. Ordinarily, when the bladder collects 285 ml ($\frac{1}{2}$ pint) or so of fluid, complex nerve signals pass to the brain and the organ is emptied. However, the bladder is very elastic and under abnormal conditions may retain even litres of fluid and greatly distend the lower abdomen.

The urethra

The urethra is different in the male and female. In the latter the urethra is simply a short tube to carry urine from the bladder to the outside.

The male urethra also performs this service, but in addition it is the passageway through which semen reaches the outside. It is about 23 cm (nine in) long, and is considered in two portions. That which begins at the bladder outlet and runs through the prostate gland is the posterior or prostatic urethra. It contains muscles that help to hold the urine in the bladder until it is ready to be expelled. The rest is the anterior urethra, and is mainly located in the shaft of the penis. It ends at the meatus or external opening.

The posterior urethra contains openings through which the surrounding prostate gland empties its secretions. Also in this tract are the openings of the ejaculatory ducts which carry spermatozoa from each seminal vesicle. During the sexual act the spermatozoa and prostatic fluid are carried into the urethra and thence to the outside. Through the anterior urethra, therefore, pass both urine and semen.

The female urethra is much shorter than that of the male, averaging about four cm ($1\frac{1}{2}$ in) in length. Since there is no prostate in the female, the urethra is practically devoid of glands, but it does pass through

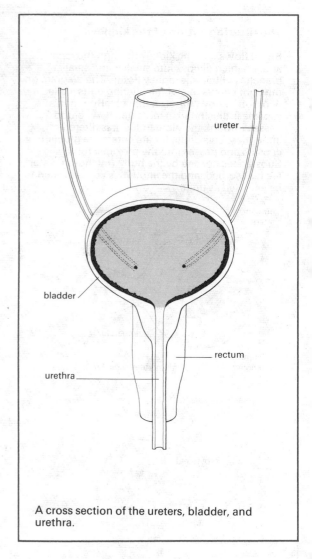

A cross section of the ureters, bladder, and urethra.

the internal and external sphincters which give control of urination. It runs close to the upper wall of the vagina and terminates in an external opening. Its function is to transport urine from the bladder to the outside.

The prostate gland

Accessory sex glands of the male, and structures intimately associated with the lower urinary tract, traditionally fall within the field of urology. The prostate is a secreting gland with three major lobes continuous with each other, completely encircling the posterior urethra. The gland has openings through which its own secretions are emptied into the urethra particularly during the sexual act. The prostate develops at puberty through male hormone.

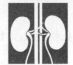

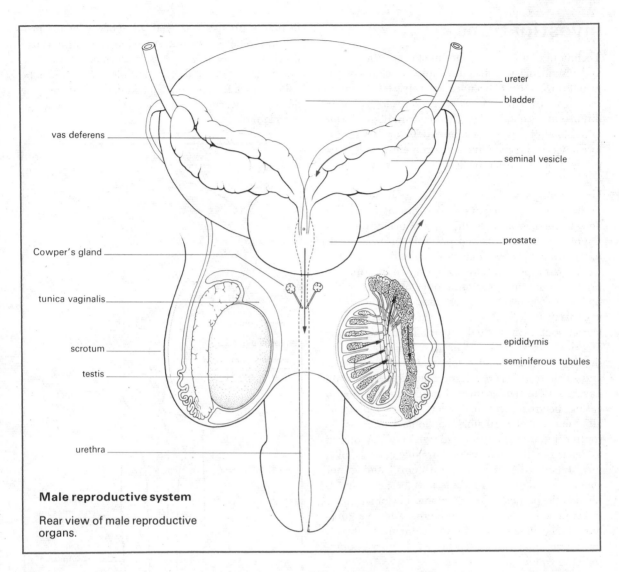

Labels on diagram:
- vas deferens
- ureter
- bladder
- seminal vesicle
- Cowper's gland
- prostate
- tunica vaginalis
- scrotum
- testis
- epididymis
- seminiferous tubules
- urethra

Male reproductive system

Rear view of male reproductive organs.

The testis

The scrotum is an external sac suspended behind the penis, and contains the male reproductive glands (testes). The testis has two important functions. After puberty it produces spermatozoa which pass by way of the seminal duct or vas deferens to reach the seminal vesicles. The first part of this tube is very convoluted and lies immediately behind the body of the testis – being called the epididymis. It then passes upwards to the inguinal region where it enters the pelvis and has a downward course behind the bladder when it becomes wider. The tube passes through the back of the prostate gland and opens into the posterior urethra.

After puberty spermatozoa are formed in enormous numbers in the testes. When mature, they travel from the testis through the vas deferens to the seminal vesicle on each side. At the climax of the sexual orgasm the seminal vesicles empty the spermatozoa into the posterior urethra through the ejaculatory ducts. Simultaneously, the prostate gland contracts and empties its secretion. The combined substance, called semen, passes by a wavelike motion along the urethra. The prostatic secretion is important in supplying substances which feed and stimulate the sperms to move after sexual intercourse into the female womb or uterus. The testis also manufactures a hormone or internal secretion after puberty. This is mainly responsible for the development of the male sex characteristics – enlargement of the penis, sperm formation, muscular development, growth of beard and body hair, and an interest in sex.

Investigations

Techniques for studying the function of the kidney and visualizing the structures and processes of the urinary tract have been extensively developed in recent years. Exact knowledge of urological conditions can be obtained by chemical analyses of urine and blood, by X-ray examination, and with the assistance of highly refined instruments, which are passed along the tract to allow visual examination.

Urine analysis   Diagnosis of disease by inspection of the urine is an ancient practice, pursued centuries ago. In mediaeval days, the flask of urine was most important for patients and practitioners who made diagnoses merely by looking at the fluid in the flask. Today, a proper analysis of a specimen of urine can provide much information about conditions of the body. A complete analysis may not always be necessary; it depends on what the doctor wants to learn about an individual patient. The mere volume of urine passed in 24 hours may for instance, be significant. Odour and colour are obvious aspects, and a colour such as red in the urine does not always have a serious significance. It is occasionally due to eating beetroot or pink sweets. Tests for sugar, albumen, and acid-alkaline reaction are more or less routine, but more sophisticated tests may be required to determine the presence of inorganic crystals, bile, pus, blood cells, bacteria, proteins, and other elements. Culture of the urine may be necessary to identify the particular germs responsible for a urinary tract infection, so that the most effective anti-microbial drugs may be used in treatment. However, urine tests alone cannot tell the whole story about a patient's condition.

Blood analyses   These may be most important in determining the degree of total function of the kidney, and in stone formation they may give a clue as to the type of stone or its cause.

Catheters   A catheter is a hollow tube for introduction into a cavity through a normal narrow outlet such as the urethra. The catheters of antiquity were made of bronze, copper, and silver; and, later, pewter, wood, and processed leather were used. Flexible catheters made of rubber came into existence in the latter half of the eighteenth century, but nowadays they are mostly made of plastic material. The catheter was first introduced to drain abnormal retention of urine and it is still used for this purpose. However, the development of smaller and more flexible catheters has enabled more delicate procedures to be carried out. An example is catheterization of a ureter which is performed through a cystoscope. This makes it possible for urine to be collected separately from each kidney, which may be of importance in assessing the relative efficiency of each kidney.

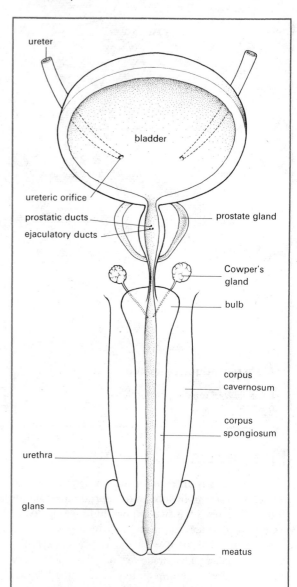

The male urethra from its beginning at the bladder to its termination at the meatus. The prostatic or posterior urethra runs through the prostate gland. The rest is called the anterior urethra. The encircling prostate gland and the ejaculatory ducts have openings into the prostatic urethra. Cowper's glands secrete lubricating fluid into the anterior urethra.

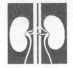

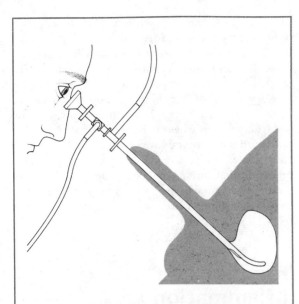

The drawing shows the passage of a cystoscope along the male urethra. This instrument is a telescope illuminated at the end allowing direct inspection of the inside of the bladder. The surgeon can pass instruments down it to crush stones, or remove portions of tissue for examination.

Cystoscopes From the catheter, the beginning of instrumentation of the urinary tract, it was a considerable leap to the modern cystoscope. This instrument consists essentially of a hollow tube with a tiny electric light bulb at its tip, and is passed into the bladder. A telescope with a system of lenses is then passed along the hollow tube and the bladder filled with water. Illuminated by the light, the interior of the bladder, the opening of the ureters and the urethra can then be inspected visually. Modern cystoscopes or endoscopic instruments are exceedingly versatile instruments. They can be used for destruction of tumours and removal of stones and foreign bodies from the bladder. They can also be used for the removal of some prostates. Recent improvements, especially in the light systems, have made it possible to see inside the ureter and kidney pelvis.

X-rays Developments in X-ray apparatus have greatly improved the study of the urinary tract and kidney function. Plain films can be made which show the outlines of the urinary tract structures and anything opaque which may be in the tract. Other details can be visualized by intravenous injection of radiopaque substances which are then excreted by the kidney, and allow the entire urinary tract to be seen. By this means normal function and shape are shown, as is any distortion or disturbance associated with a disease or abnormal process. It is also possible to introduce radiopaque substances directly into parts of the urinary tract such as urethra, bladder, ureters, and renal pelvis by a cystoscope or catheters. Recent developments in cine-fluorography make it possible to take motion pictures of the urinary tract in action, again using radiopaque media.

Congenital abnormalities

The kidney Abnormalities are common and many are not important. Others sooner or later impair function to a varying degree. Studies of function and anatomy give information on the abnormality, its influence on function, and whether treatment is necessary or not. In the process of development before birth, the kidneys, which arise in the pelvic region, migrate upwards, rotate on their long axes, and settle in their final position in the upper lumbar region. This complicated, twisting ascent is subject to aberrations which result in malformation.

An ectopic kidney Ectopic means occurring in an abnormal position. The kidney may have failed to ascend or it may have crossed to the opposite side of the body. Then, the two kidneys may lie separately but close together on the same side, or they may be fused together to form a single mass of kidney tissue. Such malformations may function well, but are prone to infection, to obstructed outflow, which causes a collection of urine to distend the pelvis of the kidney (hydronephrosis), and to stone formation.

Solitary kidney Very rarely, a person is born with only one kidney. Fused kidneys, as described above, may in effect be a single kidney, but we can do very well with only one kidney if it is functioning normally.

Horseshoe kidney As the name of this anomaly indicates, the paired kidneys, instead of being separate, are linked at their lower ends by a band of tissue, giving a shape resembling a horseshoe. The bridge may or may not contain functioning kidney tissue.

Polycystic kidneys are usually congenital and have a tendency to run in families. Usually, both kidneys are studded with grapelike cysts which fill the interior with spherical cavities and, on the surface, resemble blisters. Polycystic disease which appears in infancy has a serious outlook, but in adults the condition usually progresses slowly and is consistent with an active life for many years.

The bladder Congenital abnormalities of the bladder primarily involve failure of the bladder to close into a sac with a normal outlet. The anomaly is called extroversion of the bladder. The malformed bladder has only a back wall and no abdominal covering. Urine from the ureters comes out to the surface of the body and the patient leaks urine constantly. Correction is by surgery, and is very difficult. Most cases require diversion of the urinary stream into unnatural channels which direct the flow to the outside from the interior of the body. For example, the stream may be diverted into the rectum.

Bladder function may also be interfered with by neurological injury or disease. Inability to empty the bladder may be due to damage to nerves which may prevent sensations which normally trigger the urge to urinate.

The urethra Occasionally, a stricture – abnormal narrowing – of the posterior urethra is present at birth or may occur later in life. Congenital anomalies of the urethra usually occur in the anterior part.

Hypospadias is the failure of the urethra to close underneath, so that the tube is an open trough. This rarely extends into the posterior urethra, so control of urination is usually normal. The opening on the underside of the penis interferes with the normal delivery of the urinary stream. Plastic reconstruction may be necessary if hypospadias is present in any marked degree.

Epispadias is a comparable but less common malformation in which the upper side of the urethra remains open. The defect may be a slit or roofless channel running for a short distance from the end of the penis on the upper surface, or it may traverse the shaft of the penis more extensively, or the opening may begin and end at the base of the penis. In the last case, normal sexual intercourse is not possible. Occasionally, the posterior urethra is involved, with malformation of bladder sphincters, so that the patient cannot control urination, and is in much the same state as with extroversion. The problem is to restore urinary control and then to form a new tube by plastic surgery, from the re-formed sphincteric area to the outside. The prostate gland, testes, and scrotum are usually not involved in this abnormality.

The testis Undescended testis or cryptorchidism is a condition in which one testis or both testes fail to descend from the abdomen, where the organs arise during fetal development, into the scrotum. If only one testis is involved the defect is probably mechanical in origin, but if it is on both sides the underlying cause may be hormonal, such as a poorly functioning pituitary gland. In the latter case improving function by administering pituitary extracts will sometimes bring the testis into its proper position. Surgical correction may be necessary, however. If this is the case, it is generally agreed that the operation should be done at an early age, before the age of seven or eight, and certainly before the onset of puberty.

In order to function correctly and produce spermatozoa, the testis must be at a lower temperature than that inside the body. The scrotum has a thermostatic muscle response which relaxes and contracts in order to adjust the temperature of the testes.

Infection and inflammation

Infections of the kidney and its pelvis (pyelonephritis) are quite common. They are of great importance because chronic and recurrent infections tend to encourage changes which in time may interfere seriously with kidney function. In many ways the conditions seem to have a connection with high blood pressure. Some cases, particularly if untreated or neglected, progress to renal insufficiency – inability of the kidneys to filter toxins thoroughly from the blood. Retention of these waste products leads to uraemia or uraemic poisoning.

Infection can reach the kidney by various routes, by the bloodstream and lymphatic channels, direct ascent from the bladder, or spread from infection in surrounding tissues. Acute infections manifest themselves by pain in the kidney region, fever, and shivering, together with changes in the composition of the urine. Chronic and recurrent infection tends to be more insidious with symptoms such as headache, a general feeling of being unwell, and nausea or even vomiting.

When a specimen is examined microscopically the urine may be seen to contain pus (pyuria), microorganisms, red blood cells, and other products of inflammation. Identification of the infecting organism is made by setting up a culture in the laboratory and enables effective antibiotics or other drugs to be given. Many acute and chronic infections respond to appropriate chemotherapy, whilst rest and general care with administration of fluids may help.

However, many cases are complicated by obstruction and conditions which prevent free drainage of the urinary tract. Occasionally a focus of infection

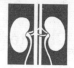

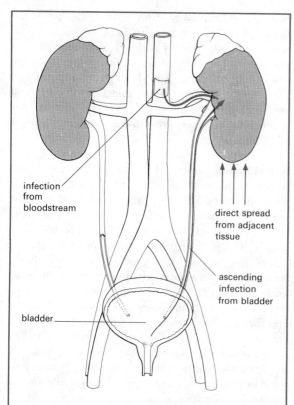

Infections may reach the kidneys by various routes. They are more common in the female due to the shorter urethra, while hormonal changes, particularly in pregnancy, reduce the tone in the walls of the ureter. Infections are common in both sexes after the passage of instruments, or operative procedures in the pelvis. Many women experience a bladder infection when they first become sexually active.

outside the urinary tract may cause reinfection. These sources of infection must be recognized and treated, and of course full urological investigation is necessary to recognize abnormalities which prevent effective drainage. Early diagnosis and treatment is important and neglect may lead to kidney damage that is difficult, if not impossible, to reverse.

Nephritis (Bright's disease) In 1827, Richard Bright of London described a disease which has since borne his name. Bright's disease is not a single condition. Several varieties are now recognized, and there is some confusion about definitions. In a broad way, the group of diseases may be called nephritis – inflammation of the kidney not resulting from infection. The blood vessels of the glomeruli and the filtering units of the nephron are commonly affected,

and when this is the case the term glomerulonephritis is used.

Although a germ may not be the direct cause of nephritis, research has identified certain strains of germs as a probable indirect cause. Acute glomerulonephritis may occur several days after a patient has suffered from an infection due to haemolytic streptococci, a germ which often causes a sore throat and also scarlet fever, although this is now quite rare. It is thought that the delayed action of toxins produced by these germs is responsible.

Salts of mercury and some other metals can cause nephritis. The kidneys, whose function is to maintain the blood's purity, filter and excrete innumerable kinds of harmful substances day and night which in their passage may produce chronic inflammation. Metabolic diseases may also produce scarring and inflammatory reactions in the kidney, such as artery-hardening (sclerotic) processes. This form of nephritis is called nephrosclerosis.

Acute glomerulonephritis usually affects young people but no age is exempt. Symptoms include loss of appetite, headache, nausea, vomiting, and passing diminished quantities of urine. There is swelling (especially of the face) due to waterlogging of the tissues (oedema or dropsy). The urine contains much albumin (protein), which is usually evidence of kidney damage. The blood pressure usually rises. The patient should be kept in bed and the diet carefully regulated, as is the intake of fluids; salt and other food elements may be restricted. The great majority of these patients recover completely and rarely have a second attack.

The outlook is less favourable in chronic glomerulonephritis. The condition may be dormant for many years during which no active treatment is required. Dropsy is not quite so common as in the acute form. There is often anaemia and a sallow complexion. Waste products tend to accumulate in the blood because of the diminished capacity of the kidneys to excrete them. There is albumin in the urine and the blood pressure rises. Although kidney impairment increases slowly, there may be a dormant period, even of many years, during which the patient may feel quite well and be able to carry on an active life. Eventually, renal insufficiency causes uraemia (the continued presence of toxic substances in the blood) together with congestive heart failure.

The relationship between high blood pressure and vascular kidney disease is of great interest because of the general high incidence of hypertension, see page 86. Special tests to reveal these relationships are now available. Arteriography (where X-rays are taken of kidney vessels) and other tests are carried out by urologists and physicians to evaluate the causes of hypertensive disease. When renal artery obstruction is found to be present, surgical correction is often possible.

Childhood nephrosis Any degeneration of the kidney without signs of inflammation is called nephrosis. The term is most often applied to childhood nephrosis. Most patients are between one and a half and four years of age when the disorder is recognized. The outstanding symptom is massive oedema (dropsy). The first signs may be a puffiness about the eyes or difficulty in putting on the child's shoes. The cause is not known. A preceding streptococcal infection such as occurs in acute glomerulonephritis apparently plays no part.

Treatment has been greatly improved by use of steroid drugs (of the cortisone family) and antibiotics to prevent severe infections to which the nephrotic child is peculiarly liable. The hopeful aspect is that many of the patients do not develop kidney failure and most children return to good health without any permanent kidney damage from the disease.

Prostatitis Inflammation of the prostate (prostatitis) is fairly common. In younger men it is more likely to be specific – that is, to be caused by particular organisms, such as those that cause gonorrhoea – and to be a spread of infection which moves up the urethra to the prostate or beyond. In middle life or later, prostatitis is not very common.

Haematuria (blood in the urine) This is always a symptom requiring immediate investigation by a physician to determine its cause. Sometimes the startling discovery of blood in the urine is followed the next day, or for days after, by clear urine, and the person may be lulled into feeling that nothing serious is happening. That may be the case, but intermittent haematuria can be serious and its first appearance is a warning to consult a doctor. There are many possible causes of haematuria, some grave, others trivial. Of the trivial variety, microscopic haematuria – presence of inconspicuous blood cells in a urine specimen – resulting from violent sports activity or exercise is perhaps the most common. The condition can occur in boxers, basketball players, wrestlers, and others subject to body blows and multiple episodes of forced forward crouching.

Albumin in the urine Albumin is a protein, like egg white, which is present in the urine of some persons, and probably at some time or other in the urine of almost everybody. Albumin is a useful substance and healthy kidneys normally do not excrete it. Therefore albuminuria (albumin in the urine) suggests damage to the filtering apparatus of the kidneys. However, some infectious diseases and even such things as violent exercise and other stresses are sometimes associated with transient and harmless albuminuria.

Renal insufficiency This is when the kidneys are unable to filter all the waste products and poisons from the blood so that variable amounts of toxic materials remain. These are harmful and as their amount increases, the kidneys ultimately fail completely. This state of uraemia is fatal unless corrected. There are of course, degrees of uraemia. Early symptoms are headache, itching, lassitude, nausea, and vomiting. The patient becomes drowsy, perhaps has convulsions, and lapses into coma and death. Insufficiency may result from some acute reversible condition, or from gradual and progressive damage and destruction of kidney tissue over some years. A major purpose of the treatment of kidney disease is to prevent insidious damage whenever possible and to eradicate such causes as infection and obstruction.

Dialysis Great advances in the treatment of renal insufficiency have been made in recent years and one of the mechanisms employed is dialysis. This is the separation of substances from the tissue fluids by passing them through a porous membrane. This can also be achieved by the technique of peritoneal dialysis, in which membranes of the abdominal cavity temporarily do the work of the diseased kidneys, but the commonest method employed is by haemodialysis.

Almost everybody has heard something about the artificial kidney. It is indeed artificial and mechanical, but can do the work of human kidneys remarkably well for short periods of time. There are several variants but all rely on much the same principle as the living kidney itself; diffusion of blood through a membrane to extract waste and then return of the purified blood to the body. An artificial kidney performs this function outside the body, and the process is called haemodialysis.

A hollow tube (cannula) is placed in an artery, in the patient's arm or leg, and blood passes through a large surface area of membranes (usually of cellophane). Dialysable waste products are filtered through these membranes into the surrounding fluid, and the purified blood is returned to the patient's circulation by a vein. Pumps, flow meters, and clot

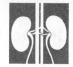

and bubble traps keep the blood moving safely. Haemodialysis is usually a hospital procedure requiring a dependable apparatus and the skills of a team of specialists, but many patients in time learn to carry it out in the home.

Haemodialysis is used to aid the body when the kidneys are not working adequately. Excellent results are obtained in reversible kidney disease, especially if this is acute and a relatively short period of outside support is required. Transfusion reactions, poisoning, and acute renal failure due to haemorrhage after giving birth, are examples of conditions in which the method may be lifesaving.

For the patient whose kidneys are irreversibly scarred, degenerated, and hopelessly inadequate, the machines are less practical because the regime of artificial haemodialysis must then be permanent and frequently and regularly repeated. Such patients may have long-term tubes inserted into an artery and vein of the wrist, or elsewhere, for easy connection to an artificial kidney, and once or twice a week these patients spend some time in hospital to have the blood cleared, or have been taught to do it at home. The alternative is to transplant a human kidney into the patient.

Successful transplantation in identical twins has focused much research upon this. Technical surgical details of transplanting a donated living kidney or that from a dead person have been mastered. The great remaining obstacle to organ transplantation is the body's rejection of donated tissue, and this is being overcome. About 60 transplantations are performed each month in this country, at the present time.

The bladder   The bladder is subject to infection. A notable difference between lesions of the bladder and many lesions of the kidney is that the former usually cause marked changes in the urine.

Cystitis or inflammation of the bladder is especially common in women. The short female urethra may be an easier pathway to invasion by infecting organisms. Occasionally infection may descend from the kidneys.

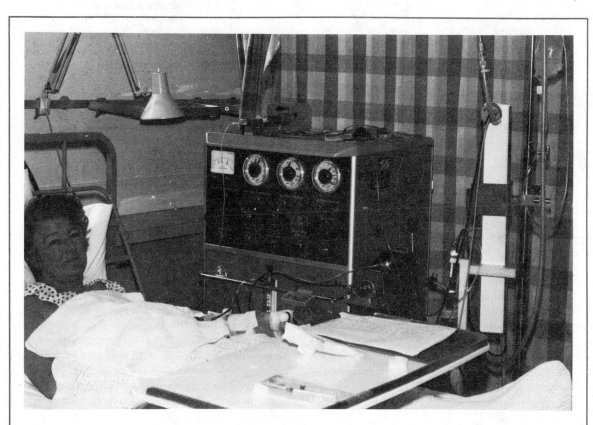

A patient in her eleventh year of dialysis.

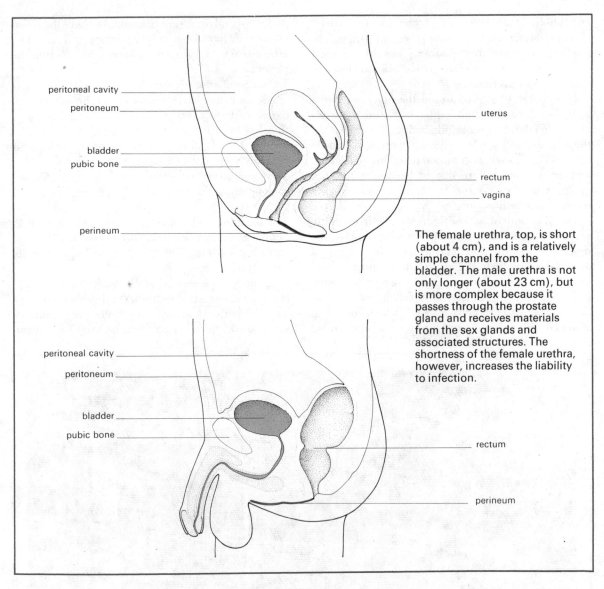

peritoneal cavity

peritoneum

uterus

bladder

pubic bone

rectum

vagina

perineum

The female urethra, top, is short (about 4 cm), and is a relatively simple channel from the bladder. The male urethra is not only longer (about 23 cm), but is more complex because it passes through the prostate gland and receives materials from the sex glands and associated structures. The shortness of the female urethra, however, increases the liability to infection.

peritoneal cavity

peritoneum

bladder

pubic bone

rectum

perineum

The urethra also may be infected and inflamed (urethritis) and the site of distressing symptoms. The diagnosis of simple acute cystitis is usually not difficult. Symptoms are pain or burning on passing urine, increased frequency, and sometimes haematuria. There is usually not much fever unless the upper urinary tract is involved. An acute infection is usually cleared up by antimicrobial drugs. A specimen of urine must be examined in the laboratory to identify the causative organism and to determine the most effective treatment.

Chronic or recurring cystitis may require a full investigation including X-ray examination and a cystoscopy to detect or exclude a cause which may perpetuate the condition.

Enuresis

Enuresis or involuntary discharge of urine is normal in children up to the age of twelve to eighteen months. Normal control of the act of passing urine (micturition) is a complicated nervous function which takes time to develop. Bed-wetting in older children often involves psychological or social factors. Nocturnal enuresis occurs in certain neurological conditions.

Incontinence of urine often occurs after spinal injury or disease and sometimes occurs in elderly people. It is then usually associated with degeneration of parts of the brain, sometimes with strokes, and is part of the general arteriosclerotic processes of advancing age.

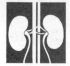

Injuries

Kidney The kidneys are loosely anchored in a bed of fat and are well-protected, so that injuries are relatively rare. Bruising may occur after a blow and produce blood in the urine (haematuria) which gradually passes. Crushing and penetrating injuries do sometimes occur, however, and usually the immediate problem is that of bleeding from the kidney which has a great many blood vessels. An operation may be necessary and then it may be possible to repair the injured structures. A kidney may have to be removed, depending upon the nature and extent of the injuries.

Bladder This is rare, is usually accompanied by serious injury to the pelvis and requires surgical treatment.

Urethra Injuries of the urethra are much commoner and are serious for several reasons. The urethra contains many blood vessels and there can be severe haemorrhage. In addition, urine may leak into surrounding tissues causing severe irritation. The after effects of these injuries may result in some degree of narrowing causing difficulty in passing urine. It may be followed by impotence and infertility. These injuries usually require surgical treatment.

Stones (calculi)

One of the oldest of surgical operations is cutting for stone in the bladder. Samuel Pepys had this operation in 1658. Cutting for stone was known even in the time of Hippocrates, who admonished fellow doctors not to cut for stone, but to leave this to the specialist. Many operative procedures for the removal of bladder stones were developed in the seventeenth and eighteenth centuries and in the absence of anaesthetics and asepsis were very painful and hazardous.

Nowadays, stones in the kidney and urinary tract are quite common and are a major problem of urology. How a kidney stone forms is reasonably well understood. Urine is a complex solution of many substances, including mineral salts. Under certain conditions, some of these substances may precipitate out, condense upon some microscopic nucleus – perhaps a bacterium or a speck of mucus – and grow larger and larger.

Stones, then, are formed of dissolved substances brought to the kidney. Why they form in some people but not in others is not understood. The incidence of stones among the population varies geographically.

Stones occur in many shapes, sizes, and colours and have differences in structure. If a stone can be obtained, analysis of its chemical composition gives valuable information. Calcium phosphate and oxalate stones are common; less so are uric acid stones. Cystine stones are rare. They are primarily due to an error of metabolism in the body's handling of amino acids from protein foods. Sometimes a tumour in the parathyroid gland increases the excretion of calcium and phosphorus in the urine and increases the likelihood of calcium phosphate stones. Other factors which influence stone formation are: an obstruction anywhere in the urinary tract which may cause lack of flow of urine; prolonged bed rest; and infection. Abnormally concentrated urine which may result from insufficient intake of water is also of importance. It is necessary to correct any abnormality in the urinary tract which might encourage the formation of stones, and to correct changes in the urinary tract which may have been brought about by the presence of a stone.

Some stones develop in acid urine, others in alkaline. Medicines and special diets, such as an acid-ash diet, may help to maintain better balances and deter future stone formation, and other medical measures depending on the patient's body chemistry and physical condition, may be helpful. It is of immediate importance to remove stones causing serious trouble such as severe pain or obstruction with infection, and this generally requires surgery. If the function of a kidney has been extensively damaged by a large stone or stones, and if the remaining kidney is functioning normally, it may be desirable to remove the entire kidney. A person who is susceptible to stone formation requires a regular medical check.

Some stones do not cause any symptoms for a long time. Some are too large to enter or obstruct the ureter, but they may move about in the kidney and injure the renal tissue. Some stones may practically fill the kidney pelvis and take on the irregular shape of the cavity, like a cast. These are called staghorn calculi from their antler-like appearance.

Many stones, however, do cause sudden attacks of excruciating pain. A bout of kidney colic is never forgotten by the person who experiences it. The pain is caused by spasm of the ureteric muscle round a stone which has entered the ureter and recurs with each attempt of the muscle to force the stone down. The pain is usually felt in the loin to start with and then moves to the front and down to the pelvic region. If the stone gets stuck in the ureter and produces back pressure on the kidney, medical measures can do little more than relieve pain, and surgery may be necessary.

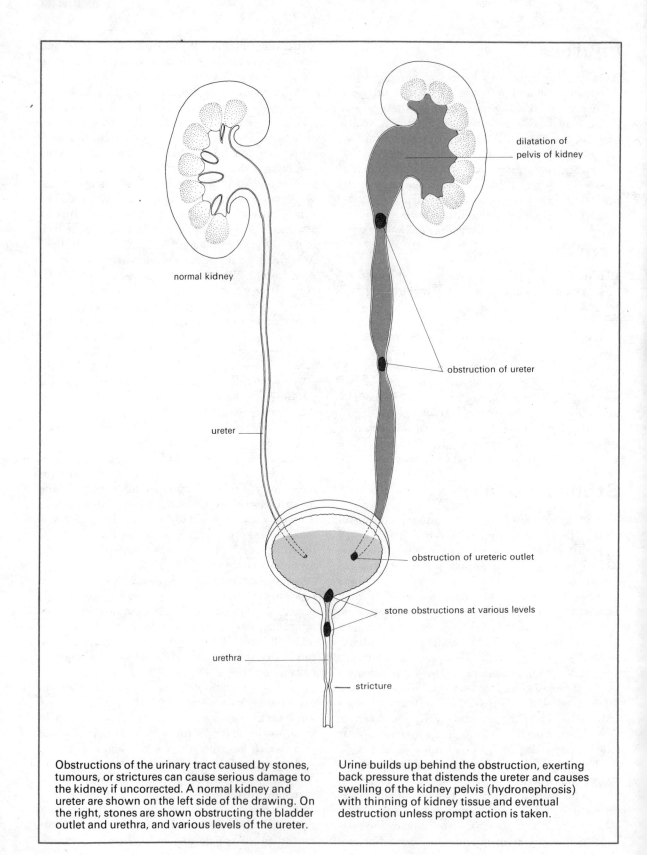

dilatation of
pelvis of kidney

normal kidney

obstruction of ureter

ureter

obstruction of ureteric outlet

stone obstructions at various levels

urethra

stricture

Obstructions of the urinary tract caused by stones, tumours, or strictures can cause serious damage to the kidney if uncorrected. A normal kidney and ureter are shown on the left side of the drawing. On the right, stones are shown obstructing the bladder outlet and urethra, and various levels of the ureter.

Urine builds up behind the obstruction, exerting back pressure that distends the ureter and causes swelling of the kidney pelvis (hydronephrosis) with thinning of kidney tissue and eventual destruction unless prompt action is taken.

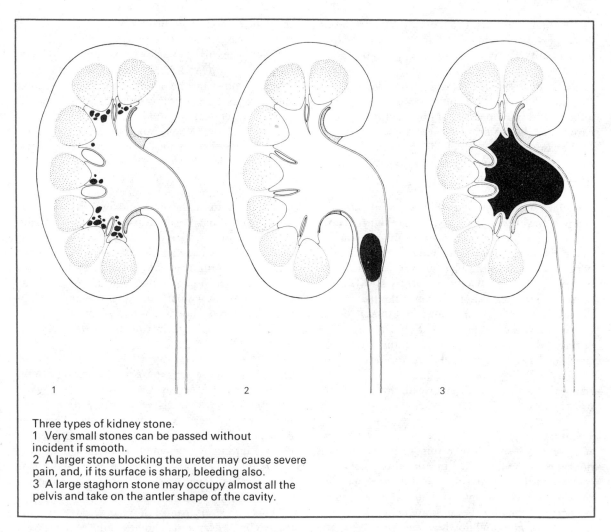

Three types of kidney stone.
1 Very small stones can be passed without incident if smooth.
2 A larger stone blocking the ureter may cause severe pain, and, if its surface is sharp, bleeding also.
3 A large staghorn stone may occupy almost all the pelvis and take on the antler shape of the cavity.

Often a stone passes into the bladder and the acute pain subsides. It is then usually passed in the urine. A small bladder stone is relatively easy to remove with instruments passed along the urethra. Occasionally, a stone will lodge in the urethra and prevent urination. Its removal is comparatively easy and is always an immense relief to the patient.

Tumours of the genito-urinary tract

Kidney and ureter Tumours of the kidney are not uncommon. They may be benign and insignificant but are often malignant – that is, a form of cancer with the ability to invade and spread to other parts of the body. Benign swellings are usually cysts of the kidney which are sacs of various sizes full of fluid. These may occur in one kidney or both and may produce a large mass in the abdomen. Malignant tumours nearly always affect only one kidney. Solid types arise in the functioning tissue of the kidney. In general, they occur in two periods of life – in infancy, and in mid-adult life. There is the so-called Wilms' tumour of childhood and the hypernephroma or carcinoma which occurs more often in persons over the age of 40. There are other tumours which arise in the pelvis and sometimes in the ureter, which look like warts with fronds like a sea anemone, and are usually malignant.

Usually the first evidence of such kidney tumours is blood in the urine. A mass is occasionally felt in the abdomen in the region of the kidney, on one side. Haematuria or the passage of bloodstained urine may not be accompanied by pain and is usually intermittent. It is always a sign which calls for full investigation although it may be due to causes other than cancer. As with all cancers, the best hope of cure lies in early diagnosis and appropriate treatment. A

195

mother may be the first to discover a Wilms' tumour, when an abdominal mass is felt in the course of caring for her baby. The tumour usually appears before the age of seven. Every child who has a palpable mass in the abdomen should be seen by a doctor. The treatment for Wilms' tumour is removal of the whole kidney and postoperative radiotherapy. A solid carcinoma also requires total removal of the kidney. In the case of warty or pimple-like growths, the ureter must also be removed since this type of tumour spreads along the tube.

Bladder Cancer of the bladder is common in this country. It is of two main types, one papillary or warty which grows into the cavity of the bladder and is relatively benign, and the other invasive or ulcerating which spreads into the bladder wall and is always malignant. The first symptom is nearly always blood in the urine which must be investigated. If the diagnosis is made early and treatment begun immediately, the results are good, but if spread has occurred the outlook is often bad. In the early stages the growth may be destroyed or removed by surgery or may require irradiation therapy or complete removal of the bladder together with diversion of the urinary flow.

Prostate

Benign enlargement. A benign tumour is one which is not cancerous and does not invade other parts of the body, but because of its situation and size it may give rise to quite severe symptoms. This is certainly true of benign tumours of the prostate – adenomatous hyperplasia. The condition is an overgrowth (hypertrophy) associated with ageing. It is rare before the age of 50, and it has been estimated that 20 to 30 per cent of men over the age of 50 have enlargement of the prostate, half of whom ultimately require operation. The outstanding symptom of prostatic enlargement from whatever cause is interference with the act of passing urine. The obstruction varies in degree and location, but the range of symptoms produced is characteristic. There is increased frequency of urination, especially at night. It may take several efforts to complete the act, the stream may be slow to start, less forceful and diminished in calibre, and then tends to end in dribbling.

The cause of benign prostatic enlargement is not exactly known but it is almost certain to be due to some upset in hormones. Treatment by hormones, however, is not at present satisfactory, so when treatment is required some form of surgery becomes necessary. Immediate intervention is needed when

the patient cannot pass urine at all, and urgent when the bladder contains a large amount of urine after the act of passing urine appears to be complete. Severe frequency at night, difficulty in starting the act, and stopping and restarting of urination, all give warning that the patient must be investigated, by X-raying the urinary tract, examination of the blood for biochemical changes, and analysis of urine. Great advances have been made in the surgical treatment of this obstruction, and the mortality rate for the operation which was at least twenty per cent half a century ago is now much nearer one per cent, and this includes patients in the ninth and tenth decades. This improvement has been achieved by good surgical technique, by advances in anaesthesia, by replacement of blood lost at operation, by control of infection and by great improvement in nursing and postoperative care. Depending on the size of the prostate and the condition of the patient, the obstruction may be removed by open operation, or by dissecting with a wire loop through an instrument passed along the urethra.

Cancer of the prostate Prostatic cancer is common and affects twenty per cent of patients who have the symptoms of obstruction. Even in the early stages it may be diagnosed by a rectal examination and in the more advanced stage it is obvious. There are certain conditions – stones in the prostate and certain chronic infections – which are sometimes difficult to differentiate from cancer by touch alone and it may be necessary to remove a small piece of tissue from the suspected area for microscopic examination.

When prostatic cancer is recognized early and treated by surgery and irradiation, the control rate is high. Unfortunately, this early diagnosis is uncommon. If the growth is limited to the region of the prostate, irradiation may be effective. If it is discovered late and spread has occurred outside the confines of the prostate itself, control is difficult. When secondary growths which are common in the bones of the spinal column and pelvis are already present, local treatment is not helpful. A large proportion of cases, however, are hormone dependent; that is, the cancer may be controlled by giving the patient female hormones. In some who respond well, life may be prolonged for many years.

Urethra Malignant tumours of the posterior urethra are rare unless they arise in the prostate gland. Malignant tumours of the anterior urethra are also extremely rare. Blood in the urine and constriction of the urethra with difficulty in passing urine are

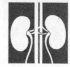

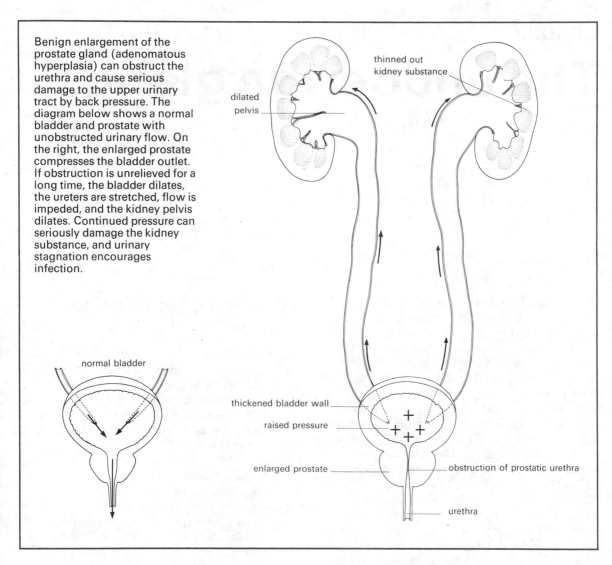

Benign enlargement of the prostate gland (adenomatous hyperplasia) can obstruct the urethra and cause serious damage to the upper urinary tract by back pressure. The diagram below shows a normal bladder and prostate with unobstructed urinary flow. On the right, the enlarged prostate compresses the bladder outlet. If obstruction is unrelieved for a long time, the bladder dilates, the ureters are stretched, flow is impeded, and the kidney pelvis dilates. Continued pressure can seriously damage the kidney substance, and urinary stagnation encourages infection.

thinned out kidney substance

dilated pelvis

normal bladder

thickened bladder wall

raised pressure

enlarged prostate

obstruction of prostatic urethra

urethra

symptoms which need to be investigated without delay. Early radical removal of the tumour combined with irradiation is the usual treatment.

Testis Tumours of the testis are highly malignant and may occur at any age, but are most common in the early teens and twenties. Any mass in the testis, especially if it is not associated with fever, should be suspected of being malignant. Treatment is by surgical removal and irradiation.

Hydrocele and spermatocele A hydrocele is an accumulation of fluid in the scrotum, in the potential sac covering the testis. The swelling is usually obvious to the patient. A spermatocele is a cyst involving the sperm-conducting apparatus. These swellings are not very significant if small but can become a nuisance if they increase in size, and should be removed.

Obstruction

This can occur anywhere between the main collecting parts of the kidneys – the calyces – and the external opening of the urethra. It may be congenital or acquired as the result of a stone, tumour, or narrowing caused by injury or inflammation. Obstructions sometimes arise at the junction of the pelvis of the kidney and ureter from a congenital physiological defect or from an impacted stone. In the ureter, the cause is often a moderate sized stone which has become impacted, or, occasionally, a tumour. The common cause of bladder neck obstruction is enlargement of the prostate, and in the urethra a narrowing, rarely congenital, sometimes inflammatory, and usually due to injury in industrial or traffic accidents. Most require surgical treatment.

Chapter 9

The endocrine glands

Revised by A. Stuart Mason, MD FRCP

We are all students of endocrinology in everyday life. Growing, maturing, loving, even being scared, or just keeping going through the day all depend on the endocrine glands. They play a large part in the development of the body and maintaining its constant chemical equilibrium against the adversities of environment.

The endocrine glands are ductless, which means that they secrete hormones directly into the bloodstream, in contrast to organs such as the salivary glands that secrete saliva through a duct into the mouth. A hormone is a chemical messenger controlling certain functions necessary for the health of the body as a whole.

The ability of man to respond and adapt successfully to his changing environment is made possible by the coordination of two controlling systems. One is the nervous system, the other the endocrine system. The nervous system connects each part of the body to the brain by a network of nerve fibres. Information and action are transmitted by minute electrical currents. This provides a system of high-speed communication. Hormones are the slower messengers of the endocrine system. Their function is related to the control of body chemistry and the long-term processes such as growth and sexual development. The two systems come together at the hypothalamus. This structure lies at the base of the brain and contains centres exerting nervous control, and nerve endings adapted to secrete hormones. The hypothalamus also receives information from other parts of the brain and from the concentration of hormones in the blood. Based on this information its action integrates the work of a large part of the endocrine system.

Location of endocrine glands

The endocrine glands are scattered about the body and have little similarity in size, shape, or structure. As the hormones they secrete travel to their target tissues by the blood, there is no need for any gland to be near the organ that it influences. The pituitary gland is situated at the base of the skull, in a small bony cavity. The thyroid lies in the neck, bridging the windpipe. The parathyroid glands are embedded in the lobes of the thyroid. The endocrine cells of the pancreas are scattered in groups throughout the organ and weigh only a few grams. The main bulk of the pancreas is concerned with making the pancreatic digestive juice that passes into the gut. The pancreas lies across the back of the abdominal cavity. The adrenal glands lie on top of the kidneys. In women the ovaries lie in the pelvic cavity on either side of the uterus, and in men the testes hang in the scrotum just below the abdomen. Ovaries and testes are known collectively as the gonads. The functions of the thymus are obscure.

Hormones

Most of the hormones manufactured by endocrine glands are small proteins (polypeptides), or steroids. Polypeptides are made of amino acids, the building blocks of all protein structures in the body. Steroids are four-ringed compounds of carbon, hydrogen, and oxygen, and are made from cholesterol. Once hormones reach the bloodstream they circulate all over the body, usually attached to a

The endocrine glands

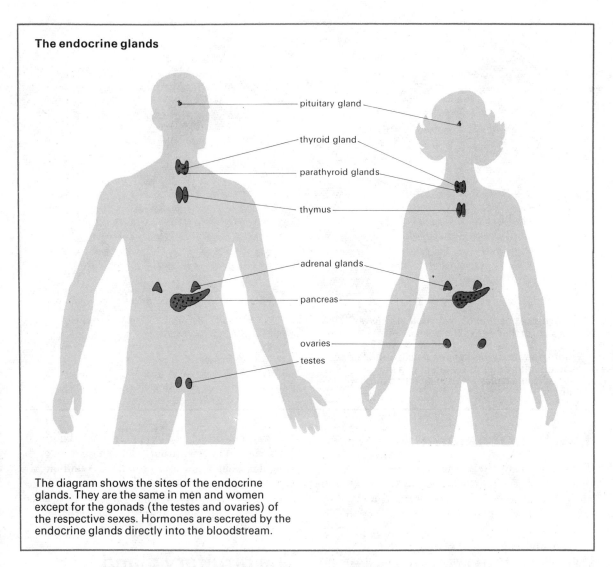

- pituitary gland
- thyroid gland
- parathyroid glands
- thymus
- adrenal glands
- pancreas
- ovaries
- testes

The diagram shows the sites of the endocrine glands. They are the same in men and women except for the gonads (the testes and ovaries) of the respective sexes. Hormones are secreted by the endocrine glands directly into the bloodstream.

specific protein in the blood. Receptors on the cell surfaces of the organs then capture the hormones as they pass, and are specific in that they capture the right hormone, letting the others go by. The hormone affects the cell's chemical activity and also alters cell shape and size. More than one hormone can act on a cell, each modifying the other's action. Without hormones cells could not develop properly. The orderly secretion of hormones keeps the internal chemistry of the body constant and, therefore, healthy. Without hormones a child does not grow, an adolescent girl's breasts do not enlarge, and a boy lives to be a beardless eunuch. On the other hand, too much of a hormone can distort the body and destroy health. Too much, or too little, of various hormones alters mood, desire, and drive.

It is a tribute to the stability of the endocrine system that its diseases are relatively rare. For this reason a doctor may not immediately think of diagnosing an uncommon endocrine disorder when it mimics the course of some common disease. The fact that an overactive thyroid makes the sufferer very nervous does not mean that all nervous people have thyroid disease. Lack of growth hormone slows a child's development, but it is a rare cause of shortness. So in describing diseases of the endocrine system it is important to keep a sense of proportion, and patients, if in doubt, should always seek professional advice. The following description of endocrine glands, their hormones, and the diseases that their disorders may cause, does explain technical terms of diagnosis, but it should also give an idea of how the endocrine system is an integrator of body function and a guardian of health.

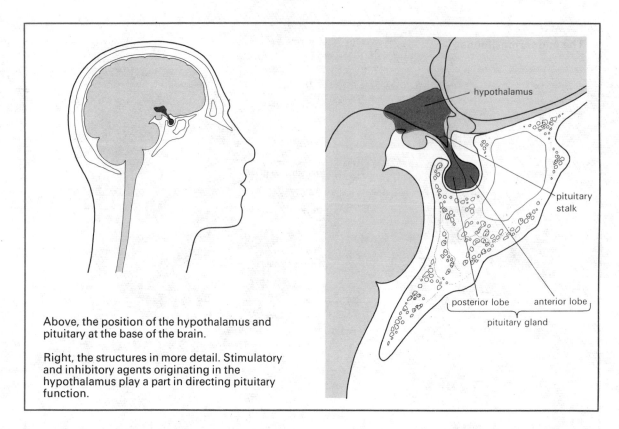

Above, the position of the hypothalamus and pituitary at the base of the brain.

Right, the structures in more detail. Stimulatory and inhibitory agents originating in the hypothalamus play a part in directing pituitary function.

The hypothalamus

The hypothalamus lies at the base of the "old brain", that is the lower part of the brain that deals with instinct and body control. The "newer brain" is the seat of intellect, memory, and voluntary action. The hypothalamus is the essential link between the nervous and endocrine systems. Within the hypothalamus lie centres concerned with sleep and waking, appetite and thirst, body temperature control, water balance, and sexual function. Some of these functions are based on nerve mechanisms, others are based on hormone secretion of the anterior (front part of the) pituitary, which is first stimulated by hormones from the hypothalamus. Special neurosecretory cells in the hypothalamus actually make the hormones that are released from the posterior (back part of the) pituitary.

The hypothalamus controls many of the automatic regulating (homeostatic) functions of the body, and any disorder may upset these functions. Changes in the hypothalamus, therefore, may cause extreme obesity because of uncontrollable hunger; failure of temperature control so that the body becomes too cool (hypothermia) or has a high fever (hyperpyrexia); or sudden attacks of sleep (narcolepsy).

Puberty may be delayed or appear at an abnormally early age. The menstrual cycle may stop or be irregular. Sometimes any one of these conditions or a combination of them are due to destructive changes, from tumours, injury, or inflammation. More often, function is disturbed without any actual structural damage to the hypothalamus.

The pituitary gland

The pituitary, twelve by eight mm ($\frac{1}{2}$ by $\frac{1}{3}$ in) in size, lies in a bony hollow in the base of the skull. It is really two separate glands. Its posterior lobe is the bulbous end of a tract of specialized nervous tissue originating in the hypothalamus and running down the stalk that connects the brain to the pituitary. The posterior lobe stores and releases two hormones made in the hypothalamus: vasopressin and oxytocin. Vasopressin is so called because it can constrict small blood vessels, but its real function is to prevent the kidney letting out too much water. Such an excessive urine flow is called diuresis, so vasopressin is often termed the antidiuretic hormone or ADH. Oxytocin promotes contraction of the pregnant uterus and is used for the induction of labour, when it is injected slowly into a

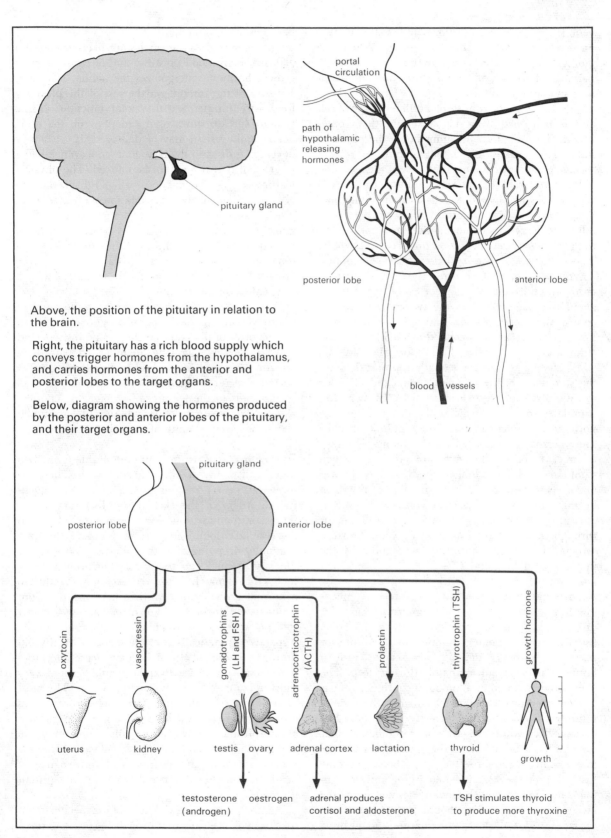

portal circulation

path of hypothalamic releasing hormones

posterior lobe

anterior lobe

blood vessels

pituitary gland

Above, the position of the pituitary in relation to the brain.

Right, the pituitary has a rich blood supply which conveys trigger hormones from the hypothalamus, and carries hormones from the anterior and posterior lobes to the target organs.

Below, diagram showing the hormones produced by the posterior and anterior lobes of the pituitary, and their target organs.

pituitary gland

posterior lobe

anterior lobe

oxytocin

vasopressin

gonadotrophins (LH and FSH)

adrenocorticotrophin (ACTH)

prolactin

thyrotrophin (TSH)

growth hormone

uterus

kidney

testis   ovary

adrenal cortex

lactation

thyroid

growth

testosterone   oestrogen
(androgen)

adrenal produces
cortisol and aldosterone

TSH stimulates thyroid
to produce more thyroxine

Chapter 9 The endocrine glands

vein. It also causes the secretion of milk so that it plays an essential part in breast-feeding. When the mother's nipple is stimulated by the baby sucking, a nervous reflex is set off that prompts the hypothalamus and posterior pituitary to release oxytocin.

The anterior lobe consists of a different type of cell and is nourished by a blood supply that comes straight from the hypothalamus down the pituitary stalk. This enables the hypothalamus to secrete specific releasing hormones that govern the secretion of hormones from the anterior pituitary. In this way the pituitary and hypothalamus form one functional unit. Most of the anterior pituitary hormones influence the activity of other endocrine glands rather than having a direct action on the body as a whole. These hormones are called trophic hormones. Thyrotrophic hormone controls the thyroid, adreno-corticotrophin controls the cortex of the adrenal gland (see page 208) and the two gonadotrophins control the gonads (ovaries and testes). Often these hormone names are abbreviated to TSH for thyroid-stimulating hormone, ACTH for the adrenal stimulator, and, for the gonadotrophins, LH for the stimulator of the corpus luteum, and FSH for the stimulator of the ovarian follicle. In men, LH stimulates the cells of the testis that secrete male hormone and FSH stimulates the tubules that make spermatozoa. Two anterior lobe hormones that have a direct action on the body are prolactin, which stimulates milk formation in the developed breast, and growth hormone, which stimulates growth in height throughout childhood and plays an important part in controlling energy balance and tissue repair throughout life. A brief account of some disorders associated with the pituitary will indicate the importance of this gland.

Acromegaly and gigantism Acromegaly, meaning large extremities, is a long-term progressive disease due to oversecretion of growth hormone, usually from a benign tumour of the anterior pituitary. Normally the pituitary secretes growth hormone in short bursts, mainly during sleep. The oversecretion caused by a tumour is continuous and is not switched off by sugar, which stops the normal pituitary from secreting growth hormone. The disease affects adults, who cannot grow taller, as their long limb bones have fused the growing ends to the main shaft. Therefore the other bones become distorted, the hands and feet enlarging and thickening. The skin becomes coarser and fleshier so that the face gets a bulldog or bloodhound look. The bones of the face broaden, the lower jaw enlarges, and the brow

becomes more prominent. The nose widens and the tongue enlarges. Acromegalics are likely to develop arthritis, high blood pressure, and often diabetes as growth hormone antagonizes the action of insulin. Pressure of the tumour on the rest of the pituitary frequently interferes with sexual function. If the tumour spreads upwards it can press on the optic nerves and eyesight may be damaged. It is a slowly developing disease, the change in appearance being so gradual that it may not be noticed. The physical features suggest the diagnosis, which is backed up by X-rays of the skull and an estimation of the amount of growth hormone in the blood after giving the patient glucose. Treatment may be by various forms of radiation directed at the pituitary, or by surgical removal of the tumour in selected cases. Control of the growth hormone secretion can be obtained with a drug called bromocryptine.

Gigantism is a diagnosis covering a wide range of disorders that make a child grow to a great height. In the majority of tall children there is no disease, and they are merely following an inherited pattern of growth. It is rare for a child to develop a growth hormone-secreting tumour, which, when it does occur, leads to the features of acromegaly coupled with an excessive rate of growth and a height much above the accepted limits of normal.

Dwarfism Dwarfism is an undesirable term. It is more realistic to talk of restricted growth. There are numerous causes, ranging from a variety of congenital disorders of the skeleton to lingering severe illness or malnutrition. Maximum rates of height increase are found in earliest infancy, the rate gradually dropping after the fifth year. So a severe illness in infancy can prevent a child from gaining inches that cannot be recovered later despite return to a normal growth rate. Average height and weight ratios in childhood are shown on page 255. Short stature, when due to childhood thyroid failure, responds dramatically to treatment with thyroid hormone. Failure of growth hormone secretion causes marked slowing of growth and the child becomes very short in comparison with contemporaries. The most usual form of deficiency, fortunately rare, is an isolated failure of growth hormone secretion, the rest of the pituitary working normally. Sometimes the child's pituitary can be damaged by various disease processes which cause widespread disturbance of pituitary function, not only a lack of growth hormone.

Human pituitary growth hormone is specific to the species, which means that growth hormone derived from the pituitaries of other animals such as the ox will not promote growth in man. Therefore treatment of growth hormone deficiency can be only with injections of the hormone prepared from human pituitaries. Such injections have no effect on growth unless the short stature is due to lack of growth hormone. It has to be shown that the child's pituitary cannot secrete growth hormone despite adequate stimulus by the hypothalamus. As this treatment is a form of substitution therapy it has to be continued throughout the normal period of growth, an onerous task for the patient.

Sexual precocity   Premature sexual development may include the whole of the sexual system so that both girls and boys are fertile or it may be confined to the development of secondary sex characteristics such as breasts or body hair, when it is called precocious pseudopuberty. Any sexual development before the age of ten can be termed premature, although it must be remembered that the age of onset of normal puberty has a wide span. In these days of contraceptive pills which contain ovarian hormones, it is not unknown for a very small daughter to grow breasts because she has eaten mother's "special sweets". True precocious puberty is more common in girls than in boys. It usually represents a slip in biological time in a perfectly healthy girl. However it is extremely embarrassing for a six year old to have an adult body and regular menstruation. The hypothalamus times the onset of puberty by initiating release of gonadotrophins from the pituitary which activate the ovary whose hormones develop the female body to adult form. Fortunately, it is possible to suppress the pituitary output of gonadotrophins with synthetic steroid hormones. This can hold the progress of puberty in check until an appropriate time. Precocious puberty in boys is frequently associated with a tumour involving the hypothalamus. Usually the sex changes are found in conjunction with evidence of deep-seated brain disease.

Rarely, tumours of the adrenal, ovary, or testis cause sex development of the pseudopuberty type. Congenital adrenal hyperplasia, in which the adrenal gland makes too much male hormone, and too little of the vital metabolic hormones, will cause virilization of a girl or pseudopuberty of a boy. This condition, which tends to run in families, is treatable with steroids that suppress the abnormal adrenal activity and provide the body with the vital hormones.

Sexual infantilism   Failure of development of sexual characteristics does not become evident until the time of normal puberty is passed. Often such late developers have no disease but suffer from a time slip of the hypothalamus and will develop in due course. The psychological trauma of remaining sexually infantile while school friends are becoming adult is serious, and it is important for such children to receive hormonal therapy which can be given effectively until nature takes over. Failure of sexual development because of organic disease ranges from primary failure of the ovary or testis to function, despite adequate pituitary stimulation, to failure of the pituitary to secrete gonadotrophins. The exact hormonal and structural problem can be, and should be, worked out by experts. The problems will involve sexual development itself which is dealt with by giving the appropriate hormones, and the problem of eventual fertility which is more difficult but, in certain cases, not insurmountable.

Panhypopituitarism   Overall loss of anterior pituitary function can result from tumours, cysts, or death of tissue (necrosis) of the gland. Necrosis due to deprivation of blood supply is most commonly seen after severe haemorrhage at childbirth. Destruction of the anterior pituitary with a loss of its secretory functions is followed by failure of the glands under pituitary control. These glands are the thyroid, adrenal cortex, and testis or ovary. Partial pituitary failure will first diminish sexual function, then growth, and finally the vital control of thyroid and adrenal glands. The combined effects of gonadal, thyroid, and adrenal failure cause severe illness with low blood pressure, intolerance of cold, collapse under stress, extreme fatigue, poor appetite, and total loss of sexual desire and function. This potentially fatal disease can be alleviated by substitution of the various hormones produced by the target glands.

Lactation   Spontaneous milk production can occur in a woman who has not just had a child and even in a man if there is excessive pituitary secretion of prolactin which governs milk production. Unlike other pituitary hormones whose release is prompted by a hormone from the hypothalamus, prolactin is held in the pituitary by a hypothalamic hormone that inhibits its release. Certain tranquillizing drugs stop this action and allow the pituitary to secrete prolactin in large amounts, thus causing milk secretion from the breast. The same can happen with direct secretion of prolactin from a pituitary tumour. Prolactin in excess prevents the gonadotrophins from stimulating the ovaries so menstruation fails. High prolactin levels can be caused by the contraceptive pill – this is one cause of failure of menstruation after the pill has been stopped. Actual milk secretion from the breast does not occur in every case of high prolactin secretion; it depends on whether the breast is sufficiently developed to give milk. Excess prolactin is a cause of infertility, and lowering the level with bromocryptine will allow conception.

Diabetes insipidus The normal hypothalamus is sensitive to the state of the body's water content. If the blood becomes too thick ADH (antidiuretic hormone) is secreted, cutting down the loss of water through the kidney. When enough water has diluted the blood to normal, ADH secretion ceases. Similarly, drinking a large volume of fluid keeps ADH secretion down until the excess water is eliminated in the urine. The mechanism is also sensitive to nicotine which prompts release of ADH and to alcohol which suppresses it. Part of an alcoholic hangover is due to dehydration from lack of ADH.

Damage to the hypothalamus can lead to loss of the capacity to secrete ADH. The kidney then lets out large quantities of water and the body's liquid is kept up only by thirst-prompted high fluid intake. The combination of huge urine volumes, the urine being very dilute and almost colourless, and intense thirst is the feature of diabetes insipidus. This uncommon disease is not to be confused with the common disease diabetes mellitus, with sugar in the urine. Head injury can cause diabetes insipidus, but in the end it cures itself. Tumours and inflammation of the hypothalamus have longer lasting effects and there is also a form in which ADH secretion fails for no discernible reason, the rest of the hypothalamus and pituitary continuing to work normally. Preparations of ADH are available as a nasal spray and as injections. The treatment of this distressing condition is effective and the sufferer is released from a life confined between the water jug and the lavatory.

There is another form of this disease called nephrogenic diabetes insipidus in which the supply of ADH is normal but the kidney is incapable of response and just goes on letting out water at all times. This is usually a hereditary condition.

The rarely seen reverse situation of diabetes insipidus is one of inappropriate ADH secretion in which the urine flow remains relatively low while the blood becomes too dilute. This lowered osmotic pressure leads to a feeling of general illness and headache, progressing to water intoxication with drowsiness and even fits. This can occur if the setting of the hypothalamus is faulty and may occur in some lung disorders and with adrenal failure.

The thyroid

The thyroid, weighing about 25 gm (one oz), lies in the neck. It has two lobes, one either side of the windpipe just below the level of the larynx. The lobes are joined by a narrow strip of thyroid tissue running in front of the windpipe. The thyroid is unique among endocrine glands in that it requires a supply of iodine to makes its hormone. Therefore its function depends on the external environment, whereas other glands obtain their raw material from substances readily available in the body. Iodine is coupled with two molecules of tyrosine, an amino acid, one of the group that forms the building blocks of all protein structures. The resulting hormone, thyroxine, contains four iodine atoms. Another more potent form is made within the thyroid and elsewhere in the body by alteration of thyroxine; this form is triiodothyronine. The whole thyroid cycle of trapping iodine, combining it with tyrosine, storing it as thyroglobulin and finally releasing the hormones is under the control of the pituitary TSH (thyroid-stimulating hormone). The release of TSH is initiated by the hypothalamus with its specific releasing hormone. A balance is kept between circulating levels of thyroid hormone and TSH secretion so that there is a constant level of thyroid hormone in the bloodstream.

The thyroid affects the metabolism of practically all the tissues of the body. Its hormones regulate the rate of oxygen consumption, that is, the rate at which the body burns up its fuel, known as the metabolic rate. The hormones are also potent growth promoters and are necessary for the full development of the brain. As the thyroid regulates the metabolic rate of other endocrine glands, it can influence the production of their hormones. Too little thyroid hormone produces a low metabolic rate and slows down all biological processes. Too much hormone speeds up metabolism until everything is working too fast and it also makes the body unduly sensitive to adrenalin. For healthy thyroid function there must be a normal pituitary, an adequate daily supply of iodine in the diet, and normal pathways of hormone synthesis and release from the thyroid.

Hyperthyroidism Hyperthyroidism, or excessive secretion of thyroid hormones, is also known as thyrotoxicosis or Graves' disease after the Dublin physician who published an account of the condition in 1835. Thyrotoxicosis means a poisoning of the body by an excess of normal hormone. Thyrotoxicosis factitia is the name given to the condition caused by taking too many tablets of thyroxine, by design or

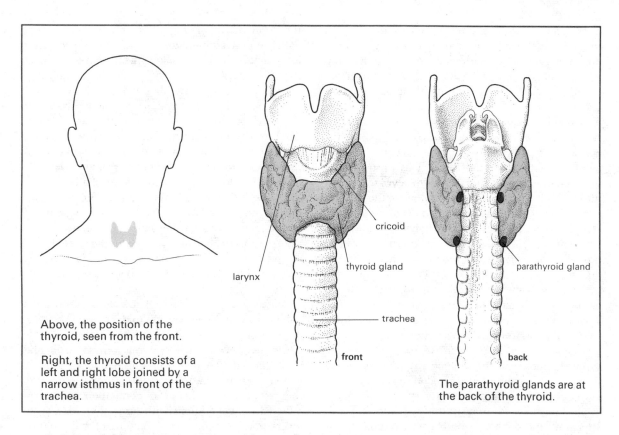

Above, the position of the thyroid, seen from the front.

Right, the thyroid consists of a left and right lobe joined by a narrow isthmus in front of the trachea.

larynx

cricoid

thyroid gland

trachea

front

parathyroid gland

back

The parathyroid glands are at the back of the thyroid.

accident. Overactivity of the thyroid is, in some cases, caused by a benign tumour, or adenoma. But more commonly the whole thyroid is overactive, being driven by a thyroid stimulator that acts like, but is not, TSH. This curious substance is formed by the immune defence mechanisms of the body and is best named "thyroid-stimulating immunoglobulin" or TSIG. It has also been known as LATS or long-acting thyroid stimulator because of its behaviour in experimental situations. In an obscure way this is tied up with autoimmune thyroiditis (see later) and with the substance that makes the eyes of some patients abnormally prominent (exophthalmos).

The increased metabolic rate of hyperthyroidism causes loss of weight despite a good or increased appetite. The skin is soft, flushed, and hot. Sufferers are intolerant of hot weather, often thirsty because of water loss through the skin, and usually very tense and anxious. The exceptional emotional instability may, of course, be an exaggeration of an anxiety state, something that many people have from time to time. The thigh and shoulder muscles become weak and the hands tremble. Everything goes faster; frequent bowel action is common and, most particularly, the heart pounds away at a great rate. So the patient is tired, breathless, distressed by

palpitations, and miserable. The thyroid usually enlarges and the eyes stare. It is a condition that affects women more often than men. Its natural history is very variable in severity of disease and in tempo; the condition tends to wax and wane. About one third of cases would probably cure themselves in the end, but treatment is necessary because hyperthyroidism can make a person very ill.

The choice of treatment depends on many factors, including the patient's age, general health, state of heart and lungs, and size of the thyroid. So-called antithyroid drugs, such as carbimazole, stop the formation of thyroid hormone, so that the right dose will keep the thyroid's secretory activity normal. However treatment has to be very prolonged and the relapse rate is high. Surgical removal of a large part of the thyroid is an effective cure but the operation is a major one. Before operation the gland has to be controlled by antithyroid drugs. Here the transient benefits of iodine are very useful. The third method of treatment is the use of radioactive iodine to destroy part of the gland. This radiation treatment is reserved for those past childbearing age, so that any genetic risk to children is avoided. Radioiodine has no immediate ill effects but is slow to work. The choice of the right treatment for the individual requires expert

Chapter 9 The endocrine glands

assessment. Apart from direct attack on the thyroid, the patient's symptoms may derive largely from increased sensitivity to adrenalin. So drugs that stop adrenalin acting may be of benefit. A great deal can be done with sympathetic guidance through a disturbing illness.

Excess thyroxine raises the upper eyelid causing a surprised stare. In some cases of Graves' disease the eyeballs are pushed forward by an accumulation of jelly-like material behind them. This protrusion of the eyes, or exophthalmos, makes the eyes water and the eyelids bulge. The muscles that move the eyes are often affected, causing double vision. This unpleasant complication can develop with hyperthyroidism, or before it, or get worse when the thyroid has been brought back to normal function. Thus it is not directly related to the excess of thyroid hormones but is linked with the disease, having something to do with the thyroid-stimulating immunoglobulins. Treatment of exophthalmos relies on keeping down its severity and waiting for it to cure itself. This may take many months or even years. Acute severe exophthalmos can be helped by cortisone-like steroids. Protecting the eye, soothing drops, and diuretics all have a place. Surgery can bring the eyelids together to protect the eye and improve appearance. If double vision becomes permanent, it can be relieved by operation.

Hypothyroidism Deficiency of thyroid hormones can arise for a variety of reasons. Children may be born with an inefficient thyroid, or none at all. Adults may develop thyroid failure because their pituitary has ceased to function; lack of TSH is one feature of panhypopituitarism. Far more commonly the thyroid itself is attacked by an autoimmune process which slowly destroys the gland. Equally slowly the hormone levels drop to cause a gradually progressive illness.

The low metabolic rate that is the consequence of thyroxine deficiency slows down all life processes. Increasing fatigue, lethargy, aching muscles, constipation, and intolerance to cold are common symptoms. The weight rises despite dieting. The most characteristic feature of hypothyroidism is the changed physical appearance of the sufferer. The skin becomes dry and puffy, like a fat mask over the face; the eyelids swell and the voice thickens to a croak. These changes are due to infiltration of the skin with a mucus-like substance, which gives rise to the name myxoedema that is often used instead of hypothyroidism. Depression, anaemia, and high blood cholesterol are other features. The onset is so slow that the vague but increasing illness and inability to cope with life may go undiagnosed. In elderly people the low metabolic rate makes them more liable to hypothermia.

Once thought of, the diagnosis is relatively easy and laboratory confirmation will demonstrate the low level of blood thyroxine and the high level of TSH, representing the pituitary's efforts to stimulate the inactive thyroid. Of course, in the rare cases of thyroid failure secondary to pituitary failure the TSH level will be low and remain so after challenge with the hypothalamic TSH-releasing hormone. Treatment is most effective; full health can be restored and maintained, provided the patient continues to take the appropriate dose of thyroxine for the rest of his, or more often her, life. The initial dose has to be low in case a sudden increase of metabolic rate affects the heart.

Congenital hypothyroidism The age-old term for a child born with a defective thyroid is cretin. The term cretin comes from old French, meaning "little Christian" because such children were so docile and well behaved. One type of cretinism, now fortunately rare, is endemic goitrous cretinism found in areas of the world where the local population had been afflicted for generations with large thyroids due to severe iodine deficiency. The infant's thyroid is enlarged at birth and hypothyroidism while still in the womb has prevented full development of the brain.

Sporadic cretinism is of two types. The first is one in which the child is born without any thyroid at all. This naturally produces a poorly infant, lethargic, often jaundiced for a long while, and just not thriving. There is grave danger of the brain failing to mature and the body remaining stunted. Hence early diagnosis and treatment are essential and can be confirmed by the fifth day of life because the blood TSH level is very high and can be measured accurately. A more common variant of this state is due to partial growth of the thyroid which will maintain the child through infancy but is insufficient to allow a normal rate of growth. The child becomes abnormally short and shows some of the signs of myxoedema. The other type of sporadic cretinism is due to an inborn error of metabolism, the thyroid being present and enlarged by excess TSH, but incapable of forming hormone. Usually the block to hormone formation is partial so that the child is short and fails to thrive, the large thyroid being the obvious abnormality. In one form the disorder is associated with congenital deafness.

Early diagnosis should avoid full-blown cretinism

which is a state of mental retardation, dwarfism, sparse hair, coarse dry skin, puffy face, and large tongue. Constipation goes with a pot belly, which often has an umbilical hernia. Treatment of cretinism must be started as early as possible. Even then mentality may be subnormal. Replacement doses of thyroxine must be taken for the rest of the patient's life.

Goitre Goitre is a term applied to all swellings of the thyroid. Most forms of generalized thyroid enlargement are due to some long-term excess of pituitary TSH, which has been attempting to stimulate the thyroid into proper functioning. The classic example of this has been mentioned under sporadic cretinism, when an inborn error prevents the thyroid from making sufficient hormone. A milder variety of this type of block can cause goitre in childhood and adolescence.

Endemic goitre This condition is due to iodine deficiency and sometimes goitre-producing substances in the diet. It has been seen in mountainous areas and other parts of the world where the water and food supplies contain insufficient iodine to allow the thyroid to make enough hormone. Women are affected more than men because the menstrual cycle and pregnancy make demands on the thyroid. So the goitre often appears during a girl's puberty. As a public health measure, the use of iodized salt or iodine in other forms has done much towards eradicating this worldwide trouble.

Nodular goitre Nodular goitres are common swellings of the thyroid occurring usually in middle-aged women. Thyroid function is normal, but the swelling causes pressure symptoms in the neck which have to be relieved by surgical removal of the affected tissue. Sometimes nodules are single, just one lump of cells in the gland. Here there is a vital distinction between benign adenoma, that is, a tumour of glandular tissue, and cancer. It must be stressed that several varieties of thyroid cancer are easily treated by surgery and irradiation, and the long-term results are excellent.

Scanning of the thyroid after the administration of a small dose of radioactive iodine gives useful information because it can depict the areas of activity throughout the thyroid.

Thyroiditis Acute virus infections may cause sudden tender swelling of the thyroid that subsides in a few days and does no damage. Most important is autoimmune thyroiditis in which the body's defence mechanisms treat the thyroid as a foreign tissue and attack it, just as in the rejection of a grafted organ.

The blood contains the marks of the battle in that specific thyroid antibodies can be detected. The process usually affects middle-aged women. The goitre may be firm and fleshy, or small and hard. Function of the thyroid may be increased, normal, or deficient. In the end hypothyroidism is likely to result.

The parathyroid glands

These glands, usually four in number, are superficially embedded in the back and side surfaces of each lobe of the thyroid. Each parathyroid is only about six mm ($\frac{1}{4}$ in) across, and one or more may be out of place, lying behind the breastbone. Parathyroid hormone (parathormone) is concerned with keeping a steady level of calcium in the blood. If the level falls, parathyroid hormone is secreted to bring calcium out of bone to adjust the level. Removal of the parathyroids results in a sharp fall in blood-calcium and a rise in phosphorus. The low calcium level increases neuromuscular excitability to cause muscle twitching or tetany (not to be confused with tetanus, an entirely different disease). Tetany can be severe, with painful contractions of the muscles of the hands and feet. When very severe it can cause convulsions. Another hormone, calcitonin, used to be thought to come from the parathyroid but is actually secreted from special cells within the thyroid. This hormone helps to reduce high blood-calcium levels and to store calcium in bones.

Hyperparathyroidism Excess secretion of parathyroid hormone, causing hyperparathyroidism, comes from a benign adenoma of one gland. Occasionally all four glands are adenomatous, a condition that often runs in families. The diagnosis is made when a raised blood-calcium level is found together with an increased blood concentration of parathyroid hormone. Primary hyperparathyroidism is usually associated with renal colic or blood in the urine indicating the presence of kidney stones. The excess calcium in the blood leads to an excess of calcium in the urine and hence kidney stones of calcium salts. Any patient who has such stones should have blood-calcium measurements made in case hyperparathyroidism is the cause. A marked rise in blood-calcium, from any cause, produces headache, weariness, thirst, and an increased volume of urine. In some instances the bones are affected by the amount of calcium drawn out by parathyroid hormone. Removal of the parathyroid adenoma removes the trouble.

Secondary hyperparathyroidism is an increased secretion of parathyroid hormone by all the glands, which enlarge in compensation for disorders that depress blood-calcium. Chronic kidney failure is the usual cause of secondary hyperparathyroidism. This is now of importance in those whose lives depend on renal dialysis.

Hypoparathyroidism This is a rare condition, apart from removal of the parathyroids as a complication of thyroid surgery. The parathyroids, like the thyroid, can be destroyed by autoimmune disease. The condition usually arises in childhood. The cramplike tetany may be confused with epilepsy. Cataract of the eyes is common, the teeth erupt like leaning tombstones and have no roots, the scalp hair is thin, and fungus infections of the skin are common. The condition can be controlled, and maintenance of a normal blood-calcium level can be obtained by using vitamin D. Treatment has to be monitored by regular measurements of blood-calcium and the amount of extra calcium taken has to be carefully assessed.

The adrenal glands

The first disease to be connected with an endocrine gland was described by Thomas Addison of Guy's Hospital in 1855. He identified the disorder caused by the destruction of both adrenal glands, a disease that still bears his name. The adrenal glands are two small triangular bodies lying just above the kidneys. The adrenal consists of two parts with distinct functions.

The medulla forms the inner portion of the gland. It is really an extension of the autonomic nervous system and secretes adrenalin. Destruction of the medulla does not affect health as there are plenty of other adrenalin-secreting cells elsewhere in the body. Adrenalin is vital in energizing the body to meet sudden dangers and alarms. The mother seeing her child run into the road and the athlete awaiting the start of a race both have a sudden surge of adrenalin. It triggers off the "fight or flight" mechanisms of the body and causes a rapid pulse, pounding heart, pale skin, and sweaty palms; it mobilizes sugar from the liver to provide instant energy. The same physical changes due to adrenalin are seen when someone suffers from acute anxiety, when the emotion is not directly related to the danger of circumstances.

The cortex forms the outer part of the gland and is composed of layered glandular cells. The cortex secretes steroid hormones, all closely linked in structure but differing in activity. Grouped according to function, the adrenal hormones are glucocorticoids concerned with sugar metabolism and stress, mineralocorticoids that control salt balance, and sex steroids which are similar in action to those of the testis and ovary. Our ability to withstand stress (in terms of injury or infection) depends on the efficiency of the adrenal cortex. The main antistress hormone is the glucocorticoid cortisol. The rate of cortisol secretion is determined by the stimulus of pituitary ACTH. The pituitary is activated by the hypothalamus which interprets the chemical and nervous information it receives from the body affected by stress. There is also a feedback relationship between the level of cortisol in the blood and the amount of ACTH. When the cortisol level drops, more ACTH is secreted until the level of cortisol returns to normal. Conversely an increased level of cortisol inhibits the output of ACTH so that the adrenal is rested. This mechanism is of major importance when patients are being treated with synthetic steroids related to cortisol. When given in an appropriate amount these steroids will stop the pituitary putting out ACTH and so the patient's adrenals become inactive. This inactivity can continue for some time after treatment has been stopped; thus the patient is liable to suffer from adrenal insufficiency.

The major mineralocorticoid is aldosterone which retains salt in the body by acting upon the kidney. Faced by salt depletion, as in heavy sweating, the adrenal increases its secretion of aldosterone which diminishes the amount of salt in the urine. Salt depletion from any cause leads to nausea, muscle cramps, low blood pressure, and general weakness.

Addison's disease Chronic adrenal destruction, as shown by Addison, is usually due to autoimmune adrenalitis or tuberculosis. The former is more common and affects women more often than men; the body's defence systems attack the adrenal tissue, a process similar to that of autoimmune thyroiditis, indeed the two disorders may be seen together. Although the destruction of the adrenals is gradual, the symptoms may be sudden and catastrophic. Minor infections can cause death because the adrenal is incapable of responding to stress. Otherwise the course of the disease is one of increasing disability with weakness, fatigue, loss of appetite and morning nausea, vague abdominal pains, and extreme helplessness in the face of minor stress. Fainting may occur due to a fall in blood pressure on standing. All these symptoms are due to lack of cortisol and aldosterone. The major physical sign is darkening of the skin, accentuated by sunlight. This is caused by excess circulating ACTH from the pituitary's vain attempt to stimulate the inactive adrenal. The pigmentation is seen as a dirty brown on the fingers and in the creases of the palms. Areas of pigmentation may appear in the mouth.

Once thought of, the diagnosis of Addison's disease is comparatively easy; there are low levels of blood cortisol that do not rise when the adrenals are challenged with injections of ACTH. The disease is rare, but infection may kill suddenly and the patient is safe only when the right substitution therapy has been started. Tablets of cortisol or cortisone combined with a synthetic mineralocorticoid (fludrocortisone) are most effective. At all times stress must be countered by immediate increases in cortisol dosage, given by injection if the patient feels sick. If the cause is tuberculosis, this must be treated with the proper drugs, even if there is no evidence of tuberculosis in other organs.

Secondary hypoadrenalism Failure of ACTH secretion is an important aspect of hypopituitarism. The patient has a pale skin due to lack of ACTH and does not lose salt in the urine as in Addison's disease, because aldosterone secretion continues. The life-threatening part of hypopituitarism is the loss of cortisol secretion, particularly in the face of stress. Cortisol is a life-saving treatment for this condition, just as it is with primary adrenal failure. More common than any disease of the pituitary is the failure of ACTH secretion that may accompany the use of cortisol-like steroids in the treatment of nonendocrine disease like rheumatoid arthritis or asthma. All the synthetic steroids used have the power to suppress pituitary secretion of ACTH just as cortisol does when present in unusually high amounts. With prolonged high dosage the adrenals wither due to lack of ACTH and take a long time to return to normal function when the steroid therapy is stopped. So the patient is at risk of hypoadrenalism and cannot face stress. To minimize this risk synthetic steroids are given in the smallest dose possible. Sometimes a dose given on alternate days is effective and safe, or local application, as in a spray for asthma, cuts down the amount reaching the circulation. When necessary, as in preparation for an operation, extra steroid is given to offset the effects of stress.

Hypercorticoidism Various disorders are associated with excess or imbalance of the hormones produced by the adrenal cortex. It must be remembered that the therapeutic use of steroid

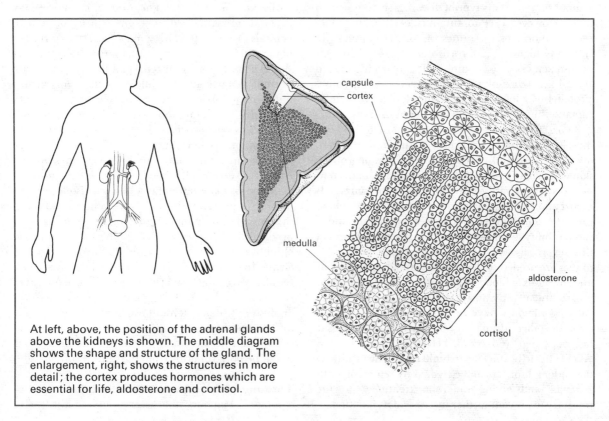

capsule
cortex
medulla
aldosterone
cortisol

At left, above, the position of the adrenal glands above the kidneys is shown. The middle diagram shows the shape and structure of the gland. The enlargement, right, shows the structures in more detail; the cortex produces hormones which are essential for life, aldosterone and cortisol.

hormones can produce a picture that closely resembles the natural disorder.

Primary hyperaldosteronism Small benign tumours, or sometimes diffuse growth of the aldosterone-producing cells in both adrenals, cause excessive output of aldosterone, the most potent of salt-retaining hormones. The result is high blood pressure accompanied by a low blood-potassium level. Sodium is retained in excess and potassium excreted in the urine. The resulting potassium deficiency can lead to extreme muscle weakness, sometimes with cramplike spasms. The bowel becomes distended with gas. More urine than usual is passed at night. Chemical diagnosis depends on finding a high blood level of aldosterone and a low level of renin, the enzyme that normally stimulates aldosterone secretion. It is usually necessary to remove the tumour, but sometimes the disorder can be controlled by a drug aldactone.

Cushing's syndrome The effects of excess gluco-corticoid secretion were described in 1932 by Harvey Cushing, an American surgeon. The excess may come from a tumour of the adrenal cortex, benign or malignant, or from excess stimulation of both adrenals by ACTH. As Cushing thought, excess ACTH is due to pituitary disorder, often coming from a small tumour. This type of disease is seldom seen in men. However certain tumours of the lung may secrete enormous quantities of ACTH causing abnormally high levels of cortisol in the blood (hyper-cortisolaemia). This condition is found in middle-aged men. Excess cortisol, the main glucocorticoid, causes protein breakdown into sugar, interference with sugar metabolism, and storage of fat in certain areas.

Thus, Cushing's syndrome is characterized by muscle wasting and weakness of the limb muscles, obesity of the trunk, neck, and face, thinning of the skin which may lead to large stretch marks, and a tendency to bruise easily. The complexion becomes reddened and women may grow excess hair. High blood pressure, mild diabetes, collapsed vertebrae, and a susceptibility to unusual infections are the features of this severe disease. Specialized radiographic techniques are needed to demonstrate an adrenal tumour and the levels of blood ACTH have to be determined.

Treatment obviously depends on the cause. Adrenal tumours have to be removed. After operation the other adrenal will be tiny and inactive as it has been deprived of ACTH stimulation, so that ACTH has to be injected to build it up. The pituitary-dependent disorder can be treated by removing both adrenals and giving radiation treatment to the pituitary to prevent further increase of its function.

Excessive sex hormone secretion At the time of puberty in both sexes the adrenal cortex changes its hormone production and makes some androgenic hormone. This can account for some hairiness and acne in growing girls. At any time a tumour of the adrenal can cause virilization of a woman; fortunately this is a rare occurrence. The commonest cause of undesired face and body hair in a woman is an inherent tendency of the skin to excess hair growth. This is exaggerated by normal or minimally raised levels of androgenic hormone.

Congenital adrenal hyperplasia This rare condition affects boys and girls. It runs in families and is present at birth, being caused by the lack of an adrenal enzyme which is essential for the manufacture of cortisol and aldosterone. The result is that, even in fetal life, the adrenals produce too much male hormone and are constantly stimulated by ACTH as they do not make enough cortisol to suppress the pituitary. Hence the adrenals become enlarged resulting in a mixture of cortisol and aldosterone deficiency, like Addison's disease, and virilization. Indeed the virilization is the price of survival with the adrenals' ineffective attempts to produce enough of its vital hormones. Infants of both sexes are in peril because they suffer from severe Addisonian crises, with extreme salt loss. The Addisonian crisis may be fatal unless treated. The girl will be born with genitals distorted towards a male pattern and the sex of the child may be wrongly attributed. If she survives she becomes more virilized. The boy's genitals are normal at birth but in childhood the penis grows, pubic hair appears, and the whole body becomes unusually muscular and large. The testes do not enlarge, as in precocious puberty. Treatment of the Addisonian crisis is life saving. Later cortisol or suitable substitutes have to be given to stop the ACTH excess and, thereby, the excess adrenal secretion of male hormone. Fludrocortisone is often needed to prevent salt loss. By keeping the adrenals suppressed but without giving enough cortisol to produce the appearance of Cushing's syndrome the child of either sex should grow up normally and be fertile. In girls the initial distortion of the genitals may require correction by plastic surgery. The diagnosis of congenital adrenal hyperplasia is confirmed by analysis of urinary steroid hormones. It is important for the mother of the patient to realize that the condition runs in families and that another child might be born suffering from the same disorder.

Tumour of the adrenal medulla (phaeochromocytoma) Tumours that secrete adrenalin (or a

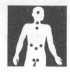

related substance, noradrenalin) arise in the medulla of one or both adrenal glands. Occasionally the tumour can arise in adrenalin-secreting cells lying beside the aorta, the great artery at the back of the abdomen. The secretion from these tumours is spasmodic, with sudden bursts of excess adrenalin. These cause sweating, apprehension, palpitations, tremor, and headache. During the attack the blood pressure rises to very high levels. Later, the blood pressure may remain elevated at all times. Treatment consists of surgical removal of the tumour.

The testes

The male gonads or testes lie just below the abdomen in the scrotal sac. This vulnerable position is necessary because the formation of spermatozoa requires a temperature slightly lower than that found in the abdomen. The testes do not develop until the time of puberty. The bulk of the adult testis is made up of the tubular system that produces spermatozoa. The endocrine portion of the testis comprises clumps of cells that secrete testosterone, the male hormone. The cells also produce small amounts of oestrogen, the female sex hormone.

The testis is under the control of the hypothalamus and anterior pituitary. Puberty is started by the biological time clock of the hypothalamus which in turn starts off pituitary activity by stimulating it with the gonadotrophin-releasing hormone. The pituitary then secretes LH which stimulates the testosterone-producing cells of the testis, and FSH which promotes the growth of the testicular tubular system that finally makes spermatozoa. The testosterone changes the boy's body into a man's. Growth of the penis and scrotum, pubic and axillary hair, increase in muscle mass, deepening of the voice, and beard growth are all induced by testosterone.

When the spermatozoa are formed in the tubules they take three months to become mature and are then stored in the seminal vesicles, beside the prostate. There they swim in the seminal fluid, the volume of which depends on adequate testosterone. The seminal fluid is ejaculated at the climax of the sexual act.

Disorders of the testes

Delayed puberty Delay in the onset of puberty is quite common and later sexual development is normal. It is a temporary disability, not a disease. But it can be a real disability as the boy feels inferior and isolated from his sexually developing companions. Therefore it is a condition worth treating with carefully gauged doses of male hormone given by mouth. Such doses sensitize the genital structures to the effect of gonadotrophins and speed up the normal process of puberty. Success is indicated by enlargement of the testes; treatment is then stopped.

Eunuchoidism Underdevelopment of the gonads (hypogonadism) in the male may be due to primary failure of the testis or to failure of the pituitary to secrete sufficient gonadotrophins. If the cause of hypogonadism is present before the age of puberty, the boy fails to develop into a man. If the failure occurs in a sexually mature male, sexual performance tails off, the amount of seminal fluid diminishes, sex hair tends to fall out, and the skin becomes smooth and dry. Lack of pituitary gonadotrophins may be a part of overall pituitary failure or it may be a selective loss – either because the hypothalamus cannot secrete its

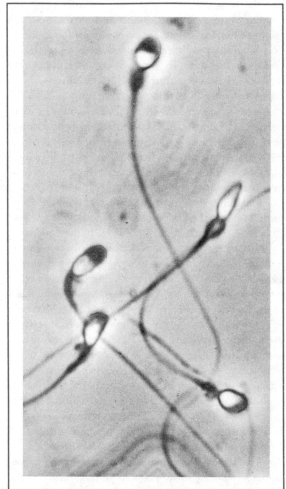

Spermatozoa swim in the seminal fluid. Over a hundred million may be ejaculated at one time.

gonadotrophin-releasing hormone or because the pituitary's gonadotrophic cells are unable to function.

The underdeveloped male frequently grows tall with disproportionately long limbs, lacks a beard, has small genitalia, and a feminine distribution of pubic hair. The voice does not deepen and the muscles are poor in bulk and strength. The emotional stresses are more severe than any sexual ones because sex drive is low or absent. Replacement therapy with male hormone can give satisfactory results but does not produce fertility. Male hormone usually has to be given by injection (every few weeks) or by implantation of hormone pellets (every few months).

Klinefelter's syndrome This syndrome is diagnosed after the age of puberty. The degree of hypogonadism is seldom severe, in fact genital growth and sexual performance can be within the wide range of normal, but the testes are very small and hard because the tubular system cannot develop and so spermatozoa cannot be made. Some breast swelling is often found and is a major embarrassment. This is a congenital condition due to faulty sex chromosomes. Instead of the normal male pattern of XY sex chromosomes there is an extra X making the complement XXY.

Undescended testes (cryptorchidism) In the embryo the testes begin to form in the region of the kidneys and usually complete their journey to the scrotum by birth. About three per cent of newborn boys have undescended testes; by the age of one year the number is down to half a per cent. However the normal descended testis may be retractable, easily pulled up into the abdomen by the muscle that raises the testis. This can be confused with the testis that cannot descend. Sometimes the failure of descent is on one side and due to an anatomical abnormality in the path of descent; this can be corrected by surgery. If both testes are undescended they may be brought down by injections of gonadotrophin. If they remain in the wrong position the tubular elements will not grow and infertility results. Therefore it is important that patients should be treated before they reach puberty, preferably around the eighth or ninth year. Surgical positioning of the testes in the scrotum is required if injections fail. It must be remembered that the testis in the wrong position may also be deformed so that success of treatment cannot be guaranteed.

Infertility A deficient number of healthy spermatozoa in the seminal fluid is a factor in male infertility. In the absence of obvious signs of hypogonadism or of Klinefelter's syndrome the endocrine system is seldom at fault. There may be damage to the testicular tubular system or a block in the ducts that should carry the spermatozoa to the seminal vesicles. Therefore hormone therapy has a limited part to play in the treatment of male infertility.

The ovaries

The ovaries, like the testes, have two functions: to provide ova and to produce hormones that alter the girl's body into that of a woman and prepare the womb (uterus) for pregnancy. The ovary is unique in that during its active life only one portion of one ovary is active at any one time. Two months before a girl is born the ovaries contain a total of seven million cells that could develop into a functional unit producing hormones and an egg. When the girl is born, the number has dropped to one million and by the time that puberty starts the number is down to 300,000. Only about 400 will develop into active follicles, the rest will degenerate. The menopause heralds the last follicle capable of developing, then the ovary sinks into inactivity.

The ovaries are awakened to activity when a girl reaches eleven to thirteen years. They are stimulated by the pituitary starting to secrete the gonadotrophins, FSH and LH. These two gonadotrophins are found in the male as stimulators of the testis. The female hypothalamus differs from that of the male in having a biological time clock that sets the rhythm of the monthly menstrual cycle. It is the hypothalamic gonadotrophin-releasing hormone that controls events. The developing ovarian follicle, prompted by FSH, secretes an oestrogen, predominantly oestradiol. Oestrogen causes feminine development at puberty, enlarging the breasts, the uterus, vagina, and the rest of the genital tract, producing feminine curves of body fat and some body hair. In mid-cycle a surge of pituitary LH is released, in response to the rising levels of oestrogen. This allows the developing egg or ovum to be released from the ovary. The follicle then changes under the influence of LH, becoming what is called the corpus luteum, and secretes, in addition to oestrogen, another hormone – progesterone. This changes the lining of the uterus (endometrium), already built up by oestrogen, to make it a suitable "nest" for the fertilized egg. This is the necessary preparation for pregnancy or gestation, hence the term progesterone. If pregnancy does not occur, the corpus luteum shrinks after two weeks of activity, the secretion of oestrogen and progesterone falls suddenly and, deprived of hormonal support, the endometrium breaks down, its bloody fragments being the menstrual flow. If conception has taken place the ovary is supported by a luteinizing hormone

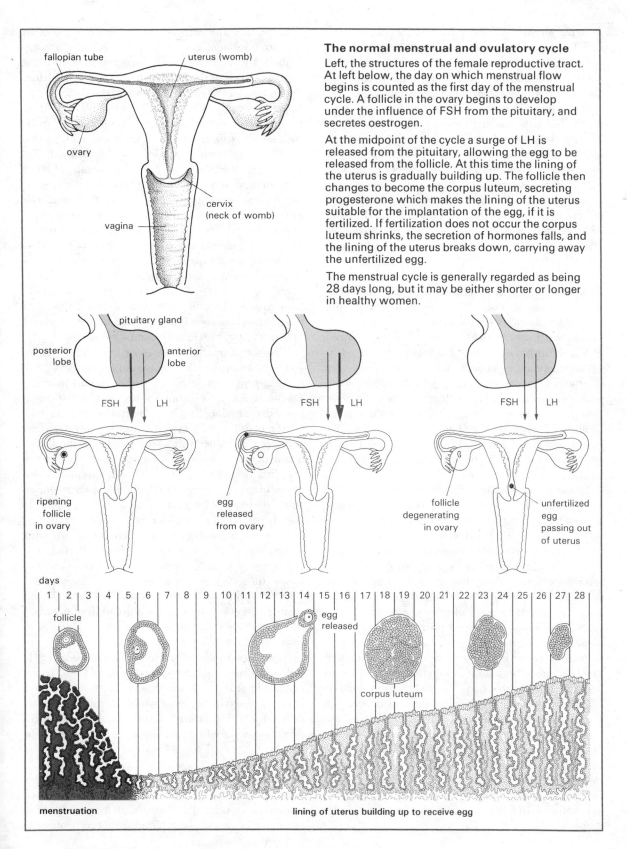

The normal menstrual and ovulatory cycle

Left, the structures of the female reproductive tract. At left below, the day on which menstrual flow begins is counted as the first day of the menstrual cycle. A follicle in the ovary begins to develop under the influence of FSH from the pituitary, and secretes oestrogen.

At the midpoint of the cycle a surge of LH is released from the pituitary, allowing the egg to be released from the follicle. At this time the lining of the uterus is gradually building up. The follicle then changes to become the corpus luteum, secreting progesterone which makes the lining of the uterus suitable for the implantation of the egg, if it is fertilized. If fertilization does not occur the corpus luteum shrinks, the secretion of hormones falls, and the lining of the uterus breaks down, carrying away the unfertilized egg.

The menstrual cycle is generally regarded as being 28 days long, but it may be either shorter or longer in healthy women.

fallopian tube

uterus (womb)

ovary

cervix (neck of womb)

vagina

pituitary gland

posterior lobe

anterior lobe

FSH LH

FSH LH

FSH LH

ripening follicle in ovary

egg released from ovary

follicle degenerating in ovary

unfertilized egg passing out of uterus

days

| 1 | 2 | 3 | 4 | 5 | 6 | 7 | 8 | 9 | 10 | 11 | 12 | 13 | 14 | 15 | 16 | 17 | 18 | 19 | 20 | 21 | 22 | 23 | 24 | 25 | 26 | 27 | 28 |

follicle

egg released

corpus luteum

menstruation

lining of uterus building up to receive egg

from the products of conception and the progesterone secretion continues and rises. This form of LH is produced in such amounts that large quantities spill into the urine and it is the detection of this hormone in the urine that is the basis of most pregnancy tests.

Progesterone is necessary, together with oestrogen, for the full growth of the female breast so that it can become a milk-producing organ. Progesterone also alters the basal body temperature, causing a slight rise. Thus the body temperature is lower in the first half of the menstrual cycle and rises after ovulation to a new plateau. So daily records of temperature indicate the date of ovulation. However this date can be ascertained only by using several months records. It is of no use as an indicator that ovulation is about to occur.

Absence of menstruation (amenorrhoea) Amenorrhoea is normal before puberty, during pregnancy, and after the menopause. Amenorrhoea is said to be primary if menstruation has never occurred although the girl has reached the age of puberty. It is called secondary amenorrhoea if menstruation ceases after a more or less regular cycle. It is important to realize that every girl has to "learn" to menstruate so that irregular cycles during puberty are common and should not cause alarm. The complete absence of menstruation is never a threat to health, it is a symptom that has to be investigated to find the cause.

Primary amenorrhoea may be due to some local abnormality of the womb. If this is the case the usual signs of body change due to oestrogen are present but no menstruation occurs. It is more likely that there is ovarian failure so that the adolescent womb does not receive its usual stimulus from the ovary, and the secondary female sex characteristics remain undeveloped. This may indicate only a delay in normal puberty from some upset of the hypothalamic time clock, which may be due to poor health from any cause. However, if a girl shows no signs of becoming a woman by her sixteenth year the ovary has failed to function either because it is inherently defective or because it has not had the necessary pituitary stimulus. In the first instance the blood level of gonadotrophins will be high, in the second it will be low. One variety of primary ovarian failure is known as Turner's syndrome. This represents an abnormality of sex chromosomes, usually with just one X, instead of the normal female XX. Associated congenital abnormalities include short stature, deformity of the neck, and a characteristic body shape.

Secondary amenorrhoea in young women is often due to emotional causes, characteristically accompanied by sudden loss of appetite and weight (anorexia nervosa). This is in the end self-curing, depending on the emotional state of the patient. The hypothalamus "switches off" and, after a normal weight has been achieved, the hypothalamus can be successfully stimulated by clomiphene. The same drug can be used to make normal menstruation return after the use of the contraceptive pill. This is a combination of oestrogen and progesterone designed to suppress ovulation by suppressing the pituitary's output of gonadotrophins (see page 201 for details). When "the pill" is stopped it is not uncommon to find that normal menstruation does not come back within the first few months. Usually the pituitary reasserts itself and normal menstruation is resumed, even if it takes a year to do so. However some disorder may have arisen while the pill was used and a thorough diagnostic evaluation is needed. Clomiphene is useful in stimulating an inactive pituitary into activity.

Absence of ovarian activity can be countered by giving oestrogens with or without progestogens (acting like progesterone). This is necessary in primary amenorrhoea if the secondary sex characteristics are not fully developed. These ovarian hormones will promote full sexual growth but the menstruation produced is artificial in that it is due to the direct action of these hormones on the endometrium and the bleeding occurs when the tablets are stopped. The same thing occurs with the pill and it is quite wrong to think that the pill regulates the menstrual cycle. It merely imposes an artificial cycle.

Recently it has been shown that excess prolactin secretion can cause amenorrhoea by interfering with the action of gonadotrophins on the ovary. Bringing down the level of prolactin with a drug called bromocryptine will allow a normal and fertile menstrual cycle. Clomiphene is useful in many cases of amenorrhoea due to pituitary insufficiency as it provides a stimulus to pituitary activity. If the pituitary is completely inactive then the use of FSH, prepared from human sources, with LH will cause ovulation. It is a difficult and risky form of therapy, only to be used in selected cases of infertility; never to be used just to produce menstrual bleeding. Superovulation and multiple pregnancy are a considerable risk.

Premenstrual tension Most women feel at their worst in the week preceding a period. Water retention, emotional tension, and a tired bloated feeling may become disabling. Sufferers from migraine may get their worst headaches at this time. Often it is a matter of the body overreacting to the normal hormonal changes of the cycle. Sometimes the disorder is associated with relative progesterone deficiency. Many patients can be helped by progesterone or by altering the hormonal changes of the menstrual cycle. It is not a condition that should be suffered as the lot of all women; expert guidance will help.

Ovarian virilism　The normal ovary does not secrete a significant amount of male hormone (androgen), but the ovary can easily form small cysts so that the follicles do not develop normally. Menstrual chaos is the result, together with a greasy skin and increased body hair growth. The crippled ovary produces too little oestrogen and too much androgen. This is called Stein-Leventhal syndrome and can often be relieved by removing the cysts to leave healthy ovarian tissue to work again. There are also rare benign tumours of the ovary that produce androgen.

The menopause　The menopause literally means "cessation of menstruation". The process is usually a gradual one. The periods become irregular, less profuse, and eventually cease altogether. Removal of the womb (hysterectomy) causes menstruation to cease, but does not cause the menopause unless the ovaries have been removed as well. The menopause is also known as the climacteric, or change of life, though life does not really change. Possible effects on general health are explained below.

The menopause is centred on the ovary and its built-in obsolescence. The events of the menopause start when the number of surviving ovarian follicles is so small that monthly pituitary stimulation cannot activate a responsive follicle. This is the beginning of natural ovarian failure and the menopause is completed when the last follicle ceases to function. This may be long after the last menstrual period. On the other hand the menopause begins before menstruation ceases.

As ovarian follicles respond more and more inefficiently to the pituitary there is a loss of ovulation and of progesterone secretion before oestrogen production is much impaired. However oestrogen secretion is likely to vary widely from cycle to cycle. At this stage progesterone therapy may help. When oestrogen deficiency takes over as the dominant feature of the menopause various things happen. The lack of ovarian activity disturbs the pituitary; LH levels increase but do not show an ovulatory surge. Later the FSH levels become raised and remain at

this high level for the rest of life. The combination of high FSH and low oestrogen levels is responsible for hot flushes. These and the other manifestations of oestrogen deficiency seem dependent on the tempo of ovarian failure. Abrupt deprivation of oestrogen, as with surgical removal of the ovaries, produces far more disturbance than the natural gentle decline in function.

When the ovary has failed, some oestrogen can be provided from an adrenal hormone (androstenedione) that is converted into oestrogen by fatty tissue; one advantage of being plump. Genital tract atrophy is caused by oestrogen deficiency, making intercourse painful. This atrophy is fully reversed by oestrogen therapy. The bladder is also affected by loss of oestrogen and an urgent desire to pass urine is sometimes mistaken for cystitis. Less well recognized are the muscular aches and pains that may be due to lack of oestrogen. What is quite certain is that the bones thin far more quickly after the menopause and this rate of thinning can be slowed by giving oestrogen.

In general the slowly diminishing level of oestrogen is well tolerated by the body and the extra-ovarian oestrogens compensate into later life. Moreover the change in emotions and family relationships in a woman's middle years can produce symptoms that have no endocrine basis. But the fact remains that many women pass through these years far more healthily if given hormone replacement therapy, either as oestrogen in small doses or as a combination of oestrogen and progesterone. The possible adverse effects of such treatment cannot be overlooked. They may have dangers in terms of endometrial cancer. Of course, this does not apply to those who have had a hysterectomy. They may also increase the risk of blood clotting. Therefore the decision to treat or not to treat requires expert guidance. By no means all women need any form of hormone therapy to help them through the menopause and the ensuing years, but many do benefit greatly from the judicious use of ovarian hormones.

Chapter 10
Diabetes

Revised by David Pyke, MD FRCP

Diabetes is a disease in which the body cannot properly use the sugar and starches in the diet. Instead of being used by all the tissues of the body to provide energy, sugar accumulates in the blood. There is normally some sugar in the blood (about one part in a thousand) but in diabetes the amount rises considerably. Most of the symptoms of diabetes come from this rise in blood sugar. The reason why the blood sugar rises is that the hormone insulin is not produced in adequate amounts by the pancreas. Normally, insulin enables the cells of the body to utilize sugar.

The pancreas is a gland which lies behind and close to the stomach; most of the gland – about 98 per cent – is concerned with making enzymes that pass into a duct which drains into the duodenum. These enzymes help us to digest the protein, starch, and fat that we eat; without enzymes these foods could not be broken down for absorption and we would starve. Only about two per cent of the pancreas makes insulin. The parts which do so are tiny specks of tissue scattered throughout the pancreas, over a million of them, called the islets of Langerhans (after Paul Langerhans, who discovered them in 1869 while a medical student). If these islets fail to produce insulin, or make too little, diabetes results.

The fact that a secretion of the pancreas was needed to prevent diabetes was discovered by accident, as so many important scientific discoveries have been. In 1890 a technician noticed that a dog, whose pancreas had been removed, started to urinate all over his cage. The urine was found to contain sugar and it was soon realized that the dog had diabetes. This started a hunt for the substance which protected normal animals and men from getting diabetes. It was thought that if this could be found, it might be possible to save diabetics, who at that time nearly all died. But it was not easy. Many people had tried, but it was not until 1922 that a Canadian doctor, Frederick Banting, had the sound idea that the substance in the pancreas which everyone was looking for might be destroyed, after the pancreas was removed from the body, by digestive enzymes produced by the rest of the pancreas. By closing off the duct which empties the pancreatic enzymes into the duodenum, Banting caused the enzyme-secreting tissue to shrivel up, and six weeks later was able to remove the tissue containing islets of Langerhans from a living animal. He then had no difficulty in extracting insulin from the pancreas. At last diabetes could be controlled (though not cured) by replacing insulin in those who could not manufacture it in their own bodies, (hormone replacement therapy). Banting was unfortunately killed in an air crash in 1942 but his codiscoverer of insulin, a 21-year-old medical student, Charles Best, lived until 1978. There can be few men who have lived to see so many people's lives saved by their discoveries.

Diabetes is common. In childhood it is rare but with increasing age it becomes more frequent, so that in the 60's and 70's about one person in 30 is diabetic. The overall frequency in the population is about one in a hundred. Some people think that diabetes is becoming commoner, especially among older persons. This may be true, or it may be that the apparently increased frequency is due merely to better methods of discovering cases in the early stages.

Diabetes is found in all countries of the world. When it has been claimed that it was unknown in a country it has usually been found, when properly looked for, to be about as common there as anywhere else. In developing countries, where many people are severely undernourished, diabetes is less frequent than in more prosperous nations, but when immigrants from poor countries arrive in richer ones the risk of developing diabetes goes up.

Diabetes is commoner in women than men. In early life there is no difference in frequency between the sexes, but after the age of about 50 or 60 it is commoner in women. No one knows the reason for this difference, and indeed it may not always have been true. Records from the beginning of the century suggest that at that time diabetes was just as common in men of all ages as in women.

The cause of diabetes

The essential disorder in diabetes is failure of the pancreas to make insulin, but why this happens is not fully understood. The remarkable feature of this failure, which may be only partial, is that the rest of the pancreas (the 98 per cent of the gland which makes digestive enzymes) is almost never affected. Even when the islets of Langerhans are completely destroyed and the patient is therefore unable to manufacture any insulin at all, the rest of the pancreas is entirely normal. This isolated failure of the islets suggests that whatever the cause of diabetes, it is specific, and something which damages the cells of the islets alone.

In most young diabetics the pancreatic islet failure is complete, so these patients are dependent upon insulin injections for their lives. If insulin were stopped for a few days they would become seriously ill and in danger of dying. In most older patients the pancreatic islet failure is not complete, and the gland still retains some capacity to make insulin. These patients, therefore, do not usually need insulin injections and can be treated by tablets or diet only. But there are exceptions; some older diabetics do need insulin to keep alive and a very few young ones can manage without it.

To some extent diabetes is inherited, that is to say it tends to run in families. But the tendency is not a strong one, and most diabetics have no relatives who are affected. Direct inheritance of the disease from parent to child is uncommon. Before having a child, a young woman (or man) with diabetes may ask about the chances of passing on the disease. The answer is that the child of a diabetic has no chance of being born with diabetes and only about a one in a hundred chance of developing the disease by the age of ten. That risk is above average, but still very small, and most prospective parents are not deterred by it.

It seems probable that diabetes is due to an inherited predisposition or tendency and requires some other cause to be added to it for the disease to appear. In some cases this tendency is strong, in most cases weak. Presumably there are some people who have the genetic tendency to diabetes but who do not encounter the external agent (whatever it is) which is needed to convert the genetic tendency into the disease.

The great question which is now occupying research workers is "What is the external agent which causes diabetes in susceptible persons?". A virus has been suspected. It is known that viruses can cause diabetes in some animals and it is possible that they may do so in man, but there is as yet no direct evidence. The noninherited cause or causes of diabetes are unclear, but it is generally acknowledged that they do exist, and that gives hope that one day it may be possible to prevent, abort, or even cure diabetes.

It has been said that if two diabetics marry each other, all their children will eventually get diabetes. This is incorrect. The true figure is probably less than one in four.

In some older diabetics it is thought that obesity may be partly responsible for the diabetes. Older patients are, on average, overweight, and if they lose weight their diabetes may get better or even apparently disappear. Having a large number of babies may also increase a woman's chances of getting diabetes in later life. Sometimes a woman may develop mild diabetes during pregnancy which then subsides after the baby is born; it may or may not recur in later pregnancies, or when the woman is middle-aged.

Symptoms of diabetes

The commonest symptom of diabetes is thirst. It can be so severe that a child can hardly stop drinking; at the same time the diabetic passes excessive amounts of urine, and may have to get up two or three times in the night to urinate. In women there may be intense itching of the vulva. Symptoms may come on acutely, that is over a matter of days; more commonly they are gradual, and it is weeks or months before the patient is driven to consult his doctor. If the condition is severe the patient will lose weight and feel abnormally tired.

Sometimes a diabetic may appear to have had no symptoms and the condition is discovered as part of a medical examination for life insurance or employment. Even in these cases, however, there have usually been some symptoms, but the patient has ignored them or feared to consult his doctor.

Occasionally diabetes is discovered through one of its complications, such as those affecting the eyes or the feet.

The diagnosis of diabetes   It is usually easy for a doctor to decide whether a person has diabetes or not. He can test the urine; in most normal people it does not contain sugar, in most diabetics it does. To be sure of the diagnosis the sugar level in the blood is measured; if it is raised, the patient has diabetes. If there is still doubt, because the blood level is on the borderline of normality, a special glucose tolerance test is done.

Once the disease has been diagnosed, all diabetics should be taught how to test the urine. A testing outfit for use at home can be prescribed on the National Health Service.

Treatment

All diabetics need treatment – it may be quite simple and consist merely of following a diet. The purpose of the treatment is to relieve symptoms, reduce the amount of sugar in the urine and blood, and diminish the risk of complications.

Anyone who has diabetes needs to limit the amount of sugar he eats. This means cutting down not only on such obvious things as sugar in tea, sweet cakes, and chocolates, but on bread, potatoes, and biscuits as well, as these foods contain starch which is broken down to sugar when it is absorbed by the body. Some foods contain no sugar, for example, meat, eggs, and salads, and these can be eaten freely.

Sugar-containing foods are not forbidden but they are limited. A diabetic is taught to recognize the starch content of foods and to choose the right amounts of each, having been given a total ration for the day by his doctor. It is not necessary to weigh foods.

It can be difficult for a diabetic to estimate how much starch there is in food when he is eating in a restaurant, and sometimes he will make mistakes. No one keeps meticulously to a diet, but it is not too difficult to keep to it reasonably well. How much starch a diabetic should have is usually decided by a doctor, or dietician, after considering his age, how severe the diabetes is, how active a life he leads, what his tastes and appetite are like, and other individual features.

If a diabetic is very fat he will be put on a strict diet, containing perhaps 100 gm (3½ oz) of carbo-hydrate a day; but in the case of an adolescent boy with a huge appetite who is very active, the amount may be three times as much. There is no one diet to suit all diabetics.

As diet is such an important part of the treatment of all diabetics it is worthwhile for the patient to spend some time learning about it. No other treatment of diabetes is likely to succeed if the patient is not keeping to the diet prescribed.

For about one third of all diabetics, an appropriate diet is the only measure needed to control the disease. In older patients the proportion is even higher. Excessive thirst subsides, urine and blood tests return to near normal, and the patient can be in as good health as anyone else.

If, in spite of keeping to a diet, the symptoms do not disappear, or if urine and blood tests still show too much sugar, tablets are needed.

Tablet treatment   There are two types of drug used in the treatment of diabetes, sulphonylureas and biguanides.

They do not contain insulin and act in a different way. The sulphonylureas cause the patient's own pancreas to make more insulin. If his pancreas is incapable of doing so, the tablets are useless. This explains why in most young diabetics whose pancreatic islets have failed, these tablets do not work.

The way biguanides work is different and not so well understood.

Sulphonylureas   These tablets are very safe but, like all other medicines, they can have side effects and in a few cases they cause skin rashes. The tablets can be taken for years and, as a rule, do not lose their effect, but they cannot control diabetes in a person who does not keep to a diet. Usually patients taking drugs need to continue doing so, but occasionally the diabetes seems to get better and the medication can then be stopped.

Biguanides   These drugs are not usually prescribed unless either a patient is very fat and his diabetes has not responded to diet alone, or diet and sulphonyl-urea tablets have not been effective, and something more is needed. Biguanides, therefore, tend to be used less often than the sulphonylureas and can sometimes cause indigestion, diarrhoea, or a bitter taste in the mouth. If such symptoms are bad, biguanide treatment must be stopped.

Insulin   Insulin is made from the pancreas of cows or pigs. The exact chemical structure of insulin from animals is slightly different from that of human insulin, but these differences do not usually matter in practice.

If insulin is taken by mouth it is destroyed in the

stomach, so it always has to be injected. Injections are made just under the skin (subcutaneously) in the thighs, hips, abdomen, or arms. Injections are almost painless although in the first few weeks of treatment red lumps which last for about 24 hours may form where the insulin has been injected and then fade. Some people, especially women, develop hollows in the skin a few months after insulin has been injected. These hollows are unsightly but completely harmless; sometimes they lessen gradually over years but more often they persist. It seems that the newer types of insulin do not cause these hollows.

There are several different types of insulin which are prepared in various ways to give shorter or longer periods of action. Short-acting insulins have to be given twice daily, or more often; long-acting insulins only once. Obviously it is preferable to have only one injection a day but unfortunately the long-acting insulins do not always control the sugar level satisfactorily, so it is still quite often necessary to give short-acting insulin twice a day; indeed many doctors think that this is still the best treatment.

Types of insulin

Short-acting	Soluble, Actrapid*, Nuso*
Intermediate	Isophane (NPH), Semilente, Semitard*, LeoRetard*
Long-acting	Lente, Protamine Zinc (PZI), Monotard*
Very long-acting	Ultra lente, Lentard*

The types marked with an asterisk are the newer, more purified preparations of insulin; they are called monocomponent, pro-insulin-free (PIF) or rarely-antigenic (RI). The difference of meaning between these terms is slight. Earlier insulin preparations (that is, those not marked with an asterisk) are perfectly effective and almost as pure as the others; the only important differences in practice are that these purer forms seldom, if ever, lead to the formation of hollows and they may need to be given in slightly smaller doses.

Injections are usually given quarter to half an hour before a meal. All diabetics on insulin need to be on a starch restricted diet and it is important that the timing of meals is approximately the same each day. If there is too long a gap between meals, the action of insulin in lowering blood sugar is not modified by the effect of meals; therefore the level sinks too low, and the patient becomes hypoglycaemic. The symptoms of hypoglycaemia are slowness of speech and thought, shaking, sweating, unsteadiness, pallor, aggressive behaviour, tingling round the mouth, seeing double, and finally unconsciousness. If the condition is very severe, there may be epileptic fits. Usually the onset of an attack is gradual, the patient realizes what is happening, and takes extra sugar so that he quickly recovers. Sometimes, however, because he becomes slow-witted and even aggressive, he may lose his normal good sense and not realize what is happening or what he should do. It may then be necessary for someone else, who recognizes the symptoms, to give him sugar even if he denies that he needs it. Occasionally a diabetic on insulin becomes suddenly hypoglycaemic and he may become unconscious before he realizes that anything is wrong. Glucose must be injected into a vein as soon as possible because it is dangerous to give anything by mouth to an unconscious person. Another, slightly less effective, treatment is to give glucagon, a substance which raises the blood sugar level.

Hypoglycaemia may be frightening to the patient or bystander, and if it occurs when driving a car it can be dangerous. It is because of the risk of hypo-glycaemia that diabetics on insulin should be aware of its features; they should not go too long without a meal, or undertake any activity where loss of control would be disastrous (such as swimming alone, flying an aeroplane, or climbing a mountain). Many activities can be undertaken if in company, which would be dangerous alone, as strenuous muscular exertion tends to produce hypoglycaemia. Driving is usually safe provided sensible precautions are taken, but a diabetic who drives a car always needs to be very careful. It is legal for a diabetic to drive a car, but if he has an accident as a result of a hypoglycaemic attack, his licence may be taken away. Diabetics who live alone are sometimes frightened that if they have a hypoglycaemic attack at night they will die (this is a common unvoiced fear of children). They can be reassured. Recovery, although slow, is almost invariable. Death in a hypoglycaemic attack is almost unknown.

If a diabetic on insulin stops his injections or if for some reason his need for insulin increases and he fails to recognize the fact, he may pass into diabetic coma. This can also happen when a person develops diabetes and the condition is not diagnosed. Diabetic coma never develops suddenly (unlike hypo-glycaemia); it takes many hours or even days to come on. One of the important causes of diabetic coma is an infection. If a diabetic on insulin develops, say, gastroenteritis, which may increase his need for insulin, the patient may think that because he does not feel like eating he need not take his insulin and stops the injections, when in fact he may need more insulin than usual because of the infection.

If a diabetic on insulin becomes thirsty, and especially if he starts to vomit, he should test his urine and if it contains sugar take extra insulin. If this does not quickly correct the symptoms he should call his doctor. If the condition is severe the doctor will send the patient to hospital where he will probably receive extra insulin and have intravenous medication.

Complications of diabetes

Sometimes, after a matter of years, diabetes may lead to complications affecting the eyes, kidneys, nerves, or arteries. Although doctors can detect these complications by careful examination, in the majority of diabetics they cause no trouble or disability. Thus a doctor may see some tiny haemorrhages in the retina at the back of the eye (retinopathy) but the patient is unaware of their existence and does not suffer from their effects. Occasionally the retinopathy is severe, and the haemorrhages are large and interfere with sight, even to the point of blindness. However, patients who go blind form a very small minority of all diabetics. Diabetic retinopathy can now be treated, or have its progress slowed, by a technique of photocoagulation in which an intense tiny beam of light produces minute burns in the retina.

Diabetic neuropathy is the term used when the nerves are affected, producing pain or numbness of the legs. Sometimes this is temporary and due to poor treatment of diabetes, so that recovery ensues after proper treatment; more often numbness of the feet persists.

The kidneys may be damaged by diabetes (nephropathy), even to the point of causing kidney failure and death. Fortunately this is the rarest serious complication of diabetes and most diabetics who do have nephropathy show no signs except an abnormal urine test. As with other forms of kidney disease, transplantation has been tried, sometimes with success (especially if a kidney from a relative can be used), but there are still many failures.

Disease of the arteries (arteriosclerosis), particularly of the coronary arteries supplying the heart, is somewhat commoner in diabetics than normal people and this is particularly true of women. In non-diabetics men are more prone to coronary disease, but in diabetics the two sexes are equally affected. If arteriosclerosis damages the arteries of the legs and feet it can lead to pain in the calves on walking, painful foot ulcers, or devitalized tissues (sometimes rather frighteningly termed gangrene). Arteriosclerosis is a process of ageing of arteries and happens to everyone as they grow older. It is therefore commoner in older than younger diabetics just as it is commoner in older nondiabetics.

Sometimes arteriosclerosis is patchy and by removing one piece of obstruction a good blood flow can be restored, but more often the process is widespread and no cure is possible. It is for this reason that it is so important for diabetics, particularly older patients, to take care of their feet. It is better to prevent an injury or infection of the foot than to treat it once it has occurred, when because of poor blood supply and neuropathy, it may be difficult to cure. Diabetics should keep their feet clean and dry, wear well-fitting shoes and, if they have any difficulty with their sight, get a chiropodist to cut their toenails. Whenever there is the slightest doubt, a chiropodist should be consulted.

In extreme cases, because of pain or infection or both, amputation is necessary. This is usually performed about fifteen cm (six in) below the knee. When the wound has healed the patient learns to walk on an artificial leg and most patients manage to do this very well; they recover their independence and lead normal lives. In patients who have had an amputation it is most important to see that the other foot comes to no harm. That foot needs special protection while the patient is in bed after the operation and extra care from a chiropodist afterwards.

Pregnancy

Women with well-controlled diabetes are as fertile as normal women and pregnancy presents no greater risk to them. But there is an increased risk to the baby. If the mother's diabetes is not very carefully treated throughout pregnancy the baby may not survive. It is for this reason that great care is taken of these patients; they are seen frequently throughout pregnancy, they may be admitted to hospital some weeks before the birth, and delivery (by the normal route, or by Caesarean operation) is brought on two or three weeks early. Results of modern care are good, and only about five per cent of babies are lost, compared to about two per cent of babies of nondiabetic mothers. The number of babies born with congenital defects (for example, heart valve disorders, or abnormalities of brain or spine) is about twice the normal for diabetic mothers. Pregnancy does not worsen diabetes, but it is generally wise, because of the extra burden of being a diabetic, for a woman to limit her family to two. A diabetic woman can usually take the contraceptive pill without any special precautions. In rare circumstances the pill may upset the control of diabetes (and the same may be true of the menstrual cycle).

Diabetics can obtain advice and help from the British Diabetic Association, 10 Queen Anne Street, London, W1M 0BD.

Diabetes insipidus

The full name of the common disease described in this chapter is diabetes mellitus (the latter word meaning "honey-sweet") so-called because of the sugar in the urine. There is also a disease with a similar name, diabetes insipidus (no sugar in the urine), a very rare disease. Apart from the fact that in both conditions the patient passes a large amount of urine, the two diseases are entirely different in origin, effects, and treatment. Diabetes insipidus is discussed in chapter 9.

Chapter 11
Pregnancy and childbirth

Revised by Dame Josephine Barnes, DBE MA DM FRCP FRCS FRCOG

A pregnancy is one of the most important events in a woman's life, and has profound physical, emotional, and social effects. It is natural and desirable for a pregnant woman to wish to know about the medical management of the pregnancy, both in her own interests and those of the baby.

For most women, the first sign of pregnancy is that the monthly period does not arrive. Shortly after, or even before the period is missed, other symptoms may appear. These may be nausea and vomiting, lack of appetite in the morning, inability to eat certain foods, or sudden distaste for smoking and alcohol. There may also be some increase in the size of the breasts, a frequent desire to pass urine, and a heavy feeling in the lower abdomen and pelvis. These symptoms should lead to a strong suspicion of pregnancy, but they are not definite and they will need to be confirmed by a doctor.

Diagnosis of pregnancy

Modern medicine has several reliable methods for the diagnosis of pregnancy. When the period is more than two weeks overdue (that is, from a medical point of view, a pregnancy of six weeks) a doctor may be able to detect a pregnancy by an internal examination, though this can be difficult if the woman is overweight or has exceptionally tense muscles.

Pregnancy tests When the fertilized egg has become implanted in the uterus (womb), the tissue surrounding the baby, the chorion, produces a hormone which passes into the mother's bloodstream and is excreted in her urine. The presence of this hormone, chorionic gonadotrophin, can be detected in the urine and this is the basis of pregnancy testing. The original pregnancy tests were performed on animals; mice, rabbits, rats, and toads were used, but these have largely been superseded by tests which can be done in the laboratory or the doctor's consulting room. Commercial pregnancy tests are available from chemists' shops and there are also do-it-yourself tests.

The pregnancy test becomes positive about six weeks after the last period. The tests are not completely reliable; false negatives and false positives occur in about two per cent of cases. There are more sophisticated and accurate tests which measure the exact amount of gonadotrophic hormones but these are available only in certain hospitals.

In recent years there has been a development of the use of ultrasound (or sonar). Very high frequency sound waves are used to outline the contents of the pelvis; by their use it is possible to see the signs of pregnancy from the sixth week onwards. It is also possible to find out if there are twins at this early stage.

By the fourth month of pregnancy it is possible to detect the bones of the baby on an X-ray, but the modern practice is to avoid all but medically necessary X-rays in pregnancy. Between the sixteenth and the twenty-second week the mother feels life, becoming conscious of the movements of the baby; the doctor can also feel and hear these. By the twentieth week the doctor may be able to hear the baby's heartbeat with a stethoscope. With ultrasound the heartbeat can be detected much earlier.

The duration of pregnancy

The duration of normal pregnancy is generally calculated as 40 weeks, or 280 days, or nine months and one week from the first day of the last normal period. This is not to say that the baby is bound to arrive on the due date. In fact only five per cent of babies arrive on the day they are expected. However about 90 per cent of babies arrive during the two weeks before or the two weeks after the expected date. Nowadays the calculation of the due date may be made difficult in various ways. Many young women are now taking the contraceptive pill, and after stopping the pill (or forgetting to take it) the monthly cycle may be irregular, thus making the calculation difficult. Some normal women have irregular periods in any case. A mother may conceive again while she is breast-feeding or shortly after having a baby or a miscarriage. However, with the modern development of ultrasound, precise estimation of the duration of pregnancy is now possible, particularly if the ultrasound examination is done at or before the twentieth week of pregnancy.

The best advice that can be given to a woman who thinks she may be pregnant is to see her doctor. They can then make all the necessary arrangements; in the cases where she may feel she qualifies for legal abortion under the Abortion Act, it is important that consultation takes place as early as possible.

Changes that may be noticed

A pregnant woman may notice a number of changes in her body and the way she feels.

Nausea and vomiting Many women suffer from nausea in the first three months, and about half are actually sick. Usually this is no more than a temporary affliction and it clears up, often quite suddenly, after the third month. Later on an abnormal appetite may result in overweight. Traditionally, pregnant women develop cravings, sometimes bizarre, for certain foods.

If pregnancy sickness is interfering with normal life, several steps can be taken to help. It is best to eat something dry such as dry toast, a biscuit, or an apple before getting out of bed in the morning. Fried food is best avoided and there may well be a distaste for alcohol. Drug treatment of sickness must be given with care and medicines taken only if prescribed by the doctor. Vitamin B sometimes helps. Dicyclomine in a dose of two tablets at night and one in the morn-

ing helps in some cases, and is available on prescription, but should be avoided in the early weeks of pregnancy. If sickness goes on all day and if the woman is losing weight or obviously becoming ill, medical advice must be sought and admission to hospital may become necessary. Neglected vomiting during pregnancy can lead to serious illness, but it usually responds quickly to appropriate treatment.

Constipation is common in pregnancy and tends to be worse in those women who suffer from pregnancy sickness; there may also be general discomfort in the abdomen with wind and distension.

Congestion There may be a feeling of congestion and discomfort in the lower abdomen and pelvis. This is associated with the increased flow of blood through the reproductive organs. The lower abdomen often feels enlarged. This is due partly to congestion and partly to the fact that the abdomen is enlarging to make room for the growing baby.

Frequent passing of urine is common in the early weeks when there is congestion and when the enlarging womb is pressing on the urinary bladder. Rarely the womb may become wedged in the pelvis and the woman cannot pass urine at all. If there is exceptional frequency or difficulty in urination, medical advice should be sought at once.

Distaste for smoking and certain food and drinks Women who smoke may find that they acquire an aversion to tobacco smoke. It is now considered that pregnant women ought not to smoke, so this is a good time to give up the habit. The pregnant woman may find it difficult to digest fatty or highly flavoured foods, or to take alcoholic drinks.

Basal body temperature Women who find it difficult to conceive may have been asked to keep a chart of basal body temperature, taken first thing in the morning. The temperature normally rises by one fifth of a degree Centigrade (two fifths to three fifths of a degree Fahrenheit) after ovulation has occurred. If the woman becomes pregnant this rise is sustained, so that if it stays up for twenty days or more this is almost conclusive evidence of pregnancy unless the woman is taking a medicine containing sex hormones.

Breast changes are a prominent sign of early pregnancy in some, but not all, women. The breasts increase in size so that a larger brassiere may be needed. The nipples become more deeply pigmented and the pigment may extend outside the normal nipple area. Enlarged glands appear in the nipple area and the veins become prominent and easily seen.

Difficulties in the diagnosis of pregnancy In some women the early symptoms of pregnancy are virtually absent; slight bleeding may occur at the time of the first two or three missed periods; very rarely a woman has apparent periods, episodes of bleeding throughout pregnancy. Bleeding, if profuse, is always a danger sign at any time during pregnancy. In the early stages it may denote a threatened miscarriage, or the embryo may have died in the womb. If a miscarriage occurs it may be necessary to remove the remains of the pregnancy by dilatation and curettage (see chapter 13).

Miscarriage in the early months of pregnancy occurs in at least ten per cent of cases. A threat of miscarriage should be treated with absolute rest in bed; in some cases hormone injections may be given to try to save the pregnancy. An ectopic pregnancy is one in which the egg is implanted outside the womb, generally in the fallopian tubes. This is a potentially dangerous condition, as rupture of the tube with severe internal haemorrhage may occur. In most of these cases there is usually pain and bleeding at about the sixth or eighth week of pregnancy. The abnormally placed pregnancy will have to be removed by an abdominal operation, and the affected tube removed as well.

Pregnancy in women using contraceptives
Pregnancy may occur in women using various contraceptive measures. The contraceptive pill is the most reliable precaution so far discovered, and pregnancies occur only when women either do not take the pill or when they suffer an internal upset with vomiting and diarrhoea which prevents absorption of the pill. Certain drugs, such as tranquillizers and antibiotics may make the pill less effective. Since many women have scanty periods while taking the pill or may occasionally not menstruate at all, the diagnosis of pregnancy may become obscure. The intrauterine contraceptives or coils afford good protection, but there is a greater pregnancy rate than with the pill. Ectopic pregnancy is said to be commoner in women wearing coils. Mechanical methods such as the sheath or cap are slightly less safe than the coil. Pregnancy can occasionally occur even when the woman has had an operation for sterilization or the man a vasectomy. A woman should not believe that there is no possibility of pregnancy.

Antenatal care and examination

Once the diagnosis of pregnancy is made and the decision is reached that the pregnancy is to continue, the parents of the unborn baby have a number of decisions to make. Nowadays many pregnant women are working outside the home and provided the woman's health remains good, and the pregnancy is progressing normally, there is no reason why she should not continue to do so. If this is a first baby the couple may have to make considerable adjustments in their way of life. The loss of the wife's earnings may upset the family budget and there will be the additional costs of providing a layette and the necessary equipment for the baby.

An early decision should be made as to where the baby is to be born. In Britain, over 90 per cent of babies are now born in hospital, so a bed should be booked, and contact made with the antenatal clinic, generally through the family doctor. A woman having her first baby will be advised to have the baby in hospital and to stay there about seven days, provided the hospital facilities permit. She will need to have special tests and to be examined regularly. This may be carried out by the hospital, or care may be shared between the hospital and the family doctor or local health clinic; midwives may also take part in her care. Some family doctors undertake the total care of their pregnant patients, generally in cooperation with the local authority or practice midwife.

A recent development has been the practice of keeping the woman and her baby in hospital for only a short time – six to 48 hours – after the birth. This arrangement is suitable for normal women who already have one or more children. However, early discharge should be booked in good time as the local midwife will want to see that conditions are suitable at home.

Antenatal care The value of routine examination during pregnancy is unquestioned and indeed has been proved to contribute substantially to the health and wellbeing of the mother and her baby. Antenatal care may be given at hospital clinics, local authority clinics, or general practitioners' surgeries. Nowadays many women receive care shared between the hospital and the general practitioner or clinic. It is realized that antenatal care can offer more than care for the physical wellbeing of the mother. It is also an opportunity for her to ask questions and to receive reassurance about any worries she may have. An antenatal record card is usually given to the pregnant woman, and she should carry it with her at all times. This contains her main medical history and details of her pregnancy and is designed to be useful in an emergency. It also provides a channel of communication for the doctor and midwives.

The first antenatal examination is carried out at the time of booking, usually at about the third month. A history is taken of past illnesses and operations, any family history of disease or twins, the history of all past pregnancies and deliveries, and the history of the present pregnancy. A full medical examination is made to exclude any general disease. A vaginal examination is usually made to check the size of the uterus and to see if there is any misplacement or abnormality. At this time also a check is made of the capacity of the pelvis. The breasts are examined and the mother told how to prepare for breast-feeding. Her height is recorded at the first antenatal visit, and her weight at each visit. Her blood pressure is taken and a sample of her urine tested at each visit.

Certain special laboratory tests are made at the first visit and some are repeated as the pregnancy progresses. A sample of blood is tested for diseases such as syphilis, rubella (German measles), and for hepatitis (a serious infection leading to jaundice). The blood group and Rhesus factor are determined and tests are done for anaemia. The urine is further examined for the presence of any infection which may lead to illness later if not treated. At the time of this internal examination a smear test is sometimes taken from the cervix. A swab is taken from the vagina to exclude the presence of infections such as thrush and trichomonas. The mother is generally examined every four weeks until the 28th week, then every two weeks until the 36th week and thereafter weekly till she is delivered.

At the follow-up routine examinations she is weighed, her blood pressure is taken, and her urine tested. Her abdomen is examined to check the progress of the baby and to ascertain its position. After the sixth month the doctor or midwife can hear the baby's heart with a stethoscope. It can be detected before that with ultrasound. An internal examination may be repeated at 36 weeks to make sure that there is plenty of room in the pelvis for the baby to pass. Iron tablets, often combined with folic acid, are prescribed to be taken regularly from the twentieth week.

Blood tests for anaemia are carried out from time to time during pregnancy. In Rhesus negative mothers the blood is also examined for antibodies to see if there is any interaction between the mother's blood and that of her baby. Special tests on the blood or urine may be performed if the growth of the baby does not appear to be satisfactory. Examination with ultrasound is undertaken in many clinics. This is helpful in determining the duration of the pregnancy and the rate of growth of the baby. It can also be used to detect twins and some abnormalities. The examination is painless and harmless.

Amniocentesis consists of inserting a needle into the uterus and removing some of the fluid (liquor amnii) which surrounds and protects the baby. It is a simple procedure done under a local anaesthetic, but to avoid the risk of infection it must be done in sterile conditions as in an operating theatre. Amniocentesis is performed after the sixteenth week of pregnancy to extract some of the baby's cells which normally float in the liquor together with the liquor itself. The cells can be cultured in the laboratory and examined to ascertain if there are any defects in the chromosomes which may indicate that the baby has some serious abnormality, the most important being that the baby suffers from Down's syndrome (mongolism). As this particular defect, which leads to mental retardation among other things, is commoner in older mothers it is usual to offer the test to mothers over 40. If such an abnormality is found, legal termination of the pregnancy can be carried out, if that is what the parents wish. Examination of the liquor or the mother's blood may also detect excess of a substance called alpha-fetoprotein. This is produced in excess in babies with defects of the backbone such as spina bifida. This test may be offered to women who have already had an affected child or in whom ultrasound examination suggests a defect. Certain rarer congenital diseases can also be diagnosed from amniocentesis. Most of these are inherited so the risk is already known. It is possible by culture of the cells to determine the sex of the unborn child and thus to assess the risk of the child having a sex-linked disorder such as haemophilia, which affects only male babies.

Amniocentesis is also used in later pregnancy to determine the maturity of the baby's lungs. Premature babies may have breathing difficulties due to immaturity of the lungs. The risk of this can be determined before birth by estimating the amounts of two fatty substances called sphingomyelin and lecithin in the liquor or by estimating the amount of palmitic acid; in some cases it may be difficult to decide the best moment to deliver the mother, but by this test it is possible to decide to wait until delivery is safe for the baby. Amniocentesis is also used in Rhesus cases to find out if the fetus is affected.

Care during pregnancy

The mother herself, with the help of her husband and her family can do a great deal to ensure a trouble-free pregnancy and delivery.

Chapter 11 Pregnancy and childbirth

Diet A normal mixed diet will provide most of what is needed for the mother and her baby. Pregnant women should not overeat but should take as much as they can get, or can afford, of fresh meat, fish, eggs, cheese, fruit, and fresh vegetables. Starchy and fried foods, and highly flavoured foods are best avoided. It is advisable to take at least a pint of milk or its equivalent in cheese every day, but there is no virtue in drinking raw milk for those mothers who dislike it. Milk can be taken in many ways. Strong tea or coffee may interfere with sleep and are best avoided.

If the diet is adequate, extra vitamins should not be necessary, but if needed vitamin tablets can be obtained through the general practitioner. Iron should be given from the fifth month onwards, but it is best avoided in the early weeks when there may be nausea and constipation. Many of the iron preparations now given contain a small amount of folic acid and this combination should prevent anaemia.

Weight gain Every woman should gain some weight in pregnancy, the normal being about twenty per cent of the pre-pregnant weight, or 9 kg (20 lb) for a woman weighing 45 kg (7 stone); in fact the total gain is generally about 13 kg (28 lb). This gain is not of course all baby. The average baby weighs about 3·5 kg ($7\frac{1}{2}$ lb). The placenta (afterbirth) weighs about 0·5 kg (1 lb) while the liquor, the water surrounding the baby, weighs about another 1 kg (2 lb). The womb (uterus) increases in size by about 1 kg (2 lb). There is also an increase in breast size accounting for a further 0·5 kg (1 lb). The volume of the mother's blood increases by a further 1 kg (2 lb). The rest is accounted for by fluid retained in the mother's tissues and by the laying down of fat.

A weight gain of about 2·5 kg (5 lb) a month is within normal limits after the twentieth week of pregnancy, but it should not be more than this. Excessive weight gain may indicate excessive fluid retention and be a warning of toxaemia of pregnancy (see page 239) or may indicate the laying down of fat which will be difficult to shed after the baby is born. It is a sad fact that in many young women, obesity begins with the first baby. On the other hand, loss of weight or failure to gain it in the last weeks of pregnancy may be a sign that all is not well with the pregnancy. Failure to gain weight or a small loss of weight often occurs when labour is imminent. This is probably due to lower hormone production by the placenta, which during pregnancy produces very large amounts of hormones, which in turn tend to promote fluid retention in the mother. For this reason, most doctors and clinics like to weigh every woman at each antenatal visit.

Table 1
Approximate weight gain during pregnancy

	Kilograms	Pounds
Baby	3·5	7·5
Placenta	0·5	1·0
Liquor amnii	1·0	2·0
Uterus	1·0	2·0
Breasts	0·5	1·0
Mother's blood	1·0	2·0
Retained fluid and fat	6·0	12·5
Total	13·5	28·0

A mother who is gaining too much weight, especially during the middle months of pregnancy, should reduce her intake of carbohydrate and fatty foods and eat mainly protein foods, such as meat, fish, eggs, cheese, and milk. She should cut down on bread, cakes, biscuits, and fried foods, and give up sugar and sweets. On the other hand a mother who is not gaining weight or is losing it, but eating normally, should seek medical advice.

Bowel action Constipation is very common during pregnancy. The best way to overcome it is by a liberal intake of fluid, fruit juices, and a diet containing plenty of roughage in the form of bran, fruit, and fibrous vegetables. There is no harm in taking mild laxatives such as magnesia or bulk laxatives. Senna may also be useful. Powerful purgatives, and laxative products containing liquid paraffin are best avoided.

Diarrhoea is less common but if persistent may lead to malnutrition and anaemia, so that special investigation and treatment may be needed.

Heartburn, a burning pain in the centre of the lower chest or upper abdomen with an acidic taste in the mouth, is an unpleasant but common symptom of the later months of pregnancy. It is believed to be caused by reflux of the acid stomach contents into the lower part of the gullet (oesophagus). It tends to be worse when lying or stooping, and sleeping with extra pillows may help. It is important not to take medicines containing sodium bicarbonate as this may cause distension with gas or fluid; for this reason women are advised not to buy proprietary digestive medicines, many of which contain bicarbonate of soda, but to obtain the appropriate treatment by prescription.

Flatulence or excessive wind in the intestines is common throughout pregnancy. It can be relieved by attention to diet, avoiding indigestible foods.

Cramp in the lower limbs, often worse at night, may cause discomfort in late pregnancy. There is no special treatment, but walking about or rubbing the affected limb may help.

Backache is common in pregnancy as the ligaments and joints supporting the back become softened and loose. The enlarging abdomen also affects the woman's posture and this may place an undue strain on the back. Antenatal exercises, which help to maintain a good posture, and relaxation will help in many cases. A firm mattress or even a board placed under the mattress will be necessary in severe cases. It is important to maintain a good position with the back well supported when driving a car or sitting for long periods.

Palpitations and fainting occur in some women and are generally not serious symptoms, though all pregnant women should be carefully checked for evidence of heart disease at their first antenatal attendance. Faintness can usually be relieved by putting the head between the knees or by lying down.

Sleep A pregnant woman may find it difficult to sleep well, especially in the later months when the large abdomen causes discomfort and the baby's kicking disturbs her. On the other hand many women feel excessively tired in pregnancy and seem to need more sleep than usual. This may lead to a vicious circle of tiredness and sleeplessness. The obvious measures such as a comfortable bed, a hot drink at bedtime, and plenty of exercise in the fresh air during the day will help in most cases. A few will need a mild sedative. The tendency nowadays is to avoid barbiturates but there are mild and safe sedatives which can be given when necessary.

Varicose veins often appear for the first time in pregnancy, usually in the lower limbs but sometimes in the outer lips around the vaginal entrance (vulva) as well. They can be prevented to some degree by not wearing tight garters or socks which tend to constrict the veins. If varicose veins appear the woman should walk where possible and try to rest, with her legs raised, for one or two spells during the day. It may also help to raise the foot of the bed about fifteen cm (six in). Support tights of various types are to be recommended for any woman even with mild varicose veins, and they should be worn throughout the day. Many different manufacturers make these garments and they are obtainable from any large hosiery store at reasonable prices. Stronger support tights are obtainable from surgical stores on prescription. If the veins are very bad, full length elastic stockings can be prescribed by the family doctor. They are now available in a variety of nylon yarns and colours, and need not be unattractive. Elastic stockings should be put on immediately on getting up in the morning. The legs should be raised and the stockings rolled on from the foot to the thigh. If a vein becomes tender, reddened, and swollen this may mean that phlebitis has occurred and medical advice should be sought immediately. Operations for varicose veins or injection of the veins are not generally recommended during pregnancy, though very large varicose veins occurring before the 26th week of pregnancy can sometimes be tied off.

Haemorrhoids (piles) are quite common in pregnancy and during the few days after delivery. There are two main kinds. Internal piles are varicose veins of the rectum. They may become very large and protrude from the anus, causing discomfort and sometimes bleeding. An external pile is a single, often thrombosed, vein frequently found in a skin tag at the margin of the anus and associated with a crack or fissure in the skin. This is a painful condition. It may be relieved by local applications or suppositories, obtainable from the family doctor. Among the best are the old-fashioned witch-hazel or hamamelis. A very painful external pile may require a minor operation to remove the clot. Piles tend to be made worse by constipation and the passage of hard stools so that prevention of constipation is the most important measure.

Vaginal discharge An increase in discharge from the vagina is common during pregnancy and it helps to lubricate the vagina during childbirth. The usual discharge is pale mucus. There are two common causes for an abnormal discharge which may cause soreness or irritation. Thrush is caused by a fungus infection called candida or monilia; it causes a thick white, often irritating discharge. There are many treatments which mainly consist of insertion of vaginal tablets, pessaries, or creams. The other common infection is caused by trichomonas parasites which give a yellowish frothy discharge, often with an offensive odour. This may be treated with tablets taken by mouth or pessaries that are inserted into the vagina. In antenatal clinics it is usual to take a swab of the vaginal discharge at the first visit to detect infection. This may need to be repeated if there is infection or if discharge appears during pregnancy. Some types of venereal disease characteristically cause vaginal discharge. These must be treated as they can have serious effects on the baby.

Vaginal bleeding is always a serious symptom during pregnancy and it should be reported immediately to the doctor. At the time of the first two missed periods there may be slight staining which is unimportant. However, bleeding in the early months may indicate a threatened miscarriage or even an ectopic pregnancy. In the later months bleeding is a serious sign, for it may indicate that the placenta has partly separated from the uterus, thus endangering the baby's survival. In such cases immediate admission to hospital is imperative. The placenta may be in the lower part of the uterus, placenta praevia, so that there is a risk to the baby. Occasionally, however the bleeding is coming from the neck of the womb (cervix) and is caused by an erosion (a type of ulcer) or a polypus. Sometimes bleeding as a result of these last two disorders is provoked by sexual intercourse.

Exercise A moderate amount of exercise in the fresh air is desirable for pregnant women. Care must be taken to avoid the more violent forms of exercise and much depends on what exercise the woman normally takes and whether she is accustomed to it. Tennis, golf, and swimming are probably harmless in most cases. The risks of skiing, skating, and riding depend on the woman's proficiency. More violent forms of exercise such as mountaineering, diving, and water skiing are best avoided during pregnancy. The risk of a fall must be taken into account. Normal prenatal exercises are recommended for all women except for those with a tendency to bleed or with a history of heart disease.

Travel A normal healthy pregnant woman can travel without risk during pregnancy, except during the last six weeks when she should remain close to the place where the baby is to be born. Long journeys by plane, train, bus, or car are best avoided as they tend to be tiring. Many airlines will not accept a pregnant woman as a passenger on long international flights if she is over 32 weeks pregnant, unless she can provide a medical certificate. If a long car journey must be undertaken, the woman should stop, get out of the car, and walk about every two hours or so. She would be wise to go straight to bed for a rest when she arrives at her destination. When there has been a threatened miscarriage, travelling is best avoided until the doctor says that the pregnancy is well-established. Care may also be needed when the woman suffers from high blood pressure, kidney or heart disease, or any other major abnormality. When travelling by car a pregnant woman should always wear a well-fitting seat belt, which should lie across the pelvic bones, and not over the abdomen.

Clothing This is generally a matter of common sense and of the woman's own tastes. Clothing should be comfortable, and tight belts and girdles should be avoided. There is certainly no need for maternity wear to look unattractive, and a new outfit can provide a boost to morale. Many fashions, particularly pinafore dresses and smocks, are suitable, and can be worn afterwards. The wearing of maternity corsets is no longer considered necessary for health,

but an elastic belt may be comfortable in the later weeks when the uterus becomes heavy and the abdominal muscles stretched. Some women with severe backache benefit from a well-fitting corset with proper support for the back. It is important that shoes should fit well, a larger size or half-size may become necessary as pregnancy progresses. It is best to wear low heels; fashion shoes and high heels may disturb posture and lead to backache, also they make the woman less stable and more liable to falls. A well-fitting brassiere should be worn; the mother will probably find that she needs a larger size and cup than she has been accustomed to. If she intends to breast-feed, the breasts and nipples will be examined. In most cases the care of the breasts during pregnancy consists of washing the breasts and nipples daily to remove crusts. A small amount of lanolin or a special nipple cream may be applied to the nipples and towards the end of pregnancy the breasts gently massaged towards the nipple to express the brownish fluid, colostrum, which forms as a precursor to milk. If the nipples are small, retracted, or inverted, special plastic shields or shells may be worn under the brassiere. These help to make the nipple protrude and make breast-feeding easier.

Drugs and medicines The thalidomide disaster emphasized the fact that any drug that the mother takes is passed on to the baby. For this reason a pregnant woman should be very careful about any drugs or medicines, especially in the early weeks when the delicate tissues of the baby are forming. There is now a long list of medicines and drugs which are not advised for pregnant women and the best advice is "if in doubt don't take it".

Medication may be needed for various reasons; some women have headaches and can reasonably take normal doses of aspirin or paracetamol as required. Others need help with sleeping. Barbiturates are best avoided, but the benzodiazepines (for example nitrazepam) appear to carry little danger in normal doses for a short period. Infections may need treatment with antibiotics. Penicillin and its derivatives are safe. Medicines containing sulphonamides may lead to jaundice in the baby, while tetracyclines may lead to yellow staining of the teeth and should not be given to pregnant women or to children under the age of seven. There is now a wide range of medicines to deal with most of the infections likely to be encountered, but expert advice should always be sought.

Sexual intercourse can continue normally in pregnancy though it is usual to advise against it in the last four weeks or so. It is important to avoid excessive pressure on the mother's abdomen, and the use of alternative positions for intercourse that are comfortable as well as satisfying may be adopted. If there is any bleeding during pregnancy it is usual to advise against intercourse, at least till there has been no bleeding for four weeks.

X-rays Exposure of pregnant women to X-rays should be carried out only when it is essential. There is a suggestion that exposure of the embryo during the first three months may cause damage. For this reason women of childbearing age should not be exposed to X-rays except during menstruation and the few days after it. An exception is made for X-rays to the chest which can probably be safely taken, with the abdomen screened by the wearing of a special lead apron, up to twenty weeks and may be necessary if serious disease of the chest such as tuberculosis is suspected. In later pregnancy X-rays may be needed to show certain abnormalities of the baby, to confirm a diagnosis of multiple pregnancy or to determine whether the mother's pelvis is large enough to allow the safe passage of the baby. Radiologists are aware of the need to cut the amount of radiation to the absolute minimum.

Smoking It is now universally agreed that smoking is harmful to pregnant women and their babies. The babies of women who smoke are smaller and more premature. Every effort should be made by husband, relatives, and friends to dissuade pregnant women from smoking and to persuade those who do smoke to give it up. Fortunately many feel disinclined to smoke in the early months; those who are seriously addicted are advised to cut their smoking to a minimum.

Alcohol Mothers who are established alcoholics need urgent treatment. Alcohol, taken in moderation and preferably with food, is probably harmless, but, taken with certain drugs, may harm the baby. If mothers do wish to drink, spirits should be taken diluted, and light wines may be more acceptable. In general, the less alcohol that is taken the better.

Infectious diseases Pregnant women are no more immune to infectious diseases than those who are not pregnant. Among the most serious is rubella or German measles which, if acquired during the first sixteen weeks of pregnancy, may affect the fetus and can lead to blindness, deafness, and congenital defects of the heart and brain. These risks are so serious that many doctors feel that a proven attack of German measles occurring in early pregnancy is an indication to offer legal abortion under the Abortion Act. The rubella (German measles) vaccine should be offered to all young girls at about the age of eleven or twelve to confer lifelong protection. However it is not considered safe to give this vaccine during pregnancy. Most clinics now test pregnant women routinely for evidence of past infection. Those not immune should be advised to avoid contact with the disease or with anyone with a rash; immunization should be given after delivery. One difficulty is that rubella is a very mild infection and many people are not aware of having had the disease.

Infantile paralysis or poliomyelitis is another serious disease during pregnancy. All adults in this country should have been immunized in childhood, but here again immunization should not be given during pregnancy. Syphilis is a disease which can lead to very serious complications; there may be a late miscarriage or the baby may be stillborn. Those born alive suffer the effects of the disease. Although syphilis is still comparatively uncommon in pregnant women in this country, its effects are so serious that a blood test for the disease should be carried out in every woman in every pregnancy. Those who are found to have the disease or who have had it in the past should receive treatment in every pregnancy. Treatment consists of a course of injections of penicillin and is effective in preventing infection of the baby.

Other infections may occur in pregnancy and these include the common cold, influenza, and other infections such as measles, mumps, and scarlet fever. Most adults have had the childhood infections and are therefore immune. However a bad cold or an attack of influenza should not be neglected, as high fever may lead to death of the baby or premature delivery. A pregnant woman who has a raised temperature should remain in bed and if fever persists for more than 24 hours she should see a doctor.

Dental care It is important that the mother's teeth are kept healthy and in good condition during pregnancy. Dental care under the National Health Service is given free to pregnant women. Decayed or septic teeth can carry a danger of infection. Normal dental treatment can safely be carried out during pregnancy. However it is wise to avoid nitrous oxide (laughing gas) anaesthesia as there is a risk that the mother may become short of oxygen and this may be dangerous for the baby. Local anaesthetics are safe, but if a general anaesthetic is needed it should be given by an expert anaesthetist who should be informed of the pregnancy.

Preparation for childbirth

Every mother hopes for an easy, safe, and normal birth, and most are willing to do what they can to prepare for the great event. Antenatal care as we

Chapter 11 Pregnancy and childbirth

know it today dates from less than 50 years ago: the concept of preparation for childbirth is even more recent. The pioneers in this field, such as Grantly Dick Read and Helen Heardman, were active in the late 1940's and the 1950's. Their methods are based on relaxation to reduce tension, and exercises to teach the mother how best to help herself in labour. In France and the Soviet Union the idea of psycho-prophylaxis developed. This came from the original idea of Pavlov that women could be trained to overcome pain and to promote normal childbirth. Hypnosis has also been used by a few obstetricians; for those who practice it regularly the results are excellent, but the technique is exacting and it is unlikely to be universally adopted. By no means all doctors are able to practise hypnosis.

Whatever method is used, most clinics now offer classes for preparation for childbirth. These may be conducted by physiotherapists or midwives and may include lectures or talks from doctors as well. The purpose of the classes is twofold. The first object is educational, to explain to the mother and father what is happening in pregnancy and what they can expect to happen in labour. Secondly, the classes can include

things such as the care of the newborn baby, practice in bathing the baby, instruction on the care of the breasts and breast-feeding. Advice may be given on preparing the home and obtaining the layette. These classes have a wide scope, and time should always be left for questions.

Relaxation and exercises form part of the physical preparation for childbirth. Relaxation helps to relieve tension and reduce pain in labour. It can be learnt several weeks in advance so that the mother is able to relax to the utmost when the time comes. Exercises are designed to strengthen the muscles of the abdomen and pelvis and to teach the mother how to bear down in the second stage of labour. The mode of breathing is important; in the first stage shallow panting breathing is combined with relaxation as the contractions become strong at the transition to the second stage. In the second stage of labour a powerful pushing or expulsive movement is required as in expelling a bowel motion. The mother is taught to take in a breath, hold it, and then push.

The exercises, breathing, and relaxation may be varied so that the mother's posture is corrected and

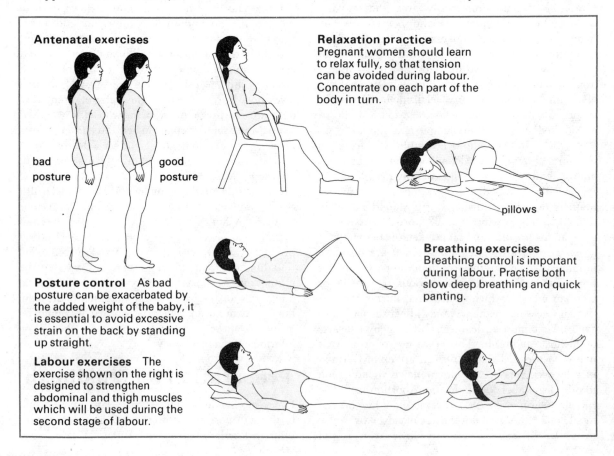

Antenatal exercises

bad posture

good posture

Posture control As bad posture can be exacerbated by the added weight of the baby, it is essential to avoid excessive strain on the back by standing up straight.

Labour exercises The exercise shown on the right is designed to strengthen abdominal and thigh muscles which will be used during the second stage of labour.

Relaxation practice
Pregnant women should learn to relax fully, so that tension can be avoided during labour. Concentrate on each part of the body in turn.

pillows

Breathing exercises
Breathing control is important during labour. Practise both slow deep breathing and quick panting.

she is taught how to carry herself and walk well. This often helps to prevent the backache so many women suffer during pregnancy. Most training for childbirth is given in classes organized in hospitals or clinics or privately, by organizations such as the National Childbirth Trust. Preparation classes are certainly to be recommended for mothers having a first labour. The experienced mother who feels that she knows the exercises and understands how to help herself in labour may prefer not to attend.

Although preparation for childbirth has the aim of normal easy labour, and though it undoubtedly contributes a great deal towards this, mothers should be warned that not all labours are normal. A forceps delivery or a Caesarean section may be needed to ensure the safety of the mother and baby. Some mothers who have anticipated normal childbirth feel cheated when they cannot achieve it, so an advance explanation of what may have to be done is essential.

Maternity benefits

A woman who is having a baby and is resident in the United Kingdom is usually entitled to certain maternity benefits and she should take advantage of these and of the practical help available. Detailed information can be obtained from local offices of the Department of Health and Social Security or from hospital or local authority clinics.

Maternity grant (as at April 1978) There is a Maternity grant of £25. The grant is paid as a lump sum provided that National Insurance contribution conditions are met. If the husband has full insurance and the woman is not working, she can claim on his insurance. If she is insured in her own right, having been working in the two years prior to becoming pregnant, she can claim on her own contribution record. A single woman can claim only on her own contributions.

Maternity allowance This is paid for eighteen weeks, that is twelve weeks before the estimated delivery date and six weeks following delivery of the baby. The basic rate of Maternity allowance is £18.50. There is now an earnings related supplement to which many women are entitled, and this supplement is normally paid from the third week of Maternity allowance.

Child benefit From November 1979 the weekly rate for all children is £4.

Child benefit increases payable to one parent families From April 1978 the rate payable for the first child is £6, and for each subsequent child £4. Like Child benefit these payments are tax free.

Milk and vitamins are available free to:
1. An expectant mother and all children (including foster children) under school age in families who are getting supplementary benefits, family income supplement, or whose incomes are low.
2. An expectant mother who already has two children (including foster children) under school age, regardless of family income.
3. All but the first two children under school age in families with three or more children (including foster children) regardless of family income.

Family planning Family planning now comes under the National Health Service and advice and contraceptives are free.

Maternity leave The Employment Protection Act, 1975, came into force in June 1976 and entitles the pregnant woman to the following rights:

She cannot be dismissed solely because she is pregnant.

She will have the right to return to work if she complies with certain conditions.

To qualify she must:

Be employed for 21 hours a week or more.

Continue to be employed until eleven weeks before the expected week of confinement.

Have two years continuous service prior to the eleventh week.

Inform her Head of Department in writing at least three weeks before leaving that she will be absent due to pregnancy.

Produce a medical certificate stating the expected week of confinement, if so requested.

Inform her Head of Department that she intends to return to work.

A woman then has the right to return to her job within 29 weeks of her confinement and must notify her employer a week in advance of her proposed date of return.

It should be added that the question of entitlement to these benefits is sometimes a complex one, and women may in fact find themselves ineligible for various reasons – girls who have not worked in the previous year, divorced women, women with so-called common law husbands, and pregnant schoolgirls.

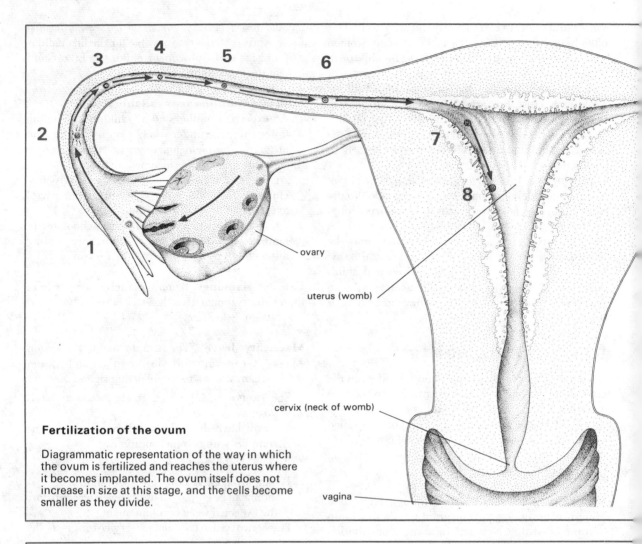

ovary

uterus (womb)

cervix (neck of womb)

vagina

Fertilization of the ovum

Diagrammatic representation of the way in which
the ovum is fertilized and reaches the uterus where
it becomes implanted. The ovum itself does not
increase in size at this stage, and the cells become
smaller as they divide.

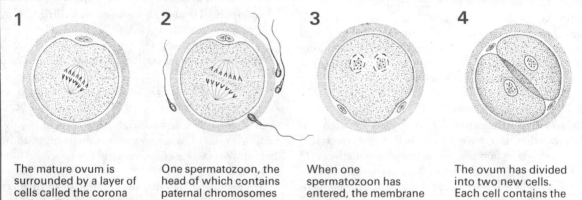

1 The mature ovum is
surrounded by a layer of
cells called the corona
radiata. The nucleus of
the cell carries the
maternal chromosomes
— one half of the full
complement.

2 One spermatozoon, the
head of which contains
paternal chromosomes
(the other half of the
full complement),
penetrates the
membrane of the ovum
to achieve fertilization.

3 When one
spermatozoon has
entered, the membrane
changes and no other
can do so.

The fertilized egg is
propelled towards the
uterus.

4 The ovum has divided
into two new cells.
Each cell contains the
full complement of
chromosomes.

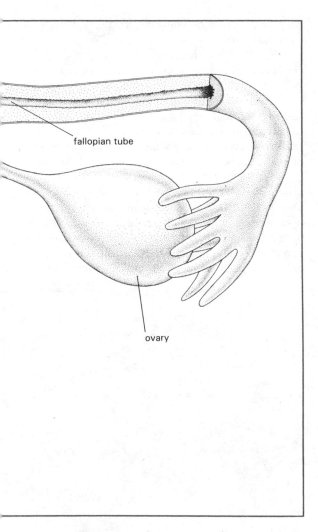

fallopian tube

ovary

The course of pregnancy

From the viewpoint of the doctor or midwife, pregnancy is conveniently divided into three parts. Each part is of roughly three months (a trimester). This is a useful division because of the particular events which tend to occur during the course of pregnancy.

The first trimester During the first three months or thirteen weeks of pregnancy the uterus enlarges to about three times its normal size and by the end of this period fills the pelvis. The doctor, and sometimes the patient herself, can feel it through the abdomen.

All bleeding in pregnancy is a serious symptom demanding immediate medical advice. Nevertheless a few women get some staining at the time of the first two or three missed periods. This may settle down but in some cases it becomes more profuse and is accompanied by cramp-like pain. This may be a threatened abortion and the survival of the baby is then in doubt. The usual management is to put the woman to rest in bed. Hormones may be needed in certain cases to try to preserve the pregnancy. The woman should remain at rest till there has been no bright bleeding for a week; normal activity should be resumed gradually and exertion and sexual inter-course avoided until it is certain that the pregnancy is well-established.

In other cases the pains become more severe like the pains of labour. Vaginal examination reveals that the opening of the uterus or cervix is enlarged and the condition is often described as inevitable abortion.

5

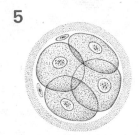

There is another cell division, producing four cells. Thereafter the cells divide and double in number at each division.

6

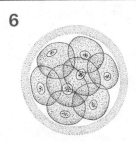

The ball of cells (morula) continues to pass down the fallopian tube.

7

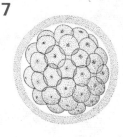

The morula develops an internal fluid-filled cavity and by this stage has entered the uterus.

8

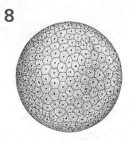

The outer layer of the implanted ball of cells develops to form the membranes and placenta. The inner cells will become the embryo.

Chapter 11 **Pregnancy and childbirth**

The products of conception are then expelled, either completely or incompletely. Usually the uterus has to be curetted to remove the remains, and the bleeding then continues for a week or so. A normal period should occur after a month to six weeks.

A spontaneous abortion – or miscarriage – is a natural process that occurs without artificial intervention. In the majority of these there is a serious defect in the development of the egg-cell, and indeed there may be no baby at all. Thus a miscarriage may be Nature's way of getting rid of a seriously abnormal pregnancy.

Sometimes the baby dies in the womb, and then it obviously stops growing. The woman often notices a persistent dark brown discharge. This may also require a curettage to remove the products of conception. When a woman has three or more consecutive spontaneous miscarriages the term habitual abortion is used.

Therapeutic or legal abortion is permitted in certain circumstances under the Abortion Act, 1967. In brief this provides that if two doctors are prepared to certify that continuation of the pregnancy would constitute a risk to the woman's life or health greater than if the pregnancy were terminated; that there is a risk to the health of the existing children of her family; or that there is a substantial risk that the child if born would suffer physical or mental handicap, then abortion is legal. The decision concerning legal abortion still has to be made by doctors, and the operation to terminate pregnancy may legally be performed only by a registered medical practitioner, in a clinic or hospital registered for the purpose. The operation must be notified to the Chief Medical

Development of the embryo

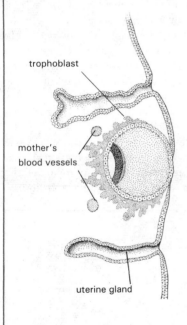

trophoblast

mother's blood vessels

uterine gland

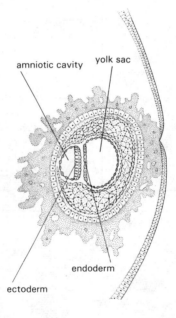

amniotic cavity   yolk sac

endoderm

ectoderm

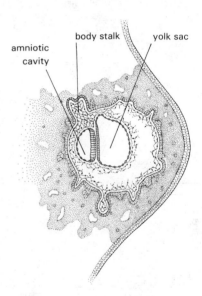

amniotic cavity   body stalk   yolk sac

Day 6

The cells of the outer layer (trophoblast) penetrate the lining of the uterus to be in close contact with the mother's blood vessels.

Day 9

The inner (germinal) layers (endoderm and ectoderm) become differentiated. The amniotic cavity appears.

Days 13 to 15

The yolk sac develops but soon shrinks away. The amniotic cavity begins to expand.

Officer of the Department of Health.

The embryo, as the growing baby is called in the early weeks, is a mere pinpoint in size at the time of implantation in the womb. By the third month it has grown to some 7·6 cm (three in) in length and weighs about 28 gm (one oz). During this time all of the vital organs, heart, lungs, intestines, brain, eyes, and skeleton are formed. It is at this crucial period when the mother may not even be aware that she is pregnant, that external events such as illness in the mother or certain drugs may have a disastrous effect on the developing baby – named a fetus from the third month till birth. After the third month, events affecting the mother have less disastrous effect on the fetus, as the vital organs have then formed.

In a very few cases the womb or uterus containing the fetus may become stuck or impacted in the mother's pelvis; the uterus at the beginning of pregnancy is retroverted or tilted backwards. Normally at the third month the uterus rights itself but occasionally it does not; this may obstruct the urethra, the passage from the bladder, so that the mother is unable to pass urine, or, occasionally, may cause a miscarriage. Impacted uterus is painful and alarming but is quite easily overcome by emptying the bladder and correcting the position of the uterus.

Hydatidiform mole is a rare abnormality of the chorion, which forms the placenta. The chorion becomes converted into tiny cysts, each about the size of a currant, and the embryo usually dies and becomes absorbed into the growing tissue. The mole may grow very rapidly, the mother be very sick, and signs of toxaemia (see page 239) may develop. Usually there is bleeding as in a threatened miscarriage and

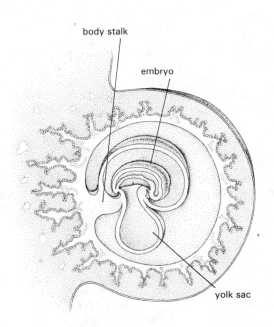

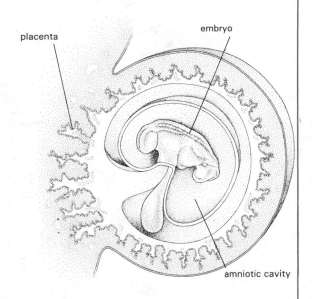

Day 20

The embryo is now a curved three-layered disc and becomes suspended on a body stalk, through which it receives nutrients from the trophoblast.

Day 28

The body stalk develops into the umbilical cord through which blood circulates between the placenta and the embryo. Oxygen, carbon dioxide, and nutrients are exchanged through the placenta, but the placental and maternal circulations do not communicate directly. The embryo now begins to show the development of organs. The amniotic cavity expands and its outer layer merges with the inner layer of the trophoblast.

235

Chapter 11 Pregnancy and childbirth

part of the mole may be expelled. Nowadays the diagnosis can be made by special biological tests and by ultrasound. The treatment is to remove the mole, generally by suction, from the uterus. There is a small risk of a malignant tumour, choriocarcinoma, developing, so the woman must be kept under surveillance for two years. During this time she should not take the contraceptive pill or use an intrauterine contraceptive, but she must take precautions against pregnancy. These conditions are found to be commoner in women of Chinese and Japanese origin than in other ethnic groups.

Ectopic pregnancy This occurs when the ovum becomes trapped in the fallopian tube, where fertilization takes place. The embryo then grows in an abnormal place. It cannot reach maturity here unless, very rarely, it is expelled into the mother's

abdominal cavity and grows there – a normal child has been born after developing in this way. However, most tubal pregnancies end before the third month. The embryo may die in the tube, forming a tubal swelling; there may be bleeding into the abdominal cavity from the tube; in about five per cent of cases there is massive haemorrhage into the mother's abdomen with collapse, which can be dangerous. For this reason if a tubal pregnancy is suspected, usually because the mother has pain and bleeding, a full investigation is undertaken. In doubtful cases a special technique called laparoscopy helps to establish the diagnosis. Laparoscopy is performed by inserting a special telescope through a small incision in the abdominal wall, enabling the operator to inspect the abdominal contents. Treatment almost invariably means the removal of the affected tube, a

Development of the embryo

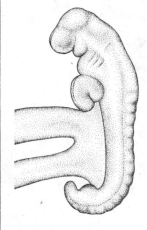 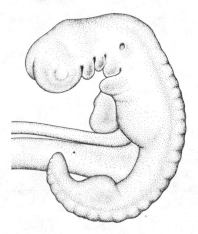 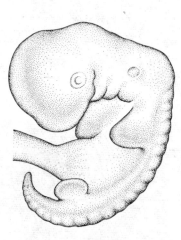

28 days

The gallbladder and liver tubules start to form, and areas of the brain begin to develop. A swelling indicates the beginning of the stomach. The heart tube becomes slightly bent, with local bulges and constrictions.

actual size

32 days

The nose parts are suggested by a pair of thickened bulges. There is a tiny liver prominence and belly stalk. Primitive head parts – mouth, brain, eyes, and ears are forming. An opening develops between the mouth and gut; a little later the anus appears. Primitive thyroid cells form at the floor of the throat. A small rounded outgrowth shows the beginnings of the larynx and trachea. The heart is under the chin, and although divisions are recognizable it still operates as a simple tube. The first heartbeats occur.

34 days

Arm and leg buds appear – also thickenings which will be the tongue. The gut elongates. Primitive blood vessels function. The eye lens, retinal layer, cranial nerves, and pancreas start to form.

comparatively simple abdominal operation similar to the removal of the appendix. Normal pregnancy is possible after ectopic pregnancy and women who have suffered this may have several subsequent children. The possibility of another ectopic pregnancy does however exist, and the doctor will be alert for this complication in subsequent pregnancies.

The second trimester This is often called the silent area of pregnancy since it is relatively peaceful with the fewest complications. The mother usually becomes conscious of the movement of the baby, feeling life from about the 16th to the 22nd week. As the baby grows, the movements get stronger and they may even disturb the mother's sleep.

Growth From a length of 7·5 cm (three in) the fetus grows to about 36 cm (fourteen in). At 22 weeks it weighs about 227 gm (8 oz) and at 28 weeks 1 kg (2 lb 3 oz). Under British law a baby becomes legally viable at 28 weeks (from the first day of the last menstrual period). Babies born before 28 weeks have been known to survive; a baby which is born dead after 28 weeks is legally considered to have been otherwise capable of survival, and therefore is referred to as stillborn. The uterus grows with the baby and by the 28th week is five to eight cm (two to three in) above the mother's navel. She now gains weight at the rate of about 0·5 kg (one lb) per week.

Miscarriage Premature delivery is the greatest hazard of the second trimester. It is still legally an abortion or miscarriage. In most cases the baby born before 28 weeks does not survive. In a case where late miscarriages have occurred in the past the doctor may advise a minor operation to stitch the cervix or neck

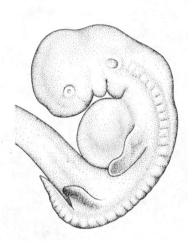

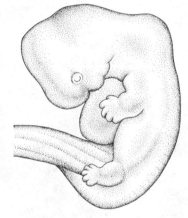

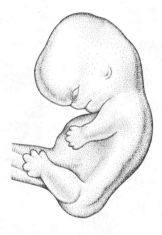

35–37 days

The arm and leg buds lengthen, and regional divisions of the brain are recognizable. The lung buds branch and kidneys begin to form. The skin and primitive eye parts develop, and the nasal pits become recognizable as nostrils.

40–42 days

The stomach has assumed its adult shape. The salivary glands become identifiable, and the milk lines from armpits to groin appear as slight thickenings from which breasts will later develop. Pre-cartilage cells are being laid down to form parts of the skeleton. The heart is at a critical stage of development – the parts grow and fuse to form the four chambers.

46–49 days

Distinct beginnings of fingers, toes, and eyelids can be seen. The autonomic nervous system is forming, together with delicate fibres that will be the muscles. The nasal openings break through, the optic nerve fibres extend, and the gallbladder elongates. Adrenal gland cells accumulate, and the thyroid cells start to move into position. The tail now disappears.

of the womb early on in the pregnancy and so prevent it gaping open as the pregnancy advances – a condition which predisposes the woman to premature labour or miscarriage. This operation is often named after Professor Shirodkar of Bombay who was among the first to describe it. Most mothers, however, find that the second trimester is the best part of pregnancy. They often feel exceptionally well.

The third trimester The last weeks of pregnancy are naturally subject to some increase in discomfort. The infant grows from a little over one kg (two lb) to over 3·5 kg (seven lb) and the uterus continues to enlarge till it appears almost to fill the mother's abdomen. Her waist measurement increases to about one m (40 in). She becomes much more conscious of the baby's movements and these may disturb sleep.

Abnormal bleeding is now a serious sign. If bleeding occurs, however slight, the mother should immediately retire to bed and send for her doctor as a matter of urgency. There are two principal causes for such bleeding, now termed antepartum haemorrhage, both serious, and both involving the afterbirth or placenta.

Placenta praevia means that the placenta is in an abnormally low position inside the uterus. If it lies completely below the baby over the outlet of the womb, birth cannot take place without severe bleeding. Bleeding may also occur if it is higher up on the wall of the womb. The typical sign is painless bleeding. It is usual to admit the woman to hospital and to keep her in bed until all bleeding has ceased. The exact location of the placenta can be determined by means of ultrasound. It is preferable, unless

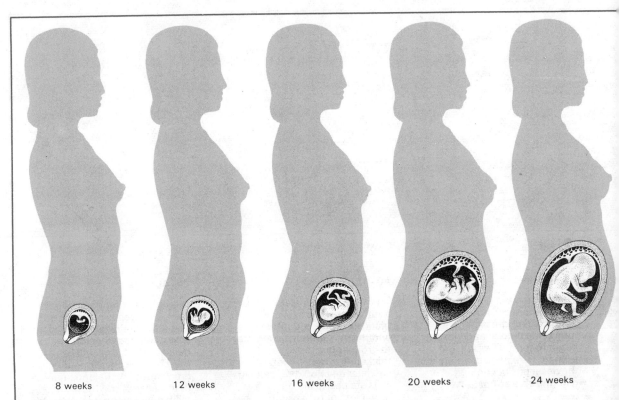

| 8 weeks | 12 weeks | 16 weeks | 20 weeks | 24 weeks |

Development of the fetus

The fetus has now developed from a minute oval body into recognizably human form, and it already possesses most of the organs and tissues. Centres of bone growth have been established at 8 weeks, and ossification of the bones begins. Human facial characteristics become more obvious as the nose and upper jaw grow rapidly, and the bilateral parts of the lips and palate meet and fuse. The buds which will become teeth appear.

At 12 weeks the eyelids meet and fuse, the eyes remaining closed until the seventh month. The inner ear structure is almost completed, and the formation of the eye lens is proceeding rapidly. The external genitals appear as swellings. Primitive hair follicles and the deeper-lying skin layers become distinct.

bleeding is severe, to keep the pregnancy going until the 38th week since every day counts in the baby's favour. If the condition is severe, Caesarean section will be the best and safest measure for both mother and baby. If bleeding is severe, blood transfusion will be needed.

Accidental haemorrhage is the term applied to bleeding from a normally situated placenta. Part of the placenta may become detached from the wall of the uterus. A large amount of blood may accumulate in the uterus and this leads to severe abdominal pain and shock. This is a grave emergency, often associated with high blood pressure. It may be dealt with in various ways. If bleeding is slight, it may settle with rest and the pregnancy continue normally. If it is severe it is usually necessary to induce labour or in some cases to perform a Caesarean operation.

Toxaemia of pregnancy is another potentially serious complication and one which is watched for carefully at antenatal visits. The symptoms that the mother will notice include retention of fluid with swelling of her ankles, hands, and face, and rapid gain of weight. The doctor will look for a rise in blood pressure. Protein in the form of albumin may appear in the urine and this is one of the reasons why a sample of urine is tested at each visit. In the most serious form of toxaemia, known as eclampsia, convulsions occur, a condition dangerous for both mother and baby.

If symptoms or signs of toxaemia appear, the mother will be admitted to hospital for rest, medical treatment with drugs to reduce her blood pressure, and a controlled diet with the minimum amount of salt. Regular observations are made on the mother and baby, and special tests may be made to make sure

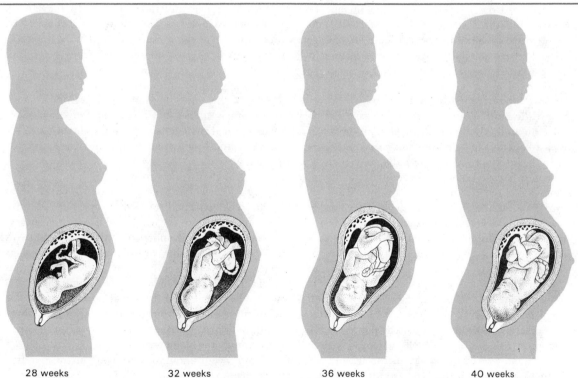

28 weeks   32 weeks   36 weeks   40 weeks

By 16 weeks the brain has become a recognizable counterpart to the adult form, in that the large bulge of the forebrain is distinguishable from the cerebellum and brain stem. The buds of what will be sweat glands appear first on the palms and soles. The outer skin thickens into distinctive layers. At 20 weeks the structures of the ovaries and testes are well established. The collecting tubules of the kidney branch out.

At 24 weeks eyebrows and eyelashes begin to become visible, and the fetus is coated in downy hair (lanugo). Skin ridges form on the palms and soles as the basis of fingerprints and sole prints. The bronchial tree continues to branch, as it does even after birth. At 28 to 32 weeks the eyelids separate. The testes begin their descent through the inguinal ring to the scrotum. Fat begins to be deposited under the skin, and the fetus becomes plumper and plumper until birth. A fetus at 28 weeks is sufficiently well developed to survive. All the vital organs have been formed and further development is mainly that of gaining size.

Chapter 11 **Pregnancy and childbirth**

that the baby is not suffering as a result of its mother's condition. In many cases the doctor may advise induction of labour because with progressing toxaemia the baby is at risk. However induction will not be done before the 38th week except in severe cases. Toxaemia is more frequent in women with high blood pressure, kidney trouble, or previous toxaemia. Good obstetrical care is essential, especially putting the mother to rest at the earliest sign of trouble. Toxaemia is more frequent in women having twins.

Rhesus factor The Rhesus, or Rh, factor gets its name from the Rhesus monkey, in which in 1940 a factor was discovered in the red blood cells. About 85 per cent of Caucasian women have the Rh factor and are Rhesus-positive, Rh-positive or D-positive (the Rhesus factor is one of a group of blood factors also known as Cc, Dd, Ee). The remaining fifteen per cent do not have the Rh factor D, but the factor d, and are described as Rhesus-negative. These factors are inherited so that if an Rh-positive man marries an Rh-negative woman they may have children who are Rh-positive. The baby, as it grows in the uterus, produces Rh-positive red blood cells and these may pass into the mother's bloodstream, causing her to produce an antibody to the factor D. This antibody may pass back to the baby and cause destruction of the baby's red blood cells. The baby may then be born with a disease known as haemolytic disease of the newborn, or erythroblastosis. This leads to anaemia, or jaundice, or both in the developing baby; the most severe form causes the baby to be distended with fluid and it is often stillborn.

Most Rhesus-negative women can produce one or two healthy babies or even more. However, a woman can be sensitized by any Rhesus-positive pregnancy, even one which ends in a miscarriage. Determination of the Rhesus factor is a normal part of routine antenatal care. If the mother is Rhesus-positive there is little if any risk, but if she is Rhesus-negative then extra care (and a series of blood tests throughout the pregnancy) will be taken. Even so the odds are favourable, as only about one mother in twenty who is Rhesus-negative will have an affected baby and this will usually happen in a third or later pregnancy.

When the baby is born, blood is taken from the umbilical cord and tested for anaemia and jaundice. If the baby is severely affected its blood can be exchanged for Rhesus-negative blood and this is generally successful; the baby then develops normally. In some cases it is necessary to deliver the baby early. Rarely, when a mother has previously lost an affected baby it may be necessary to give the baby a blood transfusion while it is still inside the uterus.

However, prevention of Rh disease is now possible. An injection of a special protein, Rhesus gamma globulin, is given to mothers at risk within 72 hours of the birth of a Rhesus-positive baby or a miscarriage. This destroys the baby's red blood cells in the mother's bloodstream and prevents her producing antibodies, so preventing haemolytic disease in subsequent pregnancies. There are other blood groups which may produce cross reactions between the mother's blood and that of her baby but these are usually mild and transfusion is rarely necessary.

Twins Twins present additional problems to the expectant mother, to the doctors and the midwives looking after her, and to the father. In the United Kingdom twins occur in about one in every 80 pregnancies; in some ethnic groups they are commoner, in others less common. A tendency to produce twins tends to run in families.

Identical twins (uniovular, from one egg) are always of the same sex and develop from a single ovum which divides into two soon after conception. One identical twin closely resembles the other. Very rarely identical twins may be conjoined, as in the case of what are called "Siamese twins". This is, however, an exceedingly rare occurrence.

Fraternal twins originate from two separate eggs fertilized by two separate spermatozoa. The eggs arise from one or both ovaries, embed in the uterus separately, and grow independently. Fraternal twins may be of the same or different sex and their relationship is no closer than that of any other brother or sister. They are more common than identical twins. Identical and fraternal twins cannot be positively identified from their appearance at birth. Examination of the placenta and membrane may help, as may the blood groups.

Triplets occur about once in 9,000 births, quadruplets once in 500,000 births, while the odds against having quintuplets are about 40 million to one. Thriving quintuplets have been born and have survived. Multiple births are commoner in women who have received so-called fertility drugs as a treatment for their previous difficulty in conceiving. The drugs stimulate the ovaries to produce several ova instead of the one or two produced normally.

The doctor may suspect twins when the uterus is larger than would be expected, when there is a family history, or when there is a rapid gain in the mother's weight. By means of ultrasound twins can now be diagnosed very early in pregnancy, even by the sixth week. An X-ray will show them clearly from about the twentieth week.

Multiple pregnancy is to some degree abnormal in the human female. The uterus is larger and much more uncomfortable so that the mother may suffer from indigestion, vomiting, shortness of breath, and insomnia. Premature delivery is common and the babies may be smaller than normal. Toxaemia can be a serious complication. In the management of twin pregnancy many doctors now advise that the mother should enter hospital for rest and observation between the 31st and 36th week of pregnancy. A carefully supervised regime of rest and diet can prolong the pregnancy and produce larger and healthier babies.

Labour with twins may be prolonged and difficult, and the risk to the second twin is slightly greater. One of the babies may be in an unfavourable position so that the birth may be difficult. The management of labour requires expert care because of the risk to the babies and the risk that the mother may have a haemorrhage.

Labour and delivery

Anticipating labour   As the expected date – D-day or Delivery Day – draws near, the expectant mother and father need to make certain preparations. Most babies in Britain are now born in hospital, but preparations for home delivery are not very different and the doctor or midwife will give advice on what is required. The mother is generally given an Expected Date of Delivery (E.D.D.) which is calculated from her last monthly period and from observations made during her pregnancy. As a matter of fact only about five per cent of babies, or one in twenty, arrives on the day it is actually due; on the other hand about 90 per cent arrive during the two weeks before or after that date. Thus the mother might be unwise to travel too far from the place where the birth is to take place during the last six weeks of pregnancy. She will have been told what to take to hospital and she should have a suitcase packed ready in good time. Most hospitals prefer to provide clothes for the baby while it is under their care, but it is sensible to pack a carrycot with the things that the baby will need on the journey home.

Twins

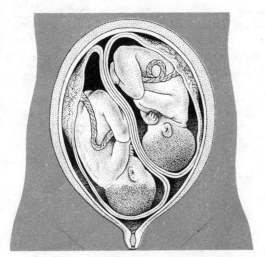

Fraternal twins develop from separate egg cells. The diagram shows fraternal twins in the uterus, each enclosed in complete and entirely separate fetal membranes, the chorion and amnion. Fraternal twins may not resemble each other very closely, may be of different sex, and do not have identical "packages" of heredity-carrying chromosomes and genes.

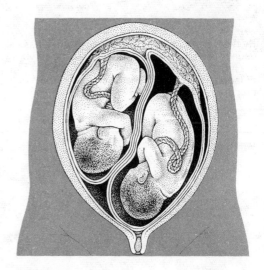

Identical twins arise from a single fertilized egg cell which divides into two independently growing cell masses, each of which develop into a fetus. Since this division occurs after fertilization, identical twins have the same genetic material, are therefore always of the same sex, and resemble each other very closely. Identical twins are contained in the same chorion, but have separate amnions.

Chapter 11 Pregnancy and childbirth

A full term fetus just before birth

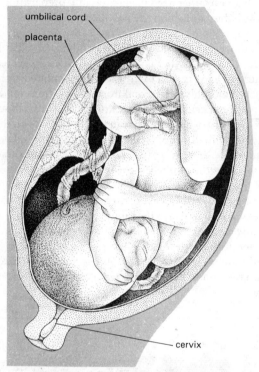

umbilical cord

placenta

cervix

By the time the baby is ready to be born, it has usually settled with the head against the cervix — the most common position for birth. The first sign of labour is likely to be the discharge of the mucous plug from the cervix. This is the "show".

During the final weeks of pregnancy, (the thirty-eighth to fortieth week) there is frequently no further increase in weight. The activity of the baby is also somewhat reduced. The mother may notice an increased sense of wellbeing, a lightening of the uterus as the baby's head drops down into the pelvis, and she often feels she has more energy than usual for her household activities. Mild, fleeting, irregular uterine contractions coming every ten or fifteen minutes and lasting ten to fifteen seconds may be noted. These contractions in fact go on throughout pregnancy, becoming stronger as labour approaches. They are generally painless but are sometimes associated with slight discomfort or backache. When labour starts, the contractions come more frequently, every ten minutes or more often, become stronger, and are usually associated with some pain or discomfort. If regular contractions become established the mother should prepare to go to hospital, or in the case of a home confinement inform her doctor or midwife. It is advisable to take no food or drink once labour has begun.

At the onset of labour the woman often notices the discharge of a plug of mucus from the cervix. This may be associated with a small amount of watery discharge or blood, the so-called "show". In a few cases the membranes rupture, releasing the liquor amnii – the fluid which surrounds the baby in the uterus. Labour usually starts within a short time of this occurring, and if the membranes are ruptured the mother is better in hospital. Normal labour lasts up to 24 hours or even more with the first baby; after the first it is usually shorter, three to twelve hours, so the mother who has had a baby before should go to

Birth of the baby

Doctors divide the process of birth into three stages – the dilatation of the cervix, birth of the baby, and delivery of the placenta. The longest stage of labour, the first, may take several hours and occasionally more than a day.

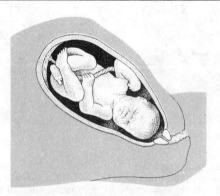

When labour commences, the walls of the uterus make rhythmical contractions and the cervix begins to dilate. This is the first stage.

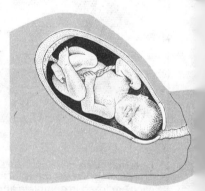

When the cervix is fully dilated the membranes often rupture and the amniotic fluid escapes (breaking of the waters).

hospital at the first sign of labour. False labour, the occurrence of contractions without opening of the cervix does happen sometimes.

Understanding labour The expectant mother ought to have some understanding of what happens in labour – literally the work – which is the bringing forth of a child. Very rapid labour is undesirable because the mother may not be properly cared for, and severe tearing of her tissues may result.

The first stage of labour is the period from the onset to the full dilatation of the mouth of the uterus (cervix), which allows the baby's head to pass through into the vagina. The intensity of the contractions usually increases as the first stage progresses. When the cervix is only slightly dilated the contractions tend to be mild or moderate, but towards the end of the first stage they become severe and many women find this the most trying and painful part of labour. These severe contractions last 40 to 50 seconds as compared with 10 to 20 seconds in the early part of labour. If the membranes have not ruptured early in labour the doctor or midwife will usually rupture them towards the end of the first stage; this improves the quality of the contractions and shortens the duration of labour.

The transition stage As dilatation is almost completed a feeling of pressure on the rectum (back passage) is felt and the mother begins to experience an uncontrollable desire to push with her contractions.

The second stage of labour is often called the expulsive stage and lasts from full dilatation of the cervix to the birth of the baby. While the mother's role in the first stage has been mainly passive, the pressure of the baby's head brings about a desire to push or bear

down as in passing a large motion. In a normal birth the baby is born by the expulsive efforts of the mother, who is encouraged to breathe in deeply, hold her breath, and push with each contraction. She should have been taught this in her antenatal classes. The second stage of labour with a first baby may last up to two hours, but with subsequent births it may be only five to thirty minutes.

The third stage of labour is the stage between the birth of the baby and the birth of the placenta. Normally it takes five to ten minutes, but if the placenta is not born within half an hour the doctor may then have to remove it in case a haemorrhage occurs. A general anaesthetic will be used for this purpose. Contraction of the muscular wall of the uterus largely stops bleeding from the raw surface where the placenta was attached.

Relief of pain in childbirth The object of the management of labour is to make it as comfortable an experience as possible. The mother who is well-prepared and who understands what is happening can often deliver herself with a minimum of pain and discomfort and this applies particularly to births after the first. It is most important that women in labour should not be left alone and here her husband or a sympathetic relative can be of the greatest help.

Many drugs have been given in the past for the relief of pain in labour. Anything given to the mother passes to the baby and may affect it after birth. For this reason in modern practice doctors tend to use pain-relieving drugs and anaesthetics with caution. In the early stages of labour when the mother is not feeling much pain, but needs to rest and perhaps to

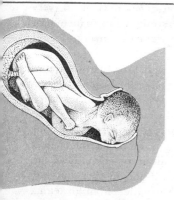

The second stage of labour is the actual birth of the baby, usually with the back of the baby's head facing the mother's front.

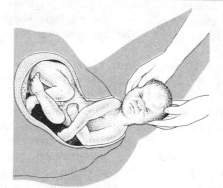

When the head is delivered it rotates so that the shoulders and rest of the body emerge quickly and easily.

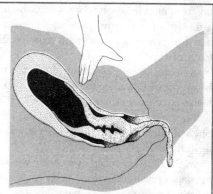

The third stage of labour is the delivery of the placenta. Contraction of the uterus stops bleeding by compressing the blood vessels.

sleep, a simple sedative may be given to her by the doctor. Pethidine is a drug much used for the relief of pain and in normal doses it is safe, though it may make the baby a little sleepy. Towards the end of the first stage the mother may be given a mixture of nitrous oxide and oxygen to breathe through a mask. Ideally she should have been shown the apparatus and how to use it during the classes for preparation for childbirth.

A local anaesthetic may be injected before making an incision, or episiotomy, in the lowest part of the birth canal to speed up the birth and prevent undesirable tearing. An anaesthetic may alternatively be given by the epidural or caudal route, the epidural into the middle of the back, the caudal at the lower end of the backbone. A local anaesthetic is injected to block the pain nerves and make the mother painfree. The only disadvantage of this is that it also partly paralyses the expulsive muscles and thus may make it difficult for the mother to push out the baby. It can, however, be given only when there is an experienced anaesthetist available who is familiar with the technique.

Hospital procedures Labour ward procedures differ greatly from one hospital to another, depending among other things on the facilities and staff available, and the preferences of individual doctors or midwives. In many hospitals in Britain medical students and pupil midwives take part in the delivery, though they are not allowed to accept responsibility except under supervision of trained staff, but their presence can help all concerned as they can stay with the mother and make necessary observations.

When a mother arrives in labour she is usually taken to an admission room where she undresses, has a shower or bath, and puts on a hospital gown. It is usual to give suppositories or occasionally an enema to empty the lower bowel. She will then be examined by a doctor or midwife. Her temperature, pulse, and blood pressure will be taken regularly and the baby's heart checked frequently. An internal examination will be made to see how far the labour has progressed. She will then be put to bed, either in a first stage ward or in the delivery room.

In the delivery room everybody wears a gown and mask to prevent infection. As delivery approaches the mother may sometimes have her legs supported in stirrups to make access easier for the doctor or midwife. The vulval area is cleansed with an antiseptic solution and covered with sterilized sheets or towels.

As the vagina distends, a local anaesthetic may be given and an episiotomy made. This is an incision in the vaginal margin which helps the baby's head to be born easily and prevents severe tearing of the mother's tissues. The baby's head is born slowly, usually facing the floor; as the full head appears it turns to left or right. The shoulders are then born, followed by the rest of the body and the legs, with the remainder of the amniotic fluid. Normally the baby takes its first breath and gives a loud cry as soon as it is completely born, but sometimes assistance is needed to start breathing. A rubber tube is put into the baby's mouth to suck out any fluid remaining in its mouth or throat to prevent this being inadvertently inhaled into the baby's lungs. The cord which attaches the baby to the placenta is cut and the baby wrapped in a towel and either put into a warm cradle or given to the mother to hold.

As the baby is born the doctor or midwife usually gives the mother an injection which makes the uterus contract firmly, thus helping to expel the placenta and prevent haemorrhage. The placenta is now delivered, generally by gentle pulling on the cord, and the mother's abdomen is examined to make sure that the now empty uterus is firmly contracted. The episiotomy is then sewn up. Nowadays fine stitches that do not have to be removed but dissolve in the tissues are used, and with a local anaesthetic the procedure is virtually painless.

The mother and father can now relax and enjoy their newborn infant. The mother is given a cup of tea and allowed to rest under observation in the delivery room for a while before she is taken to the main ward.

The condition of the baby after birth is carefully checked to see that its colour and breathing are satisfactory. Some babies take a little while to breathe normally and have to be given oxygen. A very premature baby will be put straight into an incubator and may need to go to a special-care nursery.

Induction of labour There are many circumstances in which the induction or the bringing on of a labour may be advised. In general, labour is started artificially if it is felt that the mother or baby will be safer. The danger of postmature pregnancy (one where the pregnancy has gone on much longer than its expected dates), especially in older mothers, has been recognized recently. If the mother has any bleeding during pregnancy or suffers from toxaemia, diabetes, or any other disease, then induction of labour may be indicated.

Before induction is done the mother will be examined internally to make sure that the cervix is "ripe", that is, that there is a good chance that labour will start easily. In urgent cases it may not be possible to wait for this. Drugs recently introduced make the induction of labour a much more certain procedure than formerly, and they are powerful drugs which can be given by mouth or by injection. In order to administer them by injection, a fine needle is put into a vein in the mother's arm or hand and the solution dripped slowly in through a transfusion bottle.

Induction of labour is most often begun by rupturing the membranes. An internal examination is made and an instrument passed into the uterus to break the waters and allow some of the fluid to escape. This is a simple and almost painless procedure. During labour the condition of the baby is constantly checked. This may be done by simply listening to the baby's heart with a stethoscope, but other methods of monitoring are also used. The baby's heartbeat and the contractions of the uterus can be simultaneously recorded through a small microphone like a disc which is strapped gently to the mother's abdomen. Or a small clip may be attached painlessly to the baby's scalp through the vagina and cervix to give an electrical recording of the heartbeat. If the baby's condition is giving rise to concern a sample of the baby's blood may be taken from the scalp to see how well the baby is standing up to labour.

Difficulties in labour   During the antenatal period the mother is examined to make sure, as far as is possible, that there is plenty of room for the baby to be born normally. If there is doubt an X-ray examination or an ultrasound scan in the last week of pregnancy or even during labour will help. It is possible thus to measure the baby's head and the mother's bones and so predict the likelihood of any difficulty.

Forceps delivery   Obstetric forceps are metal instruments with curved ends which are used in cases where the mother is unable to push the baby out, or where urgent delivery becomes necessary. They are designed to protect the baby's head from pressures during delivery. A local, epidural, caudal, or general anaesthetic is used when a forceps delivery is conducted.

Vacuum extraction   The idea of applying a suction cup (the ventouse) to the baby's head and pulling on it gently is over a hundred years old. It has recently been reintroduced, especially in Sweden, and it is in use in some hospitals in this country. The advantages are that it can be applied under local anaesthesia and before the cervix is fully open; forceps cannot generally be applied so early. The baby is born

Breech presentation

Breech presentation occurs when the baby's buttocks appear instead of the head at the cervix. Labour is usually longer in a breech birth. Steps are taken to deliver the head before the baby starts to cry.

unharmed but with a "chignon" or swelling on its scalp – this disappears in a few days.

Breech delivery   Most babies are born head first, but in about three per cent the buttocks or breech are lodged in the birth canal. If a breech presentation is found in the later weeks of pregnancy, an attempt may be made to turn the baby round. If this is not successful an X-ray will often be taken to make sure there is enough room for the baby to pass through. If there is any doubt Caesarean section may be advised. Breech delivery requires skilful management, the particular difficulty being that the baby's head comes last and has to pass quickly through the birth canal.

Prolonged labour   Any labour which has lasted for more than 24 hours is considered to be prolonged. There are many possible causes, among the commonest being a malposition of the baby, such as a breech, or twins. When everything is normal, labour can be accelerated by rupturing the membranes and giving an intravenous drip containing drugs which stimulate the uterine activity. The drip in itself helps the mother and the baby, as it can at the same time help to prevent thirst, and the glucose in the drip also helps to keep up the mother's strength. Nevertheless a long labour is very exhausting for the mother – and the father if he is present – and everything possible is done to prevent it. If the mother is not in sight of delivery after 24 hours a careful assessment of her condition and that of the baby is made, particularly to assess the progress made and to determine the prospects. In some cases of prolonged and difficult labour a Caesarean section will be the best solution, but this will not be done if there is a reasonable alternative.

Caesarean section   Here the mother is anaesthetized, and the baby delivered by an incision into the uterus through the abdomen. It is named after Julius Caesar who was alleged to have been born in this way. It is one of the safest of operations. In Britain about five per cent of babies are born in this way.

Caesarean section may be elective, that is performed before labour, or emergency, that is performed during labour or when an abnormal situation such as a haemorrhage occurs.

Elective Caesarean section may be performed because there is insufficient room for the baby to pass through the mother's pelvis, so-called disproportion. It will be advised in some cases of breech presentation, or where there is severe toxaemia, or where there has been repeated haemorrhage. Caesarean section may be performed in labour if the progress is not satisfactory or if the baby shows signs of distress before it can be safely delivered through the vagina. Surgeons try to avoid Caesarean section before the baby is mature, that is before the 38th week.

The operation is performed by making an incision through the abdominal wall as low down as possible; the muscle wall of the uterus is opened and the baby and placenta removed. The uterus and abdominal wall are then carefully sewn up. In modern practice it is usual to give a general anaesthetic, but the operation can be done with epidural or even local anaesthesia.

A Caesarean section is not necessarily "the easy way to have a baby". The risk to the mother is slightly higher and the first few days are painful. Gas pains and bladder difficulties may be present though they usually subside within a week or so. The hospital stay for most Caesarean patients has to be a few days longer than that for women delivered normally. How many Caesareans may a woman have? There is no theoretical limit, though most doctors feel that three or four is enough. A number of women having had a Caesarean can be delivered normally in a succeeding pregnancy; this will largely depend on the reason for the Caesarean. In such cases special care will be needed during pregnancy and labour because there is a chance, albeit very small, that the scar of the previous operation may give way, with danger to mother and baby.

The puerperium
(the six weeks after delivery)

The first week   The mother may feel tired after delivery if she has had a long labour. Most feel at peace and exhilarated that the nine months of waiting and planning are over. Some find that when they see the baby there is a feeling of anticlimax. This should be understood by all, and mothers should not feel guilty if maternal feelings are not immediately apparent. Ideally the first contact with the baby should be in the delivery room when the mother holds him, looks him over, and if she is going to breast-feed lets him suck the nipples for a moment or two on each side. There may be reasons to delay this first contact if the birth has not been normal or the baby is premature or not breathing well.

The length of time the mother and baby remain in the hospital will depend on individual circumstances and may be as short as six hours or as long as fourteen days. If the mother is to go home within 48 hours this must be a planned early discharge. She and the baby will be examined before leaving, and the local midwife and family doctor informed so that the necessary care begun in the hospital can be continued in the home. Sometimes the midwife may come to the hospital with her, deliver her with the aid of the family doctor, and then take her home.

Wherever the mother is during the first week after delivery there are certain basic things that are important in her care and that of the baby. The mother is generally allowed up and permitted to go to the lavatory and use a bath, shower, or bidet from the day after delivery. She may gradually increase her activity over the next few days but it is important that she gets adequate rest and sleep.

Breast-feeding   Every mother should be encouraged to breast-feed unless there is an important reason against it. The breasts and nipples should have been prepared during pregnancy and the mother should put the baby to the breasts for a few seconds each side as soon as possible after birth and again after twelve hours. The breasts may become heavy, swollen, and even painful within a day or so. This is the normal reaction which precedes the flow of milk. The baby should be allowed to suck for two to three minutes on each side until the milk flows freely. It is important to realize that breast-feeding can at first be quite uncomfortable, but it is well worthwhile to persevere. The milk supply may not be fully established for about a week. Most babies lose weight

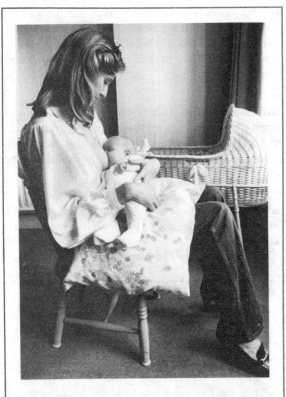

When feeding the baby, either with the breast or the bottle, it is easiest to sit in a comfortable low chair. Do not bend down to the baby, but raise it to the right level, supporting its head.

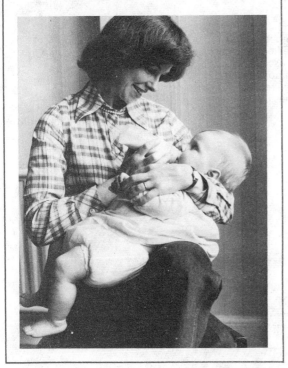

in the first week, however they are fed; part of this loss is due to the fact that the baby loses water to begin with. It should not cause alarm or make the mother abandon breast-feeding.

Before giving the baby a feed the mother should wash her hands, breasts, and nipples. She should sit in a comfortable position with her back well supported with perhaps her feet on a stool. The inexperienced mother will need a lot of help to begin with and staff do not always have the necessary time for this. Those who persist and succeed in breast-feeding for even a few weeks find it a rewarding experience. Moreover, it conveys to the baby immunity from certain diseases, reduces the chances of gastroenteritis and bowel problems, and establishes the baby's nutrition in the natural and normal manner.

Aftercare The uterus at the time of delivery weighs about one kg (two lb); by six weeks it has shrunk to its nonpregnant weight of about 60 gm (two oz), but it loses most of this weight in the first week. There is bleeding, either more or less than a normal period for the first week; in fact intermittent bleeding continues for up to four weeks. This should have ceased altogether by six weeks.

Episiotomy Sometimes the wound becomes swollen and painful during the few days after delivery. The mother should wear a pad to protect her clothing while she is still losing blood. If the stitches are painful, frequent salt baths may give relief. After a Caesarean section the stitches are generally removed a week later.

Exercises After birth the abdominal muscles tend to be soft and floppy; the abdomen, like the uterus, shrinks in the first few weeks. All mothers should be encouraged to do simple exercises to strengthen the tone of the muscles of the abdomen and pelvis. This helps the woman to regain her figure and to prevent troubles such as prolapse of the womb in later life. In most hospitals these exercises are done under the supervision of a physiotherapist.

Bladder and bowels During the first three days the mother passes a lot of urine, as the water retained during pregnancy is eliminated. After a difficult birth or a Caesarean operation there may be difficulty in passing urine for a day or two; in certain cases it may be necessary for a catheter to be put in to empty the bladder. Many women complain of constipation after childbirth and some have piles which may become very swollen and painful. A simple laxative does no

247

harm, but the use of additional bran in the diet as well as extra fluids and fruit may be effective, and certain gentle laxatives are also available from the family doctor on prescription. Piles may be relieved by frequent baths and the application of a soothing ointment, again obtained by prescription.

Rest and sleep   Both in hospital and after she goes home the recently delivered mother needs ample rest and sleep, as her nights may be disturbed by the baby. Hospitals usually insist on special rest periods for the mother, during which visiting may be discouraged. Sometimes mothers become very overexcited, or alternatively depressed. The "third day blues" are well-known to experienced mothers, but an anxious husband may be distressed to find his wife in tears. Usually this passes off quickly, but in a very few cases

the depressive reaction may become much worse and require medical help. Some women wake at night sweating profusely due to changing hormone levels similar to the "hot flushes" sometimes occurring at the menopause.

Infections   Great care is taken in the labour ward to avoid introducing infection. People with colds, sore throats, or influenza should not visit a recently delivered mother as they may pass the infection to her or her baby.

Afterpains   These are cramplike pains felt in the lower abdomen during the first few days after delivery and are associated with the contractions of the uterus. They are commoner in women who have had more

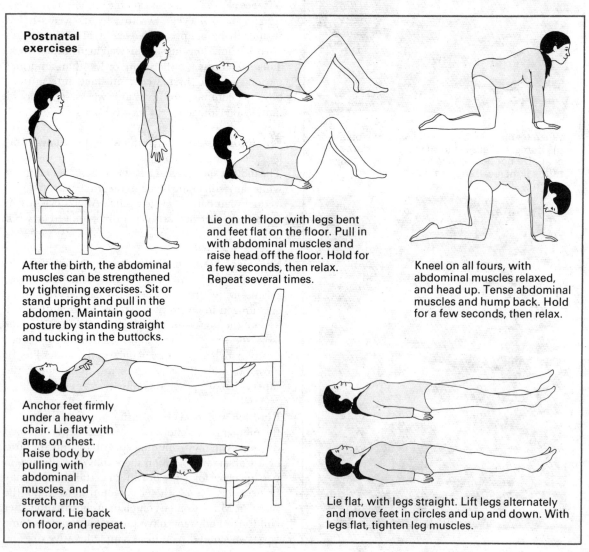

Postnatal exercises

After the birth, the abdominal muscles can be strengthened by tightening exercises. Sit or stand upright and pull in the abdomen. Maintain good posture by standing straight and tucking in the buttocks.

Lie on the floor with legs bent and feet flat on the floor. Pull in with abdominal muscles and raise head off the floor. Hold for a few seconds, then relax. Repeat several times.

Kneel on all fours, with abdominal muscles relaxed, and head up. Tense abdominal muscles and hump back. Hold for a few seconds, then relax.

Anchor feet firmly under a heavy chair. Lie flat with arms on chest. Raise body by pulling with abdominal muscles, and stretch arms forward. Lie back on floor, and repeat.

Lie flat, with legs straight. Lift legs alternately and move feet in circles and up and down. With legs flat, tighten leg muscles.

than one child and tend to be felt most when the baby is being fed, because the act of suckling makes the uterus contract. If they are very severe they can be relieved by simple pain relievers.

Going home Some babies require feeding more often than others. So before the mother goes home she should have become familiar with her baby and his needs. She should have been shown how to bath him, though in modern hospitals babies are not usually bathed until the day they go home. If the baby is bottle-fed, the mother should be shown how to sterilize the bottles. She should also be shown how to prepare the feeds.

Arriving home For many women this is the worst and most alarming part of childbearing, particularly for the inexperienced mother. In hospital she is supported and cushioned against the outside world, but now there is a baby, shopping, cooking, cleaning, and all the household tasks to be done. There may be other children to care for. It is important that the mother should have as much sensible and sympathetic help as possible. She should try to plan her day around the needs of the baby at first and be sure to get at least one hour's rest herself during the day. A small baby seems frighteningly frail, though in fact it is surprisingly tough, and, if properly fed and cared for, it will soon fit into the household routine.

Six weeks later The mother should have a postnatal examination when the baby is about six weeks old. The doctor will check her weight and general condition. The muscle tone of the abdomen and pelvis will be checked and if it is still weak the mother will be encouraged to continue her exercises. A vaginal examination is usually made to make sure that all the tissues have healed and that the uterus has returned to the normal size. At this visit birth control is discussed and a suitable contraceptive may be supplied if this is what the woman wishes. Most contraceptives can be used although the standard contraceptive pill may not be advised if the woman is still breast-feeding. This visit is also a chance to discuss any problems, difficulties, or worries that the mother may have about herself and her baby.

Monthly periods may not return while a woman is breast-feeding, but if the baby is bottle-fed the first period normally arrives about six to eight weeks after the birth. Sexual intercourse may be resumed as soon as bleeding has ceased and the stitches are no longer tender. As pregnancy is possible, though not very likely, even quite soon after delivery, contraceptives should be used unless the couple wish to have another baby soon.

Legal aspects of childbearing The birth of every child in the United Kingdom must by law be registered within 42 days in the district where the birth took place. The Registrar of Births, Deaths, and Marriages often visits maternity hospitals in order to assist the mother with this. The baby can be registered by the father, the mother, or any person present at the birth. The registrar will issue a birth certificate; this is an important document which the baby will need throughout its life, for example in applying for child allowances and many other documents, such as a passport; it is quite a good idea to ask for two copies of the certificate and to keep one in a safe place, for example in the bank. A shortened form of birth certificate can be obtained and may be issued to an unmarried mother. If the parents are not legally married at the time of the birth the child is illegitimate though it may be legitimized at any time if the parents marry. All births are notified by the doctor or midwife to the local health department. A health visitor will normally visit the home to see that the mother and baby are well and that the baby is properly cared for. She can often give much helpful advice.

About eighteen out of every 1,000 babies are unfortunately born dead (stillborn) or die in the first week of life. If the baby is stillborn it may have died during labour or before labour – a certificate of stillbirth is then issued. If the baby dies at any time after birth a doctor must issue a death certificate or report the death to the coroner. These are sad happenings but they cannot be overlooked. Fortunately many more babies now survive their birth than even twenty years ago.

Contraception

Contraception, family planning, or birth control may be simply defined as the prevention of pregnancy, except when it is desired. Most couples aim to limit the number of children they have and to plan their births. In fact all the methods of birth control in use today, with the exception of the contraceptive pill and other hormonal methods, were already known and in use by the end of the nineteenth century. It is, however, only recently that public discussion has been acceptable.

Conception and contraception

The aim of contraception is to prevent fertilization of the egg or ovum, or to prevent the fertilized ovum from being implanted in the uterus. The methods known in the past or in current use may be summed up as follows:

Methods to prevent the sperm reaching the cervical canal Intercourse without penetration of the vagina. Withdrawal or coitus interruptus. Use of a sheath or condom. Various types of barrier to cover the cervix – diaphragm or Dutch cap, cervical cap, vault pessary. Appliances worn in the cervix.

Chemical spermicides may be used with or without a mechanical barrier; they include soluble pessaries, creams, foaming preparations, soluble tablets, and jellies. Most contain spermicidal chemicals. Some similar preparations used with caps are mechanical barriers only.

Intrauterine devices ("the coil") There is now a large variety, the modern ones being usually made of plastic; copper may be added and hormone pellets have been incorporated in some devices under trial. Intrauterine devices probably act by preventing implantation of the fertilized ovum.

Combined oral contraceptives ("the pill") containing an oestrogen and a progestogen. They probably inhibit ovulation and also modify the lining of the uterus and the secretions of the cervix.

Progestogen-only pills ("the mini-pill") These act on the uterus, they may be given as pills or as long-term injections lasting 70 to 80 days.

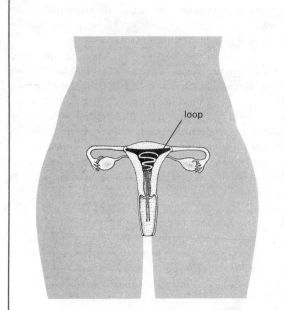

The intrauterine device (IUD), which may be in the form of a loop or coil, is a highly effective method of contraception. It must be fitted by a doctor or at a Family Planning Clinic.

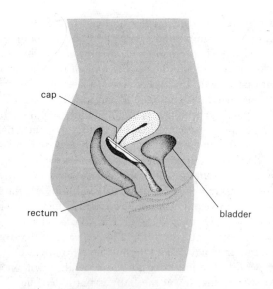

There are several forms of cap, the most common of which is the diaphragm or Dutch cap. They act by covering the cervix to prevent sperm from entering, and should be used with a spermicidal jelly for full effectiveness.

The rhythm method or "safe period". This is the only method available to those who for religious or other reasons are not allowed to use conventional contraceptives. Intercourse is avoided during the fertile period of the month, that is when ovulation may be expected to occur.

Sterilization   In men this is achieved by vasectomy which involves cutting a duct, the vas deferens, on each side; sperms do not then reach the semen.

In women sterilization is achieved by cutting the fallopian tubes, or by applying clips or rings to them through a laparoscope. Removal of the ovaries or of the uterus (hysterectomy) always leads to sterility.

Other methods not yet available or in general use include the "morning-after pill", while the possibility of a "pill" for men is being actively investigated. Immunizing women against pregnancy is a possibility which is not yet generally available or advised.

Abortion or legal termination of pregnancy is widely used as a method of family limitation rather than contraception. Since the Abortion Act 1967 a large number of legal abortions are performed every year, replacing the illegal and often dangerous "back-street" abortions of former times.

The choice of a contraceptive method

The ideal contraceptive should be simple to use, free from side effects, cause the minimal interference with the spontaneity and enjoyment of intercourse and, above all, be reliable. It should also be cheap. In Britain contraceptives are now free on the National Health Service, but in developing countries they are comparatively costly.

The hormonal contraceptives are at present obtainable only on a doctor's prescription. Intra-uterine devices should be fitted by a doctor and so should a diaphragm or cervical cap. Sterilization involves a surgical operation.

Thus contraception without medical advice is mainly achieved through withdrawal or the use of the sheath. Sheaths are easily obtained and have the great advantage that they afford the best protection against sexually transmitted disease. For maximum safety a chemical contraceptive should be used with a barrier method – sheath, diaphragm, or cervical cap, since there is a high failure rate with chemicals, pessaries, jellies, and creams used alone.

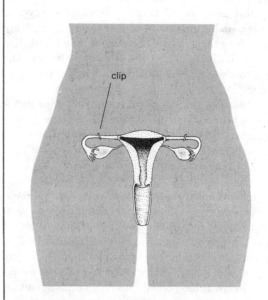

Female sterilization is achieved either by removing a section of each fallopian tube, which is likely to be permanent, or by closing the tubes by means of clips which can be removed later with possible restoration of fertility.

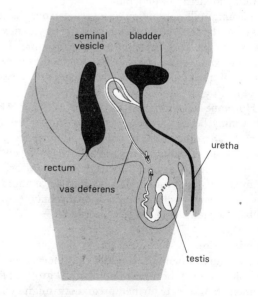

The usual method of male sterilization is vasectomy, that is severing the vas deferens in the groin. Conception does not become impossible until the man's ejaculate is found to be sperm-free.

Chapter 11 Pregnancy and childbirth

The rhythm method requires restraint on the part of the couple and careful observance of the safe period. This can be calculated if the menstrual cycle is regular, or by the use of a basal body temperature chart. It is then reasonably reliable but less so just after childbirth or in women approaching the menopause when ovulation may not occur at regular intervals.

Intrauterine devices afford reasonably safe contraception without any further action by the couple concerned. Some women do not tolerate them and they may cause pain or bleeding. They are best used for older women who have had children.

Hormonal contraception is now well established. In most cases the combined pill containing oestrogen and a progestogen is used and it is estimated that at least three million women take the pill in Britain today. Serious side effects include blood clotting, which may even be fatal if it affects the heart or if the clot moves to the lungs. It has recently been recommended that the dose of oestrogen should not exceed 30 micrograms; caution should be observed in giving the pill to women over 35, to those who are obese or have high blood pressure, or to heavy smokers. Some women with diabetes, epilepsy, or migraine do not tolerate the pill well. Minor side effects such as weight gain or depression may also occur, but these are minimized with the modern low dose pill.

The mini-pill, containing a progestogen only, is not as safe as the combined pill, which is the safest known contraceptive. It may cause irregular bleeding. It is useful for older women, for those who do not tolerate the combined pill or for women who are breast-feeding.

Hormone injections last for ten to twelve weeks. They may be given to women who cannot use or tolerate any other form of contraception. They are particularly of value in women who have recently been immunized against rubella (German measles) or in those whose husbands have had a vasectomy, because some weeks or even months may elapse before the man can be declared sterile.

Sterilization, male or female, is now chosen by many couples when they consider that their family is complete. It may be advised on medical grounds for women in whom a further pregnancy might constitute a serious risk to life or health. Careful counselling of the couple is essential as sterilization should be regarded as irrevocable, though reversal can be achieved by a further operation in a proportion of cases.

The most important advance in contraception has been that it is now freely discussed and women in particular are more able to discuss it with their family doctors. Family planning clinics are now available almost everywhere and there is a wide choice of reasonably safe methods. However it is important that the method be fully understood and that further advice is obtained if the method seems unsatisfactory. Instruction in methods of contraception is now part of the syllabus for medical students, student nurses, and pupil midwives; in addition, further training after qualification is available in family planning clinics, in hospitals, and at postgraduate courses.

Reliable contraception makes a valuable contribution to the health and wellbeing not only of women but of the family unit as a whole.

It must be added that apart from the sheath, which does afford some protection, contraceptive methods, however efficient at preventing pregnancy, offer *no* protection against the sexually transmitted diseases. It is also to be remembered that these diseases, notably gonorrhoea, have greatly increased in recent years.

Marital and sexual problems

Many novels, plays, and films lead young people to think that when a couple get into bed together they will immediately enjoy married (or unmarried) bliss. Unfortunately this is often far from the truth. The wedding day is long, exciting, tiring, and sometimes alcoholic. The couple are often inexperienced. There may well be mental and physical difficulties on the wedding night which cause one or both partners to feel inadequate and guilty, let down and disappointed. They may even be shocked and thoroughly upset by the whole business.

It takes two to make a happy marriage, and on the psychological, social, and sexual sides there is much to be learnt. The difficulties that couples may encounter are unhappily legion, and writing about them is complicated by the fact that no two people ever have quite the same problem.

It is best for those with marital or sexual problems first of all to consult their doctor, a trusted relative or friend, or a marriage guidance counsellor.

Further reading

The National Marriage Guidance Council publishes a comprehensive list of recommended books, including those on sexual techniques, childbirth, and information for young people. The list includes most of the books mentioned here, as well as many others, and gives information on prices and brief notes on each book.

The book list is available at NMGC centres all over Britain (except Northern Ireland), and books may be obtained through the Council. Book lists may also be obtained from the NMGC Book Department, Little Church Street, Rugby.

David Mace *Getting ready for marriage*. Oliphant
Eric Berne *Games people play*. Penguin
Jane Cousins *Make it happy*. Virago
Paul Brown and Carolyn Faulder *Treat yourself to sex*. Dent and the National Marriage Guidance Council
G. Dick-Read. *Childbirth without fear*. Pan
Eustace Chesser *Love without fear*. Arrow
David Mace *Sexual difficulties in marriage*. The National Marriage Guidance Council
Jack Dominian. *Marital breakdown*. Pelican
Helen Kaplan *The new sex therapy*. Ballière Tindall

Chapter 12
Infant and child care

Revised by Leonard Arthur, MB MRCP

It is good for new parents to know that a healthy baby is not so delicate or fragile as he may seem. Healthy babies are remarkably tough, but helpless in the sense that they cannot say what they want or where it hurts, and their needs must be satisfied by others who keep close watch, give loving care, and protect them against hazards.

Newborn babies have a temporary immunity to a number of diseases, passively established by antibodies passed on to them by the mother before and immediately after birth. At the same time, infants are more susceptible than older children to skin and digestive disorders and some kinds of infection. Children are the special targets of so-called childhood diseases, but are also subject to other afflictions, including rare ones, that also affect adults.

The sections dealing with child behaviour are principally intended for those parents lacking confidence on how to act, where there is no reliable grandmother or friend close by. If you look something up and decide that you have gone wrong, do not worry. It is not your fault. Do not blame yourself. A loving parent's instinct is seldom wrong, even if it goes against the advice given here. Trust your feelings. Trust your baby's feelings too – "baby knows best", especially about likes and dislikes.

Growth patterns

Never again in his life will a baby grow as rapidly as during his first year. Physical growth is easily measured in terms of weight and height. This gives a useful, though by no means exclusive, yardstick of development. Disturbances or interruption of growth may accompany or give a clue to conditions that need correction. However, individual growth is an individual matter, sudden weight gain may be as ominous as weight loss, and what a worried parent takes to be the skinniness of a child who was previously chubby may be a normal phase of development.

Weight In general, a baby weighs three times as much at the end of the first year as he did at birth. His birth weight is doubled at approximately five months of age. Continuous weight gain during the first year is one index of good nutrition and, particularly during the first few months, weight that remains stationary for a couple of months may be caused by illness or improper feeding.

Weight continues to increase during the second year, but at a slower rate. At about two or three years of age, a child may look comparatively thin and undernourished to a worried parent, although his growth rate is normal. A great growth spurt comes with puberty, which begins at different ages in different children. Rapidly growing adolescents customarily consume, and need, more food than adults.

Height In many homes, when a child is old enough to stand against something flat, there is a periodic ceremony of marking his height on a wall or door frame. If such records are kept year by year, it will generally be found that, although height continues to increase, the rate of increase after the age of three or four is slightly less each year until puberty brings a spurt in height as well as weight.

How tall will a child ultimately be? This is not only an interesting speculation, but sometimes a matter of concern to parents, one or both of whom may be unusually tall or unusually short. There are some rough formulas for predicting future height, such as the following: measure the child's height at two years

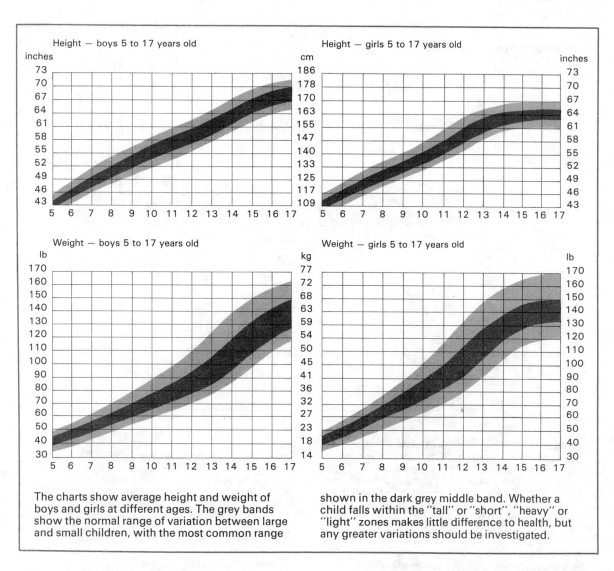

Height — boys 5 to 17 years old

Height — girls 5 to 17 years old

Weight — boys 5 to 17 years old

Weight — girls 5 to 17 years old

The charts show average height and weight of boys and girls at different ages. The grey bands show the normal range of variation between large and small children, with the most common range shown in the dark grey middle band. Whether a child falls within the "tall" or "short", "heavy" or "light" zones makes little difference to health, but any greater variations should be investigated.

of age and multiply by two. Add slightly to this result if the child is a boy, subtract a little if the child is a girl. However, the answer cannot be taken too literally.

Sometimes parents worry because a child shoots up so fast at a stage of growth that he appears to be developing gigantism, or, on the other hand, because he hardly seems to grow at all while playmates of the same age are growing out of their clothes. It must be remembered that puberty, with its great stimulus to growth, comes relatively early in some children and late in others. As a general rule, one may expect that effects of early or late maturation will level off, that the fast grower will slow down and the slow grower catch up, with ultimate height within a normal range.

Body proportions change remarkably from birth to maturity. At birth a baby's head is a quarter of the size of the body, the forehead is wider than the chin, and the lower jaw small and receding. Growth lengthens the limbs and trunk so that at about two years of age the body is longer and thinner and the head is about one fifth the size of the body. At six years, the body has stretched out further so that the head occupies about one sixth of its length. The tendency to linear growth continues until puberty when the body tends to broaden relative to height. At about the age of fifteen the head is one seventh the size of the body, and this proportion is maintained through life.

There are some sex differences in growth patterns. Boys are heavier and longer than girls at birth and up to about six years of age, when girls weigh more than boys. Because boys usually mature a year or two later than girls, on average, they are shorter and weigh less than girls until the early teens when they catch up and surpass girls (with respect to height and weight).

Chapter 12 Infant and child care

Development in early years

average height inches

| 4 weeks | 4 months | 6 months | 9 months |

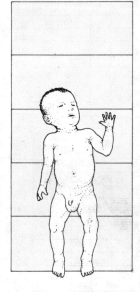 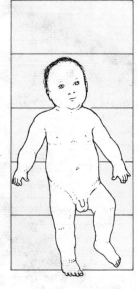 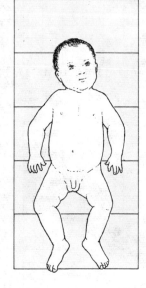 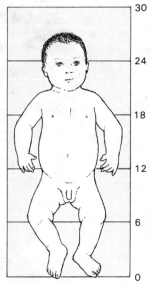

30

24

18

12

6

0

Activity
Stares at rooms, lights, faces close by.
Looks at people and is just beginning to follow.
Head sags forward on sitting.
Hands grip on contact with objects.
Will drop rattle immediately if placed in hand.
Usually enjoys bath but cries when being dressed or undressed.

Vocal
Little throaty noises.

Social
If infant cries, will usually stop crying if picked up.
Reduces activity and usually calms down when talked to — especially by deep voice of man.

Activity
Lifts head up well when lying prone.
Watches his hands and fingers. Plays with them.
Grasps rattle or squeaky toy in hand and usually takes to mouth and bites.
Interested in food.
Follows lights.

Vocal
Laughs and coos.
Gurgles, growls, squeals, often even coughs to make sound.

Social
Recognizes parents and others close to him.
Smiles spontaneously, especially at those he knows.
Enjoys people.
Interested in other children. Likes rhythm.
Enjoys being bounced on knee.

Activity
Sits up without support leaning forwards.
Bounces on feet when held by hands.
Rolls over by self.
Reaches for and grasps toy or rattle.
Shakes rattle and bangs it.
Transfers objects from one hand to the other.

Vocal
Vocalizing a good deal.

Social
Enjoys people more.
Talks to toys.

Activity
Sits up well.
Crawls.
Pulls self up on side of playpen.
Holds bottle.
Feeds self biscuit.
Often will walk with both hands held.

Vocal
Often says what sounds like "mama" and "dada".
Enjoys sounds of his voice — often laughs at them.

Social
Waves "bye-bye".
Plays patacake and peep-bo.
Likes to be with family in group.
Enjoys pram ride.
May be shy with strangers.

average
height
cm

| 12 months | 15 months | 18 months | 2 years |

91

76

61

46

30

15

0

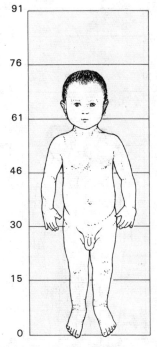
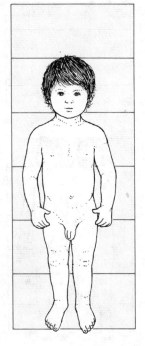
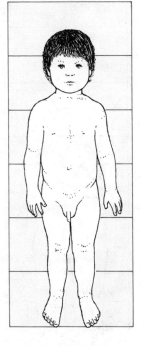
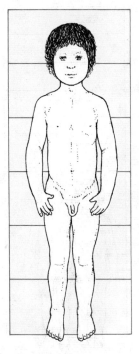

Activity
Walks held by one
hand.
Stands alone for a
moment.
Plays well with objects.
Short attention span.
Throws things out of
playpen.
Enjoys putting things in
and out of boxes.
Likes to put things on
head.

Vocal
Usually has vocabulary
of about 4 words
including "mama" and
"dada".

Social
Helps in dressing self.
Usually coming out of
shyness with strangers.
Responds to "no! no!"
but may continue, smiling.
Still enjoys pram.
Interested in dogs, cars,
other children.

Activity
Walks independently
though unsteadily.
Crawls upstairs.
Throws objects.
Looks at pictures in
book.

Vocal
Imitates sounds.
Tries to say many
things.
Much gibberish.

Social
Vocalizes wants and
needs.
Often will indicate
when wanting to
urinate or have a bowel
movement.

Activity
Walks well. Rarely falls.
Will climb into large
chair or seat
self in small chair.
Throws or rolls ball.
Builds 3 or 4 blocks.
Pulls toys. Carries dolls
and animals. Can carry
out directions.

Vocal
Has a few words as a
rule.
Often names pictures in
books.

Social
Usually sociable and
affable.

Activity
Runs well.
Walks well up and
down stairs.
Builds 6 to 8 blocks.
Carries out directions.

Vocal
Sentences of 2 to 3
words.
Starting to use
pronouns.

Social
Plays by other children
rather than with them.
Indicates toilet needs.

Development of children

3 years	4 years	5 years	6 years	
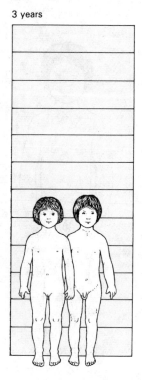	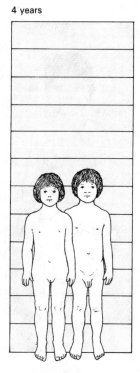	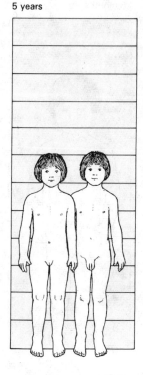	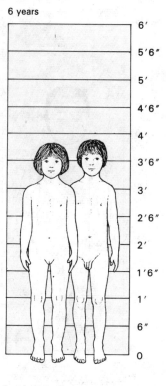	6' 5'6" 5' 4'6" 4' 3'6" 3' 2'6" 2' 1'6" 1' 6" 0

Activity
Balances on 1 leg.
Walks upstairs alternate feet.

Vocal/intellectual
Dozens of single words.
Sentences up to 6 syllables.
Gives full name on request.
Beginning to understand abstract words. For example, bigger, smaller.
Copies line, circle, cross.
Matches shapes and sizes.

Social
Negativism at its height.
Child's increasing awareness of himself as separate person.
May play with one other child.
Unselfconscious in activities.

Activity
Hops, pedals tricycle.
Fastens buttons.
Undresses.
Puts on socks and shoes.

Vocal/intellectual
Answers simple hypothetical questions.
For example, what would you do if you were thirsty.
Names objects in a complex picture.
Can draw recognizable man, a face and body with limbs but without hands or feet.
Counts to 4.

Social
Plays with 2 or more other children.
Insatiable curiosity.
"Why" rather than "what".
Beginning to be self-conscious in public.
Beginnings of self-control.

Activity
Kicks a ball.
Jumps over a rope.
Dresses.
Fastens buckle but not laces.

Vocal/intellectual
Describes pictures, not just labelling.
Can copy a square.
Can copy house with windows.
Counts up to 15.
Reproduces simple colour pattern with bricks.

Social
Much less evidence of defiance.
Accepts sharing.
Friendly.
Often vivid fantasies in play 5 to 8.

Activity
Throws and catches ball.
Increasing dexterity.

Vocal/intellectual
Sentences of 10 or more syllables.
Uses adjectives.
Copies triangle.
Can write first name.
Can match many shapes.
Uses abstract words.

Social
Boastfulness, pride in achievement.
Rules in play accepted and often insisted on.

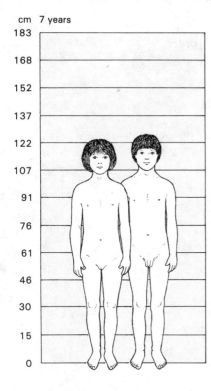

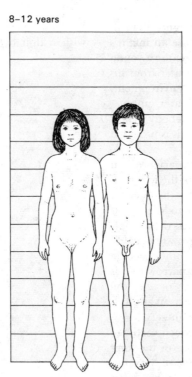

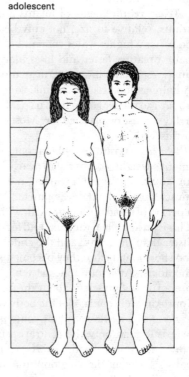

cm	7 years	8–12 years	adolescent
183			
168			
152			
137			
122			
107			
91			
76			
61			
46			
30			
15			
0			

7 years

Activity
Can skip with rope. Ties laces.
Independent dressing and feeding.

Vocal/intellectual
Describes and interprets pictures.
Describes differences between 2 familiar objects.
Can draw diamond.

Social
Children play well at simple card games (Snap,
Beggar my Neighbour) and board games (Snakes
and Ladders).

8–12 years

Activity
Consolidation and refinement of motor skills and
coordination.

Vocal/intellectual
Learns to classify and arrange in series.
Accepts more formal teaching.
Hypothetical reasoning from 12 increasing rapidly
in adolescence.

Social
Age of socialization.
Loyalty to school friends and the gang.
Conformity in dress and behaviour patterns.

Adolescent

Activity
Muscle power advances rapidly in boys and girls,
stopping at end of growth spurt in girls.
Development of adult skills at games and music.
Breasts and pubic hair develop and growth spurt
begins at mean age of $11\frac{1}{2}$ in girls, pubic hair,
growth of penis and testes, and somatic growth
spurt begin at 12 to 13 in boys.
Menses at mean age of $13\frac{1}{2}$.
Normal variation 9 to 17.

Vocal/intellectual
Voice deepens in girls (13) and boys (14).
Speaking voice falls about 1 octave in boys, less in
girls.
After this age individuals diverge into full range of
human behaviour and intellectual development.

Social
Affection begins to include people outside the
home. Self-consciousness and shyness gradually
overcome. Ideas of love at first derived from
observation of parents, "the media", fantasy.
Later discover that mature love includes
tenderness, unselfishness, generosity, and
responsibility as well as desire and passion.
Altruistic and idealistic attitudes often held.
Assertion of independence often by rebellion
against authority (parents, school), but identifies
with peer group.

Chapter 12 Infant and child care

Infant and adult differences There are considerable differences in the proportions of water, bone, and muscle in infants and adults.

Water requirements of infants are higher than in adults, relative to size, not only because an infant's body has a higher water content but because a young baby breathes faster and loses more water from his lungs, especially in an overheated dry environment. A baby cannot ask for a drink, so his water supply – about 150 ml per kg ($2\frac{1}{2}$ fluid oz per lb) of body weight a day – must be planned for. Most of this is provided by his feeds.

Muscles constitute only about a quarter of an infant's weight, compared to nearly half the weight of an adult. At about eighteen months the skeletal muscles begin rapid development. The toddler age is a period of rapid muscle growth, with loss of baby fat. This is an age when the arms and legs grow noticeably faster than the trunk, and the child's clothes become too short long before they become too narrow for his shoulders. At about nine or ten years of age, the proportion of muscle is about the same as in adults – approximately one half of the body weight.

Bones of a newborn infant contain much cartilage or gristle, and only the central sections of the long bones are mineralized. An X-ray film of a young baby's skeleton, showing only the mineralized part, looks like a collection of separate bones. One of the objective criteria of growth and development is bone age which measures the progressive mineralization of the child's skeleton.

Development in early years It is always unwise to set hard-and-fast standards of infant and child development. Growth and development are finally determined by heredity and the environment in which the child lives. Physical growth, age at sitting up, standing, walking, talking, and adolescent development, are partly inherited family traits, even though children in the same family may show differences. Development of qualities such as speech, sociability, and alertness to surroundings, is often largely dependent on the type of attention a child gets from his parents or parent substitutes.

An average normal child has ten to fifteen words in his vocabulary at eighteen months of age, but many children who are entirely normal may not start talking until after two years of age. The average child is walking at thirteen to fourteen months of age, but many normal children may not walk unsupported until fifteen or sixteen months.

The chart of development in early years on page 256 is based on studies of average children and is not to be regarded as fixed or absolute. Only large deviations from the average need investigation.

Various aspects of child care are hereafter dealt with in alphabetical order.

Accident prevention

Accidents are the leading cause of death among children from one to fourteen years of age. Sadly, it is still true that over 90 per cent of these accidents are preventable. A doctor can prevent a child from contracting diphtheria, tetanus, whooping cough, typhoid, poliomyelitis, and measles, but the prevention of accidents is almost entirely the responsibility of parents. Nothing like a complete list of hazards can be given, but if parents will remember the following, modified from recommendations of the American Academy of Pediatrics, they may save their children's lives or prevent serious accidents which could severely injure or disfigure for life.

BE SURE THAT:

1 The handles of boiling saucepans are out of reach.
2 The child does not play with electric appliances or electric plugs.
3 No poisonous medicines, including aspirin and sedatives, are available, even if on a high shelf. They should be locked away in a cupboard.
4 There are no dangerous substances on the kitchen or bathroom floor or shelves, or in unlocked cupboards; especially ammonia, paraffin (kerosene), furniture polish, paint thinner (turpentine substitute), or weed killer.
5 There are no rat poisons or insecticides around.
6 Safety gates are placed and kept closed at the top of the stairs and at the back door and driveway.
7 Bars or locked screens are placed inside or outside upstairs windows.
8 The child is not left in the bath alone; he may turn on the hot water and be scalded, or may slip under the water. Always run cold water into the bath before the hot.
9 Nonskid or rubber guards are placed under loose mats or carpets.
10 Toys, shoes, and other objects which may cause accidents at night are tidied away.
11 Small children are never given lollipops, unless they are sitting down. No boiled sweets or nuts. The child with a lollipop may fall while walking and tear the roof of his mouth. Boiled sweets or nuts should not be offered for they may be inhaled and completely close off the windpipe. If this should happen, hold the child upside down and attempt to dislodge the obstruction by several sharp blows over the upper back or chest.
12 Any firearms are locked up and the key kept out of reach.

13 Razors, manicure set, and sewing basket (with lethal scissors and needles) are put away securely.
14 You are careful of matches and cigarette lighters, a great potential danger.
15 Doors open to potential danger are locked.
16 Pools, ponds, and cisterns are fenced in or covered.
17 Toys have no sharp edges, exposed nails, small parts, or eyes that can be pulled off.

To which we would add:

18 Do not use strings, necklaces, or string fastenings to garments which go round the child's neck.
19 Always use a fireguard for electric, gas, or coal fires.
20 Make sure that nightdresses and frilly party frocks are made of nonflammable or treated material.
21 Safety belts or special car seats for children are a must. Small children should never travel in the front seat of a car. If the mother or father wishes to hold the child on a car journey, they should sit in the back. Parents should also avoid inflicting orphanhood on the child by not being too proud to do up their seat belts, even on short journeys.
22 See that the child does not play with large plastic bags. Children have been known to place them over their heads and suffocate.

Adoption and fostering

One in ten married couples have difficulty in conceiving a child and about one in twenty never have children; many such couples would like to adopt a child.* Society feels a responsibility for its children, so wants to make sure that adopted children get a fair deal. At first voluntary agencies, often church sponsored, took on the task; nowadays local authority Social Services Departments are also involved. In many areas voluntary societies and the Statutory Authority both offer a service. The local Social Services Department has information on what agencies are available locally; or it is possible to write

* A.I.D. (Artificial insemination by donor) is on the increase for infertile couples where the husband for instance has low sperm counts, especially when they learn how long they may have to wait before a baby is placed with them.

Chapter 12 Infant and child care

to the Association of British Adoption and Fostering Agencies, 4 Southampton Row, London WC1B 4AA. Most church agencies (although not the Roman Catholics) no longer make any stipulation about religious upbringing of the child.

Legal aspects The law as it applies to children is still extremely complex, in spite of a major new Children's Act in 1975. Many provisions of previous Children's Acts are still in force, and many of the provisions of the 1975 Act have still (1979) not been implemented. The following notes are written as guidelines only, and for legal advice a solicitor, Citizens Advice Bureau, or the fostering and adoption unit of the local Social Services Department should be consulted.

Private or third party adoptions will be illegal when the relevant section of the 1975 Act is implemented. All adoptions will then have to be arranged through an officially recognized Adoption Agency. Parents who want to adopt have to have a medical examination and are then interviewed by a social worker, usually on five or six occasions. If accepted, they wait for a baby. When the child is first placed with them, usually at around six weeks old, he is technically in the care of the local authority (no Child Benefit, formerly called Family Allowance, is payable to them); after a period of three to six months there is a further visit from an independent social worker appointed by the court, the guardian *ad litem* (for the suit, that particular matter). Finally the couple go before a Judge in Chambers (privately, not in open court), together with the guardian *ad litem*, and an Adoption Order is made. From this moment the child is theirs before the law, with all the rights of a natural child of the adopter, including rights of inheritance. All his former ties are excluded (with minor exceptions).

When the natural parent changes her mind Until the new Children's Act it was possible for a natural parent to object to the adoption right up to the last moment (the Adoption Order). This could place a strain on prospective adopters. The new arrangement will be the Freeing for Adoption procedure under which the natural mother gives the adoption agency powers to apply to a court for parental rights before the child is placed for adoption. If the natural parents have refused to make up their minds, or have abandoned the child, the agency may apply to the court for parental rights, and for parental agreement to adoption to be dispensed with. The father of an illegitimate child has no parental rights. Natural parents may no longer make any conditions about religion, though they may express their wishes.

Fostering A foster home is better for a child than an institution and local authorities are already closing Children's Homes. Foster parents do wonderful work for children in need and anyone willing to undertake this is urged to contact the local Social Services Department or voluntary society (again, if preferred, write to the Association mentioned above).

The strain of caring for a foster child is always heavy, and long-term fostering breaks down in 50 per cent of children under one, rising to 85 per cent for children over five. Local authorities are starting to offer more support, both financial and emotional, for foster parents, who are paid a fostering allowance depending on the age of the child. Average rates are (in 1979) – for a child up to 5 years, £10.50 to £20, increasing with age up to £15 to £30 for a 17 year old. There are, however, no nationally agreed rates and each local authority lays down its own scale of payments. Foster parents do not get Child Benefit but with handicapped children Attendance or Mobility Allowance can be claimed. Foster parents are liable for the good behaviour of a foster child; and are likewise responsible for his physical and mental wellbeing. Anyone who is not a relative who fosters a child privately for more than six days must inform the local authority, which has the power to prohibit the arrangement.

New rights for foster parents One of the aims of the 1975 Children's Act was to prevent situations where a natural parent capriciously decides to take back a child. After a child has been in care for six months, a natural parent must give 28 days notice before removing the child. After three years the local authority may apply for parental rights over the child, and after five years foster parents will be able to apply for adoption without fear of the natural parents capriciously removing the child, though the natural parents may oppose the adoption at the court hearing.

Custodianship and guardianship The 1975 Children's Act established the new legal status of custodianship. This is half way between fostering and adoption. Foster parents may apply for legal custody of a child after one year (if the natural parent consents) or after three years even without consent and will then be able to make decisions about the child's future without consulting the natural parents (relations may apply for custodianship after three months with the natural parent's consent, or a year without). Unfortunately, because of the extra resources needed to cope with this reform, (social worker time, court time) no date has yet been given for implementation and it may be a long time before it comes in.

Guardianship applies mainly to property. A parent may appoint someone to act as guardian to a child after his death; or the courts may do so. The guardian must apply the child's property to his (the ward's) benefit.

Access to natural parents One reform of the 1975 Act which has been implemented is the right of adopted children born in England and Wales who have reached the age of eighteen to be given the names of their natural parents as recorded in their original birth certificate. (This has always been a right in Scotland.) Write to the General Register Office – address given at the end of this chapter.

What sort of children are adopted In the last fifteen years there have been changes in the number of babies adopted: 17,000 in 1961, 25,000 in 1968, down to 17,000 again in 1976 (figures for England and Wales). The 30 per cent fall over eight years is due apparently to more unmarried mothers wishing to keep their illegitimate babies. It is much harder to find a healthy baby to adopt now. Great care used to be taken to offer a healthy baby to adoptive parents; there were often (and still are, but less frequently) damaging delays in placing babies because of vague fears that they might have some congenital defect. About one child in 50 is born with a congenital abnormality. It therefore seems unrealistic to attempt to guarantee an adoptive child. Counselling of prospective adoptive parents should include the fact that the child may turn out to have (or develop) a handicap which they (like natural parents) should be prepared to accept. The baby may be born with a handicap or stigma, social (such as mixed race), genetic (such as mentally handicapped or epileptic parents) or medical (such as spina bifida, cerebral palsy). These babies are even more vulnerable if reared in institutions and recent efforts to achieve adoptive or foster homes for them have been surprisingly successful, both in finding couples prepared to accept them, and in the outcome for the children. Another group which is desperately in need of a stable family life is that of older children, including adolescents, whose homes have broken down, or who have never had a home. Even when these children have a history of maladjustment, behaviour problems, and delinquency, successful placements are being made, to the enormous benefit not only of the child, but of society. The agency responsible for helping these "hard to place" children is Adoption Resource Exchange, 40 Brunswick Square, London WC1N 1AZ.

Payment for adopters and foster parents At present no allowance is paid to adoptive parents, though they are entitled to the statutory allowances (Child Benefit, and for handicapped children Attendance and Mobility Allowance). Many workers would like to see the payment of a wage for fostering; though the allowance is untaxed and worth more in real terms than a taxable income. The danger of "baby farming" abuses is negligible if foster parents are vetted. Some local authorities have pioneered extra payments for foster parents of hard to place children and it is hoped that this will become the rule.

Animal bites

Children are not infrequently bitten by their own pets or dogs which have been annoyed, hurt, or frightened. At present there is no risk of rabies in the United Kingdom. Any wounds on the child's body should be thoroughly washed with soap and water and a dry adhesive dressing applied. Most doctors also advise a tetanus booster injection after an animal bite. As rabies is spreading across Europe, never let your child play with or fondle a dog or cat in other countries. If your child should be bitten, give the owner of the animal your name and address and leave your name and address at the local police station. When you return home, report to your doctor.

It may be a comfort to know that if the dog is still alive ten days after biting it did not have rabies at the time.

Gerbil, hamster, and guinea pig bites Children are occasionally bitten while feeding pets. These bites need only be treated by washing thoroughly with soap and water and covering with an adhesive dressing.

Snake bite See chapter 29 on First Aid.

Insect bites and bee stings As a rule, insect bites and bee stings give only temporary pain and discomfort. Usually prompt relief can be given by applying a paste made from a few drops of water in a tablespoon of bicarbonate of soda, or by applying a witch-hazel dressing or a wet dressing of epsom salts. For severe reactions from bee stings the child should receive antihistamines by mouth. If this is not followed rapidly by relief from the reaction, the child should receive injections of adrenalin or ACTH from the doctor or let isoprenaline tablets dissolve under the tongue.

In addition:

Avoid feather pillows, duvets, and eiderdowns.
Use man-made fibre or cotton blankets and quilts.
Enclose the pillow and mattress in plastic covers.

Asthma

The majority of wheezing babies and children are not so severely affected as adults, though they are correctly labelled as having asthma. Young people have smaller airways than adults, so they wheeze more easily and it does not mean so much. Wheezing is usually caused by allergic airways obstruction; infection, excitement, anxiety, and exertion may increase it; and most children improve spontaneously over the years. It is often familial, and may be linked with other allergic conditions such as eczema, seasonal hay fever, or perennial rhinitis (inflammation of the mucous membrane in the nose). Allergy is an overreaction of part of the body's immune defence system. Many babies have a little eczema and a little wheezing from time to time in the first year of life. Breast-feeding at least ensures that cows' milk allergy does not occur too early in life, but no doubt the body encounters many other allergens. Skin testing, or better, bronchial provocation tests and courses of specific hyposensitizing injections are not as widely used in this country as in North America (fashions in medicine, as in other things, vary from country to country) but are sometimes invaluable. More widely used are bronchodilator drugs and local corticosteroid sprays. A new drug, sodium cromoglycate (Intal), acts by preventing release of the harmful substances produced in the bronchi by the allergic reaction.

Management of the acute attack First of all, do not panic. Calmness and reassurance by the parents reduce the anxiety component of a wheezing attack. Give the prescribed drugs immediately and in most cases the attack will subside. If the child becomes really distressed, particularly if the pulse rises and the child becomes blue (cyanosed), he will need oxygen in hospital.

Prevention, and the house dust mite Allergies to foods and domestic pets may be important (it is wise to forgo the pleasures of a family dog or cat, guinea pig or hamster) but the commonest allergen seems to be an invisible and harmless little mite which can be found in large numbers in house dust, even in the cleanest homes. Use this daily routine:

Vacuum soft furnishings.
Damp dust bedroom furniture and floor.

Autism (childhood autism)

Even in infancy, some babies do not smile back at their mothers, do not babble at four months in response to conversation, and do not learn to talk. Such a child avoids eye-to-eye contact, repels caresses, and his mood may vary from destructive energy with screaming, to vacant immobility. He (boys outnumber girls by two or three to one) may develop obsessive rituals and repetitive mannerisms, twiddling a piece of fluff or spinning a brightly coloured toy, drumming or tapping. Affection is more easily shown to objects or animals than to people. Normal habits such as nail-biting, thumb-sucking, rocking, or head-banging may worsen into self-mutilation such as punching his own face, or biting his wrists or arms.

Linguistic, social, and emotional development may be variously deficient, while motor and intellectual functions are near normal; or there may be overall delay, from birth (with hindsight – most children are nearing two before diagnosis). Sometimes, however, a child who has been normal begins at the age of two or three to withdraw emotionally, and may end up with the full syndrome.

Inability not only to create speech and gesture, but to understand those of others, is an invariable feature; such children are often misdiagnosed as deaf and fitted with hearing aids. There is a symptom overlap with the excessively shy child who prefers not to talk (elective mutism) and with a little-understood syndrome of noncommunication in West Indian children, but they lack other features of autism.

Causes Autism implies preoccupation with self. It is generally agreed that it is a psychosis of childhood which begins before the age of four and is not schizophrenia. It is not "caused" by the parents. Although childhood autism is compatible with normal or even superior intelligence, the majority of these children are of low or very low intellectual ability. The cause is unknown, but a high proportion show other neurological abnormalities and about one third later develop epilepsy. About one in every 45,000 children born becomes autistic. Affected children often look physically normal. Some features of autism are seen in normal children and many in the mentally handicapped. Both in mental handicap of prenatal origin and that which is acquired (for instance after meningitis or head injury), the same lack of brain cells and pathways that hinders normal motor and intellectual function also plays havoc with emotional responses. Although there are strong reasons against the behaviourist belief that childhood autism, like adult schizophrenia, is purely a learnt response, there is no doubt that a lot of autistic behaviour arises as a secondary handicap in mentally handicapped children, and can be prevented by enlightened handling by parents and attendants which includes plenty of stimulation, teaches children to develop social skills, and rewards even tiny achievements.

Treatment Even though it is accepted that the family is not the cause, parents need a tremendous amount of sympathy and support. The child needs psychotherapy and occupational therapy, but most of all he requires specially designed, and early, education. Most autistic children will make slow but steady progress which falls short of achieving complete normality. Parents will find the National Society for Autistic Children helpful (see page 298).

Baby battering

All mothers and fathers wish to be good parents, so it is as well to remember that there is no guarantee that any one may not find him or herself in the position of having wilfully injured or hurt a child. There may be some relatively simple steps to prevent that last loss of control. Parents who can avoid isolation, and enlist the emotional support of their spouses or neighbours, are protected. Parents who find their crying child becoming difficult to bear need not be ashamed to seek help. In emergency, telephone someone. If there is no one you know of who you can ask for help or if you think your friends would be too shocked, try the NSPCC, the Samaritans, the Social Services Department or even (in case you can't find the number) dial 999 and ask for the police. In most cases, you will find a lot of help from these agencies, who are only too well aware of the consequences of people not seeking help until it is too late. Do not feel that you are unnatural or beyond help because you feel aggressive towards your child. A good and loving relationship can often emerge even after violence has occurred.

If you see or suspect a case among your friends, relatives, or neighbours, we suggest the following:

Show your sympathy for the *parent* (not the child) by some such approach as: "Babies do make us want to slap them sometimes" or "Crying gets on your nerves". This may lead to a person accepting the need for help.

Don't keep it to yourself. Get the parents' consent to go for help if you can; if not, contact one of the agencies yourself.

Bed-wetting (nocturnal enuresis)

Bladder control in normal children develops at different ages and depends upon the individual readiness of the child. Statistical studies on normal children have shown that 50 per cent of two year olds are dry at night; 75 per cent of three year olds, and 85 to 90 per cent of five year olds. In other words, bed-wetting is not considered abnormal unless a child has passed the age of five, or when the child has been dry at night for a period and then reverts to wetting the bed.

When the child has never been dry, the condition is referred to as primary enuresis. When bed-wetting starts after a dry period, it is called onset enuresis. The child who achieves dry days, but continues to wet at night, seldom has any physical disease.

Enuresis may be caused by a urinary tract infection, or occasionally by diabetes mellitus. Rarely, the child who dribbles day and night may have an anatomically abnormal ureter (the tube carrying urine from the kidney to the bladder). A dye injection followed by X-ray pictures of the kidneys and bladder (intravenous pyelogram) will show this. A child who can achieve a dry night even occasionally is unlikely to have this abnormality. The urine should always be examined and cultured in the laboratory, but in the vast majority of cases of enuresis investigations are negative.

Although the cause of bed-wetting is not known, the following factors may influence it:

The child may be perfectly normal, but have late development of bladder control. This lateness of control is frequently familial, and is often in the history of one of the parents.

Although bed-wetting occurs in many well-adjusted children in secure homes, anxiety does

Chapter 12 Infant and child care

appear to play a part. Children who are unhappy at home and those that have anxieties are often bed-wetters. It may be seen following hospitalization, or when one or other parent has to be away from home; it was frequently observed during the last war when a child was evacuated, or when fathers left home for military service. It is often found among older children when new infants are born.

Many bed-wetters sleep very soundly. It is not known whether this is a cause of the bed-wetting, or simply an association.

Treatment As each year passes after the age of five, more and more wetters become dry; there is a strong tendency for spontaneous cure. The doctor should make sure that there is no organic disease, that facilities for emptying the bladder at night are available (a potty under the bed may make it easier for a child than a walk down a cold dark passage to the toilet), and that the child is not being punished for something that he cannot help. Beyond this, it is possible that treatment succeeds only in those who would have become dry anyway. Help for child and parents might follow these lines.

Organic causes of bed-wetting such as diabetes, kidney disease, or some abnormality of the urinary tract, can be easily determined by a doctor and necessary treatment advised.

But in the absence of organic causes the following measures may be taken to correct the condition:

The home and school environment should be investigated to determine if anything exists which produces great anxiety in the child. This should be dealt with if possible and the child should be reassured.

Lifting a child at ten to eleven p.m. may be of considerable help if it does not upset the child too much. It may accustom the child to sleep dry for long periods of time and cause him to awaken when the bladder is full.

Small bladder There have been conflicting reports on whether some bed-wetters have abnormally small bladders. The bladder is an exceedingly elastic structure, and it seems unlikely that real anatomical smallness plays a part. Irritability of the bladder nerves may cause the bladder to empty by reflex at a smaller filling pressure. Daytime clock training, where the child is taught to void at longer and longer intervals, had a vogue but its effect is doubtful.

Restriction of fluids Experience suggests that this is of little help. Excessive drinking is a habit some children fall into and, particularly if the fluid contains a natural diuretic (tea, cocoa, or coffee), may be a cause of bed-wetting. Wet beds are not unknown, for instance, among immoderately beer-drinking adults.

The star chart Behaviour modification by conditioning, in which desirable behaviour is rewarded, and undesirable behaviour is ignored (not punished, which increases anxiety) is nowadays popular. A simple method is to give the child a diary card (star chart) on which he sticks a blue star for a dry night, and an additional gold star for a run of four dry nights. For the more materialistic, a small regular money reward may be an incentive (1p or 2p is sufficient). It is wrong to speak of this as a bribe. Bribes are used to persuade people to do wrong. Rewards are given for right actions.

The pad and bell apparatus A most successful method of treating the bed-wetter who has reached the age of six is by means of an apparatus that rings an electric bell the moment a child starts wetting at night. It consists of a special pad placed under the child's sheet. This pad is connected by wires to an apparatus containing a bell or a buzzer. In some of these instruments a light turns on every time the bell or buzzer responds. As soon as the slightest amount of fluid reaches the pad the circuit is closed, the bell rings, and the child wakens at once and goes to the toilet. Some doctors have found the method effective in 95 per cent of children over six who are still habitual bed-wetters. Other reports have recorded less success. In most cases the child sleeps through the night without wetting after the apparatus has been used for only three to four weeks. A number of models are available. Parents may be able to borrow one free of charge from the local hospital or Health Clinic. Alternatively, they are advertised in newspapers and in mail order catalogues. Read the instructions carefully, as electrical burns have occasionally been caused.

The apparatus works by conditioning the child. At first, the urination causes a bell to ring and the child wakens and immediately withholds. Later he learns to awaken when the bladder is full before the bell rings. Still later, he learns to sleep through the night without bed-wetting and without awakening. This method has also been found effective even in cases of enuresis due to emotional causes. Studies of many such children have shown that no emotional harm results from this method of treatment. As a matter of fact, most of the children are so delighted with their accomplishment that they are generally happier, reassured, and much less anxious.

Drug treatment Some doctors still prescribe central nervous system stimulants, such as amphetamine, with benefit; however, amphetamine is a drug of abuse, and it may be better to discourage its use even for legitimate reasons. The antidepressant drugs imipramine (Tofranil) and amitriptyline (Tryptizol) do appear to have a specific effect on enuresis, not directly related to their action on the mind. The doctor may prescribe a trial of one of these drugs, to be abandoned if it is not immediately successful. Treatment may be required for several weeks. Drug treatment should never be continued for more than a limited period, even if leaving it off results in relapse of bed-wetting. It is undesirable for children to take drugs for long periods for an essentially harmless condition. After a six or twelve month interval they may be tried again. A word of warning: both these drugs are highly dangerous in overdosage, causing heart arrhythmias and death, so be sure that younger children cannot get at them.

Finally, there is no doubt that having a bed-wetter in the family is a major nuisance. Even the most loving mother can become extremely resentful towards a bed-wetter. Lowering the emotional temperature by encouraging her to express this resentment often helps both mother and child, and this is something which can be done by a grandmother, a family friend, or a Health Visitor as well as by the family doctor. As far as we know, group therapy has not been employed for this condition, but the success of Enuresis Clinics may depend to some extent on the informal group therapy of the parents in the waiting room.

Bereavement

No easy words can take away the grief that a parent feels at the death of a child. Losing a stillborn child is not so rare as losing a healthy infant or schoolchild, but it is still a real loss and a mother still needs to express and share her grief. A stillbirth is not something trivial and to be ignored. With the death of a son or daughter the parents are faced with a whole range of emotions for which they are unprepared. Making the grief harder to bear are the inevitable feelings of guilt which accompany the loss. These may be centred on the parents themselves – could they have foreseen it – acted differently – sought help sooner. Sometimes the guilt is projected on to someone else – the spouse, the doctor, or the hospital. It is easy to look for someone to blame. Feelings of guilt, either personal or projected, should be thought

about and talked about, but as soon as possible let go of. They cannot bring the child back to life, and they delay the transition from looking back, which is what grief is about, to looking forward, which is the beginning of recovery from it.

The mother's and father's grief needs to be accepted by family and friends. The brothers and sisters may hide their grief and need special help. Reminders of the dead child should not be consciously avoided, and yet not ostentatiously displayed. Tears are not to be ashamed of, nor is laughter at remembered foibles and funny ways of the dead child, whose life in this way gradually becomes a happy and not a haunting memory, and gives him immortality in a sense.

It is important that the doctor should not lose touch at once. In a sudden or unexpected death, discussion after two or three weeks of the postmortem findings may clear up a lot of questions that have troubled a parent's mind. In cases of hereditary or familial disease the genetic implications will need to be considered, and formal genetic counselling may well be advisable. There are now genetic counselling clinics in all parts of the country, and referral to the nearest one can be arranged by your doctor.

We can never bring a dead child back to life, but we can still do something for him by remembering him with affection, and by cherishing his survivors – his brothers and sisters, our husband or wife, and even ourselves.

Birthmarks

The Latin word for birthmark is naevus, and the medical term applies to all, not any special type of birthmark. Birthmarks are the result of enlargement of blood vessels in the skin, or of some extra pigment in the skin. Most of them occur, as the name implies, during the development of the baby before birth.

Various types of birthmark occur. Some are the dark red type, often raised (strawberry naevus), some are brown (naevus molle, mole), and others are flat, varying from pink to purple (portwine stain). A strawberry naevus, (strawberry mark, haemangioma) is not visible at birth but appears soon after and enlarges during the first eight or nine months.

Many of these shrink and lose their colour towards the end of the first year; almost all have disappeared by the age of five. Those that persist can usually be covered by cosmetic camouflage, but occasionally

267

some on the face may need tidying up by a plastic surgeon after the age of five. No other treatment should be given. Rarely, giant haemangiomas may threaten vital structures, such as throat or windpipe. Brief courses of steroid treatment may cause useful shrinkage. In life-threatening situations, radiation therapy may be necessary.

Treatment of portwine stains is difficult. The very pale portwine stains will often disappear within a few years after birth, but the darker stains remain. Marks may be covered completely by preparations especially devised for this purpose. Such preparations completely cover the mark, match the colour of the skin, are waterproof, will not come off on clothes, and remain on the skin until removed by cold cream. Several new approaches have also been reported, among which are tattooing the stains and dermabrasion.

Small children under the age of six are not as a rule bothered unduly by a birthmark and up to that age most playmates are not much concerned about it. Occasionally a great deal is made of a birthmark by those around the child. Troubled parents speak of it in front of the child. Visits are made to doctors and discussions are carried on frequently about treatment or hospitalization. Parents should avoid talk of the birthmark and warn friends also to do the same.

Moles are permanent pigment spots. If small and in a conspicuous place they can usually be removed by a plastic surgeon. If this is impossible or must be postponed for a while, the masking cosmetic may be used.

Breath-holding

Some infants and small children have a tendency to hold their breath when frightened, hurt, or when crying vigorously. They stop breathing, turn blue, lose consciousness, and occasionally get convulsive seizures. Practically all of these children cease these breath-holding attacks within a few minutes and are their normal selves again. Although the attacks are very frightening to adults around the child, they are not at all dangerous, and this is not epilepsy. The only danger is that many frightened parents tend to give in to a child to prevent such attacks. It is better to learn to avoid confrontations by foreseeing them and diverting the child's attention (except in danger, such as running across roads, or playing with fire or electricity, when confrontation should be immediate but calm). The brains and nervous systems of these children are perfectly normal, and most of them cease to have such attacks by the time they are three years

old. Drug treatment is not necessary, and indeed there is no effective drug. Occasionally a small dose of tranquillizer or sedative may tide the child (and even the parents) over a particularly difficult patch.

Sometimes after a bump on the head, not bad enough to cause concussion, the child suddenly goes pale, collapses, and is unconscious for a few seconds. This may be wrongly diagnosed as epilepsy.

Brother against brother

Battles between the young have been recorded since Cain slew Abel, and parents naturally worry about sibling rivalry. Sometimes this can jolt parents into realizing that they have been subconsciously favouring one child against another, and a re-examination of attitudes by the parents may ease things. Reticent parents may have forgotten how important it is for each child to hear "I love you" repeated to him personally, and with feeling. It is common for one child to set up another by quietly tormenting him and often acting innocent when turned upon. It is usually fair to blame both parties to a quarrel, not only the apparent aggressor. Children in a family vary in temperament, and it may happen that one child (not always the eldest, and sometimes a girl) will attempt to dominate the rest. The mother needs to uphold the rights of the weaker one, and not give in to the one that shouts loudest. But it is necessary to accept that there will always be an irreducible minimum of warfare in the family. Quarrels seem to occur especially at times of treats and holidays. Parents have to work at being fair, and being seen to be fair.

Coeliac disease

Coeliac disease is an important cause of diarrhoea and failure to thrive in this country. It is caused by a specific intolerance to one of the proteins of wheat flour, gluten, and is sometimes called gluten entero- pathy. It is most often diagnosed in the first two years of life, but may appear at any age. The infant is miserable, fails to grow, and becomes floppy and weak. The abdomen is distended and the buttocks wasted. The parents may notice a gradual fading of health a few weeks after cereal feeds are first introduced. Diagnosis usually requires hospital admission and the removal of a piece of the lining mucous membrane of the small gut for microscopic examination (jejunal biopsy). This is done by passing a capsule on a long tube by the mouth, through the stomach, and into the small intestine. Once the diagnosis is proved, rapid and complete recovery follows the permanent exclusion of wheat flour (unless the gluten has been removed) from the diet. In suspected coeliac disease, it is preferable to carry out jejunal biopsy before the gluten-free diet is tried, as afterwards the telltale signs disappear, and diagnosis becomes more difficult.

Colds and coughs

Some children seem to get an unending succession of colds. A head cold with sniffing and sneezing is often followed by a cough which may last two or three weeks. Such periods of susceptibility may continue for as long as six months, in spite of tonics, malt, or antibiotic. No method of preventing this is known to medical science. Unless the tonsils are proved to be the cause, no benefit is likely to result from their removal.

Colic and the crying baby

Colic is a condition found most often in young infants, usually during the first three months. It is characterized by a tendency to attacks of abdominal pain and as a rule, during these periods of pain, the abdomen is distended and the child's legs are drawn up on the body. However, a baby crying for any reason will tend to draw his legs up, and there are many causes of crying other than colic.

Tension in the baby Many babies cry a great deal because they have an unsatisfied need for sucking pleasure and are unable to relax until this need is met. The need for sucking varies in different infants. A great many infants with so-called colic will cease crying and relax once they are given a dummy teat (comforter). Tensions are also carried over to the baby from the people who handle him. There are many instances where a tense crying infant, handled by a tense and nervous person, will quiet down when placed in the care of a calm and relaxed person.

Swallowing excessive air during feeding The concept of wind as a cause of colic has been overstated. A few greedy feeders may swallow excessive air, which will usually be readily burped up if the child is sat up for a minute and his back or abdomen gently rubbed. Frantic efforts by the mother to get up the wind are seldom justified.

Hunger The possibility of hunger must not be overlooked in an investigation of the causes of infant crying. Hunger is not infrequently the cause among infants who are breast-fed. Many mothers rarely have accurate knowledge of the amount of milk taken by their infants. Most of these infants fall asleep at the breast, apparently satisfied, but awaken 30 minutes to an hour later crying from hunger. This crying is not relieved by a dummy but often is temporarily relieved by giving warm water. The possibility of lack of sufficient breast milk can be easily investigated by weighing a fully clothed baby immediately before nursing and again immediately after, without changing the nappies or any piece of clothing. This weighing should be repeated at four or five successive feedings before a decision is made as to the adequacy of the feeding.

Allergy Some colicky children are sensitive to cow's milk. If this is the case there is immediate relief once the baby is placed on a soya bean or meat base formula.

The crying baby Crying creates strong feelings in the parents. This is a built-in mechanism by which a baby in distress seeks help. After the above causes have been eliminated, the parent may find it difficult to tolerate the feeling of helplessness which he or she experiences when he or she cannot give comfort. There is no doubt that some strong-willed babies are able to bully their mothers into a state of weeping servitude by their demands. Parents, as well as babies, have rights, and they must not deny themselves rest when they have done their best. The mother may need support from her husband and friends; sometimes professional help from a doctor or health visitor may be needed. In an extreme case it may take a brief hospital admission to allow both mother and child to calm down and the normal loving relationship to be re-established. Excessive crying has been a prelude to baby battering. Parents who feel their control slipping should not be ashamed to get help immediately, by telephoning a friend, running next door to the neighbour, or even ringing the National Society for the Prevention of Cruelty to Children. Finally, excessive crying in a normally placid baby may be a sign of disease, such as a raised temperature, earache (otitis media), a virus infection, or (rarely) meningitis.

Congenital disorders

Any abnormality that is present at birth is congenital, but not necessarily hereditary. Many birth defects are accidents that are most unlikely to recur in subsequent children. Some defects and disorders, however, are genetic, transmitted by interaction of the genes of the parents. This does not necessarily mean that every child of the same parents will have the same defect.

Should some abnormality be present in a child at birth, or be recognized in infancy or early childhood, parents may worry and wonder about the risks of having other children. The obstetrician, paediatrician, or family doctor can frequently set any fears at rest. Some conditions do, however, carry variable risks of repetition which may make special genetic counselling advisable. Your family doctor will be able to refer you to a genetic counselling clinic in your area. The mechanisms of heredity are complicated; for fuller discussion see chapter 26.

Antenatal testing (amniocentesis)   See chapter 11.

Constipation

By constipation is meant that the child's stools are hard and that there is difficulty in passing a motion. Many normal children may have a stool of normal consistency only every other day, and this should be of no concern if it causes the child no distress. Unfortunately, there has been far too much emphasis placed on the supposed dangers of constipation. Not only have most people been brought up to believe that everyone has to have a daily bowel movement to remain in good health, but are constantly being told by manufacturers and advertisers of laxatives that the bowels must be regular. This is not true. There is no arbitrary necessity for a daily evacuation. Many perfectly healthy people normally have bowel movements every two or even three days.

Constipation in infants can usually be controlled with ease by regulating the child's diet as well as by the addition of substances that soften the faecal matter, if necessary. Constipation may be caused by a number of conditions, among which are bad diet, forced toilet training, chronic use of laxatives or suppositories, obstructive lesions, and anal tears (fissures) that cause severe pain on defaecation.

Treatment of constipation   It is a recognized fact that diet has an effect upon the consistency of the stool and regularity of the bowel movements. For instance, cow's milk is more constipating than breast milk. In early infancy, breast-fed babies who develop constipation can usually be cured by giving the mother an increase of fruits and other laxative foods. In bottle-fed babies, constipation may be treated by changing the sugar in the formula to one with more malt, by adding prune juice to the diet, or by adding malt extract to the formula. All older infants and children of all ages require bulk and roughage for adequate functioning of the intestinal tract. This is obtained through the addition of vegetables and fruits, which leave adequate residues, to the diet. The occasional use of liquid paraffin or a senna preparation may be helpful if the stools become very hard.

The chronic use of laxatives and suppositories, although originally given to counteract constipation, eventually makes the digestive system so dependent on the abnormal stimulation that it will not function without it.

Suppositories and enemas should be resorted to only on rare occasions. At times, in severe constipation, a faecal mass in the rectum becomes large and impacted. This can be softened and passed without pain either by use of a suppository or a proprietary enema which comes already prepared in a plastic bottle with an enema tip. When constipation reaches this degree, however, it is best to seek the advice of your doctor.

Toilet training   Forcing a child to sit on the potty or toilet against his will is one of the most common causes of constipation. The child tenses up and resists and often refuses to move his bowels, with resultant constipation. Parents should learn to relax while toilet training a child. It should not be attempted too early – fifteen to eighteen months is the earliest, and it can be left till two years.

If a child resists, no force should be used, but each time the child soils he should be reminded of the toilet. Although he should not be scolded for soiling, he should be praised for using the potty or toilet. There is a time of toilet training readiness for each child which varies just as the time for sitting up, standing up, walking, and talking varies from child to child. When a child is ready to be toilet trained, he will usually train easily without force or scolding.

Anal tears (fissures) frequently bring about constipation. A large hard stool distends the anal ring in defaecation and tears the mucous membrane. These tears are extremely painful whenever the anus opens, so the child, fearing this pain, withholds his motion and develops constipation, which often becomes chronic. In such cases, an anaesthetic and healing ointment is applied to the anal tear several times a day and the stools are kept soft by large doses of liquid paraffin or paraffin emulsion, using two to four tablespoons to ensure lubrication and softening of the stool.

Convulsions

One of the most frightening experiences for a parent is to see a child in convulsions. It occurs suddenly, the child becomes unconscious, the eyes are rolled up, the body first may twitch and then relax completely, so that many parents fear the child is dying. Breathing is heavy and coarse, there may be some frothing at the lips, and in rare instances soiling and urination. Convulsions are almost always more frightening than dangerous. The attack usually lasts for a few minutes at the most, and as a rule has subsided by the time a doctor arrives.

The most common cause of convulsions in young children under the age of four is high fever which can accompany infections, such as contagious diseases, sore throats, inflamed ears, and virus infections such as measles. These are known as febrile convulsions, and only certain children respond to fevers in this manner. The reason for this is not entirely clear. Some doctors feel that in susceptible children the nervous system is more irritable than in other children and adults. The tendency to have febrile convulsions is almost always outgrown by the time a child reaches four years of age. There is also the type of convulsion that occurs in children who are breath-holders (described above).

Convulsions may be caused by other less frequent conditions such as inflammation of the brain in certain infections, damage to the brain before or after birth, pressure on the brain, lead poisoning, and kidney trouble.

Treatment First telephone for a doctor. Keep calm. Remember that practically all convulsions subside without any danger to the child. But several suggestions may help in limiting the duration of the seizures. If the child has a high fever, do not wrap him up, but undress him, and sponge him with tepid water, preferably in a draught or by an electric fan. If you have a thermometer, continue cooling until the temperature falls below 38°C (100°F). Perhaps one

in twenty children will have a febrile convulsion. Although technically the convulsion is an epileptic fit, epilepsy only occurs in about 1 in 200 children, so the vast majority of febrile convulsions are harmless. Recent evidence, however, suggests that some febrile convulsions are not as benign as was formerly supposed. Severe, prolonged convulsions (more than half an hour) may cause pressure on the temporal lobes of the brain, or reduce their blood supply, producing a small scar which may act as an irritable focus for temporal lobe epilepsy in later life. Some doctors may advise you to keep the child on an anticonvulsant drug for a year or so, to prevent further febrile convulsions occurring. In any case, try to avoid further episodes by giving aspirin or paracetamol and cooling the child straight away whenever you suspect he is sickening towards a fever.

Cot death

The sudden, unexpected, and tragic death of a normal baby is one of the distressing facts that face parents today. About 1 in 500 apparently normal babies die like this, usually between the ages of three and six months. It is now the second commonest cause of death in the first year of life, after congenital abnormalities. The cause is unknown, and there are no specific preventive methods. Parents who have suffered bereavement in this way may feel the need to discuss the death and the events leading up to it with their health visitor, doctor, or a paediatrician or pathologist. Help may be obtained from the Foundation for the Study of Infant Deaths, 23 St. Peter's Square, London W6 9NW.

Cradle cap

This is a condition commonly found in young infants. It appears as a thick scaling or greasy crusting over patchy areas of the whole scalp. It is due to a secretion from the oil glands in the skin, even in those babies whose scalps have been kept clean. In most instances it may be successfully removed by oiling the scalp with baby oil, mineral oil, or petroleum jelly and then gently combing through with a fine-toothed comb. If this is not successful, the doctor will prescribe an ointment which will dissolve the scales and crusts and will soothe any irritation which may be present on the baby's scalp. Usually the scalp of a baby is shampooed twice a week. However, when a tendency to have cradle cap exists it can be washed every day or every other day.

Croup

Croup describes the noisy breathing of a child with laryngitis. The technical name for the noise is stridor. The usual cause is a virus infection which may require admission to hospital, but is seldom dangerous. A less common cause is acute epiglottitis, caused by a bacterium called *Haemophilus influenzae*, which is dangerous because of the risk of sudden airway

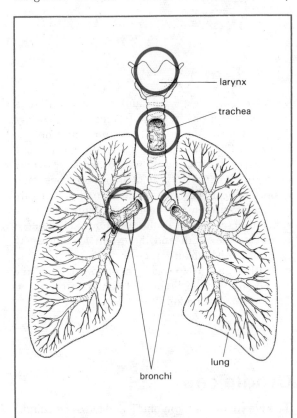

The most serious form of croup (laryngotracheobronchitis) is an emergency requiring immediate medical attention to control obstruction to breathing that may be fatal if not relieved. Thick mucus may clog the larynx, the trachea, and the bronchi, obstructing the passage of air to and from the lungs. Usually the infant has a high fever and respiratory infection preceding an acute attack.

obstruction and suffocation. You may be able to see the swollen epiglottis (the flap at the back of the tongue which folds down backwards to close off the windpipe during swallowing) like a red cherry during a bout of coughing. Acute inflammation of the epiglottis (often part of acute laryngotracheobronchitis) is an emergency, and needs hospital treatment. Viral croup is not severe, and usually settles quickly without special treatment. It is doubtful if the old-fashioned steam kettle is of any value, and there is a risk from scalding. Medical advice should be sought in case your baby has the more severe condition.

Cystic fibrosis

This is a comparatively rare familial disease characterized by serious and persistent lung infections, loose foul-smelling stools, and failure to gain weight. It affects about 1 in 3,500 children.

The onset of symptoms may occur at birth, when the meconium (see Encyclopedia of Medical Terms) is so sticky that the baby cannot move his bowels (meconium ileus). Because of the obstruction, the abdomen is distended, the baby vomits green bile, and urgent treatment in a hospital unit with facilities for neonatal surgery is required. The obstruction may be dislodged by an enema, but in some cases it may have to be relieved by operation.

The condition occurs because the fetal pancreas fails to produce the digestive enzyme trypsin which normally breaks up the sticky meconium and renders it soft and slippery.

Of babies with cystic fibrosis three quarters escape meconium ileus, but develop attacks of bronchopneumonia in the first few weeks or months of life; they fail to gain weight and produce frequent foul-smelling stools.

In the later stages of the disease the child becomes extremely thin with a large protuberant abdomen. There is a history of chronic lung infections with numerous attacks of pneumonia. As time goes on, most children with this condition develop shortness of breath and some difficulty in breathing due to the mucous plugging of the breathing tubes which makes the exchange of oxygen and carbon dioxide in the lungs extremely difficult. In hot climates, salt loss can be a problem, from the abnormally salty sweat produced, but this seldom occurs in temperate zones. The condition can be diagnosed with certainty by tests of salt in the body sweat, and by tests that show a

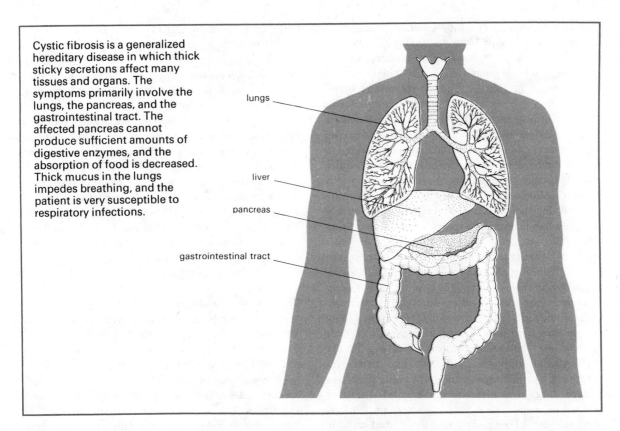

Cystic fibrosis is a generalized hereditary disease in which thick sticky secretions affect many tissues and organs. The symptoms primarily involve the lungs, the pancreas, and the gastrointestinal tract. The affected pancreas cannot produce sufficient amounts of digestive enzymes, and the absorption of food is decreased. Thick mucus in the lungs impedes breathing, and the patient is very susceptible to respiratory infections.

lungs

liver

pancreas

gastrointestinal tract

lack of digestive juices from the pancreas. Treatment entails close medical supervision for the prevention and control of chest infections, the addition of pancreatic extracts, and regular physiotherapy by the parents to prevent sticky secretions accumulating in the lungs.

Genetic risk Cystic fibrosis is inherited as a Mendelian recessive condition. That is to say, each parent contributes half the abnormal factor necessary for the disease to appear. Statistically, there is a one in four risk of subsequent children being affected. Unfortunately, there is at present no way of identifying an affected fetus during pregnancy. If cystic fibrosis is diagnosed at birth, the outlook may be improved by intensive treatment right from the start.

Developmental examinations

In many parts of the country, mothers have an opportunity to bring their babies for special developmental examinations at specific times during the first few years of life. The ages are fixed by the Health Authority in different areas. Favourite ages are six weeks, six months, ten months, two years, and five years. The purpose of the examination is to reassure the parent that the child is normal, as in the vast majority of cases; in the occasional case where a handicap is identified, to make sure that appropriate treatment is begun at the earliest possible moment. Hearing and vision checks are most important. Examinations may be carried out by either doctors or health visitors. In most large towns, there is a Developmental Assessment Unit where a child suspected of any abnormality can be fully assessed by a paediatrician or paediatric neurologist, and also by other specialists such as a speech therapist, physiotherapist, and educational psychologist. But before these tests take place, every five day old baby has a blood sample taken (heel prick) which is tested for phenylketonuria, and at about the same time is screened by a doctor for congenital dislocation of the hip. Seven months later the baby's hearing is tested by a health visitor.

Handicap Great strides have been made in recent years in the prevention, recognition, and treatment of handicapping conditions in infancy and childhood. Nevertheless, congenital and acquired disorders leading to handicap continue to arise, and such a diagnosis is a major blow to a family. Doctors' attitudes have become much more positive, so that emphasis is laid on what a child can achieve, rather than on what he cannot. Though there may be no measure that can restore full normality, many forms of help are now available. After the age of two, a Constant Attendance Allowance (in 1979 £10·40 per week for day, £18·60 for day and night) is provided to lighten the burden of parents whose children require extra help due to mental or physical handicap. A Mobility Allowance of £12 per week to compensate partially for the problems of spina bifida, severely mentally handicapped, or spastic children in getting from place to place is payable from five years upwards. Constant Attendance Allowance is not taxable, Mobility Allowance is. A Family Fund is available to assist with purchase of a washing machine, drier, car, or other aid. Wheelchairs and walking aids are supplied through hospitals. Home adaptations, for instance the building of a downstairs room, shower, and toilet, or the provision of a lift, are done by local authorities. People who find themselves parents of a handicapped child have many problems to face. They are fortunate if they find a patient listener in their doctor, social worker, or teacher, someone who is both truly sympathetic, and capable of dealing efficiently with their practical problems. Finally, since many abnormalities are inherited, they need expert genetic counselling to discover whether there is a high risk of recurrence in subsequent births, and whether there are methods of antenatal diagnosis.

Diarrhoea

By diarrhoea is meant a frequency of loose or watery stools. Breast-fed babies in early infancy usually have loose bowel movements, often with each breast-feed. This is not diarrhoea. An occasional loose movement in the average child, even if it is once or twice a day for a number of days is not diarrhoea, but frequent loose or watery stools are of significance, and treatment should be under the direction of a doctor. The first aid is to keep the child warm and give him water to drink. Infants and small children are particularly susceptible to gastrointestinal upsets. In the small infant, diarrhoea can have serious consequences. It is rarely dangerous after one year of age. There are many causes of diarrhoea, among which are infections, food allergies, laxatives or laxative foods, ulcerative colitis,

cystic fibrosis, coeliac disease, and occasionally the cutting of teeth.

Cow's milk allergy Cow's milk allergy or intolerance, is a common cause of diarrhoea in infancy and more rarely in older children, and responds well to a formula without cows milk.

Irritable colon There is a common form of toddler's diarrhoea in which the motions become loose, one or two a day, and undigested food particles may be observed. It is sometimes referred to as "the carrots and peas syndrome" since parts of these vegetables may be recognized in the stool. It may follow a bout of infective diarrhoea, and persist for many months. These toddlers continue to thrive, however, and the condition is harmless. It may be ignored, or the symptoms may be abolished by sieving the food or putting it through a blender.

Treatment of diarrhoea Most episodes of diarrhoea clear up after a few days without treatment. Antibiotics are best avoided. When acute diarrhoea is accompanied by griping pains or colic, one or two doses of kaolin and morphia mixture (NOT to be given to children under five) bring immediate relief; Lomotil tablets are also effective. Diarrhoea associated with ulcerative colitis, cystic fibrosis, or coeliac disease requires careful and specific medical care.

Disease prevention

At the present time there are inoculations or oral preparations that in almost every instance will completely prevent most of the serious infectious diseases. The most important of these preventive measures are those against diphtheria, tetanus, whooping cough, poliomyelitis (infantile paralysis), and measles. In spite of this, there are still many children lacking these protective measures, either because their parents were careless, or had a prejudice against inoculation, or believed that vitamins or diet could prevent disease. Some children may have died of these preventable diseases because of the laxness of their parents. In areas where there has been laxity in carrying out prevention, the diseases have reappeared, disproving the idea that modern sanitation alone is responsible for the present low rate of disease. This is no time to live in the past. All children should have the benefits of modern protection from these deadly but preventable diseases. It is wise to keep a family record of immunizations in some permanent form, like the record-chart shown on page 281. It is easy to forget the dates of vaccinations and inoculations, but often it becomes important at some future time to know the date accurately. Families may move to different communities, members are treated by different doctors, a doctor may cease practice, and altogether it is a wise idea to keep your immunization records where you can refer to them at any time. Remember, too, that immunizations wear off in time and need boosting or renewal at intervals recommended by your doctor.

Down's syndrome
(mongolism)

Down's syndrome (named after the London physician who first identified it in 1866) was at first called mongolism, but it occurs in all races, and the resemblance to mongoloid races disappears if the facial features are analysed accurately. The degree of mental retardation varies. Some of these children are severely retarded; all will end up with some degree of dependency, though they may be able to undertake simple tasks. In 1959 it was discovered that most of these children had an extra chromosome in all the cells of their bodies, 47 chromosomes instead of 46 (see chapter 26). Down's syndrome is sometimes known as 21-trisomy because the extra chromosome belongs to the small 21 group in which a third chromosome appears instead of the normal pair.

One fact about Down's syndrome is definitely established, and that is that older mothers are more likely to give birth to these children than younger mothers. Whereas statistically only about 1 in 1,000 are born to mothers between 20 and 24 years, approximately 1 in 50 are born to older mothers – those between 40 and 50 years of age.

These children are usually not difficult to handle since they are often affectionate and of pleasant disposition, but being retarded they are slower in development and need a good deal of extra care and help. They are generally more susceptible to respiratory infections such as colds, ear infections, and pneumonia. They may also have congenital heart lesions and often have hernias. Other severe congenital abnormalities are also more frequent, such as narrowing or blockage of the gullet, duodenum, or anus.

Amniocentesis, in which a few drops of fluid from the sac surrounding the developing embryo are withdrawn for analysis, can identify an embryo with Down's syndrome. This is done at about the fourteenth week of pregnancy and if the result is positive (after two or three weeks) the pregnancy can be terminated. This service is available to all mothers over 40, or 38 in some areas, and is also offered to mothers who have previously borne an affected baby.

Feeding

There are strong reasons for believing that breast-feeding is better for babies than cow's milk, however much it is modified. Both death rates and disease rates are lower in the breast-fed compared with the artificially fed, even when social factors are allowed for. In the first few days of life, foreign proteins are able to pass directly into the baby's circulation. This is beneficial, as breast milk contains protective maternal antibodies against disease, but cow's milk does not contain them, and absorbed cow's milk protein may be a factor in such allergic states as asthma and eczema. Breast milk, by denying iron to bacteria, interferes with their multiplication. Breast milk protects against tetany (nothing to do with tetanus), one form of convulsion in the first few days of life. Breast-fed babies seldom become overweight. Breast-fed babies do not develop salt poisoning (hypernatraemia) from putting too much powder in the feeds. Diarrhoea and vomiting and chest infections are commoner in bottle-fed babies. All these factors are even more important in the tropics and among the poor.

Having said this, a majority of babies in the West have been reared on cow's milk for at least a generation, and infant mortality has fallen sharply over this period. Children are taller, heavier (sometimes too much so), and healthier than they have ever been. An individual mother can be reassured that she can bring her baby up with great success on cow's milk; it is only in large-scale surveys that the benefits of breast milk become so obvious.

Breast-feeding is not without its problems, too. Failure of lactation is all too common, and paediatricians regularly see breast-fed babies whose weight gain has been less than adequate.

Amount of feed An infant who is on the breast may take a variable amount at each feed. There is never a standard amount of each feed. Likewise, simply because a doctor prescribes a certain measure for each feed, it does not mean that the baby must take the whole amount, or that the amount will necessarily satisfy the infant at every feed.

Cow's milk feeds   Cow's milk contains too much protein, salt, and phosphate, and insufficient vitamins; unmodified milk may make tough curds in the stomach. The government has recommended suitable proprietary brands for babies under six months. After six months it is probably reasonable to give the baby ordinary cow's milk.

Sterilization   Bottles and teats should be sterilized either by boiling for five minutes or by sterilizing solution, for example, hypochlorite (Milton). All milk residues should be removed by careful cleaning before sterilization. In an emergency, a cup is more easily sterilized than a bottle. Almost all delivered milk is pasteurized; if raw milk is supplied by the dairy, it should be boiled. It is not necessary to sterilize bottles or boil the milk after six months.

Weaning   Weaning is used both in the sense of the introduction of mixed feeding, and of discontinuation of breast-feeding. Cereals such as wheat, oats, barley, and rice are given to young babies at widely varying ages in different cultures. There has been a trend towards earlier cereal feeding. Milk alone is adequate until the age of three months, but there is no reason not to introduce cereals at six weeks if the baby seems hungry after his milk feed. Breast-feeding, as long as it is supplemented with cereal (and dinners after six months), may continue well into the second year as it does in most peasant societies, but most mothers in developed countries think of stopping at six to nine months. The eruption of milk teeth is not a bar to continued breast-feeding.

Fever

The first thing for a parent to remember is that the degree of fever is no indication of the severity of an illness. Some minor illnesses, such as influenza or a cold, can be accompanied by high fever, whereas some potentially serious diseases, such as bronchiolitis, may have only slight fever. The illness of a child should be judged more by the way he acts than the temperature registered on the thermometer. Hospitals usually measure the temperature with a rectal thermometer up to the age of two. The rectal temperature is approximately 0·5° C (1° F) higher than the mouth temperature. Generally the rectal

temperature varies between 37° and 37·7° C (99° and 100° F). The normal mouth temperature is 37° C (98·4°F). A child's temperature fluctuates during the day, between 36·7° C (98° F) and 37·2° C (99° F), usually being higher in the late day and evening. In the home, parents should not take the rectal temperature. Any warm fold of skin will do, such as the armpit, the groin, or under the chin. The temperature in a skinfold will usually be about 0·5° C (1° F) below the mouth temperature. Children of about six years and upwards usually accept a thermometer in the mouth. Occasionally, at the end of an infection, the temperature may drop as low as 36° C (97° F). This is no cause for concern as long as the child behaves normally. The temperature will usually return to normal within 24 hours.

Treatment   If the fever is high, 38·3° C (101° F), or if it makes the child uncomfortable, efforts should be made to lower it. The best means of reducing the temperature when the fever is very high, 40° C (104° F), is by tepid sponging. Use a bowl of cool but not chilled water. Damp the body with a sponge or flannel and allow it to dry near an open window; an electric fan is even more effective.

Aspirin or paracetamol can be given in tablets or as syrup. The usual dosage would be one half of a children's 75 mg aspirin tablet for infants under six months of age; one tablet (75 mg) for children six months to two years; two tablets (150 mg) for two and three years of age; three tablets (225 mg) for children of four; and an adult tablet (300 mg) for those who are five years and older. For paracetamol the same dose of tablets is used.

A warning must be given that an overdose of aspirin may be extremely dangerous to a child. Most of these preparations for children are flavoured so as to make them attractive and acceptable. Too often, children, thinking them to be sweets, will take large amounts with serious consequences. It follows that aspirin should be kept entirely out of reach of children. Keep tablets in childproof containers or use foil-wrapped packs.

Cold syndrome   Babies lose heat very rapidly in the first month of life, and if they kick off the covers, their temperature may drop. Also, small babies, particularly those born prematurely, may react to illness by growing cold rather than hot. This may mislead a parent into thinking the baby must be all right because he has no fever. Shake the thermometer right down to the bulb. The lowest mark on the scale is normally 35° C (95° F). If the temperature remains below this, and particularly if the baby feels cold to the touch, consult your doctor immediately. In cold weather, frequently touch the baby's head. If it feels cold, check body temperature.

Food refusal

Eating, sleeping, and defaecating are three particularly sensitive areas of a child's upbringing where he can hold his parents to ransom by refusing cooperation. Often parents may bring their child to the doctor complaining that he does not eat. He has no vomiting or diarrhoea, and is active and full of energy. The doctor examines the child and finds a lively healthy youngster. The easiest way for him to convince the parents that their fears are groundless is to weigh and measure him and plot his growth on a chart which will show him to be of appropriate stature for his age. Small portions of foods which he is known to enjoy should be offered at the normal family mealtime, with gentle (not frantic) encouragement; what he does not eat is removed without comment. Snacks between meals are discouraged. Special cooking and special treatment are withheld. Emotion must not be shown at refusal of food. As soon as the child perceives that he is no longer able to manipulate his parents by food refusal, he will enjoy his meals without fuss. A healthy child will never voluntarily starve himself.

"Glands in the neck"

Parents sometimes get worried about "glands in the neck" (cervical adenitis) because in bygone days this condition was often caused by tuberculosis. Lymph nodes in the neck are an easily seen part of the body's antibody defences and they drain the tissues of the mouth, nose, and throat – often infected in minor illnesses. They may be slow to disappear after a throat infection. They are harmless and antibiotic treatment is not required. Very occasionally an abscess may develop and require incision. Immigrant children may develop a tuberculous neck gland; a tuberculin test from the doctor or clinic may be positive and this needs hospital investigation and treatment.

Haemolytic disease of the newborn

Fifteen per cent of British mothers have Rhesus negative red cells. If such a woman marries a Rh-positive man, she may have a Rh-positive fetus. Leakage of the baby's red cells into her circulation may stimulate her to form anti-Rh antibodies capable of destroying red cells in the Rh-positive fetus of a subsequent pregnancy. This is Rhesus haemolytic disease. The work of Dr (later Sir) Cyril Clarke, a clinical geneticist, in the 1960's showed that antibody formation could be prevented in Rh-negative mothers by the injection of immune anti-D (anti-Rh) serum after delivery of an Rh-positive fetus. This destroys any fetal red cells that may have leaked into the maternal circulation before they have had time to stimulate antibody formation. Most of the small number of Rhesus babies now are being born to mothers who became sensitized before the present programme of prevention began in 1970. There is still a small number of newly sensitized mothers however, the result of spontaneous or induced abortions in early pregnancy. Even early (second or third month) abortions should be reported to the family doctor so that he may arrange for an anti-D injection if the patient is Rh-negative.

Another cause of haemolytic disease of the newborn is an inherited red cell abnormality, G.6–P.D. (glucose–6–phosphate dehydrogenase) deficiency. This abnormality may provide some protection against the malarial parasite. Malaria disappeared from the United Kingdom in the eighteenth century, so that the gene appears more commonly in people from tropical and Mediterranean countries. In Singapore, for instance, 40 per cent of neonatal jaundice is associated with G.6–P.D. deficiency. Although jaundice may occur spontaneously in these babies, it may also be precipitated by some drugs and foods (sulphonamides, some kinds of bean), and appropriate precautions are necessary.

Headache and migraine

Children may copy complaints, such as of headache, that they have heard from others. This is probably the commonest reason for a child to complain of headaches, and simple reassurance is all that is needed.

However, headache is occasionally a danger signal when it arises from raised pressure inside the head, and may then be part of an acute illness (meningitis, intracranial bleeding) or chronic illness (subdural haematoma, that is a blood clot over the brain, or tumour). Headache due to raised intracranial pressure is commoner in the early morning and is often accompanied by vomiting. Examination of the retina by the doctor should exclude dangerous causes.

Migraine often occurs in children, even young children, though it may not follow the adult pattern. Auras (blind spot, spots or lights before the eyes) are rarely reported. A family history is common. Duration varies from a few hours to two days. Headache which continues for longer than two days, or which recurs oftener than once a week is not usually migraine. Photophobia (avoiding the light), vomiting, and prostration may occur. Abdominal pain is common. The best advice is to reassure and comfort the child, and to let him lie down in a quiet and darkened room to sleep it off. Low blood sugar may be a factor, and making sure that the child does not miss meals (especially breakfast) and gets his snack (milk, biscuits, even a fizzy drink) between main meals helps to prevent them. Children are less suspicious and more suggestible than adults, and strong reassurance from the doctor after full physical examination, together with the suggestion that the headaches will gradually diminish and disappear, is nearly always effective. It is better to avoid starting pill-taking habits – a lump of sugar may be as effective as aspirin or paracetamol, and the powerful drugs sometimes needed in adult migraine (ergotamine, methysergide) should hardly ever be used. Migraine symptoms (headache, vomiting, and drowsiness) are common after epileptic fits.

Psychogenic headache describes "more severe, frequent and persistent headache without organic cause which does not follow the symptom pattern of migraine". Simple reassurance is valuable, but the headache may be a distress signal which needs answering by having a look for emotional causes and relieving them. Eyestrain is a very rare cause of headaches.

Headaches may be used to avoid going to school. Have a word with the child's teacher, explore any areas of special strain in school or on the way to or from school, ask the teacher if she will agree to have the child even with a headache, and then encourage the child to keep to school routine.

Head lice (pediculosis)

Infestation of the hair with head lice is a common condition, frequently found among schoolchildren, especially in large cities. The lice can pass from one child's head to another if the children are close together, or the condition can be contracted if one child wears the hat of a child who is already infested. Once in the hair the lice lay their eggs, like tiny pearls, which become tightly glued to the hairs. These eggs look like dandruff to the naked eye, but cannot be brushed or combed out. Their pearly colour can be seen under a magnifying glass. The head lice are small insects which look like miniature tiny crabs. They bite the scalp, since they use blood for food, causing severe itching and at times even infections of the scalp. There is no way of preventing a child from catching the condition. The aim should be to detect it quickly and clear it up as soon as possible. This can usually be done within 24 to 48 hours.

There are two problems to be considered in treatment. The first is to kill the living lice, the second to kill and get rid of the eggs. At present there are a number of rapid and highly successful treatments. One of the best combines two insecticides, DDT and benzyl benzoate, with a wetting agent to loosen the eggs from their attachment to the hairs. Two applications are used, twelve hours apart – the first to kill the insects, the second to kill the eggs. The dead eggs can usually be removed by combing them out of the hair with a fine-toothed comb. If any eggs remain, a second treatment is advised a week later.

In some parts of Britain the lice have become resistant to this treatment. Another preparation called Malathion is then used.

Heart murmurs

The fact that a child has a heart murmur is, by itself, no reason for a parent to be concerned or over-anxious. Such murmurs may be heard in many normal children. Between 50 and 75 per cent of all normal healthy children may have heart murmurs at some time or another during their childhood. Often these murmurs are heard only when a child is anaemic or has a fever.

Heart disease due to valve damage during an attack of rheumatic fever used to be as frequent as congenital heart disease, but it has become less and less common, and is now extremely rare. Congenital heart disease due to malformations of the heart or blood vessels occurs in about 1 in 250 births. It is usually divided into blue (cyanotic) and not blue (acyanotic) types. In the former there is mixing of oxygenated and deoxygenated blood in the heart, and insufficient blood passing through the lungs. The abnormalities vary in severity from conditions incompatible with life, to very mild forms which could easily pass unrecognized throughout a patient's life. With regular examination of babies at intervals throughout infancy and later at school, parents are frequently alarmed at being told that a murmur is present.

Parents of infants with congenital murmurs should realize that the important thing is not the murmur itself, but whether or not the defect produces cardiac difficulty. This would include blue spells, rapid breathing, extremely poor appetite, and failure to thrive and grow normally. In many instances the congenital cardiac defect may be corrected by operation, after which the child will be as normal as any child born without a cardiac defect.

In the commonest variety, interventricular septal defect (VSD), there is a high rate of spontaneous closure of the hole during the first year of life. Even if the hole persists, it is commonly so small that it causes no trouble at all. Usually a child will be asked to attend a cardiology clinic at intervals. In all but the mildest cases, the doctor will arrange a special investigation, cardiac catheterization, when a fine flexible hollow tube will be passed into the heart along one of the major veins in the arm or leg, and pressures and oxygen saturations of blood inside the separate heart chambers will be recorded. A dye injection with X-rays will then be done (angiocardiography) and this will enable a complete diagnosis to be made, and the need for operation to be assessed. In uncomplicated cases, this will probably be delayed until the child is five or six years old, but if there are signs of heart failure, it may be done in infancy, even in the newborn.

Dental hygiene All children will want to avoid the need for drilling and fillings by good dental hygiene, but this is particularly important in congenital heart disease. Bacteria dislodged from decayed teeth into the circulation may lodge in abnormal heart valves or holes and cause subacute bacterial endocarditis, a dangerous and sometimes fatal complication. Children with congenital heart disease should be taught from an early age to limit their consumption of sweets, avoid sweetened drinks, never eat between meals, and brush their teeth regularly with a fluoride toothpaste. It is to be hoped that their parents will campaign through their local authority for fluoridation of public water supplies. The dentist should be advised if a child has congenital heart disease, as scaling, dental extractions, and major fillings may need to be accompanied by antibiotic protection.

Functional murmurs Innocent murmurs (functional murmurs) are those murmurs that are heard in children and are of no significance. They may be louder during fevers or chest infections. This is one of the forms of paediatric nondisease which have been the cause of much anxiety and distress in the past. If a child has no symptoms, and the murmur has all the characteristics of an innocent murmur (an experienced paediatrician or cardiologist will be able to distinguish these), the parents may be reassured that their child's heart is normal. No restrictions of any sort are needed.

Hernia

Hernias are due to a weakness of, or an opening in, the abdominal wall. The intestines beneath push through such areas and cause a bulging or ballooning. These weaknesses or openings are almost always present from birth. But, although a weakness is there, the hernia may not push through until much later – in adolescence or even in adult life.

Two types of hernia are commonly found in infants and children. One is the umbilical hernia where the protrusion occurs at the region of the navel. Umbilical hernias are harmless. They never become strangulated. Small ones less than 2·5 cm (one in) in diameter usually close spontaneously. Larger ones should be left for a few years, after which they can be closed by a simple operation. Strapping is unnecessary and unhelpful. The other type is where the weakness is on either or both sides of the lower abdomen, causing a bulging where the abdomen is joined to the thigh. This type is called an inguinal hernia.

The danger of a hernia is greatest in situations where so much of the intestines may push through that it is difficult or impossible to push the protrusion back. This may then interfere with the blood supply of the intestine and produce a strangulated hernia, which is dangerous since gangrene may occur. It is vitally important that when an infant or child with a hernia develops abdominal pain and later vomits, the first place to look is in the region of the hernia to see if it is protruding. If so, every effort should be made to

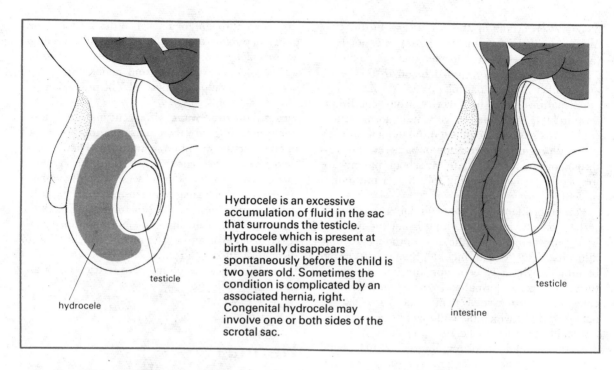

Hydrocele is an excessive accumulation of fluid in the sac that surrounds the testicle. Hydrocele which is present at birth usually disappears spontaneously before the child is two years old. Sometimes the condition is complicated by an associated hernia, right. Congenital hydrocele may involve one or both sides of the scrotal sac.

hydrocele

testicle

testicle

intestine

quiet the child and push the protrusion back, for crying forces more of the intestines through the open or weakened area. If it is difficult to reduce the hernia with gentle pressure the child should be placed in a warm bath which usually relaxes the abdominal muscles. If this is unsuccessful a doctor should be called immediately. Inguinal hernias, unlike umbilical hernias, do not close on their own, and will need to be repaired by a surgeon.

Hydrocele A good many male infants are born with a soft rounded swelling within one or both sides of the scrotal sac. This swelling is due to an extra amount of fluid in the sac around the testicle, where normally only a small amount is present. In almost every instance such hydroceles will subside and disappear spontaneously before the infant has reached two years of age. At times a hydrocele in infancy may be associated with a hernia in the lower abdominal region. Such a possibility can be investigated by the child's doctor. A hydrocele which is still present after the age of two is easily cured by operation.

Infantile eczema

Infantile allergic eczema is the most common skin disorder of infancy, with the one exception of nappy rashes. Its cause is not known, though allergies to food, particularly to cow's milk, or to contact with irritating substances may play a part. There is often a family history of allergy (asthma, eczema, or hay fever).

In infancy eczema usually starts as a scattering of red pimples on the cheeks. The eruptions become more pronounced and spread to cover the whole face unless the cause is discovered and removed. If the condition gets more pronounced, the pimples form tiny blisters which break, causing a moist eczema, and finally a crusting. Usually there is considerable itching and the child becomes very irritable. The eczema, even if untreated, tends to clear up almost entirely between one and two years of age, although some lingering eczematous lesions may continue to remain in the folds of the elbows and behind the knees.

A doctor can usually prescribe ointment that will relieve the condition. If the eczema is due to an allergy to cow's milk it is readily relieved by soya bean or meat-based milk substitute. Other foods responsible for eczema in the first year of life besides milk may be eggs, wheat, and orange juice. Where soap is suspected as an irritating agent, hypoallergenic soap or substitutes such as baby oil or baby lotion may be used, though they themselves, with baby powder, may be the offending agent. Allergic skin tests which may be helpful in diagnosing the cause of most allergies are not helpful in infantile eczema due to food sensitivity.

Immunization record

disease	date of original immunization			date of boosters			doctor
	1st child	2nd child	3rd child	1st child	2nd child	3rd child	
diphtheria							
tetanus							
whooping cough							
poliomyelitis							
measles							
rubella (German measles)							
mumps							
other immunizations such as influenza, typhoid, etc							
				retests			
tuberculin tests							

Schedule for active immunization of normal infants and children

March 1977

birth	BCG vaccine for high risk groups (see page 287)
10 weeks	First DPT injection (diphtheria, pertussis, tetanus)
	First oral polio live vaccine
4 months	Second DPT, oral polio
10 months	Third DPT, oral polio
14 months	Measles live vaccine injection
5 years	Booster DPT injection and oral polio
13 years	BCG if tuberculin (Heaf) negative
14 years	Rubella live vaccine injection (all girls)

Whooping cough (pertussis) vaccine should not be given to babies with a history of brain damage, low blood sugar after birth, or epilepsy. The risk of brain damage following whooping cough immunization is probably less than 1:50,000 and may well be less than 1:200,000. The Government has promised compensation (a cash payment of £10,000) to cases of brain damage following vaccination where definite symptoms have occurred within 48 hours of an injection.

Infectious diseases For other infectious diseases and fuller descriptions, see chapter 2 and index

Source	Mode of transmission	Incubation period	Period of contagion	Type of rash
Chickenpox Virus closely related to, if not the same as, the virus causing shingles (herpes zoster). In secretions of nose and throat of infected person, and in skin vesicles.	By direct contact with person who has the disease.	12 to 19 days (usually 13th or 14th day)	From 1 day before appearance of rash to 6 days after appearance of rash.	Rash begins as small pink spots which develop into pinhead-size pimples. Then a tiny blister forms on top of pimple which turns to scab in about 4 days. Rash covers whole surface of body including scalp.
Diphtheria Diphtheria bacillus. In secretions of nose and throat of infected person or carrier.	By direct contact with infected person or carrier, or by contact with articles infected by patient or carrier, or through contaminated milk.	Usually 2 to 6 days	Period of contagion varies – usually 2 weeks or less. Contagion considered over when 3 successive nose and throat cultures are negative at intervals of 24 hours.	None.
German measles Virus in secretions of nose and throat of infected person.	By direct contact with person who has the disease.	14 to 25 days (usually 17th or 18th day)	From start of symptoms to at least 4 days after. Contagion considered over 3 days after onset of rash.	Rash which is pink and mottled usually appears first on face and neck and works down, covering whole body in 12 to 24 hours.
Infective hepatitis Hepatitis virus in faeces and possibly in secretions of nose and throat of infected person.	Mostly by faeces of infected person. Possibly contracted by nose and throat secretions of infected person.	10 to 50 days (average 25 days)	Unknown. Virus may be in faeces 2 to 3 weeks before onset of disease and at least during acute stage.	None.
Influenza Influenza viruses. Usually Type A, Type B, or Asian type, in secretions of nose and throat of infected person.	By direct contact with infected person, or by articles recently contaminated by infected person.	Usually 1 to 3 days.	Shortly before and up to 1 week after onset of symptoms.	None.
Measles Virus in secretions of nose and throat of infected person.	By direct contact with person who has the disease.	7 to 14 days (usually 10 days)	From 4 days before until 5 days after rash appears.	Mottled pink rash appearing first on face and neck and extending down over whole body within 3 days. Then starts fading from head down.
Meningitis Viral meningitis: virus in secretions of nose and throat of infected person. Bacterial meningitis: due to variety of bacteria, only meningococcal meningitis is regarded as an infectious disease.	By direct contact with infected person or carrier.	1 to 10 days (usually 3 to 7 days)	As long as the bacteria remain in the nose and throat of infected person.	Tiny dark red spots appearing mainly on trunk and buttocks in about 40% of cases (meningococcal meningitis only).

Signs and symptoms	Treatment	Care of exposed people	Immunization (Prophylactic)
Chickenpox Usually fever and headache, followed by appearance of rash within 24 hours. Rash fully out in 2 to 3 days, followed by drop in temperature. Itching of lesions usually subsides by 4th day.	No specific treatment. Cut fingernails, apply drying and anti-itching lotion such as calamine lotion with 10 per cent phenol, anti-itching baths. Antihistamines by mouth may also be helpful.	None. Patients on continuous steroid or anti-cancer treatment should avoid contact.	None.
Diphtheria Headache, fever, and sore throat with confluent white exudate forming over tonsils, throat, and soft palate. Fever around 39°C. There may be difficulty swallowing, a croupy cough, and bloody discharge from nose.	Diphtheria antitoxin. Penicillin. Erythromycin.	Penicillin by injection and also by mouth for 5 to 7 days.	Diphtheria toxoid with booster inoculations given at periodic intervals.
German measles Symptoms usually mild, with low grade fever and occasional headache. There are usually swollen glands behind neck and on back of head. These appear either before or during appearance of rash. Eyes may be slightly inflamed.	No specific treatment.	Usually none given or desired except for women exposed in first 3 months of pregnancy. A blood test should be made to see whether or not they have immunity.	Live German measles vaccine will immunize for long periods of time but the degree and duration of immunity is not fully determined. It should be given to all girls approaching puberty.
Infective hepatitis Early signs are malaise, weakness, headache, and loss of appetite. Then right upper abdominal discomfort and pain, nausea, and vomiting usually occur. Urine is dark, faeces light-coloured. Soon afterwards jaundice appears.	None specific. In severe cases with liver damage, corticosteroids may be used.	Injections of gamma globulin usually protect for 5 weeks or longer.	Temporary immunization for 5 weeks or longer may be obtained with injections of gamma globulin.
Influenza Usually sudden onset with headache, malaise, chills, and aches and pains in arms, legs, and back. Nose congested. Hard, dry cough common. Duration approximately 3 days.	No specific treatment.	None.	Polyvalent vaccine against known viruses causing influenza. Yearly booster injection to maintain immunity.
Measles Fever usually 3 or 4 days, followed by hard dry cough, red eyes, and running nose. Tiny white spots (Koplik spots) then appear on inner cheeks, gums, and palate. Then fever rises high as rash appears and continues for several days until rash has covered body. Then fever drops, cough subsides, and eyes clear as rash subsides.	No specific treatment. Antibiotics often used to prevent complications.	Measles may be prevented or modified by injections of gamma globulin during incubation period. Treatment must be early to prevent the disease. Gamma globulin of no help once symptoms have appeared.	Live measles virus vaccine will immunize for long period, possibly for life. May develop a fever in 6 to 8 days. Killed measles virus vaccine protects for 2 to 3 years. No reactions.
Meningitis Fever, headache, vomiting. Later, delirium and loss of consciousness. Stiffness of neck is a common sign, the child being unable to put chin on chest.	Viral meningitis which is commoner than bacterial meningitis requires no treatment. Intensive antibiotic treatment directed at the specific organism causing the infection is required in bacterial meningitis.	Penicillin, sulphonamides, or erythromycin by mouth as prescribed by doctor in cases of meningococcal meningitis.	None.

Infectious diseases

Source	Mode of transmission	Incubation period	Period of contagion	Type of rash
Mumps Virus of mumps in saliva of infected person.	By direct contact with person who has the disease.	14 to 21 days (average 17 days)	Until swelling of affected glands has completely subsided.	None.
Poliomyelitis Poliomyelitis virus in faeces, and material from nose and throat of patient or carrier.	By direct contact with patient or carrier, or by contact with faeces of patient.	Usually 7 to 14 days but may be less.	Not known. At least 5 days from nose and throat secretions. Virus may be present in faeces for several weeks.	None.
Roseola infantum Virus probably in nose and throat secretions of infected person or carrier.	Not known, but probably by direct contact with infected person or carrier.	Not known.	Not known.	A mottled measles-like rash which may be faint or bright pink, usually covering the body within 24 hours after appearance.

Scarlet fever – see page 293

Source	Mode of transmission	Incubation period	Period of contagion	Type of rash
***Smallpox** Virus of smallpox.	Contact with patient, either direct or indirect. Infection may come from lesions of patient, clothing of patient, or air surrounding patient.	8 to 16 days (usually 12 days)	From first symptoms until all scabs have been shed.	First, small dark red spots which form pimples appear over body. On the 5th or 6th day fluid appears in these lesions and blisters form, each about the size of a pea and surrounded by red area. Blisters are dimpled. By the 9th day, fluid turns to pus. Then pus dries and scabs form.
Typhoid and Paratyphoid fever Salmonella bacteria	From faeces and urine of infected person or carrier, either directly or indirectly from water, contaminated milk, food, shellfish.	7 to 21 days (average 14 days)	As long as patient or carrier harbours the typhoid organisms in faeces or urine.	Usually scanty pink spots on trunk (rose spots) a few days after onset of symptoms.
Tetanus Tetanus bacillus.	Usually occurs through infected wounds.	3 to 21 days (average 10 days)	None.	None.

* Smallpox has now been almost eradicated from the world due to a tremendous effort by local health authorities coordinated by the World Health Organi

Signs and symptoms	Treatment	Care of exposed people	Immunization (Prophylactic)
Mumps Occasionally fever and vomiting, but often no signs or symptoms before tender swelling appears in front of and below ear. Usually on one side first, swelling on other side of face appearing in 2 or 3 days.	No specific treatment recommended in infants and children.	None.	Live mumps vaccine gives long immunity but is not usually recommended in Britain as the disease is mild.
Poliomyelitis Usually starts with fever, vomiting, and irritability. These may subside after several days. Then usually a flare-up occurs after 2 or 3 days, with severe headache, fever of around 39°C, and a stiffness of neck and back. Pain in affected muscles follows. Paralysis occurs in 10 to 15 per cent of cases.	None specific.	None of proved value. Gamma globulin has been used but effectiveness is questionable.	Sabin oral live polio vaccine usually protects for life.
Roseola infantum Sudden onset of high fever, often over 40°C. Usually child does not appear very ill. No physical signs as a rule, except slight red throat. After 3 or 4 days of fever, temperature drops to normal, rash appears, and child is well.	No specific treatment.	None.	None.
Smallpox Headache, backache, fever, and characteristic rash.	No specific treatment. Antibiotics may be given to lessen scarring from secondary bacterial infection.	Immediate vaccination.	Smallpox vaccine repeated every 3 years.
Typhoid and Paratyphoid fever Onset usually with fever, headache, malaise, loss of appetite, backache, and bronchitis. Diarrhoea is usually present but not always. Mild abdominal tenderness and distension also are common symptoms. Condition usually lasts 1 to 3 weeks.	Appropriate antibiotics.	None. Family contacts excluded as food handlers until 3 successive negative tests of faeces and urine.	3 doses of typhoid vaccine given by injection at weekly intervals. Booster every 2 years.
Tetanus Increasing stiffness of jaw until difficult to open mouth. Later, stiffness of back and abdominal muscles with neck thrown back and back curved in. Spasms of muscles are excruciatingly painful.	Tetanus antitoxin, sedatives, sometimes tracheostomy, and artificial respiration.	Not necessary.	Tetanus toxoid, 2 injections at intervals of 1 month. Booster every few years. For immediate immunization of those not protected by tetanus toxoid, tetanus antitoxin is given.

Infectious diseases

Source	Mode of transmission	Incubation period	Period of contagion	Type of rash
Tuberculosis Tubercle bacillus from sputum of infected person.	Cough droplets from sputum of infected person. Can also be spread through articles contaminated by such sputum or bacteria.	Approximately 3 to 8 weeks from time of infection to signs of tuberculin allergy as shown by skin tests.	Children with first infection type of tuberculosis are generally not contagious. Children who develop tuberculous lung cavities (very rare) or with draining tuberculous sinuses are contagious as long as tubercle bacilli are present in sputum or drainage.	None.
Whooping cough Whooping cough (pertussis) bacillus.	Discharges from mouth and cough of infected person. Almost always by direct contact or by objects freshly moistened.	5 to 21 days (usually under 10 days)	Contagiousness greatest in early stages before severe cough becomes paroxysmal (repetitive). Contagion is believed to last 6 weeks from onset.	None.

Infectious diseases

Communicable diseases listed in the chart are for the most part preventable by timely vaccination. Some of the diseases are relatively uncommon and immunization is desirable only under conditions of susceptibility or exposure, which should be determined by a doctor. Influenza vaccine is not used routinely but is generally restricted to high-risk patients and those with respiratory disease.

Intussusception

This is a serious condition most commonly seen in children under the age of two (the average age is seven months). It is caused by one portion of the intestine pushing inside the next segment. The pressure of the outside intestine compresses the blood vessels of the inner loop, cutting off the local blood supply. (See illustration on page 346.) If not relieved quickly, the inner portion of the loop may become gangrenous. This condition is twice as common in boys as in girls.

The child cries out suddenly with violent abdominal cramps and then starts vomiting. The cramps subside and then occur again at fairly regular intervals, generally leaving the child weak and limp. The telltale and most frequent sign of intussusception is blood in the stools. At times only a slight discharge of blood is passed by the rectum, but more frequently there is a mixture of blood and mucus which resembles red-currant jelly.

Intussusception is an acute emergency and a doctor should be called immediately, for unless the condition is relieved it may prove fatal. Often the physician can feel the mass in the abdomen caused by the enlargement of the intestine. In rare instances it will subside under manipulation by the doctor. At other times it will subside when the child is given a diagnostic barium enema before X-ray examination. If the intussusception is not relieved, an immediate operation is necessary. Time is very important, for if one waits too long and gangrene occurs, an amputation of part of the intestine may be necessary. This is a serious and critical operation for a small child who is already extremely ill and completely exhausted.

Signs and symptoms	Treatment	Care of exposed people	Immunization (Prophylactic)
Tuberculosis Usually little or no specific signs or symptoms of the first infection type of tuberculosis, the type usually seen in children. The signs and symptoms may be only those of a mild infection with low grade fever and a dry cough. Complications such as an infection through the bloodstream will produce more severe symptoms.	Isoniazid is the treatment of choice and should be given for at least a year. A newer drug, rifampicin, has shown great effectiveness in tuberculosis. In severe cases, one of the drugs may be combined with streptomycin and para amino-salicylic acid.	Repeated tuberculin tests and X-rays if tests are found positive.	BCG vaccination is at present offered to three groups of children: tuberculin negative (Heaf or Mantoux testing) contacts of active cases; tuberculin negative schoolchildren at age 13; and newborn babies born into high risk groups such as a family history of tuberculosis or immigrants (West Indians and Asians). It is then given on the 2nd or 3rd day of life.
Whooping cough Onset insidious with simple dry cough. As disease progresses, cough gets more severe at night. At about the third week cough becomes very severe, spasmodic, and paroxysmal (repetitive), during which the child may lose breath and become blue. At end of paroxysmal cough there is a long crowing inspiration (the whoop of whooping cough). Vomiting may occur.	Ampicillin or amoxycillin (which should be given early) may be helpful in preventing complications. Severe cases particularly in the first 6 months of life require hospital treatment. Improvement occurs after 3 weeks.	When a child develops whooping cough, it is probably too late to immunize his brothers and sisters if they have not already received vaccine.	3 doses of pertussis vaccine injected at intervals of at least 1 month.

Jaundice of the newborn

The child in the womb is living as if in thin air (comparable to Mount Everest, 9043 m). In order to increase its oxygen carrying capacity his blood carries twice as many red cells as it will after birth. When the lungs take over from the placenta at the moment of birth, the body sheds its spare red cells, retaining the iron and the protein. The remaining pigment is broken down through various steps to bilirubin. This is deposited in the skin, teeth, bones, and whites of the eyes, and, rarely, if the concentration is high enough, in the brain, especially in the basal ganglia where it can produce mental retardation, spasticity, and deafness. Exchange transfusion is seldom required. In 1958 it was noticed that babies in a sunny nursery lost their jaundice, and nowadays artificial daylight is used (phototherapy). The body has its own mechanisms for excretion of the bile pigment through the liver into the duodenum, where it is responsible for the normal yellowish colour of the stool. It is only when this mechanism is overloaded that phototherapy is used. Dehydration, prematurity, or bruising over the head which may occur with strong labour pains, increase jaundice. Follow-up studies have shown no adverse effects from the ordinary jaundice of the newborn.

Leukaemia and malignant disease (cancer)

Now that the former major killing diseases of childhood, acute bacterial infections, tuberculosis, and gastroenteritis, can be successfully treated, accidents and malignant disease have become the most common causes of death in children over the age of five (ten and five respectively per 100,000 per year). Acute lymphoblastic leukaemia is the commonest malignancy of childhood. A previously healthy school child becomes listless and very pale, and bruises, large and small, appear. Spontaneous bruising in an otherwise healthy nonanaemic child is much more common and is benign. The diagnosis of leukaemia is confirmed by (after anaesthesia) inserting a strong needle into a bone (usually the crest of the hipbone) and sucking some of the marrow into a syringe for staining and microscopy.

The child will then be entered on a treatment schedule which in most cases will be one of those designed by the Medical Research Council. Remission of the disease is induced by a combination of several drugs. More than 90 per cent success is achieved at this stage. After this, the child will receive two to three weeks X-ray treatment to the head, and a series of injections of methotrexate into the spinal canal by lumbar puncture (again a general anaesthetic is usually used). This is central nervous system prophylaxis and kills leukaemic cells which are not reached by the drugs already given by mouth or by injection. Finally, a twelve week repeating cycle of maintenance treatment is begun, and continued for two-and-a-half to three years. At present 60 per cent of children with acute leukaemia are alive and well at the end of their treatment.

This makes it all sound simple but it is a punishing time for parents and patient alike, and both need a lot of support. Leukaemia is regarded with morbid curiosity by many people, and it is better to keep the diagnosis strictly within the family circle. Other forms of cancer in childhood are so rare that a chapter like this cannot take account of them, but all are now treated by a combination of surgery and chemotherapy, and the outlook has improved. Joining the local branch of the Leukaemia Society may be very helpful to parents.

Low birth weight and the premature baby

About six per cent of babies weigh less than 2,500 gm ($5\frac{1}{2}$ lb) at birth. They were previously defined as premature by the World Health Organization, but now low birth weight babies are considered as either pre-term (born before 38 weeks gestation) or "light-for-dates". Both these groups of babies are at greater risk than full-term babies weighing more than 2,500 gm, but their problems are not the same. The immature baby is more likely to have breathing problems, he cannot suck or swallow reliably, has difficulty maintaining his body temperature, and is more liable to infections. For these reasons he is often nursed in a ward in a Special Care Unit. The respiratory distress syndrome is common, but the mortality is less than in the past and with skilled nursing and other measures the outlook is good. The mother will find her baby being nursed in an incubator, fed through a fine plastic tube down the nose, and she will be asked to wash her hands and wear a gown when she handles him. She may find that he is wired up to various monitoring systems, recording his heartbeat and respirations, and sometimes his breathing will need to be assisted. It is important for her to be able to see him, touch him, and smell him, handle and feed him whenever possible, and feel that he is really hers even when much of his care has to be in the hands of nurses. If she has to leave hospital without him she can keep in touch by visits and the telephone. Expressing and bringing in her breast milk for him is something she can do that the nurses cannot. In many units, not only fathers but older brothers and sisters are encouraged to visit, so that the new baby is fully a member of the family from the start. Research has shown that nowadays most premature babies who survive do just as well in the long run as full-term babies. When the baby comes home, do not be afraid to handle and enjoy him just as you would a bigger baby, but remember to give him the iron and vitamins that you will be supplied with.

Masturbation

"We all enjoy it but we do it in private". This message can begin to be got across to the child when he begins to emerge from innocence to the age of self-consciousness (say two to three) but before this age parents can be safely reassured that the habit is harmless and that attempts to discourage handling and exploring are not necessary. Let us help children to grow up feeling less guilty about it than we did ourselves.

Mongolism

See under Down's syndrome.

Nappy rash

Almost every baby has a nappy rash at one time or another. It is not dangerous but can cause considerable discomfort. A nappy rash is really an ammonia burn. The urine, which does not contain ammonia when it is passed, is acted upon by bacteria on the skin which break up the urea in the urine, causing the formation of ammonia. Prevent nappy rash by removing wet nappies as soon as possible, washing and drying the bottom carefully before putting on a clean nappy, and using a little powder or cream. If nappy rash develops, leave the bottom exposed if the surroundings are warm. A one way nappy liner is useful. This is a siliconized cotton liner through which urine passes without wetting it, into the absorbent nappy outside. The liner in contact with the baby's bottom remains dry so helping the rash to heal. Gentle antiseptics, such as benzalkonium, kill ammonia-producing bacteria and can be used as a cream and as a nappy rinse.

Parents and the law

From *Children in Britain (1976)*, **a booklet from the British Information Services**

Parental rights and duties

Rights of natural parents   In England, Wales, and Scotland the father and the mother both have equal rights of guardianship over their *legitimate* children up to the age of eighteen. They have equal rights to take decisions about the upbringing of children (for example, the education of the child or the religion in which the child is to be brought up). Consent has to be given by both parents to adoption of their child or (except in Scotland) to the marriage of a person aged under eighteen. Equal rights of guardianship were introduced by the Guardianship Act 1973; previously the father was recognized as the natural guardian.

If there is a fundamental disagreement between the mother and the father over the upbringing of the child, either may bring the matter before a magistrates court or a county court. In such a case the parent may apply either for a decision on the matter in dispute or to be awarded sole custody and/or care and control of the child. The court, when taking its decision, must have the welfare of the child as its prime consideration. It makes such orders as it thinks fit regarding custody and the right of access to the child by either parent. When hearing an application for custody, the court may also ask for a social inquiry report from a local authority or probation officer; or commit the child to the care of a local authority, if it appears to the court that there are exceptional circumstances making it impracticable or undesirable for the child to be entrusted to either parent or to any other individual.

In England and Wales the Matrimonial Proceedings and Property Act 1970 makes provision for the welfare of children of parents who become parties to divorce proceedings or judicial separation. Similar provisions for Scotland are in the Matrimonial Proceedings (Children) Act 1958. A divorce court is required to satisfy itself about the custody and care of any child of the marriage. The welfare of the child is the paramount consideration and there is no presumption in favour of either spouse. The court is not bound to commit custody to either party and may in exceptional circumstances commit a child to the care of a local authority, or order that he should be placed under the supervision of a probation officer or social worker. If custody is given to the mother, or some third person, or if the child is committed to local authority care, the court may require the father to contribute to the child's maintenance; in some cases, where custody is not given to the mother, she too may be required to contribute to the child's maintenance. Parents enjoy equal rights of application to the court on matters relating to their children.

Under the Matrimonial Proceedings and Property Act courts have wide powers to order financial provision for children. Financial remedies operate in the interests of husbands and wives equally. Payments made generally continue until the child's first birthday after reaching the school-leaving age of sixteen, although they can be extended if the child remains in education or training.

A marriage between persons either of whom is under the age of sixteen is void. In England and Wales young people between the ages of sixteen and eighteen, unless already widowed, must usually obtain the consent of the parent or guardian to their marriage and, if this consent is refused, a court may give it instead if it thinks fit. No parental consent is required in Scotland for children of sixteen and over.

Illegitimacy   A child born to parents who are not married to each other is illegitimate. There is a legal presumption that a child born to a woman during her marriage is the legitimate child of her husband, unless they are living apart under a decree of judicial separation or (in England and Wales) in accordance with the order of a magistrates court. This presumption can be rebutted only by evidence showing beyond reasonable doubt that the husband could not have been the child's father.

The mother of an illegitimate child has the right of custody of the child and the right to determine his religion. She has a duty, as long as she is single or a widow or separated from her husband, to maintain the child until he is sixteen. The mother may apply to a court of summary jurisdiction for an affiliation order against the man alleged to be the father. If the court grants the order, the father may be ordered to contribute a limited* sum to the child's maintenance up to the age of thirteen, or sixteen if the court so directs, or, in the case of a child engaged in a course of education or training, the court may direct that payments be made until the child reaches the age of 21. In Northern Ireland, the order continues in force until the child, if a boy, attains the age of fifteen years, or, if a girl, the age of sixteen.

Under the Legitimacy Act 1959, in England and Wales, either parent of an illegitimate child may bring guardianship proceedings for the custody of, or access to, the child (but the court may not in these proceedings make any order for maintenance, this being exclusively a matter for affiliation proceedings).

In England, Wales, and Scotland a child may be made legitimate by the marriage of its parents to each other after its birth. (If the child has in the meantime been adopted by one or both of its parents, they may then apply for the adoption to be revoked and the entry deleted from the Adopted Children Register). The position in Northern Ireland is similar. Throughout the United Kingdom legitimation is subject to certain conditions as to the father's domicile.

Under the Family Law Reform Act 1969 an illegitimate child and his parents have the same right to share in each other's estates on an intestacy as if the child were legitimate. Illegitimate children also have the right to apply to the court for provision out of the estate of their parents. Similar provisions in Scotland were enacted by the Law Reform (Miscellaneous Provisions) (Scotland) Act 1968.

The Births and Deaths Registration Act 1953 and the Registration of Births, Deaths and Marriages (Scotland) Act 1965 make provision for a short form of birth certificate which contains no particulars of parentage, and thus does not disclose an illegitimate birth. Northern Ireland has similar legislation in the form of the Births and Deaths Registration Act (Northern Ireland) 1967.

Offences against children The principal statutes dealing with the prevention of cruelty to children are the Children and Young Persons Act 1933, and the corresponding Acts of 1937 and 1968 for Scotland and Northern Ireland respectively. These Acts make it an offence punishable by fine or imprisonment for any person over sixteen years of age who has the custody, charge, or care of any child or young person under sixteen years of age, wilfully to assault, illtreat,

neglect, abandon, or expose him, or cause or procure him to be assaulted, illtreated, neglected, abandoned, or exposed in a manner likely to cause him unnecessary suffering or injury to health. The Acts also define other specific offences, for example, to cause or allow persons under sixteen to be used for begging; to give intoxicating liquor to children under five (fourteen in Northern Ireland); to cause or allow children under fourteen to be in bars of licensed premises*; to sell tobacco to persons under sixteen (not applicable in Northern Ireland); to expose children under twelve (seven in Scotland and Northern Ireland) to the risk of burning; and to fail to provide for the safety of children at entertainments. It is an offence under the Sexual Offences Act 1956 to cause or encourage the seduction or prostitution of girls under sixteen. Regulations made under the Consumer Protection Act 1961 require nightdresses designed for children to be made of material which meets a prescribed standard of low flammability.

The Offences Against the Person Act 1861, and other statutes and the common law also specify other offences involving harm to persons, including children. These offences are crimes such as homicide, including the special offence in England and Wales of infanticide (where a mother causes the death of her child under twelve months of age when she has not recovered from her confinement); the sexual offences of rape, incest, and indecent assault; and other assaults.

Employment of children and young people
Restrictions arising out of international conventions of 1919 and 1920 on the employment of children and young persons in industrial undertakings, including mines, factories, building and engineering construction works, railways and transport undertakings, are contained in the Employment of Women, Young Persons and Children Act 1920. They include a general prohibition of the employment in these undertakings of children below the limit of compulsory school age; this prohibition also applies to the employment of children in ships at sea, except when only members of the same family are employed upon the vessel, or it is approved work on a school or training ship.

The law on the employment of children in England and Wales is contained mainly in the Children and Young Persons Act 1933 as amended by the Education Acts 1944–62 and the Children and Young

---

* In Scotland no limit is prescribed to the amount which the court may order the father to contribute to the child's maintenance.

* In Scotland, this provision is effected by the Licensing (Scotland) Act 1962 and in Northern Ireland by the Licensing Act (Northern Ireland) 1971 which specifies an age limit of eighteen years.

Persons Act 1963 and the Children Act 1972. The responsible Government departments are the Department of Health and Social Security and the Welsh Office. In general, the legislation imposes considerable restriction on the employment of children under school-leaving age, but gives local education authorities power to make by-laws modifying or supplementing the statutory provisions in certain respects.

The employment of a child is prohibited until he has attained the age of thirteen (unless authority is given in local by-laws for him to be employed by his parent or guardian in light agricultural or horticultural work). From the age of thirteen, while still at school, he may not be employed before the close of school hours on any day on which he is required to attend school (unless local by-laws authorise his employment for not more than one hour before school hours); before seven o'clock in the morning or after seven o'clock in the evening of any day; for more than two hours on any day on which he is required to attend school or on any Sunday; nor may he be required to lift, carry, or move heavy objects likely to cause him injury.

By-laws made by local authorities may prohibit absolutely the employment of children in any specified occupation or may prescribe conditions, such as the age below which children are not to be employed (they can prescribe a later minimum age than that provided by the Act), the maximum number of hours to be worked, the meal and rest intervals, and the holidays to be allowed. Local education authorities are not compelled to make by-laws about the employment of children, but all of them have done so. The by-laws do not become law until they have been confirmed by the Secretary of State. Commonly they prohibit occupations considered unsuitable for children, such as employment in a barber's shop, in the kitchens of catering shops, as attendants in billiard saloons, in slaughterhouses, and so on. All by-laws that permit employment (usually in the delivery of milk or newspapers) before school impose a condition that the employment shall not begin before seven o'clock in the morning. A by-law widely in force requires the child to be medically examined before he can be employed. Many authorities have fixed a maximum of five hours' work a day on school holidays and a weekly maximum of 25 hours.

Under the Education Act 1944 a local education authority has power to prevent, or impose restrictions on, the employment of a child if the employment is prejudicial to the child's health or renders him unfit to obtain the full benefit of his education.

The position in Scotland is substantially the same as in England and Wales. The central authority is the Scottish Education Department, while local administration is in the hands of education authorities.

In Northern Ireland the control of the employment of children is mainly governed by the Children and Young Persons Act (Northern Ireland) 1968 and by-laws.

The minimum intervals which must be allowed for meals are specified. The employment of young persons at night is generally prohibited but young men aged sixteen and over may be employed at night in certain circumstances. In Northern Ireland no child under minimum school-leaving age may be employed in any industrial undertaking; young persons under eighteen can be so employed only if they are certified as fit for work at the particular process.

The hours of work of young shopworkers are limited under the Shops Act 1950 to 44 hours a week for those under sixteen and 48 hours for those between sixteen and eighteen. The Shops Act (Northern Ireland) 1946 limits the work of young people up to the age of sixteen to 40 hours in a week. Those aged between sixteen and eighteen are limited to 44 hours.

Prematurity

See Low birth weight.

Punishment and discipline

Rewards for good behaviour are more effective in bringing up children (and training animals) than punishments for doing wrong. Rewards need not be more than a word or pat of praise; let them come often. Punishments have their place too, but let them be few and far between. They are more effective if not used too often. Ignore minor naughtiness; this works. There can be strict discipline without severe punishment, and lots of punishment without discipline. Discipline can be strict and regimented, or it can be lax and permissive, and again normal emotionally healthy children will emerge at the end of either system, provided it is consistent and provided there is a little love with it. What leaves a child floundering is capricious punishment, being rebuked one day and getting away with similar behaviour the next. That way he can never construct for himself a view of society which makes any sense. Society, which to a young child is the family, must stick to its own rules. Mother and father should try to adopt roughly similar standards for their expectations of the child. Positive rules in a family work better than negative ones. "Tell the truth", rather than "don't lie". "Be fair", rather than "don't cheat". "Be safe", rather than "don't go near the fire". "Keep calm", rather than "don't lose your temper". Grown-ups must lead the way by keeping to the rules themselves.

Corporal punishment   This is a controversial and emotive question. Parents, doctors, and educationalists are deeply divided, for and against. Both sides can claim successes for their methods, but both have to admit failures. Fortunately, children are resilient and most come to no harm from either method. It is clearly difficult for the Family Medical Guide to come down firmly on one side or the other.* Parents should make up their minds in the light of their own experience, what they have read and heard about the problem, and all the circumstances of each case. All agree that babies under a year old should never be smacked; there is too much risk of injury.

Pyloric stenosis

The pylorus is a ring of muscular tissue and mucous membrane which surrounds the opening between the stomach and the duodenum. The pylorus opens and closes periodically to control the passage of the stomach contents into the duodenum. In pyloric stenosis the pyloric muscle is too thick and obstructs the opening at the end of the stomach so that food is unable to pass into the intestines. The food is then vomited out with great force. The condition is four times more common in boys than in girls. Vomiting usually does not commence until the infant is between eight and fourteen days of age, and from that time the vomiting becomes marked and very forceful. Medication is rarely of help. The child becomes extremely hungry and the stools become very small and infrequent. There is progressive weight loss and dehydration becomes more and more pronounced. On examination a physician can usually feel the pyloric mass. The condition is completely relieved by an operation which cuts some of the muscle fibres of the pylorus. The cause of pyloric stenosis is unknown. It does tend to run in families and there is about a one

* It is only right to add that the reviser of this chapter is not in favour of corporal punishment. (Editor)

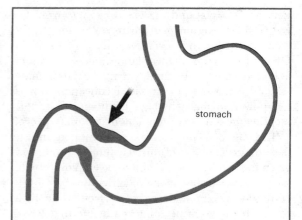

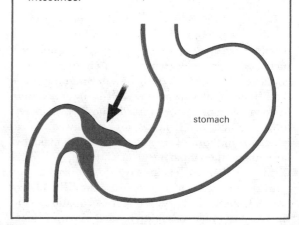

The pylorus is a ring of muscular tissue which surrounds the opening between the stomach and the duodenum. The pylorus opens and closes periodically to control the passage of some of the stomach contents into the duodenum. Above, a normal pylorus. Below, pyloric stenosis – the muscle is abnormally thick, preventing food from entering the intestines.

in eight risk that subsequent babies will be affected; there is a similar likelihood that a child may be affected if the mother or father has had the condition. Pyloric stenosis does not affect babies after the age of twelve to fourteen weeks.

Rocking and head banging

These repetitive, sometimes apparently compulsive and even obsessional habits worry parents. They are less common than formerly; they are gratification habits, among which may be included thumb sucking, nail biting, nose picking, and masturbation.

Excessive rocking is seen, for instance, in deprived and bored children in hospitals and institutions and may indicate the need for extra play and stimulation. Sometimes you may see caged animals at the Zoo doing it, and it is a solitary, inward-directed, and society-rejecting symptom. Mentally handicapped children and autistic children do it. Despite this statement parents must not immediately conclude that such a child is handicapped; of course this is not true. If a perfectly normal toddler learns to rock his cot, and drive his parents mad with the squeak, take courage and an oil can. If necessary screw the legs of the cot to the floor, for your own piece of mind, and be assured that it is a passing phase.

Rubella in pregnancy
(German measles)

Maternal rubella (German measles) during the first three months of pregnancy carries something like a 40 per cent chance of causing damage to the fetus. Deafness, eye cataracts, congenital heart disease, and mental retardation are the commonest effects, but there is a much wider syndrome affecting liver, blood-forming organs, and bones. Congenital rubella is a disaster, but fortunately women can be immunized against it and every parent should make sure that her daughters are protected before they reach child-bearing age. Rubella vaccination is offered at present to schoolgirls at the age of thirteen to fourteen. A past history of an attack of German measles is not a reason for omitting it, as many virus infections can produce a rash indistinguishable from that of rubella. A blood test can, if necessary, be carried out to show whether a person has naturally acquired resistance, and this should in any case be done as soon as a woman knows she is pregnant. If she is not immune, and comes into contact with the disease, a further blood test will show whether she has acquired the infection. If this is within the first three months of pregnancy, she can be offered an abortion. Babies born with the effects of rubella may excrete the virus in their urine for up to a year, so it is important that nurses who may become pregnant while looking after them should be protected by immunization.

Scarlet fever
(Scarlatina)

Scarlet fever is nowadays an uncommon infection. It is caused by strains of streptococcus germs which produce a toxin to which some children are susceptible and some are not. The distinctive feature is a red rash followed by peeling of the skin. Otherwise, the manifestations of scarlet fever are the same as those of other streptococcal infections such as sore throat. In fact, streptococcal throat can be thought of as scarlet fever without a rash. Symptoms of scarlet fever – irritability, fever, sore throat, vomiting – are usually sudden in onset. These are followed in a day or so by the appearance of bright red spots and a rash, usually beginning in the neck, chest, and back areas, which may spread to the entire body except the head. The skin around the mouth is pale, and the tongue bright red. After the rash fades, in about a week, the skin begins to peel off in fine flakes or in larger pieces. Thick parts of the skin may continue to peel for several weeks.

In addition to bed rest, treatment generally includes use of an antibiotic to which streptococci are susceptible, such as penicillin. The antibiotic has no effect on the toxin that causes the rash, but it does limit the infection. Most cases of scarlet fever today are quite mild. Sometimes the rash is such a slight blush that it is barely perceptible. For reasons unknown, scarlet fever has become a much less severe disease than it used to be in past generations when it was greatly feared. Nowadays, serious complications are uncommon, although proper care to watch for and prevent them is important.

Earache or inflamed glands of the neck are possible complications that parents should watch for. Rarely, scarlet fever or streptococcal throat may be followed by rheumatic fever or may reactivate the disease. Patients should be under a doctor's care. There is no prevention for such throats, but antibiotics may limit the advance of the disease following exposure and restrict its spread within the household.

School refusal and school phobia

Going to school is usually the first long-term and repeated separation from parents that children experience and it is natural for it to make them anxious. Most overcome it satisfactorily, but a few tears are usual at the start. Parents need to be particularly patient and reassuring at this time, though impatience is the usual reaction because it is always a busy time. Parents have to be ready for work, children dressed, and all the time the clock is hurrying round to nine o'clock. Sometimes it happens that a child has been going happily to school for some years and suddenly loses confidence. It may be a change of teacher, class, or school. Try to let the child see that you understand and identify with his suffering. "I know going to school sometimes makes you feel sad, but there are some hard things we all have to do", is better than: "You're going to go and that's that", or calling him a baby. It is usually best to be firm about this but the treatment is not the same for all children, and it can be a difficult problem. A preliminary exploration of possible causes with the teacher is a good idea. If the child claims to be ill, with sore throat, headache, or stomach-ache and is not obviously ill it is probably better to take him to school, mention his symptoms to the teacher, and ask her to let you know if he really cannot manage. Another time the child has genuinely been ill but even when he is physically better he feels faint-hearted about going back to school. Here again it is best to get him to school and explain the problem to the teacher. A consultation with the family doctor may help.

In older children school refusal may merge into an acute school phobia, an apparently unreasoning and disproportionate fear of school when the rest of daily living is coped with adequately. Here the help of your family doctor or even specialist psychiatric help may be needed.

Bullying in school is a different matter. It is wrong that children should suffer this and a school with a good name to maintain will not tolerate it. Usually the problem can be solved by firm action by the school authorities. Never let the child's fear of reprisals deter you from seeking help for him. Bullying which takes place outside school boundaries, for instance on the bus, will usually be accepted by teachers as part of their responsibility; but if not a direct approach parent-to-parent will often effect a cure. One father of a bullied patient was surprised at his sympathetic reception by the father of his child's tormentor, who took his side at once and could hardly be restrained from thrashing the bully on the spot. If bullying continues to occur, there should be no hesitation in complaining to the police.

Only if these measures fail should a change of school be sought, and your family doctor, School Medical Officer, and Area Education Officer would help with the decision.

Sleeping problems

All mothers (and fathers too) have some bad nights with some of their babies. Most people cope with it fairly well, but continued loss of sleep can bring a mother to the verge of breakdown. Her own distress communicates itself to the baby, and a vicious spiral is set up. Breaking this spiral is difficult, but it is helpful if she can restore herself by two or three nights of uninterrupted sleep through her husband offering to go on night duty (for example, at a weekend) and even by a small dose of a sleeping drug from her doctor. Sympathy and support from her family and health visitor are needed. A warm well-fed baby in a dry nappy usually sleeps well but some infants and particularly toddlers, can reduce their mothers to resentful servility by their demands. Such demands are particularly hard to resist in a shared house or with elderly or uncongenial neighbours. This situation may require a moment in which parents must decide not to pick the baby up, bring him drinks, or allow him downstairs – whatever the cost. It is a good idea to warn the neighbours first. The treatment succeeds within two or at most three nights and relief is usually permanent.

Speech problems (speech delay, stammering)

Learning to talk is a continuous process, and there is no normal age below which a child does not talk and after which he does. However, speech delay is a common problem for which parents seek advice. The worst type of speech delay is that due to deafness and every child should have a screening test of hearing around seven months. At a year to one and a half a child will spontaneously use words with meaning, perhaps half a dozen sounds which may not be clear words but are used consistently to refer to different objects. A two year old will probably have 20 to 30 different words and begin stringing them together. Talk to your baby. It may sound daft, but it is good to chat to him if you are alone in the house together, explaining this and that, even though much of it is above his head. You can do this right from the start, when you are feeding him. A mother who talks to her baby a lot will diagnose deafness early, when instead of babbling back to her at five to six months old, he makes no sound. Speech delay may be part of overall delay in a mentally handicapped child. Even in these cases the more speech he hears from you the better.

Do not worry if your older child (two to three) does not form his words properly. It is quantity, not quality that counts at this age. Correct him by saying his wrong words right but let him come to it in his own time. Do not inhibit him by telling him "No, not poon, *spoon*". Better: "Yes, that is your *spoon*". Later he will learn to tidy up his pronunciation, but fluency is the thing to go for at the start. Expect infantile forms till five or six; it is normal.

Stammering is another phase that many normal speakers have gone through. Here again self consciousness is a heavy secondary handicap which too vigorous correction can make worse. Never mock at or copy your child's stammer and, after explaining the reason, forbid it also to other members of the family and elicit their sympathy. This applies to school too. Children are said to be cruel but explaining a handicapped child's needs to the class usually results in a tremendous supporting effort by the others.

A persistent stammer needs professional help from a speech therapist who is available through schools, clinics, hospitals, and in many places through the family doctor. The speech therapist indeed likes to be contacted about all speech problems even in the toddler age group.

Squint

Binocular vision begins very early (five or six weeks) but it is not until the baby develops fine visual discrimination that most squints begin to appear, in the second year of life. The baby squints because he is not getting the same image from both eyes, and so he suppresses the poorer image, loses fixation from that eye, and it swings out of line. Soon the eye will lose its vision – the lazy eye – and it can never be regained. The younger the age at which a squint develops, the quicker vision is lost. At six months, substantial vision can be lost in a few weeks. At three years, loss of vision will be much slower, but the sooner treatment is started the better. Never leave a squint to see if it will correct itself. The child must be seen by an eye specialist as soon as possible, no matter at what age the squint is seen. Loss of vision in infancy, for instance by development of congenital cataract in one eye, may show itself by a squint, in both eyes by nystagmus, a rapid scanning movement of the eyes trying to see round the obstruction in the lens. Squints

due to refractive errors (shortsightedness or longsightedness) are treated with spectacles which correct the image on the retina; later an operation may be needed to correct residual muscle imbalance. Another cause of squint is paralysis of one of the eye muscles, which may be an early sign of raised intracranial pressure, due to a brain tumour; this is rare but must be excluded, particularly in the child who develops a squint after the age of six.

Stealing

Occasional stealing from the sweet shop is a common experience. Stolen apples taste sweet, and now that most children live in towns without ready access to neighbours' orchards, this pursuit has become an urban alternative. Peer group pressure allows group conscience, notoriously weak, to take over from individual conscience, which remains strong. Vandals seldom act alone. When your child is caught thieving it is not the end of the world. Looseness in family standards at home may have allowed him to assume that dishonesty is not always wrong. However, if stealing at home or at school becomes frequent or blatant and persists in spite of punishment, it can be a severe symptom of psychiatric problems. It is sometimes a symptom of secret guilt, the victim seeking punishment for the crime he dare not admit to, by setting up substitute crimes he is certain to be caught at. Skilled professional help may be needed.

Stomach-ache

There are lots of causes of abdominal pain – cramps during diarrhoea, acute appendicitis, kidney or bladder infections, and rarer ones like peptic ulcer or colitis. But the symptom we are considering, functional abdominal pain (where no physical cause can be found) is a specific complaint of childhood and it is by far the commonest. Functional abdominal pain is characterized by frequent brief attacks of central pain, lasting a few minutes, repeated a few or many times in a day and often at night. The child may go pale in an attack, and curls up mute and miserable till the pain passes off and he happily goes out again to play. There is no vomiting or diarrhoea and he does not lose weight or condition. The cause is unknown, but it is not a grumbling appendix. The child needs a full physical examination, and if this is negative, the doctor will explain that it is a recognized condition which is harmless. This explanation and reassurance is in many cases followed by a reduction in frequency and severity, and by eventual disappearance of the pain. Although anxiety and stress may be factors, it also affects children who are happy and well-adjusted at home and at school, and it is not part of the cure to identify psychopathology in every case.

Teething

Usually infants experience very little if any discomfort while cutting the first eight teeth – the middle four above and below, but the first four molars (the flat grinding teeth) that appear in the back of the mouth, usually between twelve and eighteen months of age, are likely to cause some pain and upset. The baby may be miserable and awaken during the night, crying. He may lose his appetite. Salivation, sore gums, increase in thumb-sucking, and some irritability are normal at this time, but general upsets (for example, diarrhoea) are not a result of teething and should be referred to the doctor. A small dose of aspirin (75 mg) or paracetamol (120 mg) is helpful. Occasionally infants develop fever during the course of teething. This is usually due to a throat or respiratory infection rather than the teething itself. Some physicians feel that during the period of teething an infant's resistance to illness is lowered.

Thrush

Thrush is a fungus infection of the mucous membrane of the mouth usually affecting young infants. It often occurs while the infant is still in the nursery but may appear at home as well. The inner cheeks, lips, gums, soft palate, and tongue have scattered patches of greyish white colour. The tongue is often heavily coated. These patches cannot be removed easily by rubbing, and when they are removed by greater pressure the tissue beneath bleeds. The infected mouth is painful and infants so infected have difficulty in feeding. Thrush is caused by a fungus (*Candida albicans*). An anti-fungal antibiotic, nystatin, given as ten drops of a suspension after feeds for five days, is usually effective. The older treatment of painting with one per cent gentian violet is also effective, but messy. A uniform white fur on the tongue (not the cheeks or palate) is commonly seen in bottle-fed babies, and is harmless.

Tongue-tie

Minor mutilation of human beings, especially children, from cutting of the uvula to circumcision, is a survival from primitive rituals based on superstition. Some of these have unfortunately been adopted as medically expedient. The fold of skin under the tongue (lingual fraenum) which helps to stabilize the tongue is often accused of causing speech delay but it never does. Tongue-tie is a nonexistent malady.

Tonsils and adenoids

Reasons for removal of adenoids There are only two reasons for removal of adenoids.

Firstly, *frequent infections causing deafness*. Frequent infections, which in turn cause frequent attacks of ear inflammation (otitis media) form one reason. The earaches of childhood are almost always due to infection and swelling of adenoid tissue at the opening of the Eustachian tubes (the tubes that connect the middle ear with the back of the throat). Repeated infections of the middle ear may result in so-called glue ear in which sticky mucus prevents transmission

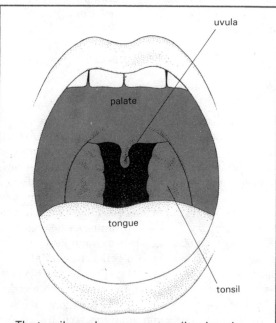

The tonsils can be seen most easily when the tongue is depressed. The small structure that hangs down from the back of the palate is the uvula, above and behind the base of the tongue. The adenoids lie at the back of the nasal passages and upper throat near the Eustachian tube opening.

of the sound waves from the eardrum across to the nerve endings in the inner ear.

Besides removal of the adenoids, the surgeon may want to suck out the glue through the eardrums and insert a grommet (tiny plastic tube) for a few months, to allow the middle ear to dry out and prevent the re-accumulation of glue.

Secondly, *tissue is so large that it obstructs breathing*. Obstruction of the nasopharynx, which is shown by constant mouth breathing and snoring at night, has a number of bad results. In the first place, the nose is important in breathing, for it not only filters the air inhaled, but moistens and warms it before it reaches the throat, trachea, and bronchial tubes. Breathing through the mouth tends to dry the mucous membranes of the throat and respiratory tubes.

One other aspect of obstructive adenoids, often overlooked, is that they tend to spoil a child's appetite by preventing the taste of food. Experience of the loss of taste when a cold blocks the nose, makes one understand just how much of the pleasure of eating is lost by lack of smell. Following adenoidectomy (removal of adenoids), most children who have had obstructive adenoids eat with eagerness and gain weight. Many paediatricians advise removal only of adenoids if necessary, leaving the tonsils intact if they are healthy and cause no difficulties.

Reasons for removal of tonsils

Size of tonsils The size of tonsils is rarely an indication for their removal. Only two conditions may be considered. When tonsils are so large as to obstruct the swallowing of food, removal of the tonsils is necessary. At other times tonsils are very large and swell up during infections to such a degree that they almost close the throat passage and make breathing very difficult. In such cases the doctor must make the choice between immediate removal or treating every infection quickly with antibiotics in an attempt at control before the tonsils enlarge too much. Many doctors prefer to try to hold off removal of the tonsils if it is at all possible, because many tonsils shrink in size between the age of three and ten years.

Repeated attacks of tonsillitis or chronic infection of the tonsils Repeated attacks of tonsillitis or chronic infection of the tonsils may be considered as justifiable reasons for their removal. In such conditions it seems obvious that the tonsils, instead of serving as protective agents have become the seat of infection. The child is not only constantly being run down by the infections but, if he is of school age, misses many days of education and contact with his companions. In these children there is usually a quick and remarkable improvement in general health following the removal of the tonsils.

It is said that children who have had rheumatic fever or kidney inflammation should have tonsillectomies. This is not a sufficient reason for the operation. There is no evidence that, if tonsils are healthy, their removal gives such children any added protection against subsequent attacks of these diseases. The prevention of recurrent rheumatic fever attacks is discussed in chapter 3.

Vitamins

Rickets and scurvy (caused by deficiencies of vitamins D and C respectively), which were two of the scourges of infancy and childhood in former times, are completely preventable by adequate amounts of vitamins, essential parts of every diet. Baby milks are fortified with vitamins A and D, but we still recommend all mothers to take vitamin supplements during pregnancy and lactation and to give their babies vitamin supplements throughout the first two years of life. These can be obtained at very small cost from Infant Welfare Clinics. They seem to be especially necessary for Asian families living in this country, and for Asians we recommend vitamin D supplements also during the rapid growth of adolescence, between the ages of ten to sixteen for girls, twelve to eighteen for boys.

Vomiting

Vomiting in infants and children is common. It may be associated with numerous conditions, among them infections, gastrointestinal infections, or milk allergy, poisons, pyloric stenosis, intussusception, coeliac disease, intestinal obstruction, psychological causes, pressure on the brain, and lack of a normal amount of sugar in the blood. Vomiting is not to be confused with regurgitation, which is simply bringing up of food after eating – generally of no significance. It is common in the newborn and young infant. It usually subsides and disappears before a child is six months of age. In a few instances it may continue as long as a year. Wind, due to swallowed air, has been the time honoured culprit, but its importance has been exaggerated. There are a number of types of vomiting. Vomiting as such is due to the expulsive force of the stomach. If the force is very marked, as in pyloric stenosis, the undigested or partly digested food is vomited out with such force that it is thrown half a metre from the body. This is called projectile vomiting. Vomiting which is immediate would signify either an irritated or sensitive stomach, an allergy to a specific food, or a marked narrowing of the gullet (oesophagus).

The vomit is usually tinged with yellow due to the normal backflow of small amounts of duodenal bile. Vomit which is green is always a serious sign of obstruction. Blood in the vomit of a very dark colour (so-called coffee ground vomit) may occur when capillaries bleed in the course of severe vomiting. It may also be a sign of a serious blood condition where capillaries are fragile. Green or bloodstained vomit is always an indication that a doctor should be called.

Treatment Simple vomiting from intestinal upsets can usually be arrested by the following steps.

Give nothing by mouth for one and a half hours after last vomiting spell.

Then start with one half tablespoon of plain water. Increase by a half tablespoon every 20 minutes until four tablespoons are reached ($2\frac{1}{2}$ hours). Four tablespoons are then given every half hour until the child's thirst is satisfied. Then cereal, biscuits, or toast may be offered. Gradually increase the diet but only if the child desires it. Do not give milk or lemonade until the stomach has settled.

Useful addresses

Adoption Resource Exchange,
40 Brunswick Square,
London WC1N 1AZ.

Association of British Adoption and Fostering Agencies,
4 Southampton Row,
London WC1B 4AA.

British Diabetic Association,
10 Queen Anne Street,
London W1M 0BD.

British Epilepsy Association,
Crowthorne House,
Bigshotte,
New Wokingham Road,
Wokingham,
Berkshire RG11 3AY.

Coeliac Society,
P.O. Box 181,
London NW2 2QY.

Cystic Fibrosis Research Trust,
5 Blyth Road,
Bromley, Kent BR1 3RS.

Foundation for Study of Infant Deaths,
23 St. Peter's Square,
London W6 9NW.

General Register Office (CA section),
Titchfield,
P.O. Box 7 Fareham,
Hampshire PO15 5RU

Leukaemia Society,
(Mr. David Harding, Hon. Secretary)
186 Torbay Road,
Harrow, Middlesex HA2 9QL.

National Association for Welfare of Children in Hospital,
7 Exton Street,
London S1E 8VE.

National Society for Autistic Children,
1a Golders Green Road,
London NW11 8EA.

National Society for Mentally Handicapped Children,
17 Pembridge Square,
London W2 4EP.

Spastics Society,
12 Park Crescent,
London W1N 4EQ.

Chapter 13

Special concerns of women

Revised by Sir John Stallworthy, FRCOG

Gynaecology is the branch of medicine concerned with the study of the female reproductive organs and the effects which their normal and abnormal function have on health and wellbeing. It covers the whole span of life from birth to death. Because the biological purpose of these organs is to reproduce the species, it follows that problems associated with pregnancy and childbearing may also have important gynaecological significance in clinical practice. One example is when a woman with a tumour in her womb becomes pregnant, or fails to conceive because of the tumour.

Obstetrics is the specialized study of pregnancy and childbearing in all its aspects in health and disease. The two subjects of obstetrics and gynaecology are so closely interrelated that in Britain and Commonwealth countries there is a joint training programme embracing both obstetrics and gynaecology for doctors wishing to specialize in this work. The Royal College of Obstetricians and Gynaecologists was founded in 1929 to improve the art and practice of midwifery, and, in this way, the standards available for the care of women. There are now Fellows and Members of the College in more than 50 countries. Because of the interrelationship of gynaecology and obstetrics to other branches of medicine, and to avoid unnecessary repetition, there will be references in this chapter to other chapters in the book.

Childhood problems

Anatomical defects The doctor or midwife in attendance at the birth of a baby will examine it for any obvious abnormality. When it is born in an institution, and in Britain most babies now are, it will usually be examined in more detail subsequently by a paediatrician. Any defect of the external genital organs will be apparent at these examinations. Fortunately, congenital malformations involving the vulva seldom occur, and when they do, can in most cases be dealt with quite simply. For example, the labia may appear to be joined together in the midline, thus concealing the entrance to the vagina and even the urethral orifice. All that the doctor needs to do in most of these cases is to exert gentle tension with a finger on either side of the midline and the labia separate to reveal a normal vulva. The clitoris, which is the female analogue of the penis, may be so enlarged at birth as to resemble a penis. When such abnormalities are found, it is wise to obtain the advice of a gynaecologist or paediatrician because of the importance of avoiding any mistake in determining the true sex of the infant. This prevents the serious implications of a female child being brought up as a boy or vice versa. There are now accurate tests, including the study of chromosomes, to facilitate sex determination in difficult cases.

The hymen is usually a thin membrane at the opening of the vagina, but it may be thick and cause difficulty at the first intercourse, or it may have no opening and so obstruct the vagina (imperforate hymen). Very rarely, examination after birth of the infant reveals a midline swelling in the vulva due to the accumulation of fluid in a distended vagina closed from the exterior by an imperforate hymen. This fluid has collected during intra-uterine life as a result of secretion from lining cells in the reproductive passages. More commonly an imperforate hymen causes no difficulty at this stage, and may remain unnoticed until puberty. When menstruation begins the blood cannot escape and month by month accumulates behind the imperforate hymen in a slowly distended vagina. For this reason, if period-type discomfort occurs at puberty without apparent menstruation a gynaecological examination is essential. In both these cases correction is by simple surgical incision with care to avoid infection. Subsequently normal uterine function can be expected.

The uterus is formed during fetal development by the union of the lower part of two parallel tubes and the disappearance of their adjoining walls. The upper ends of these tubes remain separate throughout life as the fallopian tubes. An extreme abnormality occurs when the two tubes do not merge and communicate only at the cervix (neck of womb) resulting in two uterine cavities. Many variations occur between the extremes of two completely separate uteri and one which externally appears to be normal but internally has a septum in the midline of the upper portion of the cavity. Similarly there can be a midline septum in the vagina (septate vagina). As with the uterus, there are variations ranging from two completely separate vaginas to a short septum attached to the cervix in the midline. Many women with these congenital variations lead normal lives and produce children without difficulty. If problems such as infertility are associated later in life with congenital abnormalities of the internal sex organs, gynaecological advice is necessary to assess what relevance they have, if any, to the infertility. These anatomical variations of the internal sex organs, as opposed to changes in the vulva, are unlikely to be detected at birth or in childhood because they cause no symptoms.

On rare occasions there may be arrested development, or even absence, of the internal sex organs (agenesis). There may be no ovarian tissue or no uterus, but more commonly complete or partial absence of the vagina. This is sometimes detected during examination after birth but more commonly is found in later childhood or at puberty. An artificial vagina which enables a woman to participate in, and enjoy, sexual activity, can be constructed by plastic surgery. There are a number of techniques for doing this, some of which are simpler and safer than others. For this reason, it is wise to request the family doctor to refer the patient to a gynaecologist with special experience in this type of surgery.

Tumours of the reproductive organs are uncommon in infancy and childhood. One rare condition, imperforate hymen, which may be recognized at birth and be mistaken for a tumour because of a midline swelling in the vulva, has already been described. Any apparent swelling of the vulva in early life, or discharge, particularly if bloodstained, should be reported at once to the doctor because tumours, though rare in early life, may be malignant. Early diagnosis is urgently required. Treatment is the same as for corresponding tumours in adults, with surgery, irradiation, or chemotherapy. Combinations of treatment are being used with increasing frequency. Because malignant conditions of the reproductive organs in early life are rare and serious it is desirable that the child with cancer should be given the benefit of the skills, teamwork, and equipment found only in oncological (cancer) centres specializing in this type of work.

Certain tumours, usually growing in an ovary, produce the oestrogenic hormone responsible for growth of the genital tract. Very rarely they occur in young girls and as a result there is precocious sexual development. Changes characteristic of puberty occur with enlargement of the breasts and the development of hair on the pubis and in the armpits. Vaginal bleeding may occur, suggesting the onset of menstruation. It is easy to appreciate the psychological difficulties for both the child and her parents which almost inevitably result. As will be seen later, there are other causes for precocious development and the condition requires careful investigation, including hormone tests to establish the cause. When a tumour responsible for the liberation of hormone is identified it must be removed.

The adolescent girl

The cyclical relationship between collections of cells in the hypothalamus, at the base of the brain, the pituitary gland, and the ovary is described in chapter 9. In a normal healthy child at the age of eleven to thirteen years in Britain (the age varies in different countries) the ovaries begin responding to the stimulating hormone released from the pituitary gland and start producing the female (oestrogenic) hormones responsible for the development of the secondary sex characteristics in the genital tract and the breasts. They are also responsible for the general development of the female figure as well as the characteristic female psychological attitudes. If in Britain this development takes place at an earlier age, so that menstruation begins before the age of ten, it is regarded as premature, and assessment by a specialist is indicated. This phase of change and growth which leads up to the beginning of menstruation affects not

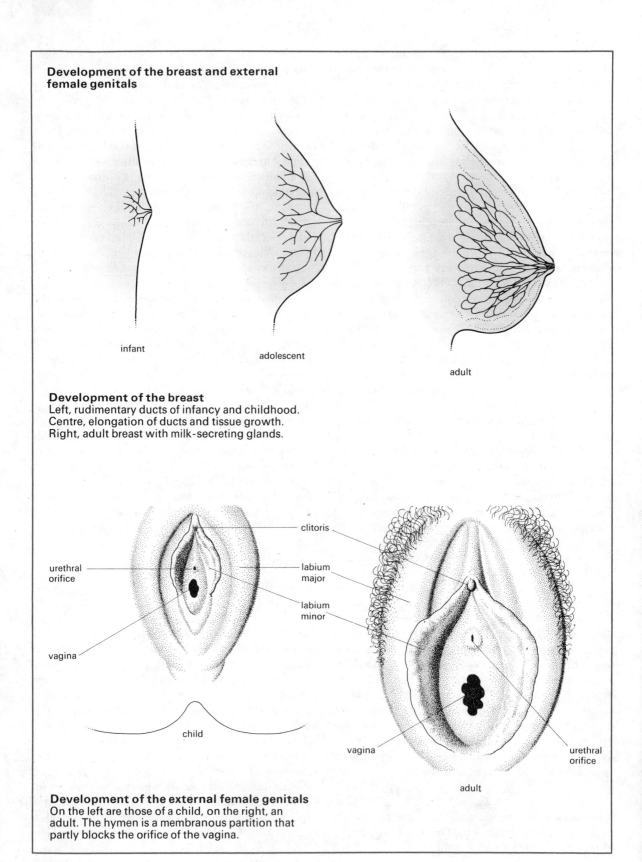

**Development of the breast and external
female genitals**

infant

adolescent

adult

Development of the breast
Left, rudimentary ducts of infancy and childhood.
Centre, elongation of ducts and tissue growth.
Right, adult breast with milk-secreting glands.

clitoris

urethral
orifice

labium
major

labium
minor

vagina

child

vagina

urethral
orifice

adult

Development of the external female genitals
On the left are those of a child, on the right, an
adult. The hymen is a membranous partition that
partly blocks the orifice of the vagina.

only the child's body but often her personality as well. Feminine contours develop, assisted by the enlarging breasts, vulval changes already described take place, and hair appears on the mons veneris, the outer aspect of the labia majora, and in the armpits. Personality changes vary considerably and careful observation will often reveal that they occur periodically. They are a manifestation of the changes taking place in the cycle of hormone production in the brain and ovary and are therefore quite natural phenomena. Nonetheless considerable sympathetic understanding is often required to help an adolescent girl through this difficult phase of her life. She tends to be emotionally unstable and at times behaves in a way which for her is uncharacteristic. She may burst into tears with minimal provocation, become recurrently difficult with other members of the family with whom she was previously on good terms, and cause not only them but herself recurring distress for reasons which she herself cannot understand.

During this phase the greatest contribution a mother can make to her daughter is to give her a sense of security and an understanding of the significance of those changes which are taking place in her body while she is passing from adolescence into womanhood. Ideally these facts should be explained at an earlier age so that the changes will not come as a surprise. If for any reason a mother feels unable to help her daughter in this way her failure is an expression of an impaired relationship between the two, as a result of which it is the more necessary that a wise mature adult friend or relation should be commissioned for the purpose. An informed, intelligent, and healthy understanding of menstruation and its implications before it begins is a tremendous help to a young woman on the threshold of her years of reproductive potential. This is particularly important in an age of changing attitudes to sexual freedom. It should not be forgotten that the effect of a good relationship between the father and the adolescent can also be very important in providing a stabilizing influence. Fortunate is the girl whose adolescence takes place with the background of a united home in which the personal relationships between all members of the family are good.

A critical appraisal of the contemporary scene in Britain emphasizes the importance of these relationships, and the need for facilities for wise counselling for those who are deprived of them. The Department of Health has found it necessary to advise doctors that they may prescribe contraceptives to children under the age of sixteen (age of consent) without the knowledge or approval of parents or guardians. But unfortunately the only age group in which the number of legal abortions has continued to rise is in those of sixteen and under. Counselling is the first priority, not contraception.

Menstruation The scientific explanation of this is described and illustrated in chapter 9. The age at which it occurs in perfectly normal girls varies within a usual range of ten to sixteen years. Occasionally development is slower and menstruation may not occur until eighteen or even later and be followed by subsequent normal menstrual behaviour. Nonetheless, just as it is wise to obtain expert advice if menstruation begins before the age of ten, it is equally advisable to have a specialist examination if there has been no period by the age of sixteen. Apart from any other reason it provides an opportunity for the necessary reassurance if the girl is found to be normal. Failure to menstruate can be a source of great anxiety to an adolescent girl when her friends and classmates have already started.

A girl's attitude to menstruation, even years before it begins, is influenced consciously or subconsciously by her mother, aunts, or family friends. Those who speak of "the curse", of "being unwell", or of "sickness" suggest something to be feared. Equally reprehensible, though less likely to occur in modern society, is the attitude of silence and neglect which results in the girl discovering one day, or night, that she is bleeding and quite unprepared for what in the circumstances may well prove to be a terrifying event. The girl who understands that menstruation can be welcomed as marking the transition from adolescence to womanhood, and is a normal process associated with the capacity for loving and motherhood, has received the preparation for life to which every girl is entitled.

There is no single uniform pattern of menstrual behaviour and recognition of this fact can save a lot of unnecessary anxiety. What is normal for one woman may not necessarily be regarded as normal by another. One may require protection for 2 or 3 days in every 21, while another has a heavier loss over a longer period of time and may require protection for 7 days in every 28. Particularly at the onset of menstruation (menarche) and at the menopause, when it finally ceases, irregularities of menstrual behaviour are common. After the first period a regular monthly sequence occurs with most women but it is not unusual, and no cause for alarm, if one or two periods are missed during the early months. The possibility of pregnancy should not be overlooked even at this early stage of the establishment of

Chapter 13 Special concerns of women

menstrual rhythm. Occasionally heavy and prolonged painless bleeding occurs at this stage. As explained in chapter 9, ovulation (the shedding of an egg cell from the ovary) does not necessarily occur every month and vaginal bleeding can occur at either regular or irregular intervals without ovulation. When this takes place, however, there may be excessive stimulation of the lining of the womb by the oestrogenic hormone without the balancing effect of the ovarian hormone progesterone. The latter is liberated from a remarkable little structure known as the corpus luteum (yellow body) which forms in the ovary within the capsule from which the egg cell has been liberated. In the absence of ovulation there is no corpus luteum and therefore no progesterone, one of the physiological functions of which is to control the amount of menstrual blood loss. When ovulation does not occur the menstrual cycle is described medically as anovulatory. Such cycles are very common at the menarche and by no means uncommon, for temporary periods, during the subsequent years of reproductive life. For example, it is usual for a woman to have anovulatory cycles following childbirth or abortion. They can also be induced by such diverse factors as emotional tension and anxiety on the one hand, or the contraceptive pill on the other. Although most anovulatory cycles are not associated with excessive or prolonged bleeding, this does occasionally happen, particularly but not exclusively at the menarche. Apart from the anxiety and inconvenience which such losses can cause, anaemia is likely to develop and for this reason medical advice should be sought. It is usually not difficult to control the loss and institute regular and more normal cycles by adjusting

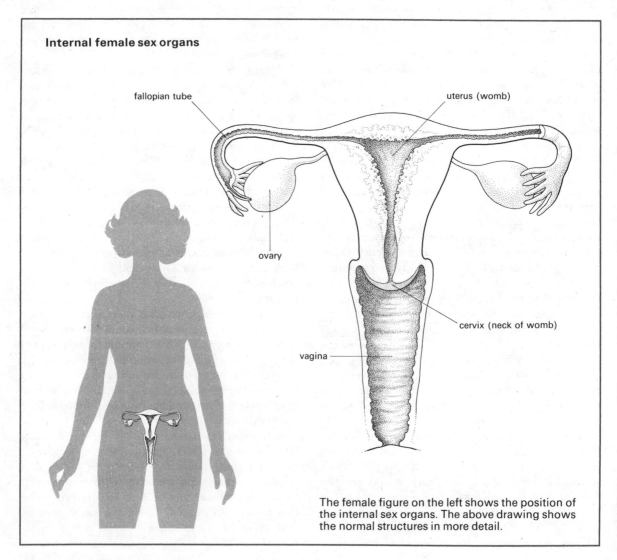

Internal female sex organs

fallopian tube

uterus (womb)

ovary

cervix (neck of womb)

vagina

The female figure on the left shows the position of the internal sex organs. The above drawing shows the normal structures in more detail.

the hormone balance. Very occasionally blood transfusion and removal of the thickened lining of the womb by surgical scraping (curettage) are required.

Dysmenorrhoea (Painful menstruation) Many women have no discomfort associated with menstruation. Strange though it may seem, some women athletes of international calibre admit to feeling better when they are menstruating, and are pleased if this coincides with an important athletic event. On the other hand, dysmenorrhoea can be a source of considerable distress to the patient and is responsible for a great loss of working hours in industries employing large numbers of women. The healthier and happier a woman is, the less likely she is to complain of dysmenorrhoea. It is not surprising therefore that some women who are troubled with it at home or at work are completely free of discomfort when on holiday.

It is uncommon for periods to be painful from the onset of the first menstruation. The more usual pattern, to which of course there are exceptions, is for them to be painless initially while the girl is at school. Later, sometimes much later, when she has found employment or is at college or university, she may have discomfort or pain with periods for the first time, though not necessarily with all of them. If she seeks medical advice she is almost certain to be told after examination that there is no evidence of disease and that she is perfectly normally developed. This fact, together with an explanation of why she is having pain, can be reassuring to her. The reason is that during the initial establishment of menstrual rhythm, as described in chapter 9, she has been having anovulatory cycles because the ovary was not releasing an egg cell each month. Now, however, ovulation is occurring, progesterone is being formed by the corpus luteum, and this hormone is responsible for altering the pattern of activity of the muscle in the wall of the womb. This is the source of the discomfort or pain. This type of dysmenorrhoea is commonly described as being primary, as opposed to secondary dysmenorrhoea which typically occurs later in life and is due to disease in the pelvis. Women taking the pill seldom complain of primary dysmenorrhoea. The simple explanation is that the pill inhibits ovulation and therefore the progesterone effect on the womb is absent. It has long been recognized that even severe primary dysmenorrhoea is usually cured after pregnancy and a vaginal delivery.

Primary dysmenorrhoea Symptoms vary from discomfort to severe pain which occasionally is associated with nausea and even vomiting. Characteristic features are that pain when present is felt in the midline of the lower abdomen just above the pubis or in the lower back. It usually occurs either with the onset of the menstrual flow or immediately preceding it. Once the flow is well-established it is usual for the discomfort to ease. In severe cases the pain is described as cramping in nature with the feeling that "something inside is trying to get out". Because primary dysmenorrhoea is not caused by disease in the pelvis but is a disturbance of function associated with hormone balance, it is not surprising that it is more common and tends to be more severe in anxious, nervous, and tense women, particularly those who are not yet adjusted to the changes which have been taking place in their bodies and the influence these may have on their future happiness. It is for this reason that emphasis has been given previously to the important contribution which can be made by sympathetic and timely instruction of the growing girl to enable her to face with optimism the problems and implications of adolescence and menstruation.

Acquired dysmenorrhoea differs from the primary type in several ways. Unlike the former, it is a symptom of underlying pelvic disease. Typically it develops later in life with an increasing incidence after the age of 30, but it can be a major source of distress even in young women. An example is when abortion or childbirth has resulted in inflammation of the womb, ovaries, and tubes, which have been left permanently damaged and instead of being able to move freely, as they should be, are fixed by past inflammation to the adjacent bowel and the walls of the pelvis. Acquired dysmenorrhoea can also occur in young, as well as in older, women as a sequel to pelvic infections from sexually transmitted diseases, which are now common.

Unlike the discomfort and pain of primary dysmenorrhoea which is localized to the midline and usually commences with the onset of the flow, or immediately preceding it, the discomfort and pain of acquired dysmenorrhoea is more generalized, and tends to be more pronounced on the side of the lower abdomen most involved by the underlying disease. For example, with the condition of endometriosis, to be described later, the pain may be entirely one-sided if the disease affects the ovary and ligaments only on that side. Another feature of the pain and discomfort is that it usually begins several days or even a week before the onset of menstruation and becomes progressively worse. It is relieved by the onset of the period but in bad cases there may be only a relatively short interval after the period before symptoms recur. A woman developing acquired dysmenorrhoea is wise to consult her doctor so that the cause can be found and treated.

Treatment From what has already been said it will be obvious that the treatment of acquired dysmenorrhoea is the treatment of the underlying cause and will be influenced by the age of the patient as well as by the nature and extent of the disease. It will vary from medical treatment (including the use of hormones and techniques such as pelvic diathermy and ultrasound used by specialists in physical medicine) to surgery. This in turn will vary in extent from removal of one ovary and tube with preservation of the womb and the other ovary and tube if the disease is localized, to removal of the womb with both tubes and ovaries when disease is more widespread. The earlier the correct diagnosis is made, the more likely it is that relatively simple surgery is all that will be required.

Primary dysmenorrhoea, although not a manifestation of organic disease, can sometimes be difficult to treat. When this is the case it is usually because the young woman was inadequately prepared both from the point of view of factual knowledge and of emotional adjustment to the physiological changes which were to take place in her body. Attempts to correct these defects are an important aspect of treatment. Any tendency to leave work or go to bed for a day or two should be discouraged. Attention to general health, including the treatment of anaemia with iron, should not be overlooked, and exercise rather than inactivity should be encouraged. This is particularly important because so many young women experience primary dysmenorrhoea for the first time when they leave school and are engaged in sedentary work. There is often associated constipation. Such physical activities as walking, swimming, dancing, and cycling can prove beneficial. The danger of becoming addicted to pain-relieving drugs should not be overlooked. The supply of tablets to relieve period pain, without a doctor's prescription, must make a considerable contribution to the receipts of drug houses.

Until a few years ago, it was common practice in severe cases for a doctor to perform stretching of the neck of the womb on the anaesthetized patient. The rationale was that as primary dysmenorrhoea was so often relieved by the vaginal delivery of a baby, the same beneficial result might be achieved by this forcible stretching. More extensive surgical procedures, including division of the nerves through which pain impulses from the womb are transmitted to the brain, were sometimes performed. Fortunately these procedures are now seldom if ever indicated. As stated already, primary dysmenorrhoea does not occur during anovulatory cycles of bleeding. Such cycles can be induced by hormones and the simplest way of doing this is by using one of the low-dose contraceptive pills. This is preferable to surgery and likely to prove more effective. After an initial period of several months of freedom from pain, during which every effort is made to restore the patient's confidence in herself and improve her understanding of the physiological explanation of her troubles, she should be encouraged to try without the pill. If she is then leading a more active healthy life, there is a reasonable chance that she will not need further treatment with it.

Sexual awakening Legislation on sex discrimination cannot alter the biological fact that as children grow up they become progressively more aware of sex differentiation as it affects their own bodies. This is the time for frank answers to direct questions and the gradual and progressive development of an informed and healthy attitude to sex as something normal, fundamental, and important to ultimate happiness and fulfilment in life. The sympathetic relationship between young and old which makes possible this type of preparation also provides opportunities of warning children about the undesirable and potentially dangerous aspects of sexual activities. The pill may prevent pregnancy, but it does NOT prevent venereal disease. The dangers must be explained in context and at the appropriate times so as not to create unnecessary anxieties in the child's mind, and possibly make normal sexual adjustment with a loved one more difficult in later life. Promiscuity, unplanned pregnancy, and sexually transmitted disease can be sources of permanent unhappiness. A child has the right to know where danger lies before being faced with the relevant personal decisions. It is equally, if not more, important for him or her to know that sexual happiness is an essential constituent of love and fulfilment in marriage. This positive and constructive approach is one to encourage.

The mature woman

Most young women, even those who embark on a career of their own, still look forward to the day when they will share a home and children with the man they love. With many this will be a sentimental dream divorced from any deep understanding of the problems likely to be encountered. Others will have been better prepared, as described earlier, during the vulnerable years of growth and adolescence. They are the more fortunate ones who will be less likely to repeat the mistakes with which all are familiar even within their own circle of acquaintances, friends, and family. Unhappy marriages, divorce, unwanted children, and sometimes the effects of sexually transmitted disease, are evidence of a great deal of disillusionment and secret suffering. It is understandable that extreme youth makes it easier for these hard facts of life to be overshadowed by sentimental dreams. Understanding parents and a wise doctor can do much to help, with an emphasis on decisions likely to contribute most to ultimate happiness. A young couple should be encouraged to consider such fundamental questions as:

As well as physical attraction, is there also mutual devotion and respect?
Do they want to share the responsibilities, as well as the joys, of producing and caring for children of their own?
Do they share common aims and interests in life?

Medical examination A premarital consultation, preferably attended by both partners, gives the doctor an excellent opportunity of helping them both and contributing to the happiness of their marriage. The time he spends in a preliminary review of personal and family backgrounds, which could be a source of great concealed anxiety, can be time well spent. An example is when the young woman reveals that her mother died in the process of bringing her into the world. The effects that this can have on her own attitude to motherhood can be far-reaching and nothing but good will come from the encouragement a doctor can give concerning progress in making childbirth safer and happier than it was when she was born. The interview also provides opportunities of discussing the menstrual history of the patient, which may be relevant to her fertility, and of learning something of the couple's mutual attitudes to marriage, contraception, and parenthood. If during this interview the doctor has not won the confidence of the young woman, and preferably of both partners, an important opportunity of helping them has been lost.

The physical examination which follows the consultation should be thorough as far as basic essentials are concerned. For example, any obvious symptoms such as pallor indicating possible anaemia should be noted and investigated. The blood pressure should be recorded and the urine examined for albumin and sugar. Examination of the breasts will often give an opportunity of reassuring an anxious

patient. Many young women are anxious lest they will be unable to feed a baby because they believe their breasts are too small. In fact, these are often the most efficient breasts for feeding as there is a minimum of fat and the breast consists almost entirely of milk-secreting lobules. Examination of the abdomen and of the pelvis by vaginal and rectal examination will provide the information necessary concerning the vulva, vagina, womb, ovaries, and tubes. The doctor will probably make on a glass slide a film from cells collected from the surface of the neck of the womb (Papanicolaou or smear test). In a young woman this is unlikely to reveal any abnormality but is a useful yardstick for subsequent periodic tests on the neck of the womb every two or three years.

Occasionally conditions are found during the examination which require further investigation or attention, either because of their possible effect on the patient's general health or because of difficulties they could cause at intercourse or during pregnancy. Examples are a raised blood pressure or albumin or sugar in the urine, all of which should be investigated before a planned pregnancy is begun, a thick hymen with a narrow opening which could make intercourse painful or impossible, or unsuspected tumours of the ovaries or womb. When a doctor can report after this examination that the patient is not only healthy but has a perfectly normal genital tract, he will have made an important contribution to the happiness of both partners. They should be encouraged to ask questions and the nature of these is usually such that a gynaecologist is particularly qualified to answer them.

There may be anxieties concerning what constitutes normal sexual behaviour, the frequency of intercourse, what can be done if there is failure to conceive, the relative safety of contraceptive techniques, and the advantages and disadvantages of breast-feeding, to mention but some of the more commonly asked questions.

Feminine hygiene This can be a problem and cause anxieties at all stages of life. From infancy until the onset of menstruation, and following the menopause, the vulva and vagina are particularly susceptible to infection. The relative immunity during the years of reproductive activity is due to the nourishing effect the oestrogenic hormone liberated by the ovary has on the cells of the skin covering the vulva and lining the vagina. Before the menarche and after the menopause this hormone is deficient and the resistance of the skin to injury and infection is correspondingly reduced.

Chapter 13 **Special concerns of women**

The external genitals of an infant girl and young child may become inflamed, swollen, and sore if they are not cleaned regularly and adequately. The best way of doing this is by washing with water and a soap such as one marketed specially for babies. Stronger soaps containing carbolic and other allegedly anti-septic compounds should be avoided as they can prove extremely irritant to the delicate skin of an infant. Where the labial folds embrace the clitoris and entrance to the vagina a secretion known as smegma, arising from glands in the skin, collects and can act as an irritant. In the infant it should be removed gently with cotton wool soaked in warm soapy water, or after the application of warm olive oil a dry cotton wool swab will usually wipe it away.

It sometimes happens that in the course of exploring their own anatomy, small children will insert various small objects into such available orifices as the ears, the nose, and sometimes the vagina. Once inserted the foreign body is soon forgotten and in the vagina it may cause no discomfort for a day or two but there will then be a vaginal discharge, yellow, greenish, or even bloodstained, often with secondary inflammation of the vulva itself. Similar discharge and evidence of local inflammation with soreness can occur in those fortunately rare cases in which venereal infection occurs in the genital tract of an infant. This is most likely to be the result of direct physical contact with an infected mother. In both cases there is certain to be secondary infection by such common pus-forming organisms as the staphylococcus, strepto-coccus, or *E. coli*. The importance of this fact is that if swabs are taken from the vulva or the vaginal entrance in an attempt to discover the nature of the infecting organism, without exploration of the vagina itself or the taking of swabs from the neck of the womb, the real cause of trouble, be it a foreign body or the gonococcus, may remain undetected. For these reasons, when there is persistent or recurrent discharge and inflammation the doctor is likely to suggest that the child should be anaesthetized and examined. Small instruments are available which will permit inspection of the vagina and neck of womb, the removal of a foreign body, and the taking of the necessary swabs for culture, without damaging the hymen.

The growing child and adolescent girl should be made aware of the importance of cleanliness to the body as a whole, including the external genitalia. For example, there is less chance of infecting the vulva and vagina with organisms arising in the bowel if, after a bowel action, the anal area is cleansed from the front backwards and not in the reverse direction.

There is also much to be said for cleansing the area with soap and water applied with a sponge kept for the purpose, always from the front backwards, after the initial use of toilet paper.

It is surprising how many women who consult a doctor because of vaginal discharge and irritation admit ignorance of the steps outlined above, designed to promote maximum cleanliness and to reduce the chance of vulval and vaginal infection.

The amount and length of vulval hair varies considerably from patient to patient. When it is long it can easily become matted by perspiration or by vaginal discharge, and particularly in the latter case it can be responsible for an unpleasant odour. This makes attention to local cleanliness the more necessary.

Whether to douche or not to douche is a question which troubles many women. In some countries it is a much used practice and in others rarely employed. No rule is applicable to all, but there are certain guiding principles which may prove helpful. The first is that if douching is necessary the best time for it is first thing in the morning after rising. The reason for this is that mucus from the neck of womb, or discharge secondary to infection, tends to collect at the top of the vagina during the night, and works its way down to the vulva once the patient gets up and about. Many women troubled in this way will remain perfectly comfortable all day if the vagina is cleansed first thing in the morning. The second point to remember is that many women do harm to themselves by using douches with preparations such as Lysol or Dettol solution which may prove irritating. Contrary to popular belief, a douche will not destroy infecting organisms, but acts only by washing away the collected discharge from the vagina. Useful and simple household remedies are one teaspoonful of sodium bicarbonate (baking soda) or one teaspoonful of common table salt to one pint of warm water. Whatever is used, on no account must the nozzle of the douche be inserted into the neck of the womb. If this is done, fluid can be forced into the uterine cavity and even through it into the tubes and from them into the peritoneal cavity. With an irritant solution this can be disastrous. As a further precaution, gentle pressure that is just enough to provide a slow return of the fluid and discharge is all that is necessary.

Finally, the position can be summarized by saying that if there is no discharge to cause annoyance there is no indication for douching, and if there is troublesome discharge it is wise to see a doctor so that the cause can be identified and appropriate treatment advised.

Coital problems

Dyspareunia This means difficult or painful intercourse and is a common cause of tension in marriage. It may be primary or develop later in life, even after many years of satisfying intercourse. In the first case it causes trouble at the first attempts at intercourse and may be due to a local cause such as a tough hymen which will not stretch easily, associated with a small opening into the vagina. This would be detected at an adequate premarital examination, at which time advice would be given on how the patient can enlarge the vaginal opening by gentle but progressive stretching with the fingers. A useful time to do this is when relaxing in a hot bath. On the rare occasions when a tough rigid hymen is detected the doctor may advise its incision prior to marriage. Another cause of primary dyspareunia is when the pelvic muscles go into spasm (vaginismus) and make penetration painful or even impossible. This unhappy complication is unlikely to occur in a mature woman adequately prepared for marriage and its implications, sharing the experience with an understanding and gentle partner. When it does, much patience and sympathetic understanding will be necessary from both partners and the sooner medical advice is obtained, the better are the prospects of success. A simple manoeuvre which many women have found helpful is to reverse the common position adopted for intercourse so that the woman is astride her husband. This enables her to control the rate and depth of penetration. If she then bears down with an expulsive movement, she automatically relaxes the muscles of the pelvic floor and finds that penetration is not now painful.

Dyspareunia is often acquired later in life and a common cause is a tender scar following operations on the vulva or vagina. Incisions made or tears sustained at childbirth can be tender for some time after healing is complete. Sometimes the entrance is either too tight or the tender scar promotes spasm when intercourse is attempted. It is wise to consult a doctor at once, preferably the one who performed the repair. It is usually a simple matter to restore normal function and this type of acquired dyspareunia should not be allowed to create marital tension. Other causes of acquired dyspareunia are certain types of uterine misplacement with prolapse of the ovaries so that they lie so low in the pelvis that they interfere with deep penetration, or inflammatory masses following pelvic infection, or certain types of tumour, particularly if fixed low in the pelvis in the region of the top of the vagina. For these reasons it is wise to consult a doctor as soon as possible so that the cause can be determined and appropriate treatment given once acquired dyspareunia develops.

Contrary to what is often believed, many women continue to enjoy a satisfying sexual relationship for many years after the menopause. On the other hand, with the withdrawal of oestrogenic hormones following cessation of ovarian activity at the menopause, regressive changes take place in the vulva and vagina. There is reduced elasticity of the tissues and progressive narrowing of the vagina itself. Unless regular intercourse takes place dyspareunia may occur with the resumption of sexual activity after a long period of abstinence. Oestrogenic hormone can be administered to restore the vulva and vagina to a more normal state and a woman, whatever her age, need feel no embarrassment in seeking the help of a doctor should this be necessary.

Orgasm When a woman responds to sexual stimulation there is an immediate and great increase in blood supply to the sexual organs. The glands in the neck of the womb and at the entrance to the vagina secrete clear mucus, sometimes in considerable quantities. The clitoris becomes engorged with blood and much harder and the sensitivity at its tip is more acute. The vessels in the labia fill with blood so that these become firmer and more prominent. The pelvic organs including the uterus are also congested. If the peak of excitement is reached the muscles supporting the lower vagina contract rhythmically and the upper portion distends. The contractions continue for several seconds during which the blood supply returns to approximately its former state with the woman feeling relief and satisfaction.

Orgasm is this phase of maximum arousal, involuntary contractions, and relief. Few women always achieve it and many women never do. For most, it occurs with varying frequency and its incidence is influenced by factors such as fatigue, anxieties, dyspareunia, ill health, and lack of understanding, sensitivity, or technique by the partner.

Some women who fail repeatedly to achieve orgasm become frustrated and suffer from chronic pelvic congestion which may produce such symptoms as excessive vaginal discharge, chronic aching in the lowest part of the back, painful periods (acquired dysmenorrhoea), and a frequent desire to empty the bladder. The physical and emotional consequences of all this can become one of the more common reasons for discontent in marriage and ultimately divorce. Both partners are involved and as ignorance and lack of understanding by one or both is usually the primary reason for failure it is very important that the

Chapter 13 **Special concerns of women**

medical advice of one skilled in handling such problems should be sought as early as possible. Much of this distress could be prevented by wise counselling before marriage.

Pelvic infections   Infection of the genital tract is very common, and many organisms can be responsible. They vary from those commonly associated with wound infections, of which the streptococcus is a typical example, to those less commonly found in this area, such as the bacteria responsible for tuberculosis or those which cause gas gangrene. Gonococcal infections are also commonly found and can be responsible for much permanent ill health when they pass through the uterus to involve the tubes and ovaries and cause peritonitis. Until relatively recent times more women died from pelvic infection after childbirth and abortion than the total number now dying from all causes associated with pregnancy. The initial advent of the sulphonamide drugs which could kill certain bacteria, followed by the discovery of penicillin and subsequent antibiotic agents has been responsible for this miraculous saving of life from infections associated with pregnancy. Nonetheless, women still die from pelvic infection and its dangers must not be forgotten. For example, if bleeding is prolonged or heavy for more than a few days after abortion or delivery, a doctor should be consulted. The trouble could be due to retention in the womb of a portion of the afterbirth which can become a focus of severe infection. Common infections, although they are distressing, are less serious if found locally on the vulva and at the vaginal entrance. These are often the result of chemical irritation from antiseptic soaps and local applications, deodorants, detergents, or cosmetic powders. The importance of vulval cleanliness has already been emphasized. Irritation from garments, particularly nylon ones, soiled by excessive perspiration or by urine in women who have incomplete bladder control, can be the source of trouble. Identification of the cause and appropriate changes of garments or habits, will usually bring relief.

Organisms responsible for sexually transmitted diseases, particularly syphilis and gonorrhoea (see chapter 2), frequently initiate trouble by infecting the vulva, vagina, or cervix. Early diagnosis and treatment facilitate rapid and complete recovery, but in the meantime these diseases are easily transmitted to other partners by sexual intercourse. Pelvic infections are potentially serious and self-medication is not justified.

Low-grade inflammation of the vulva with chronic, persistent, or recurrent irritation is not uncommon. When it occurs the urine should be tested for sugar because the condition is not infrequently associated with diabetes. Whatever the underlying cause, the resulting irritation (chronic vulvitis) can be a source of great discomfort leading to itching and disturbed sleep. If this condition is allowed to persist over a length of time, not only is the general health impaired but changes can take place in the skin of the vulva leading to the formation of white patches (leucoplakia) and even ultimately to cancer. It is the more necessary therefore that patients with these symptoms should obtain medical advice and have periodic careful examinations of the vulva.

Yeast infections   These not uncommonly affect the vulva and vagina. They are particularly likely to occur during pregnancy, in the diabetic patient, or after the use of antibiotic preparations. They are also not uncommon after the menopause. There is frequently an associated thick white discharge in which the fungus responsible can be found. There can be considerable associated irritation of the vulva and, in this case, the doctor will probably take swabs for microscopic examination in order to isolate the fungus or other organism responsible. The sexual partner is often infected and will be suffering from irritation of the penis. Once the diagnosis is made the condition can usually be cured by local medication, but it may recur.

Trichomoniasis   This extremely irritating and common infection is due to a microscopic protozoan known as *Trichomonas vaginalis*. It is very infective and usually, though not always, transmitted by sexual intercourse. There is often a profuse yellowish-white frothy offensive vaginal discharge with associated irritation and a burning feeling of the vulva and vagina. As with yeast infections the male partner is also often involved although he may be free of symptoms. Because of the acute infection of the vulva and vagina the woman is likely to complain of local soreness, irritation, burning pain when she passes urine, and dyspareunia if intercourse is attempted. The correct diagnosis is made by microscopic examination of the vaginal discharge and is essential to effective treatment. Recurrence is not uncommon, particularly if the male partner harbours the organism, for example in his bladder, and remains untreated. Until recently treatment was by local applications using creams and vaginal pessaries, but a few years ago a new drug (metronidazole) given by mouth to both partners has revolutionized treatment.

Cervicitis   The cervix is the neck of the womb. Infection (cervicitis) is common and may be caused by a variety of organisms. Sexually transmitted infections such as syphilis, gonorrhoea, and trichomoniasis have already been described. Acute and chronic virus infections by a herpes virus occur from time to time, although an acute infection causing symptoms is relatively rare. Tearing of the neck of the womb during childbirth, unless repaired at the time, is not uncommonly followed by chronic or recurrent low-grade infections. The usual symptom is an excessive vaginal discharge.

Condylomata These are benign multiple skin tumours like warts on the vulva and in the anal region. They can be painful and are caused by virus infection. Irritation, pain, and discharge can be the symptoms for which the patient consults her doctor. The condylomata sometimes respond to local applications but more commonly are destroyed under local anaesthesia by using electric cauterization.

In summary, many and varied organisms can be responsible for excessive vaginal discharge, with or without vulval pain and irritation. Because of the serious potential of some of these infections, the patient will not only be examined in the surgery, but the doctor will often make the exact diagnosis by microscopic examination and culture of the discharge. Appropriate and effective treatment can then be instituted with a minimum of delay.

Tumours The reproductive system, particularly the womb and ovaries, and the breasts, are especially susceptible to tumour formation. Tumours may be either benign or malignant and the relative incidence of these two types varies from organ to organ. In the United Kingdom, cancer of the breast is almost twice as common as cancer of the neck of the womb (cervical cancer). There are geographical differences of incidence but this is probably due to racial factors. For example, cancer in the neck of the womb is the most common malignant disease in the Bantu women of Africa. Fortunately, as discussed later, cervical cancer is almost a preventable disease in a modern developed society.

Polyps These are tumours, usually small and benign, which project from the surface of an organ to which they are attached by a narrow base or stalk. Those which arise from the neck of the womb and project into the vagina may be single or multiple and are usually small, red, vascular, and soft. They frequently cause no symptoms and are detected only during pelvic examination, but not infrequently they are responsible for discharge which may be blood-stained, particularly after contact during intercourse, after douching, or following the insertion of tampons

or diaphragms. They are easily removed, often by being twisted until the stalk breaks and the polyp comes away in the forceps holding it. This is a painless procedure, often performed without an anaesthetic. The polyp should always be sent for microscopic examination, particularly when there is recurrent polyp formation at the same site. A rare but very malignant tumour known as a sarcoma may be identified.

Fibroid (Myoma) Uterine fibroids are very common tumours. They are detected in about ten per cent of women attending gynaecological outpatient clinics and at least one woman in five between the ages of 35 and 40 has them. They consist of the type of muscle and connective tissue which normally constitutes the wall of the womb, and characteristics significant to their treatment are that they are frequently multiple and are always surrounded by a capsule from which they can be shelled out like a pea from a pod. Beginning as tiny microscopic tumours they ultimately vary in size from a minute nodule like a pin's head to a tumour larger than a full-term pregnancy. They never occur before puberty and though sometimes found during the twenties, they are most common after the age of 30. A large fibroid can have a great effect on the size and shape of the womb, particularly when it grows centrally and projects into the uterine cavity. There is symmetrical enlargement which can, if the tumour is particularly soft, be mistaken for an abnormal pregnancy with bleeding. This type of fibroid is known as submucous because it is covered by the lining of the womb. It is particularly liable to be the cause of prolonged and heavy bleeding and infertility. Its presence can be confirmed when necessary by X-rays.

Symptoms. Many women lead normal lives in every way and are quite unaware that fibroids are growing until they are discovered unexpectedly during a pelvic examination. Unless degeneration or infection occurs, which is not common, the tumours are painless. Normally they cease to grow after the menopause but if they enlarge at that stage of life they should be removed because degeneration is occurring within the tumour and occasionally this may become malignant.

Because of the position of the womb in the pelvis, its enlargement by fibroids can cause pressure symptoms on neighbouring structures, particularly the bladder and bowel, with resultant urinary symptoms such as frequency and occasionally retention. This means inability to pass urine, causing painful distension of the bladder. Menstrual disturbances, particularly excessive or prolonged bleeding (menorrhagia) are the most common of the symptoms for which a patient with fibroids consults her doctor. As already stated, the submucous fibroid is the one most likely to cause excessive bleeding and as there are many other causes for this, it does not follow that because fibroids are present they are necessarily the cause of the menorrhagia. When necessary, various tests and investigations, such as X-ray of the uterine cavity, will help the doctor to make the correct diagnosis.

Small fibroids causing no symptoms and not large enough to be felt when the abdomen is examined require no treatment. But the patient should understand that in the event of symptoms developing, or a lump being felt above the pubis, she should notify her doctor. In any case it is advisable for her to have periodic examinations, preferably twice a year. Fibroids tend to enlarge, sometimes dramatically, during pregnancy and to a lesser extent with patients taking oral contraceptives. If a fibroid can be felt on abdominal examination, as opposed to during an internal examination, it should be removed. The reason is that fibroids have a precarious blood supply received through the surrounding capsule and as the tumour enlarges, its central portion tends to degenerate. The absorption of the breakdown products of such an area can cause chronic ill health with anaemia, indigestion, loss of weight, and lassitude.

Treatment. Surgical removal is the best treatment for fibroids causing symptoms, or for those requiring removal for the reasons given above. Myomectomy is the operation of removing a fibroid from its capsule so as to preserve the uterus. This operation was perfected by a distinguished British surgeon, Mr. Victor Bonney. His aim in devising the operation was to make it safe for women to have babies after fibroids had been removed and to save them from having a hysterectomy, which was the commonly performed operation. The success of his procedure has brought happiness to countless homes all over the world.

Removal of the womb (hysterectomy) with the fibroids is the alternative procedure. Further details are given on page 321. With modern anaesthetic and surgical techniques, this is no longer an operation to be dreaded. The stay in hospital is often only a few days and the patient can return to normal life as soon as she feels like doing so, often within a few weeks of the operation.

Ovarian tumours The ovary is very susceptible to the growth of tumours. These may be hollow (cystic) or solid, and not infrequently are found simultaneously in both ovaries, although one may be much larger than the other. They can be found at any age from the newborn infant to the centenarian.

Fortunately, approximately 75 per cent are benign. In the newborn infant and in very young children, as well as in the aged patient, the proportion of malignant growths is much higher than during the ages between.

Ovarian cysts A cyst is a tumour, usually thin-walled, containing fluid. This may be watery (serous) or thick and gelatinous (mucinous). Cysts vary tremendously in size: from those so small that they are detected only when the abdomen is opened for some other operation, to those which are so huge that the patient can hardly walk.

There are many varieties of ovarian cyst, including a relatively common type, often multiple and usually benign, known as dermoids. These, derived from an ovum, may contain fatty material, hair, and even teeth, bone, and other tissues. Just as a fibroid can be removed from its capsule in the womb, so a dermoid cyst can be removed from a capsule in the ovary leaving healthy ovarian tissue, thus preserving fertility.

Solid ovarian tumours These are not as common as cysts but may also be either benign or malignant and can occur at any age.

Occasionally an ovarian tumour will contain cells which produce hormones such as those described in chapter 9. Usually the female hormone is produced, but less frequently an ovarian tumour will produce the male hormone. These both cause characteristic changes recognizable by a doctor. For example, the male hormone will produce virilism. In this the breasts become smaller; hair grows on the face, abdomen, and elsewhere; the periods cease; the clitoris becomes larger; and the voice deepens. Feminizing tumours are more common. They can cause precocious development before puberty, prolonged and heavy bleeding after it, and post-menopausal haemorrhage in the elderly. Because most ovarian tumours are painless at first, even when malignant, many are found unexpectedly during the course of a general or pelvic examination, or when the abdomen is opened for an operation not connected with disease of the genital organs. Many ovarian tumours, as they enlarge, convert · their normal attachment to the womb into a stalk or pedicle. When this happens, the tumour can twist on its pedicle, causing severe colicky pain in the lower abdomen on the side on which the tumour has twisted. The symptoms are severe and abdominal examination usually reveals the cause of the trouble. An immediate operation to remove the twisted tumour is necessary. Whatever the reasons which lead to its discovery, once an ovarian tumour has been diagnosed it should be removed, irrespective of the age of the patient. According to the nature of the tumour as recognized by the surgeon at the operation, and the age of the patient, the decision will be taken whether to remove only the tumour, or the womb and the other ovary as well. In young women, and particularly with dermoid tumours, the surgeon will examine the other ovary carefully because tumours are frequently found on both sides. Usually these tumours are easily removed and leave the womb and ovaries so that pregnancy can occur if desired.

Endometriosis The membrane which lines the cavity of the womb is called the endometrium. Its cells respond to hormone stimulation as described in chapter 9. For reasons not fully understood, some of these cells may be transplanted elsewhere in the body, usually into the pelvis and rarely above the level of the navel. They may become implanted on the surface of the womb, usually in relation to the attachment of its supporting ligaments, on the surface of the ovary, the tube, the rectum and lower bowel, or bladder. Wherever they settle they respond to hormone stimulation as though they were still part of the lining of the womb. The result is that they undergo cyclical changes of congestion, bleeding, regression and recurrent congestion. Bleeding is usually slight and occurs into the pelvic and abdominal cavity. The endometrial cells and supporting tissue (stroma) multiply, and over a considerable period of time, which may be many years, form slowly growing tumours which can be detected on careful clinical examination of the pelvis. This is the condition of endometriosis. It rarely occurs in women in the developing countries, but in the last 20 or 30 years has become progressively more common in the western world. The disease is self-limiting in that it ceases to progress or cause symptoms when the hormone stimulation responsible for its activity ceases at the menopause. Cancer developing in areas of endometriosis is extremely rare.

Symptoms. Although it is a benign tumour, endometriosis is responsible for a great deal of suffering. It is one cause of acquired dysmenorrhoea and acquired dyspareunia. It can be responsible for prolonged bleeding, rectal pain (sometimes associated with bleeding at the time of a period), bladder pain (also occasionally associated with the passage of blood in the urine at period time), and is commonly associated with infertility. An experienced doctor usually has little difficulty in making the correct diagnosis, partly from the history with its characteristic cyclical sequence of symptoms and partly from detection during vaginal or rectal examination of tender little nodules on the surface of the ligaments supporting the womb, on the surface of ovaries fixed by adhesions, or elsewhere in the pelvis. These nodules can be extremely tender if examined before a period. Although infertility is often associated with endometriosis, many women become pregnant in spite of it, and when they do, their symptoms disappear during the pregnancy and on occasions the endometriosis regresses and even disappears. In the same way, symptoms can be relieved by the administration of hormones as used in contraceptive pills. These can enable a woman to delay or even avoid surgery. If, because of the nature or severity of the symptoms, operation becomes necessary, the gynaecologist must decide whether a limited operation would suffice or whether the womb, ovaries, and tubes should be removed. This is more likely to be necessary when symptoms are severe towards the end of reproductive life. In a younger woman complaining of dyspareunia, infertility, and acquired dysmenorrhoea, every effort should be made to preserve the reproductive organs. At the operation, nodules containing tiny blue cysts filled with blood are characteristic. With removal of the ovaries, or at the menopause, activity ceases, but when operating on young women the aim of the surgeon is to preserve ovarian, tubal, and uterine function whenever possible. The surgeon will try to restore mobility to the ovaries and tubes, correct any misplacements caused by endometriosis adhesions, and either excise or destroy by coagulation with an electric needle areas of endometriosis which it would not be safe to cut out because of their relationship to bladder or bowel. Many women have had the babies they desired after this treatment has enabled them to lead normal lives again.

Uterine displacements

Retroversion Many women are caused unnecessary anxiety when they are told that they have a retroverted uterus. This means that it is lying backwards. They may have been told that the normal position for the womb is to lie forwards so as to rest on top of the bladder. Such a uterus is said to be anteverted. It is true that this is the more usual position, but approximately ten per cent of women are born with a womb congenitally retroverted. Most go through life without any difficulty and are unaware of the so-called displacement which in their case is the normal position. There are signs which a gynaecologist can detect on vaginal examination which help him to distinguish a congenital retroversion

Chapter 13 **Special concerns of women**

from one that is acquired. In approximately ten per cent of women who were born with a normal anteverted uterus, this falls backwards into the retroverted position after childbirth or abortion. In most patients this causes no difficulties, but because symptoms may develop at a later date, as summarized below, the usual practice is for the womb to be manipulated into the original anteverted position at the postnatal or postabortal examination. The doctor may insert into the vagina a plastic support (pessary) for a few months to hold the womb in good position until the ligaments stretched during the baby's birth become less relaxed.

Symptoms. A retroverted uterus is usually symptomless. If it is enlarged, as by a fibroid, and particularly if there is relaxation of the pelvic floor and vagina, a feeling of heaviness and bearing down may be reported, particularly on the eve of a period and during one. At this stage the womb and surrounding tissues are more vascular, and vaginal discharge due to excessive secretion of mucus by the glands in the neck of the womb, heavy or prolonged menstrual bleeding, and pain in the lower back may develop. When a womb falls backwards it tends to pull the ovaries with it, and if one of these lies beneath the retroverted uterus it can result in pain at intercourse (dyspareunia) on deep penetration. This can be so severe, and cause such unhappiness, that an operation is necessary. In most patients with symptoms caused by a retroverted uterus, the doctor can manipulate it forwards where it can be held in good position by a plastic support (pessary) inserted into the vagina. If the appliance is the correct size and well-fitted, the woman is unaware of its presence and it does not interfere with intercourse. In some women a retroverted uterus is the only abnormality detected when a couple are investigated for infertility. This is a further reason for moving the uterus by manipulation or, if this is unsuccessful, by operation. This is not a serious procedure, but should not be performed unless there is a clear need for it. Manipulation is usually successful, and operation is seldom needed.

Prolapse Dropping of the womb (prolapse) is one of the most common reasons why middle-aged and elderly women are referred to gynaecologists. The close relationship of the womb to the bladder in front, and the rectum behind, is demonstrated in the diagrams below. All three structures are held in their normal position in the pelvis by supporting muscles and ligaments which constitute the floor of the pelvis. Sometimes there is a congenital weakness in these tissues with the result that even a relatively

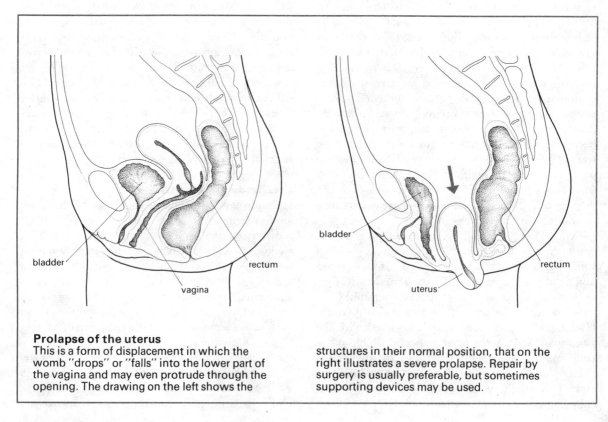

Prolapse of the uterus
This is a form of displacement in which the womb "drops" or "falls" into the lower part of the vagina and may even protrude through the opening. The drawing on the left shows the structures in their normal position, that on the right illustrates a severe prolapse. Repair by surgery is usually preferable, but sometimes supporting devices may be used.

young woman who has never borne children may complain of pelvic discomfort and a sense of dropping, and will be found to have a womb which telescopes down the vagina until the neck of the womb may even protrude at the vulva. More commonly, however, women with symptoms indicating prolapse have borne children, and stretching or tearing of ligaments and separation of muscles can result in areas of weakness in the pelvic floor. If this happens, the bladder may be pushed down so as to bulge into the front of the vagina (cystocele). If the weakness involves supports to the rectum, this may bulge forwards into the vagina (rectocele). Sometimes the defect occurs at the top of the vagina, so that the lining of the abdominal cavity bulges through this between the womb and the rectum, to form a swelling at the top of the vagina (enterocele). These weaknesses in the pelvic floor may be initiated at the time of delivery, but the conditions described above are usually noticed for the first time many years later. They are particularly liable to occur at or after the menopause, because deficiency of oestrogenic hormone at this time leads to regressive changes in the genital tract and its supports, and in this way further weakens the pelvic floor. In many patients, both young and old, there is a general weakness involving the uterus, bladder, rectum, and sometimes the peritoneal sac, so that these organs bulge into the vagina.

Because the bladder may not empty properly when it bulges into the vagina (cystocele), infection (cystitis) is a common complication, and if the tissues supporting the neck of the bladder are weakened, there is frequently the complaint of inability to control the bladder effectively. The patient states that she wets her clothing when she laughs, coughs, or strains (stress incontinence) or that she has a sudden desire to pass urine which she may not be able to control (urge incontinence). On the other hand, a bulge of the rectum into the vagina (rectocele) is often symptomless apart from the sensation of something bulging into the lower vagina or vulva, but a large rectocele can be associated with difficulty in emptying the bowel. Some women find it necessary to exert pressure on the rectocele by inserting fingers into the vagina before they are able to pass a hard motion.

Treatment of these conditions was originally undertaken by the wearing of supporting pessaries, which many years ago were so commonly worn that there were special clinics in many hospitals for fitting them. The better alternative is by surgical repair. Modern anaesthetic and surgical techniques are now

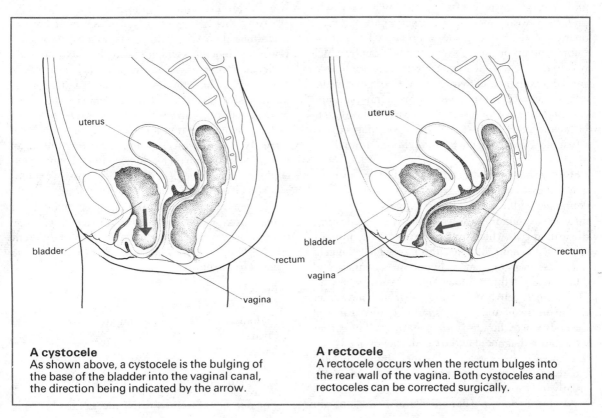

A cystocele
As shown above, a cystocele is the bulging of the base of the bladder into the vaginal canal, the direction being indicated by the arrow.

A rectocele
A rectocele occurs when the rectum bulges into the rear wall of the vagina. Both cystoceles and rectoceles can be corrected surgically.

Chapter 13 Special concerns of women

so safe that gynaecologists usually advise a surgical repair even for women of considerable age. Moreover, in younger women who wish to have further children, there is no reason against surgery and subsequent childbearing on the understanding that if obstetrical difficulties are anticipated at the time of birth, Caesarean section may have to be performed. In older women, or in those who no longer wish to have children and have an unhealthy womb, possibly with menstrual difficulties, many gynaecologists will combine the repair operation with the removal of the womb through the vagina (vaginal hysterectomy). This repairs the pelvic floor, relieves the patient of her symptoms, and leaves her with a functioning vagina, but frees her from the risk of more serious trouble, including cancer of the womb. She can of course no longer become pregnant.

Vaginal supports (pessaries) of various shapes and sizes still have a place in treatment. This is particularly so when symptoms have developed immediately after childbirth. In these cases the support can hold the womb in place during the important weeks following the birth of the baby while the stretched ligaments and muscles are returning to normal. From four to six months later when the pessary is removed many women are free of symptoms and require no further treatment. For those who prefer to wear a support rather than have an operation, the modern plastic pessaries are a great improvement on the former rubber rings which required changing at frequent intervals, sometimes caused irritation, and frequently were responsible for a foul discharge. Plastic supports are nonirritant and can often be worn for several years without needing to be changed. If a discharge develops, particularly when bloodstained, a doctor should be consulted.

Pelvic cancer A cancer is a malignant growth. This means that starting as a local tumour it is not contained within a capsule but spreads or infiltrates into the surrounding tissues while at the same time discarding cells which may be carried by lymphatic channels to chains of nodes through which the cells may pass to more remote lymphatic channels and establish a satellite tumour known as a metastasis. Other cancer cells from the original growth may enter the bloodstream and be transported to any region of the body where they also form metastases. The earlier a tumour is diagnosed and treated, the less likely it is that it will be spread by either lymphatics or bloodstream. This means that the prospect of cure is greatly increased.

A Greek doctor (Papanicolaou), working in

America, established the fact that from a study of cells on the surface of the neck of the womb, changes could be recognized under the microscope many years before a cancer of that area could be seen or felt. Fortunately these cells are constantly being shed into the vagina and replaced by cells growing from the deeper layers of the surface. The great contribution Dr. Papanicolaou made was that these superficial cells could be collected easily and painlessly from the neck of the womb, and when placed on a glass slide, could, after preliminary treatment and staining, be examined so that cells indicating either premalignant or cancer changes could be recognized. This is the basis of the cervical cytology ("Pap" or smear test) which is used extensively for screening healthy women. It has made a remarkable contribution in reducing the incidence of cancer of the cervix (neck of womb). If all women used the facilities available for a regular pelvic examination including a cervix test at least once a year until there were a minimum of two, and preferably three, consecutive negative tests, few would have the distress and dangers associated with cervical cancer. At the discretion of their doctor, subsequent examinations could be at longer intervals, initially every two years. A further development, initiated in Germany at the time of the first world war, is an instrument known as the colposcope. Basically this is a combination of a bright light to illuminate the vagina and cervix, in association with powerful binoculars which enable the doctor to study under high magnification the cells on the surface of the cervix. This enables premalignant areas, and actual cancers, which cannot be seen with the naked eye, to be recognized in their earliest phase of development. The treatment of such tumours gives virtually a 100 per cent cure. In many European countries, and to an increasing extent in Britain, well-equipped gynaecological departments use the colposcope as an additional aid in early diagnosis.

The genital tract is unfortunately a common site of malignant disease. The relative incidence of these tumours varies in different countries and in different ethnic groups in the same country. In Britain the order of frequency is:

Breast
Cervix (neck of womb)
Endometrium (body of womb) } equal
Ovary
Vulva
Vagina
Fallopian tubes (oviduct)

The number of women with cancer of the breast is

approximately equal to the total number with uterine cancer (that is, cervix and endometrium combined). The vulnerable area of the cervix and area of early local spread is illustrated below.

Cancer arising in the vagina, as opposed to spreading there from the neck of the womb, is rare, although within the last few years in America a number of adolescent girls and young women have developed this growth and it has been demonstrated that when each was a fetus in her mother's womb, the mother had been given large doses of a particular hormone, which at that time was administered as treatment for certain complications of pregnancy. No similar case has been reported in Britain, in spite of careful searches in cancer records. Nonetheless, the American reports give emphasis to the importance of women avoiding drugs during pregnancy whenever possible.

Cancer of the cervix (neck of womb) is one of the common malignant tumours arising in the genital organs. There are racial variations in its incidence although the reason for this is not yet fully understood. Fifty years ago in Britain it was nearly ten times more common than cancer beginning in the lining of the womb (endometrial cancer or cancer of the corpus). The position is now very different. The

incidence of cancer of the cervix has fallen steadily, while that of the endometrium has risen until they are now seen with equal frequency. Fortunately, not only are fewer cases seen, but they tend to be diagnosed much earlier and because methods of treatment have greatly improved the final result is that the number of women dying from this form of cancer has been much reduced. In fact, as explained earlier in reference to the Papanicolaou or smear test, if the changes taking place in the cells on the neck of the womb are recognized in the preinvasive stage, the cure rate is virtually 100 per cent. The word "preinvasive" means that the cancer cells have not invaded the surrounding tissue nor spread elsewhere in either the lymphatics or the bloodstream.

Even when the growth is not recognized at such an early stage, the facilities for treatment are now so good that thousands of women lead healthy happy lives with no recurrent trouble after cancer of the cervix has been treated.

The figures below give an indication of how a neglected growth can spread. In that on the right which illustrates the normal structures in the pelvis, there could still be early changes in the superficial cells on the neck of the womb which if not detected by the smear test, or by colposcopy, could later produce

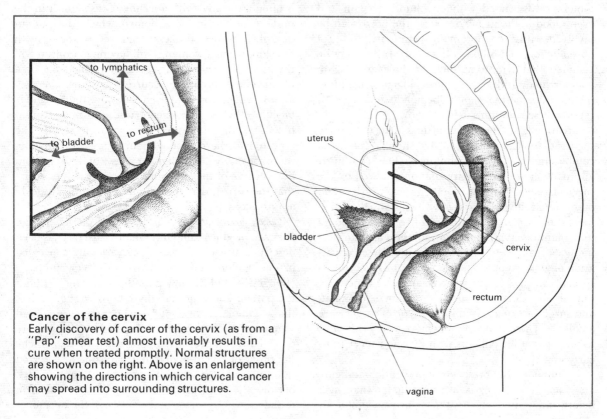

Cancer of the cervix
Early discovery of cancer of the cervix (as from a "Pap" smear test) almost invariably results in cure when treated promptly. Normal structures are shown on the right. Above is an enlargement showing the directions in which cervical cancer may spread into surrounding structures.

Chapter 13 **Special concerns of women**

spread as seen in the figure on the left. If symptoms are ignored so that the cancer continues to spread as shown, it can destroy the cervix, spread upwards into the wall of the womb above, or involve the wall of the bladder in front or the bowel behind. While doing this it not uncommonly extends down into the vagina itself.

Symptoms. The smear test will recognize the early changes at a time when treatment is simple and cure so assured that in certain circumstances the patient may even be allowed to have babies subsequently. This fact emphasizes the need for women to take advantage of the facilities available for routine screening of the cervix.

Once the malignant cells burst through the deeper layer of the mucous membrane to invade the surrounding tissues, an ulcer, which at first is painless, develops and causes a bloodstained discharge. This may be first noticed after intercourse or on the surface of a contraceptive diaphragm. It should be reported to a doctor at once. As described earlier there are simple causes for the same symptom, such as a benign vascular polyp, but it is wise not to take chances. Another indication is that bladder symptoms are likely to arise when the growth spreads to involve its wall. They are a frequent desire to empty the bladder, sometimes associated with discomfort or pain and even blood in the urine. Similarly the bowel can be involved, with discomfort in the rectum, irritability of bowel action, and blood in the stools. It must not be assumed that symptoms such as these are due to haemorrhoids (piles). A gynaecological, including rectal, examination should be made if a woman reports these symptoms to her doctor.

Treatment. This consists of destroying the growth by irradiation, removing it by surgery, or by a combination of both techniques. The combined approach of preliminary irradiation followed by the surgical removal of the womb, tubes, ovaries, and other areas involved, is now being used on an increasing scale. The treatment of this type of malignant disease by modern radiation and surgical methods requires team effort with the close cooperation of gynaecologist and radiotherapist working in special tumour centres where elaborate, expensive, but highly effective modern radiation equipment, and surgeons experienced in this type of surgery are available. These centres now achieve a cure rate of 80 to 90 per cent for patients with uterine cancer in its early stage.

In summary, the prospects of prevention and cure for cancer of the cervix are now better than ever before and women who use the facilities available for periodic examination need no longer fear this disease. Those most at risk are women who have had many sexual partners, whether they have had children or not. By contrast, cancer of the cervix is practically never seen in a virgin.

Cancer of the endometrium This disease is increasing in incidence in developed countries. The exact reason is not known, but it is perhaps significant that in developing countries the disease is beginning to occur more frequently in the affluent sections of urban communities. It is a disease which rarely occurs under the age of 50 and has a higher incidence in women who have continued to menstruate after this age, particularly where the menopause has been associated with heavy or prolonged bleeding. Unlike cancer of the cervix, this tumour has a higher incidence in women who have *not* borne children, but also occurs in those who have. The growth tends to remain within the womb itself before spreading to other areas much longer than cancer of the cervix does. For this reason the outlook is good, if symptoms are reported early. There is some evidence to suggest that the prolonged administration of oestrogenic hormone may increase the risk of this cancer.

Symptoms. After the menopause (change of life) vaginal bleeding is the characteristic symptom. This is often associated with a feeling of discomfort in the midline of the lower abdomen which the patient describes as period-like in nature. If the growth develops when a woman is still having periods, it will reveal its presence by irregularity of bleeding or a bloodstained discharge occurring between the periods. It will be apparent from the above that irregular bleeding before the menopause, postmenopausal bleeding, or bloodstained discharge should be reported to the doctor without delay. Fortunately, there are many nonmalignant causes of this symptom but because of the possibility of cancer it is essential that the correct diagnosis should be made as quickly as possible.

Cancer of the ovary The potential of the human ovary to produce tumours of many varieties has been described already. Because the ovaries are concealed in the abdominopelvic cavity they can undergo changes, including new growth formation, without the patient knowing that anything is wrong. So it is that tumours, either solid or hollow (cystic), will sometimes reach a considerable size before they are detected. If an ovarian tumour twists on its pedicle, the onset of severe abdominal pain on the affected side will lead to the correct diagnosis. Other tumours, because they produce hormones, will draw attention to themselves by virtue of the action of the hormones on the patient, as for example when there is an excessive production of the female oestrogenic hormones leading to irregular or heavy bleeding. In contrast, the rarer tumour producing the male hormone will lead to a cessation of periods and the changes previously described as virilizing, with excessive growth of hair, change of voice, and enlargement of the clitoris. If a malignant ovarian tumour spreads to adjacent structures, the first thing the patient may notice is a rapid enlargement of the abdomen due to an accumulation of fluid (ascites), or the onset of abdominal discomfort or pain. The optimum time to diagnose an ovarian tumour is before any of these complications develop, and this is a further reason for a woman having periodic examinations at, say, yearly intervals, however well she is feeling.

Treatment is by surgery, often supplemented by irradiation and sometimes by the use of special (cytotoxic) drugs to suppress malignant activity. Fortunately, approximately three quarters of all ovarian tumours are benign, but it is always important that they should be recognized early so that a gynaecologist can determine their true nature and implement the necessary treatment.

Choriocarcinoma This long name describes a tumour which fortunately is rare in Britain, but frequently seen in women in the Far East. It is always associated with pregnancy and may develop after a normal delivery, an abortion, or when pregnancy occurs outside the womb. Most commonly, however, it is a later complication of another relatively unusual but benign tumour which occurs as a complication of pregnancy itself. Both the benign and malignant manifestations arise from cells which in a normal pregnancy would enter into the formation of the afterbirth (placenta). From what has been said it is obvious that this cancer is found in women during the years of childbearing and, within that range, can occur at any age. A common symptom is continuing, or recurrent, bleeding after delivery or abortion. Diagnostic changes occur in the level of one of the hormones normally circulating in the blood during pregnancy. There are now sensitive tests for measuring this and thus confirming diagnosis. Because cells from this tumour tend to spread to the lungs there may be a cough or even bloodstained sputum. X-ray of the chest may demonstrate collections of these cells.

Treatment. The modern treatment of this rare but previously fatal cancer is by the use of powerful drugs, sometimes assisted by surgery. As with certain other cancers mentioned earlier, the relative rarity of the disease and the expertise required for its efficient treatment necessitate that this should be put into the hands of those with special experience and skills. Your doctor will be able to advise on this.

Cancer of the vulva This is not nearly as common as the tumours already described. It is seldom seen in younger women although it can occur in those aged 30 to 40. The risk of its development becomes greater with advancing years and particularly after the menopause. This is the stage of life in which regressive changes are taking place in the genital tract associated with lessening of oestrogenic hormone levels once the ovaries cease to function. There is frequently a history of prolonged or recurrent irritation of the vulva. This can be so marked that it makes life miserable for the patient, often becoming worse at night and resulting in disturbed sleep and soreness due to scratching. One result of this can be the development on the vulva of white areas due to the superficial cells in the skin undergoing changes as a result of chronic irritation. This can progress to the stage of a cancer developing, although in many patients with cancer of the vulva these white areas (leucoplakia) are not found. The important point is that because a long history of vulval irritation is often given by patients who report for the first time with a malignant tumour, it is the more necessary that any woman with persisting, or recurring, itching of the vulva should consult her doctor. He will have the affected area examined and, if necessary, tests carried out to determine the cause of the irritation. By doing this and having appropriate treatment she will reduce very greatly the chance of cancer developing at a later date.

Symptoms. The first indication of trouble is the development of a lump or ulcer anywhere on the vulva. If the lump is a malignant tumour it will form an ulcer as it progresses but sometimes a small ulcer is the first detectable sign of trouble. At this stage the ulcer is usually painless but secondary infection occurs early and there can be considerable pain and tenderness if the area is touched. Sometimes another ulcer will develop on the opposite side of the vulva (a so-called "kiss ulcer"). As the cancer grows, malignant cells can be carried by lymphatics to nodes in the groin and to others deeper in the pelvis. This is another reason for reporting the trouble early and having adequate treatment.

Treatment is by surgery. Even in elderly women there is a high rate of cure following surgery when performed by experienced gynaecologists. While it is obviously more convenient for patients to be treated as near as possible to their own homes and friends, the facilities and experience necessary for the modern treatment of cancer make it desirable that those with malignant disease should be transferred when necessary so that they can benefit from the equipment and skills which specialized cancer (oncological) centres can provide.

Malignant melanoma This is a relatively rare cancer which can occur on the vulva. It arises from a type of mole which, if seen on the face, is sometimes described as a beauty spot. For this reason it is unlikely to arouse interest when found elsewhere in the skin of the body. It is one of the tumours which, when it becomes malignant, tends to spread widely and rapidly. For that reason any change in the behaviour of a mole on the vulva, or elsewhere, should be reported to the doctor as soon as it is noticed. The type of change which may occur is that the mole becomes larger, darker in colour, raised into a little lump which can be felt, or cracks to form a little ulcer from which there will be discharge and even bleeding. Treatment is by surgical excision which if performed in the early stage of change, and before ulceration occurs, is a simple procedure.

Cancer of the fallopian tube This also is a very rare tumour. Even gynaecologists and surgeons of wide experience seldom see many patients with this disease. An unusual symptom which, when it occurs, is characteristic and should lead to the correct provisional diagnosis is that the patient develops a profuse watery discharge and on examination is found to have a tumour attached to the side of the womb. Particularly when there is no such discharge and this tumour is felt, it is likely that the diagnosis will be made of an ovarian growth. The distinction is not important for the patient because operation is necessary for both conditions and the correct diagnosis will be made when the surgeon sees the tumour.

Treatment. This is a serious disease and the best outlook for the patient will be obtained in the type of department already described in which modern radiation facilities and teams skilled in both radiation and surgical techniques are available.

SUMMARY It will have been noted how frequently in the preceding brief summary of malignant tumours of the genital organs the point has been stressed that the prospect of cure is related not only to the facilities available for treatment but to the early stage at which cancer has been diagnosed. Herein lies the justification for periodic routine examinations, including the Papanicolaou or smear test, and the reporting without delay of such symptoms as irregular bleeding, bloodstained discharge, swelling of the abdomen, a lump, ulcer, or persisting irritation of the vulva or a lump, however small, in the breast. Many women would be saved to live normal healthy lives if they treated these warning symptoms seriously and obtained medical advice with a minimum of delay.

Menopause (change of life) The hormonal explanation of this phase of a woman's life, marking as it does the end of her powers to reproduce, has been explained in chapter 9. Because there is widespread confusion concerning what is normal in changes of menstrual behaviour during the menopause, the following guidelines are given.

Some women, after menstruating normally for years, will stop suddenly as though they were pregnant. In fact, at first they may fear that conception has occurred. Any doubt can be settled quickly by a hormone test on an early morning specimen of urine. Other women will have regular periods but of decreasing duration and amount of loss until there is no further bleeding. A third group will have irregular losses of decreasing amounts and duration, sometimes for many months. They may miss a period completely and one or two months later have another, usually of short duration and reduced loss, until finally the periods cease. The point in common in all three groups is decreasing loss, with or without increasing intervals between. Any pattern apart from these three should be regarded as abnormal, although in most cases investigation will show that there is no serious trouble. In other words it can be stated that heavy or prolonged periods, or intermittent episodes of bloodstained discharge, are *not* normal at the change of life and should be reported without delay. "Don't worry about your heavy periods, it is only the change" is a dangerous doctrine.

Postmenopausal symptoms This phase of life for many women coincides with major changes in the family. Children are growing up and may have adolescent and teenage problems. Others are away at work or have married and are now making homes of their own. Some women find it difficult at first to adjust emotionally to these alterations in family life. Depression and anxiety can create tensions in the home and be associated with suspicions and fears for which there is no justification. A woman who has a career of her own, or outside interests which she finds absorbing, is less likely to have these difficulties.

The attitude of a woman, who possibly by now is a grandmother, will be influenced considerably by the bonds which have been developed through the years with the children, and by the extent to which they share their new lives and experiences with her. The time spent in caring for her own health and appearance in the knowledge that there is no need for the menopause to bring an end to these important activities, is time well spent. Because of the lessening of those direct family responsibilities which for many years have kept her occupied, she will now have more time to devote to those activities which interest her most. Fertility is greatly reduced, and rapidly declining at this stage of life, so much so that after six consecutive months without a period the chance of pregnancy occurring is extremely slight, increasingly so if the menopause is delayed until after the age of 50. Because of the importance of avoiding an unplanned pregnancy at this time, a woman should obtain the advice of her family doctor or a gynaecologist if she is uncertain whether to discontinue using contraceptives.

As stated earlier in relation to relaxation of the pelvic floor and the development of prolapse, symptoms due to the weaknesses responsible for this may be noticed for the first time at the menopause or shortly after it. The deficiency which occurs in the levels of oestrogenic hormone once the ovary ceases to function can be associated with an increased tendency for infection to occur in the vulva and vagina, with associated irritation and discharge. Medical advice should always be sought for any of these problems with the assurance that there is effective treatment available which can not only relieve the symptoms but restore the possibility of leading a normal sex life.

Treatment consists of correcting hormone deficiency by the carefully controlled administration of oestrogenic hormone, but it requires medical supervision.

In conclusion, it should be remembered that many women retain their elegance, beauty, and charm, and lead happy satisfying lives without any need for hormone replacement therapy. This is because other glands in their endocrine system (chapter 9) provide adequate supplies of hormone to compensate for that which is lost when the ovaries cease to function. Nonetheless, for those women who require its assistance, the administration of oestrogenic hormone can transform their lives. In excess it may stimulate the lining of the womb and cause vaginal bleeding which should be reported to the doctor.

Gynaecological operations Few people, male or female, welcome the prospect of surgery unless severe symptoms make them anxious to explore any possible way of obtaining relief. When an ovarian tumour twists on its pedicle, or severe internal bleeding is caused by the rupture of a blood vessel by a pregnancy occurring outside the womb (ectopic pregnancy), there is acute abdominal pain, and immediate surgery is required. However, most gynaecological operations are not so urgent, so there is usually ample time for a woman to be informed of the reason for any surgery which is advised, its probable extent, severity, and implications. The final right to give consent rests with the woman and for her subsequent peace of mind it is wise for her to remember this and be as well-informed as the circumstances will allow. It is strange but true that many women, when about to undergo a gynaecological operation, are caused most distress by their closest friends or relatives. This is the more unfortunate in that those responsible have in fact been trying to help but have failed to realize that the symptoms the patient has reported, and the facts which the doctor discovered when he made an examination, are relevant to each particular patient and influence the advice given as to the type of operation required. They will also have a bearing on whether further treatment may be necessary and how long the stage of recovery is likely to be. A woman should not hesitate to ask her doctor, or the gynaecologist who will operate on her, these important questions because an understanding of what is involved will add to her peace of mind and hasten her recovery.

Dilatation and Curettage ("D. & C.") This relatively simple procedure consists of stretching open the neck of the womb, after it has been exposed at the top of the vagina, by inserting dilating instruments of progressively increasing size. When the neck of the womb has been opened, the cavity above can be explored with special instruments, and the superficial lining of the womb removed with a curette. This is an instrument like a tiny spoon on a long handle. The material removed is sent for examination under the microscope by a pathologist and the information so obtained helps the doctor to prescribe the necessary treatment should the curettage itself not relieve the symptoms. The lining of the womb regrows from deeper layers which are not disturbed at the operation. This procedure is often performed on a patient who comes to hospital in the morning, prepared for an anaesthetic by not having had anything to eat or drink after waking, and she should be able to go home later in the day. Most women, however, stay in hospital for one night and can return to their normal activities the day after returning home. The operation can be performed under local anaesthesia but most women prefer a general anaesthetic.

Hysterectomy is the operation of removing the womb.

Chapter 13 Special concerns of women

As will be seen from the information given in this chapter, it is an operation which can be advised for many and varied reasons and the extent and type of operation will be influenced by the underlying cause for which it is performed. In modern gynaecological surgery it almost always involves the total removal of the womb (total hysterectomy) as opposed to the operation which was standard practice for many years, namely subtotal hysterectomy. In this operation the neck of the womb was left in position while only the upper portion or body of the womb was removed. Surgery is now very much safer than it was at the time when the operation of subtotal hysterectomy was developed and whereas in those days the danger of a woman dying was about the same as that of death in association with the removal of an appendix (namely one per cent or more), anaesthesia and surgery are now so safe that a thousand or more consecutive operations involving total hysterectomy may be performed without one patient dying. It must, however, be remembered that the operation is irrevocable.

When the womb is removed through an incision into the abdominal wall the operation is known as abdominal hysterectomy. Frequently a gynaecologist experienced in the necessary technique will remove the womb through the vagina without making an abdominal incision (vaginal hysterectomy). This is usually the operation advised when the need to remove the womb is associated with some degree of prolapse (described earlier in the chapter). In this way, both problems can be dealt with at the one operation. When hysterectomy is performed for uterine cancer, a more extensive operation is necessary including removal of the ovaries, part of the vagina, and the lymphatic pathways. When the gynaecologist operates for benign causes, the ovaries may or may not be removed. It is wise for the patient to discuss the possible fate of her ovaries when her doctor, or the gynaecologist, tells her that a hysterectomy is necessary. It should be noted, however, that these days, if ovaries need to be removed, the woman need not fear the onset of premature menopausal symptoms because these can be avoided by the administration of the oestrogenic hormone postoperatively just as it can be used, as described earlier, after a normal menopause. One useful way is to insert a sterile pellet of hormone at the time of operation.

Hysterectomy, whether performed abdominally or vaginally, is not the serious and debilitating procedure which it once was and which some people seem to think it still is. Many women actively engaged in professional or business activities are back at work within a few weeks of leaving hospital. Moreover they should be able to enjoy an active and full life, including normal sexual activity. While there are exceptions to every rule, it is not correct to say that total hysterectomy always interferes with sexual satisfaction. In fact most women have a satisfactory sex life after hysterectomy, particularly when persistent or recurring bleeding, pain at intercourse, discharge or other symptoms had previously interfered with their happiness. Understanding the reason for the operation, and acceptance of the need for it, will help promote postoperative peace of mind and restoration of normal function.

Prolapse repair As stated above, this may be combined with the operation of vaginal hysterectomy, but particularly in younger women the operation consists of repairing, through the vagina and without an abdominal incision, weaknesses in the pelvic floor, by strengthening the supporting tissues which normally maintain the position of the womb, bladder, and rectum. The time spent in hospital after this operation depends on its extent, which in turn is related to the severity of the prolapse. It is also influenced by the facilities available if the patient goes home. If there is no help there, she is wiser to stay longer in hospital or in a convalescent home, but a total of ten to fourteen days in one or both of these will seldom need to be exceeded. There are many women well enough to return home earlier than this. They will continue to have some vaginal discharge during the healing process which takes longer after the vaginal operation than after an abdominal one, because it is impossible to keep the vaginal suture line dry. There may be decreasing discharge for as long as two to three weeks after the patient leaves hospital. Advice should be given to avoid attempts at intercourse until after the gynaecologist makes his postoperative examination approximately a month after the patient goes home.

Sterilization It is obvious that if hysterectomy is performed a woman can no longer bear children and in carefully selected patients this operation will be advised, partly as a sterilizing procedure, when the gynaecologist considers all the details of the case. An example is when a woman, in addition to requesting sterilization, is having trouble with excessive or prolonged periods, or has enlargement of her womb due to a fibroid tumour. Generally speaking, however, sterilization is effected by causing a blockage in the fallopian tube so that sperm cells cannot pass upwards to meet the egg. Women sometimes express anxiety about the inability of these eggs to be disposed of if they cannot escape down the tube, or if hysterectomy has been performed and the ovaries and tubes have been left in place. There is no need for such anxiety because the tiny egg cell is quickly absorbed after it has been liberated from the ovary, unless it is fertilized by a sperm cell and passes into the womb to initiate a pregnancy. There is therefore no possibility of an increasing collection of eggs in the pelvis.

The tubes can be severed, or obstructed by coagulation or clips, through either a small abdominal incision, which can be so placed in a natural transverse crease above the pubis that it is not visible a few weeks after operation, or through the top of the vagina so that there is no incision on the abdominal wall, or through an instrument known as a laparoscope. This is inserted through a small stab incision near the navel and allows the surgeon to see the tubes as if he were looking through a telescope. With special instruments it is possible to block the tubes without making the incision necessary for the open operation described above. The question of which technique the gynaecologist will use depends on many factors which will be reviewed by him when assessing the best procedure for each particular woman.

When the decision to perform sterilization is made, it should be clear that both the patient and the surgeon regard it as an irrevocable step. If the patient has doubts about this, she is wiser not to give consent until she is certain. With modern techniques it is, however, often possible to restore continuity of the tubes and in this way restore fertility should unforeseen developments subsequently give rise to the desire to have another baby. Sterilization, though technically a relatively simple procedure, is an operation which should not be undertaken lightly. It has brought peace of mind to countless numbers of women and stability to their homes, but it has also brought great and lasting distress to some, who, particularly when young, took a decision which they subsequently regretted. When there is doubt it is better to defer the decision and to rely on other contraceptive techniques such as the pill or an intrauterine device.

Conclusion Health and happiness in life can be influenced a great deal by the patient herself. The intimate relationship between the development and normal function of the sex organs and the influence which these in turn have on the physical, mental and emotional growth of the girl, the adolescent, and the mature woman, are indicated throughout this chapter. Preparation for fullness of life should start in the early years of the growing child with simple guidance in personal hygiene and why this is important. Ignorance and fear are two silent but powerful enemies. They are best defeated by a growing understanding from the earliest years to the stage of mature personal experience of the normal role of the sex organs and their function. Early recognition of symptoms and signs suggesting the need for further advice, and prompt action to obtain this, will reduce to a minimum the chance of health and happiness being impaired or destroyed by diseases originating in the reproductive tract.

The breast

Revised by R. S. Handley, OBE FRCS.

The treatment of breast cancer, especially in its earlier and potentially curable stage, nearly always involves surgical removal of the breast, an operation known as mastectomy. Loss of a breast is a deeply disturbing event to any woman because she feels that it has deprived her of some of her femininity. This is not really accurate because femininity is a psychological attitude, largely conditioned by those chemical substances called the female sex hormones manufactured by glands inside the body, notably the ovaries, which are quite unaffected by removal of the breast. Nevertheless a mastectomy is a disturbing and at first repugnant change of body shape and no sensitive surgeon would undertake it unless he knew the results of not undertaking it. It is perhaps a comfort for a woman who has had to lose a breast due to cancer to realize that there are at least 100,000 women in Britain who have undergone the operation and that the great majority can conceal the fact so well that close friends and neighbours are often unaware of what has happened. Surgical breast

forms, known as prostheses, are now so good that total concealment is often possible when a brassiere is being worn and it may even be possible for a woman who has undergone a mastectomy to wear a bikini without her loss being apparent. There are glamorous personalities in the theatrical world and famous women in many walks of life whose friends and acquaintances never suspect that they have had a breast removed (in some instances both breasts).

Cancer of the breast most frequently strikes women between 40 and 60 years of age. One out of every eighteen women is likely to develop breast cancer at some time during the average life span of 72 years. At present, radical mastectomy is the best chance that medical science can offer of saving their lives. "Radical" means complete removal of the breast and of some associated tissues, particularly in the armpit area, to lessen the possibility that cancer cells might migrate to other parts of the body and establish themselves there.

While there have been significant advances in

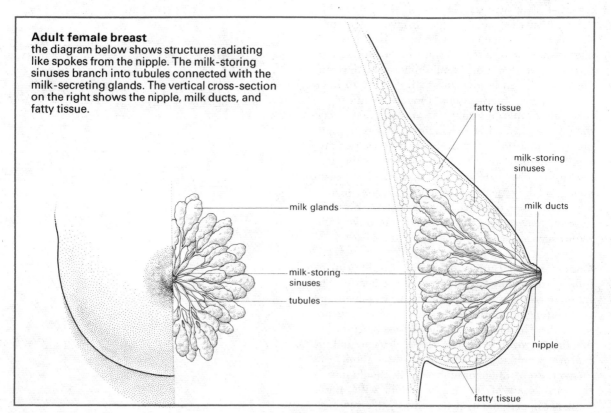

Adult female breast
the diagram below shows structures radiating like spokes from the nipple. The milk-storing sinuses branch into tubules connected with the milk-secreting glands. The vertical cross-section on the right shows the nipple, milk ducts, and fatty tissue.

fatty tissue

milk-storing sinuses

milk ducts

milk glands

milk-storing sinuses

tubules

nipple

fatty tissue

treatment made by surgery, X-ray treatment, and treatment by hormones and certain chemical drugs, there has been no decrease in the number of women who become affected by breast cancer. Early detection offers the woman with breast cancer her best hope of survival. Yet after decades of campaigns aimed at getting women to seek medical advice at the first suspicion of a lump in the breast, many months often elapse between the time a woman discovers a lump and the time when she goes to her doctor for an examination. The prime reason given by the patient for this delay is usually that the lump was painless and she thought it did not matter. It cannot be too strongly stressed that the great majority of cancerous lumps in the breast are painless in their early stages. During the wasted months of delay, a malignant growth can make disastrous progress. It can grow at the site where it started and it can send off its cells through the rest of the body, setting up satellite areas of cancerous growth called metastases.

Self-detection

Some 98 per cent of women with cancer of the breast discover evidence of the tumour themselves, usually while having a bath. The most common self-discovered sign is a painless lump, frequently in the upper outer area of the breast. Yet some women who make this discovery wait a year or more before they consult a doctor, and in the meantime the lump, should it be malignant, is spreading its dangerous cells toward other parts of the body. Ignorance and delay account largely for many deaths from cancer of the breast that would not have happened if any lump had been called immediately to a doctor's attention, when the malignant tumour was localized and chances of cure by surgical removal excellent.

It must be emphasized that not every suspicious lump in the breast means cancer. Just as there are many types of cancer cells, so are there many kinds of lumps that may appear in the breasts. Fortunately, most of these lumps prove to be harmless tumours or cysts. Yet fear that a lump in the breast invariably means cancer may provoke paralysing panic, and sad and possibly fatal delay in consulting a doctor to find out what the lump actually does mean. Discovery of a lump in the breast does not always mean that cancer is present. But it does always mean that you should see your doctor without delay.

Many doctors encourage their women patients to examine their breasts every month in a way suggested by the photographs on the next page, and give instructions in how to do so.

A woman's familiarity with the normal feel and texture of her breasts assists in recognizing changes that may occur. In some instances, self-examination procedures may perpetuate harmful cancer fears that are quite unreasonable, but there is little risk of this in intelligent women who are properly informed by their doctors.

Symptoms, other than a lump, to be aware of are:

Any alteration in the usual shape of the breast.
Elevation or sinking of the nipple.
Slight dimpling of the skin of the breast.
Discharge, bleeding, or a rash around the nipple.

As has already been stressed, pain is not a symptom of early breast cancer. Pain is nearly always a symptom of some other nonmalignant condition and seldom occurs in a cancerous lump until a late stage in its growth. It is tragic how often women with an advanced cancer say at their first consultation with a doctor that the lump did not bother them and they did not think it needed medical attention.

The doctor's examination

Diagnosis of breast cancer requires the skills of a doctor. Very advanced breast cancer is sadly obvious, but early stages are not. Examination of the breasts with a view to early detection of anything abnormal is a part of regular physical checkups. More often than not the doctor is happily able to assure the patient, to her great peace of mind, that all is well. But the nature of a small lump or other symptom, reported by the patient or discovered by a doctor, must be determined.

The doctor examines and palpates the breasts in a number of positions: with the patient standing, with arms overhead, or lying on the examining table. He also examines the armpits which contain some of the lymph channels and lymph nodes leading from the breast, a pathway which cancer cells frequently take in spreading.

A comparatively new technique the doctor may elect to use for detecting breast tumours, employing X-rays, is called mammography. Mammography is no substitute for a proper clinical examination by the doctor, but it is often useful in doubtful cases.

With the one exception mentioned in the next paragraph, final diagnosis of whether a suspicious breast tumour is benign or malignant rests upon surgical biopsy – removal of a sample of tissue from the suspicious lump for microscopic examination by a pathologist. This is done under anaesthesia in the operating room. The tissue sample goes immediately to the laboratory, and while the surgeons wait, the specimen is frozen with liquid carbon dioxide so that a tissue-thin slice may be obtained for microscopic scrutiny. Should this microscopic examination prove the tumour to be benign, the tumour alone is removed by a fairly simple operation and the breast itself is left intact with little or no disfigurement.

The one exception to the surgical removal of a lump is when the doctor thinks that what he feels is a cyst. His diagnosis (which he may make because the lump he feels is very movable and has a well-defined edge) must still be proved but many surgeons do this by inserting a needle into the lump. If fluid is withdrawn, the lump abolished, and the examination of the withdrawn fluid in the laboratory satisfactory, this constitutes proof that the doctor's diagnosis is correct. The process is called aspiration, and is easily done on an outpatient basis.

Breast self-examination

The breasts should be examined once a month, preferably just after a period. Women who no longer have periods might decide on a particular date each month.

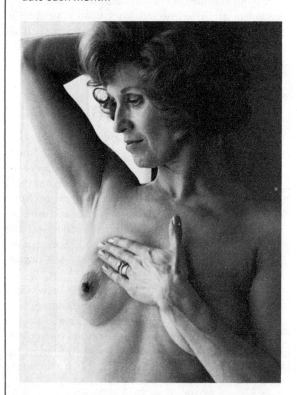

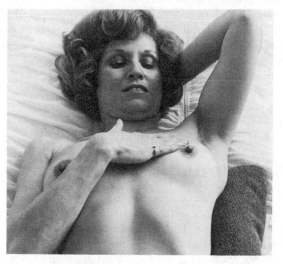

1 Place your left hand under your head, keeping the elbow flat. With the flat of the fingers of your right hand, gently but firmly examine the top inner quarter of the breast, working from the ribs and breastbone towards the nipple.

Although the bathroom is in many ways an ideal place for self-examination, it should have a good mirror in which the whole of the upper body can be seen. This is important, since by looking carefully it is often possible to detect changes (as of shape or size) in the breasts. Other changes to look for are puckering of the skin, alterations in outline, and any bleeding or unusual discharge from the nipple.

For the next stages of self-examination it is best to lie down on a bed, or sit back in the bath. A pillow under the shoulder will spread the tissues, making the breast easier to examine.

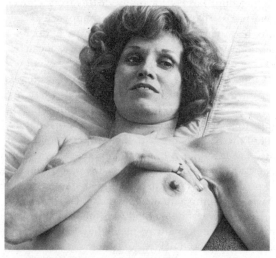

4 With your left arm at your side, examine the upper outer quarter, taking care to include all the tissue between the armpit and the nipple.

Breast cancer surgery

A biopsy specimen that proves to be malignant means radical surgery – that is, complete removal of the breast, and of adjacent lymph nodes near the armpit and collarbone. The surgeon cannot take chances. He must remove all the malignancy to save and prolong his patient's life. In the operation, the surgeon usually makes an elliptically-shaped incision and removes the breast and surrounding tissue in a single block. This technique is considered less likely to disturb and spread loose cancer cells and it also entails less disfigurement than some of the older procedures. With sutures and sometimes with skin grafts, the surgeon is able to close the incision with a minimum of scarring. As in other surgery, the pink lines of incisions become smoother and paler with the passage of time.

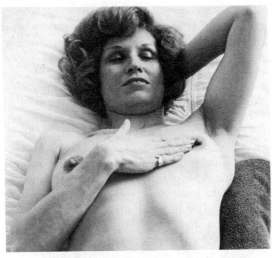

2 Next examine the lower inner quarter of the breast, paying particular attention to the area round the nipple.

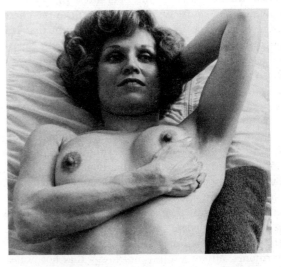

3 Then examine the lower outer quarter, starting from the ribs below and at the side of the breast.

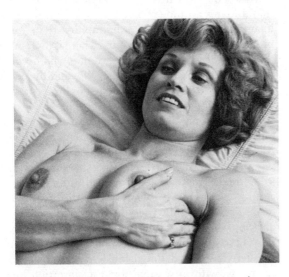

5 Finally examine the armpit, as lumps may also arise in this area.

Then follow the same procedure to examine the right breast.

It would be foolish to minimize the seriousness or complexity of this operation. Patience, delicacy, and great skill are essential. But it should be realized that it constitutes the removal of an external organ only, one which a woman can lose without major organic change or injury to her health or general wellbeing. The operation is literally superficial (by definition, on the surface). No major cavity of the body is invaded or affected.

After surgery After the operation, the surgeon may advise a course of X-ray treatment to the chest area. He may do this if he feels any doubt that his operation has not been able to remove all the deep-seated cancer cells. Some surgeons also advise a course of the new anticancer drugs but these are so new that there has not yet been time to establish whether they have a useful effect; and these drugs do sometimes have unpleasant side effects.

The so-called "magic bullet" which could destroy cancer cells wherever they hide without harming the normal cells of the body is still a hope of the future. But we do possess drugs which show heartening results against some cancers, notably of the prostate, uterus, and breast. Female breast cancer is classified as a hormone-dependent type – that is, the rate of growth of existing breast cancer is affected by female hormones, although this is not to say that hormones caused the cancer in the first place. Similarly, cancer of the prostate is affected by male sex hormones. Use of antagonistic hormones (male hormones in breast cancer, female hormones in prostate cancer), or hormone doses and removal of hormone-producing organs by castration, has proved to be of considerable palliative benefit in appropriate cases, but is not to be looked upon as a cure and never as an alternative to recommended surgery.

Unhappily, there are cases of inoperable breast cancer – disease so far advanced or so widespread that surgery cannot be curative. But even in these cases, drugs now available can usually relieve pain, delay cancer spread, and prolong a comfortable and useful life.

Dangerous fallacies

Why do so many women with breast cancer delay so long in seeking medical help that the doctor or surgeon can do little to save their lives? Fear, half-truths, phobias, and old wives' tales undoubtedly play a sad part in delaying treatment until malignancy is far advanced.

One of the most distressing of all fallacies is the mistaken belief that a diagnosis of breast malignancy is a death sentence. The truth is that more than 65 per cent of women who have had a diseased breast removed are living active useful lives. Everyone seems to hear of the occasional patient who does not do well after mastectomy, but there are no headlines for the thousands every year whose lives are unchanged or improved by mastectomy, because that is not news any longer.

Fear of disfigurement is very real and never to be treated lightly. But surgical procedures these days are done so cleanly and skilfully that even when skin grafting is necessary there is a minimum of scarring.

Deep-seated psychological fears are most difficult to abolish, and often are unexpressed and known only to the woman herself. A woman faced with mastectomy understandably shrinks from being different. Will her husband still love her? Will her family and friends view her as a freak? Actually, her femininity is not diminished. Mastectomy by itself effects no change in personality or character traits. There is no interference with hormone production and womanly functions. The patient is the same wife, the same mother, the same career girl that she was before her operation. Her physical attractiveness is not diminished; as a matter of fact, most women who have undergone mastectomy compensate by attention to make-up and grooming, making them more attractive than ever.

The young or middle-aged woman worries particularly about the attitude of the man in her life. Is she still desirable? The honest male animal will assure her that a man's attitude is based largely on a woman's image of herself, and her desirability is in direct proportion to her interest in him! There is more truth than fancy in the fact that the woman who becomes more absorbed in the man in her life, and his needs, becomes more physically attractive to him, irrespective of her surgical experience.

One must not minimize the adjustments, both physical and emotional, which the patient must make. All operations weaken patients for a time and full physical energy may take a few weeks before it returns to normal. Another aspect of adjustment lies in getting accustomed to the prosthesis, the breast form, made of various substances such as foam rubber or dacron, which fits inside the brassiere, and restores the chest contour to its normal shape when the brassiere is worn. Bathing suit designers now create garments with provision for the insertion of a prosthesis and, as has already been said, some mastectomy patients can wear a bikini without their operation being visible.

The specific cause of breast cancer (and other cancers) is unknown. We know that there is a higher incidence of breast cancer among childless women, among those who have had fewer than two children, and among those who have never breast-fed a baby. But these are admittedly negative findings, and an enormous amount of cancer research is continuing to augment our knowledge of disordered processes of cells that are involved in malignant changes. If and when some marvellous cancer drug is discovered, physicians all over the world will know about it. There are no secret cures for cancer. Unfortunately, there is cancer quackery, with promises of benefit from some mysterious medicine or treatment not employed by responsible physicians. The greatest tragedy is not the loss of money spent on worthless treatments, but that delay in seeking competent treatment may be so prolonged that chances of cure are reduced.

Early surgery is still the major means of saving the patient with breast cancer, and radical mastectomy will continue to play a dominant role in the foreseeable future. But mammography, X-rays, and the new drugs have supporting roles that continue to increase in importance.

Chapter 14
The digestive system

Revised by Sir Francis Avery Jones, CBE MD Hon.MD(Melb) FRCP

The digestive tract The human body incorporates a tube, of which the mouth is the upper opening, the digestive tract the tube itself, and the anus the lower opening. So although we speak of taking food and drink into the body, it must be remembered that strictly speaking the inside of the mouth, stomach, and intestines are outside the tissues of the body. Only when the nutrients are absorbed into the blood or tissues are they truly inside the body.

The digestive tract, although continuous, consists of sections of very different design and construction which enable it to carry out its various functions – the gullet (oesophagus), stomach, small intestine (divided into duodenum, jejunum, and ileum), and large intestine (colon). The digestive glands, salivary glands, liver, and pancreas, are in origin branches opening out from the tract. To carry out its functions efficiently the tract has marvellous coordinating mechanisms, which are partly nervous and partly chemical.

When examined after death, the intestines are about 7·5 m (25 ft) long, but in life muscular contraction of the walls makes them much shorter.

The process of digestion consists essentially of breaking down the foodstuffs into their constituent "bricks", which are then absorbed into the body and either burnt up to provide energy or built up again into the particular substances that the body needs.

Digestion and absorption The chemical processes of digestion are carried out by enzymes, complex proteins which cause or accelerate chemical reactions without themselves being consumed. Starch and compound sugars (for example, cane sugar is a compound of glucose and fructose) are broken down to simple sugars by the saliva, pancreatic juice, and small intestine juice.

Protein is digested in progressive stages by the gastric juice, pancreatic juice, and small intestine juice. Fat is rendered suitable for absorption by enzymes in the pancreatic and small intestine juices, aided by the bile.

The processes of absorption of the products of digestion are complex. Sugars and amino acids (the end products of protein digestion) pass into and through the cells of the villi (page 334) to the blood, by which they are carried to the liver and muscles. Digested fat is similarly absorbed and transmitted by the cells of the villi, but to the lymphatic vessels. These unite and lead into one large lymphatic duct which empties its contents into one of the veins at the root of the neck. So fat also enters the bloodstream, but by a different route.

The mouth and oesophagus Digestion begins in the mouth with chewing (mastication) of food by the teeth with the secretion of saliva containing ptyalin, an enzyme which begins to split starches into simple sugars. There are three salivary glands on each side of the face. The parotid gland lies in front of and below the ear, and this is the one which swells up painfully with mumps. The sublingual gland lies under the tongue. The submandibular gland is situated a little below and behind it. By carefully coordinated movement the opening to the larynx or windpipe is closed and the upper oesophagus relaxes to receive a portion of the masticated food. Waves of contraction move down the gullet and just as the food reaches the stomach, the cardiac sphincter, which is normally closed, relaxes and allows it to enter the stomach.

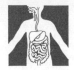

The digestive system

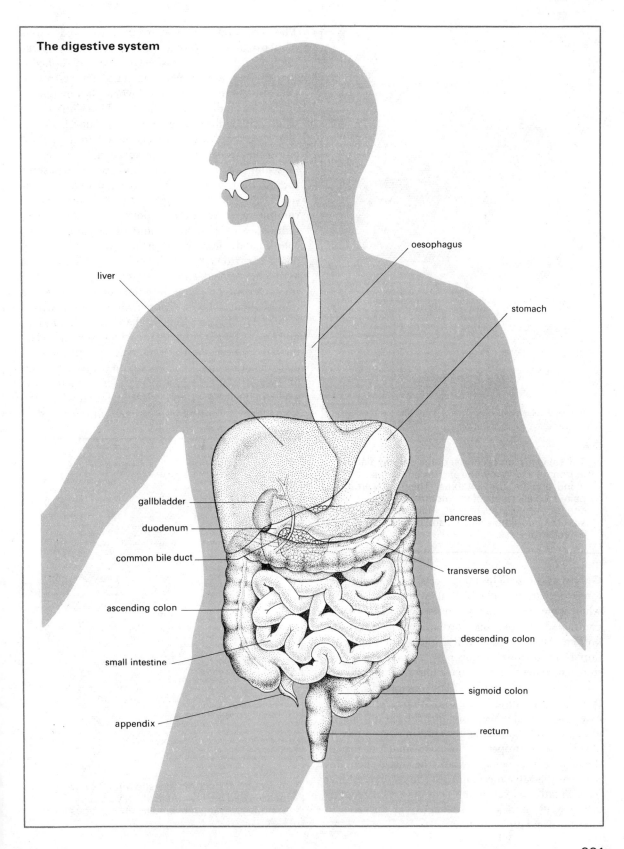

oesophagus

liver

stomach

gallbladder

pancreas

duodenum

common bile duct

transverse colon

ascending colon

descending colon

small intestine

sigmoid colon

appendix

rectum

Chapter 14 **The digestive system**

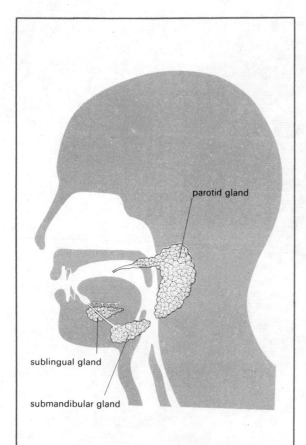

parotid gland

sublingual gland

submandibular gland

The salivary glands consist of the parotid gland in front of and below the ear, the sublingual gland, and the submandibular. The glands are paired, on each side of the mouth. Saliva contains an enzyme, ptyalin, which splits starches into simple sugars, and begins the digestive process.

The stomach The stomach is located rather higher than many people think, lying mainly behind the lower ribs on the left side. It may be described as shaped like a J. The lower end of the J represents the pylorus, and the top of the J is where the oesophagus enters the stomach at the fundus. This is the region where gas bubbles collect and may cause belching. The lower part of the stomach tapers to the pyloric end or the outlet. The short pyloric canal has a thicker muscular coat and acts as a pump gradually pushing the stomach contents into the duodenum. The stomach is a muscular organ with three muscle layers running in different directions – circular, longitudinal, and oblique – and these muscles, by coordinated contractions, make waves which sweep down the stomach, mixing its contents with the hydrochloric acid and the digestive enzymes. The stomach contents empty into the small intestine at a rate of about one per cent per minute. Emptying is achieved by an incredible mechanism, with information on movement and pressure which is registered by the sensory nerves of the stomach, being transmitted up to the brain, and then signals coming back to other fibres in the same vagus nerve, which modify the action of the pyloric sphincter. While the food is in the stomach it is continuously mixed with the hydro-

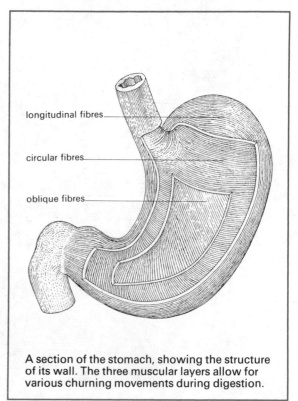

longitudinal fibres

circular fibres

oblique fibres

A section of the stomach, showing the structure of its wall. The three muscular layers allow for various churning movements during digestion.

Gravity of course helps this process, but the muscular forces are strong enough to allow swallowing even when someone is standing on his head. The ring of contracted muscle, the cardiac sphincter, at the bottom end of the gullet where it joins the stomach is important because it normally prevents the acid stomach contents flowing back into the gullet where they can cause irritation. The oesophagus passes through an opening in the diaphragm, which is an extensive muscular sheet dividing the chest from the abdomen. If this opening increases in size, it may be possible for the upper part of the stomach to slip up through it, producing a hiatus hernia. When this happens the valve mechanism at the cardiac sphincter is greatly weakened and acid may then regurgitate readily into the oesophagus, giving rise to heartburn and discomfort.

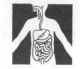

chloric acid secreted by some of the cells lining the inner wall. The main digestive enzyme secreted by the stomach is pepsin which can break down protein foods such as meat. Pepsin is active only when there is acid present and once the food reaches the duodenum, with its alkaline contents, other enyzmes take over. The hydrochloric acid produced by the special cells in the wall of the stomach is a strong acid which could burn the skin. The stomach itself is protected by the coating of mucus which is one of Nature's perfections in protection, and indeed coats the entire digestive tract, protecting the surface from the effects of its digestive secretions. Relatively few germs survive this acid bath, and the upper part of the small intestine is usually sterile. Those who have a low acid secretion may be more prone to intestinal infection such as traveller's diarrhoea. The stomach acts as a food reservoir slowly emptying its contents into the duodenum and allowing complete mixing to take place. It is possible to remove the whole of the stomach and yet the patient can continue to eat reasonably well and remain in a fair state of nutrition, showing the extraordinary adaptability of the body.

The small intestine Digestion is completed in the small intestine, and virtually all absorption occurs there. The coils of the small intestine are neatly packed together, each loop being free to glide over its neighbour, and it finally opens into the caecum, the first part of the large bowel. The small intestine is anatomically divided into three zones, the duodenum, the jejunum, and the ileum. The duodenum is so called because the early anatomists noted that the first part of the intestine which loops round the

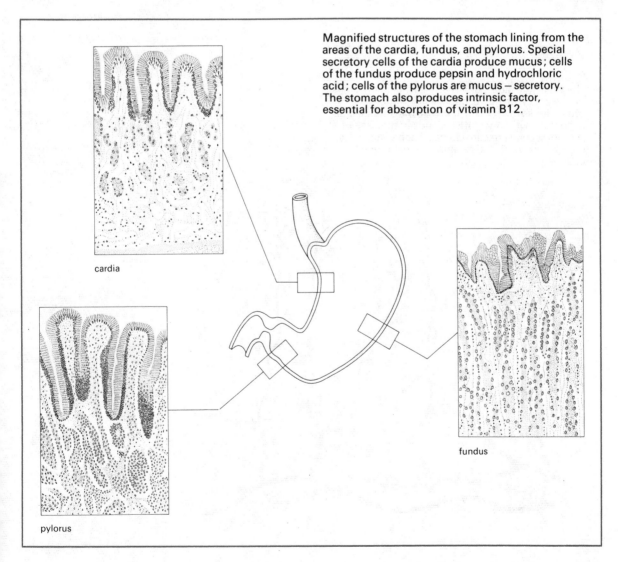

Magnified structures of the stomach lining from the areas of the cardia, fundus, and pylorus. Special secretory cells of the cardia produce mucus; cells of the fundus produce pepsin and hydrochloric acid; cells of the pylorus are mucus – secretory. The stomach also produces intrinsic factor, essential for absorption of vitamin B12.

cardia

pylorus

fundus

Chapter 14 **The digestive system**

The duodenum, the beginning of the small intestine, is an area of great chemical activity, where bile from the gallbladder and hepatic ducts enters through a common duct. Enzymes of the pancreas which split protein, fat, and carbohydrate enter the duodenum through the pancreatic duct. In the duodenum the environment is alkaline, in contrast to the acid stomach.

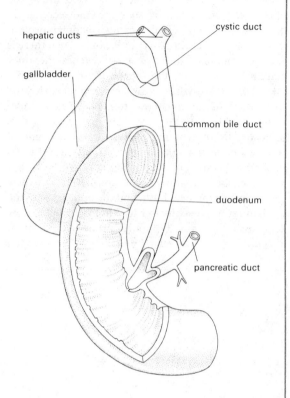

The small intestine, particularly the ileal portion, is richly lined with microscopic villi – finger-like projections which vastly increase the surface area in contact with foodstuffs. Glands at the base of the villi secrete intestinal juices. Each villus has a capillary network and a central lacteal (lymph channel).

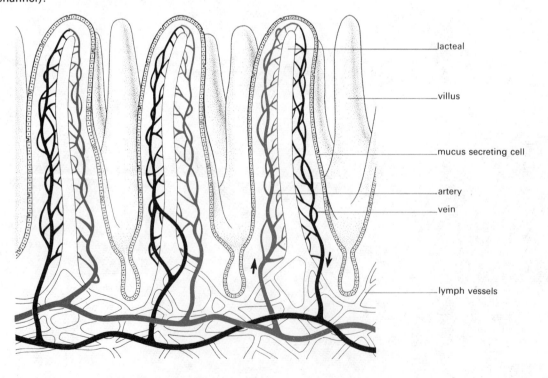

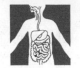

head of the pancreas was twelve finger-breadths long, twenty to twenty-five cm (eight to ten in). The contents are highly alkaline, due to the secretions of the pancreatic gland and to the presence of bile. The ducts bringing bile from the liver and juices from the pancreas open into the duodenum through a small single opening. Food entering the duodenum stimulates certain hormones produced in the wall of the intestine and these ensure the perfect coordination of the supply of bile and pancreatic juice, just as it is needed, by stimulating contraction of the gall-bladder and the secretory activity of the pancreas. The first part of the duodenum, where it joins the pylorus, is called the duodenal bulb, with the highly acid stomach contents in contact with its walls, and it is here that duodenal ulcers may form.

The first half of the small intestine is the jejunum and the second half the ileum, but the distinction is largely for anatomical convenience. The mucous lining is raised in circular folds and the surface area is further increased by the presence of rounded finger-like projections called villi which are like the pile of an exceedingly fine carpet and give the feel of velvet. Intestinal digestive glands discharge their enzymes around the base of the villi. With over five million villi in the small intestine, the effective surface area may reach the equivalent of five times the area of the body's skin surface. The small intestine is attached to and supported by the mesentery, which is a sheet of curtain-like tissue attached to the back of the abdomen, carrying the blood vessels, nerves, and lymphatic channels to and from the intestine.

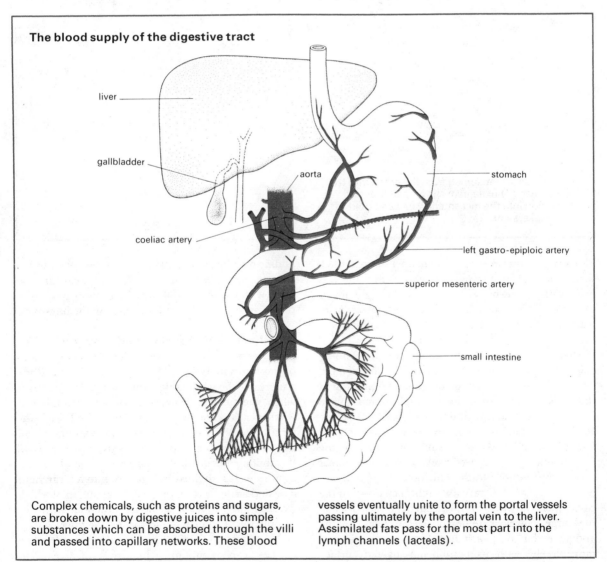

The blood supply of the digestive tract

liver

gallbladder

aorta

coeliac artery

stomach

left gastro-epiploic artery

superior mesenteric artery

small intestine

Complex chemicals, such as proteins and sugars, are broken down by digestive juices into simple substances which can be absorbed through the villi and passed into capillary networks. These blood vessels eventually unite to form the portal vessels passing ultimately by the portal vein to the liver. Assimilated fats pass for the most part into the lymph channels (lacteals).

Chapter 14 The digestive system

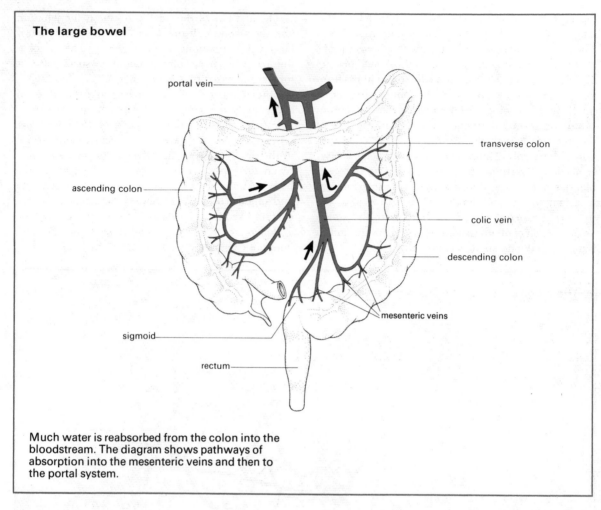

The large bowel

portal vein

transverse colon

ascending colon

colic vein

descending colon

mesenteric veins

sigmoid

descending colon

rectum

Much water is reabsorbed from the colon into the bloodstream. The diagram shows pathways of absorption into the mesenteric veins and then to the portal system.

The large intestine The ileum opens into a much wider tube called the colon. The caecum – the first part of the large bowel – starts in the right lower abdomen. The ascending colon goes upwards towards the ribs on the right side. The transverse colon then sweeps across the upper abdomen, where it takes a sharp turn downwards along the descending colon, finally taking an S-shaped turn, the sigmoid flexure, passing into the rectum, and terminating at the anus. In the colon the residual contents from the small intestine are gradually turned into faeces. It is an area of complex chemical activity. Bacteria which make up a substantial part of the faeces flourish, and indeed their metabolism makes useful contributions to the nutrition of the body. A certain amount of dietary fibre is broken down in the colon, mainly by the enzymes from bacteria. Much of the large bowel is tethered to the back of the abdomen, but part of it has a mesentery and can move freely, with its peritoneum-covered surface

gliding over loops of small intestine. The appendix is a short narrow tube branching off from the caecum and lined with lymphatic cells which probably play some protective role, as they do elsewhere in the intestine.

The liver, gallbladder, and pancreas The processes of digestion are dependent on the secretions of the associated digestive organs, the liver and the pancreas. The gallbladder stores bile and releases it when chemical messengers, hormones, stimulate it whenever fat enters the duodenum. The liver is the largest solid organ of the body, weighing about 1·8 kg (four lb) and occupying the upper part of the abdomen beneath the diaphragm, mainly on the right side. It is divided by a fissure into a large right lobe and a smaller tapering left lobe, the tip of which overlies the stomach near its junction with the oesophagus. Under the microscope the liver consists of vast numbers of minute polygonal structures called lobules, each containing hundreds of liver cells

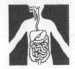

"Flow chart" of circulation of substances to and from the liver

The liver receives its own blood supply by the hepatic artery. The portal vein carries the products of digestion from the intestine to the liver, and thence to the inferior vena cava which returns blood to the heart (right atrium). Bile is manufactured by the liver, and is secreted through the bile ducts to be stored in the gallbladder.

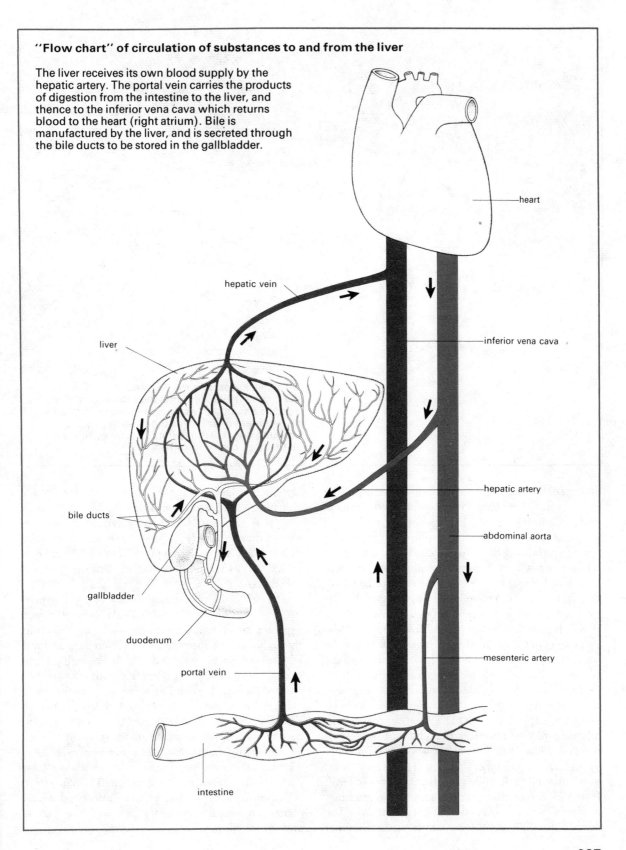

heart

hepatic vein

liver

inferior vena cava

bile ducts

hepatic artery

abdominal aorta

gallbladder

duodenum

mesenteric artery

portal vein

intestine

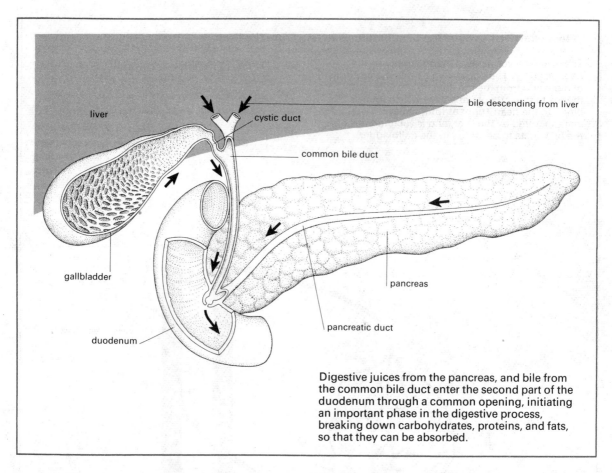

liver

cystic duct

bile descending from liver

common bile duct

gallbladder

pancreas

duodenum

pancreatic duct

Digestive juices from the pancreas, and bile from the common bile duct enter the second part of the duodenum through a common opening, initiating an important phase in the digestive process, breaking down carbohydrates, proteins, and fats, so that they can be absorbed.

arranged like fine spokes radiating out from the central vein. The liver is a very complicated chemical plant undertaking an extraordinary variety of chemical activities. It has a powerful protective effect, neutralizing the many kinds of toxic substances which reach it from the small intestine, making them harmless. It produces the bile which assists digestion. Bile is a bitter orange-yellow fluid, secreted by the liver cells, which is collected through networks of fine channels into the hepatic duct. This joins with the cystic duct to the gallbladder, where the bile may be concentrated and stored before it is released into the common bile duct which opens into the duodenum. In early days the vagaries of human temperament were reflected in the words, choleric, melancholy, bilious, jaundiced, liverish. The word "chole" means bile or gall. Our ancestors thought that depression was due to black bile – hence the word "melancholy" in ordinary language. Bile is a complex fluid containing bile salts, bile pigments, and cholesterol. It acts as a most efficient detergent in the intestine, producing fine emulsification of fatty materials. The liver is a storage organ for vitamins and for animal starch (glycogen). It is also a manufacturing site for enzymes, cholesterol, complex proteins, vitamin A from carotin, and blood coagulation factors. Its extraordinary ability to undertake so many roles depends on the rich supply of chemical enzymes which step by step build up or break down chemical substances.

The gallbladder is a storage sac about 7·5 cm (three in) long, and the bile is concentrated in it before being squeezed by muscular contraction into the duct and through into the intestine. The pancreas is a gland with many branched ducts which lies behind the stomach. It is about twenty cm (eight in) long and has a broad right end or head which nestles into the curve of the duodenum, with the tail of the pancreas narrowing off to the left side of the abdomen. The pancreas is a double-purpose gland. Its small clusters of islet cells secrete insulin, a hormone which is essential for utilizing sugars and without which diabetes may develop. The larger mass of pancreatic cells produces clear watery pancreatic juice which contains powerful enzymes for splitting fats, proteins, and carbohydrates.

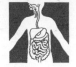

Diagnostic tests and instruments

Special instruments are used to obtain the information needed for accurate diagnosis, and some are described below. Further tests will be found in chapters 24 and 25, which discuss X-rays and laboratory tests.

Endoscopy ("looking inside") Endoscopy is one of the important developments in recent years, particularly since the introduction of fibre optics. The fibre optic system, introduced by Professor Hopkins at the Imperial College of Science, London, consists of a hundred thousand or more glass fibres, bound together, but each transmitting light separately. This means that however much the tube is curved, the image under inspection is seen with unchanged clarity at the other end. The principle is the same as with printed pictures which are made up of innumerable tiny dots. There has been rapid technological development in recent years, so that the instruments not only carry a picture and light source, but also facilities for passing probes, snares, injection channels, and cutting instruments which enable minor surgical procedures to be achieved under direct vision inside the intestinal tract. In all large general hospitals there are physicians or surgeons experienced in the use of fibre optic endoscopy. These instruments have largely but not completely taken over from the former semiflexible or rigid tubes. The present gastrointestinal fibre optic endoscopes allow complete inspection of the oesophagus, the stomach, the duodenum, and it is even possible to see the small intestine. The use of the colonoscope has greatly added to the accuracy of diagnosis in the colon, and has the added advantage of providing the opportunity of removing polyps without the patient having to be subjected to an abdominal operation. Fibre optic endoscopes are particularly valuable in giving help when there is a discrepancy between the medical history and the X-ray findings. For example, it may be possible to see small gastric or duodenal ulcers which have not shown up on the X-ray films. A further advantage of this technique is the ability to take small snips of the mucous lining to examine under the microscope – a technique known as biopsy. This may enable any cancer in the digestive tract to be diagnosed earlier.

The examination of the upper intestinal tract is normally carried out under mild sedation, after the throat has been anaesthetized with a spray or gargle.

In the majority of patients it is a simple straightforward examination without undue discomfort and can be rewarding in the extra information which it provides, enabling the most effective treatment to be prescribed.

Proctoscopy and sigmoidoscopy This is a direct visual examination of the rectum and lower part of the colon and is routinely performed with a hollow metal tube equipped with a light source. The lining of the lower part of the bowel can be inspected and biopsies can be taken to be looked at under the microscope. The sigmoidoscope enables a diagnosis of colitis (inflammation of the colon) to be established and may show up polyps, early cancers, and other disease states. The proctoscope is used to examine the anal canal and lower rectum. The instrument is much shorter than the sigmoidoscope; it enables haemorrhoids to be seen and often treated.

Peritoneoscopy (laparoscopy) This is a procedure which involves piercing the abdominal wall under local anaesthesia with a narrow metal tube carrying a light and lens system. It can also be adapted for taking biopsies. It can provide a great deal of information and avoid the need for opening the abdomen under general anaesthesia.

Liver biopsy This is a procedure for obtaining and examining a specimen of liver tissue. It is a technique which has been greatly improved in recent years and has revolutionized the diagnosis of liver disorders. The skin and tissue between two ribs is made insensitive with a local anaesthetic and then a fine special needle is inserted into the liver, suction applied, and a small core of liver tissue is obtained. In spite of its relatively small size this can provide a great deal of valuable information under the microscope and enable the exact nature of the liver disease to be demonstrated. It is usually painless but must be done with great attention to detail and with great care, and it is necessary to have the patient at complete rest in hospital for at least 24 hours. Sometimes it may be combined with peritoneoscopy which provides a visual picture of the surface of the liver and enables the doctor to biopsy individual sites under direct inspection. This will ensure that the biopsy does contain diseased tissue without resorting to opening the abdomen under general anaesthesia.

Small bowel biopsy This can be achieved by passing by mouth a thin plastic tube on the end of which is a small metal capsule. On one side of the capsule there is a small opening, and by applying suction a minute piece of small intestine can be sucked into the hole. At the same time a spring is released, which brings a minute razor-sharp blade across the opening, and this provides a small snip of mucous lining of the small intestine. It is a specialist examination which has to be done at a hospital where there are facilities for such techniques. The capsule and its tube has to be passed through the stomach into the duodenum and into the first part of the small intestine, and the position has to be checked by X-ray screening. It is relatively easy to get the tube down and the process is painless, but as with all such examinations it has to be done with scrupulous care. The patient does not necessarily have to stay in hospital overnight.

Duodenal drainage This involves passing a special multiple tube and positioning the end under X-ray control, enabling the duodenal contents to be sucked up and examined under a microscope and bacteriologically. In this way it is possible to obtain specimens of bile, and also to get a picture of the functioning of the pancreas by stimulating it with hormones. Another technique is to give the patient a fluid test meal into the stomach and to monitor at intervals the response of the pancreatic gland which will be discharging its secretions into the second part of the duodenum. The concentration of the digestive enzymes and the alkalinity can be measured in each sample which is sucked up through the tube. Microscopic examination of the duodenal contents can also provide information in certain diseases.

Gastric analysis This is a technique which involves swallowing a small plastic tube which enables the contents of the stomach to be sucked up into a syringe. The response of the lining cells and their ability to secrete acid can be recorded by analysing specimens obtained every fifteen minutes – a technique known as a fractional test meal. With a special hormone injection at the same time it is possible to achieve maximum stimulus of the particular cells which produce hydrochloric acid. This information is sometimes needed by surgeons, particularly in assessing the effects of operations for duodenal ulcer, when the vagus nerve has been cut. At one time this test was widely used in the investigation of indigestion, but it is now appreciated that the value of the test is limited.

Examination of stools (faeces) Much information can be obtained from examination of the stools bacteriologically, chemically, and under the microscope. A fresh specimen has to be collected in a clean container and delivered to the laboratory. Bacteriological examination may enable dysentery to be diagnosed. Under the microscope there may be useful evidence of incomplete digestion within the alimentary tract, evidence of inflammation, or parasitic infestation with the presence of cysts or eggs of worms. Chemical testing may show whether or not blood is present, even if there is no blood to be seen. The chemical test for blood is a very sensitive one and it is necessary for the subject to be on a meat-free regime while the stools are being collected. It is also important for the subject to avoid taking aspirin which can cause a small amount of blood loss into the stomach.

The oesophagus

Disorders of the oesophagus can give rise to difficulty in swallowing – either from some physical obstruction making the tube narrower, or from malfunction due to alteration in the normal muscular movements. Another main symptom is heartburn, a good descriptive term for the burning sensation which may rise into the chest, associated with regurgitation of acid from the stomach into the oesophagus. Normally the valve mechanism at the junction of the oesophagus and the stomach tends to prevent acid regurgitation, but under certain conditions the valve mechanism is weakened, so heartburn may occur.

Hiatus hernia The diaphragm is a sheet of muscle separating the chest from the abdomen, and the oesophagus passes through an opening, the oesophageal hiatus. Under certain conditions this may become increased in size allowing the upper part of the stomach to slip into the chest. Most are sliding hiatus hernias, in which the upper part of the stomach can slide into the chest when the patient stoops, is hunched up, or when lying down. In a few patients the herniated part of the stomach remains permanently above the diaphragm and the normal valve mechanism may not be impaired as it is with a sliding hernia. This fixed variety is therefore not associated with heartburn. Hiatus hernia is a relatively common disorder, tending particularly to come on in the obese, and in women who have had children, but with the symptoms beginning after the menopause. Often the vomiting associated with pregnancy may have weakened the diaphragm. However hiatus hernia can come on at any time of life and can be a problem with infants and old people. Sometimes a severe injury

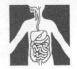

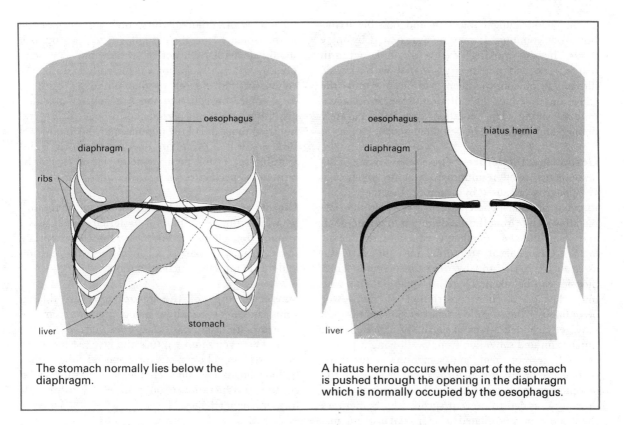

The stomach normally lies below the diaphragm.

A hiatus hernia occurs when part of the stomach is pushed through the opening in the diaphragm which is normally occupied by the oesophagus.

affecting the trunk may cause a tear of the diaphragm and allow part of the stomach to slip through. The classic symptom is heartburn on bending or stooping, when sitting in a low easy chair, or when lying flat after a meal; sometimes the discomfort may rise into the neck and angles of the jaw and even extend down both arms, simulating angina pectoris, a symptom of certain heart diseases, see page 70. Hiatus hernia pain comes on at rest and not with exercise. After a late meal some patients are woken up, particularly in the early hours of the morning by severe pain behind the breastbone. The pain may be eased by alkalis or by getting up and standing and arching the back. This pain can be prevented altogether by raising the shoulders on pillows or by raising the head of the bed. A troublesome cough at night or in the early morning may result from acid irritation extending into the back of the throat. With acid oesophagitis the oesophagus is sensitive to hot fluids or to strong alcoholic drinks, and the sufferer may find it particularly uncomfortable when bending to do housework, or when gardening. In some it may lead to spasm and narrowing of the lower end of the oesophagus, giving rise to difficulty in swallowing. Some patients may develop anaemia from oozing of blood from the inflamed mucous lining.

The fixed type of hernia is less liable to cause heartburn but does give rise to a sense of discomfort. Such patients may find they have to get up and walk about for a few minutes at the beginning of a meal, before they can continue in comfort. If the sufferer understands the mechanism of his symptoms there is much he can do to help himself. Loss of weight invariably improves the symptoms and may abolish them altogether. Care with posture is particularly important – bending at the knees and not at the hips; sitting in a high chair rather than a low chair, particularly after meals; avoiding at all times getting hunched up for any length of time, particularly in motor cars or aeroplanes; avoiding a late evening meal whenever possible, alternatively raising the head of the bed at night or having extra pillows to minimize the stomach contents flowing back into the oesophagus. It is a condition which should always be mentioned on admission to hospital so that steps can be taken to prevent acid rising into the oesophagus, particularly when patients are seriously ill and lying flat on their backs.

Oesophagitis (inflammation of the gullet) Although the usual cause is acid associated with hiatus hernia, oesophagitis can result from other causes.

341

Chapter 14 The digestive system

These include fungal infection and possible irritation from vomiting. It may be aggravated by spicy foods, heavy smoking, excess alcohol, vitamin deficiencies, and weakness associated with chronic illness. The obvious treatment is to aim to remove the cause and to reduce the irritation to the oesophageal mucous lining. The situation can be accurately defined and diagnosed by oesophagoscopy.

Oesophageal stricture This is a narrowing of the oesophagus, often resulting from acute or chronic oesophagitis, or caused by a tumour. It is more liable to occur in older people, and it is possible that the backflow of bile from the duodenum into the stomach and then into the oesophagus can be a significant factor. Oesophageal strictures must be carefully assessed by X-ray and by direct inspection, when biopsies can be taken. There are some patients who may develop a ring constriction of the lower oesophagus – the so-called Schatski ring – and they may get a sudden attack of partial obstruction with much pain and salivation from swallowing a poorly chewed piece of meat; and sometimes softer foods such as fish or bread may form a ball or bolus in the oesophagus and become lodged there. Special care is obviously needed to prevent such crises. Sometimes the stricture may be dilated using special instruments, and occasionally operation may be required.

Oesophageal diverticulum In some patients a pouch or diverticulum may form either as a result of increasing pressure or from infection of adjacent glands within the chest, and a diagnosis is easily and clearly established by means of X-rays. In most patients the condition is symptomless and no treatment is required. A pharyngeal pouch, which may form at the junction of the pharynx and the oesophagus in older people, can cause difficulty in swallowing and may require surgical treatment. This can be done successfully.

Congenital defects Occasionally congenital defects affect the oesophagus. With oesophageal atresia the oesophagus ends in a blind pouch instead of passing on to the stomach, and urgent surgical repair is needed. Congenital narrowing with a fibrous stricture can occur at any level. Webs or bands of mucous membrane may partially block the oesophagus, but these are also acquired in association with some forms of anaemia.

Achalasia (cardiospasm) This is a disturbance of the normal muscular activity of the oesophagus together with a failure of the sphincter at the junction of the stomach and the oesophagus to open up as it should do with each act of swallowing. The oesophagus gradually becomes distended until the column of fluid and food produces enough pressure to force some through into the stomach. It is a rare condition affecting perhaps only one in several hundred thousand of the population. The majority of sufferers will require an operation, which is invariably successful. Some patients, however, can be treated by special stretching techniques.

Globus sensation This is "a lump in the throat" to which the term globus hystericus used to be applied, but globus sensation is a more appropriate name. It may be part of a general nervous reaction and due to muscular incoordination.

Varicose veins of the oesophagus are dilated veins caused by backflow blood pressure from the liver and are usually associated with cirrhosis of the liver. These veins may rupture and give rise to serious haemorrhage. The passage of a special tube with a balloon on its end may enable the bleeding to be controlled. Operation is often necessary to prevent further haemorrhages.

Tumours A tumour is a growth and may be either benign, meaning that it grows locally and does not spread to other parts of the body, or malignant, which means that it may spread and involve other organs. The symptoms of a benign tumour are a sense of difficulty in swallowing and a feeling of fullness or pressure. The diagnosis will be made on X-rays and direct visual inspection with the oesophagoscope. Surgical treatment is invariably successful. The symptoms of a malignant tumour are similar to those of a benign tumour except that the former become gradually worse with increasing difficulty in swallowing. This may be associated with excess salivation and weight loss. The diagnosis is made after X-ray examination, which shows an irregularity of the oesophagus. This will have to be confirmed by endoscopic inspection and by taking a biopsy under direct vision. Examination of the surface cells removed by gentle rubbing may reveal cancer cells under the microscope. The condition is a serious one, but surgical treatment has been considerably improved in recent years. Sometimes X-ray treatment may be indicated in preference to surgery, and in some patients the best treatment is merely to insert a special plastic tube to keep the opening free for swallowing.

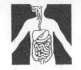

Oesophageal tear   The physical strain of vomiting may cause a small tear of the lining at the junction of the oesophagus and stomach, and this may give rise to sudden bleeding, the so-called Mallory-Weiss syndrome. Such patients may have vomited violently for some reason, perhaps on account of an acute stomach upset or overindulgence in alcohol, and then after a few hours they may vomit again, bringing up blood. Most patients will recover with simple measures, but occasionally operation may be needed. Very rarely, rupture of the whole wall of the oesophagus can occur, giving rise to sudden very severe chest pain with shortness of breath and shock, and necessitating urgent surgical intervention to close the hole. Fortunately with immediate surgery and antibiotics the outlook is now greatly improved.

Foreign bodies   Many objects can be swallowed and become stuck in the oesophagus, such as chicken bones, coins, safety pins, and dentures, but modern endoscopic techniques have helped the management of such emergencies.

The stomach

The symptoms of indigestion, or dyspepsia, are pain or discomfort in the upper part of the stomach or lower chest, and also in the back, before or, more commonly, after eating. Acid rising into the chest, belching, a sense of distension, nausea, and vomiting can be associated symptoms. These may arise in two ways. Firstly, the smooth churning activity of the stomach may be upset so that it does not function normally. This is called functional dyspepsia. Secondly, the symptoms may be due to physical change in the stomach, duodenum, or oesophagus, due to displacement, inflammation, or ulceration. This is called organic dyspepsia.

Functional dyspepsia   This may result from mental and physical stress such as anxiety, frustration, annoyance, physical fatigue from long hours of work, or loss of sleep. It can also be due to irritation of the digestive organs from eating too quickly without adequate chewing, from badly cooked or indigestible food, from chemical irritation which may be caused by heavy smoking or drinking, by aspirin, and in some people by overuse of laxatives which, as well as stimulating the colon, may upset the smooth working of the entire digestive tract. Simple commonsense avoidance of these various causes of dyspepsia may go far to relieve the symptoms, particularly if firm

reassurance can be given that there is no important underlying disease.

Organic dyspepsia   When pain and discomfort persist day after day there is likely to be some structural change. Hiatus hernia has already been discussed, and peptic ulcer is the other common cause. A peptic ulcer is an erosion of the surface of a small area, usually in the stomach or first part of the duodenum. In older people it is important to keep in mind the possibility of more serious gastric diseases such as cancer, not only in the stomach but also in other parts or organs of the body, including the colon and pancreas, which may give rise to some disorder of working of the stomach and cause indigestion. General medical conditions such as anaemia, renal failure, heart failure, or liver disease may all include indigestion as an initial symptom and this is why doctors always have to look at the patient as a whole and not just concentrate on the abdomen. Anyone who develops persistent or recurrent indigestion for the first time, at any age, should seek medical advice.

Gastritis   Acute gastritis may cause transient symptoms of indigestion, for example following overindulgence in alcohol, or the unaccustomed eating of spicy foods. Sometimes certain drugs, particularly aspirin (acetylsalicylic acid) and some of the anti-inflammatory drugs used for treating rheumatic diseases, may cause acute gastritis with heartburn, acidity, belching, and discomfort after meals. Heavy smoking is an aggravating factor. With small frequent light meals the symptoms soon clear up.

Chronic gastritis is a condition where there is a longstanding chronic inflammatory reaction in the lining of the stomach. It can give rise to varying degrees of discomfort after food, or more frequently there are no symptoms and the condition is discovered when some other condition such as anaemia is being investigated and when gastroscopy has been undertaken. Pernicious anaemia is associated with atrophic changes in the lining of the stomach, a form of chronic gastritis. It is a condition which no longer justifies its earlier name, as it responds well to treatment with vitamin B12, (see page 105).

Peptic ulcer   Peptic ulcers are found in relation to peptic secretions (pepsin is one of the enzymes in the stomach juice) and occur in the stomach, duodenum, and oesophagus. Ulcers may be small and acute, developing in a few days and healing perhaps in one to two weeks. Sometimes such acute ulcers may

343

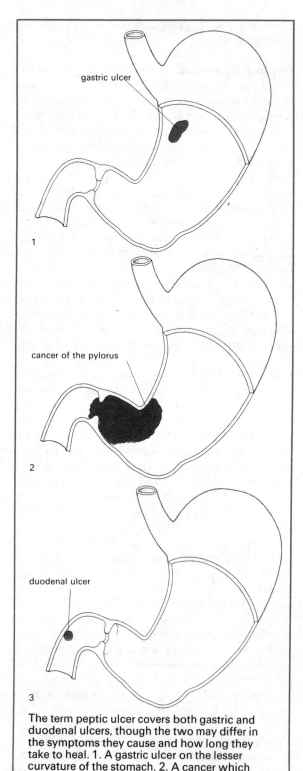

The term peptic ulcer covers both gastric and duodenal ulcers, though the two may differ in the symptoms they cause and how long they take to heal. 1. A gastric ulcer on the lesser curvature of the stomach. 2. A cancer which may obstruct the outlet of the stomach (pylorus). 3. A duodenal ulcer near the stomach outlet.

involve a blood vessel giving rise to bleeding. A chronic ulcer will tend to last for weeks or months, but there is a natural tendency for healing to take place, and some treatments may speed up the healing process. Peptic ulcers are much more common in men than in women, and women during the reproductive years seldom have a peptic ulcer. In men, nearly ten per cent will have suffered at one time or another from a peptic ulcer by the age of 50. The majority of ulcers occur in the first part of the duodenum (duodenal ulcers) and in the stomach they tend to form on the lesser curvature. Gastric ulcers seldom turn to cancer, but some gastric ulcers may of course be malignant from the beginning, and this is why careful investigation is always necessary. Duodenal ulcers never become malignant. Peptic ulcers tend to develop against a background of stress, and rapidly growing urban populations have more sufferers than those living under quieter and more peaceful conditions. Heavy smoking is an important aggravating factor and slows down the healing of ulcers, probably because the carbon monoxide present in the smoke may damage the delicate healing cells. The natural tendency to healing is increased by bed rest and small, light, more frequent meals, but strict dieting in fact is not needed, and it is not necessary to exclude fruit and vegetables as has so often been done in the past. Rich fatty foods, fried foods, pastry, spicy foods, strong tea, and coffee should be avoided, but keeping up the nutrition by a normal balanced diet will do more good than harm. Cutting down or stopping smoking is an important step. Getting a good night's rest, initially if necessary with sleeping tablets, and getting personal problems sorted out is always a great help. Today we have very useful medicinal treatments – carbenoxolone (Biogastrone or Duogastrone) which improves the defence mechanisms of the stomach and duodenum, and cimetidine (Tagamet) which greatly reduces acid secretion. Both these preparations enable ulcers to heal with the patient up and about, as quickly as if they were put to bed – a great economic advantage.

Persistent ulceration gives rise to troublesome pain. In duodenal ulcer it tends to come on before meals, waking the patient at night, and is eased by food. In gastric ulcer the pain may come on half to one hour after meals, eased by antacids. The ulcerated area of the stomach or duodenum may erode a blood vessel underlying it, and this will give rise to haemorrhage. Very dark blood may be vomited, so-called coffee grounds vomit, the change of colour being due to the effect of acid on the blood; or the blood may be partly digested and passed as a black

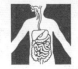

stool (melaena). Obviously such a complication demands urgent medical help and often admission to hospital. With modern treatment and, if necessary, blood transfusion the crisis can be successfully managed. Another complication may be acute perforation, when the erosive process involves the whole thickness of the wall of the stomach or duodenum. The leaking of gastric contents into the peritoneum causes a sudden onset of very severe generalized abdominal pain. Fortunately it is an uncommon complication, but one that needs urgent medical help and usually surgical treatment. With repeated ulceration – and some patients are very prone to get attacks once or twice a year – scar tissue may develop and may increasingly narrow the outlet between the stomach and the duodenum, causing pyloric stenosis. Vomiting may become a trouble-some feature and an operation may be needed to overcome the obstruction. Pyloric stenosis is also a rare congenital abnormality, particularly affecting the firstborn male child, and characterized by severe vomiting in the first month of life. Surgical treatment is highly successful.

Gastric surgery   Although in many patients peptic ulcer may be an occasional episode there are some in whom through the years the attacks become longer and more severe, causing disability and loss of work. The newer medical treatments are most helpful, but they may fail to give the necessary protection for some patients, and then operation can give great relief. Usually the surgeon cuts the vagus nerve to the stomach (vagotomy), and there are many varieties of this operation. It may or may not be combined with other procedures, such as enlarging the pylorus (pyloroplasty) or bypassing it (gastro-enterostomy). Vagotomy has the effect of greatly reducing acid secretion, enabling ulcers to heal and stay healed. In a few patients it is necessary to do a more drastic operation, removing part of the stomach (partial gastrectomy). None of the operations are perfect in the sense that they give 100 per cent protection. Usually the protection is at least 95 per cent against further ulceration, but some patients may get side effects from the operation – so-called dumping symptoms due to overrapid emptying of the stomach.

The small intestine

The main symptoms arising from disordered bowel activity are cramplike abdominal pain, diarrhoea, or weakness as a result of impaired absorption of food.

Congenital defects   As in all parts of the body there may be congenital abnormalities either in shape or position, not necessarily giving rise to any symptoms, but they may predispose towards some in the future. They may give rise to added difficulties in diagnosis, for example when the bowel is unusually sited, and acute appendicitis may cause pain on the left side instead of the right side of the abdomen. As in the oesophagus, infants may be born with total obstruction of a segment of the intestine, needing urgent operation.

Meckel's diverticulum   This is a not uncommon congenital abnormality in which there is a small pouch about five cm (two in) long, usually about 61 cm (two ft) from the lower end of the small intestine, occurring in about two per cent of the population. Acid-producing mucous lining, like that found in the stomach, may be present in this pouch and so lead to ulceration and bleeding, but Meckel's diverticulum is usually symptomless and is a condition which is difficult to demonstrate by means of X-rays. The diagnosis is usually made at the time of operation, when the pouch can be removed.

Intestinal obstruction   Obstruction of the in-testine may be due to many causes. It can be due to indigestible food residue rolling into a ball, which is particularly liable to happen in patients who have had part of their stomach removed (partial gastrec-tomy). For example, orange pith may pass quickly into the intestine causing colic or even obstruction. The green apple colic of children who raid orchards is similarly due to a bolus of indigestible food. Obstruction in older people can be due to a tumour narrowing the intestine. The commonest cause in younger people is adhesions. Normally the intestines glide over one another, but sometimes, particularly after a previous operation, loops of intestine may become stuck together, and when this happens twisting of a loop of bowel can take place causing obstruction. The symptoms are cramplike, colicky, severe pain with abdominal distension and vomiting. The diagnosis can be readily confirmed by plain X-ray of the abdomen and urgent operation is needed to overcome the obstruction. Sometimes the obstruction is incomplete and it may then respond to removal of the bowel contents by suction using a long narrow tube through the stomach and into the intestine.

After operation another type of obstruction can sometimes happen, called paralytic ileus. This is a con-dition in which peristaltic activity of the bowel ceases and the intestine becomes increasingly distended

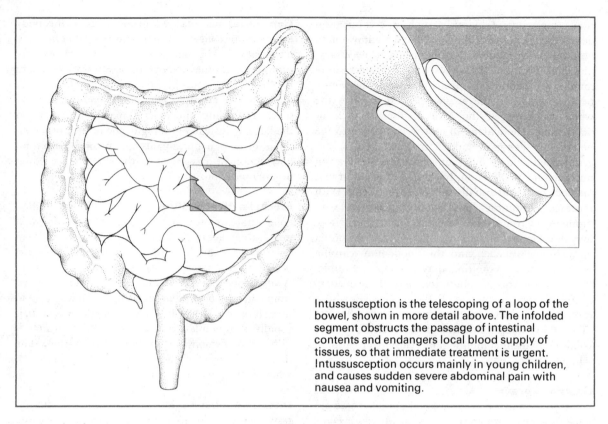

Intussusception is the telescoping of a loop of the bowel, shown in more detail above. The infolded segment obstructs the passage of intestinal contents and endangers local blood supply of tissues, so that immediate treatment is urgent. Intussusception occurs mainly in young children, and causes sudden severe abdominal pain with nausea and vomiting.

with air and fluid. Fortunately medical management will usually be successful in getting the intestine working again.

Intussusception is a condition in which one loop of bowel telescopes into the adjacent loop of bowel. In the condition known as volvulus the bowel twists on itself as a rubber balloon is twisted to keep air in it. The resulting obstruction causes sudden onset of cramplike, severe abdominal pain associated with nausea and vomiting. Sometimes removal of gas from the intestine with a long intestinal tube may be sufficient; otherwise operation is needed.

Regional ileitis (Crohn's disease) This was originally described by an American gastroenterologist, Dr Burrill Crohn. It is a condition in which a chronic inflammatory reaction occurs in a segment or segments of the intestine which becomes thickened and rigid like a hosepipe and the passage is much narrowed. Characteristically it involves the lower part of the small intestine, but it is now known that it can affect any part of the digestive tract. It is not uncommon for the colon to be involved, either on its own or in association with the small intestine. It affects perhaps 1 in 8,000 of the general population. The cause is not yet fully understood, despite a great

deal of research. It gives rise to general ill health, diarrhoea, abdominal pains, fever, anaemia, and weight loss. On examination it may be possible to feel the thickened bowel, particularly in the right lower abdomen, and X-ray examination of the small intestine will usually show a thickened segment with a narrow passage – the so-called string sign. Some patients can be treated medically, but removal of the badly damaged segment or segments is often required, particularly when there are complications arising from infection.

Acute enteritis There are a number of infections which cause inflammation of part or all of the intestine, resulting in severe diarrhoea. Some of the dysenteric and typhoid organisms, for example, cause acute infection, and cholera causes very severe diarrhoea but without inflammation. A common and irritating cause of acute enteritis is so-called traveller's diarrhoea. Many such attacks are due to a type of simple organism which may contaminate food and, when it enters the small intestine, rapidly multiplies causing diarrhoea and vomiting. It is normally self-limiting, but can have a devastating effect for a few days, spoiling a holiday. Travellers, particularly to the Mediterranean coast and the

Middle East, must take simple precautions to avoid traveller's diarrhoea. This means drinking bottled or sterilized water and not tap water, avoiding ice which may have been made from contaminated water, any uncooked fruit or vegetable that grows near the ground, such as lettuce and strawberries, unboiled milk, ice cream, and shellfish. Alcohol taken before main meals stimulates acid secretion and minimizes the risk of infection passing through the stomach into the intestine.

Malabsorption syndrome   Under certain conditions there may be failure to absorb foodstuffs fully, particularly fats, and this may give rise to the passage of bulky, offensive, greasy stools (steatorrhoea) which tend to float on the surface and which may not be flushed away easily. There are a number of mechanisms which may lead to malabsorption. There may be incomplete mixing of the digestive secretions and this is liable to occur after certain gastric operations. There may be a failure of the pancreas to produce its digestive enzymes, for example as a result of chronic pancreatitis. The bile ducts may become obstructed, but this causes jaundice as well as steatorrhoea. The lining of the small intestine may become thin and wasted (coeliac disease), and changes may also occur in the intestinal lining, for example in tropical sprue. Sometimes grossly abnormal degrees of bacterial activity may occur in the small intestine, particularly when there is partial obstruction, and greatly disorganize the digestive processes.

Coeliac disorder   This is a condition which can affect both children and adults. Patients with coeliac disease tend to lose weight, develop abdominal distension, as well as anaemia, and have steatorrhoea. Nervous irritability may be a special feature. Young children are particularly affected, but the condition can also come on in the middle years of life. It relates to sensitivity of the intestinal mucous lining to gluten which is one of the protein fractions found in wheat. This was discovered by a Dutch paediatrician, Professor Dicke, who found that coeliac children benefited dramatically when wheat and rye flour had been excluded from their food intake during the time of the German occupation, but relapsed when grain came into the country against after the liberation. This provided the clue which enabled further studies to identify the gluten in cereals as responsible for the damaging reaction that leads to thinning of the intestinal mucous lining. A diagnosis of coeliac disorder can be established by means of a special tube which enables a minute snip of the small intestinal mucous lining to be removed and looked at under the microscope. The condition is cured by keeping to a diet which rigorously excludes all gluten protein, but it is a diet that has to be kept up indefinitely. A valuable booklet has been prepared and published by the Coeliac Society, PO Box 181, London, NW2 2QY, which provides precise details of the diet and includes lists of gluten-free manufactured products.

Tumours   Tumours of the small bowel are rare, but can give rise to recurrent attacks of abdominal pain, and bleeding may occur. Sometimes there may be a congenital abnormality of small blood vessels which can give rise to intermittent or continuing slow loss of blood and consequent anaemia.

Peritonitis   Peritonitis is acute inflammation of the peritoneum which is the outer covering of the intestine and the inner lining of the abdominal cavity. Peritonitis will occur whenever inflammation can penetrate into the peritoneum either as the result of injury or perforation. The most common cause is rupture of the appendix from appendicitis. With modern antibiotics peritonitis has become a much less hazardous condition, but it is still serious.

The colon and rectum

The main symptoms relating to disorders of the colon and rectum are abdominal pain, distension, wind discomfort, diarrhoea or, alternatively, constipation and bleeding.

Megacolon   An uncommon but important congenital condition affecting the bowel is megacolon or Hirschsprung's disease. This is caused by an absence of certain nerve cells (ganglion cells) in a segment of the lower portion of the bowel. As a result the forward movement of faeces no longer takes place normally and the faeces gradually fill up the colon and greatly distend it. Patients with megacolon may not be able to have a normal bowel action for weeks. Fortunately it is very rare. Surgical removal of the segment of the colon where the ganglion cells are absent may enable normal bowel activity to be restored.

Constipation   Constipation implies that the bowels are being moved infrequently and with difficulty. The majority of people have a daily bowel action, but there are some who may have their bowels

Chapter 14 The digestive system

open two or three times a day and have done so all their lives, and others who do so only every few days but without discomfort or ill effect. Faeces in the bowel do not poison the body and there need be no anxiety if the bowels are not opened. One can have hidden constipation with more faeces than usual remaining in the bowel at any one time but with a daily evacuation, and this may give rise to some wind discomfort or a sense of incomplete evacuation. Constipation may be classified as:

Simple constipation. Absence of primary cause.

Self-induced	*Environmental*
Low intake of food	Poor toilet facilities
Low intake of fibre-containing food	Unfavourable working and living conditions
Ignoring the call to stool	Travel
Lack of exercise	

Poor toilet facilities, late rising, and the rush to get to school or to work may be as important as inadequate diet or lack of exercise. Neglect to answer the call to stool disrupts the normal mechanisms and allows the stool to become harder. Present-day eating habits particularly increase the likelihood of constipation, and the majority of persons who may feel they have a tendency to constipation will find that they can greatly improve bowel function by increasing the amount of dietary fibre or exercise. Extra fruit and vegetables help, but not as much as cereal fibre. Eating wholemeal bread instead of white bread may be sufficient, but many also need one of the bran preparations as a breakfast cereal. Natural bran obtainable from health stores is inexpensive and quite palatable as a cereal, and like All-Bran, Bran Flakes, Bran Buds, and others can be taken mixed with a wheatgerm preparation or with stewed fruit. There is increasing evidence that overrefinement of food, particularly the removal of the husk and the wheatgerm from flour, has been taken too far, and the colon appreciates wholemeal bread. The additional dietary fibre taken in this way almost doubles the volume of stool and makes it much easier to pass.

Constipation due to other factors.

Disturbances of colonic activity of unknown cause, for example, the irritable bowel syndrome.

Secondary to psychological states, for example, depression.

Caused by physical diseases affecting the colon, or due to general medical disorders.

Due to some medicinal treatments.

Where constipation fails to respond to simple dietary measures or change in habits, medical advice must be sought. This is particularly important when constipation comes on unexpectedly and for no apparent reason after 40. It can be the first symptom of a treatable disorder, such as thyroid insufficiency, depression, diabetes, and certain diseases of the bowel. The continued use of chemical laxatives is to be discouraged because, having stimulated the bowel, they merely make it lazy for the next few days, requiring further medication.

Diarrhoea Acute diarrhoea is often due to bacterial food poisoning, or it may be due to toxins formed by bacterial action in food which has been allowed to stand around in a warm temperature. (See traveller's diarrhoea, page 613). For diarrhoea treatment includes soups, fruit juices, apple juice, apple purée, but no milky drinks, together with a simple kaolin mixture, and medical help should be sought if the attack does not subside. Continuing diarrhoea, coming on gradually, or alternating diarrhoea and constipation, particularly if blood is seen, need careful medical investigation.

Irritable bowel syndrome The normal well-coordinated muscular activity of the colon can be disturbed and this may result in muscular spasms and the build-up of pressures within the bowel. Bowel rhythm is disturbed, alternating looseness or constipation may develop, and abdominal pains, particularly in the left lower abdomen, can be troublesome. These changes are particularly liable to occur when there has been a previous attack of enteritis or when there is continuing nervous stress. Heavy smoking accentuates the symptoms.

Diverticulosis This is a condition which affects the large bowel, particularly on the left side, when pouches of the colon's mucous lining protrude through small weakened areas of the bowel wall. There is increasing evidence that it is more likely to develop in persons who have a less than usual intake of dietary fibre, and it is eased by increasing cereal fibre, particularly with one of the bran preparations and wholemeal bread. It is advisable to have cooked rather than uncooked vegetables, to avoid pips and skins, and to reduce the amount of vegetables that produce flatulence, such as cabbage; spinach and carrots are well digested. Patients may suffer from a disturbance of bowel rhythm and pain particularly affecting the left side of the abdomen, but sometimes the right side, too, and this pain may be relieved by

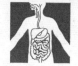

bowel action. The diagnosis is established by an X-ray examination.

Diverticulitis This is inflammation of one of the pouches – often because a small piece of hard faeces has become lodged in it. This is why sufferers from diverticulosis are advised to avoid constipation, using the diet to keep the bowels moving regularly and without difficulty. When inflammation occurs there will be localized tenderness in the abdomen and fever, and medical help should be sought. Antibiotic treatment is invariably needed. Very rarely haemorrhage or perforation of the pouch may occur, producing severe symptoms, and requiring urgent medical help.

Appendicitis The vermiform (worm-shaped) appendix is a small narrow blind tube projecting from the caecum. It is of variable length, the average being nine cm ($3\frac{1}{2}$ in). It is a vestigial structure and of no real importance to the body, but a serious risk if it becomes inflamed and infected. The inflammation may impair the local blood supply causing gangrene of the appendix and rupture, leading to peritonitis. The symptoms of appendicitis are pain in the right lower portion of the abdomen associated with malaise, fever, and vomiting, and sometimes constipation.

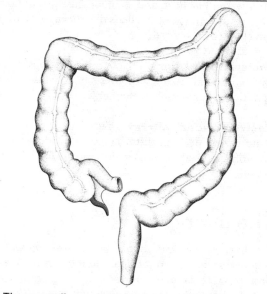

The appendix, marked in red, is a small narrow tube projecting from the caecum. A distended inflamed appendix may rupture, release poisonous material, and cause peritonitis. The appendix is served by a single artery, and inflammation may impair the local blood supply and cause death of tissues (gangrene).

The pain tends to start in the centre of the abdomen, moving down towards the right lower quadrant. The symptoms of appendicitis, particularly in infants and children, are seldom typical and the diagnosis may be difficult. Laxatives should never be given to a person who has abdominal pain of recent onset, as their use may precipitate perforation of the inflamed appendix. An emergency operation is usually needed.

Ulcerative colitis Ulcerative colitis is a condition which affects about 1 in 1,000 of the population, leading to diarrhoea with passage of blood. In some patients it may be localized to the lowest part of the bowel, where it is called proctitis, or it may extend up the bowel to involve varying lengths, and sometimes the entire bowel. The mucous lining becomes thickened and bleeding. It is not an infection in the ordinary sense of the word, but a tissue reaction in which the body seems to damage its own tissues – a so-called autoimmune reaction – and a process which can be helped by some of the cortisone-like drugs and by a drug called sulphasalazine (Salazopyrin). Medical supervision is essential, and local enema treatment with steroids is often useful. Those who have suffered from this illness should be particularly careful to avoid any extra risk of food poisoning, which may cause a relapse, and to try to protect themselves against any nervous or emotional strains which will always aggravate the condition. The use of antibiotics for any associated minor illness is to be discouraged as they can also precipitate a relapse.

Haemorrhoids Haemorrhoids are dilated veins situated just inside the anal canal. They may cause bleeding or pain, particularly if one of the veins becomes clotted. Extra dietary fibre to promote easy passage of stools is needed and may help to prevent further symptoms. Straining at stool must be avoided. If there is continuing trouble surgeons may be able to help with injections or operation. (See diagram on next page.)

Fissure A fissure is a small ulcer or break in the skin in the region of the anal canal. The main symptom is an unpleasant burning pain particularly coming on with bowel movement and persisting for some time. The first essential is to help any tendency to constipation by means of diet and to get the condition medically assessed and treated.

Tumours

Benign tumours These are polyps, which are small simple swellings on the surface of the bowel, and

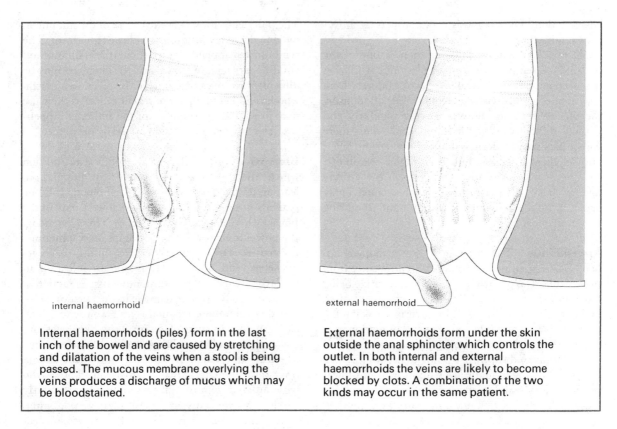

internal haemorrhoid

Internal haemorrhoids (piles) form in the last inch of the bowel and are caused by stretching and dilatation of the veins when a stool is being passed. The mucous membrane overlying the veins produces a discharge of mucus which may be bloodstained.

external haemorrhoid

External haemorrhoids form under the skin outside the anal sphincter which controls the outlet. In both internal and external haemorrhoids the veins are likely to become blocked by clots. A combination of the two kinds may occur in the same patient.

which may give rise to bleeding. Some polyps are perfectly harmless, but there is a proportion which can become larger and cause complications. They may be demonstrated on X-ray examination of the bowel. Nowadays it is possible for them to be removed with the help of the long, flexible colonoscope, and open operation is seldom needed.

Malignant tumours The symptoms of cancer of the colon depend on the site of the tumour. On the left hand side alternating diarrhoea and constipation may occur, together with cramping pains, weight loss, and sometimes visible blood in the stool. Less commonly, a tumour on the right hand side of the bowel is likely to produce diarrhoea and anaemia as the main symptoms. The majority of tumours affecting the large bowel occur in the rectum – examination by the doctor's finger may indicate their presence, and they may easily be seen through the sigmoidoscope. The results of surgical treatment are generally excellent.

Parasitic infections A number of parasites may invade the gastrointestinal tract and this is particularly common in underdeveloped countries. Amoebic infection, giardiasis, and various worms can be acquired in Mediterranean countries and in the Middle and Far East, and commonsense precautions may be needed. (See traveller's diarrhoea, page 613, and chapter 2).

Bacterial infections Bacterial infections with gastrointestinal manifestations such as nausea and vomiting are discussed in chapter 2.

Gastrointestinal allergy This may give rise to acute gastrointestinal disturbances, with diarrhoea, vomiting, and abdominal pain, and is discussed in chapter 21.

The liver

The liver is the largest solid organ in the body and is responsible for an extraordinary number of chemical processes. It is essential for the metabolism of carbohydrates and proteins, fats, and minerals, and plays a major part in neutralizing poisons and drugs. It manufactures proteins and cholesterol. It is concerned with iron storage and the manufacture of the elements necessary for blood clotting. It converts glucose to glycogen and stores the latter as a source of energy. One of its functions is the destruction of old

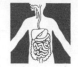

red blood cells and the conversion of the haemoglobin molecules into bilirubin. This bile pigment is yellow in colour and responsible for the yellow tinge of the skin in patients with jaundice.

Jaundice   Jaundice comes from a word meaning yellow and the common expression "yellow jaundice" is a redundancy, but nevertheless an expressive phrase. An increase in bilirubin will occur in the blood if there is excessive breakdown of red cells, if there is inflammation within the liver (hepatitis), or if there is obstruction of the bile ducts outside the liver, preventing the bile from reaching the duodenum.

Acute hepatitis (infectious hepatitis)   This is an important common liver disorder, which is described in chapter 2. It is caused by a virus infection which involves the digestive tract and this is why it is so important for anyone handling food to wash their hands carefully after going to the toilet. It can also be transmitted in some cases by injection of blood products, and can be transmitted by dirty syringes. Persons who have suffered from infectious hepatitis must not become blood donors.

Chronic hepatitis   This can be due to infection or chemical damage to the liver, resulting in fibrosis and scarring, giving rise to cirrhosis. It can be due to various chemicals, and alcohol is an important cause, but there are many patients in whom the cause remains uncertain. The early symptoms of cirrhosis of the liver are weight loss, early morning nausea, indigestion, intolerance of fats, and loss of libido. On examination the liver will have become enlarged and hardened and the spleen may be felt. Changes occur on the skin, with reddening of the palms of the hands and the appearance of small prominent vascular networks (spider naevi) on the skin of the upper half of the body. Later on there may be swelling of the abdomen due to excess fluid (ascites) and swelling of the legs. The most serious complications are liver failure and bleeding from rupture of the dilated veins which may develop in the lower end of the oesophagus. In the earlier stages abstinence from alcohol, and general medical care can much improve the patient's wellbeing. Life expectation is greatly shortened, and it is a risk that should be more clearly appreciated by those who overindulge in alcohol. A quarter of a bottle of spirits daily is probably safe for the liver. Half a bottle constitutes a real risk, and with a bottle a day almost anyone will get serious liver disease. Drinking once in a day rather than in two sessions is always safer. Disposal of alcohol by the liver

takes many hours, is a complicated chemical process, and may lead to increase of fat which can be the precursor of cirrhosis.

There are other causes of cirrhosis of the liver. Biliary cirrhosis may be associated with chronic obstruction of the bile passages. Post-necrotic cirrhosis is a form of cirrhosis which occasionally follows severe infectious hepatitis. Cardiac cirrhosis may occur in patients with chronic heart failure. Differentiation of the various forms may require detailed investigation and microscopic examination of liver tissue removed by liver biopsy.

Other liver diseases   A great many diseases may cause changes within the liver. Amoebic infection can cause an abscess, and certain parasitic infections, particularly hydatid disease, can give rise to cysts. Primary cancer of the liver is rare in western countries, but common in other areas. The liver is often affected by cancer elsewhere in the body.

The gallbladder

The gallbladder is a saclike structure seven to ten cm ($2\frac{1}{2}$ to 4 in) long which stores and concentrates bile, contracting under hormone stimulation when fats reach the duodenum. Infection of the gallbladder (cholecystitis) may develop, and gallstones may form within it.

Cholecystitis   The word is derived from "chole-" meaning bile, "cyst" for the bladder, and "itis" meaning inflammation. Acute cholecystitis is acute inflammation of the gallbladder due to bacterial invasion, as in appendicitis, and the patient is ill with fever and pain in the right upper part of the abdomen. Jaundice may develop. The condition may subside with appropriate antibiotics, but operation may be needed. Chronic cholecystitis is a chronic inflammatory reaction almost invariably associated with gallstones, and the diagnosis can be established by X-rays with a dye, which outlines the gallbladder and may show stones within it. Sometimes the gallbladder loses its ability to concentrate the dye and it will then fail to show on the X-ray film. Giving the dye intravenously may be more helpful in such patients by outlining the bile ducts and demonstrating whether or not there is obstruction in the cystic duct leading to the gallbladder.

Gallstones   In western countries gallstones become increasingly common with advancing age, and by 60 probably one in five women and one in twenty men may have gallstones present. In many patients the stones are "silent", not producing any symptoms, but it is a condition where sudden biliary pain may occur. This pain is felt in the upper part of the abdomen, often particularly on the right side, and radiating through to the right shoulder blade. It tends to come on later in the day, sometimes at night, and may persist severely for five or six hours. Sometimes the common bile duct becomes obstructed so that jaundice develops and an operation is needed to overcome the obstruction to the flow of bile.

Gallstones occur in persons who are more prone to making extra cholesterol, which becomes over-concentrated in the bile and leads to gallstones. Certain stones may be dissolved by giving a bile acid, chenodeoxycholic acid, which reduces the concentration of cholesterol in the gallbladder. The stones may gradually dissolve, if they happen to consist of pure cholesterol, but there are other varieties which may not be affected by this treatment. Gallstones which have caused pain invariably need removal, but where there is fat intolerance only, or no symptoms, it may be reasonable just to see the doctor from time to time and continue on a low fat weight-reducing regime.

Postcholecystectomy syndrome Although the majority of patients who have had the gallbladder removed do well, there is a minority who may continue to get symptoms, particularly of fat intolerance, and sometimes recurrent pain. This may happen particularly if the opening of the bile duct into the duodenum has become narrowed. These patients are also liable to get recurrent attacks of cholangitis with bacterial infection of the ducts, with fever, shivering attacks, pain in the right upper part of the abdomen, and jaundice. Treatment with anti-biotics may overcome the acute symptoms, but sooner or later it may be necessary to operate to widen the opening of the bile ducts and remove any stones which may have reformed in the ducts.

Tumours Benign tumours are mostly polyps or small swellings which may be present on the wall of the gallbladder, projecting into its cavity. They are usually an incidental finding associated with other evidence of chronic cholecystitis but are mostly unimportant.

Cancer of the gallbladder is rare. It usually occurs in elderly people who have had a history of gallstones going back many years. The risk of this possibility later in life is one of the arguments for removing the

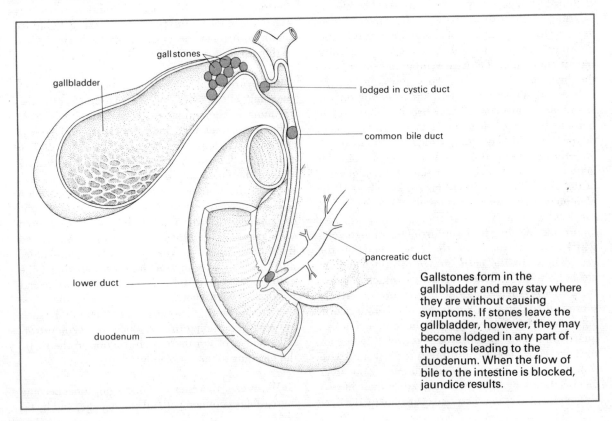

gall stones

gallbladder

lodged in cystic duct

common bile duct

pancreatic duct

lower duct

duodenum

Gallstones form in the gallbladder and may stay where they are without causing symptoms. If stones leave the gallbladder, however, they may become lodged in any part of the ducts leading to the duodenum. When the flow of bile to the intestine is blocked, jaundice results.

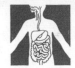

gallbladder earlier when even symptomless stones have been diagnosed.

The pancreas

The pancreas is composed of two kinds of tissue. The main mass of the gland produces digestive juices. The other part is concerned with internal secretions or hormones. This small amount of tissue is present in the islets of Langerhans where there are three types of cells – alpha, beta, and gamma – the most important being the beta cells which secrete insulin. If their activity falls and less insulin is produced, diabetes may occur. Rarely, a tumour may develop arising from these glands and then excess insulin is produced, leading to attacks of hypoglycaemia (low blood sugar), and these patients have attacks of great weakness which improve if sugar is taken.

Pancreatitis Acute pancreatitis is due to a sudden chemical reaction within the pancreas, caused by escape of the powerful pancreatic enzymes which should go down the pancreatic duct into the intestine but which may build up locally and cause an acute destructive process within the gland itself. It can occur in association with gallstones, and particularly after heavy alcohol consumption, usually starting the following day. In susceptible subjects it is liable to occur with excess alcohol together with a heavy meal. The symptoms of acute pancreatitis are sudden onset of really excruciating pain in the upper abdomen, extending into the back, associated with vomiting. The abdomen becomes very tender, and the patient may become shocked, with low blood pressure, and a cold clammy skin. The diagnosis can be established by testing the blood or urine for the pancreatic enzyme, amylase, which may be found greatly in excess of the normal amount. The majority of patients can be looked after medically, but sometimes it may be necessary to operate, particularly if there is gallbladder disease as well.

Chronic pancreatitis may result from recurrent subacute attacks of pancreatitis, or may develop gradually, particularly if there is any partial obstruction of the pancreatic duct. In this condition the fat digestion within the intestine is greatly impaired and the stools become more fatty (steatorrhoea), tending to float in water. Recurrent and sometimes severe pain may occur, and X-rays may show the presence of stones within the pancreas, or calcified pancreatic tissue. In these patients it may be necessary to join the pancreatic duct to a loop of intestine after the stones have been removed.

Tumours Benign tumours involving the pancreas are exceptionally rare, one kind being the insulin-producing tumour, causing hypoglycaemia, with exceptionally low blood-sugars leading to hunger, weakness, palpitations, and tremulousness, especially in the early morning or when a meal has been missed. Another small benign tumour may produce gastrin which overstimulates acid secretion, leading to recurrent ulceration of the stomach and duodenum. Surgical removal may be possible and the patient cured, provided the tumour is benign and not, as occasionally happens, malignant.

Cancer of the pancreas is a very serious condition, as it presents great problems in early diagnosis and in surgical treatment. The onset tends to be insidious, with upper abdominal discomfort, weight loss, and diarrhoea with fatty stools. The pain may radiate to the back and may be relieved by the patient bending forwards. If the head of the pancreas is involved, jaundice is an early symptom. The results of surgical treatment unfortunately are poor, but occasionally good results can be obtained in a tumour arising near the duct through which the secretions normally pass. However, earlier diagnosis is now being achieved with the help of endoscopic techniques to outline the bile and pancreatic ducts, and this may help to improve the results.

Chapter 15
Nutrition

Revised by Professor Ian Macdonald, MD DSc

Proper food is essential for the maintenance or restoration of health. Disease may result from lack of nutrients, from consumption of a diet which is unsuitable for a particular disease or person, or, rarely, from the ingestion of harmful quantities of unusual substances which may be contained in certain foods.

Nutrients

Nutrients in foods are chemical substances of known composition and structure. They are classified as carbohydrates (such as sugar, starch, glycogen); lipids, loosely called fats; proteins (large molecules which contain nitrogen and are built of amino acid units); inorganic elements or salts (such as compounds containing iron, calcium, and phosphorus); and vitamins. The last are a chemically unrelated group of organic compounds needed in very small quantities by the body.

Energy Carbohydrates contain carbon, hydrogen, and oxygen, and their burning is the body's usual source of energy for muscular work, body heat, breathing, and other functions. The layman may be forgiven if he is confused by the terms used for the measurement of body energy. Until recently this was measured in calories (units of heat), but there happen to be two kinds of calorie. The small calorie or gram-calorie (written calorie, with a small c) and the large calorie or kilo-calorie (written Calorie, with a capital C). One large Calorie equals 1,000 small calories. Physiological measurements are made in large Calories, so the statement that someone needs a diet of 2,500 calories a day always means large Calories.

The modern term for measuring energy (including body energy) is the joule (the unit of energy, whether from heat, or from electrical, chemical, or mechanical energy). The joule is often an inconveniently small unit, so for many purposes the kilo-joule (1,000 joules) is used.

One large Calorie equals 4·2 kilo-joules. For measurement of large amounts of energy, for example the daily requirements of a man, a still larger unit, the mega-joule (1,000 kilo-joules) is often used.

It is therefore useful to know that

$$1 \text{ small calorie} = 4\cdot2 \text{ joules}$$
$$1 \text{ large Calorie} = 4\cdot2 \text{ kilo-joules}$$
$$1,000 \text{ kilo-joules} = 1 \text{ mega-joule}$$

The joule is not a nutrient or a substance, but a unit for expressing an amount of energy.

Carbohydrates and fats are the chief sources of energy; proteins may also provide energy. One gram (one-thirtieth of an ounce) of these nutrients, when burned in the body supplies the following energy:

Carbohydrate	17 kilo-joules	(4 Calories)
Fat	38 kilo-joules	(9 Calories)
Protein	17 kilo-joules	(4 Calories)

It is evident that fat is a concentrated source of energy. Since a gram of fat provides more than twice as much energy as an equal amount of either carbohydrate or protein, it is easy to understand why reduced intake of fats is advised for those who are overweight and wish to slim. Alcohol also is a concentrated source of energy supplying 29 kilo-joules (seven Calories) per gram. Since all these categories of nutrients can provide energy, it is evident why the total food intake must be decreased in slimming diets.

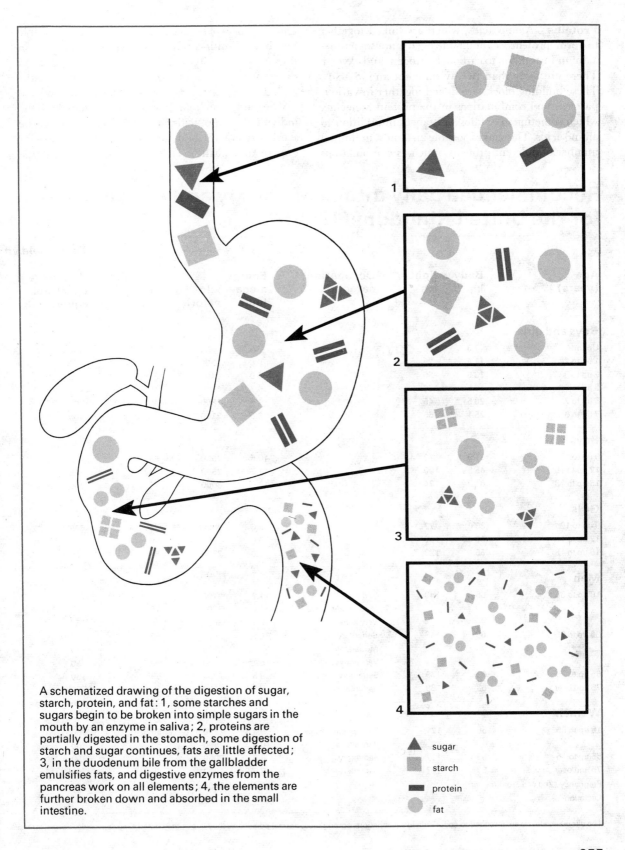

A schematized drawing of the digestion of sugar, starch, protein, and fat: 1, some starches and sugars begin to be broken into simple sugars in the mouth by an enzyme in saliva; 2, proteins are partially digested in the stomach, some digestion of starch and sugar continues, fats are little affected; 3, in the duodenum bile from the gallbladder emulsifies fats, and digestive enzymes from the pancreas work on all elements; 4, the elements are further broken down and absorbed in the small intestine.

sugar

starch

protein

fat

Chapter 15 **Nutrition**

Proteins Amino acids, which are linked together to form proteins, contain nitrogen and sometimes sulphur in addition to carbon, hydrogen, and oxygen. There are more than twenty different amino acids. These building blocks are linked together in various patterns and combinations in the protein molecule, which sometimes contains substances in addition to amino acids. This makes possible an almost unlimited number of different proteins, much as combinations and sequences of letters of the alphabet make possible an almost limitless number of words. Each protein does not necessarily contain every amino acid, just as different words do not contain all the letters of the alphabet.

The body can manufacture more than half the individual amino acids, but certain ones cannot be synthesized by the body in the amounts necessary for growth and health. These amino acids which the

Recommended daily intake of energy and nutrients for the United Kingdom (1969)

Age (years)	Body weight kg	lbs	Occupational category	Energy mega-joule	kilo-calorie	Protein (gm)	Fat soluble vitamin Vitamin A µg retinol equivalents
Boys and girls							
Up to 1	7.3	16		3.3	800	20	450
1 up to 2	11.4	25		5.0	1200	30	300
2 up to 3	13.5	30		5.9	1400	35	300
3 up to 5	16.5	36		6.7	1600	40	300
5 up to 7	20.5	45		7.5	1800	45	300
7 up to 9	25.1	55		8.8	2100	53	400
Boys							
9 up to 12	31.9	70		10.5	2500	63	575
12 up to 15	45.5	100		11.7	2800	70	725
15 up to 18	61.0	134		12.6	3000	75	750
Girls							
9 up to 12	33.0	73		9.6	2300	58	575
12 up to 15	48.6	107		9.6	2300	58	725
15 up to 18	56.1	123		9.6	2300	58	750
Men							
18 up to 35	65	143	Sedentary	11.3	2700	68	750
			Moderately active	12.6	3000	75	750
			Very active	15.1	3600	90	750
35 up to 65	65	143	Sedentary	10.9	2600	65	750
			Moderately active	12.1	2900	73	750
			Very active	15.1	3600	90	750
65 up to 75	63	139	Sedentary	9.8	2350	59	750
75 and over	63	139	Sedentary	8.8	2100	53	750
Women							
18 up to 55	55	121	Most occupations	9.2	2200	55	750
			Very active	10.5	2500	63	750
55 up to 75	53	117	Sedentary	8.6	2050	51	750
75 and over	53	117	Sedentary	8.0	1900	48	750
Pregnancy (2nd and 3rd trimester)				10.0	2400	60	750
Lactation				11.3	2700	68	1200

The allowance levels are intended to cover individual variations among most normal persons as they live in the United Kingdom under normal stresses.

body cannot manufacture are known as essential amino acids – essential because they must be supplied by the foods we eat.

The nutritional value of a protein depends on the number and kind of individual amino acids it contains, especially the essential amino acids. Dietary protein is broken down by the body into its constituent amino acids and these are reassembled to make body proteins. Clearly, the right kinds and amounts of amino acids must be present as raw materials if the body's protein factories are to put together a specific molecule.

Our many body proteins serve many functions. They are parts of the structure of muscle, skin, hair, nails, connective tissue, and the numerous other organs. Many hormones are proteins or derivatives of amino acids. The vast array of enzymes in the body are proteins.

	Water soluble vitamins				Minerals	
Vitamin D µg cholecal -ciferol	Thiamine mg	Riboflavine mg	Nicotinic acid, mg equivalents	Ascorbic acid mg	Calcium mg	Iron mg
10	0.3	0.4	5	15	600	6
10	0.5	0.6	7	20	500	7
10	0.6	0.7	8	20	500	7
10	0.6	0.8	9	20	500	8
2.5	0.7	0.9	10	20	500	8
2.5	0.8	1.0	11	20	500	10
2.5	1.0	1.2	14	25	700	13
2.5	1.1	1.4	16	25	700	14
2.5	1.2	1.7	19	30	600	15
2.5	0.9	1.2	13	25	700	13
2.5	0.9	1.4	16	25	700	14
2.5	0.9	1.4	16	30	600	15
2.5	1.1	1.7	18	30	500	10
2.5	1.2	1.7	18	30	500	10
2.5	1.4	1.7	18	30	500	10
2.5	1.0	1.7	18	30	500	10
2.5	1.2	1.7	18	30	500	10
2.5	1.4	1.7	18	30	500	10
2.5	0.9	1.7	18	30	500	10
2.5	0.8	1.7	18	30	500	10
2.5	0.9	1.3	15	30	500	12
2.5	1.0	1.3	15	30	500	12
2.5	0.8	1.3	15	30	500	10
2.5	0.7	1.3	15	30	500	10
10	1.0	1.6	18	60	1200	15
10	1.1	1.8	21	60	1200	15

Major vitamins: their names, actions and sources

Vitamin	Other names	Some things it does	Important sources
Vitamin A Large amounts can be stored in the liver. Dietary deficiency uncommon. Infants may need supplements before they begin to eat vegetables and egg yolk.	Retinol	Needed for growth of bones and teeth; for healthy epithelial cells (skin, mucous membranes); for normal vision (it is part of visual pigments of the retina). Part of an enzyme concerned with production of adrenal hormones.	Preformed vitamin A occurs only in foods of animal origin; best sources are liver, kidney, eggs, whole milk, cream, cheddar cheese, butter, fortified margarine, fish liver oils. Plant pigments known as carotenes are converted by the body into vitamin A. Best vegetable sources are dark green leafy and yellow vegetables.
Vitamin B1	Thiamine	Part of enzyme systems that release energy from carbohydrate foods. Necessary for proper function of the heart and nervous system and many tissues.	Pork, including ham, most meats, poultry, milk, eggs, peas, whole grain or bread and cereals, wheat germ, brewer's yeast.
Vitamin B2 Easily destroyed by light.	Riboflavine	Essential for normal growth and respiration of cells. Participates in protein metabolism.	Milk (rich source), offal, lean meats, fish, poultry, cheese, eggs, green leafy vegetables, yellow vegetables, bread, cereals.
Nicotinic acid Tryptophane, an amino acid of protein foods, can be converted into nicotinic acid by the body.	Nicotinamide	Participates in enzyme systems that convert food into energy. Prevents pellagra.	Liver, lean meats, bread and cereals, poultry, fish, potatoes, milk.
Pantothenic acid		Needed for synthesis of adrenal hormones, production of antibodies, healthy nervous system, and integrity of many tissues.	Widely distributed in virtually all plant and animal tissues; ordinary diet provides enough. Good sources are liver, meat, eggs, green leafy vegetables, nuts, whole grain cereals.
Vitamin B6 Human requirements not established; average diets furnish enough.	Pyridoxine Pyridoxamine Pyridoxal	Participates in metabolism of amino acids, fatty acids, and protein synthesis. Necessary for synthesis of adrenal hormones, blood cells.	Meat, liver, vegetables, whole grain cereals.
Vitamin B12 The molecule is biologically unique, in that it contains cobalt.	Cobalamin Cyanocobalamin	Needed for normal development of red blood cells, prevention of pernicious anaemia, health of nervous system, proper growth.	Food of animal origin; lean meat, fish, milk.
Folic acid Dietary deficiencies rare	Pteroylglutamic Acid	Needed for formation of red blood cells and proper intestinal functioning.	Most common foods contain the vitamin. Good sources are green leafy vegetables and meats.
Vitamin C Daily needs relatively large. Prevents scurvy.	Ascorbic Acid	Participates in adrenal gland functions, use of some protein elements, absorption of iron, formation of collagen framework of bones and teeth, integrity of blood vessels.	Found in most fresh plant foods; most abundant in citrus fruits. Good sources are fruits, juices, berries, dark green leafy vegetables, broccoli, peppers, cabbage, new potatoes.
Vitamin D Produced by action of ultraviolet rays on substances in the skin.	Cholecalciferol	Needed for normal bone growth, proper use of calcium and phosphorus. Prevents rickets.	Small amounts in eggs, tuna, salmon, sardines, herring. Substantial amounts in fish livers, and fortified foods.
Vitamin E	Tocopherol	Protects vitamin A from destruction by oxidation, necessary for normal red blood cells, appears to prevent abnormal changes in fatty tissues.	Provided in ordinary diets. Good sources are whole grain cereals, lettuce, vegetable oils, wheat germ.
Vitamin K	Phytomenadione	Enables the liver to form substances that help blood to clot.	Normally furnished by intestinal bacteria that synthesize it. Leafy vegetables are good food sources.

Fats are less complex than proteins, but are also made up of fundamental units – fatty acids and glycerol (glycerine). Again, certain fatty acids cannot be synthesized by the body and hence must be supplied by the diet. These are known as essential fatty acids. Since their chemical structure is characterized in part by various numbers of chemical bonds which contain fewer hydrogen links than they would if completely saturated, they are often referred to as polyunsaturated fatty acids. Not all polyunsaturated fatty acids are required by the body, which breaks down ingested fat and resynthesizes it into fats characteristic of its own tissues.

Carbohydrates are also broken down and rebuilt in the body. Common simple carbohydrate building blocks are glucose, galactose, and fructose. Numerous carbohydrates and derivatives exist in foods and in the body. We can synthesize all the carbohydrate we need from other available materials. The body must have sufficient nutrients to enable it to synthesize the carbohydrates, fats, and proteins necessary for proper functioning. That is one reason why a variety of foodstuffs must be consumed to feed the metabolic machinery which produces new compounds.

The body makes many chemical substances by converting constituents of foods. For example, it can transform carbohydrates into fat, or into a portion of the protein building blocks. It synthesizes milk sugar and converts certain amino acids to hormones. However, there are other substances than those already noted which the body must have and which it cannot synthesize. Vitamins and required minerals must come from the diet.

The accompanying table of Recommended Daily Dietary Allowances summarizes the major essential nutrients in foods and indicates the amount of each which is judged to be desirable for health.

Vitamins These nutrients, which cannot be synthesized by the body, are needed in such exceedingly small amounts that it is evident that they are not sources of energy. They serve instead as catalysts for bringing about many transformations and reactions in the tissues. A catalyst is a substance which initiates or promotes a chemical reaction without itself being consumed. Without a particular vitamin there occurs a given set of symptoms or a recognized deficiency disease.

There is nothing magic about vitamins. They do not possess the wondrous stimulating properties often claimed for them. A normal healthy person needs no more vitamins than he gets from a good diet, and the same applies to minerals, including trace minerals. Additional intakes of vitamins above his dietary allowances will not benefit him. Supplementary vitamins promoted for self-administration by healthy people are usually of no benefit. Critical studies of such products have shown that, in general, beneficial effects ascribed to them by persons taking them can be duplicated by giving those same people inactive pills.

Most vitamins act as coenzymes – small but essential parts of an enzyme that catalyzes some body process.

The usual source of vitamins is food. All the nutrients essential to health in the normal person are supplied by adequate diets which meet the recommended dietary allowances of the table on page 356. There are, of course, certain well-recognized medical needs for vitamin supplementation that will be discussed later.

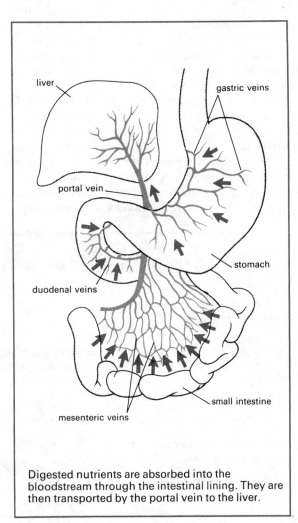

Digested nutrients are absorbed into the bloodstream through the intestinal lining. They are then transported by the portal vein to the liver.

Understanding foods

Some understanding of the nutritive value of foods is essential in planning proper meals and developing good dietary habits. But it is not necessary to remember in minute detail the amount of nutrients in individual foods or groups. It is sufficient to know that foods of certain groups are similar in their content of major nutrients, and to recognize the group to which various foods belong.

One might classify foods into many groups. But as a practical matter of diet planning and education, a convenient guide to the composition of an adequate diet is one in which common foods are divided into four basic groups, each of which has similar nutritive values. Selection of foods as indicated in the accompanying table provides adequate amounts of important nutrients more or less automatically.

This plan will supply an adult with one half to two thirds of his calorie allowance, four fifths of his iron and thiamine, nine tenths of his niacin, and all his riboflavine allowances. Other foods normally included in the daily intake but not specifically mentioned in the plan raise the supply of these nutrients to the recommended allowances and provide other nutrients as well. These foods include such items as butter, margarine, other fats and oils, sugars, desserts, jellies, and unenriched grain products.

The milk group provides abundant quantities of excellent quality protein, calcium, and riboflavine, as well as good portions of several other nutrients. Indeed, milk contains significant amounts of most of the nutrients required by man except iron and variable amounts of vitamins A, C, and D. For practical purposes one may use whole milk, buttermilk, skim milk, or cottage cheese interchangeably in a mixed diet. Hard cheeses and yoghurt may be considered equivalent for some of the milk group portions.

The meat group includes all lean red meats, fish, eggs, poultry, and dried legumes (beans, peas) or nuts. All these foods are rich in good quality protein, contain some fat, and provide good supplies of thiamine, nicotinic acid, riboflavine, and iron, among other nutrients. Meats, especially offal, are good sources of vitamin B_{12}.

Vegetables and fruits are important sources of vitamin A and carotene, of vitamin C, and provide significant quantities of riboflavine, thiamine, calcium, iron, and folic acid.

Breads and cereals provide a highly acceptable source of energy, with B vitamins and protein as well as iron.

For those who wish to know the energy and amounts of nutrients of various foods in greater detail, a table of food composition is given on page 366. Figures in this table are for foods prepared for consumption, and have taken into account the expected loss of nutrients in food preparation.

The effects of cooking on food values have been widely studied. In most cases there is relatively little loss of nutritional value when proper methods of food preparation are used. The proportion of the original nutrient retained in a prepared food varies with the nature of the nutrient as well as the food and the method of preparation.

"Food group plan" for ensuring adequate diets

Vegetable-fruit group
four or more servings

Including:
1 A dark green or deep yellow vegetable (spinach or carrots), important for vitamin A, at least every other day.
2 A citrus fruit or other fruit (orange or apple) important for vitamin C, daily.
3 Other fruits and vegetables including potatoes.

Bread-cereals group
four or more servings

Whole grain, or fortified

Milk group
some milk daily

Children	$\frac{1}{2}$ litre	1 pint
Teenagers	$\frac{1}{2}$ litre	1 pint
Adults	$\frac{1}{4}$ litre	$\frac{1}{2}$ pint
Pregnant women	$\frac{1}{2}$ litre	1 pint
Nursing mothers	$\frac{3}{4}$ litre	$1\frac{1}{2}$ pints

Cheese and yoghurt can replace part of the milk

Meat group
two or more servings

Including beef, veal, pork, lamb, poultry, fish, eggs, with beans, peas, and nuts as alternatives.

The energy, fat, carbohydrate, protein, and mineral contents of foods are little reduced by cooking unless there is excessive washing out of some of the water-soluble minerals and vitamins, or unusual dry heat which may reduce the protein nutritional value somewhat. In general, riboflavine, nicotinic acid, and vitamin D are quite stable. Vitamins A and C and thiamine may be reduced during cooking if heating is prolonged and there is free exposure to air. The loss of these nutrients is usually not greater than 25 to 30 per cent.

As a rule, cooking losses can be minimized by reducing the period of heating, using covered cooking vessels, and minimizing the amount of water that is added and discarded.

Canned and frozen foods Present day commercial canning and freezing processes consistently retain very high percentages of the nutrients originally present in the raw product. Indeed, the ability to process fresh fruits and vegetables immediately, directly from the field, allows harvesting of the crop at the peak of its nutritional value. This may produce greater nutritive value than in food which has been harvested and transported to be sold fresh.

Processed foods Procedures such as milling remove certain of the nutrients which were present in the whole grain. A similar diminution of nutritive value is caused by the peeling of potatoes, discarding of organs in dressing meat, paring of fruits, and many other acts of food preparation. The milling of wheat, for example, removes the rough outer coat and considerable quantities of fibre as well as the oily endosperm. This enables flour to be stored longer without developing rancidity, and is necessary to supply high-grade flour to our urbanized society. Properly milled flour in its commonly available form is a valuable foodstuff and its nutritional value is enhanced by enrichment.

Scientific knowledge of nutrition is not only applicable in preserving the nutritive value of foods but allows the nutritional improvement of many. Examples are the fortification of margarine and other fats with vitamins A, and D, the addition of iron to infant foods, of vitamin C to apple and other juices, the iodization of salt, the enrichment of flour and cereal products with thiamine, nicotinic acid, iron, and calcium. A considerable part of vitamin and mineral intake is derived from fortified foods.

Modern food technology Significant advances in the technology of food processing have made possible a wide variety of prepared or partially prepared foods, ranging from mixes to ready-to-eat frozen or packaged food. Common foods such as fats and bread now have much improved keeping qualities. Many of these improvements are due to new and better packaging materials and the use of safe chemical additives which prevent fat from becoming rancid (antioxidants), retard the development of moulds in breads (mould inhibitors), and otherwise improve quality. Vitamin C, for instance, is added to peaches and other fruits during the freezing process to preserve the colour of the fresh product.

Such beneficial use of chemical additives to improve foods is very different from the practices of half a century or more ago when various agents were misused in an unsafe, deceitful, or debasing manner. The present-day use of chemicals in food (foods themselves are chemical substances) is an essential part of our application of science to human betterment. Legal controls ensure constant monitoring of food quality.

Vitamin supplements

Vitamin supplements at certain periods of life, such as pregnancy and lactation, may be beneficial for healthy persons whose diets are ordinarily adequate. Certain supplementation of the diet of infants also may be desirable. Supplements may be of value to sufferers from prolonged illnesses associated with poor appetite and poor eating habits. In such instances, however, it is important for a doctor to determine the need and consider the type of vitamin preparation appropriate to the patient's needs.

Vitamin supplements differ in the variety and amounts of vitamins they contain. In some instances the formulas are designed to serve well-recognized uses, for example in pregnancy. In other instances formulas may be designed to supplement restricted dietary intakes, or to treat patients who have clearcut deficiencies, or in a few instances to be used for some non-nutritional therapeutic purpose. The latter two categories of vitamins should certainly not be taken except on a doctor's recommendation, since large amounts of some vitamins, particularly A and D, can be injurious. Healthy children who are given adequate wholesome foods need no vitamin supplements.

Overdosage Ingestion of excessive amounts of fat-soluble vitamins A and D and of carotene (an orange pigment which can be converted into vitamin A in the body) is potentially hazardous since these vitamins are not readily excreted and tend to accumulate in the body. Thus, children who receive an overdose of vitamin A may develop loss of appetite, loss of weight, become fretful and irritable, complain of itching of the skin, and develop cracks at the corners of the mouth and of the lips. Loss of hair and changes in bones may occur.

Similarly, an overdose of vitamin D continued over long periods of time may produce loss of appetite, nausea, headache, diarrhoea, and lassitude in children, and later, weakness, tiredness, and in severe cases, anaemia. Excessive ingestion of carotene, either as a carotene-containing supplement or by over-enthusiastic feeding to infants and young children of carotene-rich yellow and green fruits and vegetables (especially carrots, peaches, and greens) may result in a yellowish discoloration of the skin, most readily visible on the forehead, and on the palms of the hands and the soles of the feet. This discoloration may easily be mistaken for jaundice, but it does not appear in the whites of the eyes. It is not dangerous, but is unnecessary.

These considerations emphasize the desirability of properly selected diets as the primary basis of good nutrition and that dependence should not be placed upon one or another supplement that may be incomplete, unnecessary, or useless in a given situation, or even, at times, harmful.

Deficiency diseases

Lack of any essential nutrient over an extended period can so deplete body stores that injury results. The body normally stores enough vitamins to see it through brief periods of dietary deprivation. For all vitamins, normal stores may be depended upon to maintain an adult for several weeks and a child for a few weeks. In the case of vitamins A, D, and B_{12}, the normal stores of a well-fed person are so large that months or years may pass before deficiency signs become obvious.

Severe classic deficiency diseases, especially those due to lack of a vitamin, have largely disappeared from the United Kingdom. Important deficiency diseases which may occur in this country or are of wide international concern at present include the following:

Energy deficiency is semi-starvation and is recognizable as excessive leanness, and in children, growth retardation. It may be accompanied by other symptoms such as lack of appetite, lassitude, tiring easily, and other evidence of chronic disease. It may be secondary to chronic illness in which case its correction depends largely upon recognition and treatment of the primary disease.

Protein deficiency as it most often occurs is really a lack of both protein and energy. The most severe form, known as kwashiorkor, occurs in infants and children between the ages of six months and four or five years. It is rare in Europe. •

Kwashiorkor develops in infants and children who are fed exclusively on diets high in carbohydrate and low in protein or with protein of poor quality. Such diets consist principally of sugar, corn, manioc flour, plantain, or other single cereal or starchy tuber. Since the nutritional value of proteins depends on their amino acid composition, which varies from one protein to another, the nutritive value of a combination of proteins is greater than any one.

Scurvy A lack of vitamin C or ascorbic acid results in scurvy, a disease in which small blood vessels are easily ruptured, giving rise to small to large red spots under the skin at sites of injury and to swollen red gums which bleed easily. Scurvy is rare in the United Kingdom due to widespread use of fruits, vegetables, and the early introduction of fruits and vegetables into the diet of the infant. However, it may still be seen in the low income bachelor who lives alone, or the occasional person with unduly restricted diet.

It is more commonly seen in bottle-fed infants of six to eighteen months whose mothers have failed to supplement their diet with fruits, juices, or vegetables. Some cases have resulted from the mistaken belief that an orange-flavoured drink is identical with orange juice.

Rickets is a disease due to lack of vitamin D, which results in poor absorption of calcium from food and consequent improper mineralization of bone. In severe cases the soft bones are deformed and may even suffer fractures. Tetany (a particular kind of muscle spasm) may occasionally occur.

Foods are not the sole source of vitamin D. This nutrient is formed in the skin under the influence of ultraviolet light. These wavelengths are present in unfiltered sunlight. Hence, direct exposure to the sun increases the body's supply of this vitamin and helps to prevent rickets.

Vitamin A deficiency This vitamin is necessary for proper functioning of the light-sensitive retina of the eye, and is involved in the visual mechanism which makes it possible to distinguish various shades of grey. A deficiency of this vitamin is manifested as night blindness and reduced ability to adapt to the dark after exposure to bright light. In severe cases, the cornea of the eye (the clear window at the front of the eyeball) may undergo softening (keratomalacia), and excessive dryness of the eye (xerophthalmia) may be evident. In severe deficiency of this vitamin there may be tissue changes in the respiratory tract, but vitamin A does not have any anti-infective or cold-preventing properties as is sometimes claimed.

Pellagra and beriberi are usually associated with monotonous diets consisting primarily of maize in the case of pellagra, or white rice in the case of beriberi. Pellagra is seen only in people with bizarre food habits, alcoholics, or in rare medical conditions. Pellagra results from a lack of nicotinic acid or its precursor amino acid (tryptophan) in the diet; beriberi, from a lack of thiamine, (vitamin B_1). In both these conditions, other deficiencies are often present, as of riboflavine.

Pellagra is shown by rough, thickened, or blister-like lesions of the skin of the hands, feet, and face, soreness of the mouth and tongue, and other symptoms. Riboflavine deficiency also produces lesions of the lips and tongue. Beriberi produces changes in nerves of the limbs, especially the legs, often with some loss of motor function: oedema; and increase in size of the heart and cardiac failure. Some psychological changes may occur in either beriberi or pellagra, but neither nicotinic acid nor thiamine should be thought of as specific remedies for neurotic complaints, nervousness, or other psychological disorders.

Both these nutrients are contained in fortified flour and hence flour products make important contributions to total intake.

Nutritional anaemias There are many causes of anaemia, only some of which are nutritional in origin. For full discussion of iron deficiency and other anaemias, see chapter 4.

Iodine deficiency leads to an enlargement of the thyroid gland in the neck known as simple goitre. For details of this condition, see chapter 9.

Dental caries, or tooth decay, is associated with the quality of the diet. For full discussion, see chapter 16.

Water and salt deficiencies When loss of water from the body is excessive relative to intake, dehydration occurs. This is particularly likely to occur in infants and young children during severe bouts of diarrhoea and vomiting, especially in hot weather or in tropical climates. It is to be guarded against by offering frequent dilute liquids (tea, carbonated beverages, juices, clear soup) and water.

Patients with diarrhoea and vomiting, especially infants, may become deficient in potassium. Replacement of this salt requires careful medical supervision.

Under conditions of strenuous physical effort with profuse sweating in hot environments, sufficient salt (sodium chloride) may be lost to create a salt deficiency. This condition is characterized by weakness, abdominal cramps, and faintness, and may be relieved by taking salt. On the other hand, excessive intake of salt can be harmful. It is especially important to guard against accidental administration of large amounts of salt to young infants, as may happen by accidentally giving salt instead of sugar because of similar containers. It is safest in the home to keep salt in its original package or in an obvious container such as a salt cellar.

Overweight

Obesity is an excessive proportion of fat in the body. A practical index of obesity is body weight in relation to height and age. In a few diseases there is a tendency for the body to retain excessive amounts of water, with an increase in weight which does not indicate excessive body fat, but oedema. Such changes are readily recognized, usually by the subject, but certainly by his doctor, as being different from

Average weights for adults

in indoor clothing
applicable from 25 years of age

height cms	ft in	women kg (pounds)	men kg (pounds)
147	4'10"	47 (104)	
150	4'11"	48 (107)	
152	5'0"	50 (110)	56 (125)
155	5'1"	51 (114)	58 (128)
157	5'2"	53 (117)	59 (131)
160	5'3"	54 (120)	61 (135)
163	5'4"	55 (123)	62 (138)
165	5'5"	57 (127)	64 (142)
168	5'6"	59 (131)	65 (145)
170	5'7"	60 (134)	67 (148)
173	5'8"	62 (138)	68 (152)
175	5'9"	64 (142)	70 (156)
178	5'10"	65 (146)	72 (160)
180	5'11"	68 (151)	74 (164)
183	6'0"	70 (156)	76 (169)
185	6'1"		78 (173)
188	6'2"		80 (178)
190	6'3"		82 (182)
193	6'4"		84 (186)

Adapted from Build and Blood Pressure Study, Society of Actuaries, 1959

Chapter 15 **Nutrition**

obesity. In women of reproductive age there may be relatively small cyclic increases in body weight for a few days before the onset of menstruation, due to water retention. This premenstrual oedema does not reflect an increase in body fat.

When should weight be considered excessive? For reasons to be discussed later, the average weight of men and women in their mid-twenties – approximately 25 years of age – is a better yardstick than the changing averages in later years of life. The accompanying table does not attempt to make allowances for different body builds. Most people do not know accurately whether they have a heavy, medium, or light skeleton and musculature. Weight that is ten per cent greater or less than the figures given in the table may be quite in keeping with the physical characteristics of a given individual.

Overweight children For children, overweight of twenty per cent or more is undesirable if only because it makes them feel set apart from their social group. Gross obesity in children is frequently a sign of psychological maladjustment which itself requires attention. More important is the fact that obesity in the child is likely to lead to obesity in the adult, which is a more serious hazard.

Overweight adults A large amount of evidence points to the undesirability of following the average trend to accumulate weight gradually from the age of 25 years onward. Over the years this may result in six to ten per cent more weight than average weight at the age of 25. The weight gain reflects increased fat content of the body, and is due to failure to restrict energy intake to the level of energy expenditure.

Body fat cannot accumulate if the intake of energy equals the expenditure of energy. To gain weight one must consume more energy than is expended.

For most people, their basic expenditure of energy – maintaining body temperature, circulation, digestion, and breathing – is the largest component of total energy expenditure. The amount of energy needed to maintain these basal functions decreases with age, but often there is no similar decrease in appetite and energy is consumed in excess of energy requirements. This accounts for the most part for the average increase in weight from the late twenties onwards.

Exercise There are wide differences in the amount of energy expended in exercise. A sedentary office worker may use 1700 or so kilo-joules a day in his activities, while a man doing hard labour may expend three times that amount. The average adult in today's society seldom exercises in a manner comparable to an athletic teenage boy or manual labourer. Unfortu-

nately, the appetite-regulating mechanism does not usually reduce food intake to the level of lessened energy expenditure, and excessive energy intake is converted into fat and stored.

Vital statistics reveal that the mortality rate is lowest for adults who are five to ten per cent below average weight. This relationship is quite striking with respect to a number of specific diseases. All such evidence points to the desirability of maintaining body weight at approximately that which is standard or average for the population at age 25.

Prevention of obesity is easier and probably more beneficial to long-term health than reduction of excess weight. Prevention is accomplished by modest adjustments in diet and exercise. It is relatively easy to remove two to five pounds of body fat by some reduction of energy intake and comparatively mild exercise such as walking, swimming, or participation in sports. Riding around a golf course instead of walking, or lying on a beach instead of swimming, should not be mistaken for active participation.

Conscious efforts to increase activity should be made. For instance, make it a rule to walk upstairs instead of using the lift, to walk an additional two miles a day, and so on. At times a programme of exercise in a supervised gymnasium may be desirable to ensure regular activity. Exercise not only increases energy expenditure but improves fitness and muscle tone and, when part of an enjoyed hobby, provides mental relaxation.

A doctor can assess whether deviation from weight standards is significant. At the same time a medical examination may reveal some disorder that needs treatment. Any sudden unexplained weight gain or loss should be checked to determine the cause.

Reducing diets Reducing the amount of energy consumed daily is relatively simple, though it requires some will power. It also requires some knowledge of the energy content of different foods so that those low in joules may be chosen. This does not require a precise energy measurement of every serving. General knowledge that fats and oils are the most concentrated source of energy, alcohol is next, and that relatively pure carbohydrates such as syrups and sugars provide few nutrients other than energy, indicates that it is important to limit the quantities of these foods in a reducing diet.

At the same time, it is usually necessary to reduce the total quantity of most other foods by taking smaller and fewer servings. Energy values given in the food composition table on page 366 are helpful in meal planning.

Fruits and vegetables, for the most part, are relatively low in energy, with some exceptions (fruits canned in heavy syrup, vegetables served with oils and fats). Hence, their intake need not be greatly reduced, and may even be increased by substituting them for an energy-rich dish.

Bread and cereals should be limited to not more than four servings per day, and these should be whole grain or enriched forms to improve the nutrient quality of the diet.

Meat, fish, or poultry should be included daily, choosing foods such as leg of lamb, lean rump, lean loin of pork, lean ham, chicken, and white fish. Cottage cheese may be used as a substitute for meat.

Skim milk, yoghurt, or cottage cheese from the milk group are relatively low in energy due to removal of fat. Since some cheeses and ice creams are quite high in fat, they must be selected with care.

To be avoided are foods such as whipped cream, rich gravies, cream soups, fried foods, casseroles, creamed foods, puddings, and cakes. Butter or margarine should be limited to one serving twice a day.

Any drastic reduction of energy intake should not be undertaken without the advice of a doctor. Weight control requires personal discipline to adhere to a pattern of regular exercise and dietary limitation, restriction of alcoholic beverages, and going without between-meal and bedtime snacks.

For most overweight persons, a five mega-joule (1200-Calorie) diet gives gratifying steady weight reduction. It is of course important that the diet provides all nutritional essentials except energy. This is best achieved by a variety of well-chosen foods from the four basic food groups. A balanced five mega-joule (1200-Calorie) diet includes the following:

1 pint of skim milk
3 or more servings of vegetables
3 servings of fruit
4 servings of breads and cereals
5 ounces (cooked) of meat, fish, or poultry
2 level tablespoons of fat
4 eggs each week, not daily
Sugars and sweets to be used only as a substitute for one serving of bread or cereal

A great variety of appetizing, common, and seasonable foods can be included in this framework. Each day's menu can be varied. A sample menu for the above diet is given below. This should not be followed unvaryingly, but is used as an illustration of the principles set forth.

5 MEGA-JOULE (1200 CALORIE) DIET
Sample Menu Pattern

Breakfast
Grapefruit half
Poached egg
1 slice lean bacon
1½ oz oatmeal
1 slice toast
Tea or coffee with saccharin
4 oz skim milk
¼ oz butter

Lunch
2 oz roast beef with natural gravy
2½ oz potatoes
Grilled tomatoes, as desired
Green salad with fat-free dressing, as desired
¼ oz butter
1 apple, orange, or pear
8 oz skim milk

Dinner
3 oz chicken
2½ oz sliced carrots
Cooked vegetables, as desired
1 slice bread
¼ oz butter
4 oz stewed apples without sugar
2 oz skim milk

Beverages are sometimes overlooked as a source of energy. Carbonated soft drinks of the ordinary type contain 300 to 400 kilo-joules (70 to 100 calories) per serving. Tea or coffee with a tablespoonful of cream and a teaspoon of sugar approximates 190 kilo-joules (45 calories). Beer provides 500 kilo-joules (120 calories) per eight ounces; wines, 350 to 500 kilo-joules (80 to 120 calories) per four ounces; distilled spirits (whisky, rum, gin, brandy) approximately 350 kilo-joules (80 calories) per ounce; eggnog, 1250 to 1700 kilo-joules (300 to 400 calories) per serving. Unwise intake of beverages may make the difference between failure and success in weight control.

Energy and food composition table (composition per oz. as consumed)

Food	Energy kilo-calories	Energy kilo-joules	Calcium mg	Iron mg	Vitamin A (Retinol Equiv.) mg	Thiamine mg	Riboflavine mg	Nicotinic Acid equiv. mg	Vitamin C mg
Cereal products									
Bread									
(White)	72	304	28	0.5	0	0.05	0.01	0.7	0
(Brown)	65	278	25	0.7	0	0.08	0.02	0.8	0
(Wholemeal)	68	290	8	0.9	0	0.07	0.03	0.5	0
Cornflakes	100	427	1	0.1	0	0.32	0.40	3.0	0
Oatmeal	113	480	16	1.2	0	0.14	0.03	0.8	0
Biscuits									
Cream crackers	134	563	41	0.6	0	0.06	0.01	0.7	0
Semi sweet	122	513	36	0.5	0	0.05	0.02	0.6	0
Rich sweet	140	590	26	0.4	0	0.03	0.01	0.4	0
Dairy products									
Butter	207	853	4	0	282	0	0	0	0
Cheddar cheese	117	485	230	0.2	119	0.01	0.14	1.5	0
Cottage cheese	32	135	23	0.1	8	0.01	0.08	0.9	0
Single cream	54	222	28	0	44	0.01	0.04	0.2	0
1 egg = 50 gm	74	306	27	1.1	70	0.05	0.24	1.8	0
Whole milk liquid	19	79	34	0	10–12	0.01	0.04	0.3	0.3
Skim milk	100	426	359	0.2	1	0.09	0.49	2.8	3
Fats									
Lard, dripping	254	1043	0	0	0	0	0	0	0
Low-fat spread	103	425	0	0	255	0	0	0	0
Margarine	208	856	1	0.1	255	0	0	0	0
Oils, cooking and salad	255	1047	0	0	0	0	0	0	0
Fish									
Cod, fried in batter	56	236	23	0.1	0	0	0.03	1.9	0
Salmon, tinned	44	184	26	0.4	26	0.01	0.05	3.0	0
Sardine, in oil	62	258	156	0.8	9	0.01	0.10	3.5	0
Fruit									
Apples	13	56	1	0.1	1	0.01	0.01	0	1
Apricots, tinned in·syrup	30	128	3	0.2	47	0.01	0	0.1	1
Bananas	22	93	2	0.1	9	0.01	0.02	0.2	3
Grapefruit	6	27	5	0.1	0	0.01	0.01	0.1	11
Lemons	2	10	2	0	0	0.01	0	0	14
Melon	6	27	5	0.1	45	0.01	0.01	0.1	7
Oranges	10	42	12	0.1	2	0.03	0.01	0.1	14
Pears, fresh	12	50	2	0.1	1	0.01	0.01	0.1	1
Plums	9	39	3	0.1	10	0.01	0.01	0.2	1
Prunes	46	194	11	0.8	45	0.03	0.06	0.5	0
Sultanas	71	301	15	0.5	0	0.03	0.09	0.2	0
Nuts									
Almonds	164	680	70	1.2	0	0.09	0.07	1.4	0
Coconut, desiccated	173	712	6	1.0	0	0.02	0.01	0.5	0
Peanuts, roasted	166	689	17	0.6	0	0.07	0.03	5.9	0

Food	Energy kilo-calories	Energy kilo-joules	Calcium mg	Iron mg	Vitamin A (Retinol Equiv.) mg	Thiamine mg	Riboflavine mg	Nicotinic Acid equiv. mg	Vitamin C mg
Meat, cooked									
Beef, stewing	63	264	4	0.8	0	0.01	0.09	2.9	0
Lamb, roast	83	344	2	0.6	0	0.02	0.07	2.6	0
Chicken, roast	42	174	3	0.2	0	0.02	0.05	3.6	0
Liver, fried	70	291	4	2.5	1701	0.08	1.20	5.9	6
Luncheon meat	89	368	4	0.3	0	0.20	0.03	1.3	0
Pork, grilled chop	94	393	2	0.3	0	0.19	0.06	3.1	0
Ham	77	319	3	0.4	0	0.13	0.04	2.3	0
Bacon	127	524	3	0.4	0	0.11	0.05	2.6	0
Puddings and cakes									
Apple pie	80	336	12	0.2	4	0.02	0.01	0.3	0
Custard	26	112	31	0	10	0.02	0.04	0.2	0
Rice pudding	41	170	33	0	27	0.01	0.04	0.3	0
Ice cream, vanilla	55	228	39	0.1	0	0.01	0.06	0.3	0
Bun, currant	93	392	25	0.8	7	0.04	0.03	0.6	0
Fruit cake	104	438	20	0.5	16	0.02	0.02	0.3	0
Jam tart	111	467	14	0.4	0	0.02	0	0.2	0
Plain cake	121	506	19	0.4	23	0.02	0.03	0.5	0
Sweets and preserves, etc.									
Chocolate, milk	164	686	70	0.5	2	0.01	0.10	0.7	0
Honey	82	349	1	0.1	0	0	0.01	0.1	0
Jam	74	315	5	0.3	1	0	0	0	3
Sugar, white	112	477	0	0	0	0	0	0	0
Cola drink	13	54	0	0	0	0	0	0	0
Squash, fruit undiluted	34	146	5	0.1	0	0	0	0	0
Vegetables, cooked									
Beans, tinned in tomato sauce	17	74	13	0.4	14	0.02	0.01	0.4	1
Beetroot	12	53	9	0.2	0	0	0.01	0.1	1
Brussel sprouts	5	22	7	0.2	19	0.02	0.03	0.3	10
Cabbage	5	20	11	0.1	14	0.01	0.01	0.1	6
Peas, fresh or frozen	13	59	4	0.3	14	0.07	0.03	0.7	4
Peas, tinned processed	22	93	8	0.4	19	0.03	0.01	0.4	0
Potatoes, boiled	23	96	1	0.1	0	0.02	0.01	0.3	1–4
chips	68	294	4	0.4	0	0.03	0.01	0.6	2–6
roast	32	134	3	0.3	0	0.03	0.02	0.6	2–7
crisps	152	632	10	0.6	0	0.05	0.02	1.8	5
Sweetcorn, tinned	22	95	1	0	10	0.01	0.02	0.1	1
Vegetables, raw									
Celery	3	12	15	0.2	0	0.01	0.01	0.1	2
Cucumber	2	8	5	0.1	0	0.01	0.01	0.1	2
Lettuce	2	10	6	0.3	47	0.02	0.02	0.1	4
Tomatoes	3	15	4	0.1	33	0.02	0.01	0.2	6
Watercress	4	17	63	0.5	142	0.03	0.05	0.6	17

Chapter 15 Nutrition

Underweight

Excessive leanness is associated with increased ill health and may itself be a manifestation of illness which needs guidance from a doctor, and a planned programme for weight gain should be approved by him. To gain weight is sometimes as difficult as for an overweight person to lose it, and success requires as much discipline as weight reduction.

What has been said about reducing diets is an excellent guide to what not to do in dietary adjustment to gain weight. A dietary programme to increase weight aims to increase the daily intake of energy appreciably above caloric expenditure. This is done by eating more of all food groups, but particularly of foods high in energy.

The fundamental plan for a balanced weight-gain diet should adhere to the basic food groups outlined on page 360. From the milk group one should take four or more cups per day of whole milk, augmented by servings of cheese and ice cream. From the meat group one should eat two or more servings of meat, poultry, or fish, including the fatter cuts. One or more eggs per day and servings of the meat alternatives can add an appetizing variety.

Little can be done to enhance energy intake from the vegetable-fruit group other than to serve vegetables with sauces, butter, salad oils, and in batter. Fruits can be used with sugar or heavy syrup, with the addition of cream.

A common difficulty in efforts to gain weight is rapid appetite satiation, or a feeling of getting filled up too fast. Foods with an appetizing and appealing flavour may coax the light eater, and an interest in cooking sometimes provides additional motivation. Snacks or extra meals – mid-morning, mid-afternoon, bedtime – effectively increase intake, particularly if it is difficult for the lean subject to increase his intake at regular meals. The snacks can be sandwiches with a beverage, milk and egg drinks, milk shakes, and, for those accustomed to it, an aperitif at lunch or dinner may be a further stimulus to eating.

Harmful excesses

Overdosage of at least nine nutrients – vitamins A and D, carotene, energy, iodine, salt, potassium, fluoride, iron – is harmful. To this list may be added a number of trace elements, such as cobalt, zinc, and selenium, which are required in animals, but whose role in human nutrition is not completely defined. Even such familiar nutrients as sugar, water, and certain amino acids are toxic when taken in excess. There is an optimal range of intake of many essential nutrients, and the concept of a harmful or toxic substance must here be related to amount. It is important to consider the toxicity of even essential nutrients before taking supplements or preparations which could increase the intake of various substances far above the level of safety.

Metabolic disturbances may impair the body's ability to use commonplace and harmless nutrients, with the result that harmful breakdown products accumulate in the body and do damage. Several congenital diseases of this sort are known as inborn errors of metabolism.

In *galactosaemia*, the infant has a defective enzyme system and cannot deal with common sugars – lactose (milk sugar) and galactose (one of the sugars resulting from digestion of lactose) – with the result that these sugars do serious harm. The infant fails to gain weight, is irritable, the liver becomes enlarged, jaundice may occur, and cataracts develop if the condition is untreated. Other serious consequences include mental retardation. When recognized early this condition may be treated successfully by using special diets or formulas free of the offending sugars.

Phenylketonuria is another inborn error which can be modified by diet. Here the inherited defect is absence of a liver enzyme, which makes it impossible for the infant to handle phenylalanine, a common amino acid of protein foods. Certain breakdown products accumulate in the blood, damage the developing central nervous system, and lead to mental retardation unless the condition is detected and treated early. Treatment consists of restricting the intake of phenylalanine through use of a special digest of protein from which the amino acid has been removed, along with appropriate intake of low protein foods (vegetables, fruits) and supplements judged necessary by the doctor.

There are many other congenital inborn errors of metabolism, in most of which dietary therapy is unfortunately of little avail. A rare disorder known as *Wilson's disease* involves a defect in which copper is absorbed in excessive and harmful quantities. Treatment, by reducing the copper content of the diet and use of agents which reduce absorption and increase excretion of the trace element, is helpful.

Nutrition during growth

Growth increases requirements for dietary protein, carbohydrate, fat, vitamins, and minerals. During periods of rapid growth the requirements for basal metabolism are higher per unit of body weight than in the adult, and activity – expenditure of energy – is higher, particularly during pre-adolescence and adolescence.

To meet these large nutritional requirements, the child – especially the older child and adolescent – consumes what might appear to be inordinate quantities of food. But this also applies to infants when one considers relative body size. During early life an infant may consume 444 kilo-joules (111 calories) per kilo of body weight. If a 77 kg (12 stone) man ate at the same rate per kilo he would consume 35700 kilo-joules or 35·7 mega-joules (8,500 calories) a day – three to four times the calories that an average man of that weight actually consumes.

Growth is most rapid during fetal development. Simultaneously with rapid growth of the fetus there are growth changes in the mother's body – growth of the uterus and related structures, increase in breast size, and other increases in body tissue. After the child is born the nursing mother provides practically all the nutrients the infant requires during the first few months of life, and this accounts for her increased nutritional needs during lactation.

Infant nutrition An infant will almost triple his weight during the first year. He consumes somewhat more energy per kilo of body weight during the first half of the first year than during the second half. He tends to adjust food intake himself, refusing food when he is satisfied or being satisfied with fewer feedings. The inexperienced mother may interpret this as an indication that the baby is not eating properly and that something is wrong with him, but as long as the infant appears satisfied, healthy, and gains weight steadily, there is no cause for concern.

Rapid infant growth demands a relatively high intake of energy, protein, vitamins, and minerals. For the breast-fed infant, all of these needs will be met by an adequate supply of breast milk, except possibly for vitamin D. Neither mother's milk nor ordinary cows' milk is a necessarily dependable source of this vitamin. However, supplementation with vitamin D concentrates is simple and routine for breast-fed infants, and may or may not be necessary in bottle-fed infants, depending on whether the milk or formula has been fortified with this factor.

Foods rich in vitamin C (orange juice or other juices), or supplements, are usually introduced early, especially if the infant is artificially fed. All types of cows' milk are undependable sources of this factor, and amounts originally present in the raw products are reduced by heat-sterilization procedures.

Thus the usual pattern of infant feeding is early introduction of sources of vitamins C and D, and, usually at a slightly later period, iron-rich foods such as infant cereals, meats, and greens. Failure to provide these additions to a milk-based diet may lead to development of scurvy, rickets, or iron-deficiency anaemia.

Breast milk is considered the most desirable infant food, and the early milk (colostrum) transmits some immunological substances from mother to infant. An adequate amount of breast milk will satisfy the requirements of the infant for approximately the first six months, except for vitamin D and iron. However, it is desirable to introduce additional foods or supplementary feedings before the sixth month, to assure energy and nutritional adequacy, to develop acceptance for other foods, and to relieve the mother of regular confining nursing schedules.

Successful breast-feeding is a source of psychological satisfaction to mother and infant, and provides a safe food with less risk of infection to the infant than artificial feeding when carelessness or circumstances make proper sterilization of formulas difficult.

Artificial or bottle-feeding of infants has been greatly improved in recent years. The paediatrician has a wide choice of formulas suited to the needs of individual infants. Milk-based formulas usually use dried milk, appropriately diluted, with addition of ordinary sugar, glucose syrup, starch, dextri-maltose, or rice or barley flour, to adjust the carbohydrate and energy content. The bottled formula is commonly heated by terminal sterilization – that is, the container and its contents are heated all at once – assuring freedom from harmful bacteria and at the same time improving the digestibility of the milk.

Many varieties of prepared formulas are available and may be prescribed by the paediatrician. These are convenient and dependable, but generally more expensive than home-prepared formulas. Various specialized proprietary formulas contain added vitamins C and D, may be enriched with iron, or contain unusual amounts of iron for use in special situations. There are a number of milk-free formulas for infants who are sensitive to milk. Special formulas should be used only on the advice of a doctor.

The feeding schedule recommended by the doctor should be followed. Commonly, these are at four-hourly intervals, but there is considerable acceptance of demand feeding – giving the baby his feed when he is hungry. The time for introducing vitamin supplements and iron-rich foods varies considerably. The trend in recent years has been toward earlier introduction of a large variety of foods such as cereals, egg yolk, pureed meats, vegetables, and fruits. As the child's experience with foods is widened, the mother should continue to encourage the use of protein-rich meats, eggs, vegetables, and fruits, rather than desserts, puddings, noodles, macaroni, and pasta mixtures.

Water needs of infants must not be overlooked. Remember that a baby's requirement for water is relatively high and is greater when more concentrated formulas are used. In warm weather the requirement for water is increased. Finally, the infant is particularly sensitive to losses of water and salts resulting from diarrhoea and vomiting.

Nutrition in childhood The major nutritional problem during this period is one of developing and maintaining sound food habits despite the pressures and emotional changes which occur in the growing child and young adolescent. Difficulties include:

Deviations in eating habits induced by conflicts and jealousies, which may lead to rejection of foods and underweight, or overconsumption and obesity.

Establishment of unhealthy food habits. A child may reject meat, milk, or some other important food that he does not like. This may be an expression of negativism or revolt against parental admonition or some emotional situation, or a reflection of group pressures, such as rejection of milk by a teenage girl because her friends think milk is fattening.

Failure to eat an adequate breakfast: this may result from being rushed in the morning or poor breakfast habits in families.

Inadequate lunches and unwise expenditure of lunch money on excessive amounts of sweets, soft drinks, and other items tend to dilute the nutritional quality of the day's food intake.

Children frequently go on food binges and, for a period of several meals, enthusiastically eat some temporarily favoured food but reject others. These temporary patterns usually correct themselves unless they are overemphasized by parents to a point of conflict with the child. It is a wise parent who distinguishes between a temporary food binge that will pass and a more deep-rooted alteration in food habits that may become nutritionally harmful.

Informed adult guidance and example are very important in establishing good eating habits in the young.

Needs of the mother

Pregnancy Rapid growth during pregnancy requires a diet of high quality to avoid malnutrition of the mother, prepare her for lactation, and assure the best possible nutritional status for both mother and infant. Increased needs, in general, are met by some increase in milk consumption, regular inclusion in the diet of fish, poultry, and lean meats, use of iodized salt, and plenty of fresh fruits and vegetables. Some prenatal finding by the obstetrician may indicate the desirability of some specific supplement or alteration in the diet, such as iron supplements.

Excessive weight gain in pregnancy is not uncommon during the later months. Weight control in pregnancy by dietary restriction is the same in principle as weight control in other circumstances, discussed under obesity earlier in this chapter. It is vital that the weight control diet be of high quality, and reduced only in energy content. As a practical matter, this means avoidance of sources of energy that do not have particularly good protein and vitamin values – reduced intake of fats and oils, fat meats, soft drinks, sweet desserts, and the like. Skim milk may be substituted for whole milk.

Sometimes the obstetrician warns the patient to reduce her intake of salt, usually because of increased retention of water with oedema and rapid weight gain, changes in blood pressure, or other evidence from laboratory findings. Frequently the salt intake can be reduced sufficiently by merely refraining from adding salt to food and by avoiding obviously salt-treated foods such as ham, bacon, olives, and salted fish.

Extreme reduction of the salt content of the diet should be undertaken only under the guidance and counsel of an obstetrician, who will institute appropriate checks and perhaps prescribe a rigid special diet and a salt substitute.

Morning sickness of early pregnancy (see chapter 11) may frequently be alleviated by taking a relatively dry, small breakfast and sometimes by eating a small piece of dry toast before rising in the morning. It is not unusual for a certain amount of indigestion to be experienced even in late pregnancy. This may be helped by reducing the amount of food normally eaten at regular meals and dividing the day's usual food intake into five or six smaller, lighter meals.

Congenital defects It is unlikely that dietary deficiency in mothers in this country plays any significant part in formation of congenital abnormalities in their offspring. Certainly there is no evidence of such relationship if the mother's diet approaches the levels of Recommended Dietary Allowances, and there is no reason to believe that vitamin or other nutritional supplements during pregnancy can reduce the likelihood of a congenitally abnormal infant, in a woman taking a reasonably good diet.

It has sometimes been proposed that malnutrition, especially protein deficiency, is responsible for the toxaemia of pregnancy – a condition characterized by elevated blood pressure, oedema, laboratory evidence of impaired kidney function, and in extreme cases, fits. Carefully designed studies have failed to sustain this hypothesis. A good diet relatively high in protein is useful in treating this condition, but there is no good evidence that a poor diet is responsible for its development.

Birth size Infants born to obese women have a greater birth weight than those born to women of average weight or less. These influences on birth weight, however, are smaller and less pronounced than other influences, such as body build of the parents, except under extreme conditions.

Lactation imposes similar nutritional requirements to pregnancy except that the need for total energy and for calcium is greater. These enhanced needs can be met readily by increased consumption of the four basic food groups, with special emphasis on milk, meats, vegetables, and fruits, in keeping with appetite (unless appetite is excessive). Probably the best guide to energy intake is weight adjustment. Within four weeks or so after delivery the mother should have returned to her pre-pregnancy weight or slightly above, and should not gain additionally during lactation.

It is usually advised that the lactating woman take an additional pint of milk daily, and some increase in fluid intake is probably desirable since during lactation there is of course secretion of water in the milk.

Food fads and fallacies

There are many unsound beliefs about foods. Some of these may be associated with social groups and reflect cultural attitudes or traditional patterns. Various traditional misconceptions, though lacking in scientific validity, do no particular harm since there are many ways of compensating and adapting when a liberal choice of high quality foods in a mixed diet is available.

Quite different misconceptions are promoted by the food faddist or so-called expert, who may be sincere but uninformed, but more often has a financial rather than an altruistic motivation. The food faddist is not new, but he takes advantage of modern methods of communication and exhortation.

Frequently he is represented to be an outstanding authority or expert and does not deny it, although a check of his credentials often reveals an absence of the scientific training he professes to possess. Often he identifies himself with famous or glamorous persons by namedropping at some point in his writings.

His persuasive pitch may be aimed to convince customers of the remarkable effectiveness of his product, or on the other hand, to view with alarm the disastrous consequences to health of allegedly toxic or devitalized everyday foods other than those he promotes. The latter device leads his converts to distrust foods which by scientific evidence are beneficial and healthful.

Some fads and fallacies of the past occasionally reappear in the same or another guise, and new ones arise. Examples of fads and fallacious beliefs include the alleged production of cancer from eating foods cooked in aluminium utensils; the cure of many diseases by eating common or unusual food products; the false idea that energy taken in some particular form cannot produce body fat and hence does not count toward the total energy content of the diet; that one may remove energy from such things as potato chips; that some foods make fat melt away.

Other examples of fads and fallacies include the notion that chemical fertilizers produce foods with less nutritional value than does natural manure; the attribution to certain foods of mystic powers promoting longevity; the belief that a so-called natural food or vitamin is more healthful or beneficial than a processed or synthetic one; the promotion of capsules and preparations containing dozens of trace substances and exotic-sounding components.

Faddish misinformation interferes with building sound food patterns, and may even lead to malnourishment by excesses or deficiencies if the convert slavishly follows a rigid programme of limited special products. Damage can be done by harmless and even beneficial foods and products if faith that they will cure some condition leads to delay in seeking medical attention that may be needed urgently. Finally, faddist foods and products are almost always much more expensive than the excellent foods and products available everywhere in the open market.

Therapeutic diets

Therapeutic diets are modifications of adequate, normal diets, designed to provide for some unusual need of a particular patient. This need may be temporary, such as a period of convalescence from an

Chapter 15 **Nutrition**

operation, or it may be a permanent need that continues for years or even a lifetime.

Not all dietary instruction received from a doctor should be interpreted as placing the patient on a diet. In many instances the advised diet may be an aspect of educating the patient as to what constitutes an adequate diet and how to attain it. This is the case when a patient obviously has been following an inadequate diet or when a mother receives advice about feeding her child.

When, however, some abnormal condition such as diabetes, some types of heart disease, or other illness exists, the object is to modify a normal adequate diet to provide for an unusual need of the patient. The patient should regard such diets as redirection of his dietary habits rather than as some special therapy that sets him apart from others. The doctor or dietician is attempting to ensure adequate dietary intake with a minimum of inconvenience.

In most situations, a modified diet useful in management of a given condition is not to be regarded as a single measure of cure. Usually a therapeutic diet is only one of the therapeutic measures employed. On the other hand, diets for weight control, or for elimination of something that is harmful to an individual (as in galactosaemia or some allergic conditions) are specific therapeutic tools.

The doctor may give detailed dietary instructions himself, or he may determine the characteristics of a diet needed by the patient and indicate these to a competent dietician who is specially trained in the field of foods and diet therapy and can effectively guide the patient in establishing his new dietary habits.

Basic considerations which underlie various types of therapeutic diets may be illustrated by examples. The principle of energy adjustment has been discussed in the sections on obesity and leanness. The principle of elimination or reduction of a single substance harmful to the patient has been discussed under metabolic disturbances. The same principle is applied in diets used in the management of food allergies, the difference being that it is sometimes difficult for the allergist to identify the offending foods. This is usually done by temporary elimination diets (see chapter 21). Diets for diabetics are discussed in chapter 10.

Gastrointestinal disorders Slightly different considerations are involved in therapeutic diets for treatment of gastrointestinal disorders. Here one is concerned with the amount of food consumed at a time, the texture and physical properties of the diet, and with properties which may influence the reaction of the gastrointestinal tract to food.

In acute gastrointestinal infections with diarrhoea, the object of dietary change is to reduce the overstimulation of the gastrointestinal tract. To this end, relatively small quantities of bland foods are advised, with a liberal supply of fluids through frequent taking of moderate quantities of tea, clear soup, fizzy drinks, and the like.

In gallbladder disease with attacks of gallbladder colic and in a number of conditions in which there is poor absorption of fat from the gastrointestinal tract, the doctor may prescribe a diet with reduced fat content. Similar diets may be indicated in some cases where there is excessive cholesterol or fats (triglycerides) in the blood. The principal foods which contribute fat to the diet are meats, egg yolk, whole milk, butter, cheese, cream, margarine, lard and other cooking fats, cooking oils, and salad dressings. Any appreciable alteration of fat intake requires reduction in consumption of these fat-rich foods, in such a manner that the diet continues to be nutritionally adequate. In other words, foods such as meat and milk should not be eliminated from the diet, but lean meats, skim milk, and cottage cheese should be used to minimize fat intake from these food groups.

Polyunsaturated fats When the doctor judges it desirable to increase the ratio of polyunsaturated to saturated fats, the diet must be designed not only to adjust the total amount of dietary fat but also to adjust the sources.

Vegetable oils such as corn, soya, and safflower are rich sources of polyunsaturated fats, especially linoleic acid. Accordingly, these vegetable fats may be advised for use in cooking meats, fish, and eggs, in salad oils, in vegetables, or baked products. If it is judged desirable to reduce the saturated fat in the diet, this entails a decrease in fat derived from dairy products and meat. Only non-fat milk may be allowed, no cream, and the amount of eggs limited. To make such adjustments while maintaining the nutritional quality of the diet requires professional guidance, since uninformed dietary manipulation may cause deprivation of some essential nutrient or nutrients.

When an increase in polyunsaturated fat intake is advised it must be remembered that the polyunsaturates are a replacement of some of the other fats, not an addition to total fat intake.

Salt or sodium-restricted diets are prescribed in the treatment of some types of high blood pressure, and cardiovascular or kidney disease. Sodium (contained in ordinary salt, sodium chloride) is an essential nutrient and drastic restriction can produce deficiency symptoms. It is important that a person on a low-sodium diet be under medical surveillance.

There are three common levels of dietary sodium restriction. The first permits some 1,500 to 3,000 mg of sodium daily, approximately half the usual intake. This may be achieved by simply refraining from adding salt to foods as served and by eliminating salted foods and condiments. The lower level of 1,500 mg may be obtained by not adding any salt to foods during cooking or to foods as served. To reduce sodium intake to the lowest levels of 500 and 200 mg, it is necessary to impose strict limits on both the quantity of many common foods and the kind of foods that may be included. These low levels require careful guidance.

Unrecognized sources may increase the sodium content of a rigidly restricted diet. In some communities, the local water supply may contain significant amounts of sodium, and a number of common medicines contain some sodium.

A rigid low-sodium diet tends to be tasteless and flat. Agents which impart a salt-like flavour but add little or no sodium to the diet have been developed. These salt substitutes are primarily potassium chloride plus ammonium chloride or amino acid derivatives. The formulas vary. It is wise to check with the doctor to be sure that a particular salt substitute is suitable, since those which contain potassium may be harmful or improper in the treatment of some types of kidney disease.

Food storage

How long can perishable foods stored in a refrigerator maintain high quality? Some approximate times are given below:

1 or 2 days

Meats: minced meats, offal (liver, kidney, brains), poultry (cut-up and whole), fish, leftover cooked meats, and meat dishes.
Fruit: berries, ripe tomatoes.
Vegetables: Brussels sprouts, spinach, and other green leafy vegetables, lettuce, green onions, green peas, asparagus, and broccoli.

3 to 5 days

Dairy products: milk and cream, cottage cheese.
Fruit: cherries, grapes, peaches, apricots.

Meats: fresh meat cuts, cold cuts, corned beef, luncheon meat, sliced ham.
Vegetables: cabbage, cauliflower, celery, and carrots.

1 week

Meat: sliced bacon.
Poultry products: eggs.
Fruit: apples, oranges, grapefruit, lemons.

2 weeks

Dairy products: butter, soft cheeses other than cottage cheese.
Meats: whole cured ham.

Well-wrapped hard cheeses keep indefinitely at refrigerator temperature. Butter should be stored tightly wrapped. Fresh berries lose food value and spoil more rapidly if washed before refrigeration. Bananas, melons, avocados, and pineapples are best stored at cool room temperature. Carrots, beetroots, and radishes keep best in the refrigerator when the tops and root tips are removed.

Chapter 16
The teeth

Revised by Gerald B. Winter, MB BS BDS (Lond) FDS RCS (Eng), DCH
and M. Jeremy Shaw, BDS (Lond) FDS RCS (Eng)

Dental diseases occur throughout the world and are probably the commonest chronic diseases in the United Kingdom. Dental decay (caries) and gum disease (gingivitis and periodontal disease) are such unspectacular and slowly developing infections that they may escape notice until irreversible damage is present. Prevention is the best policy, but tooth loss may be avoided by early treatment.

On average, by the age of five years, every child has suffered over three decayed primary (milk) teeth, and by fifteen years over eight of the 28 permanent teeth have become either decayed or filled, or are missing. The National Health Service of the United Kingdom supplies 7,000 dentures to schoolchildren each year. The large proportion of people in the United Kingdom who have lost all their natural teeth is a striking indication of the impact of dental disease. The Adult Dental Health Surveys found that 37 per cent of the adult population in England and Wales had had all their teeth extracted; in Scotland the proportion was higher (44 per cent).

In the United Kingdom we spend over £260 million annually on dental treatment in general practice alone. In addition dental disease is responsible for the loss of two million working days each year. It is therefore an expensive disease to neglect. The cost of dental disease hardly reflects the immense damage it does to the quality of life. Tooth loss reinforces the awareness of ageing. Dentures can also affect taste, chewing, and the enjoyment of food.

It is easily forgotten that there is a small but never insignificant mortality from dental disease. When teeth are extracted from patients with congenital or rheumatic heart disease, death may result from infection of the heart valves.

In order to understand how dental disease occurs it is necessary to consider the development and structure of healthy teeth and gums.

The healthy mouth

Development of the jaws and teeth At the end of the first month of fetal life, folds appear at the head end of the embryo which are later to become the upper and lower jaws. These growth processes are usually completed by the end of the third month of life within the womb. By this time tooth development is well advanced. The primary (milk) teeth start as groups of cells in the developing jaws, each group corresponding to a tooth. The first evidence of mineralization of the hard tissues of the teeth (enamel and dentine) occurs in about the fourth month of pregnancy (see page 376). It is not until six to seven months after birth that the first teeth start to erupt at the front of the mouth. Eruption times vary considerably, but in general the primary teeth in the lower jaw (mandible) erupt before their counterparts in the upper jaw (maxilla), whilst the front teeth (incisors) erupt before the back teeth (molars). The full set of twenty primary teeth will usually have emerged by the time the child is three years old (see opposite).

The permanent teeth develop in a similar way but they start to form a little later. The first permanent molars often start to form hard tissues (mineralize) before the child is born, and most of the incisors and canines shortly after birth. Eruption of the first molars occurs behind the primary teeth at the back of the mouth at about six years of age; this often leads to the erroneous impression that they are members of the

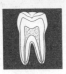

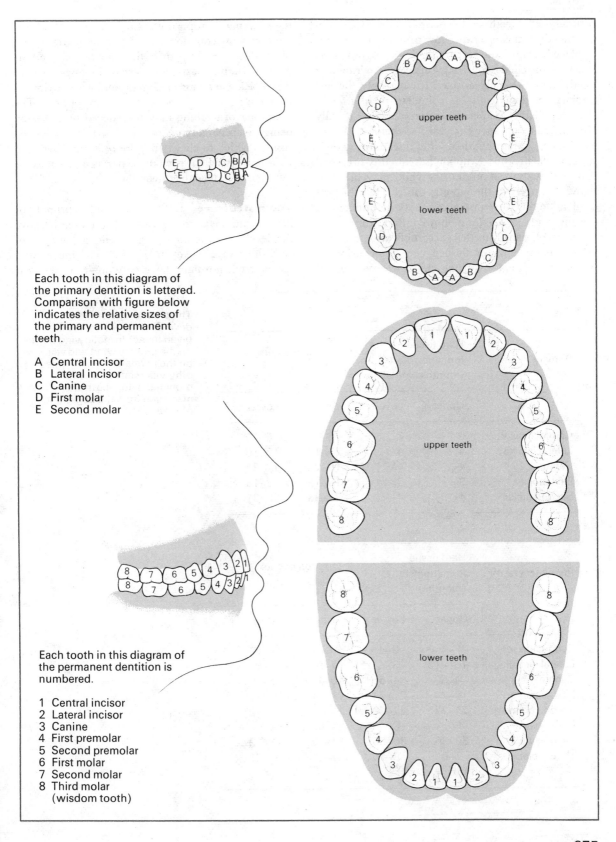

Each tooth in this diagram of the primary dentition is lettered. Comparison with figure below indicates the relative sizes of the primary and permanent teeth.

A Central incisor
B Lateral incisor
C Canine
D First molar
E Second molar

upper teeth

lower teeth

upper teeth

lower teeth

Each tooth in this diagram of the permanent dentition is numbered.

1 Central incisor
2 Lateral incisor
3 Canine
4 First premolar
5 Second premolar
6 First molar
7 Second molar
8 Third molar
   (wisdom tooth)

Chapter 16 The teeth

primary set of teeth. As the permanent teeth in front of the first molars erupt, the primary teeth they replace become loose and are shed (see opposite). By the time the child is fourteen years old, 28 permanent teeth should be fully erupted leaving only the last molars (wisdom teeth) to complete their growth. Development of the permanent set of teeth is usually completed by the age of 25 years (see below).

Teething Many children suffer discomfort as their primary teeth erupt. Eruption is frequently preceded by excessive salivation and the child may place its hand or fingers in the mouth; this is often the first indication that the eruption of a tooth is imminent. A recent study of teething showed that during the eruption of primary teeth local complications, such as gum inflammation or flushed cheeks, occurred in almost three quarters of the children observed. Of

these, a high proportion also had general disturbances; most common were loss of appetite, irritability, disturbed sleep, dribbling, or a rash around the mouth. In the past more severe illnesses such as diarrhoea, fever, or even convulsions, were attributed to teething. This association is unjustified. The symptoms of teething may be relieved by the baby being given a teething ring or hard nonsweetened rusk on which to chew. In more resistant cases mild pain-relievers such as elixir of paracetamol may be required to reduce the discomfort.

Tooth structure Each tooth, whether primary or permanent, has a crown visible in the mouth above the level of the gum (gingiva) and a longer root embedded in a socket in the jaw. The incisor and canine teeth normally have only one root, whereas

Table 1

The chronology of tooth development. All figures are given in months following birth on the primary chart and years on the permanent chart, unless otherwise stated. Figures provided before birth are measured from the beginning of pregnancy.

Primary tooth	Hard tissue formation starts (months of fetal life)		Eruption occurs (months)	
	Upper	Lower	Upper	Lower
Central incisor	3	3	8–12	6–10
Lateral incisor	4	4	9–13	10–16
Canine	$4\frac{1}{2}$	$4\frac{1}{2}$	16–22	17–23
First molar	$3\frac{1}{2}$	$3\frac{1}{2}$	13–19	12–18
Second molar	$4\frac{1}{2}$	$4\frac{1}{2}$	25–33	23–31

Permanent tooth	Hard tissue formation starts (months)		Eruption occurs (years)	
	Upper	Lower	Upper	Lower
Central incisor	3–4	3–4	$6–7\frac{1}{2}$	$5\frac{1}{2}–6\frac{1}{2}$
Lateral incisor	10—12	3–4	7–9	7–8
Canine	4–5	4–5	10–12	9–11
First premolar	18–21	21–24	$9\frac{1}{2}–11$	$10\frac{1}{2}–12$
Second premolar	24–27	27–30	11–12	$11–12\frac{1}{2}$
First molar	8*	8*	$5\frac{1}{2}–6\frac{1}{2}$	$5\frac{1}{2}–6\frac{1}{2}$
Second molar	30–36	30–36	$11–12\frac{1}{2}$	11–12
Third molar	7–9 years	8–10 years	17–21	17–21

* months of fetal life

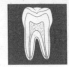

the molars have two, three, or occasionally even four. The roots tend to become more complex towards the back of the mouth. The roots of the primary teeth are thinner than their permanent successors and are consequently more fragile. Both primary and secondary teeth are similar in structure; the primary teeth, however, have relatively larger pulp chambers and thinner enamel and dentine. Enamel is the hardest tissue in the body. It is insensitive and acts as the protective covering for the crown of the tooth. It is incapable of self-repair. Dentine makes up the bulk of the tooth structure. In contrast with the enamel, there are millions of tiny cells, with extensions running in tubules through the dentine from the pulp of the tooth to the junction between enamel and dentine. Consequently it is sensitive to touch and, although an extremely hard tissue, it is softer than enamel. The

pulp chamber and canal occupy the space in the centre of the crown and root of the tooth respectively. The pulp is the living tissue of the tooth containing nerves and blood vessels which supply the cells that extend into the dentine. The nerves and blood vessels enter the tooth at the tip of the root. The root of the tooth is covered with a hard bonelike tissue called cementum. Embedded in the cementum are fibres which attach the tooth to its bony socket and allow slight movement of the tooth when pressure is applied to the crown.

Tooth support The gum (gingiva) surrounds the neck of the tooth and is attached close to the area where enamel and cementum meet, forming a firm cuff of soft tissue at the limit of the crown. There is a shallow crevice between the gum and tooth which

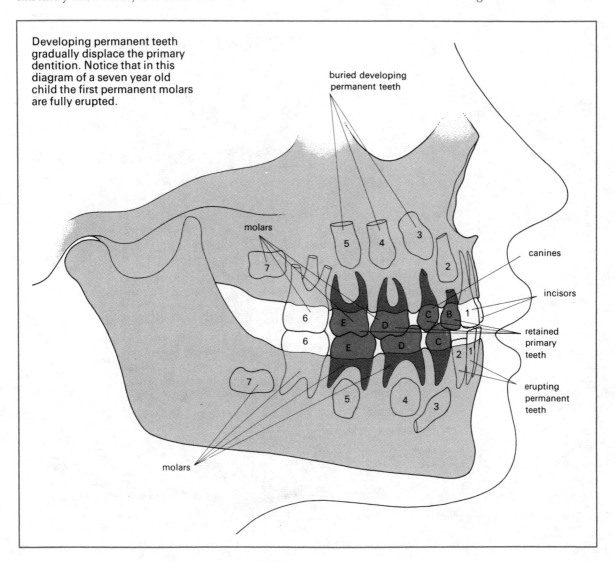

Developing permanent teeth gradually displace the primary dentition. Notice that in this diagram of a seven year old child the first permanent molars are fully erupted.

rarely exceeds two millimetres in depth when the gum is healthy. The gum should be firm, pale pink in colour, and possess a faintly stippled texture. The tissue of the gum at the base of the shallow crevice merges into the periodontal attachment which is a thin fibrous cushion between the bone of the socket wall and the root of the tooth; it is attached firmly to both. Fibres of the periodontal attachment not only support the tooth in the socket, but also hold neighbouring teeth together and bind the firm gingival cuff tightly against the tooth. The gums and periodontal attachment have a rich blood supply and nerve supply; the nerves inform the brain when the tooth is being subjected to undue pressure.

The pale pink lining material of the rest of the mouth is a soft mucus-producing tissue. It is adapted on the surface of the tongue to enable taste to be appreciated, and on the palate and gums to allow hard wear.

Disease and abnormality

Plaque dependent disease The two most common dental diseases, caries and gingivitis, are related to the presence of a soft bacterial layer known as plaque on the surfaces of the teeth. Plaque starts to form immediately after tooth brushing. It clings tenaciously to the tooth and consists of many types of bacteria and their products, together with precipitated mucin from saliva. Plaque occurs principally in the depths of pits and fissures on the grinding surfaces of molars and premolars, in the area of contact between the teeth, and in the gum crevice.

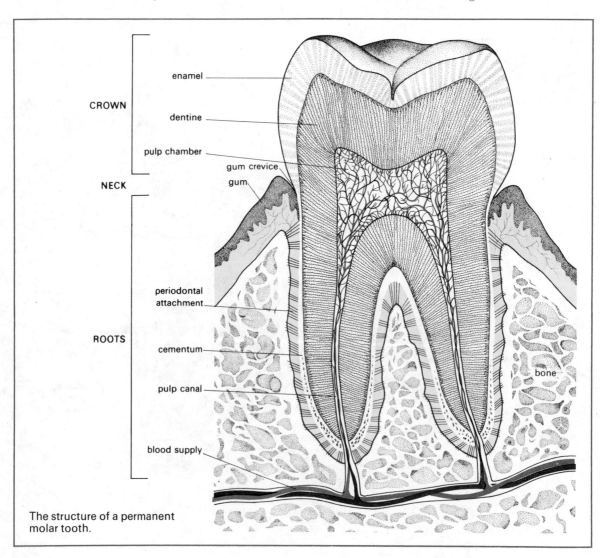

CROWN

enamel

dentine

pulp chamber

gum crevice

gum

NECK

periodontal attachment

ROOTS

cementum

pulp canal

blood supply

bone

The structure of a permanent molar tooth.

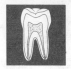

Where the salivary glands open into the mouth the reaction between plaque and the inorganic salts contained in saliva causes a hard scale called tartar (calculus) to form on the teeth. Tartar may also be found in pockets around teeth throughout the mouth in the presence of periodontal disease (see page 380).

The relationship between plaque, sugar, and caries has been established; exactly how they interreact is still under investigation. It has been shown that when sugar is introduced into the mouth the acidity of the plaque rises almost immediately; breakdown of the enamel by acid is thought to start the carious process. The relationship between plaque and gingivitis is also being studied. It has been shown that if plaque is removed from the teeth gingivitis heals, whereas if plaque is allowed to grow in contact with healthy gingiva, gingivitis follows.

Caries is a local destruction of enamel and dentine to form a cavity – otherwise known as tooth decay. Plaque accumulates in the pits, fissures, and contact areas of the tooth crown where the bacteria can live protected from removal by the tongue and toothbrush. It is in these areas that caries usually starts.

Early enamel caries In early caries there is no cavity formation. The first visible evidence of the disease is an opaque white spot due to damage to the enamel.

Later the surface breaks down and becomes roughened and stained.

Advanced caries As soon as the bacteria have penetrated the enamel they invade the underlying dentine and spread into it. The dentine is rapidly softened and the enamel undermined causing it to fracture; more bacteria are allowed into the now detectable cavity. Bacteria pass deeply into the tooth by means of the tiny tubules in the dentine. It is at this stage that pain is first experienced, particularly when sweet food and hot or cold drinks are consumed. When the bacteria and their irritant products reach the pulp, the pulp tissues become inflamed and cause more persistent pain. The blood vessels dilate, just as they do when there is a boil in the skin. Unlike a boil however, the inflamed tissues are prevented from swelling by the surrounding hard tooth structure, and the tiny aperture at the apex of the root is blocked, preventing the blood supply being maintained. The combination of impaired blood supply and rapidly spreading infection leads to death of the pulp. While this process is continuing, the enamel covering the softened dentine is continually breaking down so that the cavity increases in size. When the pulp dies, the increasingly severe toothache may subside for a time because of the death of nerve tissue within the pulp.

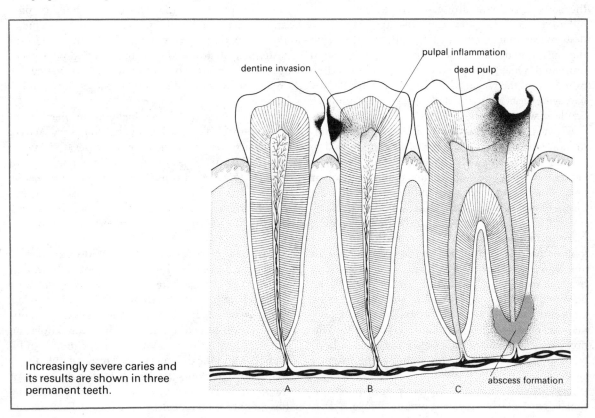

Increasingly severe caries and its results are shown in three permanent teeth.

Chapter 16 The teeth

In primary teeth, because the enamel and dentine are both very thin and the pulp comparatively large, infection and death of the pulp occur at a relatively early stage.

The dead tooth Once the pulp has died, the bacteria and their products may pass out of the root apex into the surrounding tissues and bone. The blood vessels in these tissues become inflamed, and pus may collect to form a dental abscess. At this stage the symptoms reappear, and in acute cases persistent throbbing pain is present and may disturb sleep. Pressure from the swollen blood vessels and pus pushes the tooth slightly out from the socket so that it is excruciatingly tender under pressure and is the first tooth to make contact when biting.

If the tooth does not receive early treatment, bacteria may progress further to infect the soft tissues of the face causing a considerable facial swelling. This infection may even spread further with serious consequences. In some circumstances the body defences manage to control the infection around the root of the tooth and prevent it spreading. This isolated chronic infection, if untreated, may develop into a dental cyst which can expand and lead to extensive painless destruction of the jawbone.

Periodontal disease (Disease of tissues supporting the tooth). Periodontal disease starts as a generalized inflammation of the gums (gingivitis) and proceeds to destroy the attachment of each tooth together with the surrounding bone; it results in tooth loss if untreated. One quarter of the five year old children examined in the recent Child Dental Health Survey had evidence of gingivitis, and 93 per cent of adults in Scotland were similarly affected.

Gingivitis Gingivitis is a painless gum inflammation which occurs wherever plaque is allowed to remain in contact with the gums. The disease is characterized by the gum losing its pale pink colour and becoming smooth, red, and swollen. The gum bleeds easily when subjected to pressure (particularly noticeable when the teeth are brushed) and can even bleed spontaneously. The accumulated plaque and food debris leave an unpleasant taste in the mouth and cause bad breath (halitosis). Gingivitis may become more marked in pregnancy. The altered hormone levels in the blood allow the gums to react vigorously to the presence of plaque; the tissues become more swollen and bleed very easily. This pregnancy gingivitis subsides after the baby is born but treatment is required to eradicate the original cause of the inflammation.

Acute ulcerative gingivitis This is a painful condition that is particularly prevalent among smokers. It is characterized by ulceration of the gums, especially between the teeth where the tissues are rapidly destroyed. A marked bad breath, unpleasant taste, and extreme discomfort become noticeable, and sometimes the patient has a raised temperature. The condition, Vincent's infection, was prevalent in the Armed Services during the last two world wars when it was described as Trench Mouth. Although the exact cause of this condition is not known, it is always associated with overgrowth of two microorganisms, *Borrelia vincentii* and *Fusiformis fusiformis*.

Periodontitis If gingivitis is allowed to persist, the inflammation progresses to destroy the periodontal attachment; this disease, usually quite painless, is called periodontitis, formerly known as pyorrhoea alveolaris. The fibres of the periodontal attachment hold each tooth in the jaw, the gum tightly against each tooth, and the teeth in contact with each other. As soon as periodontitis occurs, the gum becomes detached from the tooth surface and the tooth, more gradually, loses firm contact with its neighbour. This produces a pocket between the gum and the tooth in which plaque and food debris collect. The stagnant plaque hardens to produce tartar and, together with the swollen inflamed gum, prevents adequate plaque removal. As the periodontal destruction progresses the gum often regains its pink appearance; the bleeding stops and the only clue to the underlying disease is the persistent unpleasant taste, bad breath, and detectable periodontal pockets. The disease continues until it is halted by treatment or until the tooth becomes loose and is removed.

Periodontal abscess The bacteria in deep periodontal pockets occasionally become very active, and destroy tissue rapidly to produce pus (dead tissue cells and bacteria). If the mouth of the pocket is too narrow to allow the pus to escape, a gumboil or periodontal abscess forms. The symptoms of swelling and throbbing pain are very similar to an abscess on a dead tooth. Urgent dental treatment is required.

Traumatic injuries to teeth Children are particularly susceptible to injuries to the front of the mouth and teeth. By the early teens one boy in five will have damaged his front teeth, whereas girls are affected less often. Injuries vary from a simple fracture of tooth enamel to complete tooth loss. However simple the injury appears, the blood supply to the tooth can be damaged and the pulp may die. The dead pulp tissue frequently discolours the dentine so that the crown of the tooth darkens (see opposite). A tooth that dies in this manner is no longer protected by defence mech-

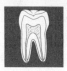

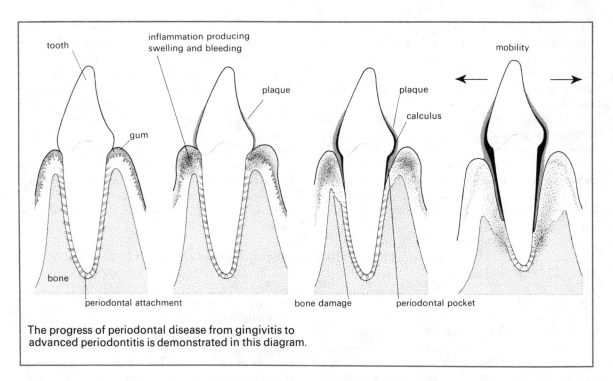

tooth

inflammation producing swelling and bleeding

plaque

plaque

calculus

mobility

gum

bone

periodontal attachment

bone damage

periodontal pocket

The progress of periodontal disease from gingivitis to advanced periodontitis is demonstrated in this diagram.

anisms in the blood and therefore is unable to protect itself against bacterial infection. Pulp infections of this type may lead to an acute dental abscess or dental cyst. More severe fractures of the tooth can expose the dentine, or even the pulp itself; these fractures require immediate dental treatment to protect the acutely painful tooth tissue. It is particularly important to keep the pulp alive in immature teeth to allow root development to be completed.

When a tooth is knocked out completely, it should

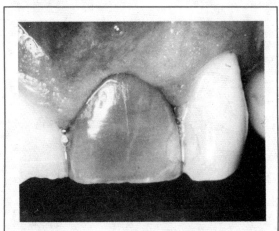

Dead pulp tissue frequently discolours the tooth.

be rinsed clean with cool tap water and immediately replaced in its socket, or wrapped in a moist handkerchief until a dentist can be reached. The utmost speed is essential if reimplantation is to have any chance of success. A dental splint is required to hold the displaced tooth in position until the periodontal attachment heals. As the blood supply to the pulp has been completely disrupted, pulp death usually ensues and the tooth will require root treatment (see page 388). Teeth that are reimplanted and treated soon after injury may last for many years.

Diseases of the lining tissues of the mouth

Aphthous ulcers These recurrent painful ulcers in the mouth are common. The ulcers vary in number, severity, and duration. Aphthous ulcers often affect the mucous membranes of the lip or cheek near the angle of the lips. In women the ulcers are sometimes associated with the onset of menstruation. The more severe, longlasting, and extensive ulcers may cause scarring when they finally heal. Whilst the exact cause of these ulcers is unknown, local steroid creams are useful in reducing their duration and the discomfort.

Denture ulcers After teeth have been extracted shrinkage occurs in the adjacent portions of the jaw support. This shrinkage occurs rapidly for the first year but has been shown to continue slowly for periods of up to 25 years. Dentures, unfortunately, do

Chapter 16 **The teeth**

not alter with the changing shape of the jaw and should be looked at every year by a dentist. Support for the lower denture is a particular problem with shrinkage of the tissues, so that the denture does not fit properly, and abrasions or ulcers are common. These ulcers heal within days when the denture is left out of the mouth, but recur quickly after reinsertion if the denture is ill-fitting. Any mouth ulcer, whether associated with dentures or not, that persists for two weeks or more requires urgent dental attention. The continuous irritation of ill-fitting dentures may cause excessive growth of the lining tissues of the mouth. The folds of inflamed tissue that form are often quite painless, but need to be removed surgically before satisfactory new dentures can be constructed.

Herpetic ulcers Primary infection by the herpes simplex virus usually occurs in childhood but its frequency in adult life is increasing. This initial infection can pass unnoticed; the only indication of the presence of the virus being recurrent blisters producing crusted sores on the lips (cold sores). The primary infection by the herpes virus can, however, be an unpleasant illness with loss of appetite, raised temperature, and extensive mouth ulceration, making eating and drinking extremely painful. For these cases maintenance of fluid intake combined with a soft bland diet, bed rest, mild pain-relievers, and local medication to reduce secondary infection are required. In most instances the acute infection is self-limiting and clears up in ten to fourteen days.

Denture sore mouth Dentures that are worn continuously night and day, even if apparently adequately cleaned, may become infected with a fungal type organism known as *Candida albicans*. The tissue upon which the denture rests becomes painlessly inflamed, whilst painful sores may develop at the corners of the mouth. If untreated, the inflamed tissue, usually in the roof of the mouth, becomes swollen and the upper denture loses its stability and drops down. Professionally prescribed antifungal ointments, day time wear and overnight sterilization of the dentures help to cure the disease. Leaving dentures in a sterilizing solution, as a routine at night time, should prevent this disease occurring.

White patches Leathery white patches can form in any area of the mouth. They are caused by an increased thickness of the lining tissue, usually in response to an irritant. Professional advice should be sought.

Developmental variations and abnormalities

Crowded teeth Modern man has smaller jaws than primitive man, and children frequently develop permanent teeth that are too large for their jaws. As the teeth erupt they become rotated, tilted, or displaced. Sometimes eruption is blocked by teeth already in the mouth, and the tooth remains totally or partially buried in the jaw. This most frequently affects the last molar or wisdom tooth (see below). Teeth that are crowded or partially erupted are difficult to clean and therefore more liable to caries and gingivitis. Crowded teeth are also unsightly and cause both child and parents concern; their abnormal position can often be corrected by treatment.

Disproportionate jaw sizes Either jaw can be too large or too small for the other. This disproportion rarely affects chewing efficiency but often causes concern for aesthetic reasons. Treatment can vary from simple tooth movement to extensive surgery, depending upon the severity of the disfigurement.

An impacted lower wisdom tooth may lead to infection of the soft tissues overlying the tooth crown. The periodontal attachment of the second molar may be damaged and caries is likely to develop.

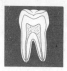

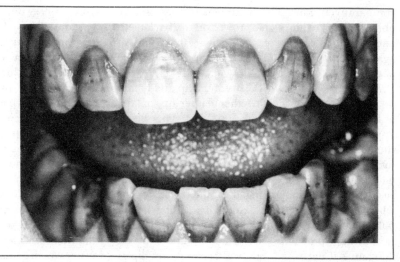

Tetracycline antibiotics administered during tooth development can produce severe discoloration.

Tetracycline tooth staining Tetracycline antibiotics administered to women late in pregnancy or to children under seven years of age are incorporated into the enamel and dentine of the forming teeth, and may lead to unsightly discoloration (see above). The colour and degree of staining depend on the type of tetracycline taken and the length of treatment; it may vary from a light yellow to dark grey-brown. Where staining of the front teeth presents a cosmetic problem, the appearance can be improved by either bleaching the surface enamel, veneering the enamel with composite resins, or providing porcelain crowns.

Developmental tooth abnormalities Structural tooth abnormalities vary from the common small white blemishes of enamel which cause little concern, to gross abnormalities of enamel or dentine which are

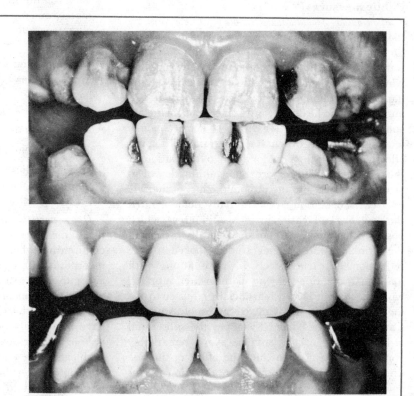

A developmental abnormality of tooth enamel is unsightly and has led to many silver amalgam restorations. The patient has been treated with porcelain crowns at the front and gold crowns at the back.

comparatively rare. The treatment of these severe abnormalities requires gold crowns on the back teeth and porcelain crowns on the front teeth to protect against tooth wear and restore the appearance (see page 383).

Hare lip and cleft palate Clefts of the lip and palate do not necessarily occur together; either lip, palate, or both can be affected in the upper jaw. They occur apparently without cause in about one child in one thousand in white races, although the frequency increases when there is a family history of the deformity. In these circumstances genetic counselling is advisable when planning a family. Clefts occur when the embryo's facial folds fail to unite in the palate and lip region; they may cause disfigurement, swallowing problems in infancy, and speech difficulties if untreated. Surgical repair of the lip is performed early in the child's life whereas repair of the palate is left until later. The palate can be covered with a removable plastic plate to assist swallowing and speech until surgical repair is complete.

Prevention of dental disease

Public measures

Fluoridation of public water supplies The report by the Director General of the World Health Organisation to the 28th World Health Assembly stated that "fluoridation of communal water supplies, when feasible, should be the cornerstone of any national programme of dental caries prevention. It is an ideal public health measure since its benefits are conferred to everyone regardless of socioeconomic level or availability of dental services. In addition it is effective without the need for active participation by the individual". This report is the culmination of 40 years of research into the profound effect of fluoride on teeth. Population studies initially demonstrated the low level of caries incidence in areas which possessed high levels of fluoride naturally present in the drinking water. Later studies looked at the reduction in caries levels in populations with inadequate fluoride content in the water supplies, when the fluoride level was artificially adjusted to one mg per litre. In the United States of America, Canada, and the United Kingdom the substantial reduction in the level of dental decay was remarkably consistent. Investigations into the effect of fluoride upon adults' teeth have shown that protection against caries extends up to the age of 65 years, but only for those people who lived in a fluoride area while their

teeth were developing. Fluoride has to be incorporated into the developing enamel and dentine to give maximum protection. In order to protect the permanent set of teeth it must be consistently available from birth, when the first permanent molars are beginning to calcify, to approximately twelve years of age when the crowns of all the permanent teeth, apart from the wisdom teeth, have completed their formation. Fluoride has the unique ability to cause the formation of a calcified tooth tissue that is more resistant to acid attack and to subsequent caries.

Fluoridation schemes function in 30 countries throughout the world providing over 150 million people with fluoridated water. In England and Wales approximately $4\frac{3}{4}$ million people receive artificially fluoridated water and a further half million receive water which contains an adequate quantity of natural fluoride. The cost of artificial fluoridation is trivial.

The Royal College of Physicians of London reported on fluoride and its effect on teeth and health in 1975. They concluded that:

Fluoride in water added or naturally present at a level of approximately one mg per litre over the years of tooth formation substantially reduces dental caries throughout life.

The consumption of water containing approximately one mg per litre of fluoride in a temperate climate is safe, irrespective of the hardness of the water.

In comparison with fluoridation, fluoride supplements such as tablets, drops, and fluoridized salt have not been shown to be as effective on a community basis.

Fluoridation does not harm the environment.

They recommended that:

Water supplies in the United Kingdom should be fluoridated where the level of fluoride was appreciably below one mg per litre.

Other public health measures Alternative public health measures to provide a fluoride supplement for children have been investigated. Fluoride has been incorporated into milk, into school drinking water, and into table salt (in the same way that an iodine supplement is incorporated into salt where there is a low intake of this element). The majority of studies have lasted only between two and four years and although some beneficial effects have been shown, problems were encountered. For maximum effect fluoride needs to be taken daily for the first twelve years of the child's life; this requires considerable enthusiasm and dedication on the part of parents; a

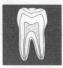

commitment that was not always maintained in these investigations. Some success has been reported with supervised fluoride mouth rinses used as a community measure in Scandinavian schools. The rinses are not swallowed and therefore provide only a limited protection for erupted teeth. As a preventive measure there is no method as effective as fluoridation of public water supplies in the control of caries.

Personal measures

Selfadministered Treatment of dental pain, following a night with toothache, can be a frightening experience for a young child. A sudden introduction to dentistry, in this manner, can dissuade a child from further treatment and is often the first step towards the early provision of full dentures. An essential part of preventive dentistry is the gradual education and introduction of the young child to the importance of dental health. Tooth cleaning should be an essential part of a baby's routine. Simple explanations about dietary restriction of sugary foods, drinks, and confectionery between meals, and the need for oral hygiene, can be understood by surprisingly young children.

The introductory visit to the dental surgery, when all the primary teeth have erupted, becomes a natural extension to the education received at home. The young child will meet the dentist and his staff, and can observe the normal examination procedure demonstrated on a parent. At the same visit or a subsequent one, the teeth can be examined and polished with a fluoride paste. Regular polishing can then take place biannually until the child is sufficiently used to instrumentation to have a successful local fluoride application. It is unusual for this to be possible before the age of four or five, as salivary control for young children is difficult, and salivation dilutes the fluoride solution or gel and reduces its protective effect. Preventive treatment introduced in this manner gives the child confidence both in his surroundings in the dental surgery and in the dentist. Should treatment for caries become necessary, it can be detected early and provided without distress to child or parent.

Oral hygiene Adequate removal of dental plaque is an essential part of the prevention of caries and periodontal disease. Plaque starts to accumulate in the gingival crevice and on the tooth and gum

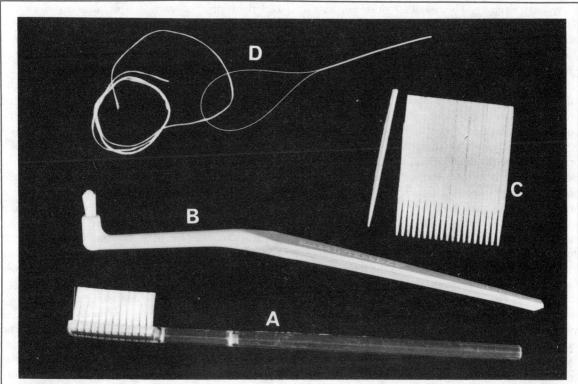

A A multitufted nylon toothbrush   C Interdental wood points   D A nylon floss threader for passing
B An interspace toothbrush   dental floss beneath bridgework

Chapter 16 The teeth

surfaces directly after brushing the teeth. It takes some time, however, for the plaque to become sufficiently abundant to cause harm. It is adequate, therefore, to clean the teeth twice a day, in the morning and before retiring to bed at night, providing all the plaque is cleaned away at each brushing. Plaque is often colourless and may be difficult to see when in limited amounts, but when plentiful may not only cause tooth discoloration but may be felt as a furry layer on the teeth. Dyes, purchaseable in tablet or liquid form, may be used to stain the plaque a vivid colour which makes it more easy to see and therefore more readily removed by brushing the teeth. Various brushing techniques have been described. However, the individual technique is unimportant providing that all plaque is removed and tooth damage is avoided. A toothbrush, if used effectively, will remove plaque except in the areas between the teeth. An interspace toothbrush (see page 385) will pass part way between the teeth, but interdental cleaners, wood points, or dental floss, are necessary to clean and massage beneath and between the tooth contact areas. Instruction on the correct use of toothbrushes, wood points, and dental floss should be obtained from a dentist or dental hygienist to avoid using them wrongly. The use of a toothbrush with a paste that is too abrasive can cause wear of the tooth surface and encourage gum recession. Wood points used carelessly can break and stick between the teeth, producing a severe gingivitis.

Choice of a toothbrush It is best to use a short head multitufted nylon toothbrush with a high density of bristles; plaque removal is more efficient when a large number of bristle tips pass across the teeth and gums. A toothbrush should be discarded as soon as the bristles become distorted; it will not then efficiently cleanse the tooth surfaces and distorted bristles may cause damage to the soft tissues. Children need a brush that is appropriate for their size and age.

Choice of toothpaste The incorporation of fluoride into toothpaste is a convenient way to apply fluoride to the tooth surface. Many investigations have shown that fluoride applied to the teeth in this way will produce a significant reduction in the rate of tooth decay. The reduction does not approach that achieved wherever fluoride has been incorporated in the drinking water from birth. Fluoride applied locally by using a toothpaste is incorporated only into the most superficial layers of tooth enamel. Pleasant-tasting and attractively coloured toothpastes encourage both children and adults to clean their teeth, and a moderately abrasive paste will assist in the removal of stain.

Fluoride tablets or drops Enthusiastic parents can provide fluoride protection for their children's developing teeth by giving fluoride in tablet or drop form from birth. Confirmation that the fluoride level in the drinking water is well below the optimum one mg per litre should be obtained from the Area Health Authority or the local Water Board before using this treatment. The tablets normally contain 2·2 mg of sodium fluoride. For breast-fed babies half a tablet (or the appropriate number of drops) should be administered until the second birthday and thereafter the dosage increased to one daily tablet. For a bottle-fed baby, the dose up to the first birthday is 0·25 mg, up to the second, 0·5 mg, and up to the third, 0·75 mg; thereafter 1 mg. For young children the tablet can be dissolved in water, whereas older children can make a local application to their teeth by chewing the tablet before swallowing. Fluoride tablets should be administered until the child is twelve years old, and if taken regularly will provide a protection similar to drinking fluoridated water.

Diet There is considerable evidence that sugar in the mouth produces a rapid increase in plaque acidity and that the number of times per day that this occurs is proportional to the subsequent caries activity. In order to prevent caries, it is wise to limit the consumption of sugar-containing food, drinks, and confectionery to meal times only. This will ensure that plaque acidity is raised infrequently and is not maintained for long periods of time. In between meals children, when they ask for a snack, should be encouraged to eat fruit, nuts, or crisps. The prolonged use of sweetened feeding bottles as comforters or pacifiers in infancy should be discouraged, as should the use of sweetened miniature feeders or dummies dipped in honey, sugar, jam, or syrup, all of which may produce very rapid caries. This form of rampant decay in infancy rapidly destroys teeth and leads to early abscess formation with consequent pain and sleeplessness. Extraction of numerous teeth under general anaesthesia may be the only treatment possible in advanced cases, a truly traumatic experience for many young children and probably the worst introduction to dental treatment.

Professionally administered measures

Oral hygiene instruction. Instruction in the use of toothbrushes, wood points, and dental floss can all be obtained from a dentist or dental hygienist. Oral hygiene techniques should be reviewed at each dental examination so that a natural tendency to lose enthusiasm can be reversed.

Local fluoride applications. Fluoride applications to the tooth surface annually or biannually have been

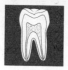

used as a caries preventive measure for over 30 years. Three main types of local fluoride application have been advocated: fluoride solutions and gels, fluoride-containing polishing pastes, and fluoride varnishes.

Fissure sealants. Fluorides are least effective in reducing caries in the pits and fissures on the grinding surfaces of molar and premolar teeth. Sealant materials which prevent plaque entering these pits and fissures have been developed in an endeavour to reduce caries in these sites. Clinical trials of these materials have shown them to be effective for periods up to five years. It has been calculated that, if a fissure sealant was 50 per cent effective in reducing caries in these sites, an average fifteen year old boy in a fluoride adjusted water area would require only three restorations in his permanent teeth. These plastic fissure sealants rely on bonding to surface enamel by etching with diluted solutions of phosphoric acid. A combination of water fluoridation and fissure sealing could provide an effective form of caries control.

Chemical plaque prevention. Daily mouth-rinsing with a solution of 0·2% chlorhexidine gluconate reduces plaque and gingivitis for periods of up to two years. A similarly medicated toothpaste is available for use under clinical supervision.

Treatment

Repair of teeth Before inserting any tooth filling material, caries has to be removed and the resulting cavity shaped to retain the filling. Pain is usually controlled during cavity preparation by using a local anaesthetic. These injected local anaesthetic agents can react with other medication. The dentist should therefore be informed of any medicines or tablets being taken at the time of dental treatment. The perfect tooth filling material should match tooth tissue in colour, strength, and wear resistance as well as react in the same way when subjected to temperature changes and chewing forces. No ideal material has yet been found; different materials have to be chosen according to the requirement of the individual tooth.

Silver amalgam This is the most common filling material for molar and premolar teeth; with certain modifications it has been used for over a hundred years. It is formed by blending a silver and tin powder with mercury to form a thick paste which is firmly pressed into the tooth cavity. The amalgam hardens quite rapidly, excess material being carved away so that it conforms to the shape of the tooth. The

mercury in the filling forms a chemical bond with the tin and silver so that it is unable to leak out of the material and be swallowed. Once the silver amalgam has set it can be highly polished and thereafter easily cleaned. The amalgam does not maintain this high polish and some surface tarnishing occurs quite rapidly. The major disadvantage of this material is that it is brittle and therefore cannot be placed where the tooth surface is being subjected to stress without sound healthy tooth tissue to support it.

Composite resin As its name suggests, this material is a mixture. A combination of quartz and other inorganic particles provides the filling with a hard surface, whilst a plastic or resin binds these constituents together. The material is readily matched to tooth colouring and is suitable for restoring front teeth; unfortunately its wear resistance is not satisfactory for premolars and molars. The surface of the material, when hard, is slightly granular and consequently plaque growth is encouraged; this, together with a tendency to shrink on setting, allows renewed carious attack around the margins of the filling. Some of the disadvantages have been overcome by using these materials with an etching technique. The enamel surrounding the cavity is first etched with acid; this removes a microscopic amount of the enamel surface to roughen it and the resin portion of the composite then sinks into the surface irregularities to bind the composite to enamel. This bond is so strong that the biting or incising edge of a fractured front tooth can be restored successfully (see page 388). Composite resins have been shown to be extremely useful in this situation as well as being used to mask discoloured front teeth.

Silicate cement Another tooth-coloured material, silicate cement, is also only used in front teeth. Carefully handled, the appearance can be quite pleasing and the life span reasonable. Plaque acidity will cause rapid breakdown of this cement; a high standard of oral hygiene is therefore necessary to prevent frequent replacement. Silicate cement has one considerable advantage; its high fluoride content tends to protect the surrounding enamel from renewed carious attack.

Aspa cement Aspa (alumino-silicate-polyacrylate) cement has been found to be extremely useful in caries-free abrasion cavities around the necks of teeth, produced by an inexpertly handled toothbrush.

Gold Dental gold is an expensive material as it is alloyed with platinum and silver. It has the dual advantage that it is both strong and does not corrode in the mouth. One principal use is to restore the more severely damaged tooth by covering the whole of the

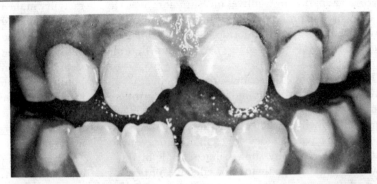

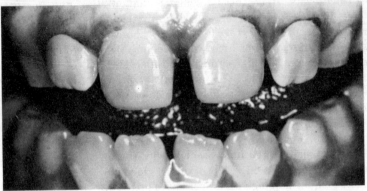

Two central incisor teeth have severe fractures involving enamel and dentine. They are restored with a composite resin bonded to the enamel using an acid etching technique. Abundant quantities of plaque can be seen adhering to the lower teeth.

biting surface and protecting the underlying weakened dentine and enamel. Inlays, crowns, and bridges are cast in dental gold and require a high degree of technical competence to achieve a satisfactory result.

Root treatment Damage to teeth by caries or injury often causes pulp death and a dental abscess. To treat this the pulp chamber and root canal in the tooth can be cleaned and sterilized and the canal closed by cementing a closely fitting seal into the tip of the tooth root. Damaged immature teeth in children can be treated and root formation allowed to continue if treatment is started before the teeth become heavily infected.

Crown repair When a tooth has been severely damaged, it is sometimes necessary to cover the whole of the tooth surface above the gum level with a replacement crown or cap. Gold is used to cover posterior teeth, where considerable strength is required, whereas aesthetically pleasing porcelain crowns are used to cover front teeth. More recently a combined crown of porcelain bonded to the surface of a gold crown has enabled the aesthetic quality of porcelain to be combined with the strength of gold. This has provided a most useful addition to the growing number of repair materials.

In circumstances where the whole of the crown of a tooth above the gum has been destroyed leaving only the root upon which to place a replacement, a post crown can be used. With this technique root treatment is carried out to seal the apex of the root; the remainder of the root canal is widened and a metal post is cemented into it with a projection above gum level onto which the final crown is cemented (see opposite).

Replacement of missing teeth After a tooth has been lost, teeth on either side of the space tilt towards it, and teeth in the opposing jaw over-erupt into the gap. The repercussions are often widespread and may encourage further caries and periodontal disease. Missing teeth should, if possible, be replaced (see opposite).

Bridges A false tooth can be joined to crowns on either side of a space. The crowns together with the false tooth are usually made in gold, or gold and porcelain. This is an expensive and time-consuming procedure that requires a high degree of expertise on the part of both the dentist and laboratory technician to provide a satisfactory result. The final bridge is cemented to the prepared teeth on either side of the space and is therefore fixed in the mouth. It requires

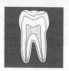

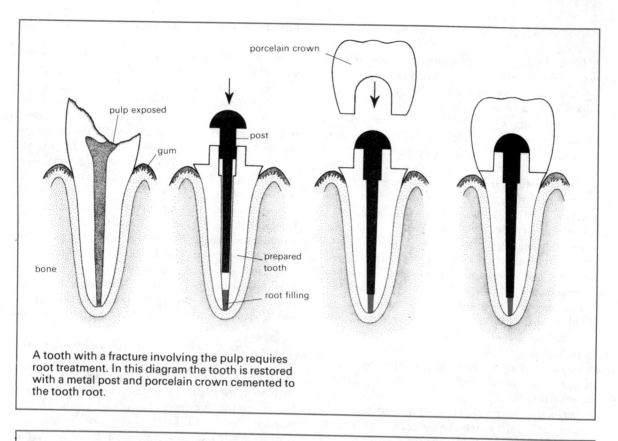

A tooth with a fracture involving the pulp requires root treatment. In this diagram the tooth is restored with a metal post and porcelain crown cemented to the tooth root.

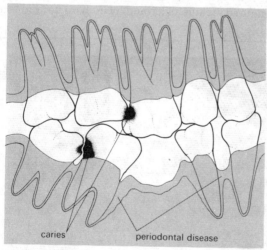

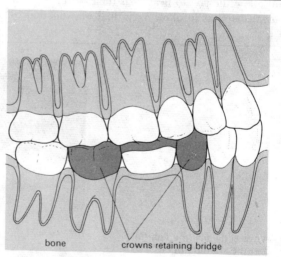

Missing first molar
The altered tooth relationships that can occur after tooth loss make oral hygiene more difficult; caries and periodontal disease may follow.

Missing first molar replaced by a bridge
A missing lower first molar is restored with a bridge. The two gold crowns are joined by a simple gold bar to replace the functional surface of the missing tooth. The bridge is cemented permanently to the second molar and second premolar tooth. This bridge design is particularly easy to clean.

Chapter 16 The teeth

meticulous oral hygiene to maintain the health of the teeth retaining the bridge.

Partial dentures   When the number of missing teeth precludes the use of bridgework a removable partial denture can be constructed in plastic, or a combination of plastic and a metal. Partial dentures can cause a great deal of damage if cleanliness is neglected since the surface area available for plaque growth in the mouth becomes considerably increased. Great care has to be taken to ensure that a high level of oral hygiene is maintained. In order to prevent a partial denture becoming dislodged whilst eating or speaking, fine metal clips and supports have to be placed on the teeth, occasionally on tooth surfaces that are visible (see below). Clips or clasps can be avoided if crowns are made for the teeth that need to be clasped, and precision retaining devices built into these restorations.

Full dentures   When all the teeth have been lost, plastic dentures can be constructed to restore both the teeth and the gradually shrinking jaw. Because of this continued jaw shrinkage, denture modifications are required regularly to maintain a close fit and prevent excessive movement which could encourage further tissue shrinkage.

Immediate dentures   If all remaining teeth have to be removed it is usual to remove the back teeth initially and allow the jaw to heal; it is then better to wear partial dentures to allow a gradual introduction to full denture wear. Immediate dentures can be constructed so that when the remaining front teeth are extracted the completed dentures can be inserted straight away and therefore avoid an aesthetically unsatisfactory toothless appearance.

Care of dentures   Full or partial dentures should be removed after each meal, where possible, and cleaned with a soft brush and soap and water; the appliance should be held over a bowl of water to prevent fracture if dropped. The success of the cleaning can be judged by using a disclosing dye, and any obstinate stains removed with a cleaner recommended by a dentist; on no account should a denture be placed in boiling water or bleach; both of these will damage the plastic. If a denture has to be left out of the mouth at any time, it should be kept in water or a sterilizing agent recommended by a dentist. Full or partial dentures should not be worn at night unless specific instructions to the contrary have been given by the dentist who is responsible for their construction.

Appearance of dentures   Teeth for full dentures are often chosen without regard to the overall facial appearance. Small white teeth are very frequently requested; they attract the attention of onlookers and broadcast the presence of artificial teeth. Dental manufacturers add to the difficulty by making denture teeth too small; very few teeth reach the required breadth of natural teeth. Both natural teeth

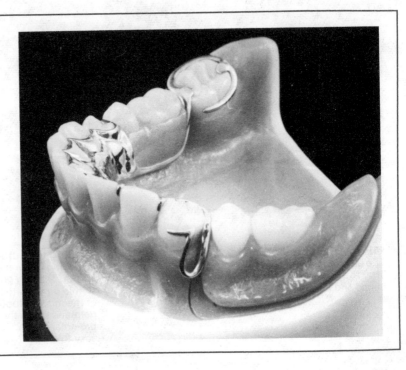

A correctly designed partial denture should not be displaced during eating and should allow chewing forces to be distributed evenly between the remaining teeth and the tissue it sits on. Clasps and rests are designed as an integral part of a cobalt chromium denture to fulfil these requirements.

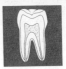

and facial complexions darken with age; it is important therefore to choose a tooth colour that blends with facial colouring.

Implants Various inert materials have been inserted into the jaws in an attempt to replace missing teeth. Considerable research into this field is continuing and reports offer hope for greater success in the future.

Treatment of periodontal disease

Scaling and oral hygiene instruction Most gingivitis can be eradicated by the removal of plaque and tartar in the dental surgery followed by oral hygiene instruction and meticulous home care. Antibacterial agents are rarely necessary except in acute ulcerative gingivitis when a combination of careful cleansing and an antibacterial drug is indicated. Plaque stagnation areas increase with the destruction of the periodontal attachment or gums by disease. Prior to correcting these defects it is necessary to improve oral hygiene so that rapid healing is ensured following surgery.

Recontouring the gums Following repeated episodes of gingivitis or acute ulcerative gingivitis the gums become misshapen and cleansing becomes difficult. After anaesthetizing the tissues with a local anaesthetic they can be reshaped with a surgical knife; a simple operation that causes little discomfort. During healing the gum is protected for one week with a pleasant tasting dressing.

Gingivectomy Periodontitis causes pocket formation between the gum and the teeth and destroys the bone supporting the teeth. In order to remove the pockets the diseased tissue is removed, the bone exposed and reshaped, and the gum repositioned further down the roots of the teeth so that the new height of the tissue is at the depth of the original pocket. Local anaesthesia is used and the operation site usually protected with a pleasant tasting dressing for one week. The repositioning of the gum exposes the tooth root which is sensitive to hot and cold; this usually settles as long as the teeth are kept thoroughly clean. The apparent lengthening of the tooth crown can be masked with a plastic shield but it is rarely necessary. Pain following these procedures is not severe and can usually be controlled by simple pain-relievers.

Orthodontics Orthodontics is the speciality within dentistry which corrects irregularities of tooth position, thus improving the appearance of the patient and helping to prevent dental disease. As crowded teeth erupt they become rotated and

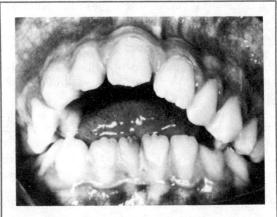

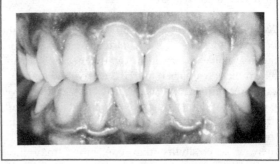

An illustration to show how thumb sucking may displace the upper incisor teeth. When the habit is discontinued, orthodontic treatment helps to realign the teeth and improve the appearance.

displaced, producing stagnation areas for plaque and increasing the opportunity for periodontal disease and caries.

Teeth often have to be removed before active orthodontic treatment is started, so that room is created to allow the crowding to be corrected. After tooth extraction a plastic plate is fitted in the mouth, bearing springs which press on individual teeth causing stretching of the periodontal attachment and slow tooth movement. The plate has to be worn continuously night and day, removed for thorough cleaning after each meal, and replaced immediately. When the teeth have been satisfactorily repositioned, the appliance has then to be worn to prevent the teeth relapsing towards their crowded position. The retention phase of orthodontic treatment is as important as the movement phase and can often occupy a similar length of time.

Complex orthodontic problems are often treated using a fixed appliance. Stainless steel bands are cemented to the teeth, and springs and wires fitted to them to allow the teeth to be repositioned accurately. More recently techniques have been evolved for directly attaching appliances to the teeth by means of acid etching of the enamel and the use of bonding agents. A course of simple orthodontic treatment rarely takes less than a year to complete; more complex problems may take two or more years, and in adults, where the teeth have to move through dense bone, treatment can be very lengthy.

Thumb sucking   Thumb or finger sucking is a habit often adopted by young children as a comforting substitute for suckling. In most instances the child gradually grows out of the habit. During the early years the primary front teeth may be tilted and a gap may appear between the upper and lower incisors. As the permanent teeth erupt they are similarly malpositioned. As soon as the sucking habit ceases, the pressure of the lip repositions the teeth in most cases. Occasionally children may require assistance in giving up the habit and in the repositioning of their displaced teeth, see page 391.

X-rays   X-rays show the contrasting densities of the body tissues. They are used in dentistry, as in other medical fields, as an aid in the diagnosis of disease. The radiation dosage required is extremely small, but as a precautionary measure protection of the lower part of the abdomen is usually employed using a lead-lined lap shield. In pregnancy it is advisable to limit the radiation exposure to essential X-rays only. If there is a possibility that conception may have occurred, it is wise to inform the dentist so that X-rays can be postponed and their necessity reappraised when the pregnancy is confirmed. Where dental X-rays are essential during pregnancy, adequate body protection can be provided by means of a suitable lead-lined apron.

Preparation for general anaesthesia   Any acute infection of the nose or throat should be reported prior to an anaesthetic appointment so that, if necessary, the appointment can be postponed.

No food or drink (even water) should be taken for six hours prior to a general anaesthetic; food or liquid in the stomach could cause vomiting during the operation.

It is necessary for a responsible adult to attend the surgery with the patient to accompany the patient home following the operation. It takes many hours for the effect of a general anaesthetic to wear off.

So, for this reason, a patient who has had a general anaesthetic must not drive a car, operate moving machinery, ride a bicycle, or take alcohol or other sedative drugs (unless under medical supervision) during the rest of that day.

Aftercare of extractions and oral surgery
After extractions or any oral surgery there will be some pain and tenderness at the site of the operation and the saliva will remain bloodstained for a few hours. An excess of exercise or alcohol on the day of operation may restart the bleeding and therefore should be avoided. If bleeding does occur it can usually be controlled quite simply by sitting relaxed and upright in a chair and applying pressure to the bleeding area for ten minutes. After periodontal surgery a thumb and forefinger can be used to squeeze the dressing on to the teeth; whereas after tooth extraction a tightly rolled clean handkerchief placed over the socket and held in place by firmly closing the jaws together will usually suffice. Rinsing of the mouth on the day of surgery should be avoided as this may also stimulate bleeding. The remainder of the teeth and any dentures should be cleaned with a toothbrush in the normal manner, care being taken to avoid the operation area. The day after surgery a mouth rinse is advisable. Half a teaspoon of salt in a tumbler full of warm water will aid healing. If these precautions are taken an infected socket will be unlikely. Occasionally, however, if an adequate blood clot does not form, infection may follow. Pain is often severe, together with an unpleasant taste and halitosis. Dressing and daily cleansing of the area is necessary and antibiotics may be required; a dentist should be consulted for this treatment.

Treatment of the handicapped and chronic sick   Handicapped people often find satisfactory oral hygiene a problem, and dental treatment difficult to obtain. Consequently dental disease tends to be severe and treatment extensive. Partial dentures, if a possibility, add to the problem of plaque control, and full dentures, particularly for the mentally handicapped, are often impossible to wear. Dental disfigurement and bad breath may hinder their social acceptability and make an already difficult life more unhappy. Sufferers from certain chronic illnesses are at risk from dental disease. Particular examples are sufferers from congenital or rheumatic heart disease who require antibiotic cover for a variety of dental operations, including extractions, and haemophiliacs who are likely to bleed severely after tooth extraction and need specialist care from a haematologist throughout the period of surgery.

Prevention of dental disease should have the highest priority, particularly for the handicapped and chronic sick. Where fluoride levels in drinking water are well below one mg per litre, supplements in the form of fluoride tablets should be provided from birth

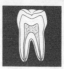

or as soon as the handicap or illness is recognized in childhood. Fissure sealants and local fluoride applications should be provided, particularly when the first permanent molars start to erupt. Those nursing handicapped children should gain instruction in oral hygiene techniques and dietary control.

Conclusion

The increase in demand for dental treatment in the United Kingdom is indicative of the greater awareness of the general public concerning the importance of dental health. Improved dental techniques and equipment have made treatment more acceptable to the patient and have helped to satisfy this growing need. Community measures to prevent disease have been less successful however; to date only eight per cent of the population of the United Kingdom receives artificially fluoridated water. The cornerstone of any national programme of caries prevention should be fluoridation of the drinking water supplies.

Chapter 17
The eyes

Revised by T. Keith Lyle, CBE MD MCh FRCP FRCS

Of the five senses, sight and hearing are by general consent the most important for our comfort, convenience, and ability to cope with the world around us. During our waking hours a continuous stream of information pours into the brain from these two sources, both of which play a vital part in all our activities and decisions. Blindness or deafness is a grave handicap. The mechanisms of vision, which we often take too much for granted, are complicated and extremely efficient. The eyes, protected from injury in their bony sockets, are self-focusing, self-lubricating, and self-cleansing. They can adapt for bright light or dim light, for distant or near vision. So sensitive is the central spot of the retina (the part which we use for reading) that it can distinguish between images only about 1/10,000 of an inch apart on its surface. The eyes deserve the best attention and care we can give them.

The eyeball

The eyeball (globe) is a sphere about 2·5 cm (one in) in diameter, distended by internal fluids and turned by muscles. The eyeball rests in a bony socket (orbit) that tapers from front to back like a cone. Beneath the eyebrows a ridge of bone gives considerable protection against frontal blows. The bony socket wall, below and on the inner side of the eye, is close to the nasal sinuses. The socket is pitted to receive structure attachments, and is pierced to allow nerves and blood vessels to enter. The tip of the cone has an opening through which the optic nerve passes from the back of the eye to make complicated connections with the brain. A semifluid mass of fat gives cushioning support to the eye and allows it to move with freedom.

Man is among the few mammals that can fix the gaze upon an object by turning the eyes and not the entire head. This movement is done by six muscles attached to each eyeball. Four straplike muscles are attached to the top, bottom, and sides of the eyeball, not far behind the visible white of the eye. Farther back, attached to the side farthest from the nose, are two other muscles. When one muscle group contracts, an opposing group relaxes.

The muscles Together, the twelve muscles move the eyes and turn them up, down, or sideways. They also hold the eyes straight. The two eyes must work together since an eye that does not follow its partner is at risk of becoming an unseeing eye. Conditions of eye-muscle imbalance are common, and in milder forms the patient may not even be aware of the condition. We are either right-eyed or left-eyed. There is always a dominant eye. One can easily determine which it is by making a circle with thumb and forefinger and looking through it with both eyes open at an object across the room. Without moving thumb and forefinger, first close one eye, and then the other. The eye which still sees the object through the circle is dominant. Dominance is unconsciously expressed in many ways, as in choosing the eye to aim a rifle.

Structures for seeing A vertical cross section (page 396) of the eye shows the arrangement of the major parts but scarcely conveys the mechanism of vision. The outer coat of the eye, the sclera, is a strong elastic tissue, visible in front as the white of the eye. At the very front of the eye, the transparent window, which bulges out a little, is the cornea, a modified continuation of the sclera. The middle coat of the eye, the choroid, is a thin pigmented layer composed largely of interlaced blood vessels, vital to the eye's nutrition. A specialized continuation of the choroid is

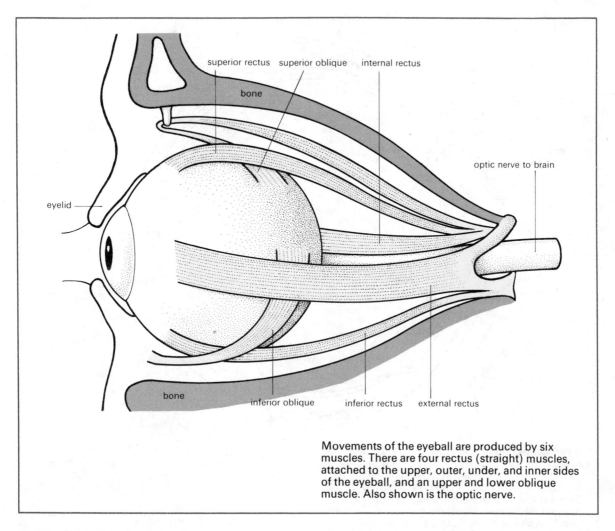

superior rectus superior oblique internal rectus

bone

eyelid

optic nerve to brain

bone

inferior oblique inferior rectus external rectus

Movements of the eyeball are produced by six muscles. There are four rectus (straight) muscles, attached to the upper, outer, under, and inner sides of the eyeball, and an upper and lower oblique muscle. Also shown is the optic nerve.

the iris, which gives the eyes their colour. The pupil is a hole in the iris, and it appears black because the inside of the eye is dark. The innermost coat is the retina, a very thin light-sensitive tissue which lines the back of the eye and curves forward like a deep rounded cup. Retinal nerves converge to form the large optic nerve. The crystalline lens is suspended just behind the iris and is attached to the ciliary body, which is principally muscle. The lens and associated structures divide the eye into two compartments. The larger chamber behind the lens is filled with semiliquid transparent vitreous humour which keeps the eyeball distended in the correct shape. The much smaller space between the cornea and lens is filled with watery liquid, the aqueous humour.

Much of the mechanical part of seeing is accomplished by structures of the front part of the eye, called the anterior segment, see page 396. The lens is delicately slung by fine ligaments connected to the ciliary body. The internal muscles of the eye are the ciliary muscles which change the shape of the lens, and the muscles of the iris which change the size of the pupil. The iris hangs from a ciliary attachment and rests lightly on the lens. The angle at the junction of the cornea and iris is an important area. Nearby, a minute passage called the canal of Schlemm permits drainage of internal eye fluids and acts as a safety valve to prevent pressures from building up and possibly damaging vision, as in glaucoma.

Focusing mechanisms The function of the eyes is to bring an image into focus on the retina, convert the stimuli of light into nerve impulses, and transmit electric currents along the optic nerves to the back of the brain. By far the most common eye defects are errors of refraction – short sight (myopia), long sight (hypermetropia), and astigmatism.

The curved cornea does a major part of the light

Chapter 17 The eyes

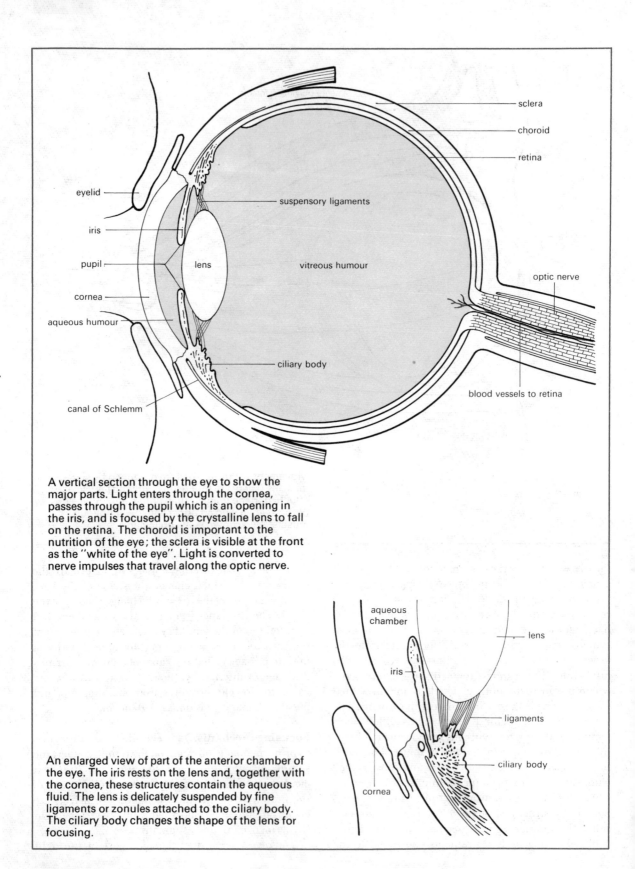

A vertical section through the eye to show the major parts. Light enters through the cornea, passes through the pupil which is an opening in the iris, and is focused by the crystalline lens to fall on the retina. The choroid is important to the nutrition of the eye; the sclera is visible at the front as the "white of the eye". Light is converted to nerve impulses that travel along the optic nerve.

An enlarged view of part of the anterior chamber of the eye. The iris rests on the lens and, together with the cornea, these structures contain the aqueous fluid. The lens is delicately suspended by fine ligaments or zonules attached to the ciliary body. The ciliary body changes the shape of the lens for focusing.

focusing. It is like a fixed lens that does not change its focus. Fine focusing is accomplished by the crystalline lens, which is made of modified skin cells that are as clear as glass. When we look at close objects, nearer than six m (twenty ft) away, focusing help is necessary to see them clearly. The lens does this by changing its thickness and curvature. This is called accommodation.

The lens is enclosed in a capsule slung by ligaments to the ciliary body. Contraction of the ciliary muscles relaxes the ligaments, makes the lens thicker and more curved, and near objects come into focus. Ordinarily, these muscles are active only when we are looking at objects closer than six m (twenty ft).

With increasing age, the lens becomes less elastic and gradually loses some of its accommodative powers.

The iris controls the amount of light entering the eye by adjusting the diameter of the pupil. The iris is a circular pigmented sheet of muscle with opposing circular and radial muscles which automatically constrict or expand the pupil in accordance with the brightness of light that strikes the eye. A fully expanded pupil exposes about seventeen times the area of a constricted one.

Making light visible   The very thin layer of the retina converts light energy that falls upon it into nerve energy that causes us to see. The retina is, in fact, part of the brain wall converted into a cup. It is about the size of a teaspoon and is a mosaic of hundreds of thousands of nerve endings with intricate connections behind them. The nerve endings are either cones or rods, each named after its shape. The

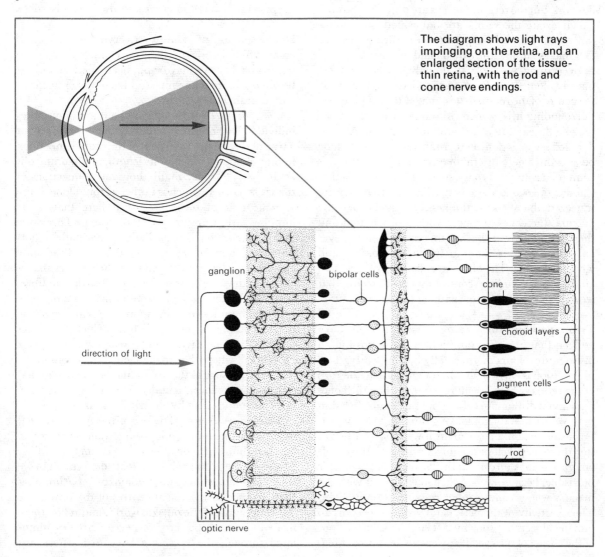

The diagram shows light rays impinging on the retina, and an enlarged section of the tissue-thin retina, with the rod and cone nerve endings.

397

Chapter 17 **The eyes**

nerve endings are pointed away from the source of light, towards the back of the eyeball. The cones are connected individually, the rods more collectively, to cells which terminate in fibres bunched to form the bundle of fibres that is the optic nerve. There are no sense receptors at the point where the optic nerve enters the back of the eye. Consequently this small spot is blind. This can be demonstrated by looking at a small object on a plain background with one eye, and moving the eye towards the nose until the object disappears. Light falls directly upon the optic nerve but this is not covered by retina so there is no vision at this point. The photochemical process is very complicated, but the result is that light energy which stimulates the rods and cones is transformed into nerve impulses. There is no difference between nerve impulses we hear as sound, or feel as pain, or taste as flavours, but the receptor tissues are different. Stimuli which excite the retina are not wiped out instantaneously; there is brief persistence of the image. This fact makes possible the cinema and television.

Everything we look at directly, to see it most sharply, comes to a focus on the fovea, an area near the centre of the retina that is smaller than a pinhead. Surrounding it is a yellowish larger area called the macula lutea (lutea is Latin for yellow). All our detailed seeing is done here. Man and primates alone possess this finely discriminating area. The fovea is composed entirely of cones, so tightly packed together – about 150,000 to a square millimetre – that they are squeezed almost to the thinness of rods. Beyond the macula, the cones are more widely distributed and there are more rods. Each retina has something over 100,000,000 rods and between 6,000,000 and 7,000,000 cones. The different capacities of these two kinds of nerve endings control aspects of seeing that we experience all the time without thinking about it.

Two systems for seeing We must all have noticed that in a very dim light it is not possible to distinguish colours or see small objects clearly. This night vision is carried out almost entirely by the rods of the retina, which are more sensitive than the cones but cannot distinguish colours or fine details. In a dim light we see best by not looking directly at an object. For example, on a clear night if we look at a bright star there may well be a faint star nearby. If we shift our gaze to look directly at the latter, it will no longer be visible, because we are then looking at it with the macula whose cones cannot respond to faint light. The sensitivity of the peripheral vision, especially to moving objects, is protective. It enables us to see "out of the corner of the eye" if any enemy is approaching.

A substance called visual purple also plays a part in night vision. It is found only in association with the rods. It is bleached by light and re-formed in the dark. That is why it takes twenty minutes or more for the eye to become fully dark-adapted. Visual purple is a chemical related to vitamin A which is necessary for its regeneration. Severe lack of vitamin A is therefore one cause of night blindness.

Cones are for bright-light seeing, and only cones can distinguish colours. The eye can distinguish about 7,500,000 barely perceptible differences of hue. Colour blindness is probably a reduction or absence of cones sensitive to certain wavelengths of light.

The visual field is the breadth of area encompassed by vision when the gaze is fixed straight ahead. The field area varies somewhat for each colour. Symptoms of tunnel vision and other distortions of the visual field are of value in diagnosing eye and also brain disorders.

Nerve paths of vision Everything we see is created from a series of signals streaming along nerve pathways. The eye may be physically perfect and yet be blind if there is any interruption of the optic nerve and its branches.

The optic nerve is a bundle of about a million fibres individually connected to parts of the retina. It is not a true nerve, but an extension of the brain, embedded in that organ for much of its length, and fanning out at the back to make many thousand connections in the visual cortex, which is in the occipital lobe at the extreme rear of the brain. It is here that nerve impulses are transformed into vision. The optic nerves from each retina partially change paths a short distance behind the eyes, in an area called the optic chiasma. Fibres from the half of each retina that is closest to the nose cross to the opposite side, but fibres from the outer half of each retina do not. The collected bundles continue to junctions at either side of the midline of the head, from which the fibres (optic radiations) fan out and spread toward the back of the head where they make their connections in the region of a fissure in the occipital lobes. It is here that the brain provides mental images of what we see, pictures conjured up by electrical impulses.

Upside-down image The eye projects an inverted image upon the retina, and the question of why we do not see things upside down is seemingly baffling. However, the problem is not a real one. We do not see the retinal image itself, but millions of nerve impulses that coalesce in the visual centres of the brain. We associate sights of the outside world, and relate them to realities, with patterns of nerve activities stimulated through the eyes. We have to learn to see.

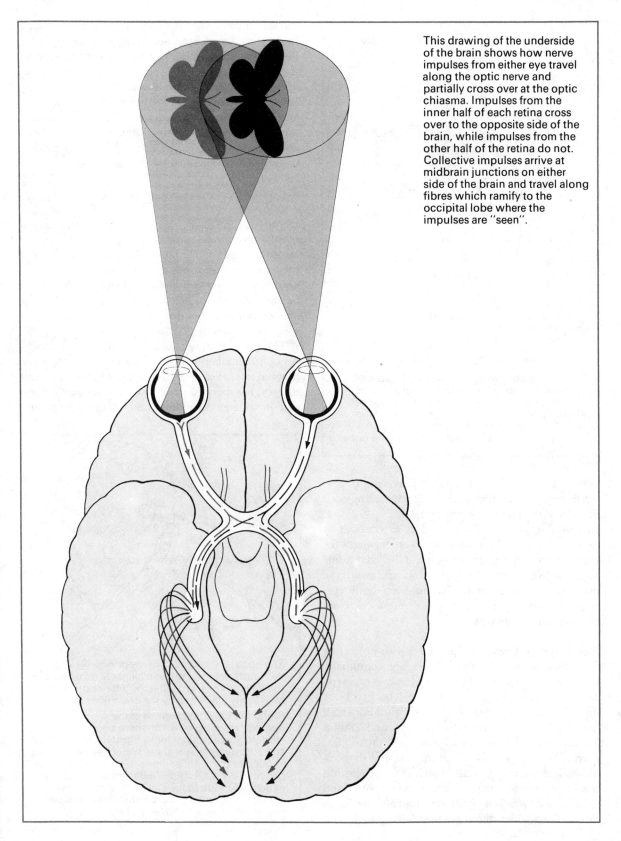

This drawing of the underside of the brain shows how nerve impulses from either eye travel along the optic nerve and partially cross over at the optic chiasma. Impulses from the inner half of each retina cross over to the opposite side of the brain, while impulses from the other half of the retina do not. Collective impulses arrive at midbrain junctions on either side of the brain and travel along fibres which ramify to the occipital lobe where the impulses are "seen".

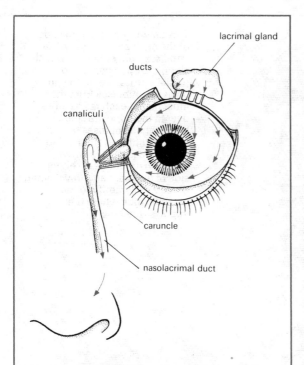

Tears are produced constantly by the lacrimal gland in the upper part of the eye socket, and they flow over the front of the eye to collect in the conjunctival sac at the inner corner of the eye. They then drain through two small channels (canaliculi) which open into the nose.

the conjunctival sac. The tears are spread by blinking the eyelids, which are lined inside by delicate tissue, the conjunctiva, which continues round to enwrap the front part of the eyeball. Some of the tears evaporate but the rest flow inwards to very small holes (the puncta) situated at the inner corner of each eye and thence through the canaliculi into the lacrimal sac and then down the nasal duct which opens into the inferior meatus of the nose. This is why profuse weeping is accompanied by a running nose.

Eye examinations

If you wish to have your eyes fully examined you should go to an ophthalmologist who can be recommended by your family doctor. Alternatively, if the latter considers your eyes are healthy and all you need is a test of vision and examination of refraction he may refer you to an ophthalmic optician who not only determines your need for glasses but also fits the spectacles required.

There is sometimes confusion about these labels. An ophthalmologist (oculist) is a doctor, who, while licensed to practise all branches of medicine and surgery, has specialized in the examination of the eye and its related structures and in the prevention,

A person blind from birth, suddenly given sight, does not immediately understand that a particular object is an orange and that a box is square.

Nerves in the retina send orders to contract or expand the pupil. Automatic nerve-orders direct the ciliary muscles to change the shape of the lens for fine focusing. We can turn both eyes inwards toward the nose by voluntary effort, but to keep both eyes straight or turning in unison is an unconscious neuromuscular function.

The tears Our eyes are provided with protection from the common hazards. Tears are continually produced by the lacrimal gland, and only in excess do they overflow and roll down the cheeks. Tears lubricate the eyes, cleanse them by flushing small particles towards the corner of the eyes, and contain an antibacterial substance (lysozyme) that inhibits germs. The tear glands, about the size and shape of almonds, are located – one to each eye – just within the upper outside part of the socket. The gland secretes tears which flow through half a dozen short ducts, along which there are accessory glands, into

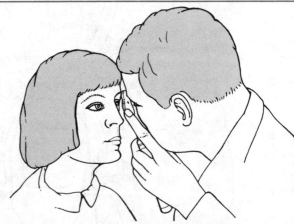

The ophthalmoscope consists principally of a perforated mirror with which light is reflected into the patient's eye, enabling the interior of the eye to be visually inspected by the examiner.

Right, the basic mechanism of the ophthalmoscope, of which there are several models. The examiner looks through the peephole and adjusts lenses for sharp focus by means of the knurled ring. A light source projects light into the patient's eye. The light is reflected back from the patient's fundus (back part of the internal eye), giving a magnified view of structures and blood vessels as shown in the large circle.

diagnosis, and treatment (including operations) of their defects and diseases, and prescribing spectacles and contact lenses. His education and training qualify him to relate findings observed in an examination of the eye to those diseases in other parts and systems of the body which may have an effect on the eye.

An ophthalmic optician is one whose education and training qualify him for the examination of eyes, without the use of drugs, for abnormal visual problems not due to disease, since he is not a medical man. He may prescribe, fit, and supply spectacles and contact lenses. While he is not qualified to diagnose or treat eye disease, if his examination leads him to suspect a defect or disease requiring medical or surgical treatment, as it may well do, he should refer the patient by his family doctor to an ophthalmologist.

Dispensing An optician is a skilled technician who is qualified to dispense and fit the spectacles as prescribed by the ophthalmologist.

Examining instruments A full examination of the eyes requires the use of a number of special pieces of apparatus. Important examining instruments are:

The ophthalmoscope, permitting the observer to study the interior structures of the eye.

A slit lamp microscope, to study with high magnification the structures in the anterior part of the eye.

A tonometer, to measure pressures within the eye.

A perimeter, to map the limits of the fields of vision.

A scotometer, to measure visual field defects.

A gonioscope, to study the angle of the anterior chamber of the eye.

A retinoscope or other instrument, to disclose any refractive aberration of the eye (for example, myopia and astigmatism), or various modifications of the above; and a set of test lenses to find which one or ones are needed to give the eyes good vision. Last is the chart for measuring visual acuity. This procedure is known as refraction of the eye and it is upon the findings of an oculist or ophthalmic optician yielded by this testing of visual acuity that the prescription for spectacles is based.

Testing for visual acuity The usual kind of chart for testing how well a person can see for distance vision consists of black capital letters of various sizes printed on a white card. The largest letter, nine cm in height, is marked 60, and the smallest, about one cm ($\frac{3}{8}$ in), is marked 6. These numbers indicate the distance in metres at which a normal person should be

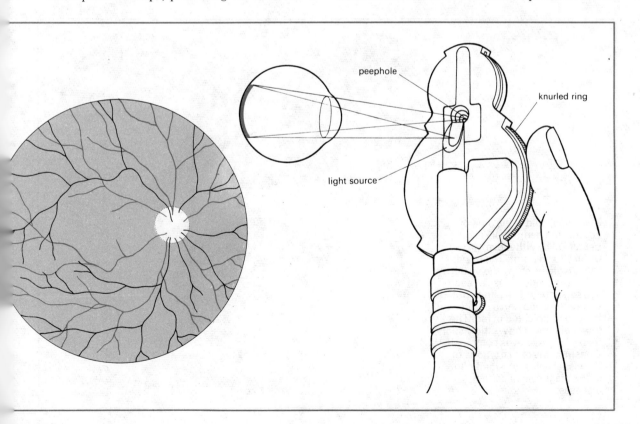

peephole

knurled ring

light source

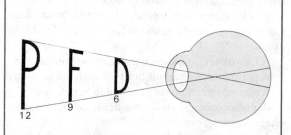

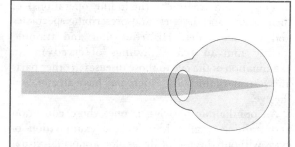

Letters of the familiar "eye test chart" are so designed that their different sizes at various distances are equivalent to a chord of identical size across an arc (5-degree visual angle). Thus a letter 6 metres away will appear to be the same size as larger letters if the latter were viewed, as indicated, from a distance of 9 or 12 metres.

Parallel light rays from a distant object are refracted into sharp focus on the retina of a normal eye. Light rays from objects closer than 6 metres are not parallel and must be brought into focus on the retina by a change in the shape of the lens (accommodation).

able to read a letter of that size. For example, if the vision in an eye is recorded as 6/9, it means that the subject placed at 6 m (20 ft) from the chart could manage to read only as far as the letter of a size that should be clear to a normal person at 9 m (30 ft). Normal vision is therefore 6/6. Some test types include even smaller letters, marked 5, so vision of 6/5 is unusually good.

For testing near vision, reading types of various sizes based on the same principles, are used. Young children and the illiterate are shown pictures of common objects (such as dog, teacup, railway engine) which correspond with the size of the letters.

Accommodation for near vision The rays of light from objects six m (twenty ft) or more away from the eye are practically parallel, and are correctly focused

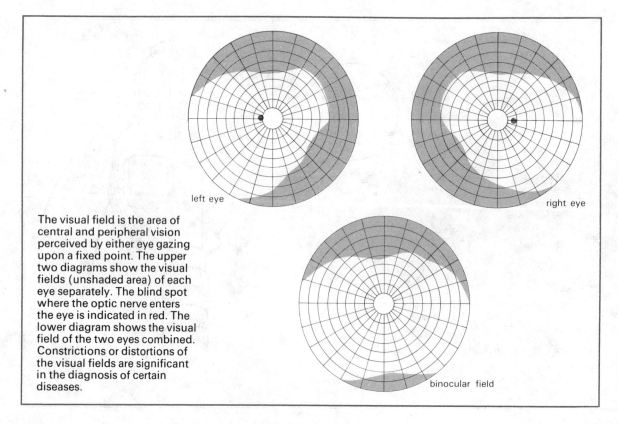

left eye

right eye

binocular field

The visual field is the area of central and peripheral vision perceived by either eye gazing upon a fixed point. The upper two diagrams show the visual fields (unshaded area) of each eye separately. The blind spot where the optic nerve enters the eye is indicated in red. The lower diagram shows the visual field of the two eyes combined. Constrictions or distortions of the visual fields are significant in the diagnosis of certain diseases.

Shortsightedness

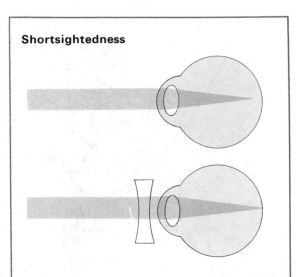

In myopia or shortsightedness, the image of an object (unless it is held close to the eyes) falls in front of the retina instead of upon it, and the object is seen indistinctly. The condition is corrected by placing a concave lens of proper curvature to bring the image into focus on the retina.

Longsightedness

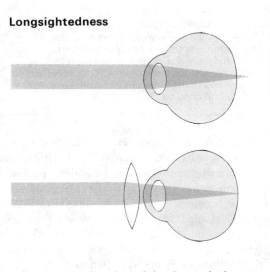

In hypermetropia or longsightedness, the image of an object is focused behind the retina of an eyeball that is too short. A convex lens brings the light rays into focus on the retina. Although hypermetropic people may be able to see things sharply by thickening the lens of the eye (accommodation) this involves effort of the inner muscles of the eye and may cause eye fatigue.

onto the retina by the cornea and lens. The rays of light from nearer objects are slightly divergent, and in order to bend the rays inwards to the correct focus the lens has to become stronger (more convex). There is a remarkable mechanism to achieve just the right amount of alteration in the shape of the lens to keep near objects in focus from distances of about six m (twenty ft) up to 25 cm (ten in) from the eye.

If the lens is removed from the eye its elasticity makes it become thicker (more convex) than when it is in its right place; in fact it assumes the correct shape for full accommodation. In the eye the lens is held in position by the suspensory ligaments (hundreds of fine radial fibres). These are elastic and so pull the lens outwards and make it thinner; it is then in the right shape for distant vision. Accommodation is brought about by contraction of the ciliary body, which makes smaller the ring of tissue to which the outer ends of the suspensory ligaments are attached. This lessens the outward pull on the lens, which therefore becomes more convex. There is a complex nervous mechanism that ensures the correct degree of contraction of the ciliary body to focus objects at various distances.

With advancing age the lens becomes less elastic, which is why most persons aged over 50 years have to wear glasses to see near objects clearly.

Astigmatism If the curvature of the cornea is irregular so that some rays of light are bent more in one area than in another, the resultant image is blurred because, if one part of the ray is focused, the other part is not. This is something like the distortion produced by a wavy pane of glass. It is called astigmatism and can usually be corrected by using a

Astigmatism

ASTIGMATISM

ASTIGMATISM

Astigmatism resulting from irregular curvature of the cornea is rather like distortion produced by a wavy pane of glass, as in the upper diagram. A cylindrical lens in the proper axis which brings light rays to even focus corrects astigmatism, lower diagram.

Chapter 17 The eyes

lens that bends the rays of light in only one plane. This is called a cylinder. A cylindrical lens can be turned in the trial frame to its proper axis to even up the focusing of the rays of light in all parts.

A prescription for glasses may look something like this:

+ (or plus) 2·0 D ⌣ + (or plus) 0·50 cyl axis 90°

What does this mean? Plus or the sign + indicates a convex lens suitable for a longsighted person. Minus or the sign − indicates a concave lens for a myopic person. The D is an abbreviation for dioptre which indicates the power of the lens. A dioptre is a unit of measurement of the refractive or light-bending power of a lens. (The normal human lens in its relaxed biconvex shape has a power of about ten dioptres.) The symbol ⌣ means combined with. Thus, the prescription given as an example means that the optician grinds a convex spherical lens of two (2·0) dioptres combined with a convex cylindrical lens of half a dioptre (0·50) situated vertically (axis 90°). Lens prescriptions may look strange, but opticians in any part of the world know what they mean.

Incidentally, it is a good idea to carry your lens prescription with you when travelling away from home, in case your glasses are lost or broken. A spare pair of glasses is good insurance, too, particularly for persons who would be handicapped without them.

Spectacles help in focusing the rays of light onto the retina. The eye is a receiving organ only and the image on the retina is carried back into the brain and interpreted there. Glasses cannot change the eye in any way or produce any disease even if they are badly fitted. Incorrect glasses can make you uncomfortable, blur your vision, make your eyes feel irritated, and by blurring your sight can cause headaches and even nausea, but in spite of this they do not produce any damage. Do not believe any rumour to the contrary. Once you have begun to wear glasses you may not always need them. You need them perhaps to see properly, but the wearing of glasses does not make things worse.

Tinted glasses and sunglasses are worn to cut down the glare of light, and it is true that some eyes are more sensitive to glare than are others. But the normal human eye is designed by nature for normal light, especially in the temperate zones. The eye also requires more light as we get older. Thus the wearing of tinted glasses is not advisable except on the beach, in high mountains, in snow, and in driving cars over concrete roads in bright light. They should never be worn after dark or indoors.

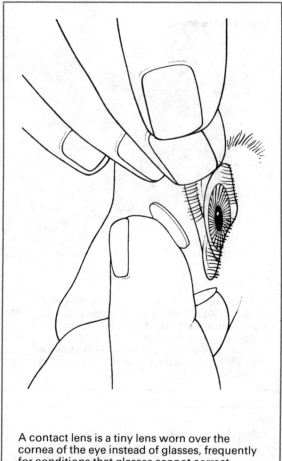

A contact lens is a tiny lens worn over the cornea of the eye instead of glasses, frequently for conditions that glasses cannot correct so satisfactorily. Contact lenses are relatively expensive, since meticulous care is necessary to shape and fit the lenses to individual eyes for safety and comfort.

Contact lenses have been remarkably developed in the past few years. When accurately fitted in the case of a person who has a strong desire and motivation to wear them, or has poor vision from ocular disease that could be benefited (such as a distorted cornea, for example, shaped like a cone), or after cataract surgery on one eye when the other eye has good vision, they can usually be worn for many hours without difficulty. However, when badly fitted they can rub against the cornea, abrade it, and lead to discomfort or even serious trouble.

Contact lenses are expensive because of the meticulous care and skill and the time required to make and fit them. They are easily lost, and sometimes get displaced under the upper lid and are difficult for the patient to remove.

In spite of these and other disadvantages, contact

lenses are effective visual aids, and as they become improved, more people are using them with delight and benefit. Newer forms of contact lenses are beginning to come into use. For instance, there are now soft contact lenses which absorb moisture from the eye and may be more comfortable to wear.

Telescopic lenses and strong magnifying glasses are useful in some cases of defective vision due to ocular disease. There are a number of these visual aids, some of them more complex and therefore more expensive than others. As so often is the case, the simplest are often the best.

Care of the eyes

Although it is remarkable how well the eyeball is protected against danger, it is still vulnerable. The fact that most eye injuries are preventable means that constant attention and awareness are required by everyone.

If you must rub your eyes, use a clean disposable tissue for this purpose, never your fingers. Wear your glasses as directed by your ophthalmologist. Read in a good light that comes from over your shoulder, preferably the left one. Remove your dark glasses after sunset and never drive your car with them on at night. If your work or your hobbies expose your eyes to the danger of flying particles, wear protective goggles.

If you think that you have something in your eye, it is likely that you have, so see your doctor or ophthalmologist right away. Irritable eyes may be caused by lack of sleep, too much drinking or smoking, or a faulty diet, as well as by the need for correct glasses or by the wearing of incorrect ones.

Home measures A simple and effective eye wash can easily be made by adding a level teaspoonful of salt to a pint of boiled water. A cotton pad soaked in the salt solution at room temperature and placed upon the closed eyelids for four or five minutes is particularly soothing for tired eyes.

After reading steadily for half an hour or so, look away at a distant object for a few moments and change the focus.

You should have your eyes checked every two or three years to see if you need glasses or a change in the ones you are wearing, but particularly to see if any disease is present or developing. This is especially important after 40 years of age.

If a chemical is rubbed or splashed into your eye, immediately hold your head, with the eyes open, directly under a gently running stream of water from the nearest tap. Do this at once, and for at least five minutes. Then go to your nearest doctor or hospital as an emergency. Chemical burns of the eyes are serious affairs and once the chemical gets into the ocular tissues, washing the eyes will not do much good, for the action continues deeper and deeper into the structures. This is an emergency.

Allergies The irritated running eyes of the hay fever victim are well known. What is not quite so well known is that allergic irritation to the eyes and eyelids can be caused by drugs or medicines, environmental dust, cosmetics, newsprint, carbon paper, foods, and many other things.

Itching and redness of the eyes or eyelids are the chief symptoms of allergy, and the tissues involved soon become swollen and watery. Do not try to treat yourself, for the job of discovering the cause can be a most difficult task even for the expert in this field, and the treatment can be as varied as the cause. (See chapter 21.)

Children's eyes

The eyes of a newborn infant do not focus or work together until five or six months after birth and then they may occasionally wander for another two or three months. If they do not appear straight or parallel by then, consult an ophthalmologist for advice and treatment.

If there is a discharge from the baby's eyes it may be due to an infection (conjunctivitis or pink eye). It may also be due to the blockage of the passage of tears into the nose. The blockage is due to a thin strand of tissue. This strand usually disappears shortly after birth, but may persist. If so, the ophthalmologist will probe the passage and open it up. Generally that is all that is needed.

The baby's pupils should be black. If not, or if there is a white pupil, it should be seen by a doctor. This may mean that there is a cataract present, or something else wrong inside the eye of a more serious nature. One should not delay in finding out what is wrong and doing something about it.

The preschool child should have the eyes examined to see if there is any ocular abnormality. Glasses may or may not be indicated. The ocular muscles may or may not be working normally together. Certain defects, congenital, familial, or acquired may be present. The parents should know about these things and take action without delay.

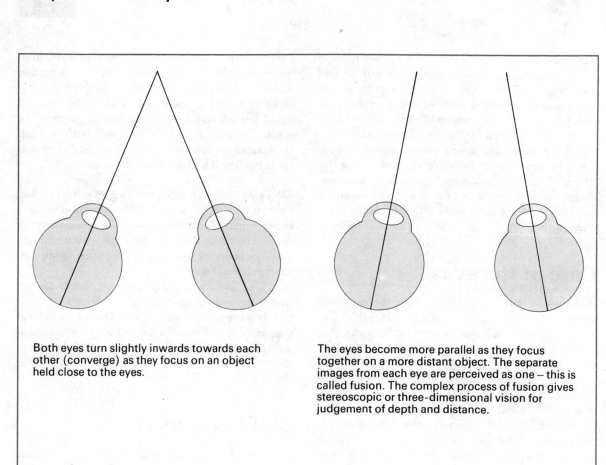

Both eyes turn slightly inwards towards each other (converge) as they focus on an object held close to the eyes.

The eyes become more parallel as they focus together on a more distant object. The separate images from each eye are perceived as one – this is called fusion. The complex process of fusion gives stereoscopic or three-dimensional vision for judgement of depth and distance.

Convergent squint

Divergent squint

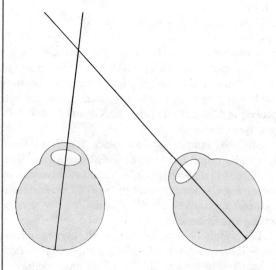

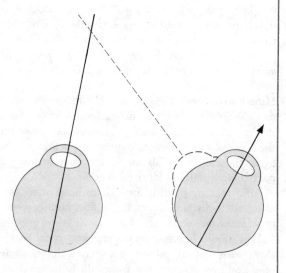

Convergent squint or cross eye. The right eye is turned in towards the left, which is properly focused on an object.

Divergent squint or wall eye, in which the right eye is turned outwards from the normally focused left eye.

Ocular muscle imbalance The eyes may be crossed or divergent from birth or become so later. These conditions require early examination, diagnosis, and care. An eye that turns in or out in early childhood may lose its vision unless treated, simply from non-use. If discovered early, much can be done to restore vision in most instances – for example, by glasses or by covering the unaffected eye, or by orthoptic treatment and other measures. It is obvious why an early examination and exact diagnosis is of the greatest importance. No child will outgrow a crooked eye (cross or wall eye) and parents should be aware of this. It is well too for the parent to be prepared for the ophthalmologist to say that surgery is necessary, for this is the case in many instances, and the earlier it is performed the better. Modern surgery differs greatly from what was done even twenty years ago, and the results are almost always satisfactory.

Squint As there are six muscles in each eye that control movement of the eyes, and the two eyes must work together as a pair, the problem of squint (strabismus) can become very complex. It is not unusual to find that in addition to the horizontal eye muscles not working together, there is a vertical imbalance as well. Also it is found in some cases that an eye squints only in a certain position of the gaze.

By fusion we mean that the image seen with one eye fuses with the image seen with the other. Fusion is essential for stereoscopic, or three-dimensional vision. Normally it is present early in childhood. But if one eye has defective vision or if there is a muscle weakness, fusion may not take place.

It happens in some instances that a child has an alternating squint even if the vision is perfect in each eye. For example, when he looks at an object with his right eye, the left turns in, and vice versa. Such patients do not have normal fusion, nor do many develop it even after the eyes have been made straight by surgery. In this instance surgery is frequently successful in making the eyes appear to be straight and cosmetically satisfactory, but the vision is still likely to be alternating between the two eyes.

It is an advantage to have normal fusion, but it is not essential in order to cope with the activities of ordinary life. It is most helpful in judging distances between objects and their relative positions in space, but a child without fusion from an early age learns to adapt himself through practical experience.

Orthoptics Orthoptic examination is concerned with the assessment of the state of binocular function and the measurement of the ocular deviations in the various directions of gaze. Orthoptic treatment consists of exercises designed to correct anomalies of binocular vision, and, by increasing the range of fusion, to help overcome deviation of the visual axes and improve binocular function.

Amblyopia, or the suppression of the vision of an eye from non-use becomes more difficult to overcome as the child gets older. It used to be thought that after the age of six, amblyopia could not be corrected. However, it is comforting to know that this is not true. Indeed, there are many instances where energetic treatment of the amblyopia even later in life has been successful. A great deal depends on the degree of the amblyopia and the age of the patient when the trouble began. Occlusion, or covering of the child's unaffected eye, may often be harder for the parent to take than it is for the child, but the cooperation of parents is essential.

Infections of the eyes

Bacteria (for example, streptococci, gonococci, or chlamydia), moulds or viruses (for example, herpes) may get into eyes. If the organism is stronger than the immunity or resistance of the ocular tissue, or if there is a break or cut in the structures, infection takes place. If the tissue covering the white of the eye and lining the eyelids (the conjunctiva) is attacked, the eye becomes red, feels sandy, and there is a discharge that varies between being watery, mucous, or full of pus. Whatever its nature, the discharge sticks the eyelashes together. This is especially noticed on getting up in the morning. The vision is not disturbed except by the discharge getting over the cornea.

Pink eye The condition is known as pink eye or acute conjunctivitis. The causative agent (a bacterium) can be transferred from one eye to the other or to the eyes of another person by fingers or cloth, because the discharge contains the contagious organisms.

Acute conjunctivitis should be treated early. Fortunately, many antibiotics and some of the sulphonamide preparations are most effective. Sometimes the organism is resistant to the drug, or may not be susceptible to it (for example, viruses), and other measures of treatment are then used for relief of this condition.

Stye If organisms, especially bacteria, get into the roots of the eyelashes a local infection known as a stye (hordeolum) takes place. If, on the other hand, the infective agent gets into one of the grease or sweat glands of the eyelids a swelling with some pus forms due to a breakdown of the greasy material. This forms a cyst of the eyelid (chalazion). Chalazions need to be opened up and drained of their contents.

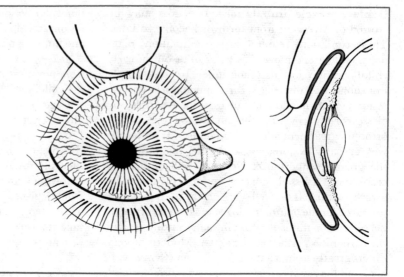

The conjunctiva is a thin mucous membrane that covers the insides of the eyelids and is reflected over the "white of the eye" and is continuous with the epithelial lining of the cornea. The cross section of the eyeball (far right) shows its location (thickness exaggerated). The drawing on the right shows the appearance of conjunctivitis, inflammation of the conjunctiva. Conjunctivitis may result from local infection, allergies, irritation, or from inflammation within the eye itself.

An embedded foreign body in the cornea can cause serious infection resulting in an ulcer that can perforate and cause loss of the eye. Or the infection may spread into the deeper structure of the eye and cause blindness.

Thus a perforating injury of the eye (for example caused by a knife or scissors wound) can cause blindness not only as the result of the direct injury, but also because bacteria have been carried into the eye.

Trachoma is caused by a bacterium (chlamydia) which attacks the conjuctiva, especially that of the upper and lower eyelids, causing a form of granula- tion. This, unless correctly and energetically treated in its early stages, becomes a chronic, steadily progressive disease which eventually leads to blindness due to ulceration and scarring of the cornea. Trachoma is rare in countries where hygiene is good, but it is a common cause of blindness today in the Middle East, Africa, and some parts of Asia. Dirt, lack of hygiene, malnutrition, close personal contact, fly infestation – all of these factors and others make fertile ground for the trachoma bacterium to grow, develop, and spread from one person to another.

Trachoma vaccines have been developed but have not given sufficient immunity. However the use of special antibiotic tablets taken regularly by mouth appears to prevent the disease process. There is also no doubt that running water, the free use of soap in each home, and the reduction of the fly population have done more to get rid of trachoma than any other measures so far.

The red eye

Without pain or blurred vision This may mean that a haemorrhage from a ruptured small blood vessel under the conjunctiva has taken place. There is no treatment needed and the condition is usually unimportant. If a person has many subconjunctival haemorrhages it is wise to have a medical examination in order to rule out some general medical condition that may be the underlying cause.

Acute conjunctivitis (or pink eye) has already been described. The eye is red and there is no pain as a rule, but there is always a gritty sensation and a discharge, and the lids are always stuck together on wakening.

A stye is an infection, usually caused by a staphylococcus bacterium, of one of the glands in the eyelid. Application of hot compresses usually brings the stye to a head, and pus escapes. If styes occur regularly a doctor should be consulted.

Unless reddened eyes result from something as obvious as exposure to smoke, the cause should be investigated.

With pain and blurred vision There are two major conditions that produce these signs and symptoms. These are acute iritis and acute glaucoma.

Iritis is an inflammation of the iris, the coloured part of the eye. The cause is frequently obscure, although it is certain that the tissues of the iris and the ciliary body as well as the choroid (these three structures are known as the uvea or uveal tract) become sensitized to a protein from some source, usually bacterial, in the body. Attacks occur, therefore, when the toxic agent comes in contact with the sensitized iris tissue. In an acute attack of iritis the eye is red and this redness is mostly concentrated around the periphery of the cornea. The eyeball is tender to touch and movement. Pain in and around the eye is sometimes severe and the vision may or may not be blurred (this usually comes later, as an outpouring of white blood cells takes place inside the eye, especially in the anterior chamber).

A RED PAINFUL EYE NEEDS IMMEDIATE EXPERT ATTENTION.

Acute iritis and acute glaucoma can cause the patient to have somewhat similar signs and symptoms. Treatment of the two conditions is different.

Acute glaucoma often begins as a reddened eye with mildly blurred vision, associated with headache in, and especially around and behind, the eyeball. A regular but not constant symptom is the seeing of rainbow rings (haloes) around street lamps at night. The attack may subside spontaneously on rest and sleep, or it may increase in severity. The congestion gets worse, the vision fades and may even disappear, the pain becomes very severe, and the patient may go into a form of shock consisting of pallor, sweating, fainting, and vomiting. Every time an acute attack occurs, more and more damage takes place. So even the mild attacks, which are always recurrent, need immediate emergency medical care.

The treatment is surgical and this is almost 100 per cent effective so that no further attacks occur and the patient is rescued from blindness. Because acute glaucoma is likely to affect both eyes in time, preventive surgery is advised for the other so far unaffected eye. This may often be difficult for the patient to understand, but is usually considered necessary by a modern ophthalmic surgeon. The mechanism of this form of glaucoma and the other form known as wide angle or simple glaucoma will be considered separately.

An ulcer of the cornea, either from bacteria or a virus, causes pain, congestion, and blurred vision.

Disease of the cornea itself, such as inflammation of the cornea (interstitial keratitis) due to syphilis, tuberculosis, or other diseases, produces pain, redness, tenderness, and blurred vision. Sensitivity to light (photophobia) which can be intense, and is usually associated with watering eyes, occurs in acute iritis and glaucoma, but is much more evident in corneal diseases.

The painless white eye with disturbed vision

A number of things, all taking place within the eyeball, may cause symptoms. The loss of vision may be gradual, as in the development and progression of a cataract or simple glaucoma. It may be due to an inflammation of the choroid (choroiditis, uveitis), with oedema and swelling – a reaction which attracts white blood cells which may fill the vitreous; or it may be caused by the erosion of a choroidal or retinal blood vessel, which may produce bleeding within the eye. It is obvious that these responses will reduce vision, sometimes gradually, at other times suddenly.

Another cause of partial painless loss of vision, gradually getting worse, is the development of a tumour within the eye.

Loss of vision may be sudden. This happens when a blood vessel within the eye, almost always a retinal one, becomes ruptured, blocked off (thrombosis), or

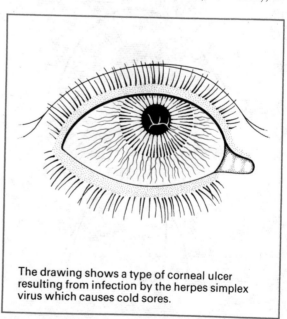

The drawing shows a type of corneal ulcer resulting from infection by the herpes simplex virus which causes cold sores.

plugged (embolus). It is also a symptom of detached or separated retina, although in this event the patient is apt first to notice a shower of black particles floating in his sight, flashes of light, followed by a developing veil or curtain which, unless treated surgically, will lead to eventual blindness. Another cause of painless, noncongestive, sudden blurring of vision or blindness, is disease of the optic nerve (optic neuritis, retrobulbar optic neuritis). These and several other conditions, some in the eye, others in the brain, all require careful study and expert diagnosis and must be considered as needing urgent medical attention.

The mechanism of glaucoma

The signs and symptoms of the two main forms of glaucoma have been described.

Glaucoma means essentially an increased pressure within the eye. Normally, the rate of formation of the intraocular fluid and its outflow are in balance. The fluid, formed by the ciliary body, bathes the interior of the eye and nourishes it and then flows forward around the lens into the anterior chamber. It is evacuated through the minute drainage canals situated in the angle of the anterior chamber. From here it goes into the veins of the sclera and conjunctiva and then into the general circulation.

If more fluid is formed than can be carried away, or if, as is most often the case, the outflow channels become narrowed with age, or blocked up by a swollen iris and dilated pupil, the pressure within the eye becomes raised.

If the blockage is sudden, as it is in acute glaucoma, it is because the angle is narrow, often genetically so. The root of the iris in these cases becomes thickened when the pupil dilates – as it does in the dark, after certain drugs, and exciting or emotional events (marital quarrel, death in the family, anger, or even after an exciting game of cards). The thickened root of the iris fills up the narrowed angle, blocks off the outflow channels and dams back the inflow. The natural mechanical result therefore is an increase in intraocular pressure (glaucoma).

In older people (about two per cent of those over 40 years of age) the blockage of the outflow is more gradual, as the outflow channels become more and

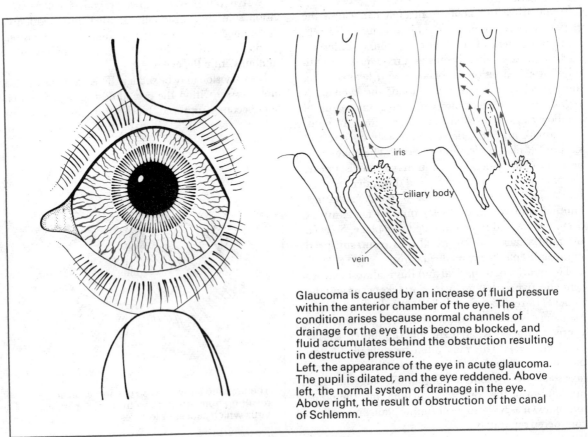

iris

ciliary body

vein

Glaucoma is caused by an increase of fluid pressure within the anterior chamber of the eye. The condition arises because normal channels of drainage for the eye fluids become blocked, and fluid accumulates behind the obstruction resulting in destructive pressure.
Left, the appearance of the eye in acute glaucoma. The pupil is dilated, and the eye reddened. Above left, the normal system of drainage in the eye. Above right, the result of obstruction of the canal of Schlemm.

more narrowed with age. The mechanics and the immediate results are quite different because of the gradual as against the sudden blockage of the outflow apparatus. This form of glaucoma is known as the wide angle (in contrast to the narrow or acutely blocked angle) form, or as chronic simple glaucoma or noncongestive glaucoma. This is a very insidious and therefore dangerous form of glaucoma. It can steal away some of the vision, by pressure on the optic nerve, retinal cells, and blood vessels, before the patient becomes aware of it. It is painless and the eye appears normal.

The increased pressure within the eye and the death of the compressed nerve fibres push back the optic nerve and depress it into a cup.

It often happens that the first thing a person with this form of glaucoma notices is a blurring of vision on the side towards the nose, which spreads to involve other parts of the field of vision until, unless recognized and properly treated, total irreversible blindness ensues (absolute glaucoma).

Owing to the insidious and serious nature of this disease, it has become routine practice by every ophthalmologist to measure the intraocular pressure or ocular tension of the eyes of every patient over 40. It is also important to examine the visual fields of such patients especially if there is any suspicion of cupping of the optic discs or any former history of glaucoma.

Ocular tension is measured by an instrument called a tonometer.

After the eye has been anaesthetized with a drop of a local anaesthetic, the instrument is placed on the cornea, and the amount of pressure required to flatten a known area gives a good reading of the ocular tension.

But tonometry is only one step, perhaps the most important one, in the study of an eye to see if chronic simple glaucoma is present. Measurement of visual acuity, the detailed examination of the visual fields to determine the presence of any blind areas, the study of the appearance of the optic nerve head (ophthalmoscopy) and an observation of the anatomy and appearance of the angle of the anterior chamber (gonioscopy) are necessary tests.

The treatment of chronic simple glaucoma is either medical (eye drops and tablets) or surgical. In the latter event a new outflow channel is made. Surgery is usually not performed until a trial of drugs is made. If

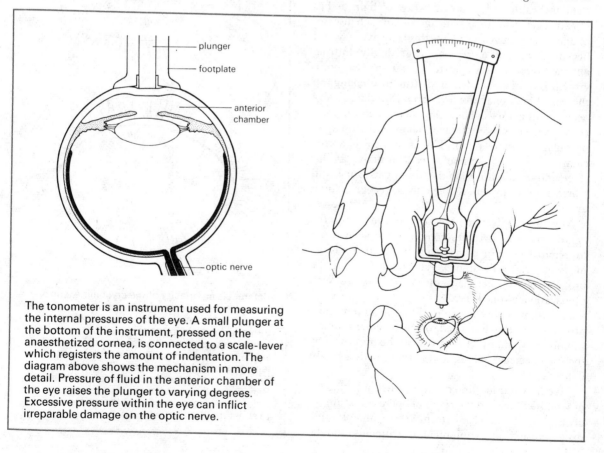

plunger
footplate
anterior chamber
optic nerve

The tonometer is an instrument used for measuring the internal pressures of the eye. A small plunger at the bottom of the instrument, pressed on the anaesthetized cornea, is connected to a scale-lever which registers the amount of indentation. The diagram above shows the mechanism in more detail. Pressure of fluid in the anterior chamber of the eye raises the plunger to varying degrees. Excessive pressure within the eye can inflict irreparable damage on the optic nerve.

medication does not relieve the raised tension, surgery must be carried out (see chapter 23). Surgery is effective in about 85 per cent of the cases of glaucoma. It will not restore the vision that is lost. If it is successful, however, it will check the progress, otherwise relentless, of the disease.

Congenital glaucoma   This is a form of glaucoma that occurs in babies and children under two. The symptoms are sensitivity to light, spasm of the lids, and watering eyes. Sometimes there may be pain which the child shows by fretting, refusing food, and being obviously miserable. An unusually large cornea, often cloudy or hazy, which increases in size, and a deep anterior chamber are signs that require attention. The cause is a faulty development of the anterior chamber angle associated with abnormal tissue that covers and blocks the outflow channels. The treatment is always surgical.

Cataract

The lens of the eye, situated just behind the pupil, is clear in health and focuses the rays of light as has already been described. With age and in such diseases as diabetes and uveitis, it loses this transparency and becomes more and more opaque, gradually shutting out the vision. This is known as cataract. It is not a growth but a biochemical and structural change in the lens. Small opacities are normal in old age and occur in all animals. They may increase in number, coalesce, and make the lens completely opaque, producing a white pupil. This is known as a ripe cataract. It may take many years to arrive at this stage and during this time the vision gets worse and worse until the patient is able only to recognize light and dark.

Nowadays it is not necessary to wait until the cataractous lens becomes completely ripe in order to remove it surgically. Incidentally, there is no medicine that will absorb, retard, or prevent the progress of cataract, and the advice to use such preparations is quackery.

It must, however, be realized that a cataract may progress very slowly indeed, or even remain almost stationary. In many cases vision can be improved by the use of correct glasses, and reading with a bright light.

Modern cataract surgery has reached a high level of sophistication and the result of operation is almost always successful. New techniques, anaesthetics, drugs, nursing care, equipment, instruments, and the

training of eye surgeons for this purpose all help. The operation itself consists of incising the anaesthetized eye, making a small hole in the iris, and removing the cataractous lens with forceps, suction apparatus, or cryoprobe through the dilated pupil. As in any operation, there may be complications, but fortunately these are usually minor in nature and yield to modern care and treatment. About one eye in a thousand is completely lost as the result of an operation. But since a cataractous eye is doomed to blindness anyway, the odds are all in favour of the patient.

Glasses after cataract surgery   After cataract surgery the lens has gone, and an eye without a lens cannot focus. It is therefore necessary to supply glasses. These are thick and sometimes heavy. At first, wearing them

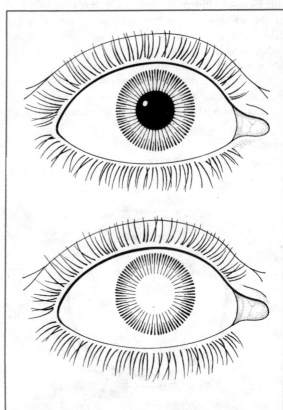

Cataract is an opacity of the crystalline lens of the eye or its capsule which acts like a curtain to prevent light rays from reaching the retina. Some forms are congenital, the more common forms occur after middle age. Opacities may be small, or they may coalesce and fill the entire lens, producing a "white pupil", as shown below, in contrast with the normal pupil above. Removal of the opaque lens restores clear vision, but glasses or contact lenses are required to substitute for the lost lens.

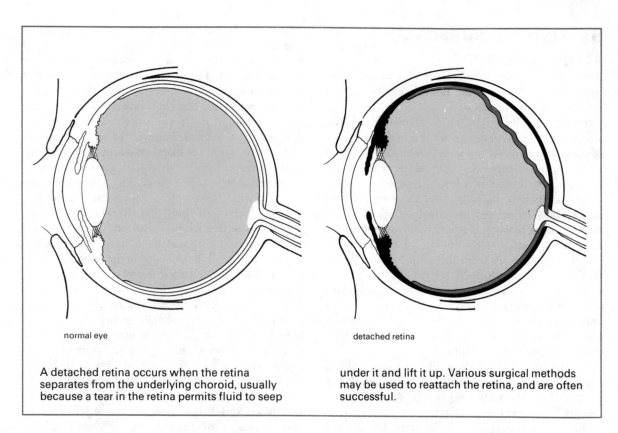

normal eye

detached retina

A detached retina occurs when the retina separates from the underlying choroid, usually because a tear in the retina permits fluid to seep under it and lift it up. Various surgical methods may be used to reattach the retina, and are often successful.

can be disturbing, because the vision is not quite the same in width, and objects seem to be bigger than they were before. The vast majority of patients, however, soon become adjusted to these disturbances and return to daily visual activities. Modern contact lenses, if properly fitted, are increasingly being used by the aphakic patient (that is, one who has had a cataract removed) with comfort and safety. Some patients cannot wear contact lenses for some reason or other, but those who can have a more efficient and wider vision than do those who wear the usual correcting spectacles.

Detached retina

The subject of detached or separated retina has already been touched upon. The condition is diagnosed by careful study of the interior of the eye by means of the ophthalmoscope. There is almost always a hole or tear in the retina. This is responsible for its separation from its bed, because the intraocular fluid gets through the hole and lifts it up. The cause of the hole or holes is not entirely known, but it is believed to be due to traction on a diseased or degenerated part of the retina by bands of tissue in the contracting diseased vitreous. Sometimes holes are the result of severe ocular concussion or perforation. The treatment is always surgical. Each hole or tear in the retina is sealed off, something like spot welding, in various ways (diathermy, coagulation, buckling of the eyeball, light coagulation). The operation is successful in about 80 per cent of cases, and the earlier the operation is performed, as a rule, the better is the chance of success.

Tumours

Malignant tumours can develop in the eye, as elsewhere in the body, either directly in the tissues or as a result of spread from a tumour elsewhere.

The usual forms seen by ophthalmologists are those arising from the retina in young children (retinoblastoma) or those of pigmented nature arising in the uvea (iris, ciliary body, and choroid), generally in adults.

These are likely to be fatal, unless the eye is removed early, although in some rare instances the tumour can be destroyed by radiant energy, or some form of cauterization, or destructive chemicals or drugs.

413

Systemic diseases that affect the eyes

Some general diseases affect the eyes. These constitute a large and growing number of cases which often lead to total blindness.

The chief of these is diabetes. Diabetics are kept alive longer than ever before because of the advances of medical treatment, but with this lengthened span of life certain changes may take place in the blood vessels of the retina. As a result, repeated haemorrhages occur into the retina and the vitreous, and with each haemorrhage the vision deteriorates. These changes in the blood vessels lead to the outpouring of exudates of various sorts and the development of proliferating scar tissue in the retina and vitreous. Cataracts may also form.

This is a complex problem and is the subject of continuous research in many countries to discover the underlying causes and mechanisms involved, to find some preventive measure, and to discover a satisfactory method of treatment.

So far efforts along these lines have not been entirely successful, but progress is being made. At the present time, the only measure of which we are certain, to prevent and to retard the advance of retinal vessel disease, is to insist that the affected patient follow his doctor's directions meticulously with regard to diet and medicinal treatment.

As one gets older, arteriosclerosis or hardening of the arteries takes place. This process also occurs in the retinal vessels. They may rupture, resulting in haemorrhages, usually small, or they may become blocked. When this happens nutrition to the retinal cells is lost and the area of the retina supplied by these vessels becomes blind.

If the arteriosclerosis is combined with high blood pressure the outlook is more serious. A particular form of this vascular disease (sclerosis) that is very common in the elderly, is the deprivation of the blood supply to the central part of the retina (macular degeneration). The vessels in the underlying choroid are the ones that are involved. This causes a blind area in the central vision, the part of the vision that is used in looking directly at an object, and results in an inability to read, recognize faces, or distinguish the colours of objects. The side vision remains good, so that patients are usually able to get about and to avoid obstructions. They do not become blind in the usual sense. Nothing can be done to restore the function of the macula. Ordinary glasses do not help. Sometimes optical aids, known as visual aids, that are essentially magnifiers, may be of some help.

Diseases of the blood, such as leukaemia, pernicious anaemia, and others sometimes lead to retinal haemorrhages. The vision can be affected to a degree compatible with the duration, extent, and location of these haemorrhages.

Congenital and familial diseases affecting the retina through its blood supply are found occasionally. A typical example of this is retinitis pigmentosa. Here the blood vessels of the peripheral part (sides) of the retina and choroid become narrowed in the course of time. The ophthalmologist sees pigment deposits in the involved zone of the retina, which come closer and closer to the macula. The latter is usually not involved, so that central vision may remain good for a long time. But the peripheral vision closes down and the sight is as if one were looking through a gun barrel (tunnel vision).

Retrolental fibroplasia The condition known as retrolental fibroplasia is rare today. In 1942 it was discovered that some premature infants who had been kept alive in oxygen incubators developed a white membrane behind the lens and were blind. In the ensuing twelve years many hundreds of babies were afflicted before it was shown that excess oxygen was to blame. Too much oxygen was toxic and led to new blood vessels developing in the anterior retina and vitreous, leading to detachment of the retina by fibrous tissue. After this discovery and the better control of oxygen delivered to premature infants the incidence of this condition dropped almost to zero. An occasional case is, however, still encountered.

Arteriosclerosis of the blood vessels of the brain may cause a stroke or cerebral vascular accident. When this happens in the areas of the fibres that conduct vision to the visual centres of the brain, sight is affected. Usually only a half or quarter of the field of vision in each eye is affected and this is most disturbing to the patient, who may feel as if he is wearing blinkers.

Tumours of the brain, by pressing on these areas directly or on the blood vessels, may give the same effect.

Headaches

Headache is perhaps the most common human symptom. It is a subjective symptom, disturbing to the patient and the doctor. There are many causes for it and its severity is no indication of the seriousness of the cause.

Eyestrain or ocular fatigue is only one of the causes. It is, however, the simplest to determine by a careful eye examination and if found, usually can be easily alleviated. In all cases of headache, therefore, it is necessary to rule out ocular conditions as a contributing cause.

Eyestrain due to refractive errors and ocular muscle defects shows itself by burning, tearing, or a sandy sensation in the eyes. The eyes may ache, and pain in and behind the eyes may be present. Patients often complain of a pulling sensation, and of becoming tired and irritable, with a distaste for reading or studying. Drowsiness and the symptoms of eyestrain are usually absent during the morning hours.

The symptoms of eyestrain are probably the result of the effort to overcome refractive and muscular defects.

Vitamins and eye health   There have been a lot of peculiar beliefs on this topic. There is no doubt that a diet deficient in vitamins can cause trouble in the eyes, some of a serious nature. But it is very rare indeed for the ophthalmologist, in this country particularly, to find definite cases of ocular disease due to vitamin deficiency. Our hygiene, living conditions, and diets are not conducive to these conditions.

When a person does not eat proper food (for example, smoking and drinking at the expense of his diet) or has a debilitating disease, or one that prevents the proper assimilation of foods, deficiency develops, which if severe enough can lead to ocular trouble such as night blindness, dryness of the eyes, optic nerve disorders, or ulcers of the cornea. A well balanced assimilated diet is essential, and if not available must be supplemented with manufactured vitamins in therapeutic doses.

Eye exercises

These words have come to have several meanings. The scientific term for exercising the eye muscles, but particularly for strengthening binocular vision, is *orthoptics*. This is a perfectly legitimate field and is often of great value.

The nonscientific term "eye exercises" usually means an endeavour to relieve myopia and avoid the need for wearing glasses, notoriously by "palming". But there is nothing that can alter the shape or length of the eyeball apart from surgery. However, it has been shown that a person can be taught to pay more attention to the shape of things and recognize them more readily, thus resulting in a sharpening of vision.

During the war it was claimed by some nonmedical technicians that colour blindness could be cured by exercises. That is, a colour-blind person could be taught to recognize the difference between red and green, for example. This turned out to be fallacious and was discarded even by the enthusiasts who had to yield to the truth that colour blindness is an anatomical anomaly of the retinal cells that cannot be altered by exercises.

Colour blindness (better described as defective colour vision) is a congenital, inherited, sex-linked defect (that is, passed down by female carriers to their sons). It is not a disease and cannot be cured. The most common form is red-green colour blindness, which affects about four per cent of males. Red and green are seen as shades of yellow, yellowish-brown, and grey. The condition does not impair sharpness of vision and the affected person is usually unaware of being colour-blind until the defect is revealed by tests involving discrimination of colours.

Red-green colour blindness is a handicap in certain occupations where discrimination of colour signals is important, as in piloting an aeroplane or driving a train, and it rules out some vocations such as mixing pigments, matching printing inks, or advising about interior decorations. But as a rule a colour-blind person is not particularly handicapped in his daily affairs, except that, if left to his own choices, he may select ties, shirts, and socks of gaudily clashing colours which to him look quite neutral and harmonious.

Since colour discrimination is a normal function of the cones of the retina, colour blindness involves some inherited and irreversible defect of these structures, probably an absence of retinal cones sensitive to particular wavelengths of light.

Floating spots

The vitreous in health is a solid transparent jelly. Ageing makes it more fluid so that cells and normal strands of tissue can float around in the vitreous when eye movements occur. As they do so, they cast shadows on the retina and these are observed as floating spots, especially in the shortsighted.

They are annoying and worrying but there is nothing to be done about it. Sometimes a more careful change in glasses will make them less obvious.

Sometimes they conglomerate and fall to the floor of the inner eye where they remain unless shaken up.

Sometimes, however, these floating spots are symptoms of trouble inside the eye, especially as a forerunner of retinal detachment. Then, too, haemorrhages and exudates in the vitreous may show themselves as floating spots, threads, or strands.

If you notice these floating objects, see an ophthalmologist to find out whether they are due merely to age or to a disease process.

Other problems

Bags under the eyes   Since the skin of the eyelids is very soft, loose fluid accumulated in the body for any reason will settle under the skin of the lids, causing bags. Loss of weight, menstruation, kidney and heart disease, overactive thyroid, disorders of other glands, hard drinking, loss of sleep, and other conditions can cause this excess of fluid beneath the skin.

Bulging eyes   These may be a familial trait where the eyes are larger or more prominent than usual. But if the condition comes on suddenly and progresses it could be a sign of a thyroid disorder (see chapter 9). If one or both eyes bulge unduly, the patient should be seen as soon as possible by his doctor for diagnosis and treatment.

All the facts pertaining to the eyes cannot be discussed here but an attempt has been made to give information that may help to explain the anatomy and function of the visual apparatus and to answer questions about the commoner ocular disorders.

Vision is so important to everyone that expert attention is always needed if it fails, and there is no likelihood that it can be taken care of by any simple "do it yourself" equipment.

Chapter 18
Ears, nose, and throat

Revised by J. Angell-James, CBE MD FRCP FRCS

The ear

Sound is a sensation that is perceived by the brain when the inner ear is stimulated by certain vibrations of the air or other media. These vibrations of the air, or of the bones of the skull, are conducted to the inner ear and cause the fluid in its cavity to vibrate. The fluid vibrations excite nerve endings which carry the impulses to the brain where sound is heard. Our hearing is one of the most sensitive and discriminating of senses, able to distinguish the vibrations of air coming from a familiar voice or from a particular instrument in a symphony orchestra. It is well protected by the location of its most delicate structures within the hard bony areas of the head. The ear is best described in three parts, each having its special function.

The external ear The external ear consists of the pinna, which assists in the collection of sound vibrations in the air and directs them in to the external auditory canal. The external auditory canal penetrates 3·5 cm ($1\frac{1}{2}$ in) into the head with the eardrum (tympanic membrane) at its inner end. The skin of the outer half contains many wax-secreting glands. The wax has a lubricating, protecting, and cleansing function and traps small particles. Some people, especially those with oily skins, tend to produce more ear wax than others. When first formed, the wax is soft and oily. Older wax is brown and may become quite hard. The wax is massaged towards the outer opening of the canal by the movement of the jaw joint immediately in front of the canal and is then washed away during ordinary face washing. Occasionally, a hard mass – literally a ball

of wax – collects close to or in contact with the eardrum at the inner end of the ear canal and does not move. The mass obstructs sound waves and the patient may think that he is losing his hearing. There may also be discomfort from pressure. Wax is easily removed by a doctor, but people should not attempt to do this themselves, because they may harm the drum. The doctor takes warm water into a large syringe, places a curved basin snugly beneath the ear, and pulls the ear upwards and backwards to straighten out the ear canal. He then presses the syringe plunger and squirts water into the ear canal along the roof in such a way that it rebounds from the eardrum and forces out the wax. In stubborn cases it may be necessary to make an opening in the edge of the wax so that water can get behind it. It sounds simple, but the washing should be done by a doctor or nurse.

The middle ear The middle ear is an air-filled cavity, sealed by the eardrum and surrounded by thin bony walls. There is an opening at the back which leads into the mastoid bone, and a tubular passage in front, 31 to 38 mm ($1\frac{1}{4}$ to $1\frac{1}{2}$ in) in length, which opens into the throat, called the Eustachian (auditory) tube. Air on either side of the pearly pink concave eardrum must be at equal pressures for the drum to vibrate freely. A partial vacuum in the middle ear, for instance, would pull the eardrum inwards and restrict its movement. Pressures are normally equalized by air which can move both ways through the Eustachian tube. Clicking of the ears when we swallow or go up in a high-speed lift is a familiar sensation. Atmospheric pressure is less as we ascend;

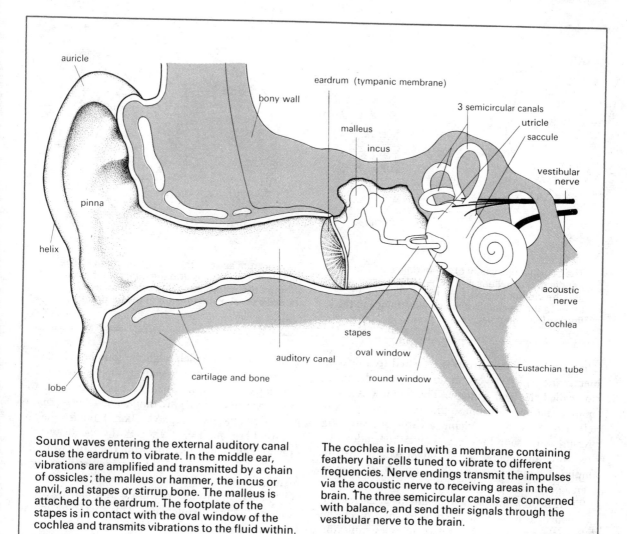

Sound waves entering the external auditory canal cause the eardrum to vibrate. In the middle ear, vibrations are amplified and transmitted by a chain of ossicles; the malleus or hammer, the incus or anvil, and stapes or stirrup bone. The malleus is attached to the eardrum. The footplate of the stapes is in contact with the oval window of the cochlea and transmits vibrations to the fluid within.

The cochlea is lined with a membrane containing feathery hair cells tuned to vibrate to different frequencies. Nerve endings transmit the impulses via the acoustic nerve to receiving areas in the brain. The three semicircular canals are concerned with balance, and send their signals through the vestibular nerve to the brain.

consequently, air trapped inside the middle ear expands and pushes its way out through the Eustachian tube. The tube is lined by a moist membrane covered with microscopic whiplike structures which waft the watery mucous secretions from the middle ear into the throat above the soft palate, after which they are swallowed. Obstruction of the tube can cause deafness, and germs travelling up it may cause infection of the middle ear which may even spread to the mastoid bone behind the ear. Such events are caused by the common cold or other virus or bacterial infections and are often predisposed to by the presence of large infected adenoids, chronic nasal sinusitis, or allergies. An extreme example is the pain and deafness suffered when descending too quickly in a nonpressurised aeroplane so that air pressures in the middle ear cannot be equalized by

opening the Eustachian tube by swallowing. This may be avoided by forcible inflation, performed by pinching the nostrils and raising the pressure in the nose by trying to blow out.

Sound waves strike the eardrum and cause it to vibrate, but the vibrations are very slight. At some frequencies, vibrations as small as 1,000,000,000th of a centimetre can be detected. A remarkable amplifying system is built into the middle ear. It consists of a chain of three tiny bones, the ossicles, the smallest bones in the body. Altogether they occupy about as much space as a small carpet tack. From a fancied resemblance to familiar objects, the ossicles are called the hammer (malleus), anvil (incus), and stirrup (stapes). The hammer handle is in contact with the eardrum. Its hammering parts vibrate against the anvil bone. In turn, the anvil moves the stirrup bone.

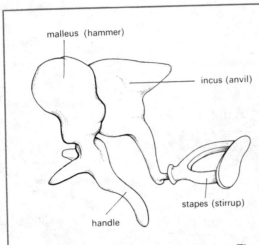

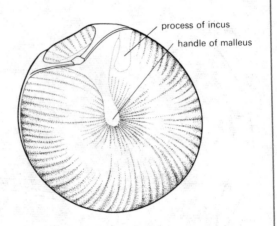

The conducting system of the middle ear. The handle of the malleus is attached to the eardrum, and the vibrations pass from the malleus to the incus to the footplate of the stapes, thence to the fluids of the inner ear.

The eardrum as seen through an auriscope. The handle of the malleus and the incus can be seen through the membrane. Tiny sets of muscles increase or relax the tension of the eardrum.

The footplate of the stirrup is attached to a flexible membrane which covers an opening into the inner ear, called the oval window. The window is much smaller than the eardrum so that this, with the lever action of the ossicular chain, greatly increases the pressure of the sound waves reaching the window. In this way, the energy of sound waves is greatly amplified – indeed, we can hear a faint whisper or even a pin drop.

There are tiny muscles and ligaments in the middle ear which assist hearing and help to protect the delicate mechanism. One set of muscles pulls the hammer bone inwards and increases the tension of the eardrum. Another muscle attached to the stirrup bone has the reverse effect and relaxes the eardrum, especially when loud noises assail it. Thus the movements in the middle ear take place in proportion to the volume of sound in order to protect hearing.

The inner ear The inner ear is a complex bony structure filled with fluid. When the sound waves reach the stapes footplate and the oval window, they enter the inner ear causing the fluids filling it to vibrate as fluid waves. Just below the oval window is another opening in the bony wall, covered also with an elastic membrane called the round window. This bulges outwards and inwards as the fluids of the inner ear vibrate and thus cushions and prevents undue pressures in an otherwise totally enclosed cavity.

Sound waves in the inner ear excite an apparatus of great complexity which might be compared in a very rough way to a piano keyboard with keys arranged in graduated steps from treble to bass. However, the inner ear console has more than 20,000 "keys" and is not laid out flat like a piano keyboard, but is coiled in a spiral like a snail shell. Indeed, the cochlea, as the organ is called, gets its name from the Latin word for snail shell. It is a tubular, bony structure lined by a membrane on which stand thousands of hair-covered cells. These are tuned to vibrate to sound waves of different pitches (frequencies). This area is the actual organ of hearing and is called the organ of Corti. Nerve endings surround each cell and the nerve fibres enter the central bony column to form the hearing (acoustic) nerve, which carries the electrical nerve impulses to the auditory centres of the brain where sound is heard. What begins as physical vibration now becomes the sound of a voice or the music of an orchestra.

If straightened out, the spiral canal of the cochlea would be about 38 mm ($1\frac{1}{2}$ in) long, but rolled up like a snail shell it occupies a space about the size of a pea. In this tiny area with its nerve lines to the brain we make billions of exquisite discriminations between infinitely complex and endlessly different patterns of sound waves that touch our eardrums. Nerve receptors for the deepest of deep bass notes – about sixteen cycles per second – are located at the very end of the innermost turn of the cochlear spiral. From here, if we imagine the spiral unwinding, the keyboard notes are increasingly tuned to higher-

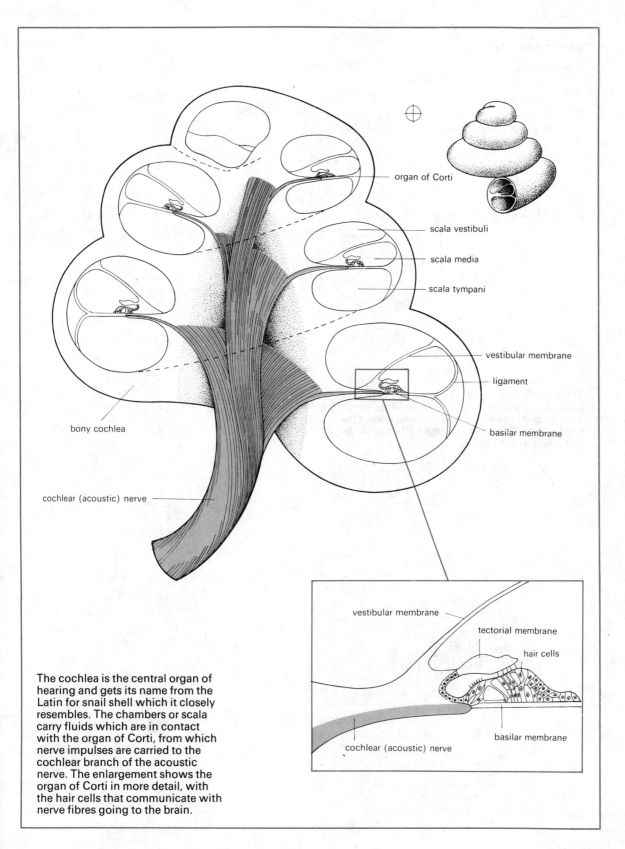

organ of Corti

scala vestibuli

scala media

scala tympani

vestibular membrane

ligament

basilar membrane

bony cochlea

cochlear (acoustic) nerve

vestibular membrane

tectorial membrane

hair cells

basilar membrane

cochlear (acoustic) nerve

The cochlea is the central organ of hearing and gets its name from the Latin for snail shell which it closely resembles. The chambers or scala carry fluids which are in contact with the organ of Corti, from which nerve impulses are carried to the cochlear branch of the acoustic nerve. The enlargement shows the organ of Corti in more detail, with the hair cells that communicate with nerve fibres going to the brain.

Chapter 18 Ears, nose, and throat

Semicircular canals

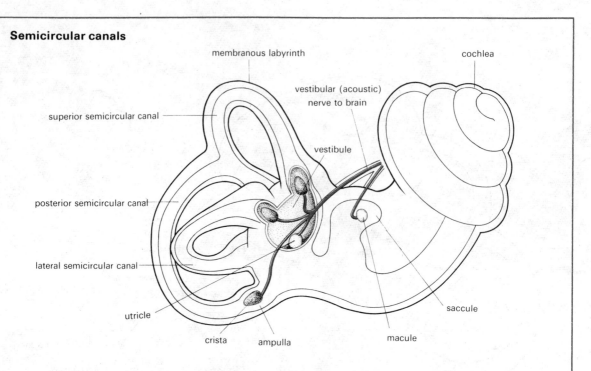

The semicircular canals are concerned with balance. They contain fluid and our sense of balance is maintained by fluid movements in the canals that affect nerve endings of the vestibular nerve going to the brain.

Macule

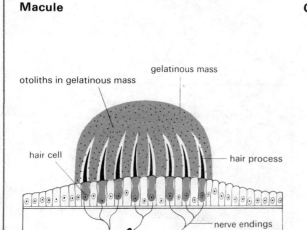

Crista

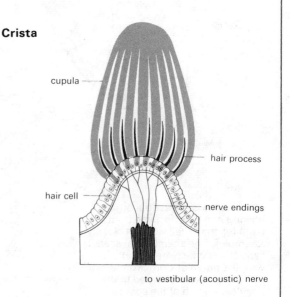

The macule and crista are sensitive to the movement of fluid in the semicircular canals and register the position of the head to the brain.

pitched sounds, until at the wider end of the cochlea we may hear very high notes with frequencies of 20,000 cycles per second or more.

Equilibrium

Our sense of balance is dependent on the organs of equilibrium. In the inner ear behind the cochlea, in the same cavity in the temporal bone, and filled with the same fluids, is the vestibular system consisting of three semicircular canals and the vestibule. The ends of the canals open into the vestibule. The canals lie at right angles to one another (mutually perpendicular). The fluid in them responds to movements of the head and minute crystals of calcite attached to hair cells like those in the hearing end organ and lying in the vestibule, horizontally and vertically, send impulses to the brain signifying the position of the head, whether upright or horizontal. These comprise an automatic governor of body balance, and the whole inner ear cavity is called the labyrinth. Inflammation of the labyrinth causes symptoms of deafness, disturbances of balance, and vomiting which may advance to severe fever, pain, and other serious complications.

Air and bone conduction

Any sound vibration that stimulates the acoustic nerves becomes audible. Vibrations can reach the nerve ends through the bony structures of the head, as well as by sound waves that strike the eardrum. We use both bone and air conduction all the time, although air conduction predominates in general listening. Bone conduction is especially related to speaking. Practically everyone is astonished, and sometimes shocked, the first time he hears his voice on a tape recording. It sounds like a stranger's voice, not at all like the voice the speaker thinks is his. The reason why our voices do not sound to us as they do to others is that a good deal of the sound we hear is bone-conducted. Auditors – and tape recorders – hear only what is air-conducted. Lower frequencies tend to be accentuated by bone conduction and the voice may sound more powerful than it really is. In voice training, recordings that reproduce the voice as others hear it are very helpful.

If our ears were a little more sensitive to low frequencies, we would constantly hear the noises of the body. If you close both ears with your fingertips, to shut out airborne sounds, you can hear a low, gentle rumbling tone – the noise of local blood circulation and tiny muscle contractions. If the ears did not have a cut-off point, we would hear some sort of thudding sound every time we took a step. We have two ears so that the brain can, by analysing the different loudness and timing of the signals from each ear, calculate the direction and distance from which a sound is coming.

Repeated exposure to loud noises may in time cause hearing impairment, such as boilermaker's deafness. Often, this is largely a reduced ability to hear high tones. Totally deaf people are relatively few, but large numbers have some degree of hearing loss. There is, indeed, a steady loss of sharpness of hearing as we grow older. The normal young ear can hear tones within a range of sixteen cycles per second – the lowest bass note of a pipe organ – up to high-pitched sounds of 20,000 cycles per second and more. A person in his sixties is lucky if he can hear sounds of 12,000 cycles per second. This loss is limited to high frequency sounds and must be considered normal since it happens to practically everybody as the years pass. It is probably related to gradual loss of elasticity from ageing, and loss of sensory cells in the organ of Corti, as well as central nerve cells. This particularly interferes with the power of discrimination between speech sounds we wish to hear and background noises of other voices, or other ambient sounds.

Ordinary conversation is relatively low-pitched, and the dampening of a screamingly shrill voice is not an unmixed blessing. Physically, if not critically, the ideal listener to high fidelity music is probably a baby. Good hi-fi sets and records can reproduce frequencies in the range of 20,000 cycles per second which are inaudible to considerable numbers of middle-aged listeners. A slight loss of perception of high-pitched sounds is not a complete catastrophe. It muffles some of the shrillness of the world. Impairment severe enough to make ordinary conversation difficult or impossible to understand is quite another matter. The pitch of human speech ranges between 300 and 4,000 cycles (wave frequencies) per second. These are the cycles most vital to the conduct of human affairs. Inability to hear well within this range is a serious personal and social handicap. Hard of hearing persons are often blamed unfairly for being crotchety, cantankerous, rude, and suspicious, if they do not answer questions, or seem to think people are whispering behind their backs, because they do not hear what is going on and have poor discrimination.

Varieties of impairment

What can be done for the person who is hard of hearing – and in most cases a great deal can be done – depends upon the nature of the impairment and its timely recognition. There are two types of hearing loss: conductive deafness and sensorineural or perceptive deafness. Sometimes there is mixed impairment involving both the conductive and nervous apparatus. There is also a sort of deafness (hysterical deafness) in which the hearing apparatus is physically intact, and the cause must be sought in psychological areas.

Different impairments affect different structures of the ear. Conduction deafness is the failure of airborne sound waves to be conducted efficiently through external and middle ear structures, so that adequate messages do not reach the inner ear. Perceptive (sensorineural) deafness is failure of the organ of Corti or the auditory nerves to accept, perceive, and transmit messages to hearing centres in the brain.

Tests of hearing

Measurement of sharpness of hearing requires some standard unit of the loudness of sound. This is the decibel. For practical purposes, we may say that a whisper is twenty decibels loud; conversation, 60 decibels; underground railway noise, 100 decibels; a jet aeroplane, 140 decibels. How much of the noise is heard depends on the ears. Standardized techniques enable hearing loss to be measured in terms of loss of decibels.

An audiometer is an instrument which emits pure tones which can be turned up louder, decibel by decibel. With it a doctor can make an audiogram which shows how well the patient hears different sound frequencies. If a sound must be made twenty decibels louder than standard for the patient to hear it, he is said to have a twenty-decibel loss of hearing for that sound frequency. If an audiogram shows, for instance, that a patient has a twenty-decibel hearing loss, it means that he probably does not hear distinctly in a theatre or meeting hall, and no doubt knows it or thinks that the acoustics are bad or that everybody has begun to mumble. A loss of more than 30 decibels usually means that a hearing aid is necessary to hear conversation distinctly, and of 50 or so that it is hard to hear over the telephone.

There are a number of other testing devices, some of them highly specialized. The latter are most likely to be used by otologists (ear physicians) and audiology clinics maintained in many large hospitals and medical centres. Devices as simple as a watch or tuning fork give valuable information to those who are trained to use them and interpret the results.

Often the family doctor is the first to be consulted about and to determine the general nature of a hearing impairment. A good deal can be learned about the nature of a hearing impairment by taking a careful history, examining, and making fairly simple tests. For instance, a vibrating tuning fork can distinguish between conduction and nerve deafness if it is placed on the bone behind the patient's ear and the results interpreted. If he hears bone-conducted sound, the difficulty lies somewhere in the sound wave conducting system; if he does not, the hearing nerves are affected.

Do you hear well?   One cannot self-diagnose ear troubles, but simple self-tests of hearing like those below may indicate that you do not hear as well as you should, and encourage you to consult your doctor who may refer you to an ear specialist.

> Do you hear speech more distinctly over the telephone than speech in a room?
> Can you hear a soft sound such as a tap dripping?
> Do you frequently miss words or phrases that others listening in to the same radio or television programme seem to catch?
> Can you – literally – hear someone who is talking behind your back?
> Do you often ask someone to repeat what they have just said?
> Do you have to strain to hear what is being said?

Deaf infants and children

Early recognition of deafness in infants is extremely important. Some infants are born totally deaf or with serious hearing loss. Surprising numbers of preschool children are handicapped by defective hearing. Unless deafness is detected and treated early, it can become an unnecessary handicap for the child. Normal development of speech and understanding of language require adequate hearing. Sounds not heard cannot be imitated and no meaning can be associated with the special sounds we call the spoken word. If no help is given at the proper time, the child may be thought to be – and in fact behaves as if he were – stupid, inattentive, listless, disobedient, or mentally retarded.

How does one suspect loss of hearing in an infant? The most obvious sign is that there is congenital absence or abnormality of the external ear. There may also be abnormality of the middle ear and the inner ear. Such abnormalities may be due to the mother having developed German measles or some other virus infection or having taken certain drugs in the first three months of pregnancy. When the external appearance is normal, the first obvious sign is absence of the startle reflex. That is, a sudden loud noise does not startle the baby or make him cry. This sign can be detected quite early, certainly by the age of six months. By the time he is nine or ten months old, a normal baby localizes sound quite well, and turns his head or otherwise indicates that he knows where the sound is coming from. A deaf infant does not. A supposedly good baby who sleeps undisturbed through all sorts of household din and clatter may simply not hear the noise. Loud voices do not awaken or disturb him. Another important sign is that the child does not develop speech at the normal time. A deaf infant may go through the babbling stages like any other baby, but he soon gives it up if he cannot hear the sounds he makes. He is shut out from the meaningful world of sound, and unless he has early speech training can communicate only by grunts and gestures as he grows older.

A baby may be born with normal hearing but acquire deafness after birth as a sequel to scarlet fever, mumps, measles, and other infections or injuries. The family doctor who attends the child is alert to such possibilities of deafness. Observations by the family that a baby or child apparently does not hear well should be reported at once to the family doctor. He will examine the child, give tests, and if the hearing defect can be treated medically, he will do so. If not, he will refer the patient to an otologist and provide reliable sources of help and information.

As in adults, impaired hearing in children may be conductive or sensorineural. The conductive type of loss can often be improved by surgery or a hearing aid. The problem is more serious if the infant has sensorineural deafness with total or almost total inability to hear any sounds at all. It is important that the situation be recognized early, because the child can never learn to talk in the normal way. He cannot imitate sounds he has not heard. He can see a dog, but cannot learn that a certain pattern of sound waves always mean dog when spoken.

But the situation is by no means hopeless. The child can be taught to speak, by special and difficult training techniques. Training is a long slow process which requires patience, love, and cooperation on the part of the parents. The role of the parents is of the utmost importance. Instruction in the methods which they can employ should be obtained from a qualified teacher of the deaf as soon as the disability has been discovered. Later, costly types of equipment, training aids, and teaching skills are necessary, and facilities generally are available only in large urban centres. The earlier the handicap is discovered, the earlier the child can be referred to a specialist teacher of the deaf, a school for the deaf, or a speech and hearing clinic. The ideal time to start training is in the second year of life when children are best able to learn and to cooperate.

Conductive impairment of hearing

Conductive impairment may be due to such a simple thing as a lump of wax blocking the external canal. Infections of the skin of the canal such as boils or fungus infections causing swelling will also block the passage of sound waves. But the most important conductive defects lie in the middle ear.

Middle ear defects

Middle ear defects include congenital malformations which may be due to infection of the mother with German measles or taking drugs such as thalidomide during the first three months of pregnancy. The commonest cause is middle ear infection from nasal infections ascending by the Eustachian tubes. These tubes are very short and wide in the young. Blows and skull fractures may damage ear structures and dislocate or fracture the ossicles. Infection of the middle ear causes pain and deafness by swelling of the lining membranes and the filling of the ear with fluid, which obstructs the movements of the drum and the ossicular chain. If it clears up completely there may be no impairment of hearing, but if it is severe or untreated it may cause perforation of the drum or erosion of the ossicles, or later, fibrous bands may develop which lock their movement, causing permanent deafness.

Earache

Earache is a pain localized in the ear, but when severe it may radiate to surrounding areas. It is a warning sign that something is wrong. Most types of earache are not dangerous, but some are. It is not a symptom to be treated for long by homely measures such as dropping warm (not hot) olive oil into the ear canal. This may possibly ease the pain a little, but it cannot correct the cause. If pain in the ear does not subside in 24 hours, disturbs the patient's sleep at night, and makes him conscious at all times that he has an earache, a doctor should be consulted.

Causes in the external ear (otitis externa) Few things are more painful than boils in the ear canal.

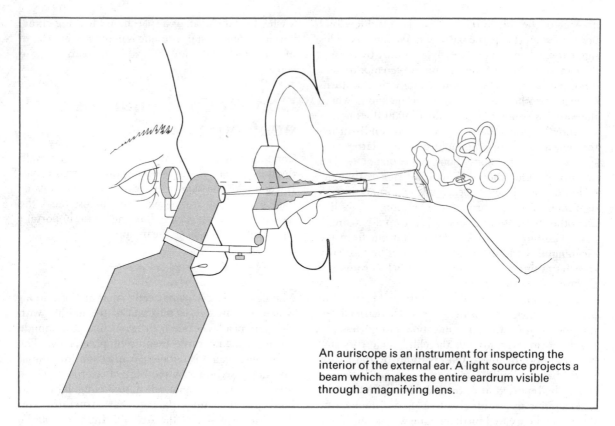

An auriscope is an instrument for inspecting the interior of the external ear. A light source projects a beam which makes the entire eardrum visible through a magnifying lens.

These are of the same nature as boils elsewhere in the body. Swelling within the narrow, confined ear canal may be extremely painful and seem to radiate to nearby parts of the face. A doctor may have to drain the boils to relieve pressure, and at the same time give treatment to control infection and prevent recurrences. The habit of poking and picking at the ear opening with a pencil, match, hairgrip, or anything else is undesirable and may be dangerous. Delicate skin may be damaged, introducing infections of various sorts, and the eardrum may be punctured. Infections and inflammation may also come about from foreign bodies lodged in the ear.

Fungus infections of the ear are not uncommon. The condition is sometimes called swimmer's ear since contaminated water and incompletely drained water tend to set up moist and soggy conditions favourable to fungal growth. The normal condition of the ear canal is to be filled with air, not fluid, and it is best to keep it dry at all times. A fungus infection of the external ear is rather like misplaced "athlete's foot". It affects the skin, is usually itchy, crusted, and weepy, and can be painful if there is swelling of the ear canal. Various ointments and solutions are effective in controlling external ear infections, but there are different kinds of organisms that may be involved and

selection of the proper medicine should be left to the doctor. Whenever water gets into the ears, it is important to drain them properly.

Middle ear infections (otitis media)   Otitis media varies greatly in severity, and mild cases require little or no treatment. In general, the condition is less severe nowadays because of better social conditions, better general health in the population, and because some of the usual organisms are, at present, less virulent. In acute infections the pain may be severe and if pus forms and is not relieved by drainage through the drum, it may spread to the spongy mastoid process behind the ear or directly to the inner ear, and later reach the coverings of the brain and the brain itself. Great danger lies in these complications.

A doctor using a viewing instrument (auriscope) can see the eardrum bulging from pressure of fluids behind it. Middle ear infections are not so common as they once were because timely treatment with antimicrobial drugs prevents many infections from progressing to this stage. Antibiotics and similar drugs usually cause an acute middle ear infection to subside uneventfully if treatment is begun in time.

Pus may break through the eardrum and drain from the ear canal. This relieves feelings of pain and pressure, but a doctor's care is necessary to be sure that the infection is completely cleared up and that there are no after effects which need attention. The broken eardrum may heal satisfactorily or it may not, depending on the extent and location of the break and other factors. If the doctor sees the patient when perforation of the drum seems imminent but has not yet occurred, and symptoms indicate that infection is advancing towards the mastoid cells, sometimes he may have to make a small incision in the eardrum (myringotomy) for drainage. Healing and hearing after this carefully placed surgical incision for drainage are usually good, but a spontaneous perforation does not always turn out so well.

Recurrent otitis media   Recurrent acute attacks often follow colds, especially when there is lingering infection of adenoids and tonsils or nasal sinuses, or allergies. In one form, which may be painless, the middle ear fills with sterile fluid, sometimes so thick that it resembles glue, and drainage down the Eustachian tube fails to clear it. The only symptom is deafness. The otologist may have to drain the ear for weeks or months by inserting a minute plastic tube through the drum.

Chronic suppurative otitis media   A chronic ear discharge – often called a running ear – is a warning to consult the doctor. This condition does NOT require a cotton wool plug.

Perforated eardrum   The drum may be perforated by direct injury through the canal or by skull fracture or explosive blast or deep diving, or even by a box on the ears. Most commonly, however, it is due to infection of the middle ear, with pus formation, which softens and finally ruptures the membrane. After the infection has cleared up the perforation may heal. However, there may be a delay in healing because the perforation is too large or the infection becomes chronic and there is persistent discharge from the ear. The symptom is easy to ignore because it is usually painless. But a draining ear is a hazard. Infection may extend at any time into the mastoid area. Low-grade infection produces just enough secretion to prevent the eardrum from healing completely but usually not enough to stimulate the patient to get urgently needed medical help. Constant drainage irritates the tissues and may cause polyps to grow, and the skin of the ear canal may grow through the perforated eardrum into the middle ear, with the formation of a fatty mass (cholesteatoma) which requires fairly radical surgery. In addition, the middle ear is directly accessible to bacteria through the perforated drum.

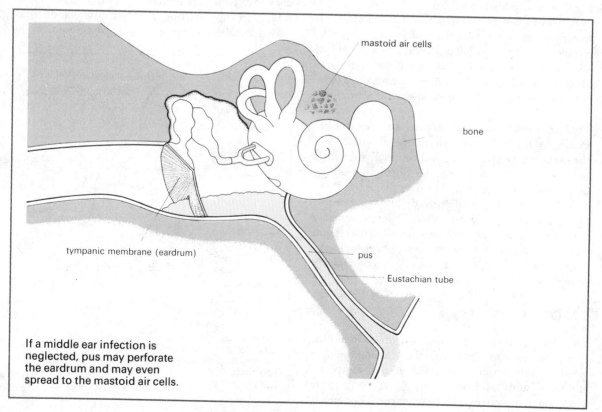

mastoid air cells

bone

tympanic membrane (eardrum)

pus

Eustachian tube

If a middle ear infection is neglected, pus may perforate the eardrum and may even spread to the mastoid air cells.

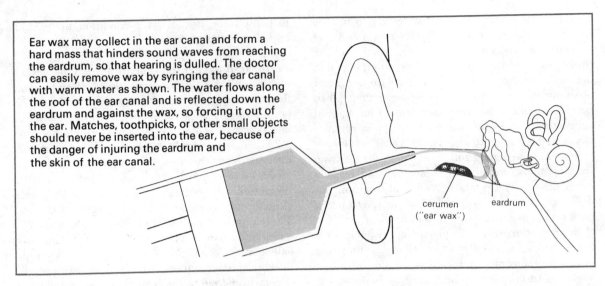

Ear wax may collect in the ear canal and form a hard mass that hinders sound waves from reaching the eardrum, so that hearing is dulled. The doctor can easily remove wax by syringing the ear canal with warm water as shown. The water flows along the roof of the ear canal and is reflected down the eardrum and against the wax, so forcing it out of the ear. Matches, toothpicks, or other small objects should never be inserted into the ear, because of the danger of injuring the eardrum and the skin of the ear canal.

cerumen ("ear wax")

eardrum

The doctor may take a swab for culture to decide which is the right antibiotic to eliminate the infecting organisms. A draining ear must be kept clean and dry at all times. It is especially dangerous for the patient to go swimming, even in heated indoor pools in the winter. Ear plugs cannot be depended upon to protect the ear completely. Nature did not really design the human ear for submersion, and a perforated eardrum is an added handicap.

A hearing test of children who have middle ear infections, or after they have had scarlet fever, measles, or other childhood diseases often associated with such infections, is important in order to discover abnormal conditions of the middle ear which may be corrected in time to avoid permanent loss of hearing.

Plastic repair of the drum and ossicular chain When all infection has been eliminated but the perforation has not healed, or conductive deafness persists, the perforation may be closed by grafting fascial tissue, or sometimes skin, over the drum. If the ossicular chain has been destroyed, it is often possible by means of an artificial device to restore continuity between the drum and the oval window, so that sound waves may reach the inner ear. These operations are known as myringoplasty and tympanoplasty respectively.

Otosclerosis

Otosclerosis is a common cause of deafness in adults. A painless overgrowth of bone forms inside the oval window and impinges on the stapes footplate, stiffening and later fixing it, so that airborne vibrations cease to pass into the inner ear. The cause is unknown, but it often occurs in several members of a family. Symptoms commonly appear between fifteen and 40 years of age. The first symptom may be some difficulty in understanding whispers, or voices at a distance. The patient usually hears his own voice well by bone conduction, and in fact it seems quite loud to him so he tends to speak softly. The same bone conduction mechanism exaggerates the sounds of chewing, so the patient may hear poorly at the dinner table, feel shut out from family chatter, and tire of asking members to repeat what they have said. As the

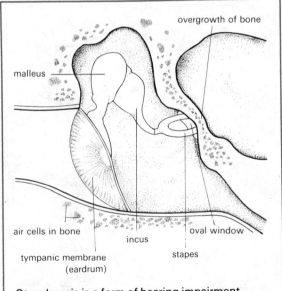

overgrowth of bone

malleus

air cells in bone

incus

oval window

stapes

tympanic membrane (eardrum)

Otosclerosis is a form of hearing impairment caused by overgrowth of bone which prevents the footplate of the stapes from vibrating freely to the fluid beyond.

condition worsens the patient tends to become more withdrawn and secluded. The deafness of otosclerosis can usually be corrected with hearing aids. It is also the one common form of impaired hearing that is possible to correct by surgery. Candidates for surgery must be carefully evaluated and selected. Little benefit can be expected, for instance, if there is associated sensorineural deafness.

Operations are now available which aim to restore the conduction of sound by removing the fixed stapes (stapedectomy), opening the oval window, and inserting an artificial stapes attaching it to the incus and sealing it into the oval window, allowing free movement once more. This is successful in as many as 90 per cent of cases. In an earlier type of operation, hearing was restored, though not completely so, by making a new window to the inner ear (fenestration). The stapedectomy operation is not simple and requires great skill. It has been made possible only by the introduction of the binocular operating microscope enabling the surgeon to see the area with magnification from six to 40 times the normal size. He has to operate in an area the size of a pea containing the very delicate hearing mechanisms.

Inner ear and sensorineural or perceptive deafness

A perceptive deafness may be sensory or neural or combined as sensorineural. Its causes may be congenital or due to injury, such as concussion or fractured skull, or to excessive noise as in boiler-maker's or gunner's deafness, to poisons or virus infections affecting the organ of Corti or the nerves going to the brain. Quinine, nicotine, and some antibiotics such as streptomycin, neomycin, and gentamicin may cause damage in this way. Infections causing general inflammation of the labyrinth may result from the spread of infection from the middle ear directly to the inner ear, damaging or destroying both the hearing and the balancing mechanisms and causing giddiness as well as deafness and tinnitus. Some toxic agents affect only the organ of hearing, causing deafness, some affect only the semicircular canals and vestibule, causing vertigo, while others involve both of these organs. In newborn children, Rhesus blood incompatibility, jaundice, or complications of labour are often associated with inner ear defects. The inner ear, unlike the middle ear, has little power of recovery and regeneration, so that deafness in such patients is often incurable.

Tinnitus (head noises)

Some sounds which do not originate from ordinary sound waves but are nevertheless heard may be imaginary, but usually they are real and quite distressing to the person who hears them. Such sounds, heard by the patient but not by others, are called tinnitus – ringing, roaring, clicking, or hissing sounds in the ears. Strictly speaking, tinnitus is not a disease of the ear, but is a feature of various ear diseases. It may occur in the absence of any demonstrable disease. For instance, a person with a perforated eardrum may experience tinnitus until the drum heals. Tinnitus is a common symptom of otosclerosis and many other middle ear conditions or infections, and persons with impaired hearing often complain of it. But tinnitus can arise anywhere along the nervous pathways of hearing and the tissues serving them, and it is exceedingly difficult, and often impossible, to pinpoint the site of trouble.

Sometimes head noises can be cured by simply removing hard masses of wax from the ears. Other local causes may be found. Clicking and ticking noises may be produced by contraction of small muscles, or in the Eustachian tube by sticky mucoid material which can snap like a rubber band when the tube opens and closes. Drugs such as quinine and aspirin, and abuses of alcohol and tobacco, may cause tinnitus. Various treatments are used to remove the local causes of head noises – medicines to reduce mucoid secretions, unblock the tubes, control allergies, or remove fluids from the middle ear. Often specific causes of head noises cannot be found, but a search should always be made. Frequently, the symptom accompanies ear disorders which themselves require treatment. Head noises sometimes disappear spontaneously or after various forms of treatment, none of which is successful in all instances. Tinnitus associated with hardening of small blood vessels in the auditory system is likely to be permanent.

Vertigo and dizziness, deafness and tinnitus (Menière's syndrome)

There are many causes of dizziness or vertigo which may arise from disorders of the end organ (semicircular canals and otoliths) or from the vestibular nerve and tracts and centres in the brain. In young people, viral infections can cause severe giddiness which usually settles in a few days. In the middle-aged and elderly they may be attacks of obscure origin. One disorder of the labyrinth which affects both cochlear and vestibular systems, is known as Menière's syndrome or disease, after the French physician who described it. It is not uncommon in middle age. It is now known to be related to a distension of the inner membranous chamber of the bony labyrinth. There are three classic symptoms – deafness, head noises, and attacks of vertigo. The vertigo is often accompanied by nausea and even vomiting and the attacks last from a few minutes to a number of hours. Expert evaluation is important and special tests required to assess the interference with the functions of the cochlear and vestibular systems. The cause is unknown, but appears to be related in some cases to migraine. Usually one side only is affected, but both ears may be involved. Various medical treatments are based on different theories as to the causes of the disorder. Among these measures are diuretic drugs and low-salt diets, to reduce swollen fluid pressures in the inner ear; motion-sickness and antihistamine drugs; sedatives and blood vessel dilators. One or other measure may be successful in an individual patient, but no single measure is successful in all cases. If medical measures fail and the disability is severe, the endolymph system may be drained by major surgery behind the ear, or the vestibular system selectively destroyed by ultra-sound or by cutting some fibres of the vestibular nerve, thus retaining some hearing. If there is no useful hearing, the whole inner ear can be destroyed, or both nerves cut by surgery through the ear and mastoid. The remaining labyrinth can then work alone without interference from the diseased side.

Hearing aids

When hearing impairment cannot be restored a hearing aid is often of great value. Well-fitted modern hearing aids could benefit more hard of hearing people than they actually do. There may be several reasons why a hearing aid is never tried or is kept unused in a drawer. Often the affected person does not want to admit that he does not hear well, and is reluctant to advertise it by wearing an instrument that he fears is conspicuous. He may buy a hearing aid of sorts because someone in the family insists on it, but will wear the instrument only under duress. A poorly fitted aid may not actually improve his hearing, so he cannot be blamed for not using it. But even an excellent aid may seem bad to him because he has forgotten what sounds are like and so has difficulty at first in interpreting many overlapping noises.

Modern hearing aids are remarkable and extremely compact electronic devices. Essentially, they are amplifying devices that make sounds louder. However, if the wrong sound frequencies are intensified and the right ones are not, the results will be anything but ideal. Hence there is no such thing as a hearing aid that is perfect for everybody. Selection, and assurance that the aid is working properly after it has been tried for a while, require the counsel of a specialist who knows all about a particular patient's trouble. In buying a hearing aid, it is important to deal with a responsible company servicing the product of a responsible manufacturer.

Hearing aids are usually of great benefit in simple conduction deafness. Air-conduction types are worn in the ear, bone-conduction types in contact with bone. The otologist will advise which is better in a given instance. There are ingenious ways of making the devices inconspicuous, such as incorporating the mechanism into the side frames of eyeglasses. Girls are said to prefer devices which are worn in the ear, which permits them to remove their glasses for the sake of appearance when out in society. Often, one ear is better than the other and an aid need be worn only in one ear, the poorer one. But sometimes the opposite is the case, and hearing is better and sounds are more natural if devices are worn in both ears.

Sensorineural deafness, with or without conduction deafness, makes the selection of the proper hearing aid more critical. Frequently, the patient hears certain sound frequencies quite well and others poorly. It is as if groups of keys of a piano keyboard were muffled so there would be gaps in a composition played on it. A suitable hearing aid should fill in the gaps and not magnify sounds that are already loud enough.

Sometimes, even with an excellent and well-fitted aid, sudden return of long-forgotten sounds may disturb the wearer temporarily. Patience and a period of relearning may be necessary (as when a person first puts on bifocal glasses) until it becomes comfortable to wear the aid. In extreme cases, hearing may have been impaired so long that some training in recognizing the sounds of speech is necessary. The combination of an appropriate hearing aid and the explanation, counsel, and assistance of an otologist can often reopen a wonderful world of sound.

The nose, sinuses, and throat

The nose and throat together with the mouth comprise the upper respiratory (breathing) and upper digestive (alimentary) tracts. Apart from acting as a simple passage for the air we breathe, the nose is an air-conditioning and filtering organ and also contains the organ for the special sense of smell. The mouth, in addition to its functions for ingestion and mastication of solid food and for taking liquid food, is also the site of the organ of taste as well as being a supplementary airway. In the pharynx or throat, air and food are separated and directed selectively into different channels. Air is directed into the windpipe (trachea) by the voice box (larynx) while food is directed behind and on either side of the larynx into the gullet (oesophagus).

The external nose

The external nose guards the openings of the vital air passages and by means of the small muscles in the wings of the nostrils slightly controls the volume of air entering the system. It also protects the very delicate organ of smell. Because of its exposed position it is susceptible to injury.

Only the upper part of the nose is underlaid with bones. There are two of them, one on each side of the midline. The bones help to form the bridge of the nose, which supports the nosepieces of glasses. The skin in this area is quite thin and the outline of the underlying bones can be felt easily by a fingertip. The framework of parts in front of the bone, including the tip of the nose and flares around the nostrils, is mostly built of tough cartilage, with some small muscles and fatty cushioning, covered with skin. Between the two nostrils is a fleshy part, called the columella, which feels soft if pressed between the fingers. Immediately behind it is a flexible but harder structure, the septum, which runs between the two nostrils to the floor of the skull at the back of the nasal cavity. The septum is largely cartilage but has a bony segment farther back. The septum is a wall which divides the nose into two chambers, a right and left cavity, each served by its own nostril. Most of the structures of the nose are paired so, for purposes of discussion, a description of one is a description of its partner.

Injuries of the external nose are quite common. The nose is part of the bony structures that surround and protect the eyes, and there may be some consolation in reflecting that some injuries are better absorbed by the nose than by the delicate eyeball. Damage to the nose should have the prompt attention of a doctor, for even injuries that seem slight and heal without much trouble may result in distortions of parts, leading to discomfort in breathing and sometimes to mouth breathing.

The nasal cavity

The main cavity of the nose lies between the floor of the brain cavity and the roof of the mouth. On the outer sidewall are three scroll-shaped bones called turbinates, which are covered by soft spongy tissue

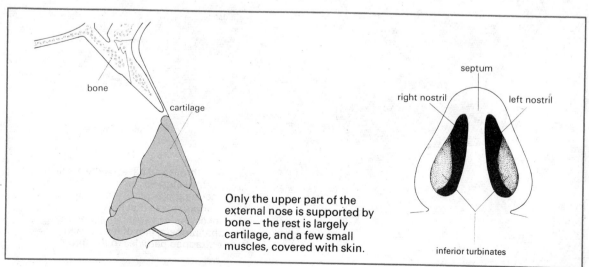

bone

cartilage

Only the upper part of the external nose is supported by bone – the rest is largely cartilage, and a few small muscles, covered with skin.

septum

right nostril

left nostril

inferior turbinates

with a rich blood supply. These shelflike projections enlarge the surface with which air is in contact on its way to the lungs. Their air-conditioning efficiency is remarkable. Incoming air picks up moisture from surrounding moist membranes; at the same time the air is almost instantly warmed to the temperature of the lining membrane which is usually 3° to 4° C (5° to 7°F) below normal blood heat, 37°C (98·4°F). These air-conditioning benefits are largely lost by mouth breathing.

The membranes that line the nasal passage secrete mucus and fluids continuously. Dry membranes are not only uncomfortable, but dryness impairs important protective functions of the nose, hence the desirability of adding moisture to room air, which tends to become excessively dry when homes are heated in the winter. Nasal secretions have two main functions – to humidify air as it is breathed in, and to help keep the nose clean.

The outer thirteen mm ($\frac{1}{2}$ in) of the passage where the hairs are sited is lined with skin and not a mucus-secreting membrane. On this skin staphylococcal bacteria are frequently found in normal people. Coarse hairs inside the nostrils, called vibrissae (the same name is given to cats' whiskers) filter relatively coarse particles from inhaled air, and finer hairs trap many smaller particles, as is obvious from the nasal secretion produced after one has been working in dusty or smoky surroundings.

The sticky mucus of the internal nose traps fine particles and many bacteria, and moves them to the junction of the nasal cavity and throat (nasopharynx) by means of tiny whiplike structures called cilia that cover the mucous membrane. The cilia keep the film of mucus and entrapped particles flowing towards the back of the nose with beating, sweeping movements. Normally the secretions are unconsciously swallowed and disposed of harmlessly in the stomach. The bacteria are destroyed by stomach juices. Nasal secretions also contain an antibacterial substance, lysozyme, from the tears, which run into the nose. Lysozyme acts against the more common forms of bacteria inhaled with the air.

It takes half an hour for particles entangled in the mucous sheet to reach the nasopharynx. In this time the relatively large bacteria cannot usually penetrate to invade the underlying membrane. If a patch becomes dried, however, the cilia are paralysed, the mucous sheet is arrested, and the bacteria infect the membrane. On the other hand, viruses are such minute bodies that they can penetrate easily even through an intact moving sheet of mucus. The deeper

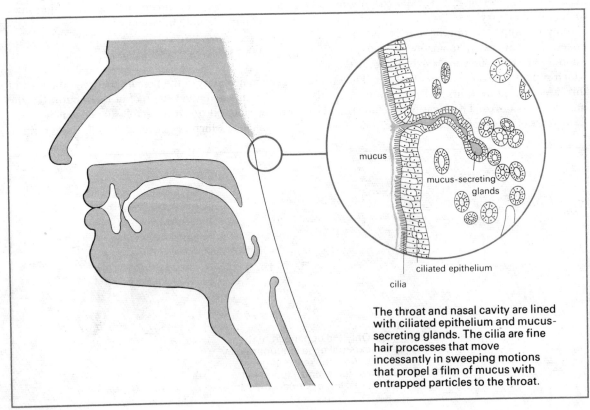

mucus

mucus-secreting glands

ciliated epithelium

cilia

The throat and nasal cavity are lined with ciliated epithelium and mucus-secreting glands. The cilia are fine hair processes that move incessantly in sweeping motions that propel a film of mucus with entrapped particles to the throat.

areas of the nasal membrane are normally sterile and no bacteria can be cultured from them, except during the course of a common cold or certain other infections.

The tissue of the lowest turbinates is erectile – that is, in certain circumstances it becomes engorged with blood and swells up. This also provides some heat regulation. When engorged more heat is lost from the body, and hence in a hot room the nose becomes stuffy, while a walk in cold air shrinks the engorged turbinates to decrease the heat loss, and thus improves the airway.

When the nose is infected by viruses and bacteria, there is general engorgement of the nasal mucous membrane, with excessive outpouring of mucus and fluid and the airway may become completely blocked. If the secretions are too copious or sticky, the normal movement of the cilia-driven mucous sheet cannot cope and the nose must be cleared by sniffing and hawking or blowing. The correct way to blow the nose is to hold a tissue in front loosely, press the side of one nostril to the septum and blow out the nasal contents from the opposite side. The second side is then blown clear in a similar manner. Do not close both sides simultaneously, or infected mucus may be forced up the Eustachian tube and infect the ear, or in through a sinus opening to infect the sinus cavity.

Sneezing This is usually due to irritation of the lining of the nose by some dust or chemical, but sometimes it indicates allergic trouble (see below) or the beginning of a common cold.

Postnasal drip This is the normal route for the clearance of nasal secretion, but we should not be conscious of it happening. However, if it becomes excessive and unpleasant there is coughing and clearing of the throat, and some people ease their embarrassment by attributing matters to an affliction popularly known as postnasal drip. We all have some back-of-the-nose drainage of which we are normally unaware. However, a patient may be excessively aware of a drainage system that is not abnormal.

Causes of exaggerated postnasal drip include simple colds and infections, allergies, obstructions, irritation of the membranes by smoke, dust, or fumes, emotional disturbances, and excessive and prolonged self-medication with various nose medicines.

Excessive postnasal drip is a symptom which, unless caused by something so obvious as a cold, should be investigated to determine and remove the causes if possible. Very often the patient is constantly aware of and worried about a condition that is not serious, and needs reassurance that postnasal drip,

though unpleasant, is harmless. Some persons are so aware of an irritation that causes them to cough or clear their throats frequently that they fear they have cancer. Assuring them that they have a simple postnasal drip removes this worry.

One can do several things to minimize postnasal drip. Overheating and poor ventilation in winter result in low humidity and drying of the nasal membranes. Secretions tend to become thicker, are not carried off normally, and droplets fall into the back of the throat. Vaporizers or devices which add moisture to overheated dry air help to keep the nasal membranes normal. Sleeping with a high pillow instead of a low flat one, often helps to reduce postnasal drip. Some people have a persistent habit of sniffing secretions back into the throat. This actually stimulates the nasal glands to produce more secretion. Sometimes, this can be stopped by simply telling the patient to blow his nose instead, though violent blowing congests the nose.

Nasal allergies At least ten per cent of the population have some degree of nasal allergy (that is, altered reactivity). The symptoms are well known and include sudden attacks of nasal irritation, sneezing, obstruction, and clear watery discharge. Nasal allergies are usually due to inhaled particles, but sometimes certain foods are responsible. Even change of temperature or emotional stimuli can start an attack of this type.

Nasal obstruction The commonest cause is infection with the common cold. At least 80 different viruses causing colds have been identified. Allergy is another very common cause. Both these conditions are usually transient. Chronic or persistent obstruction is commonly due to a bending of the nasal septum or the presence of nasal polyps, or persistent swelling of the turbinates due to lingering sinus infection. In children, the common cause of persistent nasal obstruction is enlarged adenoids. These fleshy masses of lymphoid tissue are found in the roof of the postnasal space, just behind the nose and above the soft palate. They usually diminish after puberty. Their surgical removal is one of the commonest and most satisfactory of all operations.

Young children sometimes place beads or other small objects up the nose. Removal of the obstruction should be performed by a doctor, and not by parents.

Deviated nasal septum The septum, or wall, that divides the nose into two equal parts, normally extends in a straight line from the front between the two nostrils to the floor of the skull at the back, but it is not at all uncommon for the septum to deviate from a straight line. A deviated septum may be congenital, but is more often caused by blows, injuries in contact sports such as soccer or rugby, and crushing fractures suffered in automobile and other accidents.

A crooked deviated septum may not be apparent on the outside. Its effects vary with the nature of the deformity. The air passages may be partly or wholly stopped up, making breathing difficult. If mouth breathing results, inhaled air is not cleaned, warmed, and moistened as it would be by normal passage through the nose. Air currents in the nose may be slowed or deflected so that sinus outlets do not have the benefits of air passing over them, an action which normally helps to drain their secretions. These deformities deflect the air currents and may cause excessive drying and predispose to infections. To correct deformities of the septum it is often necessary to cut out the bent portion so the rest may fall into a straight line. The operation is done inside the nose and does not leave any external scar.

Nasal polyps   Persons with allergies are especially likely to have nasal polyps – soft, moist, pendulous growths from mucous membranes which line the nose. Whether the underlying cause is an allergic reaction, some inflammatory process in the membranes, or both, is not positively known. Common nasal polyps may be small and numerous or large and single. The usual symptom of their presence is obstruction of the nasal airway on one or both sides. Severe obstruction encourages mouth breathing, with undesirable consequences. Obstructive polyps should be removed. Common nasal polyps are almost always benign, that is, not cancerous, and a pathologist's confirmation of this from examination of removed tissue is reassuring.

The nasal sinuses

The nasal sinuses are a series of air spaces which nearly surround the nasal cavity within the skull. They make the skull lighter than if the bone were solid; possibly they serve as honeycomb insulators of the nearby brain cage, perhaps limit the excursion of local fractures, and give resonance to the voice. In animals with a highly developed sense of smell, they form part of the large olfactory organ. But the nasal sinuses are not essential to life. A few people, who may never know it, lack certain sinuses, but this does no harm and may even do good; they cannot get sinusitis in those areas.

The sinuses are normally paired, one on either side of the midline of the face. These empty irregular air spaces are surrounded by thin bony walls, and are lined with mucous membrane which is like that of the interior of the nose and is continuous with it. Secretions of the sinuses normally drain through small passages into the nasal cavity. In ordinary circumstances, the interiors of the sinuses are free of germs, but it is possible for germs to enter from the nasal cavity and cause infection, or for obstructed outlets to dam up secretions, or for other variants of what is loosely called sinus trouble to arise.

There are four major pairs of sinuses – the frontal sinuses in the forehead, the maxillary sinuses in the cheeks, and the ethmoidal and sphenoidal sinuses at the side and back of the nose.

Sinus trouble   Sinusitis is due to infection with viruses or bacteria and is nearly always the result of direct infection from the nose through the sinus drainage openings (ostia). The sinuses are lined by a thin membrane secreting watery mucus which is wafted into the nose through the ostia by whiplike cilia growing from the lining cells similar to those in the nose itself. The ostia are small and may easily become blocked by thick plugs of mucus or by simple inflammatory swelling. The sinuses become infected during a cold only if the organism is very virulent or there is some predisposing mechanical obstruction or allergy, or if the patient's resistance is lowered by such factors as chill, fatigue, and general ill health.

Acute sinusitis   That such an event has occurred is suggested by acute pain, fullness and tenderness over the nasal sinuses, a raised temperature, and general malaise. The pain is characteristically worse during the morning and at midday and declines during the evening. The activity of the nasal sinus membranes is greatest in the morning and they are relatively quiescent and inactive at night during sleep. After the sinus opening has been unblocked, a copious discharge of pus comes from the affected side of the nose and the pain is relieved.

Chronic sinusitis   If the infection persists in a sinus after the acute attack appears to have passed, there will be a persistent discharge from the nose in front or at the back, together with stuffiness of the nasal airway, due to swelling of the mucous membranes from infected pus draining over them. Frequent colds may follow, as the resistance to viruses is depressed. The final diagnosis depends on the appearance in an X-ray. The immediate concern in treatment is to provide free drainage for sinus secretions. In general, simplest measures are tried first, such as steam inhalations and nose drops which constrict the tissues and unblock the obstructed openings. Antihistamine

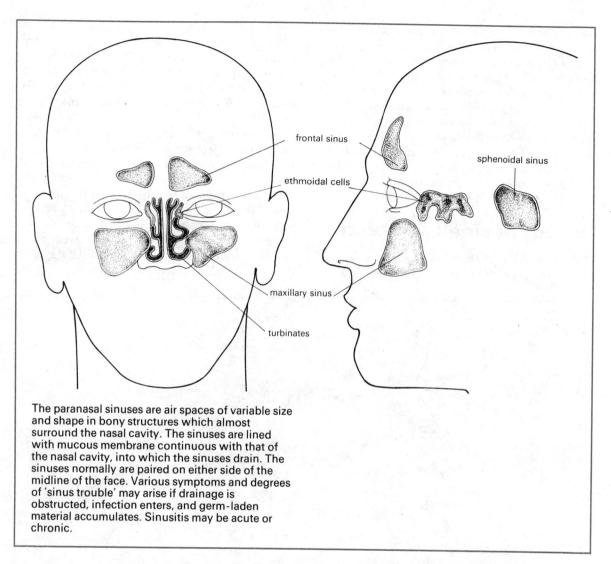

frontal sinus

ethmoidal cells

sphenoidal sinus

maxillary sinus

turbinates

The paranasal sinuses are air spaces of variable size and shape in bony structures which almost surround the nasal cavity. The sinuses are lined with mucous membrane continuous with that of the nasal cavity, into which the sinuses drain. The sinuses normally are paired on either side of the midline of the face. Various symptoms and degrees of 'sinus trouble' may arise if drainage is obstructed, infection enters, and germ-laden material accumulates. Sinusitis may be acute or chronic.

drugs may help if there is a history of allergy. If there is fever or evidence of extension of infection, antibiotics may be used. Occasionally, irrigation of the sinus with a saline solution is helpful in the chronic stage, but it is rarely necessary. Correction of conditions which lead to chronic sinusitis is usually undertaken after the acute stage is over.

Sinusitis in children There are about as many runny noses in children as there are noses. Generally the running subsides uneventfully, but sinusitis may occasionally result from neglect. Simple measures are worth applying to any child whose nasal discharge persists for more than ten days. Warm packs and steam humidification help to ventilate the sinuses so that drainage can take place. Warm packs can be prepared by soaking thick cloths in hot water and wringing them out, taking care that the pack is not too hot to be applied to the skin. A vaporizer which delivers large amounts of warm steam is a good investment. Homemade measures of delivering steam are valuable too, but care must be taken to make sure that there is no danger of direct contact with a hot vessel or with scalding vapour that can cause serious burns. Antibiotics will be needed to cut short such attacks. If recurrences occur or nasal obstruction persists, examination should be made of the postnasal space for enlarged infected adenoids, and for these surgery may be required. The sinuses may require irrigation at the same time.

Nasal sprays Medicines that are sprayed, inhaled, or dropped into the nose can be very effective in shrinking swollen membranes, but the drugs are quite potent and it is important to follow carefully a doctor's directions for their use. For instance, doses should not be taken too close together. This is apt in time to cause rebound congestion which makes matters worse and invites more frequent and more closely spaced doses. Overuse or unnecessary use of medicinal sprays can also cause postnasal drip, by forcing secretions backwards into the throat. Nose drops with oily bases should always be avoided. Fine droplets may be inhaled into the lungs, especially by infants, and oils which cannot be absorbed by tissues can cause a stubborn form of respiratory tract disease known as lipoid pneumonia.

Organs of smell and taste

Early mammals were shrewlike creatures with noses close to the ground. The sense of smell, in pursuing food and detecting dangers, was vital to the survival of many primitive types, and it is still very important to most creatures, with the notable exception of man. Our smell apparatus is greatly inferior to that of dogs, but good enough to warn us of a gas leak or decayed food, and to sustain a considerable market for perfumes and deodorants.

Our smell receptors are located in a small patch of tissue, about thirteen mm ($\frac{1}{2}$ in) square located at the very top of the nasal cavity. The patch has a yellowish tinge, in contrast to the surrounding pink tissue, and it consists of several million tiny endings of the olfactory nerve whose bundles pass through the cribriform plate (literally, perforated like a sieve) and enter the elongated olfactory bulb of the brain, lying on it. From there the olfactory nerve carries the signals to the rhinencephalon (nose brain) in the centre of the

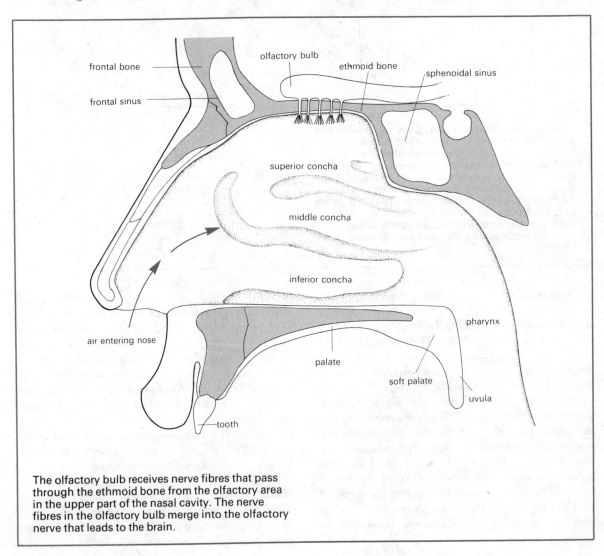

The olfactory bulb receives nerve fibres that pass through the ethmoid bone from the olfactory area in the upper part of the nasal cavity. The nerve fibres in the olfactory bulb merge into the olfactory nerve that leads to the brain.

base of the brain, where smells are recognized and analysed. A substance can be smelt only if its molecules can be drawn into the nose and dissolved in the secretions of special cells found only in the olfactory area of the nose. Therefore only relatively volatile substances can be sensed. Inspired air currents are directed upwards as well as horizontally backwards through the nose. Expired air currents are directed along the lower half of the nasal airway. The act of sniffing carries the odoriferous particles forcibly up to the olfactory organ. The sense of smell tires quite rapidly for one particular smell. Upon entering a room in which some strong odour is present, we are at first very much aware of it, but in a little while we almost cease to perceive it. There are subtle differences in people's abilities to detect different odours. Substances which have definite odour to some people may be odourless to others. These are normal variations; the rare inability to smell anything at all (anosmia) is abnormal but of itself carries no threat to health or life. Except, of course, when the smell of a gas leak or smoke is a warning to take urgent action.

Much of what we think we taste, we smell. Anybody who has a heavy cold notices that flavoured foods of many kinds seem bland and tasteless, but the taste organs are not affected. What happens is that congestion prevents air-swirls, created by chewing and swallowing, from reaching the smell-patch high in the nasal cavity. Taste buds, which are cells that are chemical receptors of taste sensations, are located in the tongue, but are not spread about evenly. Taste buds are not the minute pimples or papillae we see when we look at the tongue, but flask-shaped structures in the walls of the papillae. There are about 250 taste buds per papilla, diminishing to 90 in old age. Unlike

the sense of smell, which is so complex that no system of classifying stimuli has been successful, taste is compounded of only four sensations, bitter, salt, sweet, and sour. A particular taste bud is sensitive to only one of these. The four kinds of taste receptors are concentrated in different regions of the tongue. There is also some decrease of taste bud sensitivities with increasing age, which may explain why a wife's pie does not taste like the pie that mother used to bake.

The senses of smell and taste are chemical senses. What is perceived in the brain as an odour or flavour is the presence of certain molecules in fluids that are in contact with the receptor organs of smell and taste. Thus there is some direct contact with whatever we smell or taste. A bone-dry nose or tongue would be unable to smell or taste anything. Chemicals have to be dissolved in local mucus or fluids to become tastable or smellable, but in the case of some substances, such as mercaptan (exuded by skunks) a very few molecules are quite enough to produce a disagreeable smell. In human beings the rhinencephalon is very small and is quite overwhelmed by the massive cerebrum, but it is relatively large in many animals and reptiles that depend a great deal on the sense of smell to tell them what is going on in their environment. Dogs, for instance, can obviously see and hear, but they depend a great deal on their noses for reliable information and undoubtedly can smell things we cannot. Badgers can smell a nest of rabbits 50 cm (twenty in) below ground.

Although each taste bud is capable of registering only a single sensation – sour, salt, sweet, or bitter – all taste buds look alike under the microscope. How an individual taste bud can be so exclusively discriminating is not known, but it is probably a matter of

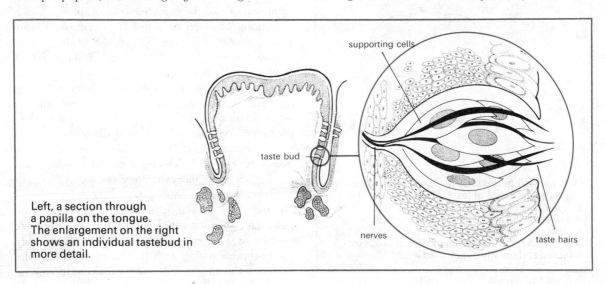

Left, a section through a papilla on the tongue. The enlargement on the right shows an individual tastebud in more detail.

supporting cells

taste bud

nerves

taste hairs

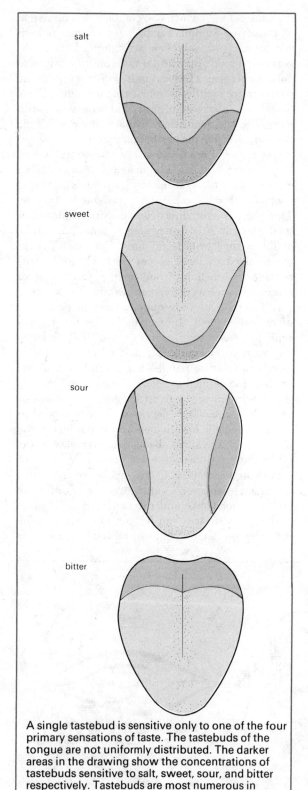

salt

sweet

sour

bitter

A single tastebud is sensitive only to one of the four
primary sensations of taste. The tastebuds of the
tongue are not uniformly distributed. The darker
areas in the drawing show the concentrations of
tastebuds sensitive to salt, sweet, sour, and bitter
respectively. Tastebuds are most numerous in
children and greatly diminished in old age.

different enzymes produced in the different buds. We
taste (or gourmets think they do) countless subtle
flavours, but all are compounded of the four basic
sensations, greatly enhanced and subtly refined by
the sense of smell.

Plastic surgery of the nose (rhinoplasty)

Many deformities of the nose do not interfere
seriously, if at all, with the health of the owner. Some
deformities are conspicuous, but many are departures
from some ideal or desired shape of the nose rather
than true deformities. Probably few human beings
are completely satisfied with the shapes of their noses.
A competent plastic surgeon can correct gross
deformities of the nose well enough to revolutionize
the lives of persons who have felt the shape of their
nose to be a handicap. He can also resculpt noses so
slightly misshapen that hardly anyone notices them
except the owner, who may be unhappy and
depressed about a nose that dominates the face.

Surgery for cosmetic purposes needs no justification. At the same time, there are a few persons who
feel that the entire course of their lives would be
miraculously changed for the better if their noses were
straightened, shortened, or otherwise modified. Since
even a perfect result cannot guarantee romantic,
social, and vocational conquests, a surgeon sometimes
rejects a neurotic patient who clearly expects
unreasonable miracles from correction of a cosmetic
defect so trifling as to be virtually unnoticeable. With
models, sketches, photographs, physical examination, and measurements, the surgeon explains what
an operation may be expected to accomplish.

A quite common objective is to remove a bony
hump, shorten the nose, narrow the bridge, lift or
narrow the nasal tip, in varying combinations. A
bony hump (a small hump is more difficult for the
surgeon than a large one) is cut down from within the
nose and excess tissue removed. At the same time the
bridge of the nose must be narrowed to accommodate
the new shape. Pieces of bone or cartilage may be used
like sculpting materials. The nose tip may droop or
overhang too much. The tip is mostly cartilage and
can be shortened, narrowed, or given a pert tilt.

The operation requires a stay of about a week in a
hospital, and probably another week before the
patient feels like returning to the daily routine of work
and living. For one thing, the operation inevitably
leaves some swelling and discoloration around the
eyes, and the patient temporarily looks as though he

has been in a fight. In about six days the patient goes home from the hospital, but returns to see the surgeon for aftercare until dressings are removed around the twelfth day. On the whole, it is best to plan for a fortnight's "holiday".

Other plastic procedures, such as correction of saddle-block deformity (conspicuous depression of the bridge of the nose) require addition rather than subtraction of tissue and involve extensive grafting, sometimes even as extensive as providing a new nose in cases where the organ has been largely destroyed by disease or injury.

The mouth and throat

The mouth, opened wide as for a dentist, is easily inspected with the aid of a mirror. The hard palate, or roof of the mouth, merges with the soft palate at a point which can be felt with the tip of the tongue. A small peninsula of tissue, the uvula, hangs down from the soft palate into the throat. These soft structures can be set in vibration by air passing over them during sleep, producing the phenomenon of snoring, which frequently causes a good deal of distress to other persons but never to the snorer.

The tonsils can usually be seen as oval, flattened bodies on either side of the passageway into the throat. Their exposed surfaces are covered with mucous membrane in which there are a number of small pits that open into saclike cavities called crypts or follicles. The deep unexposed surface of the tonsil is covered by a fibrous capsule which attaches the tonsil to the muscular wall. This arrangement makes its surgical removal relatively easy. By cutting through the mucous membrane, it can be shelled out.

Tonsils and adenoids   The tonsils and adenoids are normal accretions of lymphoid tissue in the form of a ring around the air and food passages at the level of the roof of the postnasal space and the back of the mouth. They serve the purpose of a first line of defence against organisms invading the body by these routes. As such, they have an important part to play, particularly in the early years of life when the infant is acquiring antibodies and immunity to the viral and bacterial infections in its immediate surroundings. When children first go to school, they are exposed to infections which they have not met before. It is common for the tonsils to enlarge between the ages of three and seven for this reason, and they usually return to normal size. For reasons which we do not entirely understand, they may become overwhelmed with infection owing to their spongelike conformation

and the crypts and channels which penetrate deep into their substance. If they become grossly enlarged in response to these infections, they may cause mechanical trouble by obstructing the airways, or the openings of the Eustachian tubes. They may also become the site of lingering infection. When this stage is reached, there is a danger that they may harbour organisms which can flare up and cause recurrent acute attacks of inflammation whenever resistance becomes lowered. If all medical measures fail to eliminate these infections and to reduce the size to a safe degree, surgical removal has to be considered. Great care must be taken in the final assessment, requiring experience and clinical judgment, but the results are most rewarding.

Throat   For descriptive purposes, the pharynx, or throat, is divided into upper, middle, and lower regions. It is, in fact, a membrane-lined muscular tube which is continuous with the back of the nasal cavity, where it forms a blind pouch and turns downwards to merge with the voice box (larynx) and gullet (oesophagus).

A special structure in the upper part of the larynx contains delicate folds of elastic tissue separated by a narrow slit. These folds are the vocal cords, which

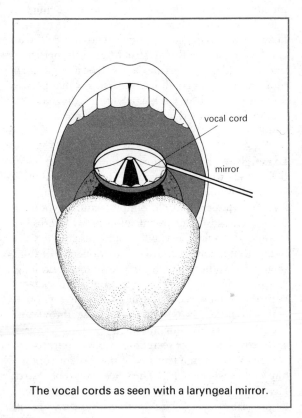

The vocal cords as seen with a laryngeal mirror.

stand out from the walls rather like shelves. Muscles control the tension and so the rate of vibration of the cords as air passes through them, modifying the sounds of the voice. This part of the larynx is called the glottis and is closed to protect the lungs during swallowing.

Just behind the opening into the larynx, and continuous with the back wall of the throat, is the upper end of the oesophagus which connects the throat with the stomach. Both air and food travel through the pharynx, but it is vital that food be kept out of the windpipe and lungs. Nature takes care of this automatically – except when we "swallow something the wrong way" and choke and splutter until we get rid of it – by an ingenious lid or trapdoor, the epiglottis. This tonguelike structure in the upper rim of the larynx opens as we breathe, and permits air to enter the windpipe, but when we swallow, food passes over it into the nearby oesophagus without falling into the larynx. Swallowing is accomplished not by gravity but by muscles. We can swallow quite as efficiently if we hang upside down.

The larynx

Hoarseness   Hoarseness is a symptom which may mean no more than that one has shouted too much at a football match. Most often the cause of temporary hoarseness is simple and obvious, such as a cold with congestion of the throat structures, but persistent unexplained hoarseness may at times be a symptom of some more serious condition. Hoarseness that persists for longer than three weeks is a warning that a doctor should be consulted without fail to determine the cause.

Laryngitis   Inflammation of the larynx or voice box is known as laryngitis. The predominating symptom is unmistakable. The patient cannot speak above a whisper, if at all. Simple acute laryngitis is usually caused either by infection or by overuse or strain of the voice. Laryngitis from abuse of the voice is an occupational hazard of auctioneers, orators, singers, and others who use the voice loud and long. The other form of simple acute laryngitis is associated with the common cold and has the same sort of re-action in the larynx as occurs in the nose, throat, and bronchi in a cold – inflammation, swelling, redness, and increased flow of secretions. Complete recovery can be expected in a few days if the patient confines himself to a whisper only. The voice should be rested. Heat and inhalations, drugs, or other measures may be prescribed by a doctor as circumstances warrant.

Smoking and dusty atmospheres are irritating to the injured larynx and should be avoided if possible.

Chronic forms of laryngitis which recur frequently without respiratory infection or voice strain have the same symptom, hoarseness, but a variety of possible causes. Loss of the voice may occur without physical disease of any nature of the larynx, as from hysterical states, remote affection of nerves serving the voice, or some other disease not localized in the larynx.

Benign tumours   Benign tumours of the larynx are not uncommon. They may be polyps, cysts, or fibrous growths. Nodules may form where abused vocal cords strike too vigorously together. These are not unlike corns or callouses produced by pressure and friction, and at times become ulcerated. Surgical removal of benign tumours may sometimes be necessary and results are usually excellent. The application of the binocular operating microscope to this surgery in recent years has now added great accuracy.

Cancer of the larynx   Cancer of the larynx is not rare. It accounts for about two per cent of malignant disease. Early cancer of the throat causes little more than a slight huskiness of the voice; no pain, no bleeding, no loss of feelings of wellbeing. Hoarseness may be the only symptom indicating cancer of the larynx at an early stage when it is most curable. All diseases of the larynx produce the characteristic symptom of hoarseness. If you are hoarse, there are two important things to remember: whisper, and see your doctor.

Bad breath

Most often the cause of bad breath will be found in the mouth or upper respiratory tract. Decaying teeth and unhealthy gums are common causes. Longstanding mouth breathing due to nasal blockage may cause offensive breath by drying out normal secretions and facilitating the entrance of microbes. Infection in the nasal cavity can cause bad breath. Chronic low-grade inflammations of the nose and upper throat can lead to loss of normal ciliary action with unpleasant breath odour. In such cases bad breath can be stopped only by locating and correcting the underlying condition. Rinsing the mouth with a solution of a teaspoonful of salt mixed in a glass of water is a simple hygienic measure. There are some people who have a quite unwarranted obsession about bad breath and some who are not aware that their breath is so unpleasant.

Hare lip and cleft palate

When a child is born with this malformation the parents may ask "Why did this happen to us?", and often develop guilty feelings that they are somehow responsible because of something done or left undone during pregnancy. They can be reassured that they are not guilty of omitting some specific measure for preventing this abnormality, since no such measure is known. It is conceivable that some infection or injury of the mother around the sixth to eighth week of pregnancy when fetal structures are being formed might have some effect in production of cleft palate, but there is much more evidence which implicates hereditary factors. In many cases, if family histories are traced, it is found that an uncle or cousin or grandparent or someone else on one side of the family or the other had a cleft palate. However, if neither the mother nor the father of a cleft palate baby has a cleft palate, there is about a 95 per cent chance that children subsequently born to them will be born with a normal palate.

Hare lip or cleft palate results from failure of the lip and palate structures to fuse properly during fetal development. There are many variations of the deformity. The lip may be cleft only on one side, or on both sides, and the lower part of the nose may be involved. The defect may involve the soft palate or the hard palate as well, with varying degrees of separation. There may be difficulties in feeding the handicapped baby, because milk easily comes back through the nose, but with patience and special feeding devices this can be overcome.

Correction of the defect requires surgery. Operations may be done in several stages as the child grows older, depending on the surgeon's appraisal of the individual case. Usually the hare lip is repaired quite early, when the baby is in good general condition and gaining weight. The results usually give a needed boost to the morale of the parents, when the unsightly deformity present at birth is dramatically lessened.

Later closure of the cleft palate, which often has to be done in stages, aims to restore structures so that normal speech will be possible. Formation of distinct speech sounds, especially certain consonants, requires complex coordination of muscles and structures of the lips, hard palate, and soft palate, and a proper air pathway so the voice does not escape in an unintelligible way through the nose. Defects of the teeth may appear and dental prostheses may be needed as the child grows older. Speech therapy may be required. Today, the end results of expert care are often excellent.

Parents of a baby with hare lip or cleft palate can be reassured that there is an enormous amount that can be done to help in this condition.

There are several societies concerned with the welfare of sufferers from some of the diseases described in this chapter.

The Royal National Institute for the Deaf,
105 Gower Street,
London WC1E 6AH.

The Swallow Club (for laryngectomy patients),
Royal National Ear, Nose, and Throat Hospital,
Gray's Inn Road,
London WC1.

Chapter 19
Bones and muscles

Revised by A. M. Cooke, DM FRCP

Everybody knows that bones furnish admirable support for the body.

They do more than that. They are busy every instant with vital activities of astonishing variety. They contain blood-forming elements that turn out millions of new red cells every minute. They furnish levers for muscles to pull on to control our movements. They contain cells which maintain, construct, and repair bone, and others that dissolve and sculpt it. They are warehouses which receive mineral salts for deposit and send them out to the rest of the body in never-ending transactions. Bone is one of the most biologically active tissues in the body.

Considering the vicissitudes it surmounts in a lifetime, it is not surprising that bone is liable to certain troubles and that people who never see their skeletons are sometimes made uncomfortably aware of them by discomforts, cricks in the back, dislocations, fractures, and aching feet.

The skeleton

Bone for bone, the human skeleton is very similar to that of other mammals, except that our upright posture and other aspects that make us human have brought about certain modifications. In broad design, we have a major (axial) skeleton and an appendicular skeleton which consists of the limbs. Arms and legs are very convenient but not absolutely essential to life. But the axial skeleton which includes the skull, backbone, and ribs is indispensable.

The spinal column or backbone is built of a series of blocklike bones, called vertebrae, stacked on top of each other. A normal backbone is not straight but has four curvatures. Individual bones of the body are securely bound to each other and to associated structures by tough bands or ligaments. Tendons connect muscles to bones. Cartilage covers the ends of bones, and ensures smooth movement of the joints.

A single vertebra is a flat, roughly drum-shaped bone with backward-projecting knobs (spinous processes) to which muscles are attached. These knobs are what you feel when you run your fingers along the backbone. There is a hole in each vertebra which serves as a protective bony canal for the great nerve trunk, the spinal cord.

Between the vertebrae are pads of elastic cartilage (intervertebral discs) which absorb shocks and permit overlying vertebrae to bend and twist a little without grating upon each other. Cartilage has a certain amount of springiness and give (pinch the top of your ear or the tip of your nose and you pinch cartilage). It is also slightly compressible and the fluid content of discs slightly reducible, so that a person who is on his feet all day may be a little shorter at night than when he got up in the morning.

Skull, ribs, and lower back Doctors have special terms for the curves and areas of the spine, although these structures are continuous. The cervical or neck region has seven vertebrae, the topmost and smallest of which has the job of carrying the head. Below is the thoracic segment of twelve vertebrae which carry the ribs, of which the topmost ten are attached in front to the breastbone. Below these at the back are two other pairs which do not have frontal attachments and hence are called floating ribs. Deviations from the standard pattern of twelve pairs of ribs are not uncommon. Some people have only eleven pairs of ribs and some may have thirteen pairs by possession of an extra pair (cervical ribs) at the top.

Next below the thoracic section is the lumbar area (from which comes the related word, lumbago).

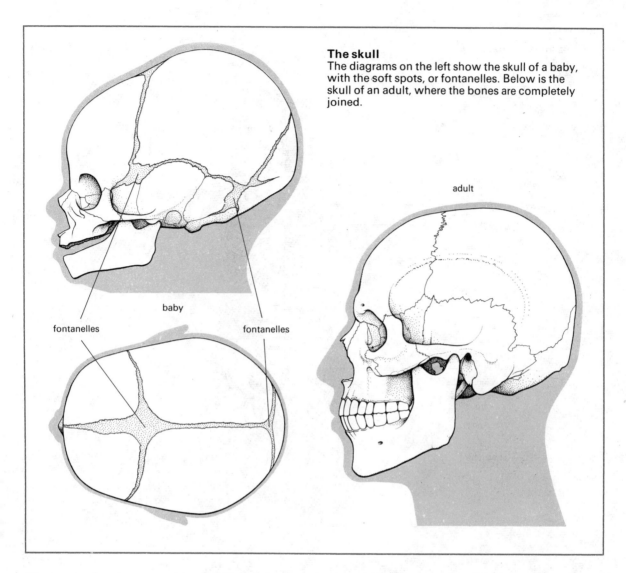

The skull
The diagrams on the left show the skull of a baby, with the soft spots, or fontanelles. Below is the skull of an adult, where the bones are completely joined.

adult

baby

fontanelles

fontanelles

There are five large lumbar vertebrae, and the general region is popularly called the "small of the back". It is a sort of pivot for rocking movements of the upper part of the body upon lower parts and, like a fulcrum, is subject to concentrated stresses at times. The prevalence of low back pain around the thoracic-lumbar junction indicates that there is room for improvement in nature's engineering. Actually, man brought it upon himself by learning to walk erect on a spine designed to be slung between four legs.

The lowermost parts of the spine embody bones that we have lost by growing up. That is, bones that were separate at birth have become fused together. Five original vertebrae fuse into a single large bone, the sacrum, and four other fused vertebrae form the coccyx. The latter is a vestigial tailbone that is tucked under the surface. Babies begin life with 33 vertebrae;

adults have 26. We lose something like 60 bones by fusion as the skeleton matures and reduces our adult complement to 206 bones, with occasional variations.

The skull, perched on top of the spinal column, contains 22 bones (plus six more if one includes the tiny ossicles of the middle ear). The brain cage or cranium is composed of eight flat bones, knitted together in irregular suture lines. A newborn baby's skull is quite pliable, and the familiar soft spots or fontanelles are cranial areas where true bone has not yet formed. Suture lines are points at which bone continues to grow as the skull develops to accommodate the enlarging brain.

The head is almost perfectly balanced on top of the spine, so it is easy to keep it erect without fatigue. This is one of the advantages of man's adaptation to upright posture.

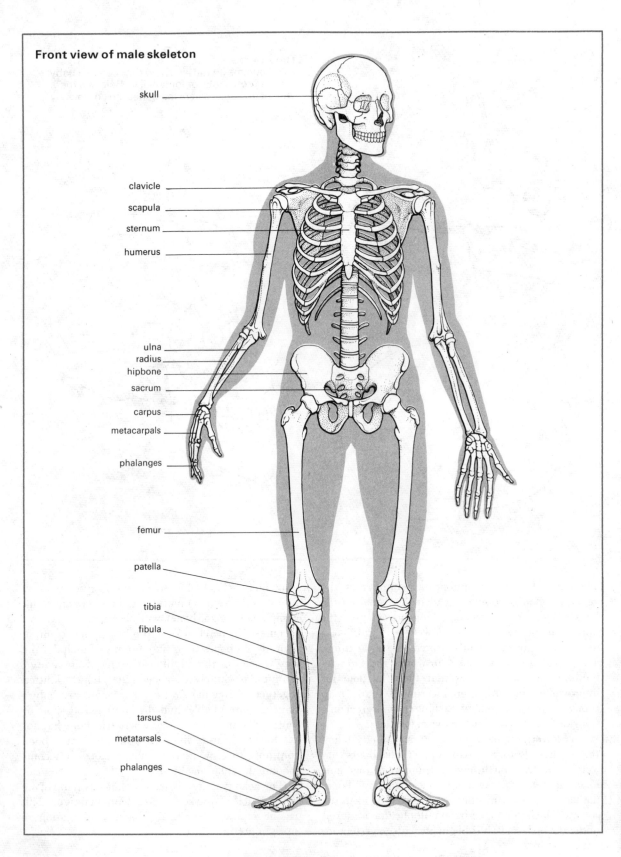

Front view of male skeleton

skull

clavicle

scapula

sternum

humerus

ulna
radius
hipbone
sacrum

carpus

metacarpals

phalanges

femur

patella

tibia

fibula

tarsus

metatarsals

phalanges

Back view of male skeleton

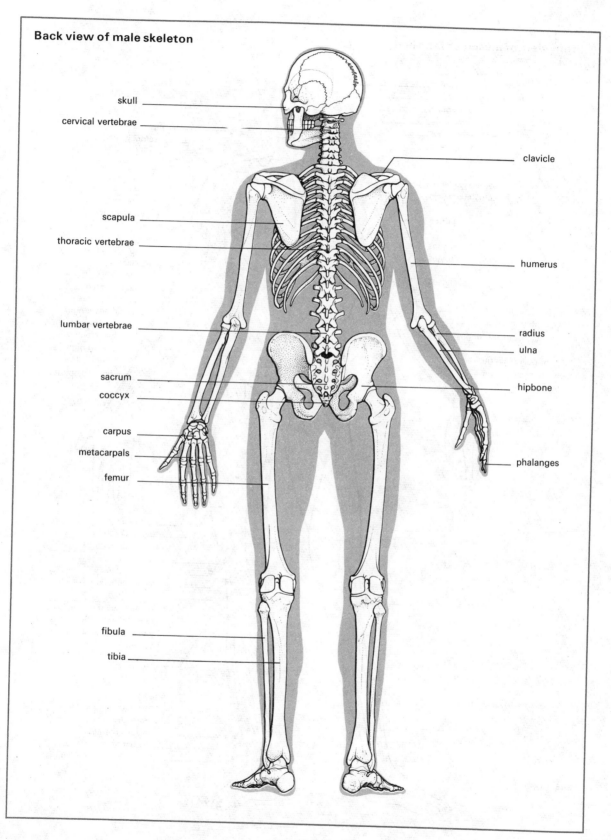

skull

cervical vertebrae

clavicle

scapula

thoracic vertebrae

humerus

lumbar vertebrae

radius

ulna

sacrum

hipbone

coccyx

carpus

metacarpals

phalanges

femur

fibula

tibia

Front view of muscles of the body

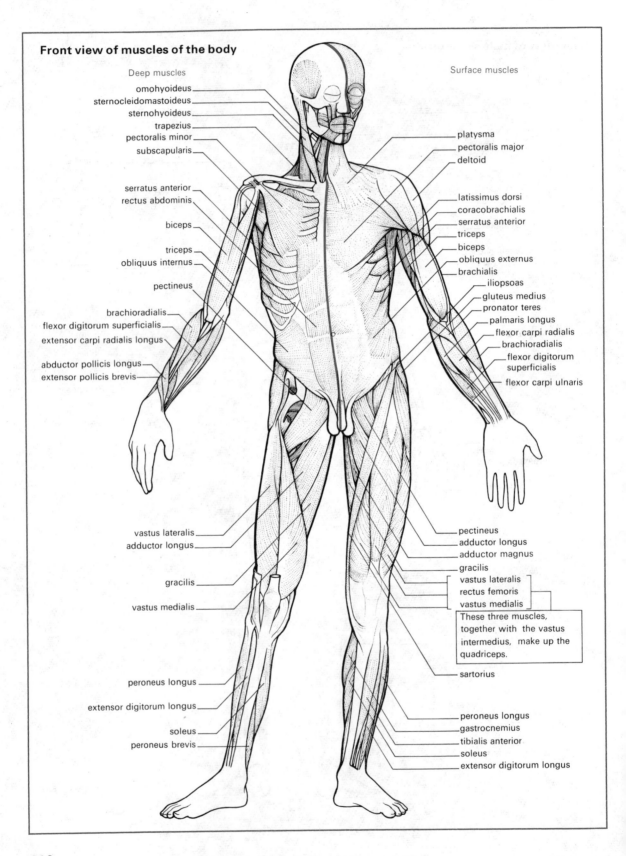

Deep muscles

Surface muscles

omohyoideus
sternocleidomastoideus
sternohyoideus
trapezius
pectoralis minor
subscapularis

serratus anterior
rectus abdominis

biceps

triceps
obliquus internus

pectineus

brachioradialis
flexor digitorum superficialis
extensor carpi radialis longus

abductor pollicis longus
extensor pollicis brevis

vastus lateralis
adductor longus

gracilis

vastus medialis

peroneus longus

extensor digitorum longus

soleus
peroneus brevis

platysma
pectoralis major
deltoid

latissimus dorsi
coracobrachialis
serratus anterior
triceps
biceps
obliquus externus
brachialis
iliopsoas
gluteus medius
pronator teres
palmaris longus
flexor carpi radialis
brachioradialis
flexor digitorum
superficialis
flexor carpi ulnaris

pectineus
adductor longus
adductor magnus
gracilis
vastus lateralis
rectus femoris
vastus medialis

These three muscles,
together with the vastus
intermedius, make up the
quadriceps.

sartorius

peroneus longus
gastrocnemius
tibialis anterior
soleus
extensor digitorum longus

Back view of muscles of the body

Surface muscles

Deep muscles

semispinalis
splenius capitis
levator scapulae
rhomboideus minor
rhomboideus major
supraspinatus
infraspinatus
sacrospinalis
teres minor
teres major
serratus posterior inferior
serratus anterior
triceps

sternocleidomastoideus

trapezius
teres major
teres minor

deltoid
latissimus dorsi

erector spinae

triceps
obliquus externus
obliquus internus
gluteus medius
gluteus maximus

obliquus internus

gluteus medius
piriformis

extensor carpi radialis longus
flexor digitorum profundus
extensor carpi ulnaris
extensor communis digitorum

flexor digitorum profundus
flexor carpi ulnaris
extensor carpi radialis longus

extensor metacarpi pollicis

extensor metacarpi pollicis

extensor primi internodii pollicis

extensor secundi internodii pollicis

extensor primi internodii pollicis

extensor minimi digiti

extensor indicis

extensor carpi radialis brevis

gemellus superior
gemellus inferior
obturator internus
iliotibial tract and vastus lateralis
adductor magnus
gracilis
semitendinosus
biceps femoris
semimembranosus

sartorius

plantaris

gastrocnemeus

sartorius

soleus
peroneus longus

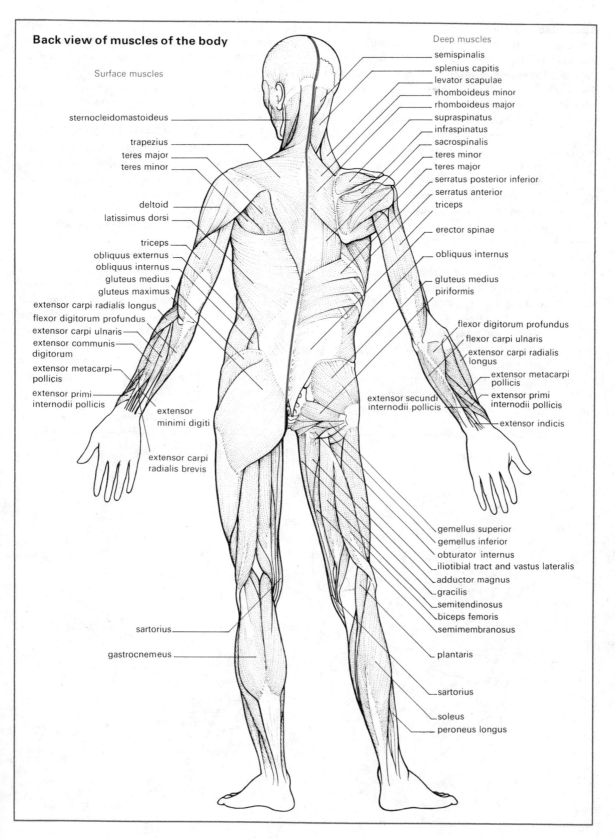

447

Chapter 19 Bones and muscles

Appendages The other part of the skeleton, concerned with locomotion and manipulation, is integrally related to the axial skeleton. The engineering design is simple in principle if not in execution. The backbone may be likened to a telegraph pole which has a crossbar at the top and another near the bottom. The top crosspiece is the shoulder girdle and the lower, more massive one, the pelvic girdle. Appendages – arms and hands, legs and feet – are connected to these structures.

The shoulder girdle consists of two collarbones (clavicles) and two shoulder blades (scapulas) which at a point of union form a socket in which the arm hangs. The pelvis is composed of three pairs of fused bones. The easiest to recognize is the ilium – which has a crest that serves as a useful ledge for balancing bulky loads on the hip – or perhaps the ischium, on which we sit. The sacrum connects with the ilia at the back, at the sacroiliac joints, and the pubic bones complete the circle in front.

Joints are the places where the bones of the skeleton connect with each other. There are several types, and they vary greatly in size and range of movement. At one extreme are the joints between the bones of the skull, which are immovably united by a thin layer of fibrous material. At the other extreme is the shoulder joint, with a very wide range of movement. In the joints with slight or no movement the bones are united by ligaments or by cartilage and ligaments. Those with free movement all have a common kind of structure. The knee is a typical hinge joint. The end of each bone is covered by a layer of smooth transparent cartilage. The joint is enclosed in a fibrous capsule which is thickened at the sides to form inextensible ligaments which prevent lateral movement. Inside the joint, where the cartilages are not in actual contact, the joint contains a membrane (the synovial membrane) which secretes a very efficient lubricant. There are also two very strong internal ligaments in the knee which prevent the joint from being overstraightened.

The hip is a typical ball-and-socket joint. The head of the thighbone is nearly spherical and fits into a deep socket in the pelvis. This makes a very strong joint. The shoulder is also a ball-and-socket joint, but of a different kind. The head of the upper armbone is also ball-shaped but the socket on the shoulder blade is very shallow. This permits a very extensive range of movement. The joint is held in position as much by the surrounding muscles as by ligaments. Consequently, the shoulder is the joint most easily dislocated.

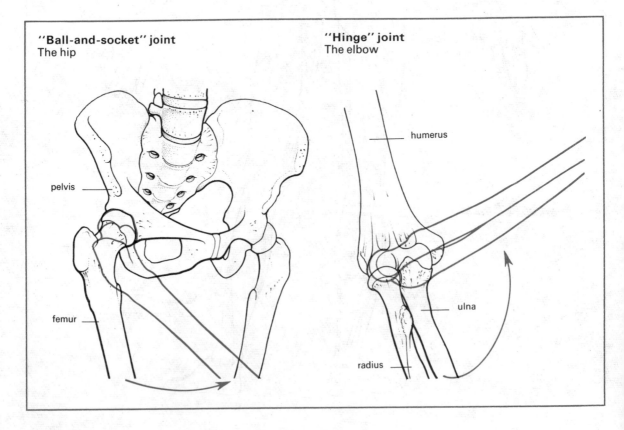

"Ball-and-socket" joint
The hip

pelvis

femur

"Hinge" joint
The elbow

humerus

ulna

radius

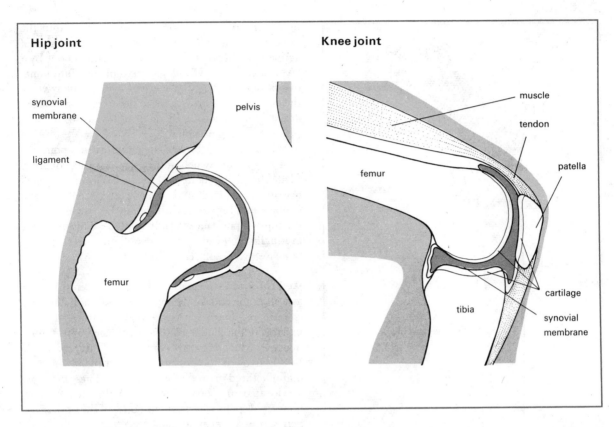

Hip joint

synovial
membrane

ligament

pelvis

femur

Knee joint

muscle

tendon

patella

femur

cartilage

synovial
membrane

tibia

We have so many bones, each with its medical name, that it is hardly possible, or even useful, to try to remember them. It is better to refer to the drawing on page 444 if you wish to locate certain bone structures in your system or remind yourself that the tibia is the same bone as the shinbone.

The structure of bone

A long bone is much stronger than reinforced concrete, much lighter, and more flexible. Two types of bone exist together – compact or hard bone, and spongy or cancellous bone. Bones are commonly classified as flat, as in the skull, or long and hollow, as in the legs.

A long bone like the femur, between the hip and knee, has a hard tubular outer layer and an internal cavity filled with marrow. Flat bones have two layers of compact bone enclosing a spongy middle. The bulging ends of long bones are honeycombed with spongy bone. The thin walls of this type of bone are arranged along stress lines to give the greatest weight-bearing strength.

Disregarding water, bone is about two thirds mineral and one third organic matter. The organic foundation is chiefly collagen. Elements are so

intimately mixed that if minerals are dissolved out by acids, leaving the organic material, the bone retains its shape but is too soft to support stresses. Similarly, if the organic material is removed by heating, the remaining minerals preserve the original shape, but the bone crumbles to ashes at a touch. In the body, bone is a community of living cells impregnated with mineral salts.

Nearly all bone surfaces are covered by a tough membrane, the periosteum. Bone cells receive nourishment from blood vessels which weave through the periosteum and reach the spongy interior directly or through an intricate network of tiny canals. Nerve fibres follow similar routes; the periosteum conveys sensations of bone pain and pressure.

The red marrow of certain bones is the manufacturing site of blood elements. Yellow marrow predominantly contains fatty material, but when necessary can also make blood cells.

Growth and repair Bone grows and repairs itself in very complicated ways. In essence, certain cells secrete the bony matrix and many become imprisoned in it. At the same time, other cells dissolve away bits of bone and help to sculpt materials to the proper shape. This simultaneous bone-building and bone-

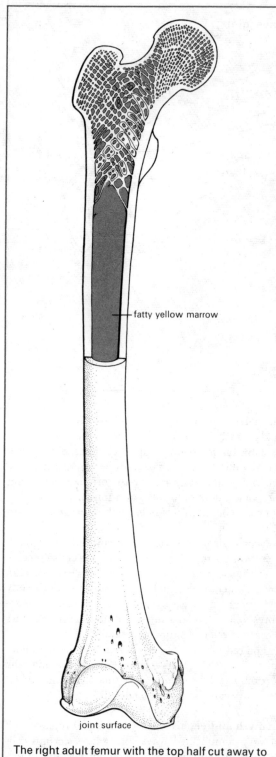

—fatty yellow marrow

joint surface

The right adult femur with the top half cut away to show variation in the thickness of the wall, and arrangement of the honeycombed interior along stress-bearing lines.

destroying process goes on continuously within the bone itself. The ends of long bones of children, sites of active growth, are separated from the main bone by a layer of cartilage. Cartilage does not turn into bone, but is replaced by it. At about the age of twenty, the cartilaginous growth plate becomes a part of the larger bone. Then the bone ceases to grow and the person becomes no taller.

When a bone is broken, lacerated tissues pour out sticky exudates which stiffen into a bulgy deposit. Little by little, bone-making cells from the periosteum and fractured bone ends penetrate the exudate and replace it with spongy bone which holds the injured parts more firmly in place. This in turn is gradually removed by bone-dissolving cells as spongy bone is slowly replaced by hard bone.

Red cells and minerals   The hollow central shafts as well as the ends of the long bones of small children contain red marrow. As the bones mature, the red marrow in the shaft is gradually replaced with yellow marrow, which is mostly composed of fatty material. Red marrow is the site in which red blood cells are manufactured in prodigious numbers. These factories are located in spongy bone, as in the ends of long bones and spongy parts of flat bones of the skull, ribs, pelvis, breastbone, and spine.

We need a certain amount of calcium to keep the heart beating, contract muscles, and help blood to clot. Most of our calcium is stored in the skeleton, in complex combinations with phosphorus and tiny amounts of a few other minerals. But this warehouse is not a mere storing place. Its salts are constantly seeking an equilibrium with the rest of the body. There is consequently a continuous movement of traffic into and out of the skeleton – now, a deposit of calcium received; next, a withdrawal of calcium to be delivered to the blood.

The concept of bones as dull inert girders and pillars, as unchanging and uninteresting as concrete, is far removed from the truth. Bone is living tissue that is constantly undergoing changes and being re-absorbed and reconstructed. It may seem rigid, but is in fact remarkably plastic, and any continued pressure can cause bone to be absorbed and to disappear very quickly. The bones of children are especially pliable and usually respond to any measures necessary to correct defects.

Osteomyelitis is an infection of bone resulting from the growth of bacteria within the bone. It is one of the dangerous diseases of childhood, but can also occur in adults. In children, the long bones are usually

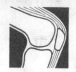

affected; in adults, the infection is more common in the bones of the spine and pelvis.

In children the infection is caused by organisms such as the staphylococcus and less commonly by the streptococcus or pneumococcus. The germs usually reach the bone through the bloodstream from a focus elsewhere in the body. Osteomyelitis can also be caused by direct spread from infected tissues in the vicinity of bone, or as the result of a wound or open fracture.

The first symptoms are usually pain and tenderness near a joint. The pain increases rapidly in intensity and jarring of the bone is painful, so that the child refuses to move the affected limb. The child is obviously ill and the temperature is usually between 39° and 40°C (102° and 104°F). In the early stages there is usually little or no swelling, and although there is great tenderness of the bone, the adjacent joint can usually be moved passively without causing additional pain.

These signs and symptoms are usually sufficient to make the diagnosis. It may take ten days before signs of infection show in X-ray films. To wait for X-ray signs to confirm the diagnosis is to wait too long.

Treatment A few years ago, acute haematogenous (blood-carried) osteomyelitis was a danger-ous and crippling disease. Antibiotics have revolutionized the treatment and mortality has been reduced to less than one per cent. However, unless osteomyelitis is treated with adequate doses of antibiotics, the symptoms may be masked, the signs suppressed, and the infection become chronic.

Surgery can be postponed as long as there is progressive improvement as a result of antibiotic therapy. But if there are signs of abscess formation, or if local signs do not begin to subside within a day after starting antibiotic treatment, the site of inflammation must be opened for drainage. If pressure from pus is not relieved, large areas of bone may be destroyed. Usually the wound can be closed after all the infected material has been removed, and with immobilization and continued antibiotic therapy, healing should proceed normally.

Cases of acute haematogenous osteomyelitis which are diagnosed late show extensive local destruction of bone and associated soft-tissue abscesses. The abscesses must be evacuated by incision as soon as possible. Unfortunately, extensive infection may not be completely controlled and chronic osteomyelitis with sinuses (suppurating tracts) draining through the skin may be present for years.

Suppurative arthritis can occur as a secondary

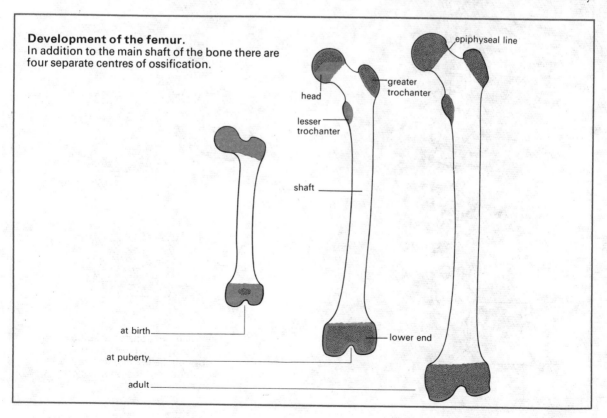

Development of the femur.
In addition to the main shaft of the bone there are four separate centres of ossification.

epiphyseal line

head

greater trochanter

lesser trochanter

shaft

lower end

at birth

at puberty

adult

The spine

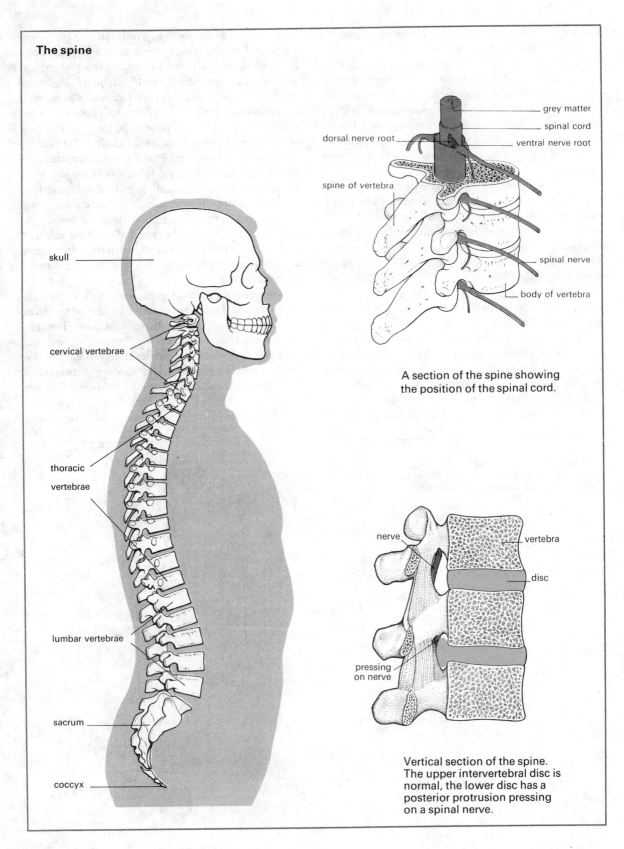

grey matter

spinal cord

dorsal nerve root

ventral nerve root

spine of vertebra

spinal nerve

body of vertebra

A section of the spine showing the position of the spinal cord.

skull

cervical vertebrae

thoracic vertebrae

lumbar vertebrae

sacrum

coccyx

nerve

vertebra

disc

pressing on nerve

Vertical section of the spine. The upper intervertebral disc is normal, the lower disc has a posterior protrusion pressing on a spinal nerve.

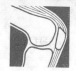

result of acute osteomyelitis. The knee joint is usually affected. Fluid from the joint should be aspirated and an antibiotic injected through the same needle into the joint cavity. This treatment fails if the primary source of infection near the joint is not treated.

Other possible complications of acute osteomyelitis are septicaemia (blood poisoning), retardation of growth, and development of chronic osteomyelitis.

Chronic osteomyelitis The chief symptom is usually a discharge of pus from an opening in the skin over the affected bone. The discharge may be continuous or intermittent. Pain is often present and is frequently associated with a flare-up or reopening of a previously healed discharge channel. The bone feels thickened to the touch and is usually covered by scarred skin showing several open drainage tracts. X-rays show that the bone is thickened and irregular. Pieces of dead bone or sequestra may be seen. It is difficult to remove completely all the pieces of dead bone which are the source of the pus draining through the sinuses. Extensive operations and many months of hospital treatment are sometimes necessary.

The spine

Posture People vary in shape, size, and occupation, and so do their postures. There is no such thing as an identical perfect posture for all people. There is a normal range of variation.

One of the key factors in posture is the angle of inclination of the pelvis, the foundation on which the spinal column stands. The hip joint and the position of the feet are other key elements of posture.

The spine is a long flexible structure with characteristic curves. At birth a baby's spine shows a continuous backward curvature from pelvis to skull. With growth, the spine develops subcurves in response to the demands of upright posture. The adult spine shows a forward curvature in the neck region, a backward curvature in the chest area, and a forward curvature in the lower back. Balance is maintained during standing by tilting the pelvis forwards. This tilting tends to flatten out the curves of the spine.

Muscles of the abdomen and spine hold the latter over the body's line of gravity. Movement of the spine is greatest in the lower back and this region is subject to the greatest degenerative changes. Bad posture can result from laziness, poor muscle development, and general debility. However, there is usually a more important local cause for a significant posture defect. Any marked change in the posture of a child or adult requires a thorough medical examination to determine the cause.

Low back pain Pain in the back can be caused by a variety of mechanisms. The main causes are injury or degeneration of the joints, ligaments, muscles, or intervertebral discs. Pain can be felt in the back as a result of nerve root irritation. Muscles which are contracted because of attempts to protect some local injury can also cause secondary pain.

Acute back sprain is usually produced by a sudden bending of the spine, as in a fall or a "snatch lifting" motion. The force is sufficient to tear the ligaments or joint capsules, producing pain and protective muscle contraction. These injuries usually heal in three weeks, if they are protected against further sprains during the healing period. Initial treatment consists of bed rest, analgesics, and local heat.

Chronic back strain is a different condition, in which there is no violent, sudden, precipitating incident, but the structures are subjected to prolonged tension greater than they can resist. Symptoms usually come on gradually and become progressively worse. They are made worse by fatigue and are improved by lying down and by physiotherapy.

Treatment is difficult since causes are varied and not always possible to eliminate. The main cause of chronic strain must be discovered and removed if a cure is to be obtained. The outlook is not always good, particularly if it is not possible to change an occupation which appears to be the main cause of the strain.

Helpful measures for aching backs not caused by a slipped disc or disease:

Sleep on a firm bed; avoid very soft chairs or sofas; use straight chairs as much as possible.

Arrange work surfaces (for example, ironing boards) to avoid leaning-forward positions that put strain on the small of the back.

Do postural exercises twice a day, such as:

In standing position, contract buttocks and abdomen, head up; hold for five seconds.

Sitting: clasp arms behind back, bend forward, raise head and bring shoulder blades together, sit erect while pulling backwards and downwards with hands.

Lie face down, arms at sides, contract buttocks and abdomen, bring shoulder blades together.

Facet syndrome is the name for a condition in which a sudden catch in the back virtually fixes the victim in a position from which he cannot move. Usually he is caught in a stooping position and cannot straighten from it. Pain is felt around the injury but does not radiate to other parts. Careful manipulation can give relief, leaving only some soreness which will last for a few days. Bed rest and sedation, however, can give relief in the same length of time without the risks inherent in manipulation. Attacks tend to increase in frequency and duration over the years, until eventually there may be chronic backache. This is particularly likely if the patient continues to perform stooping actions which tend to bring on the attacks.

Disc trouble The intervertebral discs are semi-cartilaginous buffers or shock absorbers between the bony vertebrae. After twenty years of age, it is normal for discs to age and degenerate gradually. Movements through the altered disc change, so that in varied motions of the spine, one vertebra moves on another, producing a forward or backward shift. As degeneration progresses, the symptoms, if any, are likely to change.

Early degeneration of the disc does not usually cause symptoms unless some strain is added. The strain can be slight but prolonged, as in sitting during a long drive without getting out frequently to stretch. There is usually only mild local tenderness in the back and X-rays show nothing abnormal. Treatment should be rest, followed by muscle-strengthening exercises, and education to make the patient aware of avoidable mechanical strains that are unkind to degenerating intervertebral discs.

Ruptured disc or *slipped disc* is a diagnosis commonly made by neighbours whenever someone has an aching back or sciatica. The terms properly refer only to a specific condition in which the pulpy body at the centre of an intervertebral disc (nucleus pulposus) protrudes through a tear in the surrounding ligament.

In this condition the sciatica is a dull, aching pain

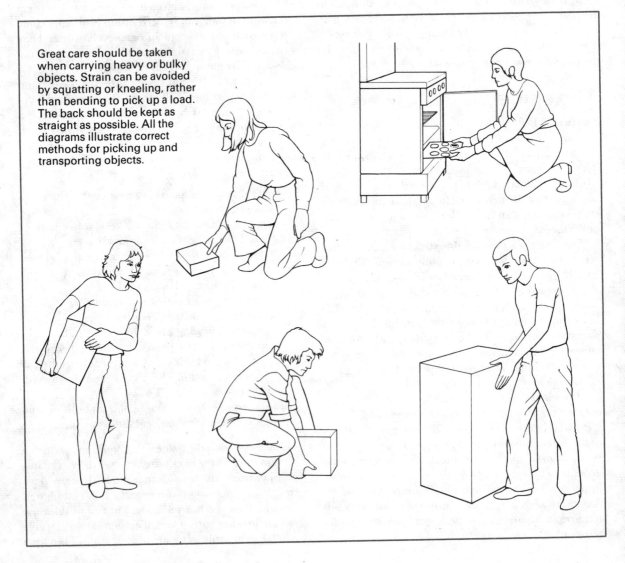

Great care should be taken when carrying heavy or bulky objects. Strain can be avoided by squatting or kneeling, rather than bending to pick up a load. The back should be kept as straight as possible. All the diagrams illustrate correct methods for picking up and transporting objects.

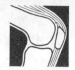

which is sufficiently bad to mask the low back pain. It is made worse by coughing, sneezing, or jarring movements. Raising the straightened leg on the painful side is often limited to an angle of 20 to 30 degrees. X-ray films may show nothing abnormal or may show narrowing of the disc space. Sometimes a myelogram (X-ray of the spinal cord after injection of a contrast medium) is necessary to establish the diagnosis and the exact position of the disc rupture.

Complete recovery usually takes several weeks, but most cases of slipped disc respond to bed rest, traction, or the wearing of a lumbar corset. Occasionally a local anaesthetic may be injected into the spine. An operation to remove the protruded section of the disc and clear the degenerated disc space is considered only when the above measures have been ineffective.

Spondylolisthesis is the term applied to a spontaneous forward displacement of a lumbar vertebra upon the bone below it. Predisposing factors are a congenital or early developmental defect. Nearly five per cent of spines show such displacement. Spondylolisthesis can exist without any sign of backache and is often discovered accidentally during a routine medical examination.

When symptoms do occur, they are usually manifested as low lumbar backache with or without accompanying sciatica. Symptoms arise from degenerative changes in the disc. If conservative treatment of symptoms of disc degeneration fails, or if the forward slip of a vertebra is of a great degree, an operation for joining the vertebrae together (spinal fusion) may be necessary.

Symptomless spondylolisthesis should not be made a reason for gross restriction of activities. Many teenagers and young adults lead perfectly normal lives despite their spondylolisthesis.

Scheuermann's disease is a common cause of backache in teenagers. For unknown reasons, certain vertebral bodies undergo changes resulting in their becoming wedge-shaped. Usually several vertebrae of the back are affected at the same time. In the active stage of the disease there is pain associated with a round back.

The diagnosis is easily made from the history, physical signs, and X-ray findings. This so-called disease is not serious. It is a self-limiting condition which lasts about two years. Treatment usually does not involve more than restriction of activity and back muscle exercises. In severe cases a period of bed rest followed by the wearing of a spinal brace may be necessary.

Scoliosis is a term used to describe a lateral curvature of the spine. There are several types of scoliosis.

Idiopathic scoliosis begins in childhood or adolescence and becomes progressively worse until growth ceases. Treatment is unsatisfactory because the cause of the condition is unknown, The deformity is usually worse in the upper back and least in the lumbar region. The earlier the onset, the worse the ultimate curvature.

It is not possible to prevent the deformity from increasing by using exercises or external splints. Several different surgical methods are employed but no particular method is outstandingly better than another.

Structural scoliosis is secondary to an underlying cause such as muscle weakness after polio or abnormally shaped vertebrae. Usually the only evidence is the visible deformity. In severe cases, spinal fusion is the corrective treatment.

Sciatic scoliosis lasts only as long as some primary painful condition of the spine produces a spasm of muscles to protect the area that hurts. By far the most common primary cause is the protrusion of an intervertebral disc. Abnormal posture occurs quite involuntarily as the body attempts to minimize painful pressure upon a nerve root. The trunk is often tilted well over to one side. Treatment of this form of scoliosis consists of treatment of the underlying condition.

Scoliosis sometimes occurs as a compensation for a sideways tilt of the pelvis, produced by a true short leg, or by an apparent shortening of the leg caused by a hip joint contracture. The spine itself is normal and the scoliosis will disappear when the pelvic tilt is corrected.

Degenerative arthritis of the spine Various degenerative changes frequently occur in the intervertebral joints of the upper and lower back and are particularly common in persons who do heavy manual work. Quite marked degrees of arthritis can exist without causing any symptoms, but if symptoms are triggered by some relatively minor stress they are likely to be persistent. Even without acute aggravation, symptoms will eventually arise in the affected area. Usually there are periodic attacks of discomfort lasting a few weeks, followed by periods of freedom from pain. In mild cases treatment is unnecessary, but in the more severe low back cases physiotherapy and some form of supporting garment give good relief.

Torticollis or **wryneck** is a rotational deformity of

the neck which causes tilting and turning of the head. The commonest form occurs in infants and is associated with a swelling in the muscles of the neck. In very early cases, gentle manipulation is enough to correct the deformity. In established cases, division of the contracted muscle at its lower end is usually performed.

An uncommon form of adult wryneck is called spasmodic torticollis. The cause is not known. This condition does not respond to ordinary therapeutic measures and is often associated with symptoms of mental strain.

Whiplash injury is a phrase which has fallen into disrepute among doctors because it does not describe any specific abnormality or anatomical derangement. It is a general descriptive term like dyspepsia or lumbago, but unfortunately is still used as if it had a specific meaning.

The injury is usually sustained in a car accident which causes the head to be thrown forward suddenly and suddenly jerked backward, or *vice versa*, like cracking a whip. The brunt of the injury is borne at the level of the fifth cervical vertebra where muscles and ligaments can be torn and strained. Rarely there may be associated bone or nerve damage.

The injury is similar to a badly sprained ankle, and treatment is similar. The neck should be protected by a soft felt or sponge rubber collar for two or three weeks. Aspirin, heat, and massage are helpful in relieving symptoms. Occasionally patients have persistent headaches following this injury.

All the symptoms appear to be aggravated by emotional factors and a nervous tense person generally takes longer to recover than a placid person.

The shoulder

The shoulder joint, like that of the hip, is a ball-and-socket joint, but with a difference. In the hip the socket is deep and the joint has strong ligaments to hold the bone in place. In the shoulder the socket is shallow and the ligaments less conspicuous, so the joint has to be held in place largely by the muscles that move it. That is why the shoulder is the most commonly dislocated joint.

Pain in the shoulder can be caused by many conditions not originating in the joint itself. For instance, pain may be derived from the lung membrane (pleura), the diaphragm, or the tissue surrounding the heart. Shingles, disturbances of the spinal cord in the neck region, and muscular dystrophies can also produce shoulder pain.

Most varieties of arthritis can occur in the shoulder joint, but degenerative arthritis is not common, probably because the joint is not weight-bearing. Most shoulder disabilities are caused by conditions peculiar to the joint.

The supraspinatus is a fan-shaped muscle attached to the upper part of the shoulder blade and ending in a tendon which is attached to the head of the humerus. Its function is to lift the arm away from the body. The tendon is sometimes inflamed or nipped as it passes under the acromial process of the shoulder blade, producing the so-called supraspinatus syndrome. The typical complaint is pain in the upper arm and shoulder when the arm is raised. The pain occurs in the middle third of the arc described when the arm is raised. There is usually little or no pain during motion on either side of this middle arc of movement. In the normal shoulder there is very little clearance between the undersurface of the acromion (the bone at the tip of the shoulder) and the upper end of the armbone when the arm is partly raised. If there is swelling and tenderness in this narrow space, pain is produced mechanically by pinching of the swollen tissues between the bones.

The most common cause of such shoulder pain is inflammation of the supraspinatus tendon (tendinitis), but it can also be caused by injuries to the tendon, injury to bony parts, deposits of soft chalky material within the tendon, or subacromial bursitis (inflammation of the protective fluid sac beneath the acromion). Whatever the cause, the symptoms are the same. The patient has pain in the middle third of the arc both when raising and lowering the arm, and often twists the arm in different ways in attempts to avoid painful movement. In some cases there is severe pain, frequently produced by a chalky deposit in the tendon.

Treatment employs either sound of very high (inaudible) frequency or the passage of high-frequency electric currents through the tissues (diathermy). Exercising the joint is also often successful, and injections of steroids may help. If calcium deposits cause severe pain, immediate relief can be given by removing the deposit through an aspiration needle or through a small incision into the tendon. In patients who suffer chronic pain and do not respond to limited forms of treatment, surgery should be considered.

Bursitis of the shoulder (subdeltoid or subacromial bursitis) A bursa is a sac containing lubricating fluid which diminishes friction between adjacent structures. When a bursa becomes inflamed the condition is termed bursitis. The bursa which lies between the acromion at the end of the collarbone and the ball end of the upper armbone is large and extends under neighbouring structures. Its inner surface which permits parts to glide freely is smooth and glistening, and it is unusual for the bursa itself to be the originating point of inflammation or infection. Virtually every case of this kind of bursitis is caused by some injury to one of the structures lying in contact with the deep layer of the bursa. Treatment should therefore be directed towards the primary cause which may be single or repeated injury, infection (whether short-lived or lingering), and other conditions that may produce bursitis-like pain that originates outside the bursa itself.

Injuries to tendons and muscles around joints are common causes of pain. An incomplete tear of the tendinous part where muscles are attached to bone is one of the causes of the supraspinatus syndrome described above. A rupture (complete tear) greatly hinders the raising of the arm throughout its range of movement. Ruptures are often produced by a relatively minor accident, such as a fall on the outstretched hand. There is immediate pain in the shoulder which increases during the next few hours and is frequently so great that drugs are necessary for its control. The patient, who is usually over 60 years of age, is unable to raise the arm and there is great tenderness to pressure on the point of the shoulder.

The outlook is good if the rupture is repaired surgically within a few days of its occurrence. If operation is unduly delayed it is unlikely that good shoulder movement will return. After the operation, the arm is usually held away from the side in a plaster cast for several weeks.

Frozen shoulder is an ill-understood condition, also known as pericapsulitis or adhesive capsulitis (inflammation of a membranous sac enclosing a part). Patients with this condition complain of moderate pain and marked limitation of movement. The pain is aching in character and comes on gradually in the shoulder and upper arm. There is restriction of movement in all directions of the joint.

Usually the stiffness gradually disappears, but it may take at least a year. The pain disappears sooner, but in early stages the arm needs rest in a sling. Occasionally manipulation of the shoulder joint is necessary when all pain has gone and some movement has returned. Manipulation can cause fractures if the bone has been weakened by inactivity, and should be performed only by someone skilled in the procedure.

Recurrent dislocation of the shoulder This is a condition in which repeated dislocations occur at the glenohumeral joint where the humerus (upper armbone) meets the scapula (shoulder blade). These usually happen when the arm is being raised or extended without any great force, as when stretching, swimming, putting on a coat, or even brushing the hair. Dislocations may be rare or so frequent as to interfere with daily activities. Often the patient is able to replace the limb himself or with the help of a friend.

The reasons why some primary dislocations of the shoulder heal without further trouble and others go on to repeated dislocations are not fully understood. However, there is no doubt that if the original dislocation is not properly put back into place (reduced) and adequately immobilized, there is a high risk of recurrent dislocation.

No abnormalities will be found if the shoulder is examined when it is not dislocated. X-rays will not usually show anything abnormal but a bone defect may sometimes be seen when a view is taken from a particular angle.

There is no effective nonsurgical treatment. If the dislocations occur frequently and are troublesome, an operation should be performed. There are several different procedures, but all try to strengthen the capsule of the joint and slightly limit its range of external rotation. A successful operation can result in a shoulder that can be used for hard work.

The acromioclavicular joint connects the collarbone and the acromion process of the shoulder blade. Changes in this joint produce pain which is usually confined to the area of the joint. The pain is made worse by excessive use of the joint, particularly for overhead work, such as painting a ceiling.

Examination of the joint does not show any thickening of the ligaments or capsule, but bony outgrowth can be felt at the margins. The arm can be raised to a horizontal level without discomfort, but raising it above this level causes pain. X-rays will show narrowing of the joint space and bony outgrowth at margins.

Treatment with diathermy is usually satisfactory, but operation is occasionally necessary.

This joint is also prone to persistent dislocation, as a result of injury. In most cases the displacement is minimal and the symptoms slight. Examination shows that the outer end of the collarbone sticks up beneath the skin. Hence the rest of the shoulder girdle hangs down lower than the collarbone. An operation is rarely necessary and a sling gives sufficient rest for occasional attacks of discomfort.

The sternoclavicular joint is where the collarbone (clavicle) is joined to the breastbone (sternum). The collarbone is occasionally dislocated, either permanently, or when the shoulders are braced back. This displacement can be troublesome, but does not usually require operative treatment. There is no effective nonsurgical treatment, and if an operation is performed, attempts are made to hold the collarbone in its normal place by reconstructing the torn or stretched ligaments.

The elbow

When the arm is held straight by the side, the elbow is bent slightly outwards, at an angle of about ten degrees in men and fifteen degrees in women. This is known as the carrying angle, and if it is greatly increased, the resulting deformity is known as cubitus valgus.

This condition usually occurs because of poor union of a fracture of the lower end of the humerus, or because local growth has been affected by disease or injury. In itself the deformity is harmless and usually not very noticeable. Function of the arm is not disturbed, but a possible complication which can arise is inflammation of the ulnar nerve.

The ulnar nerve which supplies most of the muscles of the hand passes around the back of the elbow joint on the inner side and is exposed to direct injury at the point of the elbow commonly known as the "funny bone". When the carrying angle is greatly increased, the nerve will be bent sharply around the angle and repeated injury may do damage. Scarring around and within the nerve will produce tingling in the hand and weakness and wasting of the muscles of the hand supplied by the nerve. When symptoms of nerve damage are present, it is wise to have the nerve transposed by an operation which removes it from danger by placing it at the front of the elbow.

The opposite deformity to cubitus valgus is cubitus varus, in which the normal carrying angle is reduced or even reversed. The causes of the deformity are the same as those of cubitus valgus. There is usually no disability from this but it may be unsightly.

Tennis elbow is a name commonly applied to any disorder causing pain on the outer side of the elbow joint. Only in a very few people is it caused by playing tennis. Any activity that requires rotary movements of the forearm and a firm grip of the hand (using a screwdriver, for instance) can cause the symptoms. There is pain and tenderness at the outer side of the elbow where the extensor muscles originate. The pain

often spreads down the back of the forearm, and can develop into widespread aching in all the forearm muscles, particularly if excessive gripping is involved.

Many mild cases require no treatment, but a variety of limited measures are available, of which the most common is diathermy combined with massage. Injections of local anaesthetics, with or without cortisone derivatives, are also often used. Immobilization in a sling or even in plaster is often helpful in early cases. Operation is occasionally necessary in severely disabled patients who have not responded to the other treatments. Results are not always predictable, but usually the pain disappears after healing has taken place.

The elbow is second only to the knee as a site of osteochondritis dissecans (see page 465). This is a condition in which a fragment of cartilage and bone becomes detached, and occurs most often in teenagers. Pain is moderate and movements are usually somewhat limited, but complete rigidity does not occur until the fragment is completely detached. X-rays will show an area of irregularity in early stages of the condition. In late stages, a cavity and the bony fragment lying free within the joint may be seen.

Conservative treatment which may entail several months of immobilization is used in early cases. If the fragment has separated or is ready to separate, it must be removed through an incision.

Degenerative arthritis of the elbow is not very common since this is not a weight-bearing joint. When it does occur it is usually secondary to injury or disease of the joint surfaces. Relatively minor stresses, repeated over a period of years, are just as damaging as a major injury to the joint. For instance, workers using compressed air drills are liable to develop degenerative changes in the elbow joint.

Symptoms are pain and limitation of movement. The joint aches for a considerable time after heavy use. In some patients the first abnormal sign is the seizing up of the joint by a detached fragment or loose body in the joint.

Massage and diathermy or other forms of heat are useful, particularly if use of the joint can be curtailed. Restriction of use is often sufficient treatment. Operation may be needed; loose bodies should be removed, and in exceptional circumstances the joint can be stiffened in a functional position. An alternative to stiffening of the joint is an operation in which the destroyed surfaces are removed and the joint left movable.

Ruptures of the biceps This muscle can rupture

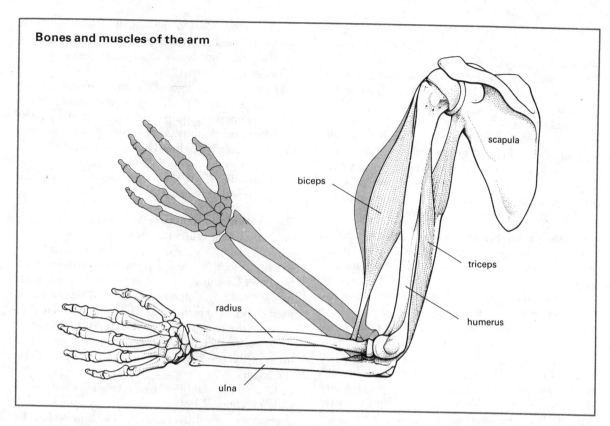

Bones and muscles of the arm

biceps

scapula

triceps

humerus

radius

ulna

at either end, but it is much more common for it to rupture at the upper end. The rupture usually affects a middle-aged person during a lifting or pulling effort, and is only slightly painful. Many men wait months before seeking medical aid. There is little loss of power or interference with customary work. When using the arm, the muscle fails to harden, and bulges lower down in the arm than is usual. Operation is seldom necessary, but when it is the results are usually good.

The wrist and hand

Sprained wrist is a common lay diagnosis, but is almost invariably misapplied. The true sprained wrist is very uncommon. Symptoms in this area are usually caused by a fracture, dislocation, or arthritis.

Persistent pain in the wrist after an accident is a serious symptom that needs thorough investigation. X-rays are essential. Fracture of the scaphoid bone below the thumb is quite common and if left untreated can produce crippling arthritis of the wrist long before normal degenerative changes could be expected to occur. Falls on the back of the hand can chip off small flakes of bone which may cause troublesome symptoms for weeks.

If such varied causes of symptoms can be excluded, then a sprained wrist can be safely diagnosed and successfully treated by strapping or temporary immobilization in a plaster cast.

DeQuervain's disease A common cause of pain in the thumb side of the wrist is a thickening of the sheaths covering two of the tendons which pass to the thumb. This stenosing tenovaginitis, or DeQuervain's disease, is most common in women. In general, repetitive actions such as typing, or strenuous actions such as wringing out the washing, produce the symptoms, which come on gradually. There is pain at the base of the thumb spreading to the nail and up into the forearm. There is usually pain when pressure is exerted over the thumb side of the wrist.

Sometimes the condition cures itself if the wrist can be immobilized and excessive action avoided. Injection of steroids can also cure. However, since operation is simple and satisfactory it is usually advised if the disability is severe. A simple stripping away of part of the tendon sheath is all that is necessary.

Ganglion of the wrist A ganglion is a saclike swelling enclosing fluid and occurring in association with a joint or tendon sheath. There is no known cause of its occurrence. There is always an attachment between the swelling and a joint capsule or tendon sheath, but rarely if ever is there any communicating passage with the cavity of the cyst. Ganglia occur most commonly on the back of the wrist, but can also arise on the palm or fingers.

Usually there are no symptoms except occasional slight discomfort. Since they are harmless, ganglia can safely be left untreated and many will disappear spontaneously. It may be necessary to cut out large ganglia or those which cause pain or pressure. Recurrence is uncommon if the whole ganglion including its root (pedicle) is removed.

Median nerve compression or carpal tunnel syndrome. A common cause of discomfort in the hand, especially in women over the age of forty, is pressure on the median nerve where it enters the carpal tunnel in the wrist. The median is one of two large nerves in the arm, passing along the middle of the arm and forearm, and entering the hand at the front of the wrist joint together with all the tendons which flex or bend the fingers. Thickening of the tendon sheaths and swelling of the joints of the wrist tend to reduce the size of the tunnel through which the nerve passes. Since the nerve is softer than the tendons, it will be subjected to considerable pressure with accompanying discomfort.

Symptoms are tingling, discomfort, and even numbness in the thumb, index, and middle fingers. If pressure has been present for some time there will be clumsiness in fine movements, objects may be dropped, and wasting of the thumb muscles may be apparent. Often, patients are especially troubled at night; shortly after going to sleep they are awakened by intense discomfort in the hand, which does not go away until the hand is exercised. Men can suffer from the same condition, and younger women may notice similar symptoms during late pregnancy, but these symptoms usually disappear after delivery of the baby. Other conditions which can cause similar symptoms must be excluded before the diagnosis is finally confirmed.

Rest occasionally helps, but usually the only lasting treatment is an operation which relieves pressure on the nerve. Recovery from the operation is rapid and relief of symptoms occurs overnight.

Degenerative changes of the wrist are quite common because of the frequency with which the joint surfaces are damaged. The symptoms are tenderness around the joint, pain on use, and limitation of movement. Relief can be given in mild cases by resting the wrist with a moulded leather or plastic splint. Most patients will not wear splints indefinitely and prefer to have an operation. The only reliable method is an operation for complete stiffening of the wrist.

Degenerative changes of the finger joints are quite common in elderly people. In most cases this is not serious enough to require treatment, but the joint at the base of the thumb may be quite seriously affected. Localized pain is produced by movement, the joint is prominent and thickened, and the range of movement is reduced. If the symptoms are severe, an operation will be necessary.

Dupuytren's contracture is a thickening of tissue of the palm which causes the fingers to be pulled down onto the palm. A similar condition may occur in the sole of the foot. There is a hereditary predisposition, but the cause is unknown. Changes are more common in the little finger side of the palm. The condition, most common in men, usually starts as a small nodule opposite the base of the ring finger. As the condition progresses, other nodules may tend to appear and areas of thickened tissue may gradually spread into the fingers.

All sorts of nonsurgical treatments have been tried without effect. The only satisfactory treatment is operative removal. In elderly patients in whom the condition is not progressing, operation is usually not necessary, but the younger the patient and the more extensive the disease, the more operation is justified.

Trigger finger is a result of constriction that prevents free movement of tendons in the sheath that surrounds them. The tendons develop a narrowing opposite to the constriction, tend to swell, and the swollen segment often develops into a nodule which has difficulty in entering the sheath when the finger is extended. Usually a click is heard as the finger bends or extends. Injections of steroids can give relief, and an operation to divide the constriction is usually effective.

Boutonnière deformity, also known as buttonhole deformity, is the result of the cutting or rupture of the tendon which extends the middle joint of a finger, so that the centre joint stays bent when the other two are extended. Treatment should be an immediate operation to reattach the tendon to the bone. Satisfactory treatment is extremely difficult if the deformity is neglected for many weeks after the original injury, and in such cases it may be necessary to fuse the joint in a better position.

Mallet finger This deformity, in which the tip of

Bones of the hand and wrist

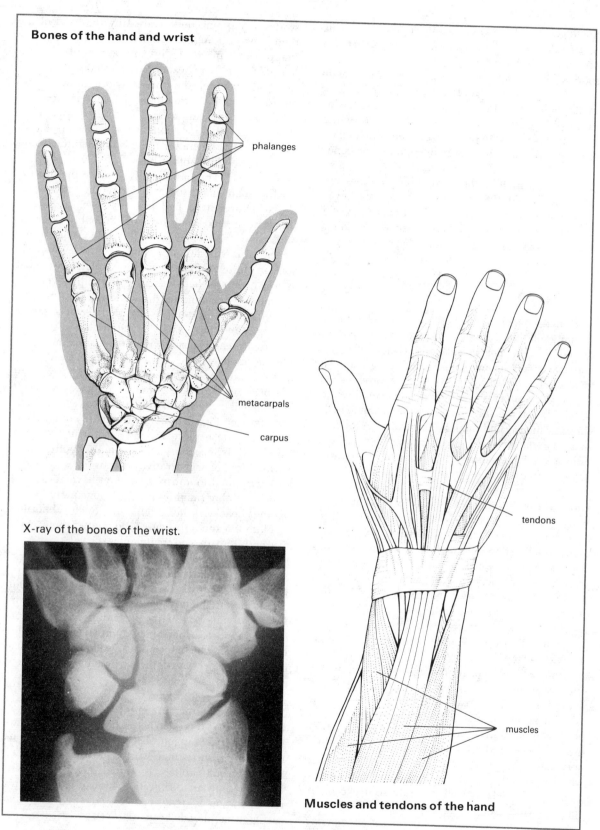

phalanges

metacarpals

carpus

X-ray of the bones of the wrist.

tendons

muscles

Muscles and tendons of the hand

the finger dips down, is caused by rupture or tearing of a tendon from its insertion (the point where it is attached to the bone it moves). The force to do this is a sudden violent blow on the tip of the finger, as in miscatching a cricket ball. Immobilization of the joint in plaster for about four weeks immediately following injury gives good results. Old injuries or those which have not responded to plaster treatment should have surgery to reattach the ruptured tendon to the bone.

Heberden's nodes These knobbly swellings that occur on both sides of the terminal joints of the fingers are a normal but sometimes painful part of ageing. This kind of arthritis is strictly confined to these joints, and never spreads to other joints. See pages 476–7.

The hip

The hip is a major weight-bearing joint and is subject to many conditions directly connected with the thrust of body weight. It is a ball-and-socket joint with a very strong capsule surrounding and strengthening it.

Most children with hip troubles are brought to a doctor when parents notice some abnormality after the child starts to walk. There is a wide variation in the time at which a child should start to walk. A hip limp in a very young child is usually caused by congenital dislocation if it is painless, and by acute suppurative arthritis (that is, where pus is present), if it is painful.

Congenital dislocation of the hip This spontaneous dislocation occurs before or shortly after birth as a result of a congenital abnormality of development, usually a flattening of the acetabulum (the cup-shaped cavity in which the head of the thighbone rests). Heredity plays a part; a woman with this condition has an increased chance of giving birth to a child with the same condition. Girls are affected at least five times more commonly than boys. The congenital dislocation is usually in one rather than both sides of the hip.

The most useful diagnostic signs are limitation of outward motion from the hip, particularly when the infant is lying on the back with the knees bent to 90 degrees, and asymmetry of the skin folds of the leg. The buttock, groin, and thigh folds on the affected side are usually deeper and higher up on the leg than on the normal side. Thigh folds can be asymmetric in infants who are perfectly normal, but asymmetry of the groin and buttock folds as well is rarely seen except in congenital dislocation of the hip.

Examination of the affected hip often demon-strates a snapping noise caused by the head of the thighbone entering the socket. After the head has snapped into place the hip can be moved within a normal range. X-ray examination usually shows that the bony roof of the socket slopes upward and outward, so that the thighbone slips out of place.

The key to successful treatment is early diagnosis. Physical examination alone is not sufficient. An X-ray is essential whenever there is the slightest doubt about the condition of the hip.

Treatment The basic aim is to place the head of the thighbone in the socket and to retain it there until the structures have had time to develop. Several different methods may be used. Probably the most satisfactory is to reduce the dislocation under general anaesthesia and immobilize the leg and hip joint in plaster. Often, after removal of the cast, a bar is attached to the baby's shoes to limit hip movement. In infants with minimal dislocations, splinting may be sufficient. Operation is occasionally necessary if the hip cannot be replaced by manipulation.

If treatment is started within the first six months of life the results will be excellent in nearly every case. The critical time is when walking starts; if treatment has been started by this time the outlook is good. If treatment is delayed until the age of two years or later, the prospects for a satisfactory result are not nearly so good. In late neglected cases, reconstructive operations will be necessary and the hip will often show various signs of degenerative arthritis.

A very small number of children have additional associated abnormalities such as congenital absence of the head of the thighbone. Such abnormal conditions cannot be cured no matter how early diagnosis is made and treatment is started.

Acute suppurative arthritis Pyogenic (pus-producing) arthritis of the hip is uncommon, but occurs most frequently in infants and young children. In infants it is usually secondary to infection elsewhere, such as pneumonia, impetigo, or middle-ear infection. The baby is obviously ill, has a sudden onset of high fever, holds the hip joint bent, and resists examination.

Usually the infecting organism is sensitive to antibiotics and the proper drug should be given without delay. It is often necessary to allow matter to escape from the hip joint because if pus is allowed to build up pressure, there will be local destruction of bone. When treatment is started late it is usually necessary to drain the infection surgically. Sometimes the operation is performed too late and the joint cartilage has already been destroyed.

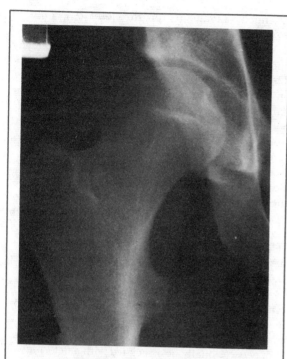

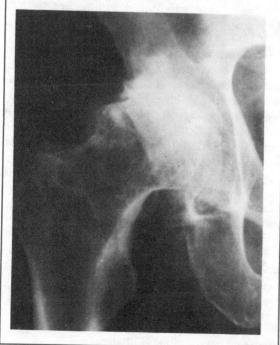

Above, an X-ray of a normal hip joint. Note the smooth rounded head of the femur, and the clear space between the head of the femur, and the hipbone due to the layer of cartilage covering the joint surfaces.

Below, an X-ray of an osteoarthritic hip. The head of the femur is flattened and irregular, and the joint space is reduced.

Perthe's disease is now one of the commoner diseases of children between three and eight years of age. It is three times as common in boys as in girls. Usually only one hip is affected, but sometimes both are. The child's general health is excellent but he usually complains of pain in the thigh or groin and has a limp so slight that it may be difficult to detect.

The specific cause of the condition is not known, but a local disturbance of blood supply leads to death (necrosis) of part of the tissue of the head of the thighbone. The condition goes through three stages – onset, activity, and healing; the last may take up to three years. During the active stage the femoral head softens and becomes deformed, and is left with some irregularities after the healing phase is over. These irregularities may lead to degenerative arthritis of the hip joint later in life.

The diagnosis of Perthe's disease is made principally from X-ray pictures. If diagnosis and treatment are late, the femoral head may already have become fragmented.

The objective of treatment is to try to prevent the soft femoral head from being squashed and fragmented into a grossly distorted shape. Every attempt to protect the femoral head by limiting weight-bearing through the affected limb should be made. No medicine or other known treatment will accelerate healing, nor is there any way to restore the femoral head after it has been destroyed.

Adolescent bent hip or coxa vara (coxa means hip joint) is a condition which occurs in later childhood. The rounded top of the thighbone slips from its cartilaginous connection with the rest of the bone and is displaced downwards and backwards, leaving an unstable joint. Usually this is a gradual development, but a fall or injury can cause a sudden displacement. In the past it was thought that all cases were associated with a disturbance of the secretions of the endocrine glands, but it is now known that in many instances the child is of perfectly normal development.

Symptoms usually begin with gradually increasing pain in the hip, associated with a marked limp. Examination shows a characteristic limitation of movement of the hip joint. X-rays are necessary to confirm the diagnosis. Treatment is by operation.

Degenerative arthritis of the hip occurs in later life and causes pain, stiffness, and deformity. In younger people, degenerative arthritis is secondary to congenital or acquired mechanical abnormalities.

463

The basic cause is wear and tear and no medicine can halt or repair this process.

Many patients have such mild symptoms and slight limitations of movement that minor modifications of work activities, local deep-heat therapy, massage and exercises, and possibly aspirin are all that is necessary.

When symptoms do not respond to these treatments, various operations may be considered. Some that are designed to stiffen the painful hip are usually reserved for younger people with strenuous jobs, such as farmers and construction workers. Other operations are designed to retain movement in the hip joint. Another operation leaves the femoral head in place but alters the thrust of body weight through the pelvis, and a further common operation is the replacement of the femoral head and neck with a metallic substitute (prosthesis). None of the operations are suitable for all cases and the choice depends upon the age of the patient, the state of disease in the affected hip, and the condition of the other hip and spine. Usually there is effective relief from pain and restoration of function but it is not possible to give absolute assurance of results in all cases.

Total hip replacement A relatively new form of hip surgery (low-friction arthroplasty), sometimes called the Charnley operation, after Sir John Charnley, a British surgeon who developed it, is made possible by the use of an acrylic cement which glues prefabricated metal and plastic joint parts to living bone. No screws or pins are used. It is well-suited to the physical conditions surrounding the surfaces of the socket and head of the thighbone.

In selected elderly patients operation is generally satisfactory. Many severely handicapped patients have been restored to normal activity, comfort, and excellent gait by the operation. Usually the pain disappears immediately after surgery and the new joint is capable of supporting weight almost immediately. The operation is a major piece of surgery which must be done with great precision and aseptic techniques to guard against possible complications such as wound infection and dislocation. A search for other, possibly better, joint cements is in progress.

The knee

The knee is the largest joint in the body. It is the hinge in the middle of a long limb and is constantly exposed to injury. Stability of the joint depends primarily on the strength and tone of the quadriceps muscles on the front of the thigh which hold the joint extended. Ligaments of the joint are only of secondary help compared with the muscles.

When the knee joint is affected by accident, operation, or disease, wasting of local muscles occurs. This wasting can be very rapid and can be countered only by many hours of hard active exercise by the patient. Physiotherapy, massage, and drugs do nothing to build up vital muscle bulk. Only hard work by the patient, using recommended exercises, can accomplish this muscle build-up.

Bow-legs (genu varum) show an outward bowing of the knee joint. A mild degree followed by a period of straightening, and even slight overcorrection which may produce knock-knees, is the common developmental pattern in children. No treatment is necessary unless the condition persists into later childhood.

Knock-knees (genu valgum) are produced by inward angulation of the knee joint. This deformity is commonly seen between the ages of three to five years. It may occasionally be associated with a deformity of the hip. But in the absence of any bone disease, the deformity usually corrects itself spontaneously in a few years.

No treatment is necessary in young children, but a shoe wedge is often fitted. Knock-knee that is present at the age of ten needs treatment by operation, either by removing a wedge from the femur to correct the angulation, or by selectively retarding the growth of the bones so that future growth straightens the legs.

Chondromalacia patellae is a degenerative condition in adolescents that is limited to the joint between the kneecap (patella) and thighbone. The condition probably arises from repeated minor injury caused by the kneecap moving on a surface that it does not fit exactly. It is not a true degenerative arthritis, but does increase the likelihood of later degenerative changes.

Patients usually complain of pain under the kneecap, slight swelling, cracking in the joint during extension, occasional catching of the joint, and stiffness after sitting. Late teenage and early adult life is the time when symptoms usually become troublesome; young mothers with much carrying and housework to do are often affected.

Treatment is difficult but if the diagnosis is made early, firm bandage support, physiotherapy, and restriction of activities are often sufficient. If diagnosis is delayed or the symptoms get worse despite treatment, an operation is advised.

Osteochondritis dissecans is a fairly common condition occurring in late adolescence, in which there is local death of a section of the joint surface of a bone and its overlying cartilage. Eventually the fragment may separate and form a loose body in the joint. The knee joint is most often affected. Injury is probably a contributing cause.

In early stages the symptoms are vague aching and feelings of weakness in the knee. These are made worse by exercise and may persist when the knee is at rest. Examination will show wasting of muscles, possibly a slight escape of fluid into the joint, but a full normal range of movement. X-rays show a well-defined crescent-shaped excavation in the bone substance.

Treatment consists of surgical removal of the fragment if it has separated and is loose in the joint. If it has not separated, the fragment can often be encouraged to regain its blood supply by an operation which drills small holes in the fragment to allow new vessels to grow in from the depths of the bone.

In young patients, the knee can be bandaged, strenuous activities curtailed, and operation avoided. Often a plaster cast is a more satisfactory method of protecting the knee. Weight-bearing is permissible but the cast may have to be worn for six months or longer.

Recurrent dislocation of the kneecap This condition is usually congenital, but is occasionally caused by injury. The congenital form, which usually affects both knees, occurs mainly in teenage girls. The dislocation always takes place sideways, with the kneecap sliding over the femur when the knee is bent.

The dislocation occurs for no known reason when walking or running, and is often experienced by girls walking up or down stairs. There is severe pain in the knee and the victim is unable to extend the joint. Someone else, however, can easily extend the joint passively and the patella slips back into position. X-rays do not usually show any abnormality, but the kneecap may be seen to be at a slightly higher level than usual.

Dislocation of the kneecap does not always become recurrent, but repeated dislocations increase the likelihood of later degenerative arthritis. If the patient is seen after the first dislocation, limited forms of treatment and exercises may prevent further dislocation. If exercise is not effective and the dislocations recur frequently causing severe disability, an operation to transpose a tendon to realign the kneecap in a more normal position will be necessary.

Torn cartilage A tear of one of the knee cartilages is quite common in young men, though not so frequent as many people think. A tear occurs when a twisting force passes through a bent or half-bent knee. Sometimes the diagnosis is easy to make because the injury is one that typically produces a tear.

There is usually pain in the joint when the tear occurs, and the patient cannot fully straighten his knee or continue what he was doing. Swelling of the knee is noticeable the next day and persists for at least two weeks. The patient often says the knee is locked, but not in the sense that doctors use the term. The physician thinks of locking as a sudden, definite inability to extend the knee fully; unlocking of the joint occurs with equal suddenness.

Treatment is decided by two factors. The torn part is made of cartilage which does not have a blood supply and therefore cannot heal. Weight-bearing through a knee joint which contains a torn cartilage will lead to strain of the knee ligaments, deterioration of the joint, and eventually to degenerative arthritis. Once the diagnosis of a torn cartilage is made, the correct treatment is removal of the cartilage.

Knee ligaments There are four principal ligaments of the knee joint, one on each side and two within the joint. These ligaments may be strained or torn in sporting injuries and accidents. Such injuries can be serious and must be promptly and properly treated if disability is to be avoided. For complete tear of a ligament the best treatment is early surgical repair. Moderate sprains can be treated by immobilization in plaster, and minor injuries by wrapping the knee and avoiding strains during healing.

All degrees of ligament injuries will lead to wasting of the quadriceps muscle, and intensive exercises will be necessary to provide future protection for the joint.

Degenerative arthritis occurs more commonly in the knee than any other joint. This is because it is a weight-bearing joint and is exposed to injury of all sorts. This kind of arthritis is common in obese women. The basic cause is wear and tear, but usually some other factor accelerates this – overweight, previous fracture or disease which has damaged the joint surface, and misalignment of the bones of the joint.

The principal symptoms are limitation of movement and gradually increasing pain, often made worse by relatively trivial strains or twists.

Treatment is nearly always started too late, because structural changes in the joint are irreversible, but weight reduction and injection of steroids can both help to alleviate symptoms. Physiotherapy, local heat, massage, and supervised exercise enable patients to carry on for many months in moderate comfort. It is wise to avoid climbing stairs and walking over uneven ground whenever possible, since these activities impose strains on the joint.

Occasionally an operation is justified, since if a loose body is present in the joint, its removal often alleviates symptoms. Stiffening of the knee can be performed for patients crippled by severe pain and marked difficulty in bending, giving complete relief of pain and a minimal handicap if the opposite knee is not seriously affected.

The foot

A comfortable, properly functioning foot is essential for the wellbeing of the whole body. Painful or abnormal feet can lead to bad posture, fatigue, muscular cramps, and backache.

The foot contains 26 bones and 33 articulations joined together by over one hundred ligaments. Nineteen muscles provide power and control of the foot. The bones are arranged in two arches – one running along the foot and the other across it. The arches are supported by the shape of the bones, the ligaments of the joints, and indirectly by tendons and muscles. The arches have a certain degree of springiness and movement between the bones and elastic supporting structures, essential for proper functioning.

The feet support the weight of the body, and act as levers to raise the body and move it forward in walking or running. In normal walking, body weight meets the ground at the heel, moves along the outer border to the ball of the foot, and thence across the line of metatarsal heads (where the long bones connect to each toe) and is transferred into the big toe. This rolling, progressive shift of body weight cannot occur in a foot that is rigid. A properly functioning foot alters its shape with every step to accommodate forces passing through it.

Foot strain The arches and supporting structures in the foot can be affected by either acute or chronic strain. *Acute strain* is usually caused by some isolated incident, such as prolonged standing or excessive use, that grossly overtaxes the foot. Symptoms usually respond promptly to rest and strapping of the foot. Unfortunately, the sprained foot, unlike the sprained hand, cannot be placed in a sling and it takes a longer time to heal.

Chronic strain of the foot can be caused by overweight, excessive fatigue, occupational demands, abnormal gait, and faults or diseases within the foot. Most of the symptoms occur in the hinge area (midtarsal) between the hindfoot and forefoot, where ligaments have to resist all the weight of the body as it is transmitted to the forefoot.

Treatment, which is usually immediately successful, is the provision of a support for the longitudinal arch to make it sufficiently high to halt downward motion before the ligaments become strained enough to be painful. Such support does not cure since it does not remove the cause of the original strain of the foot. Every effort should be made to remove the primary cause since it is bad for the foot to become permanently reliant on arch supports. Sometimes the wearing of a permanent support is inevitable because of the difficulty in controlling the primary cause of the strain.

Flat feet (pes planus) Flat feet are rarely if ever troublesome. Many Olympic athletes have flat feet. However, feet that are becoming flat are painful and should be treated. Babies' feet are always flat and it is wrong to diagnose flat feet in infants and toddlers before the arch of the foot has had time to develop. Nature provides a big fat pad in all young feet to support the inward side of the foot before muscles and ligaments develop sufficiently to support the longitudinal arch.

Even when a child first begins to stand, the foot is very mobile and flattens on bearing weight. It is wrong to force these tiny feet into supporting shoes. Rather, the child should be encouraged to go barefoot to allow muscles and ligaments to develop normal strength. The surface the small barefoot child walks on should not be hard and unyielding, but resilient, like grass, a thick playpen pad, or cushioned carpet.

True flat foot in children is very uncommon, but when it exists the deformity is usually acquired rather than inherited. Some believe that the deformity can be produced if a baby sleeps on his stomach in a spread-eagle position which puts pressure on the big toe and pushes the feet outwards.

Many people tolerate the pain of flattening feet for astonishing lengths of time because of a misconception that it is normal for feet to hurt. It is not. The pain of flattening feet is primarily produced by stretching of the ligaments, and in late cases pain can arise in bones that have fallen sufficiently to make contact with weight-bearing surfaces.

When the foot is strained it becomes weak and easily tired, and the arch droops when weight is

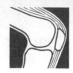

Structures of the foot
Right, some of the tendons and ligaments.
Lower right, the bones of the foot seen from
the outer side.
Below, the bones of the foot from above.

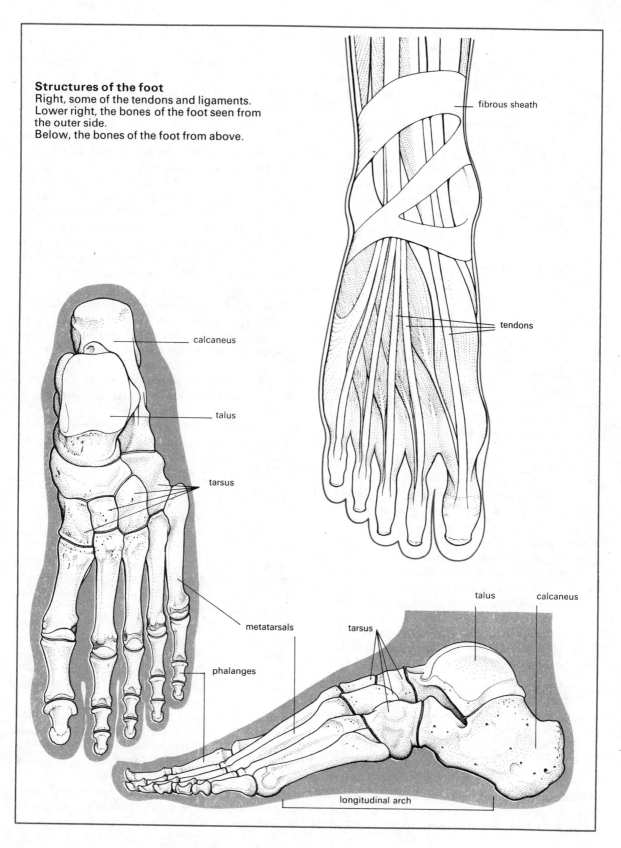

fibrous sheath

tendons

calcaneus

talus

tarsus

metatarsals

phalanges

tarsus

talus

calcaneus

longitudinal arch

borne. When the foot is raised, the arch recovers its normal shape, but in late stages the altered shape becomes fixed and the foot may be permanently flat.

Early treatment props the structures with a resilient arch support made of leather, cork, or plastic. It is important that the support should be sufficiently flexible to adapt to the changing shape of the foot during walking. Supports should be used only until the foot no longer hurts. Long-term use of a support means that the foot will become dependent on it and muscles will weaken. Later treatment consists of exercises, sensible footwear, and correct posture which is especially important because the foot is used all the time.

Flattening of the transverse arch occurs almost invariably in women. The symptom is pain in the instep area (metatarsalgia). Usually the primary cause is weakness in the muscles within the foot, and the wearing of high-heeled shoes is responsible for the persistence of symptoms. The ideal treatment is permanent abandonment of high-heeled shoes, but this therapy is almost universally rejected. Symptomatic relief can be given by placing small domed supports within the shoes. When correctly placed, these domes will restore the normal transverse arch and relieve pressure on the metatarsal heads.

Pain spreading into the toes, caused by a small growth on one of the nerves, sometimes resembles the pain of metatarsalgia caused by a fallen transverse arch. This condition can be relieved by surgical removal of the tumour.

Corrective foot exercises Foot-strengthening exercises are excellent in themselves, but too much should not be expected if exercises are done briefly and sporadically, as is often the case. It is particularly difficult to get children to do exercises they have no interest in, and even resent, and foot troubles, like others, should have the benefit of a doctor's skills. Dancing is an excellent foot exercise; so is walking barefoot on a suitable surface.

Useful special exercises are:
Picking up marbles with the toes.
In a sitting position with legs slightly bent outwards, bending the foot strongly upwards.
Walking on the outer borders of the feet.
Walking on tiptoe.

Children's feet The greatest difficulty in dealing with the developing foot lies in persuading parents to allow their child's feet to develop unhindered by rigid shoes or so-called corrective orthopaedic shoes. The growing foot is intended to move around unshod, thereby allowing full opportunity for muscles and ligaments to develop. True flat feet are so very uncommon that the diagnosis should be made by an orthopaedic surgeon rather than a shoe salesman or neighbour.

Pigeon toe, or toe-inturning, is very common in the early stages of walking, probably from the efforts of the child to improve his balance. At this stage of walking there are often signs of bowlegs, knock-knees, or internal twisting of the tibia (shinbone). In the vast majority of cases all these abnormalities correct themselves as the child develops. Occasionally there are more serious causes such as congenital deformities and those which occur in a spastic child, which need competent medical care for their correction.

Clubfoot There are two usual forms of clubfoot, congenital talipes equinovarus and calcaneovalgus. Both deformities respond well to treatment, provided it is started shortly after birth. A series of corrective plaster casts will usually restore a normal contour to the foot, although sometimes minor operations may also be necessary to relieve tightness in tendons and ligaments.

It is vital to long-term success that the children be examined at regular intervals to be sure that the correction has been maintained. It is often found that so-called relapsed clubfeet have not been checked often enough for any tendency to recurrence of the difficulty to be recognized early.

Webbed toes Webbing (a connecting membrane between digits) is not uncommon. When it occurs between the fingers, correction is necessary, but symptoms rarely develop in webbed toes. There is usually no difficulty in fitting shoes, normal function of the foot is rarely if ever affected, and surgical treatment is usually unnecessary.

Elevated little toe Occasionally there is a hereditary tendency for the little toe to be elevated above the others. There is no disability or discomfort as long as the child goes barefoot, but symptoms develop when attempts are made to force the foot into ordinary shoes. Amputation of the toe is mutilating and a poor solution. Nonsurgical treatment cannot be applied since the basic fault is a deficiency of tissue. When symptoms develop, the most satisfactory treatment is an operation designed to lengthen the shortened tissues.

Ballet dancing is often falsely accused of being harmful to growing feet. When properly controlled it is beneficial to the feet, since it produces excellent development of muscles within the feet and the calf muscles. Dancing also improves the general tone and posture of the body. Structural changes of the foot can occur only if the amount of dancing is excessive or if the child goes "up on points" too early. Ballet dancing should be moderate in amount until about the age of twelve or thirteen years, and "points" should certainly not be allowed until the age of thirteen years.

Shoes Except for fashion, the only reason for wearing shoes is to protect the feet from the weather and injury. A shoe does nothing to help the development of the muscles or arches of a normal foot. Barefoot walking is the best possible treatment for growing feet.

Children's shoes Loose-fitting cloth bootees are all that are necessary for infants before they start to walk. When the time comes to fit shoes to a baby's foot, the shoes must conform to the shape of the foot and must be large enough to allow normal movement of the foot within the shoes. The soles and uppers should be of supple leather, and neither arches nor heels are necessary. It is injurious to force a baby's foot into a miniature adult-style shoe which is wrongly shaped for infant feet.

Young feet grow at an astonishing rate. The average child outgrows a pair of shoes in three months, and generally needs a larger pair at the end of this time even though the old shoes are not badly worn. Small boys tend to demolish their shoes in three months or, as it seems to some parents, three weeks, but girls who are not so hard on their shoes may continue to wear a pair that has become too small. Inspect a child's shoes regularly to be sure he has not outgrown them.

The most important aspect of shoe fitting is adequate length. There should be a space of one half to three quarters of an inch between the end of the big toe and the end of the shoe. The widest part of the shoe should correspond with the widest weight-bearing portion of the foot. Shoes which are too short will gradually cause the toes to turn down, and persistence of this position may lead to weakness of muscles within the foot and further deformity of the toes.

Tips on shoe fitting When buying shoes it is a good idea to purchase them in the afternoon, since the foot can increase one size in length during the day, particularly if you have been standing for a long time and the day is hot. When standing in a new pair of shoes, there should be enough room to wriggle the big toe. Walk around in the shoes; if they slip at the heel, try a narrower heel width. One particular style

of shoe may be unsuitable; a good fit may require a different style. One foot is usually bigger than the other and this is the one that should be fitted.

Old shoes often give clues to poor fit or gait. Shoes may be worn excessively at one side or the other instead of under the ball of the foot which is the natural weight-bearing pivot. The shoe lining may be worn at the toes, indicating too short a shoe, or at the side or back of the heel, indicating a loose fit in this area. Socks that are too short can also constrict the feet. When a growing child needs larger shoes he usually needs larger socks as well.

Women have much more foot trouble than men, principally because of the shoes they wear. Pointed shoes cramp the toes together and produce pressure troubles such as corns and calluses. Shoes of this shape force the foot into an abnormal posture which leads to poor distribution of body weight, often resulting in backache. Constant wearing of such shoes may produce distressing deformities that cannot be completely corrected.

A reasonable justification for high heels – to help retain the shoes in stirrups when riding – has been invalid for years. Their survival among women has no relationship to practicality, but is a source of considerable foot trouble instead. A heel is high if it measures two inches. Any heel of this height or more will force the full weight of the body onto the metatarsal heads and squeeze the toes into the pointed forepart of the shoe. This crowding will lead to destruction of the transverse arch, produce calluses on the sole of the foot, and varying deformities of the toes. Calluses on the ball of the foot are not uncommonly mistaken for verrucas, which are quite different.

In young people these deformities are reversible. For example, when pregnant women wear low-heeled shoes their foot symptoms improve and they lose the calluses on the soles of their feet. Women who constantly wear high heels may suffer shortening of the calf muscles to such an extent that walking barefoot or in low heels is extremely uncomfortable. There is nothing good from a medical point of view that can be said about high heels, and next to nothing that will discourage their use.

Adult foot problems

Bunion or hallux valgus (hallux is the big toe) is a common deformity of the adult female foot, but can also occur in men. The defect is an obvious thickening and swelling of the main joint of the big toe which forces the big toe towards the other toes. There is a protuberance on the inner side of the foot where the

469

hinge bends in walking and, instead of being straight, the big toe bends towards the other toes.

Bunions are more common in the adolescent foot than is generally recognized, because children rarely complain of the pain. If the condition does give trouble in young adult life, it is unlikely that splints or sensible shoes will do any good or be tolerated by the patient. Foam rubber pegs between the first and second toes do not force the big toe into a correct position. They are more likely to force the second toe into the same deformity as the big toe.

Once the deformity is established, it is self-perpetuating and will get progressively worse if untreated. In elderly people with bunions, surgery is not warranted and shoes should be made to fit the deformed foot. In younger people there is no real alternative to surgical correction of the causes and results of the deformity. Operations which merely trim the bunion are not usually of lasting benefit since they do not treat the causes which produced the bunion.

Hallux rigidus Pain and stiffness in the large joint of the big toe is quite common in young adults. It is usually produced by repeated minor injury or a single major accident that overextends the toe with great force. The symptoms usually subside if the joint is protected for a few weeks or months, usually by fixing a small steel plate within the sole of the shoe. In a small number of patients the condition persists, and if the pain and limitation of toe movement are particularly troublesome, relief can be obtained by surgery.

Hammer toe is usually caused by cramping the toes into too small a shoe, although it can be produced by muscle imbalance in a well-shod foot. Usually this clawlike deformity affects the second toe. Symptoms are usually produced by pressure, and may be alleviated by padding. If not, surgery can give relief from the deformity.

Ingrowing toenail usually affects the big toe. The edge of the nail is driven into soft tissues by the pressure of tight shoes, or a crushing blow may inflict local injury. The forward edge of the nail as well as the side may cut into soft tissue if the nail is trimmed too short. If the area is not infected, the patient may be able to draw the overgrown tissue away from the nail after soaking the foot in hot water. In this way the cutting edge of the nail may be freed, and a wisp of cotton wool placed to cushion the contact area. This should be done daily after the bath until the corner of the nail has grown beyond the point where it cuts into the flesh. However, if the condition was caused by tight shoes it will recur unless looser shoes are worn.

When infection is present and large amounts of new tissue have grown over the nail, removal of a portion of the nail by simple surgery is usually necessary and successful. To prevent ingrowing toenail, the nail should be trimmed squarely, with enough projection at the corners to prevent gouging and the possible infection of underlying tissues.

Diseases of bone

Osteoporosis is a condition of abnormal thinning of bone, due to insufficient production of the protein foundation substance in which calcium salts are deposited. The most common type is postmenopausal osteoporosis, which occurs in a large proportion of women after a natural or artificial menopause. There may be no symptoms until some local area of fragile bone fractures from slight provocation, such as a crushed vertebra resulting from bending or a relatively minor jolt. Senile osteoporosis occurs to some degree in all ageing people. In advanced stages, deformities of the spine caused by collapsed vertebrae are not uncommon.

Hormone deficiencies are primarily involved but there are many contributing causes: poor nutrition over a period of many years or poor absorption of nutrients although the diet is good; the menopause and ageing; prolonged bed rest, immobilization, or inactivity; impaired blood supply to the bone; and various diseases such as forms of rheumatoid arthritis.

Treatment depends upon the stage and nature of the osteoporosis and the remedy of underlying factors where possible. Sex hormones are commonly prescribed, and a substantial protein diet, sometimes with minerals, though this requires careful supervision by a physician since excessive mineral intake may harm the kidneys, especially of an immobilized patient. Activity, to the extent that it is tolerated, is encouraged, with precautions to prevent further fractures. In osteoporosis of the aged, the patient should be regarded as being marked "fragile, handle with care".

Osteomalacia (softening of the bones) is also called adult rickets. Bone changes are similar to those of childhood rickets, except that they are more diffuse since there are no special areas of growth in adults. In its simplest form, osteomalacia is a deficiency disease, rare in civilized countries, but it may also result from impaired absorption of nutrients. Treatment with a high calcium, high phosphorus diet and adequate amounts of vitamin D usually gives relief from the disease.

Paget's disease (osteitis deformans) is a relatively common bone disease in people over 40 years of age. It is a long-lasting process of bone thickening, destruction, and new bone formation. In the course of time the bone involved becomes deformed and its architecture disordered. The patients often have arteriosclerosis and impaired blood supply to the bones. The disease most often affects the bones of the spine and pelvis, skull, and lower leg. The onset is gradual and patients may not seek medical assistance for many years. The disease may become arrested, or progress slowly. Fractures may occur, but heal normally. A hearing aid frequently becomes necessary.

Calcitonin A new hormone called calcitonin, discovered in 1962, is associated with bone and calcium metabolism in ways that may have therapeutic value when synthetic supplies become available. The hormone tends to decrease the amount of calcium excreted in urine, and to increase absorption of calcium by the intestines, and thus to preserve bone strength by decreasing mineral losses. The hormone has given excellent results in a few cases of Paget's disease of bone and may be useful in the healing of fractures and treatment of bone-wasting diseases such as osteoporosis.

Sprains, dislocations, and fractures

Sprains and strains A sprain is an injury to a ligament, and a strain is an injury to a muscle or its tendon. All the joints in the body are held together by ligaments powerful enough to resist all normal forces. When violent force is applied a stretched ligament will tear and a sprain occurs.

Mild sprains do not weaken the joint and usually only need support. The great majority of sprains are successfully treated with a firm supporting bandage. Severe sprains usually produce a complete tear of a major ligament and are best treated by surgical repair of the torn tissues. Sometimes the ligament remains intact and tears away from its attachment to the bone, even carrying a small piece of bone with it. X-rays will show if the bony fragment is near its original site or if the ligament is curled upon itself. If it is curled it cannot heal satisfactorily and should be repositioned surgically.

A dislocation occurs when the force applied to a joint is greater than that necessary to produce a strain. Dislocations must be reduced (returned to proper position), and usually an anaesthetic is necessary to relax the painful contraction in surrounding muscles. Occasionally, manipulation does not succeed, usually because some torn tissue or an adjacent tendon is caught between the joint surfaces. In such cases an operation may be necessary to achieve the reduction. After reduction the torn tissues must be given time to heal before allowing movement in the joint; three weeks is usually the minimum time necessary.

A *fracture* is a break in a bone. The strength of bones varies from person to person and according to age. In elderly people the bones are relatively brittle, in children, more flexible.

The surgeon who treats fractures is concerned with obtaining the best functional result for the fractured bone. This does not require perfect anatomical juxtaposition. Bone is a living tissue and is perfectly capable of uniting fractured parts that have not been exactly replaced in their original position. Because of this capacity for repair it is possible to treat most fractures by manipulations which place the broken ends close enough together for good union to occur. A good blood supply at the fracture site is necessary for repair to occur, and it follows that repair is usually more rapid in children and slower in the elderly.

During healing the fracture area must be protected from excessive movement. Various methods of immobilization are used. The most common is a plaster cast which is easily applied and removed. Some fractures need to be treated in the early days after injury by various methods of traction on the limb. A pulling force can be applied to a limb by adhesive tape stuck to the skin, or by a metallic pin placed through an unbroken part of the bone or an adjacent bone. By such means the fracture can be controlled throughout the healing process and minor adjustments of position of the broken bones can be made.

Some closed fractures, which are so grossly unstable that they constantly become redisplaced, need to be immobilized internally by some form of metallic fixation. However, this procedure adds the risks inherent in any operation. Most surgeons treat fractures without operation, if possible, because of the risk of such complications and because in fact few fractures need to be operated upon.

Different names are given to the type of break in a bone, such as greenstick, transverse, oblique, spiral, or comminuted (see illustration). But all types of breaks are treated on the same general principles: setting of the fracture into a satisfactory position; maintenance of the fracture in position until healing is sufficient to prevent redisplacement; restoration of normal function to muscles, tendons, and joints.

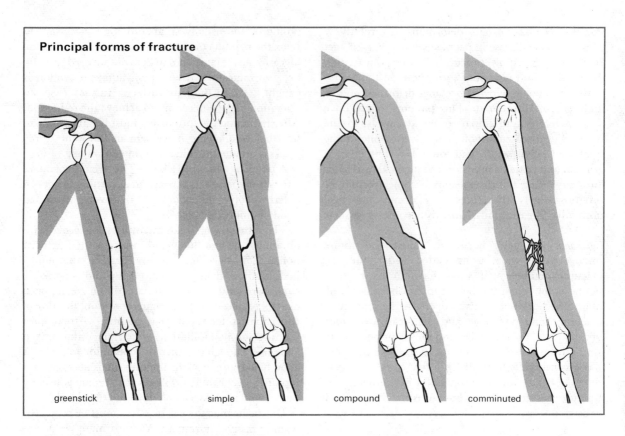

Principal forms of fracture

greenstick   simple   compound   comminuted

Restoration of function after the fracture has united is a vital part of treatment. It is usual for some joint stiffness and muscle wasting to be present after the cast has been removed. The stiffness and atrophy are directly proportional to the age of the patient and the length of time of immobilization. It is often hard to decide how soon a cast can be removed from an elderly patient in order to prevent gross stiffness and yet allow time for the fracture to heal.

Physiotherapy is of great help in the restoration of use to a stiffened limb, but active movements and active muscle contractions by the patient are the key to success. Most functional return occurs during the first three or four months. After this period, recovery slows and may not be complete for a year or even longer.

Disorders of muscles

Muscles may suffer injury, be the seat of infections, be wasted by disease of the nervous system, or be affected by a group of diseases called the muscular dystrophies.

Injuries and infections require surgical treatment and the appropriate antibiotic.

One type of muscular wasting from nervous system disease is that caused by acute anterior poliomyelitis, usually shortened to polio, and formerly called infantile paralysis. Here a particular virus damages certain cells in the spinal cord, cutting off the motor nerve supply to muscle fibres. This results in wasting and weakness. The management of the resulting paralysis and possible deformities is the province of the orthopaedic surgeon. More important is the fact that polio can be completely prevented, and in fact eradicated, by an appropriate vaccine, which is given by mouth.

Another nervous system disease is progressive muscular atrophy and its variants which cause slow damage to motor cells in the nervous system, and slow wasting of muscle groups, with consequent weakness. There is no satisfactory treatment.

The muscular dystrophies form a large group, some affecting children and some adults, but fortunately many types are rare. Myasthenia gravis causes very rapid and abnormal fatigue in groups of muscles. It cannot be cured, but it can be controlled by modern drugs. Hypertrophic muscular dystrophy produces very large, strong-looking muscles which are in fact very weak. Myotonia congenita (often called Thomsen's disease from the doctor who described it and himself suffered from it) causes muscles to contract normally, but to be very slow in relaxing. Other types of muscular dystrophy cause wasting and weakness in groups of muscles, for example in the shoulder girdle, the pelvic girdle, or the lower leg. The trouble progresses slowly and eventually results in disability and deformities, which can to some extent be helped by surgical appliances. Many of the dystrophies occur in more than one member of a family and are genetically determined. In some it is possible to demonstrate a chemical abnormality. Moreover this can be detected in apparently normal relatives, which enables the doctor to estimate the chances of any offspring being affected.

In Britain, the Muscular Dystrophy Group exists to study and encourage research in these diseases. It will not give advice to individual patients, but will help by communicating with the general practitioner, giving the location of special clinics for the dystrophies. Its address is: Muscular Dystrophy Group, 35 Macaulay Rd, London SW4 oQP.

Chapter 20

Arthritis and rheumatism

Revised by D. R. L. Newton FRCP

Confusion occurs in this field because of the many terms that are used to describe arthritis and allied diseases.

Rheumatism is not a diagnosis but a vague term which is used to describe aches and pains which seem to the patient or to his medical adviser to arise in the joints, muscles, ligaments, or tendons, or in the connective tissues – the structures and substances in the body which bind all the component parts together. *Rheumatic diseases* is the general term used by doctors to denote all those disorders that cause pain and disability affecting the joints and their supporting structures and the connective tissues. *Rheumatology* is the specialized field of medical practice which devotes itself predominantly to the study and treatment of these disorders.

Arthritis is a word which strictly should be used only to indicate actual inflammation in joints and their surrounding structures but unfortunately it is also used by doctors and laymen as a convenient term to denote all sorts of rheumatic disorders. Everybody knows someone who suffers from arthritis and who may be disabled: to be told that one has arthritis, or to imagine oneself that this is the probable cause of one's symptoms, naturally leads to fears of crippling, which in the great majority of cases are unfounded. Therefore arthritis should never be used as a blanket term to describe any rheumatic disorder other than inflammation of a joint.

Nonarticular rheumatism is a term that describes conditions in which the soft tissues related to movements of the joints are involved – for example, ligaments, tendons, bursae, and muscles.

There are over 100 conditions which are commonly grouped together as rheumatic diseases. Their medical classification presents great difficulty not only because of complex interrelationships but also, in spite of extensive research devoted to them, there remain gaps in our knowledge of the causes and mechanisms of many of the disorders. The object of research in the rheumatic diseases is a better understanding and management of these conditions in the form of new drugs to reduce the effects of inflammation, new techniques to prevent damage occurring, and surgical replacement of joints which have been damaged beyond repair. One of the advances in this field in the last few years has been the free communication of knowledge between many scientific workers including physicians, surgeons, medical research workers, and bioengineers.

In this chapter there is little point in attempting to classify the various types of arthritis and rheumatic disease, and it is proposed to discuss the broad categories of commonly occurring disorders under the following main headings:

Nonarticular rheumatism disorders which primarily affect the soft tissues of the musculoskeletal system rather than the joints.

Osteoarthrosis the degenerative disorders of joints.

Gout the most common of the disorders caused by an abnormality in body chemistry.

Rheumatoid arthritis the most common form of joint inflammation and damage.

Seronegative polyarthritis a group of disorders which resemble rheumatoid arthritis but with important differences which influence correct management.

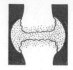

Spondylitis a condition causing active inflammation of the joints of the spine.

The diffuse connective tissue disorders conditions in which arthritis and involvement of soft tissues and connective tissues may be intermingled in a variety of ways.

Infective arthritis in which joints are infected by bacteria or other pus-forming microbes.

Nonarticular rheumatism

These disorders are not primarily due to arthritis, though many occur as a result of widespread connective tissue disorders of which joint inflammation may be a part.

Tendinitis refers to inflammation of tendons or ligaments where they arise from or are inserted into bone, or where they move in relation to other structures.

Tenosynovitis implies inflammation occurring within the lubricating sheath which envelops some tendons in their course, for example, in the palm of the hand. These lesions may arise because of local strain or injury or as a manifestation of a generalized rheumatic disorder, for example, in rheumatoid arthritis or gout. Treatment may include the use of drugs, various forms of physiotherapy, rest with or without splinting, injections of a local anaesthetic or a locally-acting corticosteroid drug, or surgery. Some anatomical sites are particularly prone to the development of tendinitis. Possibly the most important of these is the shoulder where normal function depends upon the perfect action of muscles and tendons. Other types of tendinitis occur in relation to the elbow (so-called "tennis elbow" and "golfer's elbow"); in relation to the hips and thighs (occasionally caused by horse riding); in relation to the knee, often associated with unaccustomed physical stresses; and around the heel involving the large Achilles tendon at the back of the heel and caused, for example, by wearing new or unsuitable footwear.

"Frozen shoulder" is a condition, known medically as capsulitis, which may result from uncontrolled tendinitis or may occur less commonly in association with other conditions where movement is limited such as rheumatoid arthritis, disorders of the nervous system, for example a stroke, or some forms of heart disorder. The frozen shoulder may also complicate fractures and other severe injuries around the shoulder, often despite attempts to prevent it. Some cases of capsulitis of the shoulder may be complicated by the "shoulder-hand syndrome" in which the hand on the affected side becomes swollen and painful. The natural history of the frozen shoulder is one of increasing pain and stiffness and then persisting stiffness with lessening pain before a gradual spontaneous recovery of movement. Treatment is aimed at encouraging the natural process of recovery, which is full in most cases, though it may take up to three years.

Bursitis means the inflammation of a bursa. A bursa is a small pouch with lubricating surfaces to allow ease of motion between muscles, tendons, and bony surfaces. The cause of bursitis is usually excessive use or other abuse of the structures concerned. The involved area becomes painful and locally tender, and redness and swelling may be seen if it is close to the skin surface. An example is the so-called "housemaid's knee" in which the bursa at the front of the knee becomes inflamed and swollen from excessive, and often unaccustomed, kneeling. The treatment of bursitis usually involves rest of the joint, perhaps with splinting, and the use of simple pain-relieving and anti-inflammatory drugs. Sometimes local injections or surgical operation may be required.

Fibrositis is not a distinct disease but is a term applied by some doctors to irritative processes occurring in muscles, fascia, ligaments, and tendons. Symptoms include stiffness and tenderness which may arise at the site of involvement or, more commonly are referred to a point some distance away from the actual site. Diagnosis may reveal, for example, that pain felt in the region of the elbow in fact arises in the neck which is the structure to which appropriate treatment should be applied. Precipitating factors include injury which may be single or repetitive, major or minor. Symptoms may follow strenuous or unaccustomed sporting activity. Chronic neck or low back strain are both well-known causes. Fibrositic pain often accompanies generalized infections such as common influenza-type illnesses, or it may be a manifestation of generalized rheumatic and arthritic diseases. In most patients fibrositis is a self-limiting disorder which may cause a great deal of annoyance but is never crippling unless it is the initial feature of one of the more serious forms of generalized rheumatic disease. The treatment may include the prescription of simple pain-relieving and anti-inflammatory drugs, the injection of local anaesthetic or other agents to "trigger spots", or the application of heat and deep massage and other forms of physiotherapy. Following an accurate diagnosis skilled manipulation may have a part to play in the treatment of this condition, particularly where the fibrositis arises from a condition of the spine.

Osteoarthrosis (degenerative joint disorders)

This condition was formerly called osteoarthritis. Changes in the joints due to degeneration have been found in the skeletons of early vertebrates, including the dinosaurs. Joint changes detectable by X-rays are almost universal in people in the middle and later years of life and microscopic evidence of degeneration in the weightbearing surface cartilage of joints is detectable by the third decade of life, or earlier. The problem posed here is what constitutes natural wear and tear and what constitutes abnormal degeneration. Both may produce symptoms. Even mild changes of degeneration in the joints as seen by X-rays may be regarded as arthritis and this may give the false impression that the patient is suffering from one of the active forms of joint inflammation which could cause widespread damage with resultant crippling. Therefore it is now customary to refer to the wear and tear changes which occur with age, even if prematurely, as "osteoarthrosis". Only ten to fifteen per cent of people with degenerative changes in the joints shown by X-ray have significant symptoms and it is important to appreciate that their severity is not necessarily connected with the extent of the joint changes as seen on X-ray. This is because thickening of the capsule – the binding envelope – of the joint may occur to a greater extent than wear in the weightbearing cartilage surfaces and produce quite severe symptoms. X-rays will show only loss or reduction of weightbearing cartilage. Conversely, severe X-ray changes may be accompanied by much less pain and restriction of movement than would be expected.

The underlying process in osteoarthrosis is a gradual thinning and, in some cases, eventual disappearance of the cartilage which forms the smooth inner surface of the joints. Throughout life this cartilage, like other tissues, is being constantly replaced but there may be genetic and other factors which determine that its quality may be deficient. Thus the changes which give rise to osteoarthrosis may be caused by the relatively poor functioning of the cells responsible for producing the cartilage

substance, or by a fault in the nutrition of those cells by the joint fluid which has lubricating and nutritional functions. The process of degeneration may be hastened by injury, either single or repetitive; by malformation of a joint by some congenital defect; by a previous injury causing misalignment; by some other previous damage to the joint, such as an infection or active arthritis; or by the laying down of chemical materials which should not be present, such as occurs in gout. If the cartilage is shed at an abnormal rate and eventually disappears in patches or in its entirety, the underlying bone becomes thickened, and creaking may be felt by the patient and sometimes even heard by people nearby. Some degree of loss of movement is an invariable accompaniment of this condition either because the joint is mechanically defective, painful, or limited by protective muscle spasm as well as by thickening of the joint capsule.

It must be appreciated that the rate of natural wear and tear in joints is very much an individual matter and may occur quite early in some subjects while never occurring at all in others. When symptoms arise in the presence of osteoarthrosis they need to be carefully assessed because, although they may be due to the condition, there is no reason why someone with wear and tear changes naturally occurring should not develop a more active rheumatic process as well. For example, a patient with symptomless osteoarthrosis may suddenly develop joint pain, swelling, and stiffness which on investigation may be found to be due to some other form of rheumatic process, perhaps an active arthritis, unconnected with the previous condition.

Not all joints are equally involved by osteoarthrosis and the ones most commonly affected are those which are subject to the greatest stresses, particularly in bearing weight, notably the lower spine, the hips, the knees, and the great toe joints. Other smaller joints which are commonly involved, particularly in women, are the joints at the base of the thumb close to the wrist.

Heberden's nodes are a manifestation of a common form of osteoarthrosis occurring in older people, usually women, and are named after the physician who first described them. They are knobbly firm lumps at the sides of the end joints of the fingers and may appear separately, enlarging slowly over the years, or come quite quickly, involving a number of fingers, and producing significant pain and discomfort as they develop. Because of the bony enlargement, the end joints of the fingers become less mobile, which may result in some loss of precise function such as threading needles and picking up small objects. However, the most common complaint is of the unsightliness of the knobbly finger ends. There is no treatment for Heberden's nodes, but fortunately the osteoarthrotic condition does not usually spread to other joints.

The most usual symptoms of osteoarthrosis are stiffness and aching pain in the joints, which on the whole are worse during or after activity and tend to be relieved by rest. However, many patients complain particularly of quite severe stiffness after rest following activity; for example, having rested in an armchair for an hour or two after going for a walk there may be considerable stiffness on attempting to move about again, whereas following retirement to bed for a good night's rest there may be complete relief of symptoms by the morning. Sometimes osteoarthrotic joints produce severe night pain and this applies particularly to the hip and the knee. Following a strain an osteoarthrotic joint may become swollen and acutely painful.

The mechanisms involved in osteoarthrosis are becoming better understood but the disorder is not yet preventable. Treatment therefore is directed towards relieving stress on the affected joints. A patient who is overweight imposes unnecessary stresses upon weightbearing joints and adequate weight reduction is therefore important. There is no way in which the clock can be put back to return an osteoarthrotic joint to a youthful state, but attempts can be made to slow down deterioration by correcting poor posture and removing unnecessary mechanical stresses; for example, the use of a walking stick can do much to relieve the stress on a hip, knee, or ankle in walking, provided that the stick is used correctly in the opposite hand for optimal effect. The muscles which act upon a joint which is limited in movement or is the site of pain will lose bulk and become flabby. Therefore an important principle of management is an exercise programme to rebuild these muscles in order to achieve a better control of joint movement within the least painful range of movement. The patient has to learn the difference between exercise which places stresses on the weightbearing surfaces and results in the production of more pain and more muscle inhibition, and exercises which are properly controlled to build muscle bulk and tone without placing extra stresses on the weightbearing surfaces; hence the importance of skilled physiotherapy. Physical activities which place severe stresses on the affected joints, particularly court ball games which involve sudden starting, stopping, and changes in direction, should be discouraged, whereas swimming which involves good overall movement, and muscle work without weight bearing can be encouraged.

Drugs play an important part in the management of osteoarthrosis. Simple pain-relievers may be used as needed and anti-inflammatory agents taken regularly will reduce the painful reaction to stress in affected joints. These drugs are discussed in the section dealing with the management of rheumatoid arthritis.

Patients with osteoarthrosis, particularly if weight-bearing joints are involved, may benefit from admission to hospital for a short course of treatment which combines the use of drugs and physiotherapy, perhaps with local joint injections, to settle an excessive reaction to stress within individual joints. The period under expert observation allows the patient to learn a proper exercise routine. Corticosteroid (cortisone) drugs are never used in the management of uncomplicated osteoarthrosis except by local joint or soft tissue injection.

A human joint has to be in a very bad way indeed to be bettered by a man-made substitute, but there is now a place for surgical treatment of severe osteoarthrosis in particular joints. Many patients think that it is a relatively simple matter to have a joint replaced but this is always a major procedure which no thoughtful surgeon will undertake lightly. The results obtained from certain joint replacements in the right patient at the right time are now extremely good but it must be emphasized that many artificial joints are still in the developmental stage and patients must be encouraged to discuss their individual problem with their family doctor and with the physicians and surgeons concerned.

It should be emphasized that for the great majority of patients osteoarthrosis is a mild disorder which may require some moderation of normal activities but which rarely causes severe disability. It does not affect the general state of health, and symptoms can be adequately controlled by the measures which have been outlined.

Gout

This condition is perhaps the best understood of all the rheumatic diseases and is now curable. The disorder is due to a biochemical abnormality which leads to the accumulation of uric acid salts (urates) in abnormal amounts in the body. All persons produce uric acid as an end product of protein chemistry in the body and the substance is excreted by the kidneys into the urine. We now know that there are some people who overproduce uric acid due to some aberration in the chemical processes concerned. There are other people whose kidneys do not get rid of uric acid as efficiently as they should. This seldom has anything to do with serious kidney disease in which there is failure of the kidney to cope with all its functions, which of course includes the elimination of uric acid from the body and in which a condition known as secondary gout may occur. Whatever the underlying cause, if urates build up in the body there may, in certain circumstances, be a deposition of crystals in and around joints which will provoke a sudden attack of gout – one of the most painful conditions known. The attack is characterized by sudden acute inflammation of a joint with pain, tenderness, and swelling, very often involving first the joint at the base of the big toe. The surrounding skin becomes tight, shiny, hot, and red and the patient fears the slightest movement. Without treatment recurrent attacks occur during the years and each one tends to last a little longer. As the concentration of urates builds up in the body, deposition of the substance occurs around the affected joints such as the elbows, knees, and feet and may also occur in some soft tissue sites including the ears and some tendons. Such a visible deposit is known as a tophus (plural – tophi).

Contrary to the popular opinion that gout is a penalty for high living and overindulgence in rich foods, the condition occurs throughout the population. Alcohol in any form and diets rich in certain protein materials known as purines may temporarily raise the body uric acid level and can therefore provoke an attack in a susceptible person but such habits are not in any way responsible for the underlying chemical abnormality which determines whether a person will have a high uric acid level in the blood (hyperuricaemia). It is known that other illnesses, injuries, and operations may provoke an attack of gout.

It will be readily appreciated that once the diagnosis has been established treatment falls into two categories; firstly, the treatment of the acute attack; and secondly, the management of the underlying chemical abnormality to prevent attacks of gout occurring in the future. If a patient is overweight and indiscreet in dietary and alcoholic habits, these must be suitably modified as a normal principle of sensible attention to general health. The acute attacks are treated with a suitable anti-inflammatory agent, usually by phenylbutazone or indomethacin, and occasionally by the time-honoured remedy of colchicine if there is intolerance to the others. Once the acute attack has been treated, attention can be given

Gout in foot and hand

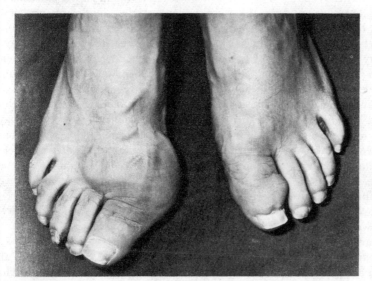

Acute gout of the right big toe joint.

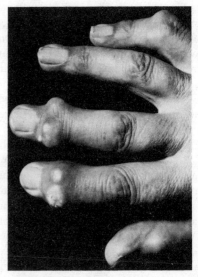

Chronic gout of the hand showing uric acid deposits and commencing ulceration on the index finger.

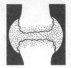

to the long-term management of the chemical abnormality which allows the excessive accumulation of urates in the body. There are two sorts of drug to do this. One group, the uricosuric drugs, are so-called because they increase the output of uric acid through the kidneys. The ones commonly used are probenecid and sulphinpyrazone. The dosage must be controlled by the doctor. An adequate fluid intake must be maintained. The other group of drugs used in the long-term control of the high level of uric acid in the body interfere with the chemical pathways by which uric acid is made in the body, so reducing the amount of uric acid which is produced. The best known drug in this group is allopurinol. It should be understood that sudden changes in the concentration of uric acid between the blood and the tissues may precipitate attacks of gout and therefore any long-term treatment must be introduced slowly and drug dosages increased gradually under medical observation. The doctor may well warn the patient that the long-term treatment may start by precipitating an attack of acute gout, though this is likely to be the last one the patient will ever have. Careful attention to detail produces good results and many doctors like to keep a patient on one of the "anti-attack" agents, such as phenylbutazone or indomethacin, during the first few weeks of the introduction of long-term treatment to guard against the possibility of discomfort associated with changes in the uric acid balance between the blood and the tissues. It goes without saying that any long-term treatment by either uricosuric agents or by allopurinol involves regular tablet taking, probably as a lifetime's measure. Some patients cannot tolerate one or other of the long-term drugs, perhaps because they have a skin sensitivity or stomach intolerance, but these difficulties can usually be overcome. In these days, therefore, the manifestations of gout can be virtually eliminated.

Rheumatoid arthritis

Rheumatoid arthritis is a generalized disease of the body involving the connective tissues and many organs and is therefore better described as rheumatoid disease even though the primary manifestations, so far as most patients are concerned, are in the joints. The disorder occurs in many forms and may show itself as pain and swelling in a single joint or more usually with involvement of a number of joints at the same time, typically in a symmetrical distribution. The cause of rheumatoid disease is not yet known, but a great deal has been revealed about the many manifestations of the disease and their control, and a number of the factors which influence its onset and development. Meanwhile attention is given to all those methods of management which limit the progress of the disease and minimize its ill effects on the patient.

Rheumatoid arthritis occurs in both sexes at all ages but is commoner in women than men. It is often possible to make a reasonably accurate estimate of the way the disorder will develop and how its manifestations may best be controlled. The onset of the disorder may be sudden, involving one joint (monoarthritis) or many joints (polyarthritis) and perhaps accompanied by general constitutional disturbance; in other words, it first appears as an acute illness. In other cases the onset may be gradual, only one or two joints may be involved, and the whole process may settle down leaving no serious consequences. The disorder should not therefore be regarded as one definable disease but as a spectrum of disorders varying greatly from one patient to the next. At one end of the spectrum is a disorder which is so mild that the patient does not perhaps realize that he has it, while at the other end of the spectrum, fortunately very rare, the disease may be of devastating severity causing an illness, which is occasionally fatal, and very serious joint damage which cannot be prevented despite the application of all the methods known to medical science.

Most people know someone who has rheumatoid arthritis. Many of those sufferers developed the disorder many years ago before present methods of management were available and it can be said that the results of their treatment would have been much better had modern measures been available to them.

Early signs of rheumatoid disease may be persistent tiredness, general malaise, aches and pains, and, most typically, morning joint stiffness of varying degree which improves as the day goes on. Symptoms may occur in episodes lasting for a few days or weeks, and these may recur. Such symptoms should be regarded by any patient as a warning that he should consult his doctor so that the cause can be determined, since symptoms of other disorders may be similar to those of rheumatoid disease. So far as the joints are concerned in rheumatoid arthritis the inflammatory process initially involves the soft tissues of the lining of the joint (synovial membrane) which swells and thickens and may produce an excess of the fluid which normally lubricates and nourishes the joint tissues (synovial fluid). This leads to joint swelling, stiffness, and pain on movement. Later the local disease process may progress to invade the joint surface with destruction of the lining cartilage and the

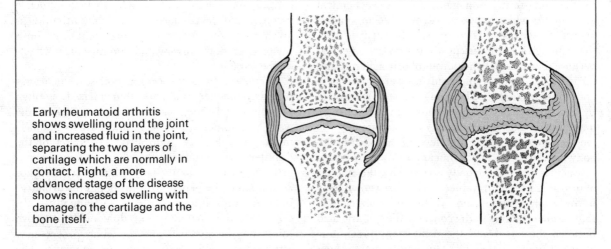

Early rheumatoid arthritis shows swelling round the joint and increased fluid in the joint, separating the two layers of cartilage which are normally in contact. Right, a more advanced stage of the disease shows increased swelling with damage to the cartilage and the bone itself.

underlying bone. If the disease is untreated the two surfaces of the joint may eventually fuse to make it totally stiff.

Although the disease may cease spontaneously at any stage it is wise to assume that it will pursue a slowly progressive course. In the majority of cases the tendency ultimately is for the process to become inactive and it is up to those treating the patient to ensure that as little damage as possible occurs.

The diagnosis of rheumatoid disease is based primarily on the history and clinical examination of the patient supported by various laboratory tests and X-rays. Patients should realize that there is no specific test for rheumatoid arthritis. There is a blood test which determines the presence or absence of so-called "rheumatoid factor", and although this is positive in a high proportion of patients who have what is medically termed classical or definite rheumatoid arthritis, there is a significant proportion of normal people in the population which gives this positive result, while at the other extreme there are some patients with severe and obvious rheumatoid arthritis who have a negative test.

In the management of rheumatoid arthritis, it is likely that many medical and paramedical people will be involved – general practitioner, rheumatologist, occupational therapist, physiotherapist, orthopaedic surgeon, social workers, and members of the Employment Advisory Service. The coordination of this team is likely to be carried out by the rheumatologist.

It may be useful at this point to consider in more detail the various forms of management which are used alone, but more often in combination, in the management of a patient suffering from rheumatoid disease.

Rest and exercise Some degree of local rest for individual joints and more general rest, particularly in the case of an overworked housewife, is usually helpful in the early stages of the disorder or in the presence of flare-ups. Few housewives with family commitments can achieve physical and emotional rest in their own home but it may be easier for a man to do so. Great benefit usually follows admission to a specialized unit in the early stages of the disease so that the overall situation can be assessed and the response to combinations of rest, graduated activity, exercise, drugs, and other therapy monitored. The position of maximum comfort for an inflamed and swollen joint is not necessarily the best in the long run and for this reason "resting splints" are often prescribed for use on individual joints, to be worn at night or at intervals during the day. The use of a pillow comfortably placed behind the bent knee is strictly taboo because it may lead to permanent deformity. Yet rest does not mean immobilization. Nobody readily moves a painful joint if they can avoid it and it needs careful instruction to show a patient how movement can best be accomplished, the right way to go about it, and the frequency with which it should be done. The muscles acting upon any painful joint tend to become inhibited and lose strength and bulk; additionally in rheumatoid disease the majority of the muscles show some degree of inflammation which is a further inhibiting factor.

Drugs A number of drugs are well established as useful in the management of rheumatoid disease. The patient should be absolutely honest about the effects which drugs seem to have. It is impossible to predict with accuracy what effect any particular drug will have on any one patient. The patient must not try to

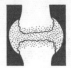

please the doctor by agreeing that something is useful when there is doubt. Equally important, any symptom which might be a side effect of a drug which is being taken should be reported, however irrelevant that symptom may appear to be at first sight. Thirdly, patients must be truthful about whether they are taking their drugs as prescribed or indeed taking them at all.

It may be helpful to categorize the different types of drug used in the management of rheumatoid disease according to their action.

Firstly there are simple analgesic (pain-relieving) drugs with no anti-inflammatory activity, such as paracetamol and codeine. Secondly there are analgesics which exhibit minor anti-inflammatory activity, such as flufenamic acid and ibuprofen which are relatively free of side effects. Thirdly there are those analgesic drugs with major anti-inflammatory activity and these include indomethacin, phenylbutazone, oxyphenbutazone, and the aspirin group of drugs provided they are taken in high enough dosage.

The purely anti-inflammatory agents are the corticosteroid drugs (the cortisone group) which suppress inflammation very strongly, but unfortunately also produce a number of unwanted side effects. These substances make the patient feel much better because they suppress the inflammatory processes in the joints and tissues which give rise to the pain, swelling, and stiffness – but they do not halt the underlying process. The important point about these potent drugs is that although they may have a part to play they must never be used without consideration

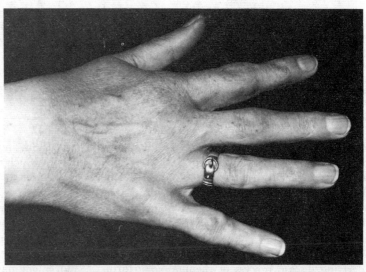

A hand showing early rheumatoid arthritis, with spindle-shaped swellings of the fingers, but no general deformity.

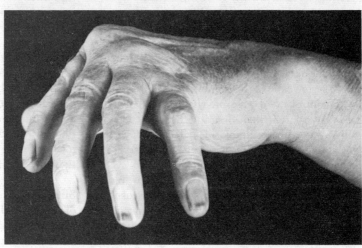

In more advanced disease there is permanent deformity of the hand with deviation of the fingers away from the thumb.

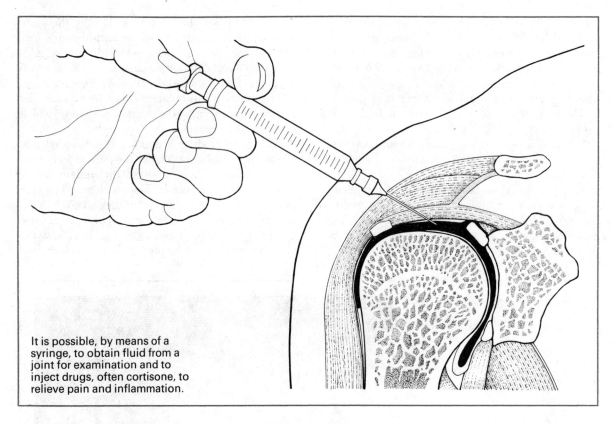

It is possible, by means of a syringe, to obtain fluid from a joint for examination and to inject drugs, often cortisone, to relieve pain and inflammation.

of every aspect of the case and they must be used only when essential. Patients should keep to the prescribed dose and not vary it, because of the danger of side effects and because there may be danger in stopping the drug suddenly. Patients who are being treated with corticosteroid drugs should carry a card stating this fact.

Drugs with a long-term suppressive effect on the underlying disease process of rheumatoid arthritis include gold, chloroquine, and D-penicillamine. All have their advantages and disadvantages.

Finally, in some cases it may be necessary to use one of the so-called immunosuppressive drugs such as azathioprine or cyclophosphamide. These are used in the more severe cases of rheumatoid disease where, in order to control the disease process, the patient has had to take a larger than desirable dose of corticosteroid drugs with resultant side effects. By introducing the immunosuppressive drug it is possible to reduce the steroid dosage and so side effects.

In a case of rheumatoid arthritis where a few joints remain inflamed despite other general measures aimed at reducing activity in the disease process, it may be possible to settle down the local inflammation by injecting a corticosteroid drug into the joint cavity. This may produce sufficient remission to allow

movement and muscle control to be regained and for a joint which is the site of commencing deformity to be restored to a more normal position.

Physiotherapy has many techniques but is chiefly devoted to regaining lost movement, retaining existing movement, and re-educating the patient in the proper use of the joints and muscles. Graduated movement may be assisted by the application of heat in various forms. One of the most valuable adjuncts in this field is the use of exercise in water.

Occupational therapy The occupational therapist assesses disability and the application of various means to enable a patient to overcome problems of daily living, such as dressing, toilet, bathing, eating, and working in various situations. The occupational therapist and the physiotherapist work closely together since their expertise overlaps even though they have their own skills to offer.

Surgery The place of surgery in the management of rheumatoid disease varies greatly according to the type and severity of the arthritis, the situation and the number of joints involved, and the degree of damage present. Some surgery is performed early in the course

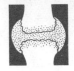

of the disease in order to try to prevent damage. Representative of this group of operations is synovectomy where the swollen, potentially damaging synovial membrane of the joint is taken out, to be replaced naturally, it is hoped, by a normal joint lining. The other main group of surgical procedures consists of reconstructive operations which may be used to stiffen hopelessly damaged, painful, and unstable joints in a good functional position; to repair tendons which have been ruptured by the rheumatoid inflammation; or, where possible, to replace badly damaged joints by artificial ones.

Diet No special diets are required in the management of rheumatoid disease, though on basic principles a patient who is overweight would be better off thinner, thus placing less strain on the weightbearing joints.

JUVENILE CHRONIC POLYARTHRITIS is the term used to denote an inflammatory arthritis, sometimes resembling rheumatoid arthritis, occurring in childhood. It used to be known as Still's disease but four or more separate conditions are now recognized as occurring in this group of diseases. The care of these children necessarily differs from that of adults, not least because specialized facilities, including good quality schooling, are necessary at the residential hospital units in which a number of patients have to spend many months or years. A proportion of these children may be left with severe disabilities which demand special care as they grow up.

Seronegative polyarthritis

This term is used to denote a group of disorders, of which the main feature is an active inflammatory arthritis of one or more limb joints and sometimes involvement of the small joints of the spine. The distribution of the joint involvement is in many cases different from that of rheumatoid disease. This group of joint disorders may appear coincidentally with psoriasis, which is a skin condition; with certain disorders of the bowel, notably ulcerative colitis; with certain diseases of the eye, notably iritis; or with chronic or recurrent genitourinary tract infections.

Spondylitis

This is a condition where active inflammation occurs in the small joints of the spine. It is sometimes called ankylosing spondylitis or bamboo spine, because if the disease runs a full course, it may result in total spinal stiffness (ankylosis). However, the process may stop at any stage and, as in the case of rheumatoid disease, there is a wide variation of involvement. This ranges from something very mild, consisting perhaps of only slight backache, to a severe spinal disorder which may require the most energetic treatment and which may unfortunately, in spite of modern methods of management, produce total spinal stiffness. Spondylitis is much more common in men than women, and may appear at any time during life, though most commonly about the third decade. Typical initial symptoms are low back pain—worse after rest, particularly first thing in the morning and relieved by getting up and moving around, and pain which alternates between one buttock and the other. Tenderness of bony points, such as the "sitting bones" or the heels may be noted, and chest tightness and soreness may occur as a manifestation of the involvement of the joints where the ribs meet with the spine. A recent finding of considerable significance is that approximately 90 per cent of patients who suffer from spondylitis belong to a certain tissue type which only approximately six per cent of the general population have.

The treatment of spondylitis is largely with the more potent nonsteroidal anti-inflammatory agents, and indomethacin and phenylbutazone are particularly useful. Patients are instructed in a regular routine of mobility and posture-correcting exercises for the spine and chest cage.

The diffuse connective tissue disorders

These form a group of diseases which often, though not invariably, occur with joint pain and stiffness as their manifestations. The so-called polymyalgia rheumatica syndrome tends to occur in both sexes, usually after the age of 60, sometimes causing severe pain and stiffness of the shoulder and pelvic girdles. It may also be accompanied by considerable constitutional disturbance, illness, and loss of weight. Treatment is almost invariably by the use of corticosteroid drugs and since the process is naturally self-limiting these drugs can usually be withdrawn within a year or so with the patient fully recovered.

Systemic or disseminated lupus erythematosus (SLE) is another generalized inflammatory disorder affecting the connective tissues and, in addition to joint involvement with active arthritis which may be damaging and deforming, other body systems are frequently involved, including the skin, kidneys, liver, heart, and lungs.

Progressive systemic sclerosis is an uncommon connective tissue disorder in which progressive scarring may occur in the skin and certain internal organs such as the gullet. However, as in other diffuse connective tissue disorders, the usual features are rheumatic with diffuse aches and pains or arthritic with pain and swelling of various joints.

Polymyositis is the name given to an ill-defined group of disorders characterized by inflammation, weakness, and degeneration of muscles. The condition may be accompanied by active arthritis or by nonarticular rheumatism. The early diagnosis of these disorders may be difficult and may require the examination of samples of skin and muscle under the microscope, a procedure known as biopsy.

Infective arthritis

Arthritis due to infection of a joint with a pus-forming organism such as the staphylococcus requires prompt attention with the use of the appropriate antibiotic therapy and, frequently, urgent surgical intervention. An acute infection of a joint does not necessarily follow a local penetrating injury and the infecting organism may have come from elsewhere in the body and have been carried to the joint by the bloodstream. Antibiotics and other chemotherapeutic agents have made septic arthritis much less of a problem than in the past provided that diagnosis and treatment are prompt. Delay can result in rapid and severe joint destruction leading to severe degenerative joint disease or a totally stiff joint. Tuberculosis as a cause of chronic joint infection has become rare in this country because of the high standards of public health and hygiene which have done so much to eliminate tuberculosis from the human and animal populations.

Investigations in arthritis and rheumatic diseases

Radiology The majority of patients going to see their doctor with rheumatic complaints require X-rays, usually a standard chest film to exclude any unsuspected lung disease and X-rays of the hands and feet. Additional X-rays may be taken of any joints which the doctor thinks might give useful information. Even if they are normal such films may be of

importance when matched against repeat films at a later date.

Special X-rays may be required in certain circumstances. Tomograms give information about the part being X-rayed at various depths from the surface. Arthrograms are performed by the injection of some form of contrast medium into a joint to show the outline of the joint cavity or to indicate the extent of any leakage of joint fluid which may have occurred into the surrounding tissues.

Pathology At first consultation most patients will have some routine blood counts performed, notably to determine whether or not they are anaemic and to give information about the number and type of the blood cells present. The ESR (erythrocyte sedimentation rate) is an important index of the activity of inflammatory disorders of the body. Certain biochemical tests are likely to be performed, such as estimation of the uric acid content of the blood and the concentration and nature of the plasma proteins. *Immunological tests* will be performed in most cases, the most important screening test being the so-called rheumatoid factor tests which have already been discussed in the section dealing with rheumatoid arthritis.

In certain circumstances excess synovial fluid may be withdrawn from a swollen joint so that it may be examined for cell content, chemical composition, general characteristics, and, if infection is suspected, the presence of microbes. *Biopsy* may be carried out on various tissues, notably skin, muscle, and the synovial membrane which lines the joints. The last examination may be done either by a small open operation or by the insertion of a special needle under local anaesthetic or by arthroscopy. This is a relatively new technique which has been made possibly only by the development of the science of fibre optics. A small telescope is inserted into the joint cavity which can thus be inspected directly, and at the same time a small piece of the lining membrane of the joint may be removed for examination under the microscope and by various immunological techniques. For the moment arthroscopy is necessarily limited to large joints such as the knee, but future technological advances may make it possible to inspect smaller joints.

Other specialized investigation techniques include radioisotope scanning in which the patient is given a dose of a short-lived radioactive substance which will be concentrated in areas of active inflammation and shown up by scanning apparatus. Thermography is a technique by which temperature changes can be

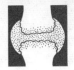

plotted on an anatomical basis, indicating the presence of active areas of inflammation.

Rehabilitation in arthritis and other rheumatic diseases

Rehabilitation implies the restoration to a patient of maximum functional capacity – physically, emotionally, psychologically, and socially. The principles of rehabilitation are similar irrespective of the nature of the patient's disability. They require team work and consultation; and of necessity such consultation must include the patient and his or her close relatives or companions. The special expertise and facilities provided by the hospital and community medical and paramedical services, by the social services, by the employment advisory services, and by voluntary organisations will be coordinated by the consultant in charge of the case.

Arthritis and rheumatism and fringe medicine

The number of specialized rheumatic clinics in this country is still too small to deal with the vast number of patients who consult their doctors. Therefore the family doctor necessarily has to be selective in the cases he refers. Thus many patients with real or imagined rheumatic disorders feel obliged to seek advice elsewhere. The rheumatic diseases with their often unpredictable course, with periods of spontaneous remission, lend themselves to the promotion of questionable methods of treatment. Many products which are advertised in the press are of no value or of unproven value. Doctors on the whole will not be too critical of patients who seek relief from dubious remedies provided that these are harmless and that the patient is not incurring financial distress thereby. However, doctors will always be greatly concerned if a patient delays consulting the family doctor whilst obtaining treatment from a nonmedical source thereby postponing the early diagnosis of a condition which is curable or for which skilled treatment can at least mitigate the most serious effects. The rheumatic sufferer and his family should be aware that there are no magic remedies for rheumatism and arthritis, that effective measures are known, and that any new measure of proven effectiveness or which is likely to be useful is known to rheumatologists long before the general public comes to hear about it. Sensational claims which appear in the lay press should be judged very critically and when a patient has doubts he should seek an honest opinion from his medical adviser.

Any rheumatic sufferer who requires information about the availability of medical or voluntary services should contact the British League against Rheumatism, c/o The Arthritis and Rheumatism Council, 8 Charing Cross Road, London WC2H oHN.

Chapter 21

Allergies and hypersensitivity

Revised by A. W. Frankland, MA DM

One man sneezes and his nose and eyes water at a certain season of the year. Another man never has such symptoms. One woman wheezes and has difficulty in breathing when dust is stirred up in the house. Another woman never does. People who react abnormally to ordinarily harmless substances are said to have allergies. Familiar examples are hay fever, asthma, allergic conjunctivitis, nettle rash (urticaria), and gastrointestinal allergies. To people who do not have allergies, the condition may seem trifling, but allergies can cause much discomfort and are sometimes serious. Allergies should not be ignored or neglected in the hope that they will disappear. Much can be done for them.

Allergy means an altered capacity to react. The thing to which a person reacts differently is called an allergen. An allergen need not be, and generally is not, harmful to the vast majority of people. There are hundreds of allergens, chiefly foods, dusts, pollens, medicines, or other chemicals. An antibody is a protein made by the body in response to an antigen. Allergy-causing antigens are known as allergens. If the allergen re-enters the body, the antibody combines with it. This may cause allergic symptoms. A person who is made ill by eating food to which he is allergic will avoid the food and may dislike it.

Anaphylaxis is derived from Greek words meaning "removal of protection", and refers to sudden, life-threatening forms of allergy.

Relationship of allergy to immunity

For each allergen there is one antibody which reacts only on contact with that allergen. However, most substances which cause allergic reactions are complex materials which may contain more than one allergen. Horse scurf, grass pollen, and milk, for instance, contain several different proteins which may act as allergens.

Allergic diseases may be said to result from deranged immunity machinery. The body goes to the same effort to rid itself of harmless or even nutritious materials as it does to rid itself of harmful substances. The effort expended is totally out of proportion to need. It is normal for a person to feel a tingling sensation and to sneeze if a small insect gets into the nostrils. But a few microscopic grains of pollen in the nose of a person with hay fever cause explosive bouts of sneezing and excessive outpouring of fluid.

Mechanisms of allergy

There are two characteristic features of allergic symptoms. Certain body cells pour out fluids. Smooth muscle (the kind concerned with automatic actions) contracts. The combination of these effects produces an allergic reaction. How the substances in the fluids are freed from cells which contain them is not clear. Of these substances, histamine is probably most familiar to the public because of the extensive use of antihistamine drugs, but a number of other chemicals – serotonin, acetylcholine, kinins, and prostaglandins – are also involved. Histamine plays some part in all allergic reactions of the immediate type. It dilates small blood vessels, causing local reddening (erythema) and a central weal, a raised, sharply delineated swelling caused by excess fluid. Histamine also causes contraction of smooth muscle.

These actions may result in symptoms that differ according to the nature of the affected organ. The effects of weals and swelling, for instance, vary with location. Weals on the skin are nettle rash (urticaria). In mucous membranes of the nose, the process produces stuffiness, and fluids pour out in excess. Swelling in the throat or tongue may interfere with breathing. In asthma there is swelling of mucous membranes with increased secretion accompanied by contraction of muscle around the bronchioles. The combination constricts the air passages and interferes with breathing. Similar changes in the intestines may produce colic and diarrhoea. Allergic swellings may interfere with joint function.

Who gets allergies?

It is difficult to estimate the proportion of people suffering from allergic diseases. About ten per cent of the population have recurrent allergic attacks, usually subacute or chronic; about half have transient episodes. Estimates of the occurrence of particular allergic disease vary greatly.

Heredity is an important factor in predisposing people to allergic diseases. Parents and relatives may be unaware of allergic diseases or may conceal them. What is inherited is not a specific disease, but a tendency to develop sensitivity. A parent with asthma may have a child with hay fever. Allergy may begin at any age, though most people who are likely to develop allergy do so before their fortieth year, simply because by then they have been exposed to many allergens and have had an opportunity to become sensitized.

The effect of pregnancy on allergic disease varies from complete relief to extreme exacerbation. Asthma often worsens at the time of the monthly period. Some women have nasal congestion at this time, and this adds to obstruction already present from allergic rhinitis. Allergic dermatitis (see page 124) often worsens with menstruation or pregnancy.

Allergens

Allergens enter the body in various ways. They may be inhaled as dusts or pollens, or may come into contact with the skin, or be contained in food and drink.

Inhalant allergens Hay fever is the best known example of an allergic reaction caused by pollen (pollinosis). Pollen grains are formed in enormous numbers in the male sexual organs of plants. Windborne pollens, which arise from grasses and certain types of tree, are potent allergens, and these pollens have been found 5,200 m (17,000 ft) up in the air and 800 km (500 miles) out at sea.

Flowers in the garden hardly ever cause hay fever symptoms. Plants with brightly coloured flowers which attract insects have heavy sticky pollen which clings to the insects and is transported by them to the female flower. Heavy sticky pollen is not significantly airborne. Allergists always question patients as to the time when symptoms occur. Plants do not deliver pollen into the air at a constant steady rate, but in spurts during certain periods of the day. More pollen is shed on a sunny day, and a brisk wind stirs more of it into the air and carries it farther. Pollen counts are made by exposing glass slides covered on one side with sticky material to air, protected from wind and rain, for 24 hours, and then the number of grains in a given area is counted under a microscope. Pollens can be identified by shape and size.

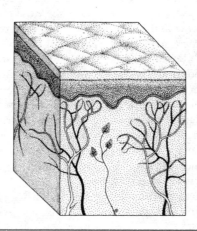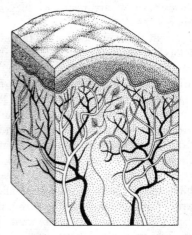

Left, normal skin. Right, an allergic skin reaction, such as nettle rash, showing increased blood supply and leakage of fluid from capillaries into the spaces between the cells.

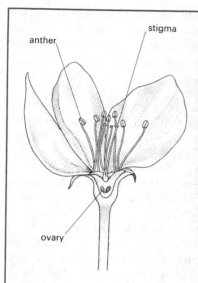

anther

stigma

ovary

Simplified diagram of a flower, showing the pollen-producing anthers and other parts of the reproductive apparatus.

Right, a photograph of grass pollen grains seen through a microscope.

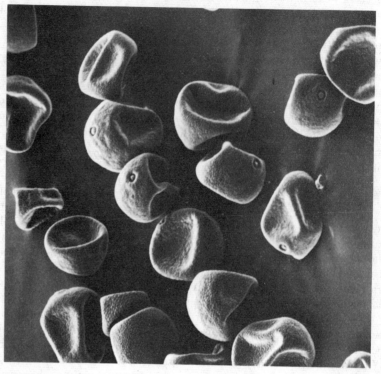

Trees Woodland trees produce much windborne pollen, in contrast to fruit trees and shrubs with colourful blossoms which are pollinated by insects.

Spores Mushrooms, green bread mould, and wheat rust are examples of fungi which shed buoyant airborne spores. Fungus spores are an important cause, and a frequent complicating factor, of respiratory allergy. In agricultural regions, mould spores are a more frequent cause of respiratory allergy than animal scurf, and rank behind pollens and house dust. Several circumstances suggest mould spore allergy.

At all times of the year, both indoors and out of doors, mould spores are in the air. These spores can cause symptoms like hay fever and also can cause asthma. The late summer mould spores are called cladosporium and alternaria. The former grows on anything that is green and the latter particularly grows on cereal crops. The dust coming off the grain from a combine harvester contains many millions of spores, particularly of alternaria. Indoors, particularly in damp houses, a musty smell indicates a high spore count. Nonseasonal allergic symptoms arise from mould spores of the penicillium and aspergillus species. There are many mould spores in the bottom of a bird cage.

House dust A frequent cause of asthma is house dust. It is present in every house, and is derived from the materials of mattresses and bedclothes, furniture, carpets, rugs, curtains, chests, paper, books, and clothing. It is entirely different from street or earth dust.

The house dust mite Mites particularly like heat and moisture and they live on human skin scales, especially those shed in bed. They are therefore plentiful in and on the mattress, in feather pillows, in blankets, and in carpets. The housewife must remove dust she cannot see. Vacuum cleaning the mattress each day is a good idea. Mites may be particularly plentiful in caravans, especially if they are used only occasionally. Asthma on the first night of holidays is not due to excitement in the allergic subject, but to mites. Uncarpeted hospital wards containing beds that are frequently completely changed will suit the dust mite allergic patient. Although dust allergy occurs all the year round, the dust mite allergic patient tends to be worse during October, November, and December.

Animal allergy All mammals can give rise to sneezing, eye irritation, and wheezing. The scurf or hair, or indeed any part of an animal can cause symptoms. A dog licking a child can cause local nettle rash. Poodles may not shed much scurf but they are popular dogs and are the cause of a great deal of asthma. Cats are stronger sensitizers than dogs. Siamese cats cause more symptoms than tabby cats. The girl devoted to horses may have to give up her hobby because of the severe allergic symptoms that horses cause. There is no animal that does not sensitize man. Asthma can be caused by elephants (in the zoo keeper), camels, goats, deer, rats, mice, gerbils, guinea pigs, and hamsters.

Ingestant allergens Sensitivity to foods may produce all the manifestations of allergy, and may be a complicating factor in patients sensitive to inhalants. Attacks of asthma can be caused by inhaled food allergens, as in bakers or flour millers, but the usual route of invasion is by ingestion.

Methods of detecting foods responsible for individual allergic reactions will be discussed later.

Albumen or white of egg, and yolk proteins to a lesser degree, are common causes of allergy. Cooking the egg denatures the protein enough to prevent symptoms in mildly sensitive persons. Persons allergic to egg should not only avoid it as such, but also the many varieties of foods that contain it. An allergy clinic often has lists of foods containing eggs, and suggested egg-free menus.

Milk is an important allergen, both on its own and as an ingredient of a great variety of foods. It causes more symptoms in children than adults and shows a tendency to decreasing potency as age advances. Denaturation of milk by heating or drying decreases its allergic potency. Cream contains some milk protein and a hypersensitive person should avoid it. There is much less milk protein in butter, perhaps one per cent. Unless their sensitivity to milk is great, allergic people may eat reasonable amounts of cheese without symptoms. It should be remembered that goats' milk is no better than cows' milk for a milk allergic child. When there is a family history of allergy it is most important that the baby is breast-fed. Cows' milk is for calves, not infants. Milk substitutes with a soya bean base may be given to infants who are intolerant to cows' milk, and milk-free diets are available from allergy clinics.

Fish, especially shellfish, are potent allergens and may produce severe allergic reactions. Any kind of edible fish may cause allergy.

Cereals Wheat flour is by far the most important offender in this group. It is used in such a variety of ways that complete elimination is almost impossible, and symptoms may persist in a wheat-sensitive patient. Rice is an important cereal that has so little tendency to cause allergies that it is a common constituent of trial elimination diets given to allergic patients. Maize ranks high as an allergic factor, but its oil, syrup, and starch seldom cause trouble. Rye may produce the symptoms of asthma.

Vegetables Almost any vegetable can produce allergic symptoms in sensitive persons, the most common being legumes (beans, peas, lentils, peanuts), potatoes, tomatoes, and celery. Other vegetables which may cause asthma and other allergic symptoms, though less frequently, are asparagus, beetroot, Brussels sprouts, cauliflower, cucumber, garlic, green peppers, mushrooms, olives, onions, radishes, rhubarb, spinach, and turnips. Sensitivity to chocolate is quite common and may cause allergic rhinitis and asthma. Tea occasionally causes trouble, but to a lesser extent than coffee. Walnuts and other nuts can cause an allergy which is sometimes severe. Allergy to fruit is commoner than to vegetables. Citrus fruits head the list, but apples may also cause severe symptoms. Strawberries are a well-known cause of nettle rash.

Alcoholic beverages All types may cause allergic symptoms due to traces of denatured protein of raw materials or substances used in manufacture. Whiskies are made from grains, rum from fermenting molasses, malt beverages from cereals. Maize, malt, rye, barley, yeast, fruit, and even vegetables are variously involved in distilling and brewing processes and may evoke symptoms in sensitive people. Wine is an offender. Fish glue, egg white, and isinglass are used for clearing beer, wine, and champagne. They are all allergens.

Contactants Acids, strong alkalis, and similar substances which cause trouble the first time the skin comes in contact with them are called primary irritants. No one is immune to them and allergy is not involved. Contact allergens are materials which are harmless to most people but produce allergic symptoms in sensitive skin.

Fur, wool, and leather often occasion contact dermatitis, but the condition is primarily caused by dyes or substances used in processing these materials. Dermatitis of the hands can result from preparation of fish, meat, and poultry dishes, or from handling flour.

Plant contactants Any of the ornamental flowers can sensitize, particularly the primrose family and tulip bulbs. Some weeds can cause dermatitis. All vegetables are capable of causing contact allergy.

It is impossible to list all contactant allergens because of the increasing number of synthetic materials, plastics, dyestuffs, and chemicals. Paints, insecticides, polishes, waxes, detergents, and other household chemicals have ingredients that can cause contact dermatitis. Metals, chiefly nickel and chromium, can cause dermatitis but the precious metals – gold, silver, and platinum – are rarely allergenic.

Detection and diagnosis

Diagnosis of allergic diseases is generally easy and will be discussed later in considering the symptoms of various allergies. Identification of the offending substance is more difficult and at times taxes the skill of the doctor and the patience of the sufferer.

History Time of onset (month and year), character (sudden or gradual), and probable precipitating factors are important clues in tracing allergens. Most of these patients tend to date the onset from their first major episode, but questioning often discloses earlier minor episodes, and the time of onset dates from the first symptoms. Recognition of the month or time of year when symptoms first appeared helps to narrow the search. For example, a housewife's eczema may be related to the birth of a baby, with increased immersion of the hands in water and detergents. Insidious onset suggests gradual sensitization to any everyday allergen of the environment, whereas acute onset suggests the provocative role of something unusual such as an infection, unusual food, new cosmetic or garment, insecticide or rug, or a seasonal pollen. A rapidly appearing dermatitis suggests a potent sensitizer such as primula or a hair dye.

Mild episodes as well as major attacks should be noted. This may help to pinpoint the cause. Some examples are the farmer who has mild hay fever daily when feeding his livestock but severe hay fever and asthma when harvesting hay and threshing; there is also eczema which is aggravated by hot water or cold air. Duration of the attack may indicate severity of the allergy, or duration of exposure to the allergen, as in the housewife who sneezes a few minutes after making beds, or the victim who has hay fever during the entire pollen season.

A clue to the cause of an attack is often given by the way a patient is able to obtain relief from it. For example, outdoor exercise or fresh air will help the patient with asthma due to house dust. Hot drinks relieve allergy to cold. From such clues, attacks can frequently be attributed to pollens, bedding, occupational exposures, or food. The next stage is to identify as many specific allergens as possible. Any

food believed to produce symptoms should be recorded, as well as any intense dislikes. Dislikes of children are sometimes protective and should not be considered whims until so proved.

Inhalants and contactants should be discussed in detail. Common causes of trouble are exposure to plants when out in the country – hiking, fishing, or picnicking. Questions should be asked about sprays and fumes of fresh paint, perfume, disinfectants, formalin, and insecticides, all of which can affect the skin or respiratory tract. What is the effect of face and bath powders, flour, soap flakes, or animals? Is there a room, sofa, chair, or bed which causes trouble? Are there any new clothes, furniture, pets, or hobbies?

Skin tests There are two chief methods of skin testing. One is designed to detect the presence of antibodies which are found in the immediate weal and flare forms of allergy, for example, hay fever and asthma. Here a scratch or prick test is made. The other type is used for the identification of substances responsible for delayed type allergy, that is, the contact dermatitis group. Here the patch test is used.

Scratch tests are usually made on the forearm. There are many variations in making scratch tests, but certain fundamentals are always adhered to. The skin is broken in a way that gives a slight oozing of serum but no actual blood. A different allergen is applied to each scratch. A positive reaction takes place promptly, within fifteen to twenty minutes. Such tests are most accurate with pollens or inhalant allergens. Unfortunately, with foods the reliability is less. Errors here are in both directions, that is, a positive reaction may be given to a food which can be eaten with impunity, or a negative reaction may be present to foods to which the individual is allergic.

The patch test, when positive, duplicates the dermatitis from which the patient is suffering. In the open patch test the material in question is applied to the skin and allowed to remain uncovered. In the closed method, which is more widely used, some of the test material is placed on a piece of fabric secured by sticking plaster, which in turn is applied to the skin. Reactions are looked for in the following 48 hours. Patients are told to remove the patches if there is any burning, stinging, itching, or other discomfort.

These tests are useful but, as in the case of all tests, must be interpreted with some skill. Even when everything has been done properly, the positive reaction tells only that the patient is allergic to that material. It does not prove that the material is causing the allergic condition being investigated. Not only must the person be allergic to the substance being tested, he must also have come into contact with it prior to the development of the eruption.

Elimination diets When symptoms are present daily, one approach consists of using elimination diets. These diets are made up of foods supposedly low in allergenic values. A useful diet is one consisting of nothing but lamb, rice, butter, sugar, canned pears, and water, these being selected because they are easily prescribed and are seldom offenders. No condiments, flavouring, or sauces are used. If the patient is not sensitive to one of the foods used, relief should be obtained within about twelve hours, but if there is no relief, the diet is maintained for another 36 hours. If after that time there is still no relief, it means either that the symptoms are not due to foods, or that the patient is sensitive to one or more foods in the diet. In the latter case, an entirely new diet of beef, carrots, and string beans is tried.

Food diary If symptoms are intermittent, offending foods may most easily be recognized by the use of a food diary, in which everything that is eaten is written down. It is not sufficient to write down a list of the foods in a notebook, for this is difficult to interpret. A record form must be used in which the foods are listed when they are eaten.

Asthma

See chapter 6.

Allergic rhinitis
(hay fever)

Allergic rhinitis (Greek "rhinos", of the nose) is generally characterized by seasonal sneezing, nasal congestion and blockage, and copious flow of watery mucus from the nose, which usually itches. Hay fever (pollinosis), the seasonal form, generally is induced by windborne pollens or fungi. The spring type is almost always due to tree pollens (oak, elm, hazel, plane, birch). The summer type is usually caused by grass pollens (timothy, rye, cocksfoot) or fungus spores (alternaria, and cladosporium, for which there are no common names).

Every year, and indeed often on the same day, persons affected feel a mild itching of the eyes, a tickling in the nose and throat, and a burning or sore sensation of the mouth. These patients can recognize by these signs that their seasonal attack has started. During the next few days, as there is increasing pollen in the air, symptoms become more uncomfortable.

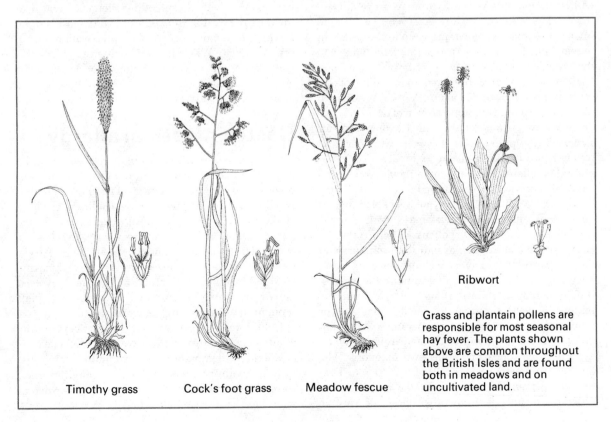

Timothy grass   Cock's foot grass   Meadow fescue   Ribwort

Grass and plantain pollens are responsible for most seasonal hay fever. The plants shown above are common throughout the British Isles and are found both in meadows and on uncultivated land.

There is now reddening and swelling of the conjunctivae (the membranes lining the eyelids and covering the white of the eye), a burning feeling in the eyes, and excess production of tears. In the mouth the burning and sore sensation persists, but the nose swells to cause partial or complete blockage; its membranes are intensely inflamed. In place of the earlier mild itching and occasional sneezing, there is now an uncontrollable flow of irritating watery fluid with sneezing. The bloodshot eyes are made more uncomfortable by light, which is consequently avoided. Hay fever may be associated with allergic symptoms of other parts of the respiratory tract such as the larynx (laryngitis), trachea (tracheitis), and bronchi and bronchioles (bronchitis, asthma). The patients' sensitivity to light and sound is intensified. They attempt to protect themselves, for example, by wearing dark glasses, or resting in a quiet darkened room. Headache is common, and aching in the back of the neck adds to the discomfort. Many patients complain of itching of the skin or even eczema during the pollen season. The duration of the symptoms corresponds to the flowering period of the causative plant.

Perennial allergic rhinitis differs from hay fever in that it is not seasonal but runs a continuous course with variations in severity. Symptoms are similar to those of hay fever, but usually less severe. Inability to smell (anosmia) is much more common than in seasonal hay fever. There is no permanent damage to the smelling (olfactory) nerves, but the passages leading to them are obstructed by swelling of the mucous membranes or by polyps. As the sense of smell plays a large part in our appreciation of taste, patients often say they cannot taste – an exaggeration, for sensing of the primary tastes (sweet, salt, sour, and bitter) is not impaired. There is usually a return to normal function after treatment, although sometimes removal of polyps may be required. Perennial allergic rhinitis can be caused by many allergens. Household dust, foods, and animal scurf may be the factors responsible, as well as pollens. There may be occupational causes, such as industrial vapours and dusts. Contributory factors include lingering nasal infection, sinusitis, nasal malformation, and polyps. (Often perennial rhinitis is not allergic, and the patient is very sensitive to smells, pleasant or otherwise, or to change of temperature. The condition is called vasomotor, and not allergic, rhinitis.)

The patient often makes his own diagnosis. The finding of numerous white cells of a particular kind (eosinophils) in the mucus from the nose helps to differentiate allergic from other forms of chronic rhinitis. The allergen which may be responsible for the symptoms is identified by means of the patient's history and skin tests. Treatment includes avoiding exposure to allergens, specific desensitization, antihistamines, and steroid drugs. Nose drops and inhalants are sometimes helpful, but their prolonged use may cause the nasal membranes to become persistently swollen even after the particular offender is out of the air.

Allergic conjunctivitis Conjunctivitis of an acute or chronic form is usually part of a wider allergic condition such as hay fever. Acute conjunctivitis is often associated with contact dermatitis of the eyelids which may be caused by overflow of various drugs placed in the eye for treatment. Conjunctivitis may occur on its own through direct contact with airborne substances such as pollens, fungus spores, various dusts, or animal scurf. Food allergy has been demonstrated as an occasional cause. Vernal conjunctivitis is a variety that typically appears in the spring. There are other nonallergic forms of conjunctivitis caused by infection with bacteria or viruses. Itching is common. Patients with hay fever have congestion of the eye vessels, giving a bloodshot appearance. The usual allergic tests are employed to help in identifying the offending allergen. Treatment includes removal from exposure and desensitization. Ophthalmic adrenocorticoid preparations give prompt relief. When itching is intense, eye baths, compresses, or an anaesthetic solution may be employed. If sunlight is offensive to the eyes, dark glasses are necessary as a temporary measure.

Gastrointestinal allergy

If the degree of sensitivity is high enough, even the briefest contact of a food with the lips or mouth will produce an allergic response. The most common reactions are itching and burning, leading to swelling of the mucous membranes. In general, the disturbance disappears when contact with the food is ended. The eyelids, lips, and tongue often take part in the reaction, but the severe swelling, in which the enlarged tongue fills the entire mouth and may even impair breathing, is usually caused by materials brought to the tongue by the bloodstream.

Cold sores (herpes simplex) and ulcers in the mouth may be activated by food allergy. Other causes of allergic inflammation of the mouth (stomatitis) include tooth powders and pastes, mouthwashes, cosmetics, medicaments, dentures, and other dental material. Denture stomatitis may be due to ill-fitting plates, but it is not uncommonly due to allergy to the plate itself. This may be tested by applying some of the material from which the plate was made, or the plate itself, to the skin, for example, on the upper arm. The test substance is held in place with adhesive for 24 to 48 hours. If a positive reaction occurs, some other denture material should be employed.

Anaphylactic shock, extremely rare, is the most startling and severe response to allergenic foods. It consists of a severe reaction following ingestion, with nausea, vomiting, diarrhoea which is sometimes bloody, violent pains, often nettle rash, collapse of the circulatory system, and even death within minutes or hours.

Colic and allergies Colic in infants is common but is rarely caused by food allergy.

Henoch-Schönlein purpura This disease, for which there is no common name, attacks the skin, gastrointestinal tract, joints, and kidneys. About half of all cases follow a streptococcal sore throat and a few are due to food allergy, but usually no cause is found.

The disease may begin with joint or abdominal pains, followed by a skin rash within hours or days. Sometimes all occur simultaneously, less frequently the rash starts first. There is generally malaise and a low grade fever. The skin changes begin as nettle rash. After a varying interval a pink or red spot appears in the rash. When the rash disappears, usually within 24 hours, a purplish spot remains. This spot is caused by haemorrhage into the skin (purpura) and the subsequent changes are those seen in bruises. The skin lesions appear in crops and do not itch. Involvement of the joints, usually of the knees or ankles, is found in about two thirds of cases. There may be mild pain or swelling, or both. Movement may be limited. The joint changes are temporary and do not result in permanent deformity. The kidney is attacked in about half the cases. If a specific food can be shown to be responsible, the patient should avoid it. When the disease follows an infection, vigorous measures will be used to ensure that the streptococcus is eliminated.

Indigestion Allergy to specific foods is occasionally a cause of indigestion.

Skin tests are so unreliable as to be valueless in many instances. More helpful information can be obtained from elimination diets or the food diaries already described, or from a careful history in which the patient is questioned about his experience with all the common articles in his diet. There should be an improvement or recovery within a reasonable time after elimination of the suspected allergen. Treatment consists of avoidance of the offending foods, as desensitization is impracticable.

Nettle rash (urticaria) Nettle rash is familiar to most people because of its frequency. Its diagnosis offers no difficulty to the doctor, in contrast to the efforts often required to identify the cause. Usually there is an abrupt appearance of weals, which vary in size from a few millimetres to several centimetres across. There is usually intense itching, which may be associated with a mild burning pain. The duration of a lesion varies from a few minutes to one or two days, but the attack as a whole seldom runs its course in less than a week. Generally the eruption is white or pink. The surface is smooth, and damage by scratching to the skin is rare in spite of the intense itching because the eruptions continually change location. A characteristic feature of the eruption is the simultaneous presence of fresh and of disappearing lesions. These are not confined to the skin. There may be involvement of the lips, mouth, and tongue.

Ordinary nettle rash is superficial, but if the changes are deeper, it is usual for a larger area to swell, producing giant nettle rash or angioneurotic oedema, which does not itch. There is also a rare form of hereditary angioneurotic oedema which can threaten life because of swelling in the larynx. The swellings are usually preceded by acute abdominal pain. The cause is due to a deficiency of one of the components of the blood serum.

The incidence of nettle rash is such that fifteen per cent of the population have at least one attack. No age is spared. About 60 per cent of cases are seen in the second and third decades of life. Women are afflicted about twice as often as men. An attack of nettle rash, even a severe one, is in the majority of instances a solitary event. But in about one third of the cases, especially in the middle years, there may be repeated attacks, or the disorder may persist for weeks, months, or even years, continuously or intermittently, with an ever-increasing disturbing influence on wellbeing.

In contrast to the transient nettle rash of some young people, the chronic form causes problems in diagnosis and treatment. Often in spite of the most painstaking efforts the factor responsible is not identified.

The following causes of nettle rash are recognized:

Antigens coming from without:
Medication and cosmetics
Foods and other substances eaten
Inhalants
Insects, parasites, and worms

Chapter 21 Allergies and hypersensitivity

Antigens coming from within:
Chronic and acute infections
Internal diseases, especially cancer
Physical factors:
Heat, cold, light, pressure, sweating, overexertion, and fatigue
Nonallergic factors:
Insects and plants
Psychogenic disturbances

Drugs are a very important cause of nettle rash. Studies indicate that of all instances of nettle rash, 30 to 35 per cent can be attributed to drugs. If only acute nettle rash is considered, this rises to 53 per cent. An important kind of drug nettle rash is the serum sickness which may follow the administration of foreign (horse or other animal) serum in the treatment of tetanus or diphtheria. The same reaction may also occur to other medicines, especially penicillin. Of particular significance, in addition to the usual signs and symptoms (nettle rash, joint pains, enlarged lymph nodes, fever) is the latent period of five to twelve days between taking the drug and developing the allergy. With a skin reaction of any kind it is important for the patient to mention to the doctor any drugs taken up to a fortnight before the rash appeared.

The chief agents causing nettle rash are probably protein-containing materials such as pollen extracts. There is scarcely any drug, even the most harmless, which cannot at times cause nettle rash. In addition to the sensitizing potential of a drug, the method of administration or the frequency of use also play a role. Paradoxically, antihistamine drugs, of value in treating nettle rash, may at times cause it. Aspirin can cause nettle rash, and if the condition is already present will make it worse. It should never be taken by a patient with this complaint.

When the time lapse between eating a food and the appearance of symptoms is short, the cause and effect relationship is obvious, but usually the diagnosis of food-caused nettle rash is more difficult. Frequency of various foodstuffs as causes of nettle rash varies with geography, socioeconomic status, and racial origin of the patient. In general, the ordinary nutrients are the commonest allergens. The following list groups foods in an approximate order of importance:

Milk and milk products, especially cheese
Eggs and egg products
Fruits (strawberries, gooseberries, pears, bananas, oranges, and other citrus fruits)
Fish, crabs, shrimps, lobsters, and occasionally, oysters
Nuts of all sorts
Vegetables, especially legumes (peas and beans), tomatoes, celery, and cabbage
Meat, primarily pork, but also mutton, beef, and poultry
Grains, especially wheat, rice, oats, and rye
Spices, coffee, and chocolate (rarely tea)

Inhalant allergens in general are not of great importance in causing nettle rash, but some seasonal cases are due to pollen. About five per cent of bakers and millers have an inhalant nettle rash due to flour. Animal scurf, house dust, barn dust, and perfume are occasionally responsible. In contrast to drugs and foods, positive skin tests to inhalants are reliable in nettle rash. There are many causes for the itching or nightly nettle rash which may appear shortly after going to bed.

Certain worms in their life cycles pass through the blood or tissues, and these (roundworms, hydatids, hookworms) can lead to allergic symptoms. The purely intestinal parasites (tapeworm, whipworm) rarely do so. Thus the exclusion of worm infestation by microscopic stool examination is desirable in nettle rash. The absence of eggs in the faeces does not exclude the presence of worms in the intestines. Other tests must be employed. There are a number of effective drugs (see chapter 2).

Occasionally allergic reactions, especially nettle rash, may be caused by protozoa (single-celled microscopic animals). These include trichomonas, malarial parasites, amoebas, and *Giardia lamblia* (there are no common names for these). Nettle rash may be present in any acute infection, but it is especially frequent in streptococcal disorders. Nettle rash is not uncommon in acute gastroenteritis (food poisoning), either during the active stages or during convalescence. It is the chronic types of infection that are most likely to cause nettle rash, and evidence of disease of tonsils, teeth, sinuses, gallbladder, gastrointestinal and genito-urinary tracts is sought for in the study of longstanding nettle rash. Sites of infection are found in ten to twenty per cent of such cases.

Nettle rash, especially of the chronic form, may accompany a number of diseases or may be a herald of an unsuspected systemic disorder. This is based on autoantibody formation, in which the patient makes antibodies against some of his own body substances.

There can be no doubt of the existence of nettle rash of psychological origin. Its frequency seems to depend on the point of view and the ability of the investigator. The more carefully the patient is questioned and examined, the less frequently is this diagnosis made. In the majority of persons who have other varieties of nettle rash, emotional factors can precipitate or worsen attacks already present but are not themselves the cause.

As elsewhere, the basis of control of allergy consists of elimination of the allergen when possible. This is easy when drugs are concerned, less easy for foods or household allergens. Ubiquitous allergens such as pollens, and occupational allergens cannot be avoided. Internal allergens are removed by antibiotics, or when these fail, by surgery of diseased tissue and by elimination of intestinal parasites. The antihistamine drugs are of value in the treatment of nettle rash.

Insect allergy

Many kinds of insects bite: mosquitoes, bedbugs, fleas, lice, midges, horse flies. Other insects, chiefly hymenoptera such as the wasp, honey bee, and hornet, sting.

Insect stings Allergy plays a role in causing the distressing effects of insect bites, and is a component of the changes which follow insect stings. No one knows how many severe reactions occur from hymenopteran stings, but the problem is large. It is probable that these stinging insects cause more deaths than is realized, because of the tendency to attribute all sudden deaths to heart attacks. People who are known to be allergic to stings should always carry an antihistamine tablet and a pressurized atomizer such as asthmatics use. It is often advised that adrenalin and a syringe should also be available at all times when stinging insects are about. It is important that help be obtained as soon as possible, because a patient may become unconscious after a sting. A doctor will give an injection of adrenalin and an antihistamine.

Bees leave their stings and venom sacs attached to the site of the sting. Prompt removal of the sting, performed carefully so as not to squeeze the venom sac, by scraping with a knife blade, finger nail, or tweezers will reduce the amount of venom which enters the sting site. Cold packs applied to the sting site will help control discomfort.

How not to be stung Bees are more likely to sting on bright warm days if interfered with while they are busy gathering nectar. Highly scented hair dressings, perfumes, and other cosmetics should not be used on picnics since they have a tendency to attract bees.

Insect bites Local reactions to insect bites are different from the reactions to stings. Initially, nothing is seen to occur, but soon a small elevated lesion appears, not earlier than 24 hours after the bite.

In subsequent bites, the interval between bite and reaction gradually decreases. With this change in the incubation period an increase in the size of the reaction at first occurs, followed by a gradual decrease until finally there is no reaction to the bites. This has led some people to believe mistakenly that they are not bitten by mosquitoes. Bloodsucking insects develop a venom to which people may become allergic. Their bite may induce allergy, and most, if not all, of the results of insect bites are to be explained on this basis. For the most part, insect bites and stings do not demand or receive much attention. Local applications of lotions such as calamine, cool compresses, or cool baths usually suffice, although the antihistamine drugs can be valuable.

Drug allergies

The extraordinary developments of new drugs in the last 25 years has led to specific treatment hitherto impossible, but the use of powerful medicines carries with it the possibility of side effects. The toxic symptoms produced by small quantities of drugs in hypersensitive patients are the same as the toxic symptoms produced by large quantities in normal persons. For example, for centuries quinine was given to cure malaria. Anyone who took enough of the drug developed ringing in the ears and deafness. In the majority of cases "enough" consisted of 500 grains (32 gm). An occasional patient developed these features from five or ten grains, but nettle rash or asthma would occur, without these symptoms, from small doses of quinine taken by persons allergic to it.

Many people are allergic to medicines. In the case of proteins, for example horse serum or insulin, the mechanism is straightforward. The preparation itself is allergenic. A modification of the process takes place with nonprotein medicaments. Here the medicines are not allergenic by themselves. They must combine first with one of the body's proteins. The resulting complex of drug and protein now acts as an allergen leading to antibody formation. When next the patient takes the medicine, the previously formed antibodies react with it immediately without the necessity of its combining again with protein.

Symptoms of allergic drug reactions are very varied and can mimic other diseases. The usual allergic diseases may be produced – hay fever, asthma, nettle rash – but in addition every organ and every tissue in the body may be the site of a drug reaction. Thus the appearance of the allergy depends more on the particular organs and tissues taking part in the reaction than on the allergen.

Chapter 21 Allergies and hypersensitivity

Preparations containing horse serum, or indeed any foreign serum, may produce serum sickness. This is an allergic reaction that appears up to eight to twelve days after serum is injected. Other drugs, notably penicillin, given by needle or by mouth, may produce a condition indistinguishable from serum sickness. Following immunization in infancy, diphtheria is now a rare disease, but antitoxin from a horse is still used in its treatment. Human antitoxin is now available for immediate protection against tetanus in someone who is not fully protected and is at risk of developing the complaint.

Nettle rash is the usual skin manifestation, and fever occurs in one third of patients. It is usually mild and lasts only for a day or two; in more severe cases, the temperature may reach 40·5°C (105°F) and last seven to ten days.

Enlargement of the lymph nodes near the area injected is usual, but all lymph nodes may increase in size. The reason for this is that lymph nodes are important sites of antibody formation. Mild to severe joint involvement, at times with intense pain, often occurs. Not uncommonly, weals form in the intestine, larynx, and bronchi, with resultant local symptoms.

If drug reactions take place while the patient is under treatment for some other condition, they are ordinarily recognized and diagnosed, for it is known what medicines are being taken. A careful history is important, for not all drugs are prescribed by doctors. Many proprietary medicines are sold for self-medication. Furthermore, drugs are often added to various toilet articles, soaps, and even to foodstuffs as preservatives. The regular or occasional use of these household products seems so harmless to the patient that, unless the doctor specifically inquires about them, they may not be identified as causing the allergy.

When a medicine comes under suspicion, it should be withheld. If the symptoms then disappear, the medicine may be taken again but in a reduced amount. If this leads to a return of the symptoms, the case is proved. Certain drugs lend themselves to the usual skin test methods, for example, foreign serum and penicillin, as well as various endocrine preparations. The majority of medicaments cannot be so tested, however, and in fact such testing may be hazardous.

If skin testing seems imperative because no substitute drug will work as well as the one under suspicion, there is a device called the passive transfer technique in which some of the patient's serum is placed in the skin of a nonallergic person. This site can then be tested with entire safety, and as much information can be obtained as if the patient were tested directly.

Cosmetic allergy Cosmetic dermatitis, a form of contact dermatitis resulting from applications of various agents to the skin, is discussed in chapter 5. Cosmetic allergy is more an all-inclusive term. Any odour, pleasant or not, can trigger off an attack of hay fever or asthma, and perfumes in cosmetics are in this category. Any cosmetic substance (such as perfume, rice powder, oatmeal powder, bath salts, hair tonic, soap, skin cream, and various lotions) is capable of producing allergy of the respiratory tract. Persons with respiratory tract allergy should purchase so-called hypoallergenic cosmetics which eliminate known allergens from their formulas as much as possible.

Physical allergy

By physical allergy is meant the development of allergic symptoms such as asthma or nettle rash after exposure to physical factors such as heat, cold, or light. Physical allergy may be spontaneous, or secondary to food or drug allergy; it may be hereditary, or it may be an aspect of some general disease.

Cold urticaria Provoking factors include serum sickness, measles, scarlet fever, chickenpox, childbirth, and emotional disturbances. Cold nettle rash may occur only after eating certain foods, or when intestinal worms are present, but in the majority of instances no precipitating or underlying causes can be determined.

Nettle rash is usually limited to areas of exposure, but generalized nettle rash may follow. Should much of the body surface be in contact with cold water, as in swimming or cold showers, generalized nettle rash may occur, with signs of histamine shock – considerable drop in blood pressure, rapid pulse, flushing of the face, and loss of consciousness. When bathing in such circumstances the danger of drowning is obviously great. Diagnosis is easily confirmed by applying an ice cube to the skin for a few minutes. Nettle rash appears over the area covered by the ice. Although the symptoms of cold nettle rash can be controlled effectively with antihistamine drugs, treatment of the basic condition is difficult and usually fails. Familial cold nettle rash is a less common inherited condition. Nettle rash is present from birth or shortly thereafter and continues throughout life. Cold air is more likely than cold foods or drinks to bring on attacks. The condition appears shortly after birth in those affected. The attack is brought on in every case by cold wind or extreme changes in temperature. In addition to the nettle rash, which usually is free from itching in contrast to other varieties, there is a burning sensation, pain and swelling of the joints, and mild fever. Drinking cold fluids has no effect. Members of affected families learn the remedy for an attack. They go to bed and keep warm.

Hypersensitivity to heat There are known examples of attacks of asthma brought on by exposure to heat, but urticaria is more common. It occurs in two forms, generalized nettle rash produced by heat, exercise, and emotional stress, and localized nettle rash produced by heat alone and only on the exposed area. The second type is rare and of little importance. The first is more common and is of interest to doctors in that it represents the one skin disease where the mechanism is known whereby an emotional stimulus can produce a lesion in the skin. In the generalized type, nettle rash is produced by the heat of a warm room, hot foods, hot weather, clothes, fever, or a hot bath. Emotional stress and exercise produce identical reactions. In some cases a combination of all three, as in dancing or competitive sports, may be necessary to bring out lesions. The weals are characteristically small, two mm ($\frac{1}{12}$ in) in diameter, but are surrounded by a large flare. When these merge, large blush patches appear, the more striking because of the tendency of this disorder to affect young redheaded women. At times there are only bright red flares. Any part of the skin may be involved except the palms and soles. In about half of these patients such general symptoms as abdominal cramps, diarrhoea, faintness, sweating, salivation, and headaches can occur.

Antihistamines give partial relief. The treatment of choice is the application of cold or iced water to the hands and arms. This, plus rest, will quickly end the episode. Of great practical importance is the fact that after an attack there is an unresponsive period. After a moderate outbreak this may last for some hours, but after a generalized severe attack produced by warming the legs for an hour, the period of freedom may last for a day or two, rarely longer.

Hypersensitivity to light In spite of man's centuries-old worship of the sun, damage can result from injudicious exposure. Apart from burning the skin, causing crow's feet and cancers, sunlight also produces hypersensitivity reactions which are being seen with increasing frequency.

Specific treatment

Avoidance Elimination of the allergen is the treatment of choice when possible. This may require a change of diet, occupation, or residence; withdrawal of a drug; or removal of a household pet, or certain articles of furniture, cosmetics, or clothing. Pollen can be avoided by taking, if possible, holidays at certain times of the year, and in certain places. Further information can be obtained of individual pollen counts in Europe in the book by Charpin, Surinyach, and Frankland entitled *Atlas of European Allergenic Pollens*. Various air-conditioning devices help in reducing exposure to pollen grains by filtering them from the air.

Desensitization Pre-seasonal pollen desensitization is used when the patient consults his doctor in the winter time. It affords relief in about 80 per cent of cases, particularly when the patient has an associated pollen asthma. This method of treatment requires three to eighteen injections of gradually increasing amounts of the pollen extract. In the past a large number of injections of the appropriate pollens in water were given. The modern tendency is to give fewer injections using slow release vaccines. Each doctor probably has his own particular preference for different extracts. Desensitization against pollens other than grasses is unusual, but silver birch pollen in Britain causes symptoms of hay fever starting in mid-April. In the Scandinavian countries it is the commonest cause of seasonal hay fever. In Europe we do not have ragweed pollen which causes so much allergy in parts of North America. Fungal spores, particularly those that grow on ripe cereal crops, can cause seasonal hay fever and asthma in August. Desensitization may be necessary in patients who are mould spore allergic.

House dust desensitization is now rarely undertaken but house dust mite desensitization is commonly done. Dust mite allergy tends to cause an exacerbation of allergic rhinitis and asthma in October to December. The first cold of winter going to the chest may not be anything to do with infection but be caused by allergy to the dust mite. Desensitization is given on an annual basis. First the injections are given weekly and then once a month or less often. The same methods are used when attempting desensitization towards animal allergies. Theoretically any known allergen should be eliminated but this is often difficult in the horse-loving girl or the cat and dog-loving family.

Reactions Local reactions during the course of desensitization are common. They resemble nettle rash or angioneurotic oedema and vary from pinhead size to involvement of the whole arm. They indicate that increase in dosage is being made too rapidly. The generalized reactions vary from malaise to severe anaphylaxis. The most common are widespread nettle rash, cough, and wheezing.

Drug treatment

Drugs for allergic disorders can be applied locally to the skin or mucous membranes. They may be swallowed as a medicine or tablet. They can be given by injection or inhalation or by some other route. Although histamine is a substance which is produced in an allergic reaction, causing local symptoms, the antihistamine drugs are disappointing in their beneficial effects in allergic reactions. Many hay fever patients become too sleepy when using these drugs. Also they should not drink or drive. It must be remembered that these drugs do not help allergic asthma but they are excellent in relieving the itch of acute or chronic nettle rash.

In asthma there is a wide range of antispasmodic drugs available.

A great advance in dealing with allergic complaints is Intal (sodium cromoglycate). It is available as eye drops, in various nasal preparations, and for inhalation to prevent allergic asthma or that induced by exercise. It has no known side effects. Any or all allergic symptoms can be controlled by the cortisone drugs. They stabilize and reverse allergic inflammation. They are used by application on the skin, in tablet form, by injection, and by inhalation using a pressurized atomizer. By the last method they have been an outstanding advance in the treatment of all kinds of asthma. Except for a sore throat due to yeast overgrowth these preparations when used for a short time have so far not been reported to cause any hazards. So long as a patient remains on any cortisone preparation, he must be under the surveillance of his doctor.

Chapter 22

Emotional and mental illnesses

Revised by Professor Michael Gelder, DM FRCP FRC Psych

It is often difficult to decide when to consult a doctor about emotional difficulties. Sometimes it is a straightforward matter of judging the seriousness of the problem. Depression can be a perfectly normal response to worry or to unhappy events, but it can also be an illness. It is not always easy for a person to decide when his feelings have passed beyond what is normal and to judge that help is required. At other times the problem is more complicated. Some people are ashamed to admit to emotional disorders or are afraid of treatment, although fortunately this is not as common as it used to be. Others find difficulty in acknowledging openly a problem which they know privately, such as growing dependence on alcohol, a difficult marriage, or a way of living which relieves their own emotional distress at the expense of the feelings of other people.

For these and other reasons the decision to see a doctor about emotional difficulties is seldom quite as straightforward as a decision about symptoms suggesting physical illness. Moreover, once the decision has been taken, it is not always clear what kind of help to expect. Will drug treatment be enough, or is lengthy psychotherapy required? Because patients are uncertain, they may suggest the wrong solution to their doctors. They may request drugs to bring relief from tension or unhappiness which is no more than a normal response to an unhealthy or unhappy style of life, an overdemanding job, or an unsatisfactory marriage. If that is the case, the patient needs not drugs but assistance, if possible, in changing his way of life. On the other hand, when suffering from severe depression a patient may believe that he has brought trouble upon himself and that no one can help him. Yet antidepressant drugs may be the first essential step on the way to recovery. All these

decisions become easier if they can be taken with some understanding of the problems, and a degree of knowledge of the occasions when medical advice can be of help.

Although it is generally agreed that emotional disorders and mental illness are common problems it is not easy to obtain exact statistics. The less severe an emotional disorder the more difficult it is to separate it clearly from the distress and unhappiness which is part of human existence. Therefore, statistics are more reliable for the severe forms of mental illness; for the minor forms the estimates will depend, in part, on the definition which is adopted. With these cautions in mind, we can observe that in this country ten to fifteen per cent of the patients who consult a general practitioner have significant emotional disorders. At the next stage, a little under one per cent of the population of countries with well developed health services are referred for specialist psychiatric care in the course of one year. Looked at in another way, a recent survey of prescribing in general practice in this country has shown that drugs which are mainly used to treat anxiety and depression were prescribed at least once during a year for one third of all middle-aged women, and one fifth of women of all ages. The most serious forms of mental illness are fortunately less common; about one person in 100 will develop a schizophrenic illness at some time in life, and two to three times this number will suffer from manic depressive psychosis.

These last figures were given in terms of psychiatric diagnoses. Some people feel that though attaching diagnoses to emotional disorders may help in the collection of statistics it leads the doctor to lose sight of the individual and his personal problems. This school of thought sees diagnosis as at best useless, and at worst a dangerous attempt to label as ill, people who are suffering from the demands which an unreasonable social order makes upon them. A diagnosis is neither of these things if used properly. A diagnosis summarizes the ways in which the patient has problems which the doctor has met in other patients before and it enables him to draw upon knowledge accumulated by other doctors. Diagnosis is obviously most useful in serious disorders which are amenable to specific treatment. To decide that a patient is suffering from manic depressive psychosis goes a long way towards an effective decision about treatment. With less serious problems such as anxiety states, diagnosis has less to contribute but is still useful. In this case, treatment will depend to a much greater extent upon a knowledge of the patient's unique personality and circumstances, but the diagnosis will still indicate the general direction that treatment should take. Moreover, in both minor and serious disorders, a clear diagnosis helps the doctor to advise his patient about the likely course of the condition with and without treatment. Anxious patients may fear secretly that if they continue to experience severe anxiety they will eventually lose control and become mad. A careful examination leading to a diagnosis allows the doctor to give his patient well-founded reassurance that this will not happen. The account which follows describes conditions in the groups used by doctors as major diagnostic categories.

Situational reactions

This is a convenient name for those common and short-lived emotional disturbances which do not reflect any serious disorder of personality and are not as severe or as long lasting as the neuroses (which are considered later). A common example is the distress which follows difficulties between partners in marriage, the breakup of a relationship, or the serious illness of a child. This distress may be experienced as depression, tension, anxiety or irritability, and as sleeplessness. Distress in adverse circumstances is, of course, quite normal. However, the reaction may become so intense that it is intolerable. It may also be so intense that it prevents the person from taking essential steps to resolve the problems which led to the intense feelings in the first place. In these circumstances the first step is always to talk about the problems; however, the prescription of a drug can sometimes be of considerable help. By reducing anxiety or depression and by restoring sleep, drugs can help the patient to take the further steps he needs to help himself. Sometimes such measures are of a

practical kind. If the original problem was financial or if active steps are needed to overcome difficulties in a marriage the family doctor may refer the patient to social agencies, such as the Citizens Advice Bureau or Marriage Guidance Council. Often, however, they are of another kind: the patient has to think over his attitudes and opinions, to accept what is inevitable, to look at the positive side of his life as well as its problems, or to question whether his own attitudes are justified. All these things can be done better with a calm mind. Drugs, properly prescribed, can produce this. Sometimes the steps should be taken at once; at other times the distress is so great that major decisions are better delayed for a few days or weeks. Often it is appropriate for those who live with the patient to join him in seeking a solution, so the doctor may ask to see the husband or wife as well as the person who comes to him as a patient. He may suggest the help of a social worker or a marriage guidance counsellor.

Used in this way, tranquillizing drugs can have great benefits. Unfortunately patients sometimes misunderstand the role of medication and this may have two opposite but equally undesirable consequences. One person may conclude that, because drugs have been prescribed, the doctor has not realized that he has social or psychological problems as well. Thinking this, he may give up hope of further help from his doctor. Others may take the opposite view and assume that to take the tablets is all that is required of them. They see their situation as similar to that of a patient with an infection whose task it is to wait passively until antibiotics take effect. If this happens, prescribing may be prolonged unduly while potentially soluble problems are left unresolved. Therefore, when seeking medical advice it is important for the patient to make sure that he understands what part, if any, the drug is to play in his treatment and what part – usually it will be the larger part – he needs to undertake for himself.

Suicide The most distressing situational reaction is a suicide attempt, nowadays often in the form of an overdose of drugs. Some of those who take overdoses are seriously depressed or have other reasons for being determined to end their lives. They have tried to do so but failed, usually because of an accidental but timely discovery by a relative or friend. However, many do not actually wish to kill themselves but seek a period of oblivion, to express desperation, or show that help is needed; these are some of the motives which lead to the overdose. Once physical recovery has been ensured, treatment follows the principles which are used for other situational reactions. Sadly, the number of attempts is increasing, particularly in younger people, and the final solution must lie in changing public attitudes to the use of medical drugs as well as in better medical and psychological treatment for people in crises.

What should the layman do when faced with a person who is threatening suicide? Remember that there is always some lingering wish to live even in those who express the strongest wish to die, and a friend can help to strengthen this wish to survive. Remember also that although suicide can sometimes be an apparently rational response to unbearable circumstances, nearly all those who are restored to life by medical treatment after a suicide attempt say that they are glad to be alive. Apart from taking commonsense steps to remove the person from danger, a friend can help most by patient and sympathetic listening. In the course of this, the suicidal person can usually be persuaded to seek more expert advice; to see his general practitioner (the best step because suicidal ideas may be an expression of a depressive illness), or a social worker, or the Samaritan organization whose trained counsellors are available for 24 hours of the day in many places (their telephone number is listed in the local telephone directory). Finally, remember that suicide is an expression of loneliness and of the feeling that other people have ceased to care. The very act of listening is therefore the first step in putting matters right.

Personality disorders

Personality refers to those characteristics·of people which are relatively enduring throughout life. While no two people are the same, it is possible to identify characteristics which people have in common. In everyday speech we talk of a person being conscientious, or of having a warm personality. In more technical terms we can divide people into introverts and extroverts. If people deviate from what is considered normal on these characteristics, they are usually said to have a disorder of personality. People with personality disorders are also very different from one another, but again it is convenient to group together those who have certain common features. Examples are the abnormally aggressive and the inadequate. The word "psychopathic" is sometimes used as if it were a synonym for abnormally aggressive personality, but the word has more than one meaning. Although psychiatrists find it convenient for some purposes to classify personality disorders in this way, it is often more helpful to try to understand the patient as an individual, and learn how he reacts to the people about him.

The boundary between normal and abnormal personalities is of course impossible to set precisely. The concept of abnormality has two aspects: a deviation from the normal range (which implies the ability to measure personality in some way) and a departure from the social norm. When the deviation is extreme the two sides usually coincide. A highly aggressive man who does not show affection will be abnormal in both senses. Even with extremes, however, there are problems. Highly original and creative people are abnormal in the statistical sense. As we consider less extreme cases the problems become progressively more difficult because abnormality has to be seen to depend on the demands which are made on the person by society as well as on the make-up of the person himself. A man or woman may live contentedly enough in one society but not in another which is, for example, more competitive.

The matter is further complicated because disorder of personality may show itself in two ways. It may cause the person to suffer, for example with recurrent anxiety, or unhappiness; or it may cause suffering in those around him if he is aggressive or lacks ordinary concern for the welfare of other people.

What help is available for personality disorders? The question can be answered only by referring to the distinction between personality disorders which cause suffering to the person himself and those which cause suffering to others – persons of the latter type are often called psychopathic personalities. Help of two kinds is available for someone who suffers from a personality disorder. First he needs to adjust his way of life to accord better with the strengths in his personality and conflict less with the sensitive areas. He may also need to talk about the ways in which he habitually deals badly with everyday problems, how he acts when he feels angry or frustrated, whether he demonstrates the affection that he feels inwardly, and so on. This approach shades into the second, psychotherapy, which helps him to modify his outlook and reactions in a more fundamental way. Because it is directed to lifelong patterns of behaviour, psychotherapy for personality disorders must necessarily be lengthy, so that a period of six to nine months of weekly treatment is usually the minimum requirement. Psychotherapy may be given to an individual patient, but increasingly group methods are being used. The patients in the group help each other to re-examine ideas and attitudes and try out new ways of relating to other people. There are many different technical approaches to psychotherapy, some of which are considered in a later section. For the moment it is sufficient to observe that there is no evidence that any one school of treatment is better than another. The methods used for all but the most intensive treatment, by practitioners with different kinds of training, have much in common and it seems that these common features have considerable importance.

Psychopathic personality disorders in which suffering is felt more by others than by the patient, are less easy to modify. In part this is because the patient is less likely to be motivated to change, and in part because the disorders respond less well to most methods of psychotherapy. In general, group methods are more effective than individual psychotherapy, and encouraging results have been reported with an extension of group methods which is usually known as the therapeutic community. In this, patients live and work together in hospital, and spend several hours each day in group meetings in which the behaviour, attitudes, and reactions of members are discussed in a constructive way. Because the personality problems are lifelong, treatment cannot be short and benefits seldom appear until several months of treatment have been completed. Personality disorders often lie behind the problems of people who drink excessively and become alcoholic, or are addicted to drugs. Of course not everyone who is alcoholic or addicted has a serious abnormality of personality; there are other causes as well. Other people with personality disorders figure in the statistics for crimes of violence. Again it must be stressed that not everyone who breaks the law in these ways has a treatable personality disorder or, indeed, a psychiatric illness.

Neuroses

From one point of view the neuroses can be thought of as more severe forms of the conditions we have referred to already as situational reactions. They consist of the same mixture of anxiety, tension, or depression and they often begin at times of personal stress, but they go further than this. Distress is more intense and prolonged, and other symptoms may appear. Moreover, the reactions do not necessarily subside when the stress has passed. Neuroses often occur in people who have some degree of personality disorder which makes them unusually vulnerable to the ordinary stresses of everyday life. However, if stress is sufficiently intense, or if there is an accumulation of problems in a short space of time, neuroses may develop in well-adjusted people.

The neurotic patient is usually dominated by the mental experience of anxiety, often accompanied by bodily sensations such as palpitations or breathlessness. Anxiety may be present all the time or it may be related to specific events, often of a quite ordinary kind such as the prospect of a bus journey or a visit to the shops. Some patients also experience insistent intrusive thoughts which they know to be without foundation but which cause great distress and cannot be dispelled. Such obsessional thoughts may take a form which makes a mother think repeatedly that she may harm her baby, or a housewife fear that she has germs on her hands that could spread disease to her family. Both know that this is not true, but neither can rid herself of the repeated intrusive idea. Like other neurotic symptoms these obsessional ideas find a faint echo in the ordinary life of many people who are not neurotic. It is not an uncommon experience to be nagged by the repeated thought that a tap has been left on or a door left unlocked, even though it is certain that it has not. Some mothers have occasional "contrary thoughts" that they might hurt their child, when they know with certainty that they will never do so. It is frequency and intensity which distinguish the two conditions, and the best guide for the person who is deciding whether to seek help is that if the feelings cause distress advice should be sought. It may be that the condition will subside without special measures, but if treatment is needed it will be started early with better prospects of success.

Neuroses take various forms. Anxiety states are dominated by anxious thoughts and feelings. Those in which anxiety is felt only in certain limited circumstances are called situational, or, more usually, phobic anxiety states. Of the latter, the commonest is agoraphobia, a condition which centres round fears of leaving home, of travel on public transport, and of visiting shops or other crowded places. Obsessional neuroses are less common and are characterized by the intrusive thoughts that have been described above. Hysterical reactions (sometimes known as conversion reactions) appear as disorders of bodily function without physical disease. A hysterical patient may have difficulty in seeing though the eyes and brain are healthy, or find difficulty in moving a limb though the muscles, nerves, and other parts are physically sound. One theory of these hysterical states supposes that anxiety has been replaced by, or converted into physical symptoms, an explanation which fits in with the suprising lack of distress which is often shown by these patients. It is for this reason that the name conversion reaction is often used. The idea is not universally accepted but the name is widely used as an alternative to hysteria.

Although three types of neurosis can be described in this way, there are far more patients whose neurosis does not fall neatly into any one of these categories. There are symptoms of more than one kind, usually accompanied by complicated problems in regard to relations with other people. For some these take the form of shyness, or a general difficulty in making intimate relationships. For others there may be more specific problems in sexual relationships or in controlling feelings in particular circumstances. In the latter case the circumstances often repeat some difficult aspect of their childhood, such as rejection or rivalry.

It is among the neuroses that there is most variation in the treatment that may be offered. For this reason it is particularly important to take the advice of a general practitioner so that if specialist help is required it will be of a kind that will be most suitable for the patient. At its simplest, treatment may resemble that which has already been described for the acute situational reactions, though it may have to be pursued more vigorously. It may include help from a social worker to enable the patient to deal with life's problems, and interviews with the patient and marital partner or relatives together to help them arrive at less stressful ways of living in the family. For other patients the methods known as behaviour therapy may be appropriate. These are directed to the control of specific symptoms such as anxiety or obsessional thoughts, or to circumscribed patterns of behaviour such as shyness or sexual difficulties. Unlike psychotherapy, they are not concerned with the origins of symptoms or with the general discussion of feelings and problems but rather with experiences which will counteract the neurosis. Thus agoraphobia often improves if the patient persistently encounters in planned treatment the situations which provoke fear. This must be done every day in an organized and graduated way. It is often necessary to teach special procedures which help patients to tolerate anxious feelings while they are practising. Specific techniques have been worked out which counteract other neurotic symptoms. Like psychotherapy, behaviour therapy is a way of helping the patient to help himself; unlike psychotherapy it pays most attention to doing rather than talking. Each has its part to play, depending on the balance of the patient's problems.

The various methods of psychotherapy are outlined later in the chapter. However it is important to observe here that the judgement when to use psychotherapy is not an easy one and that there are differences of opinion among doctors about the matter. There are also broad differences in practice between countries; for example, in some parts of the United States of America many more neurotic patients receive psychotherapy than is the case in this country. Whether this more extensive use of psychotherapy leads to better long-term results is a matter on which there is still insufficient evidence. All this is a further reason for seeking the advice of a trusted general practitioner so that the best use can be made of the services which are available.

Psychosomatic disorders

Although widely used, this is an unsatisfactory term for it has more than one meaning, Its most common usage is to denote physical disorders in which emotional factors are thought to play an important part either in provoking or in maintaining the condition. Opinions differ about the exact list of conditions which should qualify, but most would include certain cases of peptic ulcer, asthma, hypertension, ulcerative colitis, and some diseases of the skin. The words "certain cases" are important for it is not only unjustified but at times also dangerous to put too little emphasis on the physical components of these disorders. For this reason the patient who suffers physical symptoms which suggest one of these conditions should always consult his general practitioner who is usually well-placed to decide their nature and make the further judgement whether emotional factors are important in a particular case, and if they are, whether treatment is required. If treatment is indicated, it will follow the general direction that has been indicated for the neuroses. It is in this area in particular that we see the value of the system adopted in Britain by which the patient sees a specialist only after he has first seen a family doctor. The latter is in the best position to weigh up all the features of the case – medical, social, and psychological – and make the difficult judgements that are required.

Anorexia nervosa Many teenage girls try to lose weight by dieting. Usually this is harmless but occasionally it passes into a serious condition called anorexia nervosa. Dieting becomes extreme and, if forced to eat, the girl may make herself sick in order to remain thin. As a result she becomes extremely – sometimes dangerously – underweight. Yet, despite her emaciated appearance she continues to feel as if she is plump and continues her efforts to diet. At the same time the menstrual periods cease. Although this self-induced starvation might be expected to lead to great tiredness and lack of energy, the opposite is often seen: there is continuing restless activity, which adds to the relentless decline in weight. The causes of this condition are not known with certainty, but it seems unlikely that there is only one. In many cases there are emotional problems which the girl cannot put into words; sometimes these relate to the pressures of academic work, or perhaps to anxieties about physical development after puberty. In all cases it is important to seek the advice of the family doctor at an early stage, not only because he may be able to help with these emotional difficulties, but also because a number of serious medical conditions can cause a similar progressive loss of weight.

Depressive illness and manic-depressive psychosis

There must be few people who have not experienced feelings of depression in response to unhappy events in their lives. At times such feelings can be intense, especially after a bereavement, but there is a further degree of severity which indicates that what began as a normal reaction to circumstances has passed into a state of disordered function. It is the latter which is called a depressive illness. One common way that depressive illness may start is an unusually profound reaction to unhappy events which are intense or prolonged. For example, it has been shown that depression is particularly common in women who have young children and are tied to their homes, and that this is worse when they do not have a happy marriage. However, there is a minority of people who develop severe depression in the absence of severe or continued stress. Instead, the depression arises from an internal disorder, a failure of normal mood regulation, which is possibly related to changes in the chemical substances which transmit impulses between nerve cells in special areas of the brain. Because it arises from inward causes, such depression is called endogenous. Some of those who suffer from this form of severe depression also experience periods of overactivity, inappropriate elation, or irritability. This opposing state is known as hypomania and it too seems to be a failure of the internal mechanisms which regulate mood. In this condition the person becomes overactive, restless, and sleeps badly but seldom feels ill. Indeed he often feels unusually well and is overconfident in his abilities so that he may make serious errors of judgement in his work or his personal affairs. The combination of the two states in the same

person is known as manic-depressive psychosis (the word psychosis denoting a severe form of mental illness in which the patient has limited or no insight).

There is one common circumstance in which even the less intense degrees of depression can arise partly from internal causes. This is the short-lived disturbance of mood which follows immediately after childbirth in up to half the women who are delivered of a baby. At a time when one might expect them to feel happy, they are instead tearful, easily upset, and downcast. The condition usually goes away in a few days, but may occasionally persist for weeks and months and require treatment. The exact cause of this disorder is still elusive, though it is generally supposed that it has some relation to the profound changes in the woman's hormones which take place as soon as the baby is born.

People who have experienced both mild and severe depression often observe that there is a qualitative as well as quantitative difference between them, and it seems likely that this difference may turn out to be related to the development in severe depression of the changes in brain chemistry to which we have referred. Patients with severe depression experience extreme despondency, which may be accompanied by unshakeable ideas that they have no worthwhile future, or that they have done wrong or let others down. Such ideas may precede a determined suicide attempt. Sleep is disturbed in a very characteristic way. The patient usually falls asleep without too much difficulty but wakes unusually early, often at three or four in the morning, and cannot sleep again. In these early morning hours he feels at his worst; miserable, hopeless, and often agitated and restless. This profound disturbance of sleep rhythm is often accompanied by an equally characteristic pattern in the daytime, with the worst symptoms in the morning. This is in sharp contrast to the milder reactive forms of depression in which depression typically increases as the problems of the day unfold. Severely depressed people often lose appetite, and may lose weight. Women often report that their menstrual cycle is disturbed, and in both sexes sexual drive is reduced.

It is fortunate that depression is among the psychiatric disorders which can be treated most readily. Psychological treatment and a lessening of social stress will help and there is now a large number of antidepressant drugs of proven effect. Within a week or two these usually arrest the progress of the depression and gradually turn its course towards recovery. It seems that these drugs act on the disordered chemical processes which occur in the brain in severe depression, and they are, indeed, most strikingly effective in the severest depressions, in which a chemical basis for depression is most likely. In a proportion of cases drugs alone are sufficient. However, in the majority there is a mixture of internal and external causes and a need for a combination of drugs, discussion, and attention to problems in living.

Occasionally depression is so severe that it is not safe to wait for the antidepressant drugs to work and with a small number of other patients the drugs do not act effectively. In either of these circumstances electroconvulsive therapy (ECT) will often produce dramatic and sometimes lifesaving changes. The name electroconvulsive therapy may be a source of unnecessary worry to some people. It originates in the medical practice of thirty or more years ago when this treatment was first given. Today there are no major convulsive movements of the body because patients who receive ECT first have an anaesthetic which lasts for the few minutes that are required to administer treatment, and at the same time another drug is given which relaxes all the muscles of the body for the same short period. While the patient is unconscious and relaxed an electric current is passed between electrodes applied to the scalp. This sets off the simultaneous activity of large numbers of brain cells. It is indeed the kind of brain activity that can be recorded during an epileptic seizure, but only the smallest bodily movements accompany it. This brain cell activity subsides quickly and the patient wakes after a few minutes. As a rule about six treatments are required over a few weeks to treat even the most severe depressive illness. There has been much public concern that ECT may cause lasting impairment of memory. There is often a transient disturbance of memory afterwards, but there is no good evidence that lasting memory disturbance is caused.

Prevention is always better than any treatment. In the last decade evidence has accumulated which shows that manic-depressive psychosis and some of the related severe depressive illnesses can be prevented by the giving of a very simple drug, lithium carbonate. Although it is a simple chemical substance, lithium carbonate has to be taken with care because if the dose is too high it can produce other effects that are unwanted and occasionally harmful. For this reason treatment is accompanied every few weeks by measurement of the level of lithium in the blood. With this precaution the treatment is safe and effective. It constitutes a major advance for the patients who suffer severe and repeated depression and hypomania arising mainly from internal causes.

Before leaving the subject of depression, a little more needs to be said about bereavement. Grief proceeds by stages. At first, especially if the death has been sudden, emotions may be numbed. This is soon replaced by intense feelings of anguish and despair, accompanied by weeping and often by an overwhelming feeling of restlessness. Sleep is broken and thoughts are filled with images and memories of the lost one, which may be so intense that there is momentary feeling that he or she is in the room. The bereaved often blame themselves without reason for failing to do enough for the deceased before he or she died and at times they may blame their friends or doctors and nurses as well. These feelings subside slowly over the course of weeks or months, often returning in waves of intense distress throughout this time. In many countries the customs of mourning encourage the expression of emotion, and this, together with an elaborate funeral ceremony, probably helps many people to work through their feelings of grief. In our own country these things are usually arranged otherwise and many people lack religious beliefs to sustain them. For this reason it is even more important for friends and relatives to give support to the bereaved person.

At times this normal process of grieving is disturbed. Emotions may be bottled up – for example when a young widow has to continue to sustain her children. When this happens, it may appear that the bereaved person has coped very well, but the emotions return in full force weeks or months later often provoked by another, less important loss. In others, grieving may become so intense that it passes into a severe depressive illness, or it may be unduly prolonged. In all three cases, medical help can usually restore the process to normal. It is important for relatives to recognize this and encourage the bereaved to seek help. See Further reading. (page 511).

Schizophrenia

Although schizophrenia is a serious disease, knowledge of its treatment has advanced to the point that it need no longer give rise to all the fears that have been associated with it for so long. Like the severe depressive illnesses, schizophrenia may turn out to be associated with a disorder of certain chemical processes which transmit messages within the nervous system. It is almost certainly a different set of chemical processes from those which are disturbed in severe depression and it probably affects different parts of the brain. Which chemicals and which brain areas are still a matter of dispute between experts, but the general point is sufficiently well established to make it a promising line of enquiry for research workers. It appears that the tendency for these processes to break down is in part inherited. However, while the predisposition may be inherited, there is also much evidence that this predisposition is modified by factors in the environment in which the patient grows up, and in which he lives in adult life. When the breakdown comes it is often preceded by an accumulation of problems in the patient's life. While the broad outlines of this scheme are well established, the details have proved hard to fill in. Experts differ about the kind of influences which modify the inborn predisposition. Some point to occurrences in the family when the patient is very young, others put emphasis on later events. The problem is particularly difficult to study because many of the potentially important events take place many years before the patient becomes ill and also because schizophrenia is, fortunately, a rather uncommon condition. For these reasons more progress has been made with research into the ways in which established schizophrenic illnesses can be treated than with the causes. However, before outlining the principles of modern treatment, it is necessary to indicate some of the ways in which schizophrenia may affect the patient.

Schizophrenia can produce profound disturbance of thinking, feeling, and perception but it does not affect memory or intelligence. It is this effect on some mental processes with sparing of others which is the split to which the name refers. Schizophrenics are *not* "split personalities"; that is quite another disorder, a rare form of hysteria. The most striking features of schizophrenia are hallucinations, usually experienced as voices, and delusions, that is firmly held morbid ideas which often centre round themes of persecution. At the same time the patient usually has difficulty in thinking in a clear and logical way. These problems are accompanied by emotional difficulties. Sometimes these take the form of excitement or other excessive emotional responses, sometimes of apathy or emotional coldness. In older people the disturbance is characteristically of a more limited kind with the development of delusions of persecution without marked disturbance of other mental functions. These symptoms combine into various types of schizophrenia but these need not concern us here.

The treatment of schizophrenia has been revolutionized by the discovery of drugs which can control the acute symptoms. They cannot, of course, be the whole treatment but they make possible the essential social psychological measures which it is difficult or impossible to implement in an acutely ill

patient. Fortunately some schizophrenic illnesses subside within a few months and their treatment with drugs can be correspondingly short. Others, however, require drug treatment for many years with careful medical supervision. Nowadays the drugs are often given by an injection every two to three weeks which saves the patient the trouble of remembering to take tablets every day. Once the acute symptoms have been brought under control in this way, psychological and social measures can begin. Most normal people find that they are distressed by the extremes of solitude and social contact. Left entirely to themselves they tend to dwell too much on inner worries; thrown into ceaseless contact with others they feel under strain and wish for occasional solitude. The schizophrenic person reacts in an essentially similar way but can tolerate only a much narrower band of social stimulation. Left too much alone he retreats into an inner world of delusions and hallucinations; brought too much into contact with others, for example in a busy office or a lively family, his condition worsens in other ways. Much of the skill in rehabilitation after a schizophrenic illness lies in helping the patient to steer a course between these extremes. Part of the advantage of drugs appears to be that they enable the patient to tolerate more social stimulation than he could otherwise accept without becoming ill. In this way they make it possible for him to enter a rehabilitation programme, to return home, and to work again.

Relatives need advice from a doctor or social worker to decide how to arrange family life in a way that will help the patient in what may be a long illness, and they are often puzzled how best to respond to any remaining symptoms. Family members sometimes enquire what help psychotherapy can give. Simple counselling is certainly needed to help the patient to make sense of the experience of his illness and to guide him in re-establishing his life. However, most psychiatrists believe that intensive psychotherapy is hardly ever indicated. Although, as stated above, schizophrenia is an uncommon condition, its long duration causes patients to occupy a large proportion of hospital beds.

Mental disturbance associated with physical illness

It used to be common to see high fever accompanied by delirium. Advances in medical treatment have made this much less common, but rather similar states of delirium are still seen in the course of other medical illnesses. A feature common to all is confusion, that is the patient is incompletely aware of his surroundings, he may mistake the place he is in, the time, or the people he sees. At the same time he may also see things that are not there and become restless and afraid. With the treatment of the physical illness these symptoms disappear quickly, though they are alarming at the time for the patient and for his relatives.

Operations are occasionally followed by similar mental disorder, and so is childbirth, because both can be complicated by infections or by disturbance of the blood chemistry. However, operations and childbirth are sometimes followed by disturbance of another kind. They can provoke depression, less often a schizophrenic or hypomania state. Such disorders are of course especially puzzling and distressing after a successful operation or when a woman has been delivered of a healthy and wanted child. Fortunately they usually respond well to treatment and have a better outlook than the corresponding conditions occurring at other times.

So far we have considered conditions which are provoked by physical disease outside the brain, but disease of the brain itself is even more likely to lead to mental disorder. If it starts quickly it is likely to resemble the confusional states we have just discussed, but often it progresses more slowly. In that case the striking features are usually a gradual loss of memory or other intellectual functions. They may be the first signs of a localized disease, such as a brain tumour, or result from some widespread degenerative process. The latter may occur when the blood vessels which nourish the brain cells are diseased (arteriosclerotic dementia) or when the brain cells degenerate in middle age instead of old age. Treatment of these conditions is still difficult, but early diagnosis is important. Memory problems in the middle-aged are therefore a good reason for seeking a medical opinion.

Disorders in the elderly

There is no space here to discuss the many social problems which contribute to the psychological difficulties of old people. Changes in the extended family, dwindling membership of churches, and increasing social isolation have all contributed to the loneliness and loss of self esteem which are important causes of depression in the elderly. However some of the mental troubles of the elderly arise because the brain is ageing. We are all familiar with the difficulties of remembering and the slowing of mental

processes which beset the very old. At times the brain cells or the blood vessels which supply them age more quickly than the other organs of the body and the picture of dementia appears in old people who are otherwise well-preserved. In general, dementia is deterioration, usually progressive, of the mind, for example by confusion, impairment of memory and reason, or disorientation in time and space. Dementias sadly are all too familiar conditions, but they are not the only mental disorders of the elderly. Old people can be affected by any of the conditions we have considered in younger people. They may develop severe reactions to stress – and the problems of retirement, bereavement, and loneliness are, of course, especially likely to affect them – they may suffer from neurosis, the effects of a lifelong disorder of personality, or develop severe depression and, occasionally, schizophrenia. Both the last two conditions may take a somewhat different form in the elderly. Depression sometimes brings about changes which closely resemble dementia but which respond quickly to treatment. Schizophrenia often appears as unfounded suspicious ideas which may make the old person feel that he is being persecuted by his neighbours, or in danger from people who are plotting against him. Such ideas are often kept hidden so that relatives and friends may notice only an increasing social withdrawal and mistrust. Most of these conditions can be treated quite effectively in the elderly, although dementia is unlikely to respond to treatment, because it results from processes of ageing which cannot be reversed.

People who are worried about the health of their elderly relatives should ask the advice of the family doctor. Even if cure is not possible, he may be able to arrange social measures which improve the patient's life, and it may turn out that what seems to the layman to be the signs of an ageing brain is really a treatable depression, or a confusional state resulting from physical disease which can be cured. Even if the diagnosis of dementia is confirmed the doctor can often give good advice about ways in which the old person's life can be reordered and simplified so that he is better able to cope with it, and he may be able to arrange help from social or voluntary services.

Psychological treatment

In each part of this chapter a brief indication has been given about treatment. When this entails the prescription of drugs or the use of social rehabilitation it is not difficult to understand, for it resembles the more familiar treatment of physical illness with medication and graded physical activity. Psychological methods of treatment are less familiar and there are a bewildering variety of different techniques. This is not a matter which can be dealt with easily and briefly without oversimplification. Some guidance can be given but it should be supplemented and made more accurate by further discussions with the doctor who recommends this course.

Behaviour therapy Behaviour therapy uses principles taken from laboratory studies of human psychology and not from clinical observations such as those of Freud. It is concerned with conditioning, with the effects of rewards, with the practice of behaviour which will eradicate unwanted patterns and with learning new behaviour. As a broad, and rather inaccurate, generalization it can be said to be concerned with doing things rather than with talking about them. Behaviour therapy therefore has obvious uses with patients who do not find it easy to talk about their difficulties – people of below average intelligence or some patients with chronic schizophrenia. However, its most successful application has been to the problems of neurotic patients, who can talk about their difficulties easily enough. It has proved to be particularly useful for some of the symptoms of the neuroses, for example phobias, obsessions, and social anxieties, symptoms which are often resistant to treatment with drugs or psychotherapy. Now that these uses are becoming well-established, behaviour therapy is increasingly concerned with thoughts and attitudes as well as with symptoms. There are many techniques available and a number of popular accounts of the field which give details for which space cannot be found here.

Extreme views are usually more thought-provoking than those of the middle, and often easier to expound. Partly for this reason some popular accounts of behaviour therapy often suggest that it is a rival to psychotherapy. It need not be. Sometimes it is an alternative, and clinical trials are beginning to demonstrate in which conditions one or the other is superior. Sometimes the two are required for the same person, each helping a different aspect of the patient's difficulties. It is just because the two are rather closely related in this way, that the name behaviour psychotherapy has been suggested.

Individual psychotherapy By individual psychotherapy we mean all the methods in which a therapist treats one patient at a time. The word therapist is convenient because treatment may be given by a general practitioner, a psychiatrist, a social worker, or a psychologist, depending on the patient's needs and the therapist's special training. The term individual psychotherapy therefore excludes the large and growing body of group methods in which one therapist guides the treatment of several patients at the same time. Individual psychotherapy can be conveniently divided into three levels according to its aims.

Supportive treatment and counselling have the most limited aims. Many people can be tided over crises in their lives by allowing them to obtain relief by talking about their problems. At the same time the patient is encouraged to work out effective ways of solving the problems which contributed to his distress and to consider how future difficulties can be prevented. Much psychotherapy is of this simple kind. At its most elementary it shades into the help that any good doctor – or indeed any good friend – will offer at times of crisis, but there are special skills to be learnt about ways of helping the patient to help himself so that he does not become too dependent on the therapist. The aim must not only be to surmount the present problems but also to leave the patient better at solving future problems himself. Treatment of this kind usually lasts for between a few weeks and three or four months.

Re-educative psychotherapies attempt to do more. They are appropriate when the problems are to a significant extent a reflection of the patient's personality, and are therefore likely to recur even if he does not encounter major stresses in his life. There are, of course, many different schools of psychotherapy based upon the theories of Freud, Jung, Klein, and others. Patients are often confused by this and find it difficult to decide whether a practitioner of one or other school would be best. Fortunately, these distinctions become important only when the therapist is engaged in the most intensive forms of psychotherapy (which we are about to consider in the next section). They are of less consequence when the re-educative level of psychotherapy is being used. Working at this level, practitioners of different schools adopt similar techniques, and there is no evidence that the small differences between them have any important effect on the outcome. The broad principle which they share is essentially that the patient is helped by understanding his present patterns of behaviour by reference to his past. Thus it often becomes apparent in the course of treatment that the present difficulties are being encountered because the patient persists in applying in adult life some pattern of behaviour which protected him, albeit inadequately, from painful emotions at a difficult time in childhood, but which are no longer appropriate in his adult life. Understanding of this kind is not enough by itself. The patient must also be enabled to work out better ways of dealing from then on with relationships and problems. He has to learn to see himself as other people do and to discover which of his ideas and attitudes are realistic and which require revision.

The therapist's role in all this is to guide the patient (not to direct him), to draw his attention to problems but encourage him to solve them, to help him to look in profitable directions, and above all to make sure that at the end he is self-reliant rather than dependent on the therapist. This level of treatment requires special training. A few family doctors have had this, most psychiatrists can offer help at this level, and many social workers and psychologists also have the required skills. Treatment is usually once a week for between nine to eighteen months. It can seldom be faster than this for the problems are usually lifelong.

Reconstructive psychotherapy is a convenient, though not universally accepted, term for the most prolonged and involved forms of treatment. Freudian psychoanalysis is the best known example but there are others, based on the theories and methods of other psychotherapists. The aim is more ambitious; not merely that the patient should learn how to deal better with a limited set of problems in his life but rather that he should experience a much more radical reorganization of personality. For treatment of this kind patients are usually seen more often than in re-educative therapy. Sessions may take place three or four times a week, and continue for several years. It is in these intensive treatments that therapists of different schools use their special methods. Because treatment is so lengthy and expensive it should not be undertaken lightly, and it is usually best to obtain the opinion of a psychiatrist who practices all branches of his subject before going to a specialist psychotherapist for analysis. Most patients can be helped effectively without such intense treatment; a few can actually be made worse by extreme self-scrutiny. Unfortunately the value of these intensive treatments is hard to determine by the usual methods of clinical evaluation and as a result there is considerable controversy about their effectiveness. It is as wrong to say that the methods have no value as it is to apply them to almost every patient. It appears that there are a small number of patients who do gain more from these techniques than from simpler measures. However, the selection of these few is difficult and somewhat controversial. Anyone who thinks he might need

intensive treatment should certainly obtain the advice of a family doctor or a psychiatrist whose opinion he respects before making up his mind.

Psychotherapy with couples and families A patient's emotional problems often involve other people in his immediate family. Sometimes difficult relationships between husband and wife have contributed to the original problems. Sometimes the family members suffer as part of the patient's difficulties. More often there are both elements in the situation, a complicated interweaving of causes involving the husband or wife and sometimes the children as well. It is for this reason that therapists often work with patient and partner together to help them understand each other's feelings and needs, and to work out better ways of living together.

Treatment in groups It is, of course, an advantage of group treatment that one therapist can treat several patients at the same time, but this is not its main advantage. Treatment in a group gives the patient many opportunities to understand his behaviour with, and feelings towards, other people, which he cannot experience in the same direct way in individual therapy. The group usually has about eight patients as its members. Sessions are once a week and each lasts about an hour and a half. In the course of a series of group meetings most of the patient's problems should come into view through his reactions to other members of the group. The members can then help each other to see themselves as others see them, to understand the effect which each person's behaviour has on the others, to work out the origins of feelings and responses, and to arrive at better ways of responding. In all this the therapist guides and balances the discussion, but he does not direct it. He makes sure that the needs of individual patients are met, that no one is made the scapegoat of other people's problems and that the group as a whole completes its work in a reasonable time. Patients need time to identify and solve problems which have been present for many years, often since childhood, so the group usually continues for about a year to eighteen months.

Encounter and other groups. The last decade has seen the development of large numbers of other forms of group experience. These have different aims and methods from those of the therapeutic groups which we have just considered. It can be said that encounter groups are directed not to patients with serious neurotic or personality problems but to people who have less serious dissatisfactions with their lives, people who would often say that their aim is to expand their awareness of themselves and others. Of course, the dividing line between these two groups is not an easy one to draw. The methods differ also. Encounter groups usually meet on fewer occasions though sometimes the individual sessions are much longer than those of a therapeutic group. When they meet, the experience is intense and the interchanges direct. Many involve activities other than the discussion of problems which is the hallmark of the therapeutic group. Some use role-playing, others encourage physical contact between members. Such measures make the group experience more intensely emotional and many who attend regard it as a significant event in their lives which alters the way they respond to other people for long afterwards. Such intense experiences can be assimilated by healthy people but for those who have serious emotional problems they can be painful and at times even damaging. An experienced leader of an encounter group is aware of these problems and takes steps to exclude unsuitable members. Nevertheless it is a safe rule that anyone who believes that he has emotional difficulties should seek the advice of his family doctor before joining an encounter group.

Conclusion

It is inevitable that a brief account of a large and complicated subject must be incomplete. This chapter has made no mention of drug addiction or the common sexual difficulties which cause distress to many people, since both are dealt with in another part of this book. In this chapter also, attention has been given mainly to the medical aspects of mental disorders, and the role of general practitioners has been stressed. There are, however, many ways in which social workers and psychologists can help people who have emotional problems – an account which was written from their viewpoint would have given more space to social problems and to the psychological differences between healthy people. This account also omits any reference to the important subject of emotional disorders in childhood and adolescence. Rather than attempt a cursory account of these and other important topics within the space of this chapter, a list is appended of books which are written for the layman and can be obtained easily. Such books can be important sources of information but, as in other branches of medicine, self diagnosis is seldom objective and reading is no substitute for the advice of an expert. A good family

doctor is usually the best source of such advice because he can take account of bodily as well as mental health. However there are many ways in which qualified social workers or clinical psychologists can help as well. Nowadays a visit to an expert need no longer be attended by fear or regarded as a stigma. With the advances in knowledge of recent years, help will usually be available.

Further reading

Bromley, P. (1974) *The Psychology of Human Ageing.* 2nd Edition. Penguin Books.

Delvin, D. (1974) *The Book of Love.* New English Library.

Dominian, J. (1968) *Marital Breakdown.* Penguin Books.

Dominian, J. (1976) *Depression.* Darton Longman & Todd Ltd.

Kenyon, F.E. (1978) *Hypochondria.* Sheldon Press.

Kenyon, F.E. (1978) *Sex.* Sheldon Press.

Parkes, C.M. (1975) *Bereavement.* Penguin Books.

Pitt, B. (1978) *Feelings about Childbirth.* Sheldon Press.

Pitt, B. (1979) *Midlife Crisis.* Sheldon Press.

Ryle, A. (1973) *Student Casualties.* Penguin Books.

Sandstrom, C.I. (1968) *The Psychology of Childhood and Adolescence.* Penguin Books.

Storr, A. (1964) *Sexual Deviation.* Penguin Books.

Tyrer, P. (1978) *Insomnia.* Sheldon Press.

West, D.J. (1968) *Homosexuality.* 2nd Edition. Penguin Books.

Chapter 23
Your operation

Revised by Selwyn Taylor, DM MCh FRCS

The prospect of a surgical operation is to most people a frightening experience, often made worse by ignorance of what really happens. True, the operating theatre is a strange place with different sights, sounds, and smells. The patient is alone without relatives or friends, although he has usually met the surgeon and anaesthetist beforehand. At least, he will probably know the nurse who accompanies him from the ward. He can be sure that all the preliminary procedures followed, some puzzling, are done for some good reason. Modern surgery is a precise craft, and every detail counts. Also, modern anaesthesia has robbed surgery of most of its terrors for the patient. Usually, there is a prick in the arm for an injection, and the next thing the patient knows is that he is waking up back in the ward.

Pre-operative preparations A stomach operation provides an example of the routines that are performed before the patient reaches the operating theatre. The day before the operation the doctor orders a liquid supper, an enema, a sleeping pill, preparation of the skin, no breakfast the next morning, a nasogastric tube, and an injection in the arm.

The liquid supper ensures that the stomach and intestine will be empty the next morning. A nasogastric tube (a thin tube of soft plastic) is put in the nose and gently pushed into the stomach to drain out the natural digestive fluid that forms in the night. The tube is connected to a suction bottle that draws liquid and gas from the stomach, or the nurse may use a syringe. Any residue of food eaten before the liquid supper is removed by the enema which flushes out the lower intestine and rectum. The surgeon wants the stomach to be empty in case there should be vomiting.

This would be dangerous in a sleeping person because the vomit could well up in the throat and enter the windpipe and lungs.

The sleeping pill helps to relax the patient, and along with the injection the next morning paves the way for the anaesthetic. Less anaesthetic gas is required for a relaxed patient, and the less required the better. The skin of the operative area is shaved and cleansed with detergent. With stomach operations, this extends from the middle of the chest to the hips, but the incision does not extend as far as this.

Routines A great many things happen as a matter of routine. Certain tests (for anaemia, blood group, and so on) are made on all patients, no matter what the reason for their admission to hospital. Someone will take a specimen of blood, either by pricking a finger or with a needle from the bend of the elbow. A specimen of urine is collected. These are analysed in the laboratory before morning. Other tests that are not routine may be made when ordered by the doctor according to individual problems.

Every part of this routine has been worked out very carefully. These procedures are not just old customs that the hospital staff follows unthinkingly. They are the checks that ensure safety during the complexities of modern surgery. The anaesthetist examines the patient beforehand to check his fitness for the anaesthetic. When a general anaesthetic is required, the patient is anaesthetized in the anaesthetic room which adjoins the operating theatre.

The length of time each operation takes may vary. People often judge the seriousness of an operation by how long it lasts, but seriousness is not related to the time required. A very grave operation may take only a short time, whereas several hours may be needed for a slow-moving procedure of less gravity. Although

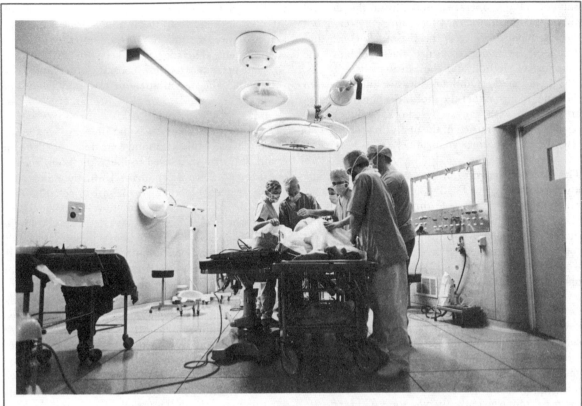

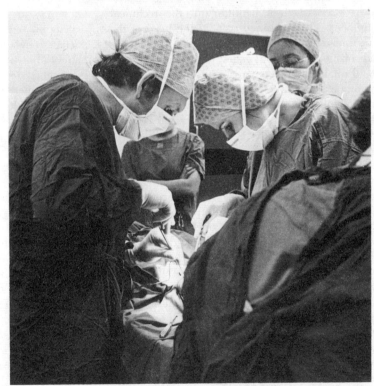

Modern operating theatres
contain a great deal of
sophisticated equipment to
ensure optimum working
conditions for the surgical team
and the safety and comfort of
the patient.

Chapter 23 **Your operation**

isolation of the operating suite from the general public adds mystery to the proceedings, mystery is not the intention. Sterility is the reason. Bacteria and dirt must be excluded, hence the scrubbing, the changing of clothes, and the putting on of gowns, gloves, and masks. Outdoor shoes are not allowed in the inner rooms; either the shoes are changed or they are covered with canvas overshoes. Only surgical personnel are permitted in the operating rooms. This is why the patient must go in alone.

The surgical team   There may be several people involved in surgery. Firstly there is the consultant surgeon who is responsible throughout for surgical care. Often he has a deputy, called a registrar, who shares his duties. However, the doctor who has most contact with the patient is the house officer, and it is he who will write case notes and see the patient after the operation. He also assists the surgeon in the theatre. In the operating theatre the surgeon is in charge, but he is only one member of a team. He has another doctor assisting him – his first assistant – and on some occasions there may be a second assistant. There is the nurse who also scrubs up and hands instruments, and another nurse who acts as runner, fetching further sterile supplies as required. There is also an operating room assistant who may take over some of these duties and is also skilled in handling all the technical equipment. The anaesthetist sits at the head of the table and is responsible for giving any intravenous fluids or blood. Surgeon, anaesthetist, and assistants are all qualified doctors and in addition undergo a long and arduous course of specialized training with very difficult examinations. It requires about fifteen years to train a surgeon from the time he enters medical school.

Recovery   Immediately after the operation the patient is still in a deep sleep. After being lifted from the operating table, he is wheeled to the recovery ward where he receives special attention. There is an experienced nurse here for every one or two patients. Each bed is in a small area partitioned on two sides but open at the end. This enables close observation, and the medical staff are close at hand. Each patient stays in the recovery ward until he is fairly well awake. This may mean an hour or several hours. As soon as the patient swallows when there is something in his mouth, or coughs when there is something in his throat, or makes some kind of motion or sound when anything hurts, he is ready to return to the ward. The nurse checks that blood pressure is stable, that the pulse is strong, and that breathing is normal.

If special attention is required for a longer period, the patient may go to the Intensive Care Unit. The set-up here is similar to that in the recovery department. The idea is to keep the ratio of one patient per nurse to allow constant observation and attention. The stay in intensive care may be for one day or several days.

Postoperative care   Naturally an operation wound would hurt if nothing were done to relieve the pain, but drugs are used to make the postoperative period easier for the patient. Until the stomach is ready to accept food, medicines are injected into the arm. Because pain-relievers have a tendency to depress body functions, excessive doses slow down the recovery process. But if a patient is in pain, he should say so, and make sure that the nurse is aware of it. Sleeping pills are given to assist relaxation under the unusual circumstances of a hospital – the bodily discomfort, restricted movement, new sounds, interruptions, and other people in the room – but patients should not expect to be drugged to sleep every night from the time of the operation until they are ready to go home.

Deep breathing is very important after surgery. When the lungs do not expand fully, the small air sacs at the edges of the lungs remain collapsed and the folds may stick together. This could encourage the development of pneumonia. The mucus in the air passages tends to become sticky after surgery and it clings to the bronchial tubes. For this reason it has to be coughed out.

Simple measures used to overcome the tendency to shallow breathing include moving about in bed, from side to side, or up to a sitting position. Other means are used when these simple measures do not work well enough. A physiotherapist may come to show the patient how to cough up phlegm most effectively.

Moisture is restored to the bronchial tubes by breathing oxygen that comes bubbling through a solution. There are machines, operating by oxygen pressure and fitted with a breathing mask, that can make the patient cough forcibly and yet without pain.

Emptying the bladder may be difficult for a patient in bed, because of the unusual position, and the control muscle of the bladder may not relax. When the bladder wall becomes stretched, the force for expelling the urine is weakened. This situation is relieved by passing a small soft tube (catheter) into the bladder.

Intravenous feeding   If the patient cannot take food or drink, he must still be fed. The common method is to drip a nourishing liquid through a hollow needle placed in a vein in the arm. Other chemical compounds are sometimes added, depending upon the requirements. This method of feeding is seldom required. The fluids are run in slowly to prevent overloading of the circulation and to allow a good mixture with the blood. In addition to nourishment, the patient receives fluid which is necessary to vital functions. The human machine must have water to humidify or air-condition the air in the lungs, to discharge heat through the skin as perspiration, and to eliminate waste chemicals.

Bowel movements may be irregular and sluggish after an operation because the patient's usual routine has been interrupted and he is not physically active. In addition, he may be trying to have a bowel movement lying down instead of sitting up.

Since the muscle wall of the intestine is weak after surgery, even normally swallowed air is not pushed along. Thus air builds up in some sections causing gas pockets. Because of this some liquids that produce more gas than others are forbidden.

There are no hard and fast rules about getting out of bed because the condition of each patient and the kind of operation are so variable. Movement prevents complications of surgery by improving breathing, circulation, urination, bowel movement, and general muscular tone of the patient.

The fewer visitors the better, except for long-term patients who are not seriously ill. Acutely ill patients who will be home shortly need only the immediate family, and this means those who live in the same house. A get-well card will do more good than a visit. Illness is a time for privacy.

The stitches or sutures in the skin may be removed before the patient leaves the hospital, or the surgeon may prefer to delay this. This is not the ordeal many patients think it is going to be. The skin sutures are not holding the incision together, because this is the job of other sutures placed in the depths of the wound. Only the skin sutures are removed.

The patient is given instructions on what he can eat and what he can do before he goes home. If there are any questions about wearing a support, going up and down steps, going outside, lifting, driving a car, taking a bath, or washing hair, they should be answered before leaving hospital.

Stomach operations

Although most stomach operations are for ulcers or tumours, other troubles also call for surgery. One such is hiatus hernia. Here, part of the stomach is dislocated into the chest cavity through a hole in the diaphragm. In the operation for correction of this condition, the stomach is returned to its natural position in the abdomen and the hernial hole is repaired.

Just the opposite is the case when the surgeon has to put the stomach up into the chest cavity after fashioning it into a tube to replace an oesophagus that has been removed. The stomach is sometimes opened out onto the skin surface of the abdomen so that feedings can be put into it directly. This is called a gastrostomy.

A fairly common operation in infants corrects an overdeveloped stomach outlet muscle that does not allow food to pass through it. The outlet muscle or pylorus is split lengthways.

Ulcers Although ulcers are referred to so often as stomach ulcers, most of them are not in the stomach but are located in the duodenum. Some ulcers cannot be healed by medicine and diet and therefore they must be treated by surgery. The conditions that make surgery necessary in ulcer cases are:

Bleeding The ulcer erodes deeply into the stomach or duodenal wall and cuts into a blood vessel.

Perforation The ulcer erodes to form a hole and then bursts into the abdominal cavity.

Obstruction The dense scar tissue around the ulcer shrinks, narrowing the outlet of the stomach.

Intractability Despite strict observance of dietary regulation, the ulcer will not heal.

Location in the stomach Occasionally an unhealed ulcer located in the stomach cannot easily be distinguished from a cancer of the stomach. Ulcers in the duodenum do not present this problem. Disappearance of an ulcer of the stomach should be demonstrated by endoscopy or X-ray after several weeks of treatment, or the condition should be corrected by an operation.

Surgical operations for ulcer accomplish one of the following objectives:

Removing the lower part of the stomach.
Bypassing the lower half of the stomach.
Enlarging the stomach outlet.
Cutting the stomach nerves.

In a normal person, the vagus nerves stimulate the stomach glands when food is taken. The glands secrete digestive fluid for about two hours; then the mechanism is shut off. The stomach outlet muscle opens at intervals to let the mixture of food and

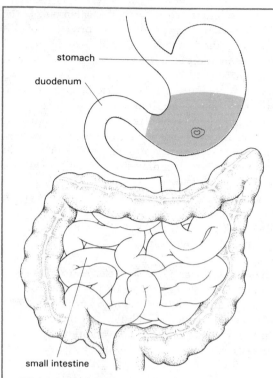

stomach

duodenum

small intestine

When operating for a gastric ulcer the surgeon may cut out the lower part of the stomach, so that the upper part of the stomach can then be joined to a healthy loop of the jejunum, below, thus bypassing the food stream from the duodenum.

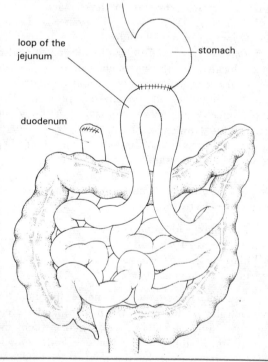

loop of the jejunum

stomach

duodenum

stomach fluid pass out into the intestine. This goes on for about four hours. During the night when no food is taken the stomach is at rest.

In some people, the vagus nerves stimulate the stomach glands continuously, day and night. Because of this the stomach lining is in continuous contact with digestive fluid, which is acid. This is one important factor in the production of ulcers. In the same way, the sensitive lining of the duodenum just beyond the outlet of the stomach is bathed by discharging jets of acid stomach fluid day and night.

Removing the lower part of the stomach   The normal acid of the digestive fluid is produced in response to a hormone released in the lower half of the stomach. In cases of ulcer the acid is produced in excessive amounts. Therefore, this section of the stomach is removed. In this type of operation the ulcer itself may or may not be removed. Even if the ulcer is not removed, the area should heal because acid exposure has been limited. This operation is called gastric resection.

Bypassing the food stream   This operation is used for duodenal ulcers when obstruction of the stomach outlet is the chief problem. In these cases the stomach is joined to a loop of intestine a little farther along than the duodenum, allowing food to go directly into the new loop and to bypass the duodenum. This is called gastroenterostomy.

Enlarging the opening   This is an operation that corrects obstruction at the outlet of the stomach, an obstruction caused by contracting scar tissue. The operation is a permanent enlargement that refashions the outlet of the stomach; it is called pyloroplasty.

Cutting the stomach nerves   The excessive volume of acid stomach fluid is reduced sufficiently to permit ulcer healing by cutting the nerves that stimulate the stomach glands. This is a vagotomy. Cutting of these nerves is often combined with gastroenterostomy or pyloroplasty, either of which will allow the stomach to empty faster.

Nothing is needed to replace the portions of the stomach and duodenum that have been removed. The digestive process is still essentially the same. Stomach fluid (now without the excess of acid), bile, and pancreatic juices still act upon food as they did before.

After some operations, such as the resections, the size of the stomach is reduced, but this reduction in size is not usually noticeable after about six months.

After this time, partly because of stretching of the remaining stomach and partly because of adjustment, the diminished size is not noticed.

Diet after a stomach operation will vary from one patient to the next. A very restricted diet is not necessary, but it is important to be careful about eating habits. Restrictions are lifted gradually and progressively.

Persons with certain types of body make-up must exercise caution in respect of foods, stimulants, and nervous tension. Nervous tension may play a larger role than irritating foods. This means that control will probably be necessary for a lifetime, not necessarily through medicine, but by reasonable control of diet, stimulants, and emotional irritations. Tobacco and spirits should be avoided.

Although it is probable that ulcers do not cause cancer, it is sometimes difficult to tell by testing before the operation whether the diseased area is ulcerous or cancerous. This is particularly true of the stomach. For this reason it is often considered safer to operate in the case of stomach ulcer. Should the condition prove to be cancer, the likelihood of removing it at an early and favourable stage is increased.

Cancers are not the only tumours of the stomach. Benign tumours also occur there. In operations for cancer of the stomach more tissue may need to be removed than in those for ulcer or for benign tumours. In a case of cancer the surgeon aims at removing every part of the stomach to which cancer cells might spread even though he cannot see or feel any spread.

Intestinal operations

Diseased parts of the intestine must usually be removed, and the sooner the better, for nourishment and elimination can be disturbed very quickly. An accurate diagnosis of the nature of intestinal disease is often impossible, except by direct observation by the surgeon or by analysis of the removed specimen.

Only rarely is the entire length of intestinal tube involved by a disease. Ordinarily it is just a section. The defect might be repaired, but more often the better solution is to cut out the diseased part. Sometimes it is necessary to remove only a short segment of a few centimetres. At other times a section of as much as a metre must be taken.

The removal of sections of the intestinal tube is better understood if one pictures the intestine as hanging from the back of the abdomen by an apron-like skirt called the mesentery. Although the intestine is quite long, about 3·7 m (twelve ft), the attachment of its apron is gathered into about ten cm (four in), and thus the intestinal tube hangs at the hem of its mesentery. Blood vessels to and from the intestinal tube fan out from the waist of the mesentery to the intestinal tube at the hem. When a part of the intestine is removed, a wedge-shaped piece of the mesenteric skirt is taken with it. The blood vessels of the diseased part are in this wedge. The freshly cut ends and their blood vessels are fitted together as the sides of the wedge are sewn.

Diseases that affect the intestine may require surgery because they cause the following: bleeding; obstruction of the intestine; telescoping of the intestine; weakening of the intestinal wall to bursting point; strangulation of the intestine by twisting; or an infection in a segment of intestine.

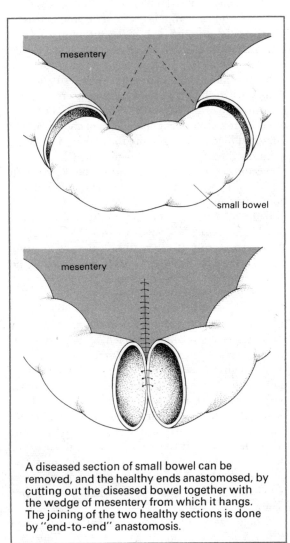

A diseased section of small bowel can be removed, and the healthy ends anastomosed, by cutting out the diseased bowel together with the wedge of mesentery from which it hangs. The joining of the two healthy sections is done by "end-to-end" anastomosis.

Chapter 23 **Your operation**

The passageway (lumen) through the intestine can be blocked by plugging, squeezing, or twisting. Very few objects that can get into the intestine are large enough to plug it, although some things can, such as an enormous gallstone that breaks out of the gallbladder, a hair ball that forms in the stomach, or a tumour that grows on a stalk. Objects that might be swallowed accidentally, such as a pin, a plum stone, a fish or meat bone, or a broken tooth, will not plug the intestine. They may cause inflammation or perforation but they will not directly plug the tube. A tumour squeezes by growing around the intestine. Twisting is caused most often by adhesions that interfere with free motion of the normally moving coils and thereby cause angulation, knotting, or locking, and consequently obstruction.

Telescoping is called intussusception. In this condition the intestinal tube is telescoped into itself. A ball-like tumour hanging by a stalk and partially plugging the intestine will make the muscle of the intestinal wall work so hard that it will telescope itself over the tumour.

Disease may erode an area in the intestinal wall, thinning it to breaking point, like rust eroding the bottom of a pan. As pressure builds up, the tube bursts or perforates at the weak spot. This, of course, allows intestinal fluid to spill out into the abdominal cavity, irritating the sensitive lining membrane.

Bleeding occurs if disease erodes the blood vessels in the intestinal wall, and the blood comes out with the bowel movements.

If the mesentery of the intestine becomes twisted the blood vessels are also twisted and blocked. Without a supply of blood, the section of intestine dies. This is called gangrene, and the twisting of the mesentery that chokes the blood vessels is called strangulation.

The disease in the intestine may be of an inflammatory nature and is called an infection. The intestine becomes red and swollen, and the swelling may be severe enough to cause obstruction.

Although diseases of the intestine differ in their nature, they produce similar effects like bleeding, obstruction, or strangulation. It is the nature of the disease that the surgeon must bear in mind when he makes his incision to repair the defect, or to bypass it, or to cut it away. It is the nature of the disease that determines how much of the intestine must be removed, how much of the mesentery must be taken with it, and how the healthy parts will be put together again.

A hole caused by an injury might lend itself to simple patching, the hole in an eroded cancerous part requires removal of an extensive area of intestine and mesentery, while a hole in the swollen and infected tissues of a badly inflamed appendix might permit nothing more than drainage of the abdominal cavity because the manipulations of cutting and sewing would spread the infection.

Tumours If the surgeon discovers a tumour, he determines by analysis at the time of surgery whether it is cancerous or benign. A long section of intestine must be removed for cancer and with this a large and deep wedge of mesenteric apron. The purpose is to remove all the primary drainage filters, the lymph nodes, that drain the affected part of the intestine through the mesentery. Only a short section of intestine is removed, and very little mesentery, if the tumour is benign. The cells of benign tumours do not wander away from the immediate area and therefore the removal need not be so extensive.

Appendicitis When the appendix becomes inflamed, it may burst, allowing pus to escape into the abdominal cavity. The lacelike curtain of fatty tissue that hangs from the colon and is called the omentum then sticks to the appendix, gathering around it and sealing it into a corner or pocket.

The operation for appendicitis is carried out as soon as the diagnosis can be proved. If the appendix has already burst and an abscess has been formed around it, the surgeon may find it preferable to drain the abscess and leave the appendix for removal at a later date, usually four to eight weeks. The appendix is often removed when the abdomen has been opened for another operation. The decision depends upon the location of the incision and the gravity of the primary operation.

Diverticula are pouchlike protrusions through weak spots in the gut; they are usually found in the colon. An inflamed diverticulum may burst and thus open up a passageway from the intestine into the abdominal cavity, the final result being peritonitis or an internal abscess. If a diverticulum has burst and formed an abscess, an emergency operation may be necessary for drainage only. Drainage means that a channel is made from the abscess to the skin outside. A rubber tube is placed in the channel to keep it open for drainage. If the section of intestine with diverticula is not badly inflamed, the section may be removed and the cut ends joined together. It is sometimes necessary to do this in stages, that is, over a course of two or three operations, using an artificial opening in the abdomen (colostomy) to bypass the bowel movement away from the recently joined ends of the intestine until healing has taken place.

There is a type of diverticulitis that occurs in a single pouchlike tube that hangs from the lower part of the small intestine. The diverticulum is a defect present at birth. When this diverticulum becomes inflamed, the reaction is swift and severe and the symptoms of the patient are very much like those of appendicitis. When it is necessary to remove a Meckel's diverticulum, as this is called, the coil of intestine containing the diverticulum and measuring a few centimetres in length is usually removed.

Regional ileitis A chronic form of inflammation affecting the ileum, which is the lower part of the small intestine, is called regional ileitis. Sometimes the portion of intestine with ileitis is removed, and at times the diseased area is bypassed so that the intestinal stream does not flow through it. In this resting condition the ileum can heal. The bypass is inside the body and does not open to the outside. It is permanent.

Mesenteric thrombosis is a condition in which the arteries to the intestine passing through the mesentery become closed by blood clots that are called thrombi. The mesenteric arteries are said to be thrombosed. Losing its blood supply, the intestinal wall becomes gangrenous and may burst. The effects of this condition are so severe that the patient collapses into a state of shock and may die if the thrombosed section of intestine cannot be removed quickly.

Defects in the intestinal arteries are demonstrated by X-ray examinations made when radiopaque solutions are injected into the abdominal arterial system. For this kind of testing a fine plastic tube is threaded into a thigh artery and up the main artery (the aorta) to the level of the navel. The injected solution mixes with blood in the intestinal arteries to show their outlines clearly on the X-ray films.

Ulcerative colitis affects the entire colon, causing ulcers inside the tube. The entire length of colon becomes thick and stiff. Almost all the colon may have to be removed for ulcerative colitis, and this removal usually includes the rectum because the ulceration is more severe in this area. Since the entire colon and rectum are removed, bowel movements must be diverted out onto the abdominal skin through an artificial opening that is called an ileostomy.

Either the right half or left half of the colon may be removed without a great change in the bowel movements. The colon has the job of taking water out of the liquid intestinal material after it leaves the small intestine. When more extensive sections of the colon must be removed, the usual amount of water absorbed in the colon will be passed in the bowel movements, which therefore may be loose.

Long sections of the first half of the small intestine may be removed without noticeable effect on digestion, but the loss of a lengthy section of the second half may interfere with the absorption of fat or iron or some vitamins. A drop in weight, or anaemia may appear several weeks or months after removal of this part of the small intestine, and medicine has to be taken to counteract this.

Colostomy When it is necessary to remove the rectum, usually for cancer, the lower colon is cut across and its contents diverted through an artificial hole made in the skin of the abdomen. This is called a colostomy. The idea of having an artificial anus opening is naturally alarming. Fortunately, there are appliances and techniques that make it possible to live with this artificial opening in comfort, and to conceal its existence from other people. A special apparatus is placed over the opening to collect the bowel movements.

A temporary colostomy may be needed to protect a surgical suture line that reconstructs the lower colon or rectum. This puts the intestine at rest for healing. At the end of this time the colostomy is closed and normal bowel movements through the rectum are resumed. Temporary colostomies may also be life-saving for gunshot wounds and the tearing wounds of serious road accidents.

Intestinal operations may be performed in stages. The first step in correcting a tumour of the colon that is obstructing the passage may be a temporary colostomy. In the second step the tumour area is removed. As a third step the colostomy is closed, thus restoring the normal continuity of the intestine and rectum.

Gallbladder operations

If a patient is found to have gallstones the probability is that the doctor will advise removal of the gallbladder. There is not much point in removing just the stones, because the stones are formed in the gallbladder and if the gallbladder has formed stones once, it will do it again. Also, the stones will have damaged the gallbladder. The general rule is that anyone in average physical condition under the age of

60 should have gallstones removed, and this involves losing the gallbladder.

A stone may slip from the gallbladder into the duct that leads from it to the main bile duct. The main duct runs from the liver to the intestine. The gallbladder is a reservoir off to the side. Once the duct is blocked, the gallbladder swells and becomes inflamed because bile cannot get out. If the blockage persists, the gallbladder swells to twice its normal size, pus forms, and the gallbladder may burst. When infection is so severe it may be that the gallbladder cannot be removed immediately, but can only be drained to the outside. There will be a second operation at a later date for removal of the diseased gallbladder.

A stone embedded in the gallbladder duct may block it only partially but not completely. From time to time the gallbladder may swell because of this blocked passage. This is the condition for which surgery is performed most frequently.

Removal of the gallbladder does not interfere with digestion because the bile then flows directly down the hepatic duct to the intestine. In most instances this work was taken over before the gallbladder was removed; it was not working and had ceased to play a part in digestive function. Removal of the gallbladder has no important physical significance, and there is no special restriction of diet subsequent to its removal.

Surgical procedures   In each gallbladder operation the main bile duct is examined for stones. If such evidence is present, the duct is opened and cleaned out all the way to its termination in the intestine. This is called choledochostomy.

If there is no evidence of stones in the main duct, it is not opened. This determination may be made by X-ray examination on the operating table. Sometimes it is necessary to open the intestine to dislodge a stone embedded at the termination of the main bile duct. This is called duodenotomy. In this procedure the main bile duct can be cleaned out in both forward and backward directions.

A drain is used after most gallbladder operations. A soft plastic tube is inserted leading down to the space that was formerly occupied by the gallbladder. The purpose is to drain away serum and a small amount of blood that oozes from the raw surface of the gall-bladder bed under the liver. The drain is drawn out gently and shortened by cutting away part of it, usually on the third, fifth, and seventh days after the operation.

When the main bile duct has been opened for removal of stones, a second kind of drain is inserted through a second small incision. It is a hollow plastic tube in the form of a T. The short top of the T is placed inside the bile duct; the vertical part leads to the outside. T-tubes are removed ten to twelve days after operation. Rarely, the patient is allowed to go home with the tube in place and it is removed at a later date. This does not interfere with normal activity. When T-tubes are removed, the opening in the bile duct usually heals within 48 hours.

It is unlikely that stones will cause trouble again once the gallbladder has been removed and the bile ducts have been checked. Virtually all gallstones are formed in the gallbladder. The reason for removing the gallbladder rather than just emptying it or draining it is to prevent a second formation of stones. In rare instances stones form in the liver ducts or in the main bile duct that leads to the intestine. This can happen even after the gallbladder has been removed.

Spleen operations

The spleen is located high in the left upper part of the abdomen, almost at the back. The front surface of the spleen is about the size of the hand. Enormous amounts of blood are pumped through the spleen, coming in through a branching system of arteries and leaving through a similar system of veins. The spleen is not essential to life and can be removed with safety. If the spleen is removed, its duties are assumed by other organs, particularly the bone marrow, the liver, and the lymph nodes.

The reasons for removing the spleen fall into four broad classes:

Overactivity of the spleen and destruction of some elements of the blood.

Injuries to the spleen.

Tumours, cysts, and abscesses.

Other rare diseases of the spleen.

A few minor changes in body physiology occur after removal of the spleen but they are not serious. For several weeks or months there is a decrease in the total number of red corpuscles and an increase in the number of white corpuscles. The increase in the number of white corpuscles is of no significance. Children, however, have lower resistance to infection.

For several weeks after the spleen has been removed, the blood platelets, which assist in the clotting of blood, accumulate in increased numbers. The concentration of these platelets is measured at frequent intervals by blood tests.

Any alteration in the blood clotting mechanism can be controlled if tests indicate that this is necessary.

Hernia operations

A hernia, also called a rupture, is a bulge of the lining membrane of the abdominal cavity through a weak spot in the muscles. These muscles, together with the skin, form a casing for the abdomen. The lining membrane is thin and stretchable. If a gap develops in the muscle casing, the muscle fibres separate, and any increase of abdominal pressure brought about by coughing, lifting, or straining will push the lining membrane through the gap, separating the muscles still further.

There are several weak areas in the abdominal muscles, the groin being the weakest in both men and women. In men, the cord from which the testicle hangs occupies a passageway between the several layers of the abdominal muscles in the groin. In women, the suspending ligament of the womb runs out of the abdominal cavity and through a similar canal, to its attachment at the front of the pelvic bone. These natural passageways through the muscles are weak spots. Another passage subject to hernia is below the groin where the large blood vessels to the thigh leave the abdominal cavity. Muscles may become weak around the incisions of previous operations. The navel is another weak spot.

Once the lining membrane has bulged out through the muscles, it will remain stretched and will protrude as a bag or pouch. This is called the hernial sac. Whenever a patient with a hernia stands, the intestine slips out of the abdomen into the sac and the bulge is visible. When the patient reclines, the intestine will fall back into the abdominal cavity and the bulge will disappear; the sac collapses.

As long as the bulge disappears with reclining, the hernia is said to be reducible. Here the intestine slips readily in and out of the sac. If the hernia does not disappear when the patient lies down, it is called incarcerated. It is caught. The intestine, slipping into the sac, may twist, and if it does this it will swell to such an extent that it cannot slip back even in the reclining position.

The real danger of a hernia is strangulation. When the intestine is trapped in the pouch, it will swell so tightly that its blood vessels become obstructed and blood cannot flow through them. The intestine becomes gangrenous and dead. The hernia is then painful and swollen. Strangulation is a real emergency, always requiring immediate operation for removal of the gangrenous intestine.

Hernial repair When a hernia is repaired by operation, the sac is removed completely and the stretch in the lining membrane is pulled together by stitching. The muscle and fibrous layers are rearranged by overlapping and then drawn up around the cord (in men) or the ligament (in women). A new canal is formed and the back wall is reinforced. When the muscles are of poor quality and are thin and frayed, a screen or mesh of fine nonirritating wire or plastic may be sewn in as an extra supporting layer. The screen is very flexible and is not noticed by the patient no matter what movement he makes.

After a healing period of six weeks the newly reconstructed groin is of normal strength. There is no further need to curtail activities or lifting.

The possibility of a new hernia breaking out in the same place is very slight.

Lung operations

During lung operations the chest cavity is opened. This exposes the lungs to the pressure of outside air, whereas normally they are sealed in a partial vacuum in the chest cavity. Opening the chest breaks the vacuum.

It is the vacuum that allows the alternate up and down movements of ribs and diaphragm to act as a bellows on the lungs, inflating and deflating them. Since the lungs are elastic, they would remain collapsed like a deflated balloon if it were not for the vacuum drawing them out and expanding them to the size of the chest cavity. During the operation there must be a substitute for the vacuum.

Gas exchange will continue for as long as the lungs can be made to suck in air and blow it out again. To accomplish this, the lungs are assisted by a bellows arrangement. The anaesthetist inserts an intratracheal breathing tube into the windpipe (trachea), and then connects this tube to a rubber bag that is filled with oxygen and anaesthetic gas. Each time the rubber bag is squeezed, the lungs are inflated with gas from the bag. The lung cells then exchange oxygen for carbon dioxide. When the bag is let go, the elastic recoil of the lungs pushes carbon dioxide gas out through the tube to the bag and the bag expands.

As a further refinement, the intratracheal tube can be inserted still further to fit into either the right or left main bronchial tube. This allows one lung to be inflated and deflated for breathing while the other lung remains collapsed. Sometimes the surgeon can work better on a collapsed lung. The collapsed lung can be inflated by rearranging the intratracheal tube.

When the operation within the chest cavity has been completed, the anaesthetist inflates the lungs to full capacity by squeezing the rubber gas bag. He keeps the lungs in this expanded condition until the ribs have been drawn together and the muscles and skin have been closed tightly by stitches. A long rubber tube is brought out from the inside of the chest cavity through a hole in the skin and is connected to a glass bottle on the floor. The bottle contains about four cm ($1\frac{1}{2}$ in) of water and the tube coming from the chest cavity is securely anchored under the water.

Each time the lungs are inflated to full capacity by the anaesthetist's air bag, a little air is pushed out through the tube and bubbles up under the water in the bottle on the floor. No air can go back in because the end of the tube is sealed by the water. In this manner, the vacuum inside the chest cavity is re-established. The air tube to the bottle on the floor is left in place for several days. By the end of this time the surface of the lung has become sealed to the lining of the chest cavity and from this point on will not collapse, nor will the vacuum be broken. The chest tube is then removed.

Removing segments of the lung   It is possible to live normally with only one good lung, and this is fortunate, because some patients must be treated by removal of an entire lung. The major loss in this event is that of reserve breathing capacity. This is the reserve we use for running, climbing, heavy exercise, and exertion. In carrying out our usual routines we use only a small part of the full lung capacity. A person with one lung can do all these usual things.

Many lung diseases are confined to just a part or segment of one lung and are not scattered throughout both lungs. The surgeon may therefore eradicate disease by removing only one or two subdivisions of one lung.

All of this comes about because each lung, right and left, is divided into separate units, called lobes. The surgeon can cut out one lobe without disturbing the others.

Each lobe is subdivided further into smaller independent units. These units, called segments, varying in number from two to five in a lobe, are not visibly separated from each other but are partitioned off. Each segment has an independent blood supply and an independent air duct system through its own bronchial tube, coming off the main tube.

When the surgeon must remove a whole lung, he works close up against the heart, disconnecting the main inlet arteries and the outlet veins to the diseased lung. The main bronchial tube is then cut across where it branches off from the windpipe. The open cuts across these structures are sealed by suturing.

This operation is called pneumonectomy (removal of a lung).

When only a lobe is to be taken out, the blood vessels and the bronchial tube to that lobe are isolated and severed. This is a lobectomy. The same principle is used for the removal of one or more segments, but this time the blood vessels and the bronchial tube are severed farther out along the line. This type of removal is known as segmental resection.

Heart operations

If blood flow is stopped for more than a few minutes, death occurs. An artificial pump is necessary to maintain blood flow when the heart has to be stopped and opened for surgery. The patient's blood is bypassed through the pump. The pipe and valve connections between the lungs and heart are so short and complex that a bypass around the heart calls for a bypass around both the heart and the lungs. A combination of a pump with an artificial lung, called a heart-lung machine, is used for this purpose. (See photograph, page 81.)

Open heart surgery   A heart-lung machine is made up of a pumping system and an artificial lung that breathes oxygen into the blood. Plastic tubes are connected to the vein system to carry blood out of the body, through the machine, and then back to the main artery, bypassing the heart and the lungs. Blood is pumped through the machine as a thin film over wide screens in a container rich in oxygen. Blood cells pick up oxygen from the enriched atmosphere.

Hypothermia   Not all surgery on the heart is "open". Some heart operations that require opening the heart for only very short periods can be performed without passing the blood through the heart-lung machine. The brain can take two periods of five minutes each without any oxygen-filled blood coming to it if the body temperature is lowered to 30 degrees centigrade. At this low temperature the brain needs less oxygen. The technique of lowering body temperature is called hypothermia, sometimes referred to incorrectly as freezing.

Heart action can be stopped temporarily by putting iced water in the sac (pericardium) that encloses the heart. Lowering the temperature of the heart decreases the oxygen requirement of the muscle.

Heart operations correct:
Defects in the main blood vessels   These are the vessels that connect directly to the heart.

Defects in the valves, between the chambers of the heart and at the main outlets from the heart.

Defects in the partition walls, the walls that separate the chambers from each other.

Coarctation of the aorta

The aorta is the main blood vessel leading out from the heart – the vessel that carries blood full of oxygen all over the body. Some infants are born with a narrow section in this tube, a section that varies usually from 5 mm to four cm ($\frac{1}{4}$ in to $1\frac{1}{2}$ in) in length. This is a coarctation and it looks like the section between two sausages.

As the faulty section is usually very short and the blood vessels have a surprising elasticity, most often the narrow part is cut out and the freshly cut ends of normal diameter are joined together directly by sutures. If the coarctation is longer and there is not enough elasticity in the aorta, a length of plastic tube is sutured in place as a graft.

To accomplish this operation the aorta is squeezed shut and clamped, upstream and downstream from the coarctation, during the period of cutting and rejoining the vessel. Since the narrow section is downstream from the brain arteries, the clamps do not interfere with the flow of blood to the brain. The other organs can stand longer periods without flow. If it appears that the time required for making the repair will be unusually lengthy, a plastic tube is connected to the aorta above and below the working area and blood is bypassed around it to all the lower organs of the body.

Patent ductus arteriosus

The ductus is a short blood vessel, about 5 mm ($\frac{1}{4}$ in) in length and diameter, that bypasses blood away from a baby's lungs when in the mother's womb. The baby's blood in the womb gets oxygen from the mother and not from the baby's lungs. As soon as the infant is born and its lungs begin to work, the ductus closes, shrinking away in time to a small cord.

If the ductus fails to close after birth, some of the oxygenated blood goes through it and back through the lungs again. This puts an extra load on the lungs and heart. The defect is called a patent (open) ductus arteriosus. To correct this defect the ductus is cut across and the two ends are sutured shut. If the pressure in the lung circuit is too high, the condition cannot be corrected. The operation for the correction of this defect does not require a bypass through the heart-lung machine.

Pulmonary stenosis

Another malformation that may be present at birth is pulmonary stenosis.

Stenosis means narrowing. Here the channel that carries venous blood to the lungs is too narrow. Blood cannot get through the opening fast enough and is dammed back in the heart. This throws a strain on the heart wall. The problem is handled in several different ways, depending upon how severely the channel is narrowed. The constriction may either be stretched or cut.

The mitral valve

The mitral valve is between the left atrium and ventricle. Disease, particularly rheumatic fever, attacks this valve more often than any of the other valves, and it becomes so scarred that it will not open wide enough to let blood through at a normal speed. This is mitral stenosis. On the other hand, disease may so affect the valve that it becomes flabby and stretches to a diameter that is so great that the valve flaps cannot close tightly. When the valve is supposed to be in the closed position to hold blood in the chamber, the blood leaks out. This is called mitral insufficiency.

Mitral stenosis is corrected by one of two methods, either by replacing the valve with a plastic substitute or by splitting the tightened and narrowed valve ring to open up its channel.

Mitral insufficiency, likewise, can be corrected by replacing the stretched and leaking valve with a plastic substitute. Or the flaps can be adjusted by taking a tuck in them with a permanent suture or by grafting on a small piece of heart sac membrane (pericardium).

The aortic valve, located at the heart exit into the aorta (main artery), may also be subject to excessive tightening (stenosis) or leaking (insufficiency). The prime causes are rheumatic fever in young people and arteriosclerosis in older patients.

A severely malfunctioning aortic valve is removed by cutting it out completely and replacing it with a plastic substitute in an open heart operation.

Septal defects

The partition walls between the heart chambers are known as septa and the defects in these walls are called septal defects. A septal defect is an abnormal hole in a wall. These are congenital malformations present at birth. The hole in the wall between two chambers allows oxygenated blood in the left side of the heart to pass into the right side and recirculate through the lungs. This puts a strain on both heart and lungs. If this defect occurs in combination with pulmonary stenosis, the leak is from right side to left side. In this case, venous blood is recirculated in the body and with exertion the patient becomes blue.

Small defects can be closed by suturing, larger ones are covered with a graft of plastic material. Several different methods are used. The method chosen depends upon which septum is involved, the size of the hole between the two chambers, and its position in the septum.

Combination defects In general, heart abnormalities are due either to faulty formation of the heart before birth and are called congenital defects, or they are the result of disease later on and are then called acquired defects. Only the more common defects are described here. A heart may be faulty in more than one way; for example, a septal defect may be combined with a faulty valve channel or an abnormal placement of an intake or outlet blood vessel. A person with a congenital heart defect may be stricken with rheumatic fever so that a valve, faulty at birth, becomes additionally defective as a result of disease. In such instances of congenital heart defect the repair requires a combination of surgical procedures.

Coronary sclerosis The small blood vessels that lead back from the aorta to the muscle of the heart wall, the coronary arteries, may become hardened and narrowed. The linings of these vessels can be scraped out by an operation known as endarterectomy. More often the narrowed portion is bypassed using a length of vein taken from the leg, a coronary bypass operation. These operations are performed usually on older people.

Genitourinary surgery

Prostate surgery The prostate gland is a small chestnut-sized organ, straddling the urethral tube that leads from the bladder through the penis to the outside. Since the channel for urine passes through the prostate, it is understandable that enlargement of the organ may obstruct the flow of urine. Back pressure of urine from the bladder up to the kidneys damages the kidneys to the extent that they cannot eliminate waste products of the body, and thus poisoning from these waste products, called uraemia, occurs. The obstruction at the bladder outlet must be relieved.

Slender telescopic operating instruments called cystoscopes can be inserted through the penis into the bladder, permitting a direct look at the interior to determine the nature and extent of the obstruction caused by the prostate gland.

Open and closed procedures There are four kinds of prostate operations. Three of these operations are called open procedures, because they are performed through an incision made either in the lower abdomen or between the legs. There is one closed operation accomplished through the penis with the cystoscope.

Kidney and bladder stones

Kidney stones are fairly common. Bladder stones are rarer, being limited for the most part to older persons. Most of the stones are found within the pelvis of the kidney. The stone may remain there or it may slip out of the pelvis and become lodged in the thin muscular tube (ureter) that conducts urine from the kidney to the bladder. When the ureter becomes obstructed, urine accumulates in the kidney pelvis to such a degree that the kidney itself becomes swollen and stretched. Obstruction to the flow of urine at any level in the urinary tract leads to infection.

If infection can be prevented and if the obstruction to the outflow of urine is not severe, the patient, under supervision of his doctor, may wait a while for the stone to pass. However, if infection sets in, or if the obstruction builds up enough pressure in the kidney to keep urine from filtering through it, surgery will be necessary. Complete obstruction which continues for several weeks causes damage to the kidney.

There are closed and open operations for removing stones. Small stones at the lower end of the ureter may be removed by a thin catheter with a loop at its tip.

Stones that are wedged in the ureter often must be removed by an open operation. The nature and location of the incision depend upon the location and size of the stone.

The slit made in the ureter for removing the stone is closed by sutures placed very loosely to avoid scar formation and narrowing of the slender ureter. Therefore after stone operations a drain is passed from the ureter to the outside because it is anticipated that there will be some leakage for several days.

Stones of considerable size remain in the pelvis of the kidney for a long time, often without causing symptoms to make the patient aware of their presence. Such stones are too large to pass down into the ureter and therefore they cause no obstruction to the flow of urine. Eventually, however, infection or bleeding may occur and the stone is discovered, but the kidney harbouring the stone may have been damaged to such a degree by this time that it will be necessary for the surgeon to remove the kidney. This is done through an incision in the flank, and the whole kidney is removed. The surgeon first determines by examination that the other kidney is present, healthy, and capable of performing the task of eliminating waste from the body.

Stones in the urinary bladder, now rare, are removed by opening the bladder through an incision in the lower abdomen. Small stones can be removed through the normal channel of the urethra by instruments that are equipped with small crushing devices at their tips. These instruments crush the stones into tiny pieces that can be washed out through the cystoscope.

Cancer may appear at almost any place in the urinary tract, the kidney, the ureter, the bladder, the prostate, and in other structures of the urinary system. Most often the organ affected must be removed. A diseased member of any of the organs that come in pairs, such as the kidneys, can be removed without impairing body functions if the remaining organ is healthy.

If it is necessary to remove the urinary bladder, a substitute bladder is formed from a length of intestine, and the ureters that bring urine down from the kidneys are transposed into the new bladder. This type of bladder opens directly to the outside and is without voluntary muscular control. It is necessary to use a plastic container to collect the urine.

Tonsillectomy

Tonsillectomy is not a minor operation. It is therefore undertaken only when the seriousness of recurrent attacks of tonsillitis clearly indicates that the patient would be healthier without his tonsils. The operation is done in the hospital where safety devices and precautionary measures are available. Children are given a general anaesthetic; occasionally tonsils are removed from adults under local anaesthesia.

Very occasionally, bleeding may occur after the operation. This may be within a few hours or as long as ten days later. Most often such bleeding is caused by a collection of clotted blood in one spot of the operated area. If this is the case, the haemorrhage is stopped by washing out the blood clots. Sometimes bleeding is persistent and the patient may have to undergo a second anaesthetic for control of the bleeding point. It is like a nosebleed; it stops or it has to be stopped. Parents are always instructed to notify the surgeon if there is the slightest bleeding after the child has returned home.

The patient's throat can be very sore for a day or two, but is usually completely healed in about a week.

Adenoids consist of the same type of tissue as the tonsils. They are located high in the back of the throat and at the back of the nasal cavity. They become infected along with the tonsils so the adenoids and tonsils are often removed at the same time.

Surgery of head and neck

Tumours The complexity of the face, jaws, nose, larynx, and neck is such that tumours may involve several organs or organ systems at the same time. When they are treated in their early stages, surgical removal is simpler because fewer organs and structures are involved. Fear of possible disfigurement by surgical removal causes many people to delay unnecessarily. If the tumour is benign, and many are, delay will necessitate removal of more tissue than would have been necessary. If the tumour is malignant, the patient who procrastinates is increasing the odds that the tumour will be fatal.

Small tumours of the larynx, for example, can usually be eliminated by the removal of a small amount of tissue. The same tumour, on the other hand, allowed to grow and expand and involve other portions of the throat, requires a far more extensive removal of tissue with much less chance of cure. Tumours of the head and neck carry a better chance of cure by early treatment than other tumours hidden in deeper regions of the body, as they quickly become noticeable. When extensive removal of tissue is required for far-advanced tumours, synthetic prostheses are used to mask the removed areas. The fabrication of these prostheses has developed into a fine art to the extent that it is hard to distinguish artificial from natural.

Techniques have been developed not only to restore appearance but to substitute for function. The patient whose larynx has been removed for cancer of the larynx, for example, can be taught to speak by swallowing air in a way that will be satisfactory for normal communication.

Thyroid operations Partial or complete removal of the thyroid gland may become necessary because of goitre, although not all goitres have to be removed.

It is seldom that the entire thyroid gland is removed. Whenever possible, enough thyroid tissue is left to supply the body with the natural thyroid secretion and to conserve some of the parathyroid glands. Sometimes almost all of the gland is diseased. In this case the surgeon recognizes that the small amount of healthy tissue he will leave will not be adequate. However, he must make a choice between healthy and diseased thyroid gland tissue. It is possible for the patient to take thyroid hormone by mouth as a replacement.

Thyroid operations require an incision in the neck. This runs across the lower part of the neck in a curve. The thin straplike muscles of the neck are separated to bring the gland into view and the diseased areas are removed. The thin scar from the wound is, of course, in a prominent place and this makes it somewhat annoying. Like all scars, it remains reddened for six to twelve months and this adds to the prominence. After this time the scar fades and is less conspicuous. In men it is usually below the collar line of the shirt. Women sometimes cover it with a necklace.

Recovery from the operation is usually rapid. Breathing and swallowing are seldom impeded, and the stitches are usually removed within four days. Usually there is a small plastic tube to allow excess serum to escape. A thin serum frequently accumulates in the wound but it is not painful and rarely persists for more than a week or two.

Operations for removal of what is known as toxic goitre are usually performed only in women of child-bearing age, and men. Older women are treated with radioactive iodine. Antithyroid drugs are available for control of the symptoms of overactivity or toxicity at any age and are also often used in conjunction with an operation or radioactive iodine. Large goitres which are toxic or do not respond well to antithyroid medicine also require removal by surgery.

Cancers may develop in the thyroid gland. They are relatively rare but it is because of the possibility of development of cancerous tumours that any lumps in the thyroid gland are carefully watched by the doctor. Every lump that is removed is examined. If it should happen that cancer is present, it may be necessary to perform further surgery, and X-ray treatment is sometimes ordered.

Tracheotomy Blockage of the upper air passages by foreign objects is relieved by tracheotomy. This means putting a temporary hole in the front of the windpipe just below the Adam's apple so that an obstruction higher up can be bypassed. A silver tube is placed in this opening to allow air to enter the windpipe directly. Small soft tubes can also be passed through the silver tube and down into the windpipe and bronchial tubes to draw out obstructing secretions.

An incision is made in the front of the neck and, after pushing the muscles and other tissues aside, the windpipe is opened and the tube is inserted. When the tube is put in the windpipe for this purpose it is temporary. So long as the tube is in place it must be kept clean and open. This can be done by the patient himself after receiving instruction from the nursing staff. After a tracheotomy tube has been removed and the wound has healed the voice will be as normal as it was before and there will be only a small scar in the front of the neck.

When the structure of the larynx (voice box) must be removed because of benign or malignant tumours, a tracheotomy tube is placed in the windpipe and it remains there permanently.

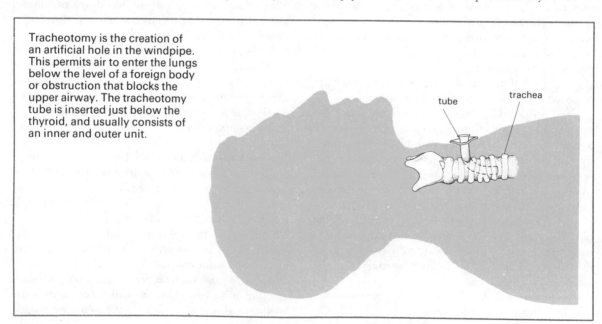

Tracheotomy is the creation of an artificial hole in the windpipe. This permits air to enter the lungs below the level of a foreign body or obstruction that blocks the upper airway. The tracheotomy tube is inserted just below the thyroid, and usually consists of an inner and outer unit.

tube

trachea

Surgery on the ear

The development of surgical techniques for correcting ear troubles has brought relief for a number of disabilities that were formerly regarded as almost incurable. These troubles include loss of hearing, chronic discharge of pus from the ear, sudden attacks of dizziness, and noises in the head.

Ear infection is usually located in the middle ear. It may erode through the roof of the middle ear to make its way into the mastoid bone and through this bone into the skull cavity to cause meningitis or abscess of the brain. Hearing loss is caused by disease in the conducting mechanism that crosses through the middle ear or by disturbance of the inner hearing nerve.

A defective conducting mechanism can often be corrected by surgery, but a damaged nerve cannot be restored. The outcome of surgery may be good, poor, or no hearing, fair hearing with the use of a hearing aid, or improvement of the benefits already obtained by a hearing aid.

Some head noises are caused by a hardening condition of the third and innermost of the small conducting bones in the middle ear. This bone, shaped like a stirrup, and called the stapes, touches a membrane which, when vibrated, sets up motions in the fluid around the inner ear nerve. The condition is called otosclerosis, and begins as a hearing loss which becomes progressively worse. As the attachment of the stapes to the membrane becomes hardened, the hearing nerve is irritated and it is this that sends impulses to the brain. Since the sound impulses are abnormal and caused by irritation, they are interpreted as ringing, roaring, or buzzing noises.

Myringoplasty   This is an operation for repairing a hole in the eardrum. A small graft of skin or vein is used to seal the hole. This separates the middle ear from the outside and prevents ear infection. In many cases hearing is improved.

The operation is performed through the ear canal with local anaesthesia. A hospital stay of several days is necessary. Healing is complete in about six weeks, at which time hearing improvement should be noticeable.

Myringotomy is a relatively simple surgical incision of the eardrum.

Tympanoplasty   Tympanum is the Latin word for the eardrum. Tympanoplasty is the name for an operation in which the middle ear, including its roof in the mastoid bone, is completely cleaned out. All infection is eradicated. This type of operation is necessary when both the eardrum and the conducting bones are diseased. The extent of the surgery depends upon how much normal structure is left after all infection has been cleaned out. The destroyed parts of the eardrum and ear bones have to be replaced by skin or vein grafts and by plastic or wire substitutes.

The operation can be performed through the ear canal under local anaesthesia, or, if the infection is severe, an incision behind the ear may be necessary and this requires a general anaesthetic. The improvement in hearing is noticeable within eight weeks. The hospital stay is less than a week. Infection may be so severe that two operations are required. At the first session all infection is cleaned out and at the second session the eardrum and the bones are reconstructed with substitutes.

Mastoidectomy   Acute inflammation of the mastoid bone is no longer common, but operations for chronic mastoiditis are still sometimes required. Chronic infection in the mastoid and middle ear must be eradicated because of the potential danger of abscess of the brain. All infection here must be eradicated before any of the reconstructive operations for restoration of hearing can be accomplished.

Fenestration   In this operation the mastoid bone is opened and the balance canals of the inner ear are exposed. A tiny hole, called a fenestrum, is made in one of the balance tubes. A paper-thin piece of skin taken from the ear canal is then placed over this hole. This allows sound waves from the air to vibrate the piece of skin at the small opening and in turn the fluid in the balance tube will transmit sound vibrations to the hearing nerve.

This was the first of the modern ear operations and was designed for otosclerosis. Its purpose was to bypass the hardened stapes that was stuck to the membrane that normally vibrated the fluid of the hearing nerve. For the most part, fenestration has been replaced by the stapes operation. Fenestration is now reserved for patients who are born without an external ear canal or for those who have suffered extensive destruction of the bone around the hearing nerve.

Stapes operation   The stapes is removed together with the membrane upon which it rests. A small section of vein is grafted over the opening and a section of wire or plastic material positioned to bridge the gap between the membrane and the bone next to the stapes. This restores the conducting mechanism.

If stapes surgery is not successful, hearing may be about the same as it was before. It is possible that it might be worse but this does not often happen. In some instances, fortunately not many, head noises can be worse than they were before. Because of the possibility of a poor result, the ear with the greater hearing defect is usually operated upon first.

Surgery for Menière's disease Formerly only the most severe and disabling forms of this disease were treated surgically because the operation for relief of the disease required destruction of the hearing nerve. Until microsurgical instruments were developed it was impossible to separate the hearing and balance filaments in the main nerve. Now that these can be separated it is possible to clip only the balance filaments. It is possible also to use selective ultrasonic beams for destruction of the balance filaments without damaging the sensory filaments.

Breast operations

A lump in the breast is occasionally due to cancer, so the first task is to prove whether or not the lump is malignant.

This entails a biopsy; the lump is removed and examined microscopically in the pathology laboratory. The usual practice is to remove the lump in the operating room with the patient asleep; most often the analysis is made in a few minutes by frozen section.

If the examination shows no cancer, the small wound is sutured and the patient can be sent home the next day.

If the analysis shows cancer, the breast must be removed, and this is done immediately. The extent varies from removal of the local breast tissue only, to removal of the underlying muscles and all the tissues under the armpit, along with the breast. The more extensive operation may be performed in case cancer cells have entered the lymph drainage paths from the breast. It is sometimes necessary to remove both breasts.

Postsurgical measures X-ray treatments may be given after surgery for breast cancer. These sterilize, so to speak, a further area around the breast. There are exercises to re-educate the adjoining muscles to give strength to the shoulder and arm. Within months shoulder motion is free and strong. Bowling, golf, tennis, and swimming can be resumed. Adjustable prostheses are available, and have been developed to a high degree of comfort, with realistic

texture. The texture and mobility of these forms will relieve many anxieties.

Benign growths Most benign lumps arise from milk ducts that have become blocked and then filled by a fluid made by the breast cells. In this manner it becomes a cavity filled with fluid and is called a cyst. Every woman has hundreds of pinhead-size cysts in the breasts, the natural result of the swelling and activity of the breasts that occurs before each menstrual period. It is only the larger cysts that show as lumps. Sometimes a hollow needle is put into a cyst to draw out the fluid and collapse the cavity.

The lump may be a noncancerous tumour, a growth that is enclosed in a capsule and that is not capable of getting into the bloodstream and spreading. In this case, only the fluid-filled lump is removed, not the breast.

Neurosurgery

Operations have been devised for a variety of troubles that affect the brain. In serious head injuries the skull must be opened for removal of bone splinters and blood clots and for the removal of brain tissue that has been damaged.

Tears in the brain capsule are repaired to protect underlying brain tissue.

Tumours, when they are enclosed in a capsule, are removed by shelling them out, or by directly cutting through brain tissue when there is no capsule around the tumour. Some areas in the brain are said to be silent, meaning that the cells in these areas can be removed or damaged without producing paralysis, blindness, or deafness, and so on.

Defects in the fluid canals inside the brain may be cured or the canal may be rerouted. Special nerve pathways in the brain are sometimes severed purposely to reduce abnormal impulses that cause convulsions, paralysis, or pain. Locating devices are combined with special X-ray equipment to pinpoint the seat of the trouble.

Spinal cord operations The spinal cord may be exposed for surgery at any point along its course.

Common operations are for tumours of the spinal cord, for injuries to the cord, or for removal of a dislocated spinal disc. Spinal cord tumours are similar to brain tumours; some may be shelled out, others must be cut away. In disc operations the spinal cord is found intact and the surgeon moves the cord to one side of the disc. There may be an indentation in the cord from the pressure of the protruding disc. The discs are soft cushions between the vertebrae. The capsule in which a disc is encased may break open, allowing the disc substances to protrude into the canal and to press upon the cord. The surgeon does not replace the disc, he removes the protruding portion of it.

In order to expose the spinal cord, it is necessary to remove part of the bone of one or more vertebrae (laminectomy). This interferes only very little with support or movement of the spine. For this reason disability following an operation on the spinal cord is usually only temporary.

Orthopaedic surgery

A bone fracture can be reduced (set) by pulling and bending motions that will manipulate the broken ends into a good position for healing. This is called closed reduction, closed because it is not necessary to cut open the limb. X-rays may show beforehand that a closed reduction will not work, either because the bone is splintered into many pieces or because the break is on a slant. Splintered or slanted ends will slip away from each other.

If the ends cannot be positioned properly, or if they will not stay in position, an operation is necessary to open the fracture to full view, to reduce it with bone levers and bone clamps, and then fasten the fitted ends together (open reduction) with some fastening device.

All kinds of devices are used to fasten broken bones – pins, nails of many sorts, wires, metal plates, and even long rods that extend the entire length of the bone through the marrow canal. All of these are made of special alloy metals that usually do not irritate body tissues. Sometimes there will be irritation of the bone and the muscle, even to the extent that the appliance will have to be removed before the bone has had a chance to heal. Some of these metal devices remain in the bone permanently, some are removed after healing is complete.

The use of appliances fixed into the bone to heal a fracture is called internal fixation. This may be all the support that is needed, but more often a plaster cast is put round the limb for additional external fixation. Metal pins can be passed through the skin and into the bone under X-ray guidance to secure internal fixation without making an incision to expose the fracture to view. This is internal fixation combined with closed reduction.

The time required for fracture healing, called union of the bone, will vary with the size of the bone, the extent of splintering, and whether the bone bears any of the body's weight, as is the case with bones of the spine, the pelvis, and the lower limbs.

Occasionally a fracture, whether set by closed reduction or by open reduction, may not heal. This will happen if the broken ends become too hard without knitting to each other. In this case, an operation will be necessary to open the fracture for removal of the hard callus. At the same time, bone chips are put around the fracture to stimulate knitting, or a solid piece of bone shaped like a stick is grafted into the bone across the break. Bone used for the stimulation of knitting is obtained from another bone in the body.

Compound fractures demand special surgical attention because of contamination of the exposed marrow of the bone by dirt and bacteria that can get in through the torn skin and muscle. This calls for immediate surgery to clean out the wound, and it may require removal of some muscle and skin tissue if dirt has been ground into it. If the wound can be cleaned satisfactorily, the fracture may be reduced at this time. If the surgeon judges the contamination to be too severe, he will pack the wound with gauze and place the limb in a plaster cast, delaying the reduction of the fracture for as long as a week, during which time any contaminants in the wound will drain out into the gauze packs. As soon as the wound is clean, the fracture can be reduced and secured in place by whatever means are necessary.

Fractures of the femur The upper end of the thighbone, the femur, is a common location for fractures among people in their 60's and 70's. This common fracture is sometimes referred to as a fracture of the hip, but this is not a good name for it because the pelvis, which is a part of the hip joint, is not usually broken. The fracture is a serious one because it will not knit unless the bone ends are held still by some method for as long as three to six months. Any method that keeps an elderly patient in bed for this length of time may lead to pneumonia, bladder infection, pressure sores, and death. This was the case years ago when these fractures were held in place by weights over the end of the bed or by plaster casts.

Unless the patient is too frail, an operation will give the best chance for survival and restoration of normal walking. The fractured ends are reduced into a good position under anaesthesia and the bone is secured by large nails or screws and possibly by a plate that is attached to the long end of the bone. With the bone secure, the patient can be moved about in bed

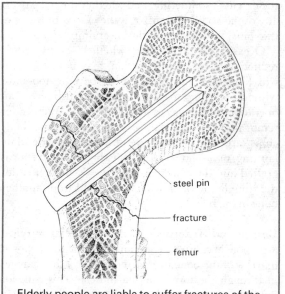

Elderly people are liable to suffer fractures of the upper end of the long bone in the thigh (femur). The fracture is reduced and fixed using a steel pin to avoid the complications of prolonged bed rest with the leg in plaster.

immediately and within a short time he can be helped to a chair and to a walker.

The higher the fracture occurs in the bone, the worse it is, because the ball-like head at the top end of the bone is nourished only by a small artery that is usually torn with the fracture. If the head of the bone dies after the fracture, it may have to be replaced at a later date by a metallic ball anchored to the bone.

Arthroplasty If the ball-shaped head of the thigh-bone (femur) has been shattered or if it has become disintegrated as a result of disease, it can be replaced with a metal ball. The ball is attached to a stem that the surgeon can seat into the hollow marrow canal of the shaft of the thighbone. The operation is called arthroplasty. The same operation – with variations – is used for reconstruction of a painful hip joint caused by arthritis. Hip arthroplasty is a serious operation and is reserved for patients who are in fairly good physical condition.

Smooth surfaces can be fashioned for smaller joints – elbow, fingers – that are stiff and motionless. The roughened cartilage at the ends of the bones is removed and the bone ends that form the joint are replaced with ones made of plastic.

Amputations The artistry and mechanical genius of today's substitutes for limbs and joints (prostheses) have brought a new world of rehabilitation to patients who are faced with amputation of a limb. The medical term prosthesis includes not only limbs and joints but false teeth, wigs, and artificial breasts. The moving fingers and hands of a prosthesis can thread needles, hammer a nail, or quiet a baby; the ankle and knee joints can dance or hike; the feet can stand at a lathe all day.

When forced to amputate, the surgeon considers the wide variety of available prostheses as they relate to his patient's age, training, occupation, and pattern of life. This is necessary because the site, or level, of amputation and the manner of shaping the bones and muscles of the limb, bear directly on the different types of prostheses the patient will be using. Some prostheses require special rearrangements of the muscle bundles in the limb for their most effective use. This is called a cineplastic amputation. The condition of the blood vessels is a major factor in determining the site and type of amputation. The surgeon always tries to remove the minimum of tissue, compatible with the requirements mentioned above.

The time required for adjustment, both physically and emotionally, to amputation and to the prosthesis again depends upon the patient's particular problem. Retraining, education in physical adeptness, and financial assistance are open to the amputee.

Amputations are necessary for a number of reasons. Limbs are sometimes mangled and damaged beyond all possible restoration in road or rail accidents, by explosions, or in mishaps with heavy machinery. It is younger people who are involved more frequently in accidents. Farm machinery is particularly dangerous if it is not used with great caution. Hardened blood vessels, especially in diabetic patients, often become clogged, shutting off the supply of blood to the limb with the result that the tissue of a foot and even part of the leg become dead (gangrenous).

Rectal operations

Pockets (crypts) and mounds (papillae) are natural structures just inside the rectum. They are part and parcel of the pleats and folds which are gathered in the rectal membrane by the circular muscle that closes the rectum. They cause trouble when inflamed and swollen. Infection in a crypt may spread through the rectal wall and burrow in the soft tissue about the anus to form an abscess. When the abscess breaks through to the skin a few centimetres distant from the natural opening, a tunnel remains as an abnormal passageway from the rectum. This is called a fistula.

The kind of operation for a fistula depends upon the contour of the tunnel and upon whether it runs a straight course to the outside or has ramifications and more than one opening. All tissue over the fistula is cut away, even a part of the muscle.

Rectal polyps These are soft fleshy outgrowths that are encountered frequently during examination with a proctoscope. A piece is taken for examination – biopsy – and the growth is removed, either by snipping it away with a scissor-like instrument or with a diathermy needle. This is done through the proctoscope. The patient is not always confined to hospital. An anaesthetic is not required.

Pilonidal cyst A tiny opening may lead to a small cavity in the fat over the coccyx. When swollen from inflammation, it may have a depth of four cm ($1\frac{1}{2}$ in). A short tunnel leads to a sometimes invisible opening in the skin.

If it becomes infected, the cyst may have to be lanced to let out the pus. Later, the cavity must be removed, usually by cutting away all the tissue around the cyst and down to the covering of the coccyx.

Cancer An operation for rectal cancer may or may not require an opening in the side for bowel movements (colostomy, see page 519). If all the rectum must be removed, including the muscle – a very small percentage of all colon and rectal cancers – this will be because the malignant growth lies within a few centimetres of the muscle at the natural anal opening. Otherwise, the involved part of the rectum can be removed through an incision in the abdomen and the cut ends of the colon and rectum sewn together. Thus the muscle at the anus will be preserved so that bowel movements can take place in the normal fashion.

Haemorrhoids, also called piles, are varicose veins in and around the rectal opening. Varicose means permanently stretched in both length and breadth.

With each bowel movement, the rectum is stretched open to let the stool come through. A straining effort to force the stool will, of course, increase the stretching force. The membrane, the muscle wall of the canal, and the veins embedded in it are all stretched in this process. After the stool has passed through the anus, all the parts recoil to natural size, and the circular muscle of the canal tightens to close the opening. The canal is about $2\frac{1}{2}$ cm (one in) in length and stretches to a diameter of four cm ($1\frac{1}{2}$ in).

The thin walls of the veins do not tolerate this repeated stretching as well as the membrane and the muscles. If the veins are weaker than normal, and this is the case in many people, they will be stretched permanently to become haemorrhoids. Veins dilate to the extent that they bulge and even hang out of the opening. Once the process has started, it tends to get worse because the stool pushes the bulging veins still further outwards as it is forced through the canal. Usually there are three, but no more than four, of these bulging veins formed into clusters. In time the membrane that covers the veins becomes stretched and lax.

Larger, hanging clusters of haemorrhoids lose their elasticity and they are then unable to recoil back inside the opening after the stool has passed through. Now, when the circular muscle closes, the haemorrhoids are squeezed halfway in and halfway out. Patients with haemorrhoids hanging out of the anus find it necessary to push them back into the canal after a bowel movement. Such haemorrhoids are also called prolapsed piles.

When subjected to the pushing force of the stool, the thinned membrane over the haemorrhoids is easily torn. Blood leaks out of the veins and they are then said to be bleeding haemorrhoids. With rare exceptions, bleeding occurs only with bowel motions. Usually the bleeding is not great and it stops within a few minutes after the bowel action.

The circulation of blood in these tortuous haemorrhoidal veins becomes stagnant and the blood in them is subject to clotting.

Pain comes in attacks that last ordinarily no longer than a few days. After this there is a quiet and comfortable spell that may last for months before there is another attack. The painful attacks may arise from swelling that is occasioned by prolonged squeezing of prolapsed haemorrhoids that have not been pushed back in after a bowel movement.

Types of haemorrhoids Haemorrhoids are classified as internal or external, or as combined internal and external. These terms have to do with the location of the bulkier portion of the haemorrhoidal mass of veins in relation to the circular muscle that is called the rectal sphincter. Those veins that are situated well up inside the canal and further in than the sphincter muscle are internal haemorrhoids. External haemorrhoids are in the skin around the opening and are outside the sphincter muscle. Although haemorrhoids may be solely external or solely internal, in most instances the stretched veins run the whole length of the canal, including the entrance and the exit. These are referred to as combined internal-external haemorrhoids.

Haemorrhoids will not become cancerous nor will they cause cancer. However, since bleeding from the rectum is one of the signs of rectal cancer, bleeding that supposedly comes from haemorrhoids must be investigated to make certain that the haemorrhoids are the sole cause of the bleeding. This does not make the patient safe for the rest of his life. If bleeding continues, it must be checked frequently, as often as every six months, for if a cancer does develop, it may hide behind the bleeding that is assumed to be due to the piles.

Rectal examinations are made with a finger and an instrument called a proctoscope. This is a tube open at one end and equipped at the other end with an electric light and a window through which the surgeon can see the interior of the rectum. The instrument, handled gently and well lubricated, can be inserted into the rectum with no pain.

Large haemorrhoids that are giving trouble from bleeding or pain should be removed. This rarely calls for emergency action. Many patients are relieved by stretching the anus under anaesthesia.

Removal of haemorrhoids is called haemorrhoidectomy. It is performed in hospital and most often under a general anaesthetic. From three to six days hospitalization will be sufficient in most cases. In a haemorrhoid operation, the varicose veins are removed. They are cut away along with the stretched membrane over them. For each haemorrhoidal cluster, a double incision in the form of an ellipse is made the full length of the rectal canal to include both the internal and the external portions of each haemorrhoid. There may be as many as four incisions along the length of the canal.

A clotted (thrombosed) haemorrhoid may be relieved by a small incision through which the clot is removed. This is accomplished with the help of a local anaesthetic, and hospitalization is not required. Most often an incision is not necessary because the clot will dissolve on its own and the haemorrhoid will shrink.

Patients are generally apprehensive about the first bowel movement after a rectal operation, but they are often surprised when the actual experience proves far less uncomfortable than anticipated. As a general rule, the bowels will move on the third or fourth postoperative day with the assistance of mineral oil or some other soft and lubricating laxative that is started on the first or second day after operation. Sitz baths (sitting in warm water) are used two or three times daily and they are initiated again on about the second postoperative day. If a bowel action is not forthcoming by the fourth day, 50 to 100 ml of warm oil are introduced into the rectum as an oil enema. This usually brings on a reasonably comfortable bowel movement for the patient.

Recurrence A patient who has had a haemorrhoidectomy may wonder whether haemorrhoids will recur. They probably will not, but it is possible for other rectal veins to enlarge even after the main veins have been removed surgically.

The rectal sphincter muscle is not cut to any extent in a haemorrhoid operation. Therefore there is usually no danger that the muscle will be injured to the extent that it will not be tight enough. On the other hand, if the surgery has been very extensive because of the extremely large size of the haemorrhoids, it is possible for scar tissue to form in the canal and thus stiffen the muscle so that it does not stretch for a bowel movement as easily as it did before. This unusual complication is ordinarily overcome without much difficulty by stretching the opening with a lubricated dilator, something the patient can easily do himself.

Plastic surgery

Plastic surgery is concerned with remodelling and restoring. It revises parts of the body that have been malformed in the growing process before birth or it restores parts that have been deformed or destroyed by injury and disease. The name does not imply that synthetic plastic materials are used.

Although plastic methods and principles govern more than half the things surgeons do, the name plastic surgery is used ordinarily for operations on areas that are visible. A cleft lip in a newborn baby can be closed by plastic surgery. A limb crippled by rigid and constricting scars may be restored to full function. Disfiguring and incapacitating injuries to structures of the face are moved back into proper alignment for healing.

A severe burn may destroy all of the skin in and about an armpit, leaving a thick mass of scar tissue that fuses the arm to the chest and prevents any motion in the shoulder. Arm motion is restored by removing the scar to allow the arm to swing out freely and up over the head. In this extended position the large denuded area of the chest and underarm is covered with a skin graft.

Skin grafts It is the plasticity, or pliability, of skin and muscles that allows the surgeon to mould and reshape the skin coverings of the eyes, nose, and lips when structures and skin have been torn away by injuries. For extensively damaged areas that cannot be covered by shifting and realigning the torn flaps, skin must be moved from another area of the patient's body to the injured area. There is no substitute for skin. Methods for storing skin in banks, as in blood banks, have not been generally satisfactory. Transfer of skin from one person to another for permanent replacement is very seldom satisfactory, therefore the surgeon must rearrange the patient's own skin.

Healthy skin can be detached, lifted out, and fitted into a raw area. This is called free grafting. The graft is completely free from its attachment and derives its nourishment from the raw surface on which it is laid. There is no nourishment from the edges. The outer layers of skin can thrive on this kind of nourishment, absorbed from the raw surface, but the deeper skin layers do not do so well.

The outer layers therefore are split away from the deep layers with an electrically driven sharp blade. This is a split graft and is in contrast to the full thickness graft described above. The depth of the split graft varies but it averages about 0·025 cm ($\frac{1}{100}$ in). The sheet of outer skin is transplanted and a new outer skin will sprout up quickly from the deep layers which are still in place and intact. Thus, the outer layers are skimmed off in a solid sheet about the depth of a bad graze, and the deeper layers grow a new cover in about the time it takes that graze to heal.

A whole sheet of split skin, removed by the grafting instrument, can be laid in the denuded area as a single sheet shaped to size, or it can be cut into small pieces the size of a postage stamp. The latter are called stamp grafts. The instrument can cut sheets 7.5 cm (three in) wide and as long as fifteen to twenty cm (six to eight in). Stamp grafts are advantageous for the larger raw areas of burns, because they can be spaced at one cm ($\frac{1}{2}$ in) intervals. The edges of the grafts, still taking nourishment from the undersurface, will grow out to meet each other.

Small full thickness pieces of skin can be free grafted, but larger sizes must be attached by a pedicle through which intact blood vessels can bring nourishment to the raised flap of skin. This is known as pedicle grafting.

For pedicle grafts the skin is elevated as a broad flap joined to the body by a pedicle. If the flap can be raised in such a fashion that its pedicle is adjacent to the area to be covered, it can be fitted by rotating its pedicle. Neither the flap nor the pedicle should be stretched; extreme twisting or tension will choke the blood supply in the pedicle.

If the distance between the donor site and the bare area is too great for a rotating pedicle, a longer skin flap is raised and fashioned into a tube, but attached at both ends by pedicles. After a rest period of several weeks during which the blood vessels in the pedicles grow larger, the pedicle farthest from the bare area is cut across. The tube is then rotated to bring the cut pedicle to the site for grafting.

Sculpturing and reshaping the face and neck require intricate realignments of the bones that frame the face and jaws. This phase is combined with muscle transplants and skin grafts. Delicate facial bones, shattered in road accidents, or removed with tumours, can be reconstructed with wires and splints that are made from synthetic materials. Flaps of muscle are used in the reconstruction of vacant spaces left by destroyed or removed bone.

Eye surgery

Cataract operations In a cataract operation the lens of the eye is removed because it has become hardened and opaque to the extent that light rays cannot pass through. Although there are many varieties of cataract, occurring at all ages, the most frequent form is seen in persons over 50 years of age, usually in both eyes, with one cataract forming more rapidly than the other.

Formerly, surgery was delayed until the cataract ripened. This meant that the hardening process had finally involved the entire lens and loosened it from its capsule. In this condition the lens could be separated from its capsule without leaving bits of cataract that would later become opaque and again block the light rays. The ripening process might come about in a few months or it might take years.

It is current practice to remove the lens as soon as useful vision has deteriorated to the point that the patient cannot carry on with his usual occupation. Modern techniques ensure that all the lens substance can be removed. Even with this trend towards earlier operation, extraction of the lens from the first eye is delayed as long as there is still good vision in the better eye. The reason for this is that there would be a refracting difference between the operated eye, now without a lens, and the unoperated eye, so long as this eye retained good vision. The good eye, being the stronger of the two, would dominate and take over all of the seeing.

There is no emergency about the usual cataract operation. The cataract is a mechanical impediment and not a disease that will spread to other parts.

Cataract operations are performed under local anaesthesia. A half circle incision is made in the white portion of the eye above the clear cornea. The upper half of the cornea and the upper half of the coloured rim around the pupil, the iris, are cut open at their

Chapter 23 **Your operation**

edges. This gives access to the lens which is drawn out by a small cup-shaped instrument that holds onto the lens by a vacuum suction. The incision is then closed.

Detached retina The retina is normally held against the blood vessel layer behind it in the wall of the eyeball by pressure within the eyeball fluid. The retina becomes detached when a crack in the retina allows eyeball fluid to seep between the layers. With no contact between the layers there is no vision.

Eight of every ten patients who are treated for detachment are helped, although frequently the retina may be jarred loose again and require further treatment.

Anaesthesia for surgery is local, by surface application and by injection of an anaesthetic solution behind the eyeball. A hollow needle is inserted into the eye to drain out the fluid between the retina and choroid layers. Then the contact is sealed with a freezing rod (cryoprobe), a laser beam, or an electric needle.

Another successful surgical method for this condition buckles the outer layer of the eyeball in the detached area and thus pushes the choroid blood vessel layer against the retina. The buckling suture remains in the outer coat of the eyeball permanently.

Corneal scars If the cornea is scarred in its central portion from a scratch or infection, light rays will be blocked from the lens, like putting a finger in front of the lens of a camera. The scarred portion can be removed and replaced with the cornea of a donor eye. If the scar does not extend the entire depth of the cornea, the outer layers can be removed down to clear cornea and replaced by a corneal graft of the same thickness. It is also possible to replace the full thickness of the cornea if the scar is this deep. The defective cornea is bored out and removed as a plug in a single piece. A plug of the full thickness of cornea is bored out of a donor eye with the same instrument. The graft cornea of the same size and shape is fitted exactly into the hole and is sutured in place.

It is also possible to obtain vision in the eye without removing the scarred cornea. This is done by removing a portion of the iris at the edge of the pupil. The iris is opened at its lower inner edge. The effectiveness of this technique can be estimated before operation by paralysing the iris with a drug. This allows the pupil to open up widely behind the scar to let in the image outside the edge of the scar.

Eye muscle operations Disturbances of the coordinated action of the eyeball muscles are corrected by operations that change the position and the length of the muscles. Usually this will amount to relocating or altering one or two muscles of one eye or perhaps both eyes, depending upon the nature of the trouble. To be successful these operations must be done at an early age.

Each eye has six muscles. For each coordinated movement of the eyes, several muscles of each eye pull at the same time, but each muscle has its particular field to cover.

The eyeball is a globe seated in a bony socket. The muscles are all attached at the back of the bony socket and reach around the globe to be inserted in front about one cm ($\frac{3}{8}$ in) from the top, bottom, and sides of the cornea. Four of these muscles (recti) run a straight course around the globe. Two of them come in at an angle (obliques). The muscles of the two eyes are controlled by the coordination centre in the brain so that the proper muscles for the left and right eyes move at the same time.

After a determination has been made of the basic one or two directions that are out of balance, the surgeon can make a correction by altering one or two muscles concerned in each eye. Frequently only one eye is out of balance.

One can visualize the six eye muscles in terms of tautness as though they were rubber bands reaching around from a central point at the back of the socket to separate points on the front of the eyeball. A weak muscle is compared to a loose rubber band, attached too far back on the ball and therefore not taut enough. A muscle pulling too strongly is like a rubber band attached too far forward and therefore too taut. Either situation prevents good teamwork.

At operation, a strong overacting muscle is detached from its position on the front of the eyeball and is reattached some millimetres farther back. This is called recession of a muscle. A weak or under-stretched muscle is advanced by relocating its attachment farther forward. Sometimes the correction in tautness is made by cutting out a short piece of the muscle and then sewing the two cut ends together. This is a resection. Another method shortens a muscle by sewing a pleat into its length.

Glaucoma Glaucoma is a condition of increased pressure within the eyeball. Although it is possible to control this pressure by drugs that open up the natural drainage channels from the eyeball, drugs may not work. The situation then demands surgical drainage. If the pressure is increasing rapidly and cannot be brought under control by drugs, an emergency operation is necessary.

Operations for control of glaucoma are many and varied. The simplest is called iridectomy. It is performed if there is rapid and severe blockage of the drainage channels. A piece of the iris is cut loose to deepen the drainage channels by correcting the forward ballooning and swelling of the iris.

Sometimes, in long-standing cases where there is damage to the outflow channels, a filtering operation is used. This form of operation is chosen when the field of vision has been reduced by damage to the optic nerve and when medicines have failed. The object is to promote drainage through the tough outer coat of the eye by drilling a small hole through it. This is called sclerectomy. Aqueous humor, draining through the hole into the subconjunctival space, is absorbed into the blood vessels as the pressure builds up. The drill hole is covered by the conjunctiva, which is the membranous veil that lines the eyelids and covers the white sclera.

Sometimes a piece of iris is cut in a fashion that will allow it to be drawn into the sclerectomy hole, where it functions as a wick. The wick keeps the hole from scarring and thus helps keep the hole open. This is iridenclesis. The tags of iris, drawn through the hole, are covered by conjunctiva to seal over any communication with the outside.

Organ transplantation

The chances of having an organ transplantation are remote, simply because the total number of such operations is quite limited. Transplants of less than a whole organ are commonplace – skin grafts, bone grafts, corneal transplants. But surgical operations for transfer of entire organs are less common.

First of all, the supply of transplantable organs runs far behind the number of patients who need them because removal of healthy organs from willing donors is risky.

As for organs from the dead body, consent by grieving relatives for their removal is not easily obtained within the short time allowable – an hour. Nor are proper facilities generally available on short notice for the speedy and surgically satisfactory removal of organs from any deceased persons.

Lastly, rejection of a transplanted organ by the sick patient's body (the recipient) presents a difficult and, for the most part, an unsolved problem.

The ethical aspects of transplantation are complicated and still under debate.

Kidneys The most frequently performed transplantations are kidneys. Thousands of these operations have been performed with a better than even chance for success. Most successful are kidney transplants between identical twins where there is practically no chance of rejection. Then, in order, are brother and sister and parent to child. Last in line are kidneys from deceased persons.

Two thousand young adults and children in Britain die each year from kidney diseases. Half of these victims have healthy organs except for their kidneys. Thus, one thousand patients annually become candidates for kidney transplantation. The supply of new kidneys, either from living donors or from deceased persons, is a problem.

There is no emergency about kidney transplantation as far as the patient with kidney disease is concerned. Such patients with kidney failure can be maintained – and will be able to work – indefinitely by kidney dialysis (kidney machine) with treatments two or three times weekly. Arrangements for transplanting a living kidney can be arranged for a time that is generally suitable to the patient, the donor, and the surgical team. By contrast, transplantation of a deceased person's kidney must be arranged for quickly – within an hour. Storage of organs for transplantation at a later date has not been satisfactory.

The operation A kidney transplantation operation moves along swiftly once everything needed for surgery has been made ready. Three connections are necessary – a single artery for the entrance of blood into and through a kidney's screening and filtering system, a matching vein to return filtered blood to the circulation, and finally, the kidney tube (ureter) that drains the solution of filtered wastes (urine) to the urinary bladder for discharge from the body through the urethra.

The new kidney does not have to occupy one of the natural kidney positions in the small of the back on each side of the spine. The transplant is placed in the lowermost part of the abdominal cavity (the pelvis) to the right of the urinary bladder. Usually the donor's left kidney is taken for the transplant because the left kidney is more accessible surgically. The open end of the new kidney's intake artery is joined to an opening made in the side of the large artery that leads to the recipient's right thigh and leg (iliac) artery. The kidney's vein is attached to the main vein returning from the thigh (iliac vein). The ureter (exit tube from the new kidney) is joined to an opening made in the right side of the recipient's bladder. All of these connections are made by suturing with fine silk thread.

Urine passes from the newly transplanted kidney

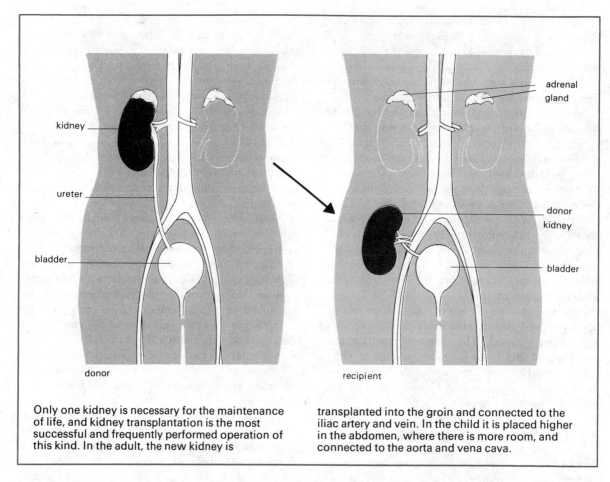

kidney

ureter

bladder

donor

adrenal
gland

donor
kidney

bladder

recipient

Only one kidney is necessary for the maintenance of life, and kidney transplantation is the most successful and frequently performed operation of this kind. In the adult, the new kidney is transplanted into the groin and connected to the iliac artery and vein. In the child it is placed higher in the abdomen, where there is more room, and connected to the aorta and vena cava.

within ten to fifteen minutes after the artery and vein connections have been completed, even before the kidney has been joined to the bladder.

The sick patient's diseased kidneys are removed a week or more before the transplantation. Elimination of waste from the blood is accomplished by dialysis on a kidney machine until the time of the transplantation operation. The dialysis machine can also be used to assist the new kidney if necessary. The recipient needs only one kidney.

Heart transplantation is reserved for patients who are beyond all hope of treatment with medicines. Unfortunately, in such patients, other organs have usually deteriorated because of the heart's failure to maintain an adequate circulation of blood through them. This is especially true of the lungs. Thus, of the 150 persons (up to 1971) who had received transplanted hearts, only a third had lived for more than six months, and many only for a few days. A few of these had survived for a full year. The Cape Town dentist, Doctor Blaiberg, first to receive a heart transplant,

lived 594 days. Rejection is the prime cause for failure.

It is difficult to estimate the number of persons who could benefit from heart transplantation.

Everything must be in readiness for a heart transplantation because the operation is performed on an emergency basis immediately after the death of the donor – a young person who has died as the result of injury or from a brain tumour and, hence, has generally healthy organs.

Almost all of the patient's diseased heart is removed. The back walls of the patient's right and left intake chambers (the atria) are left in place because the six veins that drain into the heart open through the walls of these chambers. Thus, only two sutured connections are made – the two chamber walls – to accommodate six vein connections. There remain only two more blood vessel unions, both arterial, one with the pulmonary artery to the lungs and the other with the aorta which is the main trunk line for circulation to the body in general.

A transplanted heart may start beating on its own

or an electric shock may be necessary to stimulate its muscle. The sewing time on the heart itself – two atria and two arteries – may be less than thirty minutes. A heart-lung machine is used to maintain a supply of oxygen and blood circulation, the same as in open heart surgery.

The problems beginning immediately after surgery are wound healing and control of infection, both of which are natural functions of the body that are weakened by the medications used to stave off rejection.

Liver   More than one hundred livers have been transplanted, but here again rejection has been a major stumbling block. Few of the recipients of new livers have lived for more than a year.

Among the possible candidates for liver transplantation are infants with a malformed or absent bile drainage system, children and young persons whose livers have been ravaged by infection, cirrhosis (not alcoholic), abscesses, cysts, or liver tumours called hepatomas. The liver is responsible for numerous functions.

Liver transplants are performed on an emergency basis – within minutes after a deceased accident victim's liver becomes available, because a removed liver deteriorates rapidly. As a part of the emergency procedure the recipient's diseased liver is removed and the new one connected almost simultaneously, for there are no machines to maintain a patient deprived of his liver.

Liver connections are complex, with oxygenated arterial blood and venous blood from the intestines flowing to the liver, and with venous blood flowing out of the liver to the vena cava – only 7.5 cm (three in) from the right heart intake chamber. Bile flowing out of the transplanted liver is routed to the intestine, either directly by way of the main (common) bile duct or roundabout through the gallbladder.

Other organs   Spleens, responsible for several blood conversion functions, have been successfully transplanted into the lower part of the abdomen like kidneys – connected with the iliac blood vessels. The new spleens supply substances that clot blood for haemophiliacs or supply leukaemia victims with antibodies that reduce the production of white blood corpuscles. The pancreas has been transplanted to overcome diabetes. Lungs have been transferred on more than twenty occasions with at least one patient surviving more than a full year. Most major organs, with the exception of the brain, have been transplanted with at least one long-term survivor.

Rejection remains a major problem. The capability of rejecting a foreign substance is a characteristic of all living tissues and organisms. Although this capability is a defence against bacteria and viruses and foreign substances such as steel, glass, splinters, or dirt and gravel, it is also the defence mechanism that makes successful transplants next to impossible. The major defenders are the white blood corpuscles and chemical substances called antibodies. Various methods such as radiation with X-rays and injections of cortisone-like substances and anti-white blood corpuscle serum have been used to hold these defence mechanisms in check.

Another approach has been to match tissues and cells in the fashion of blood typing and matching. In this manner, certain groups of donors of organs, whether living or deceased, are found to have compatibility with similar groups of recipients.

Anaesthesia

The thought of having to take an anaesthetic worries many people.

Before the days of ether, patients for surgery were merely stupefied with alcohol. Even with the innovation of ether the idea was to render a patient unconscious as quickly as possible and then rush through the operation with all possible speed. The choices besides ether were chloroform or nitrous oxide (laughing gas). The essence of surgery was speed because this kept the anaesthetic time to a minimum and reduced the likelihood of poisoning the brain, liver, and kidneys.

Modern anaesthesia is a complex science that employs a number of drugs, with each serving one or more purposes. Today the term anaesthesia includes four separate components, and going to sleep, which pertains to the patient's mental state, is only one of them. The other three components have to do with pain sensation, muscle relaxation, and paralysis of the reflexes.

Herein lies the great change in anaesthesia, the use of several different drugs at the same time. Each drug is used in the amount necessary to control one of the components of an overall anaesthetic mixture.

Unconsciousness is held in a safe range by using one drug for control of the mental state and separate drugs for control of the other components. Thiopentone given into the arm produces sleep quickly and naturally. However, in its safe range this drug will not obliterate pain sensation nor will it paralyse the muscles into the state of relaxation required for many operations. Thiopentone may even stimulate reflexes rather than depress them, and this could create difficulties. This drug therefore is used only in amounts that will block out consciousness, and at that stage other drugs are used to bring about a complete anaesthetic balance.

Another type of drug is succinylcholine, which does not produce unconsciousness but is highly effective for paralysing the muscles temporarily. This drug encourages the larynx muscles to open widely so that a breathing tube can be slipped easily into the windpipe of the patient.

A variety of inhalation or gas anaesthetics can be used to block pain sensation, and also to produce unconsciousness, though more slowly than thiopentone. They are used to block pain sensation after thiopentone has brought on unconsciousness. Spinal anaesthesia is excellent for handling pain, muscle relaxation, and the reflex components, but it has no effect on the mental state.

Anaesthesia includes more than just giving an anaesthetic. Blood transfusion, nourishing fluids, supportive and corrective drugs are all administered and controlled by the anaesthetist. Discriminating attention to all these factors makes it possible for most patients to be operated on with complete safety.

Anaesthesia may be classed as general, in which consciousness is lost; spinal, in which nerves are blocked at their exit from the spinal cord; regional, in which the nerves entering the field of operation are blocked; and local.

Spinal anaesthesia   A needle is inserted between the vertebrae to pierce the meninges below the level of the cord. The anaesthetic solution is then injected into the tube and mixes with the spinal fluid, which in turn bathes the nerve roots of the spinal cord. The level of anaesthesia depends on the amount of anaesthetic solution, the position of the patient, and the speed of injection. Anaesthesia lasts from one to several hours, again depending upon the type of drug.

The anaesthetist checks the patient's general condition during the operation by means of continuous monitoring devices. Among them are instruments for continuous electrocardiographic tracing of the heart action, stethoscopes that can be slipped down the gullet and into the stomach for continuous listening, thermometers that record continuously, and instruments that keep a constant record of the oxygen saturation in the blood.

The anaesthetist and surgeon consider every aspect of a particular patient's condition and medical history in choosing the most suitable approach.

Operations on children

Children accept operation and hospital routines on faith and trust which reflects the conversations and actions of their parents. Anxious parents should guard against any display of their worries.

A child's intellect does not demand any detail of anatomy and physiology. Most of the child's curiosity will be satisfied secondhand through the parents. The doctor's explanation to the child is best given in the parents' presence, thus giving the child a point of reference for further inquiries. The simplest explanations are best, relating chiefly to the need for correcting an abnormality. Timing is also very important. Discussions far in advance of the time for hospital admission may cause anxiety.

Children are naturally curious about the hospital environment and if this aspect of the operation is emphasized, an interesting experience can relegate pain and discomfort to the background. The Paediatric Department of a hospital is a children's world where all the attention is directed toward them: eating in bed, riding in wheelchairs, wearing pyjamas all day.

Children can tolerate pain and discomfort even better than adults, so long as there is affection and kindness, but they have a hard time bringing themselves to face up to it. More so than adults, they are procrastinators when it comes to pain. They will try to persuade anybody that anything uncomfortable would be less so if it were put off until just a little later. Their natural optimism leads them to believe that if something unpleasant is postponed, things will take care of themselves in the vague future. After an unpleasant experience has passed, such as a blood test or removal of adhesive plaster, they appreciate the gentle firmness that got things done right away and quickly.

Infants and children tolerate surgery and anaesthesia exceedingly well in comparison with adults. They require special attention with respect to fluid replacement for they may become dehydrated and over-hydrated quickly. Their air passages are narrow in comparison with those of adults and their cough reflexes are relatively weak. Children are sensitive to infections but they also respond readily to antibiotics.

Age is not a deterrent to surgery. Even premature infants, weighing only as little as two kg, stand up very well under extensive surgical procedures that must be done immediately if they are to survive. A tiny infant's heart is remarkably stout.

Chapter 24
X-rays and you

Revised by L. S. Carstairs, MB FRCR

This chapter will try to describe the diagnostic procedures undertaken by radiologists and the treatment procedures carried out by radiotherapists. First, it is necessary to explain what is meant by radiology and radiotherapy, and how they can help.

Radiology and radiotherapy

These are branches of medical practice using forms of radiant energy to diagnose or treat disease. Diagnosis and treatment can be performed by one doctor, but with the increasing complexity of diagnostic and treatment procedures, it is becoming less common for a doctor to undertake both types of work. In Britain the division is now virtually complete. A doctor who uses X-rays and other forms of radiant energy to diagnose disease is known as a diagnostic radiologist, or radiologist for short. Doctors who treat patients with X-rays or other forms of radiant energy are called radiotherapists.

Training in diagnostic radiology and radiotherapy usually commences not less than three years after the doctor has qualified and many will already have obtained specialist qualifications in medicine or surgery. Control of entry into diagnostic radiology and radiotherapy, in Britain, is exercised by the Royal College of Radiologists. The course leading to specialist qualification lasts three to four years and consists of practical training and lectures in the many subjects involved. It would be unusual, in Britain, for a radiologist or radiotherapist to achieve a position of full clinical responsibility, either in a National Health Service hospital or in independent practice, in less than fifteen years after having commenced studies as a medical student.

Radiation

Radio waves, visible light, heat waves, X-rays, and gamma rays are all radiations. They are packets of energy moving at the same speed (the speed of light) but distinguished one from the other by their wavelength and frequency. The power, that is the energy, needed to produce short wavelength radiation is greater than that for longer wavelengths. This power is usually derived from electrical apparatus and described in terms of its voltage. We are all acquainted with visible light. X-rays, which are not visible, have the power to penetrate objects and also to darken a photographic plate.

Although man has been aware of the fundamental properties of some forms of radiation for several centuries, the discovery that one type of ray could pass through objects which normally would not transmit light, was made in 1895, by Wilhelm Conrad Roentgen. The apparatus that he used consisted of a glass vacuum tube into which had been placed the terminals of an electrical circuit, working at high voltage. The stream of electrons flowing from the negative terminal hit the positive terminal and in so doing altered some of its atoms. The electrons in these atoms became more highly charged and then, in returning to their original state, gave off energy. This was the high energy radiation which became known as X-rays or Roentgen rays.

Another important discovery was made in 1899 when Pierre and Marie Curie isolated the element radium, a substance whose atoms decay or break down, giving off both radiant energy and particulate radiation.

How does all this affect the patient? Let us first look at the work of the diagnostic radiologist.

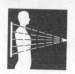

A tube of the type used by
Wilhelm Roentgen who
discovered X-rays in 1895 when
experimenting on the passage
of electric currents through
tubes containing rarefied gases.

A tube developed in 1911, with
a device to regulate gas
pressure.

X-ray tube in an oil-filled
protective casing.

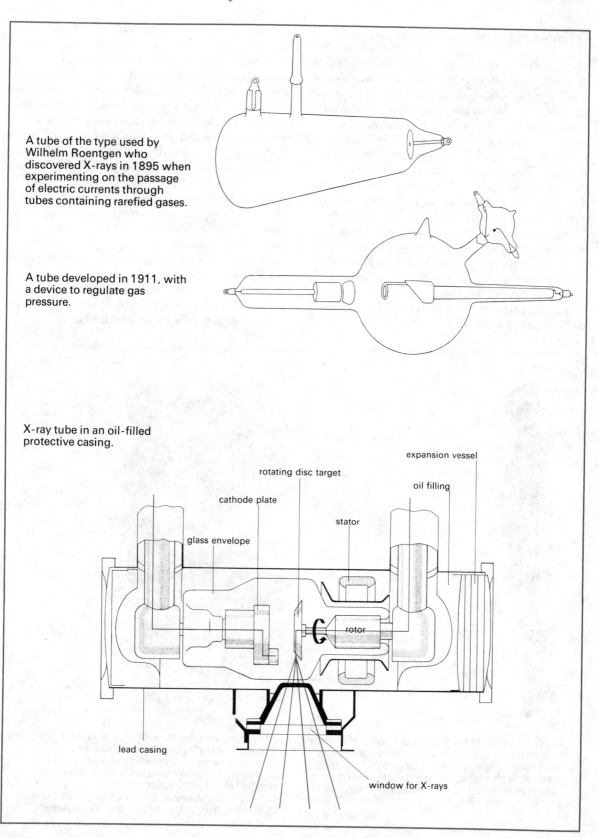

Diagnostic radiology

The key to treatment of an illness is accurate diagnosis. Many illnesses, of course, are diagnosed by relatively simple means while others require extensive laboratory investigation or even the removal of a small portion of tissue (a biopsy) for examination by a specialist in tissue abnormalities (a histopathologist). Radiology can help by showing whether the structure and function of an organ is normal or not.

Radiology is a part of the training of all doctors so that many X-ray examinations are routine, and the doctor refers the patient to the radiologist for a specific examination. This may be relatively simple, as in the case of a wrist injury, or it may be much more complex, as for example in the examination of the urinary tract or the digestive tract. Frequently, discussions occur between the doctor and the radiologist, regarding the best type of examination for the patient's problem.

Nearly every organ in the body can be explored by X-rays. To some extent, therefore, the range of radiological investigation which may need to be undertaken during a particular illness is very large. One function of the consultation between the doctor and the radiologist is to ensure that the minimum number of examinations is performed. The examinations selected should, therefore, directly contribute to the diagnosis of the illness. Many specialists are themselves expert at the interpretation of X-ray films in their own field. The final responsibility for the result of the X-ray examination is, however, that of the radiologist. He may even be regarded, in the courts, as being responsible for errors made in the preparation of the film. For this reason, he maintains close control of the work undertaken, on his behalf, in the X-ray Department.

Most major hospitals provide a 24 hour, seven day a week X-ray service, so that if the patient is admitted to the hospital as an emergency, the basic X-ray

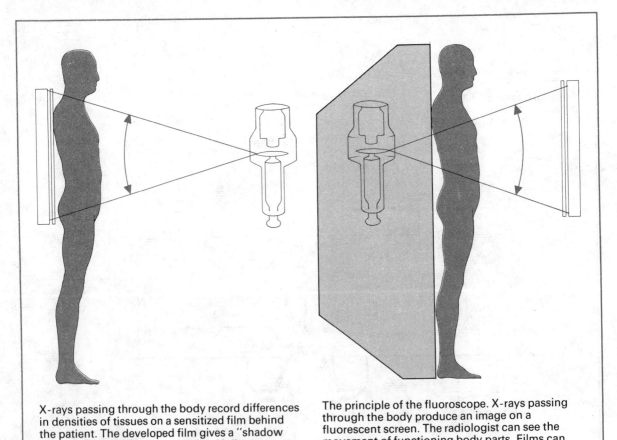

X-rays passing through the body record differences in densities of tissues on a sensitized film behind the patient. The developed film gives a "shadow picture", a photographic negative. Hollow organs can be outlined by filling them with a radiopaque material, as in a barium meal.

The principle of the fluoroscope. X-rays passing through the body produce an image on a fluorescent screen. The radiologist can see the movement of functioning body parts. Films can also be taken for later study. Nowadays, to diminish the dosage of X-rays to the patient, the image is often transferred to a television screen.

investigation can usually be undertaken very quickly. During the night or evening, there may be some delay because the radiographer may need to be called in to the hospital or he or she may be working elsewhere on other emergency examinations, for example in the operating theatres, the intensive therapy unit, or in the wards.

Appointments An appointment may be made for a patient to have an X-ray investigation following consultation with the family doctor or with a specialist in hospital. Different types of X-ray examination require differing forms of preparation and, of course, the examinations themselves take a very variable length of time. The examination of the chest may be over in five minutes but if the digestive tract is being examined the patient may have to attend the hospital for most of one day followed by short appointments on the second and possibly the third day. The appointments office or the radio-

logist's secretary will give out an appointments slip, together with a note of the preparation needed before the examination. When, for example, the stomach is being examined, it is important that the examination should commence with the stomach empty. Various medicines may have to be taken on the day before the examination, and other medicines or materials may need to be given by the radiologist before or during the examination.

It is usually necessary for the patient to remove clothing from the area to be examined because some clothing is partially opaque to X-rays and this may cause difficulties in interpreting the film. Similarly, when the skull is being X-rayed, it is necessary to remove hairpins, earrings, and dentures.

When the patient goes into the X-ray room, he will meet the radiographer who takes the X-ray film. The radiographer is a highly skilled paramedical auxiliary who has had a long training in radiography and all its allied subjects. The quality of the films obtained and

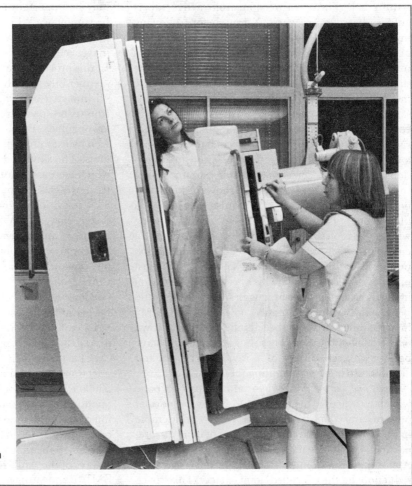

An X-ray table. Here the image-receiving film is beneath the patient, and the X-ray tube above him. Tables usually tilt at any angle from the horizontal to the vertical. The patient may lie on the table or stand in front of it. In this way the patient can be positioned precisely to obtain the desired X-ray.

Chapter 24 **X-rays and you**

the whole functioning of an X-ray service in hospital largely depend on the radiographers and the superintendent radiographer who organizes their work.

The type of apparatus used varies, depending on the examination to be performed. In some the patient is in the sitting position, in others the patient is on a flat table or on a table which can be tilted. If the examination involves the needling of an artery or the use of a general anaesthetic, the procedure will be discussed and the arrangements made will be similar to those for a surgical operation. The patient may have to be admitted to the hospital for an overnight stay or a short stay of a few days.

Let us now look at some of the diagnostic examinations in more detail.

Diagnostic examinations

Chest Almost everyone will have a chest X-ray at some time. Many employers now require a normal chest X-ray before engagement and many countries require a certificate of freedom from active tuberculosis, based on a chest X-ray, before allowing immigration. The X-ray taken shows the shadows of abnormal tissues in the lungs superimposed on the normal shadows of the lung vessels. It also shows the shape and size of the heart. Although it is one of the most frequently performed X-ray examinations, satisfactory interpretation of the film requires considerable experience. Not infrequently further radiography of the chest may be needed to ensure that a feature noted is of no significance. These investigations may include screening. In this examination, a small quantity of X-rays is used to show the lungs and heart on a fluorescent screen (also known as a fluoroscope). The effect is to show the parts moving with respiration and the beating of the heart, like a cine film rather than a snapshot. The illumination produced by the X-rays is faint and the radiologist may have to accommodate his eyes to this low level of light by wearing special goggles for ten minutes beforehand. More commonly, nowadays, the X-ray image is intensified by a special tube and then thrown onto a television screen. These image intensifiers have become an essential part of X-ray Departments and are now also in use in operating theatres.

Bones and joints An X-ray examination of a bone will show whether or not it conforms to the normal pattern and density and this is of considerable importance in diagnosing some forms of bone disease, particularly bone infections and bone tumours. Abnormalities in joints are shown on the X-ray by a reduction in the so-called joint space. This space represents the width of the cartilages which form the rubbing surface in a joint. When the cartilage begins to wear out, it becomes narrower and changes also occur in the bone beneath the cartilage and at the sides of the joint. The type and distribution of the joint changes and the nature of the alteration in the structure of the bone tend to fall into distinct categories which are related to the type of joint disease. It is often possible, therefore, to distinguish one type of joint disease from another at an early stage. In some joints, particularly the knee, it is helpful to inject a small amount of opaque fluid before undertaking X-ray studies of the cartilages. This is called arthrography.

Spine Inevitably, advancing age causes the spine (and other bones) to degenerate in the same way as other organs and tissues. These ageing changes can give rise to symptoms, and a decrease in the elasticity and thickness of the disc substance between the bodies of the vertebrae may cause loss of height. Apart from these changes, there are other conditions which may be important to discover so that treatment can be commenced. Lesions in the neck and in the lower part of the spine resulting in compression of nerves may need special investigations called myelograms. In this procedure, a liquid which is opaque to X-rays – either oily (nonabsorbable) or watery (absorbable) – is injected by the radiologist into the spinal canal (the tissue space around the nerve structures in the lower spine). Deformation of this space can then be seen by examining its dimensions and shape on X-ray films. The slipped disc is a portion of disc substance which has passed out through a rupture of the fibrous tissue which surrounds it so that it compresses a nerve. This condition is now commonly examined using the watery material. When the patient's symptoms could be due to an abnormality anywhere in the middle or upper part of the spine it is usually necessary to use the oily opaque liquid.

Skull and brain The examination of the bony portions of the skull can be undertaken by plain radiography in just the same way as an X-ray of a wrist or ankle. Some specialized examinations may need to be carried out on the mastoid areas behind the ears, particularly in the assessment of chronic mastoid infections and in finding out the causes of deafness. The nasal sinuses, which normally have a thin lining membrane and contain air, may be shown to be infected by the presence of a thick lining membrane or fluid. The brain, apart from one small speck of calcium in the pineal gland, is not visible on ordinary X-rays of the skull. It may be examined by using the EMI Scanner (page 548). This will provide a cross

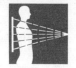

section of the soft tissue structures within the brain. The examination subjects the patient to no more radiation than is required by ordinary skull X-rays and no operative procedure is needed. Air can be introduced into the spaces within the brain (the ventricles). This can be done in the operating theatre by direct puncture through a burr-hole made in the skull or in the X-ray Department by injecting air into the lower part of the spine while the patient is sitting in the erect position. The air bubbles upward through the spinal fluid and enters a small space in the midline from which it is then distributed into the ventricles. In this way, some alterations in the shape and thickness of brain substance can be seen. Water-soluble opaque material may also be injected directly into the arteries supplying the brain (carotid arteriography). This examination is performed in the X-ray Department frequently with the patient under general anaesthesia. Alterations in the calibre and position of the vessels inside the brain may give essential information regarding the nature of a lesion or tumour in the brain substance and also, of course, show any abnormal formation of the blood vessels. An ultrasound examination may be used to assess the position of the midline of the brain.

The kidneys and urinary tract Stones in the kidney or bladder can often be seen on plain X-rays but although they may be visible, it is sometimes difficult to distinguish between them and other opacities such as calcified lymph glands. The way in which the kidneys function and also their shape can be shown by injecting a chemical containing iodine which the kidneys selectively pick out of the bloodstream and excrete. In this way, it may be possible to confirm that an opacity is due to a stone blocking one of the ureters (the tubes leading from the kidneys to the bladder) and the nature of a lesion in one or other kidney can often be accurately determined by this means (intravenous pyelograms, or IVP). The examination lasts for over an hour and, at the end, the bladder shape is seen and its ability to empty can be shown. In men who have enlargement of the prostate gland, this too can be seen and the extent to which emptying of the bladder is impaired can be assessed. Examination of the bladder by filling it through a catheter introduced through the urethra (the tube carrying the urine from the bladder to the exterior), is often an important test in female patients with repeated urinary tract infections. Special examinations can also be undertaken to show the pressure dynamics of the bladder and to exclude or confirm the presence of obstructions in the urethra.

Digestive tract This term includes the gullet (oesophagus), stomach, duodenum, the small bowel (jejunum and ileum), the appendix, and large bowel (colon and rectum). One of the commonest examinations undertaken by radiologists is the barium meal. A less common examination is the barium enema. In the barium meal, the patient is asked to drink a suspension of barium sulphate. This smooth flavoured suspension is not absorbable. It is opaque to X-rays so that the shape and functioning of the gullet, stomach, and duodenum can be seen and recorded. The recording may be on X-ray films, cine film, or videotape. It is by this means that tumours of the gullet and stomach, and ulcers of the gullet, stomach, and duodenum are most frequently shown. Another investigation which may be undertaken by either a radiologist or an endoscopist is optical examination of the upper digestive tract. An endoscope, or fibrescope, is a tube passed into the body, usually through one of its normal openings, to enable the operator to view what goes on inside. This examination is of great value in the management of sudden haemorrhage of the upper digestive tract. It is also valuable for the discovery of tumours in the stomach because small portions of the stomach wall (biopsies) can be taken through the flexible instrument for subsequent examination by the pathologist. The instrument may also be used to introduce an opaque fluid into the ducts of the pancreas to show whether it is affected by chronic inflammation or, in some cases, by a tumour.

The barium enema examination is performed after preparation of the colon. It is essential for the colon to be clear of faecal material and for this reason the patient is usually asked to take a laxative for one to three days before the examination and a colonic lavage is performed about two hours before the barium enema. The barium suspension is run into the colon through a catheter placed in the rectum. Air may also be used to enhance the quality of the films obtained. The purpose of the examination is to show the state of the lining membrane and to demonstrate or exclude the presence of small pouches (diverticula) which may be a site of infection or bleeding. Tumours of the colon and rectum may also be seen. An endoscopic examination of the rectum and the lowest portion of the colon (sigmoidoscopy) is often performed by the physician or surgeon who refers the patient for the barium enema, see next page.

Pregnancy With the increasing awareness of the radiation hazard to the developing fetus, the number of X-ray investigations performed during pregnancy has decreased. In general, X-rays of pregnant patients are not performed, unless unavoidable, before the third month. After this time, and with complete lead screening of the abdomen, a single film of the chest may be taken if there is a risk of tuberculous infection being present. X-rays of the abdomen are not now performed during pregnancy unless there is an extremely important reason for doing so. The obstetrician may need a radiological estimation of the age of the baby if, when he examines the abdomen, he feels that there is a discrepancy between what he finds and the mother's dates. This examination will usually be confined to a single film taken with the minimum of X-ray exposure. In the last stages of pregnancy, it may be necessary to assess the size of the pelvis and the position of the baby's head, and for this, a film is taken with the patient standing (standing lateral pelvimetry), preferably using an intensifying screen which will reduce the X-ray exposure by three quarters.

Children On general grounds, the X-rays taken of children are kept to a minimum. Some children's illnesses must be investigated by radiology and because of the need to keep radiation exposure down, it is essential that great care is taken during the procedure to obtain the best quality films compatible with this limitation.

In the infant, acute abdominal emergencies may require special X-rays and this can include a barium enema examination to exclude lesions in the colon and barium meal examinations to exclude abnormalities in the gullet or stomach. In very young male infants, the muscle of the valve between the stomach and the duodenum may become thickened (hypertrophic pyloric stenosis), producing severe vomiting. Most children who have vomiting do not have this condition and a barium meal is of value in excluding

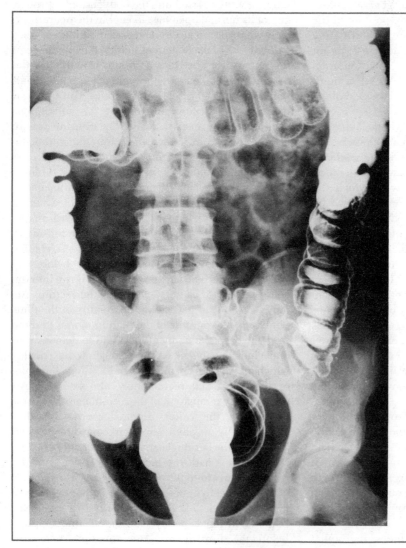

A normal barium enema.

it. In the condition known as intussusception, where one portion of the bowel telescopes into the adjacent portion, the diagnosis can be made on a barium enema examination.

Congenital heart disease presents a particular and highly specialized problem in radiological diagnosis. In such conditions, the heart specialist (cardiologist) and radiologist cooperate in the performance of examinations involving the injection of opaque material into the heart (angiocardiography), so that the size and shape of the heart chambers can be shown.

Gallbladder The liver produces bile and this passes through the bile ducts into the duodenum. The gallbladder is a small muscular bag which communicates with the main bile duct through a narrow (so-called cystic) duct. The gallbladder's function is to store some of the bile from the liver so that it is available in quantity when a meal is eaten. Eating stimulates the gallbladder to contract and discharge its bile into the bowel. The main bile duct and the duct from another important organ (the pancreas), enter the duodenum at the same point. Gallstones may form in the gallbladder. Some can be seen on an ordinary X-ray. Others are no more opaque to X-rays than ordinary tissues and therefore they are not visible. These so-called radiolucent gallstones may be shown if the bile within the gallbladder can be made opaque. This bile then surrounds the gallstones which show up as areas of decreased density. At the same time, the size, shape, and contour of the gallbladder can be shown as well as its response, or lack of response, to eating. The bile in the gallbladder is made opaque by giving the patient an iodine-containing chemical which after being absorbed from the bowel is concentrated by the liver and further concentrated by the gallbladder. If the gallbladder does not concentrate this material, then, provided the liver is known to be functioning normally, this indicates that there is either an obstruction in the cystic duct or that the gallbladder is diseased. Sometimes, it is necessary to examine the main bile duct either when the patient has had the gallbladder removed surgically or when the gallbladder does not concentrate the opaque medium taken by mouth (oral cholecystogram). An examination called an intravenous cholangiogram is then performed. Special material is injected into a vein and films (including tomograms – page 548) are taken to show the shape and size of the main bile duct and whether or not it contains stones. During operative removal of the gallbladder, many surgeons now use an X-ray examination in the theatre (operative cholangio-graphy) to ensure that there are no gallstones in the main bile duct.

Breasts An X-ray examination of the breast (mammography), using special apparatus to get films of very high definition and quality may be of great help in deciding whether or not a lump felt in the breast is due to a cyst, an area of inflammation, a nonmalignant tumour, or a malignant tumour.

Mammography can also be used, in conjunction with clinical examination, as a survey procedure in an attempt to pick up possibly important changes in the condition of the breasts before they either become felt as lumps or produce symptoms.

Infertility An examination of the shape of the uterine cavity and the state and freedom from obstruction of the fallopian tubes may be of value in the investigation of infertility. The investigation consists of the injection of an opaque fluid into the uterine cavity through the neck of the uterus (the cervical canal). The time of performance of the investigation is closely controlled in relation to the menstrual cycle.

Special examinations After the discovery of X-rays, periodically new discoveries increased the range and scope of the examinations. First there was the use of opaque substances in the bowel (bismuth followed by barium) and then came the discovery of the iodine-containing materials which could be injected to show the kidneys or given by mouth to show the gallbladder. The use of air in the central nervous system either by the spinal canal (air encephalography) or by direct puncture (ventriculography) was soon followed by carotid arteriography – the injection of a radiopaque liquid into the arterial system of the brain. This was the beginning of an enormous advance in the ability of radiology to investigate and throw light on disease. The new methods were rapidly applied to the investigation of the main arterial vessel in the body, the aorta, and to the main arteries of the limbs. A further development of the technique whereby a catheter could be introduced into an artery resulted in selective arterial catheterization with demonstration of the small arteries supplying single organs. These techniques have now become standard throughout the world. In association with these developments, X-ray study of the heart's action and structure has advanced considerably.

Initially, this examination was confined to the four chambers of the heart. Great advances in the techniques of intracardiac surgery have meant that very detailed examinations of the arteries in the walls of the heart (coronary arteriography) have become essential. Meanwhile, the need for some special examinations has declined. For example, bronchography, in which an opaque liquid is introduced into the bronchial tubes of the lungs in order to show whether or not they are diseased, is now performed less often than previously as a result of a decline in the number of patients requiring this investigation because of improved treatment of lung infections in childhood.

Other methods of investigation New and improved methods of investigation in medical diagnosis are introduced every year. The requirements are that they should be harmless or carry very few risks, should not be painful, and should improve the accuracy of diagnosis. The X-ray film is, as we have seen, a record of the shadow cast by the structures of the body when a beam of X-rays is passed through it. The record is made on ordinary photographic emulsion containing silver salts. Many refinements have been introduced to improve the quality of the photographic image but basically this principle has not changed since Roentgen discovered X-rays in 1895. Recently, the use of a silver-containing emulsion has been superseded by using an electrostatic method of recording the image (Xerox). This also has some additional advantages in the way the image is presented. The image may be intensified using a special type of intensifier tube. The radiologist then sees the image on a television screen. One piece of apparatus now always found in X-ray Departments is called a tomograph, which produces pictures of a thin section of the body. This is done by linking the X-ray tube and the film and then moving them in opposite directions so that all detail is blurred out apart from one thin layer.

EMI Scanner (computerized axial tomography, or CAT) Developments in radiology in the last 30 or 40 years have always been faced with the same problem. When X-rays pass through the soft tissues of the body, minute differences in absorption occur but until recently no method has been available for recording these minute differences satisfactorily. An apparatus is now available, the EMI Scanner, which analyses by computer the results of passing a very fine beam of X-rays through the body. The minute differences in the densities of the tissues can then be found as a result of this analysis and a picture can be created of these tissue densities on a television screen. This remarkable advance has opened a new door in radiology. Having demonstrated that such very fine differences in density can be measured and knowing that such measurements can be of enormous benefit,

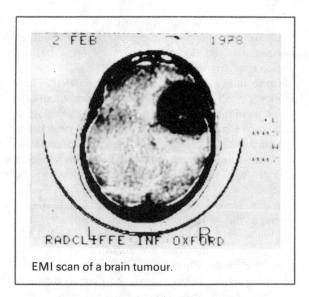

EMI scan of a brain tumour.

worldwide research is now under way to find alternative methods of achieving the same result and one such laboratory research project does not even require the use of X-rays (nuclear resonance).

Radioisotopes and organ imaging Some of the 92 or so elements of which matter is composed are radioactive and many others can be made so by artificial means. A radioactive substance is one whose atoms undergo spontaneous disintegration, with the emission of various particles and gamma rays (akin to X-rays), and finally end up as another element. For example, radium in time will end up as lead, which is a stable nonradioactive element and will not change further. The rate at which the radioactive process takes place is measured by the time it takes for half the material to disintegrate (its "half-life"). This varies from days, hours, or even seconds, to thousands of years.

In medical work small amounts of radioactive elements which have a suitable length of half-life (usually a few days) can be administered to patients, either as the element itself, or one of its salts, or in combination, for example, with a nutrient. These substances can be identified by their radioactive emissions and their progress followed as they are absorbed, digested, concentrated in some organ, or are excreted, by apparatus which measures and records the amount and pattern of the emissions (gamma cameras and scanners). Some examples are iodine which is concentrated in the thyroid gland, strontium or fluorine which are taken up by bone, selenium for the pancreas, and various compounds of technetium for study of the heart, liver, or kidneys, or for measurement of the blood flow through the lungs. Chromium can be used to "mark" the red cells.

There is also a device called a "total body counter" which measures the total amount of a radioactive substance in the body, usually a few days after its administration. In this way the amount of material absorbed and retained can be measured more easily and more accurately than by measuring what has been excreted in the breath, urine, or excreta. These procedures are usually undertaken in a hospital's Nuclear Medicine Department by hospital physicists, radiologists, and physicians working together.

The risks of investigation by radioactive isotopes are very small because the short half-life of the substances, and the minute quantities used, mean that the radioactivity disappears altogether very quickly.

Ultrasound Sound waves are not radiation. They consist of vibrations of the substance through which they are passing. We feel these sound waves in our ears. The frequency of sound waves can be so increased that we cannot hear them and it is in this range that they become usable in diagnosis. A small emitter of ultrasonic waves is placed on the skin. Tiny reflections of these waves will occur at all the tissue planes through which the beam is passing. These reflections are picked up by a sensing device. By passing the combined emitter and sensing device over the skin surface, a picture of the tissue planes below an area of the skin can be built up and recorded on a television screen. This method of showing the structure of the inside of the body is particularly important because the beam used is considered to be harmless to tissues in the quantity and strength employed. The principal use of ultrasound in general medical work today is in obstetrics. The growth of the baby, its position, the position of the placenta, and even the movements of the heart and of the chest wall can all be recorded with great accuracy and a permanent record can be made by photographing the television screen. Ultrasound is also of importance in the diagnosis of liver and kidney conditions and in some conditions affecting the brain. One very important application is the assessment of the flexibility and movement of the valves of the heart. Ultrasound apparatus is often but not always sited in the X-ray Department.

Thermography This is in effect a photograph of the body taken not with light waves but by using the heat waves produced by the body. Various disease conditions may cause areas of higher or lower temperature than normal. The method has been applied specially in the diagnosis of breast tumours. It is of course harmless and painless.

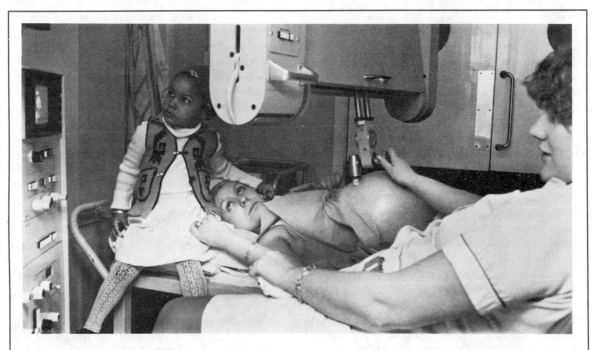

Ultrasound scanning is a new development, by which the growth and position of the fetus and placenta can be safely determined.

Radiation hazards Patients are naturally concerned about the possibility of an X-ray examination in some way causing harm either to themselves or to children they may subsequently have. In the very early days of radiology some patients and a number of radiologists developed changes in the skin. The reason for this was, of course, gross overexposure of the skin to X-rays. Some workers, for example, might have had their hands exposed to X-rays for several hours each day. Not only was the total quantity of radiation excessive, it was also low voltage. This means that its penetrating power was low and much of its energy was absorbed by the skin. These dangers are now greatly reduced by the precautions taken and by strict control of the quality of the X-rays used, in order to protect the population and its genetic potentialities, the individual patient, and the X-ray worker.

All nations are rightly concerned that the total level of radiation received by the earth's population should be kept as low as possible. Background radiation from the earth itself, cosmic radiation which escapes the filter of the atmosphere, and residual radiation from atomic and hydrogen bomb explosions all exist now. Diagnostic radiation adds to this load. The fear is that a progressive increase in radiation dosage might affect the rate of gene mutation and that this might have harmful consequences. At present the load is not excessive and it is up to us all to minimize any additions to it.

Even in the last twenty years, considerable advances have been made in reducing the X-ray dosage received by patients. The dosage may now be as little as one quarter of that used for the same examination performed twenty years ago. This has been achieved by using faster films and intensifying screens to record the X-ray image. The most careful attention to detail remains essential, particularly when the patient is a child, or a man or woman in the reproductive age. There is some statistical evidence that children who were X-rayed before birth may have been very slightly more at risk to the development of some types of cancer in later life than children who were not X-rayed. For this reason, a marked reduction in the number and extent of radiodiagnostic procedures during pregnancy has been instituted. The risks may be higher for the fetus during the early stage of pregnancy. For this reason, it is now the usual practice, in Britain, to apply what is called the "Ten Day Rule" when appointments are being made for the non-emergency examination of the abdomen or pelvis in women of childbearing age. The examinations are performed in the ten days following the first day of the last menstrual cycle, when there is no ovum in the uterus. If the patient is due to have an examination outside these days, then, if the examination is not urgent, another appointment is made.

Of course, when a patient is ill, the complications which may result from a diagnostic or therapeutic procedure have to be weighed against the risks attached to the illness. If patients are concerned about the risks of an X-ray, they should discuss them with the examining doctor. Equally, it may be advisable to accept the doctor's advice not to have an X-ray if, on balance, the symptoms being investigated do not justify it.

Radiotherapy

The treatment of disease by radiation is now almost entirely confined to the treatment of cancer. In the past, X-rays were used to alleviate some chronic, but quite benign, conditions. New methods of treatment are now available in most instances and, because of the possible risks, X-rays are no longer used. The radiotherapist now has at his disposal a whole range of weapons against cancer. The commonest still in use are, of course, the machines which produce X-rays at voltages varying between 250,000 and 2,000,000. Additionally, he can use the gamma radiation emitted by cobalt or caesium and he can use the particulate radiation produced by a machine called a Linear Accelerator. All these sources of radiation are housed in large machines which can deliver a well-defined beam of X-rays with great accuracy at the tumour site. The radiotherapist can also direct radiation into or very close to the tumour using radioactive material contained in needles or small, seedlike capsules. In this way, a very high but localized dose of radiation can be given. For superficial lesions, he can also use radioactive materials giving off particles which penetrate only for a minute distance into tissues.

These methods of radiation treatment all depend on ionization occurring in the tissues. This atomic breakup can affect the life of a cell in a number of ways. Cells which are dividing more frequently than normal are more sensitive to ionization than ordinary cells. This is one of the reasons for cancer cells being more sensitive to radiation than normal cells.

For deep-seated tumours, it is necessary to build up a dosage of radiation by passing the beams through several different portals of entry so that the dose received by the tumour is very much higher than the dose received on the skin or in the adjacent organs. This is often achieved by rotating the apparatus around the patient. It may sometimes be necessary to treat the possible pathways of extension of a cancer as a precaution.

The use of radioactive material for direct or very close application to tumours is now well established. These local applications usually consist of radium (in needles) or the radioactive gas which it gives off, radon (in so-called seeds). Additionally, many radioactive isotopes have now been discovered and because of their properties they have a number of specialized uses. Material such as radioactive tantalum can be made into wire to provide an accurate grid of high dosage in or close to a tumour mass. A quite different use for radioactive isotopes is also possible if the isotope can be joined to a chemical which the affected organ uses selectively. In this way, for example, it is possible to obtain high concentrations of radioactive iodine within the thyroid gland.

It may be wondered what is the essential difference between the radiation given when an X-ray film is taken and the radiation given for treatment. There is no essential difference in the quality of the radiation but there is a vast difference in its quantity. The amount of radiation administered to a tumour may be 4,000 to 6,000 times the radiation received during an X-ray examination of the same area.

Chemical methods of treatment The radiotherapist and his colleague the oncologist (tumour specialist) have other methods of helping to treat patients with cancer. These consist of a whole range of chemicals which affect the growth of certain types of cells. They can be used to supplement radiation treatment, or in some cases they can be used alone. They are of particular importance in the treatment of cancers affecting the blood-forming cells in bone marrow and in tumours of the lymphatic tissues.

Some tumours are also partially dependent on hormones so that they can be made to regress by altering the hormonal state of the patient. This can be done by giving an excess of one or other type of hormone or, in collaboration with a surgical specialist, the organs which produce certain of the hormones can be removed or their functioning changed.

A course of treatment The patient whose cancer is going to be treated may already have had a surgical operation or may, indeed, have a surgical operation after the treatment. The radiotherapist and the physician or surgeon concerned consult together on the best form or combination of treatments for each individual patient. The decision depends on many factors, and consultations take place between the radiotherapist and his colleagues before he puts the plan of treatment to the patient. The radiotherapist needs to discuss the nature of the tumour, as shown on biopsy, with his pathologist colleague, the findings at operation may need to be discussed in detail with the surgeon concerned. The patient's general physical condition has to be borne in mind at every stage of the treatment and will probably require further consultations with the physician in overall care of the patient. There may also be discussions with specialists involved in various forms of tumour treatment and with other doctors concerned with drug therapy, immunology, diagnosis, and specialized investigations.

In some centres, these discussions are held at regular conferences during which the treatment procedure is also discussed. It is at this stage that the physicist who is in charge of the planning of radiation treatment starts to calculate, on the basis of all the information available to him, the best ways of applying the radiation. This work is carried out in a Physics Department.

The course of treatment given may be very short, lasting only a few days or it may be lengthy, lasting up to six weeks, depending upon the type of lesion and the treatment recommended for it.

A skin reaction similar in many ways to sunburn may occur in the treated area. This can subside leaving very little trace or there may be some residual pigmentation or small vessel dilatation. The rate of disappearance of the cancer will depend on its sensitivity to the radiation. This process is carefully monitored during and after the treatment and the patient needs to be seen at intervals.

Do cancer cures occur? Yes, in many instances, they do. The rate of cure for some forms of skin cancer is now virtually 100 per cent. The prospects of a permanent cure for many other types of cancer are steadily improving. Some forms of the disease, which only a few years ago were almost uniformly fatal, are now responding well to the combinations of treatment now available. In the meantime, research into the causes of the various types of tumour continues.

The recent developments in diagnostic radiology with their combination of technical complexity and simplicity have produced startling results. In the treatment of cancer the combined attack of many different specialist groups and the added weapons of chemotherapy, hormone therapy, and immunotherapy promise equally encouraging developments in the future.

Chapter 25
Laboratory tests

Revised by Professor D. N. Baron, MD DSc FRCP FRCPath

Why do we do laboratory tests? Are they a necessary part of medical care and examination? Cannot the doctor find out all he needs to know without the help of the laboratory? Medical examination using the doctor's unaided senses does not always give the necessary information, especially in the earliest stages of many diseases; laboratory tests are also usually more sensitive in detecting the first stages in improvement, or worsening, of a patient's condition. Most of the organs are located deep in the body, inaccessible for study by bedside examination.

All testing procedures in medicine – X-rays, blood counts, chemical analyses, electrocardiograms, skin tests, and microscopic examinations, to name a few – are designed to enable the doctor to learn more about his patient than can be found out by questioning to establish the history of the disorder, or is evident externally by examination. The physical examination reveals only those signs which are manifest to the physician through his senses – things he can see, hear, feel, or smell. X-rays, ultrasonics, and scanning tests permit the doctor to observe the form and movements of internal organs. Pathology laboratory tests let him study what might be the reason for the patient's troubles, and how the disease is affecting bodily functions. A recent survey of 80 medical outpatients at a number of British hospitals showed that seven required laboratory tests to make the final diagnosis.

Pathology

Pathology has been defined as the study of the nature and cause of disease. A pathologist works mainly in a laboratory, and uses scientific methods, and a microscope or other equipment, to examine samples of blood, tissues, infectious material, and so on. A pathologist acts as a clinical pathologist when he is responsible for tests on patients, in contrast to being an experimental pathologist when he is doing research, for example into the causes of cancer, independent of individual patients and not for their immediate benefit.

Modern medicine depends heavily upon the pathologist to bring the advances of the research laboratory, in biochemistry, biology, immunology, physiology, and other basic sciences, into general practice, hospitals, and public health. A large hospital department will have a staff of several pathologists, who specialize in the various disciplines, whilst in a small department one pathologist will cover all the fields. The modern clinical pathologist advises the physician on the choice and interpretation of laboratory tests; he may take responsibility for direct patient care in a special branch of medicine. To take examples from different fields of pathology, a bacteriologist may examine a patient with an infection and decide on the best antibiotic to use, a chemical pathologist take part in an outpatient clinic for diabetes, a haematologist look after inpatients with severe anaemia, or a histopathologist go to the patient's bedside to discuss problems such as biopsy with the clinician.

The pathologist and his skilled staff of medical doctors, science graduates, and technicians, are qualified by training and experience to provide clinical laboratory services of dependable quality. This is important because laboratory procedures that are not subject to quality control and careful scrutiny may easily go wrong and give misleading results. Pathological tests that are not done in properly staffed and professionally supervised laboratories are particularly liable to error.

Laboratory tests are used by the medical profession in three different ways, to safeguard health, to diagnose disease, and to guide treatment. In addition, critical analysis of the results of laboratory tests is part of clinical research, adding to our knowledge of disease for the benefit of future patients.

Tests to safeguard health

The public health For many years the staff of the Public Health Laboratory Service has worked to promote public health. They have done this by testing drinking water for evidence of bacterial contamination, by analysing milk and other dairy products for purity and nutritional value, by checking food handlers for evidence of communicable disease, and conducting other similar investigations.

Chemical tests to safeguard health are done, for example, on water supplies or in respect of industrial hazards: these may be the responsibility of scientists other than pathologists.

Screening tests It would be valuable if periodical medical examination of apparently healthy persons, with or without appropriate laboratory tests, could enable doctors to detect disease in its earliest stages before obvious complaints had developed. Then appropriate medical treatment, or change of diet or way of life, would alter the progress of the disease and help the patient. The general current view of most doctors in Britain is that, except in special instances, such annual checkups or routine screening tests are not worthwhile; in some countries, particularly the United States of America, they are common practice. Such screening is expensive in terms of time and facilities of the doctor and laboratory, and shows overall benefit neither to the patient nor to the taxpayer who pays for the National Health Service. There are very few diseases in which it is both possible to make a reliable early diagnosis before the disease is causing the patient any trouble, and when early treatment would do the patient good.

Of course the appropriate medical and laboratory tests are performed on apparently healthy patients when there is an indication in the patient's own history or family history. An example is measurement of the serum cholesterol if the patient's father has died at the age of 60 of a heart attack, or tonometry in relatives of patients with chronic simple glaucoma. It is important to keep a watch on the blood pressure of the middle-aged, but this can usually be done when

the opportunity arises, at a patient's visit to his general practitioner for any complaint. People who are exposed to toxic hazards (such as lead) in their work must be tested at intervals to see if they are affected before obvious disease develops, but here there is an indication for the screening.

A laboratory test of proven value is the Guthrie test on the blood of all babies at about a week old, for phenylketonuria. This inherited condition occurs in about one in 15,000 births, and leads to mental retardation. If diagnosed early, its bad effects can be prevented by a special diet. The microscopic examination of cells (cytology) in a cervical smear should be done on all adult women at three to five yearly intervals. This detects many patients with cancer of the cervix at an early enough stage for successful treatment. Much research is going on into the possibility of doing prenatal laboratory tests on the blood or amniotic fluid of pregnant women to diagnose fetal disease (alpha-fetoprotein assay).

Tests to diagnose disease

When a patient goes to his doctor because of illness, his symptoms – such as cough, weakness, fever, weight loss – give the doctor a clue as to what the trouble is. The investigation is then directed towards following up the clue. The modern doctor ordinarily does not treat symptoms without attempting to learn their cause. Thus, when headache is severe and persistent, it is not enough to give a headache remedy; the cause of the headache must be sought, and treatment must be directed at that cause. The questioning must be detailed, and the examinations and laboratory tests must survey specifically those parts of the body and those diseases which may cause the symptoms in question.

Diagnostic laboratory tests are based upon a number of different principles. For example:

In infectious diseases, the tests ordinarily depend upon finding and identifying the germs which cause the particular disease or detecting antibodies which result from the presence of these germs in the body.

In diseases of the blood, the tests are mainly based upon direct microscopic examination of the blood cells and counting the different types of cells in a measured quantity of blood.

In cancer, the diagnostic procedure is based upon microscopic examination of a small piece of tissue removed from a suspicious lump or ulcer.

In other instances the tests are based upon the assumption that each organ in the body has a certain job to do, and that if the organ is healthy it will do that job; these tests require specimens that can in some way reflect organ function.

The range of laboratory tests that may be used to diagnose diseases is almost without limit. No list of tests can be considered final, complete, or authoritative. New tests are added every year, and old tests fall into disfavour. The following list of tests, grouped by organ systems and by diseases, covers most of the commonly used clinical pathology tests.

References to particular tests appear in many chapters of this book, in discussions of functions and disorders. Definitions (page 556) may aid in understanding the methods and purposes of tests that may be ordered for individual patients.

Some laboratory tests to diagnose disease, by organ systems

Heart and blood vessels

rheumatic fever: anti-streptolysin O; sedimentation rate.
bacterial endocarditis: blood culture.
coronary thrombosis: transaminase (and other enzymes).
arterial disease: cholesterol; triglycerides.

Lungs and bronchi

tuberculosis: sputum microscopy and culture.
pneumonia: sputum microscopy and culture.
cancer: sputum cytology; bronchoscopic examination and biopsy.

Stomach and duodenum

ulcer: gastric analysis.
cancer: gastric analysis; gastric cytology; occult blood.

Intestines

colitis: stool microscopy and culture.
cancer: occult blood; biopsy.
worms: stool microscopy.
coeliac disease: stool analysis for fat; calcium; vitamin studies.

Liver and gallbladder

cirrhosis: needle biopsy of liver; proteins; BSP; transaminase; alkaline phosphatase (and other enzymes); bilirubin; Australia antigen.
jaundice: same as for cirrhosis.

Pancreas

pancreatitis: amylase; lipase; calcium.
cystic fibrosis: sweat test; stool analysis.

Kidneys and urinary bladder

nephritis: urine analysis; urea; creatinine; creatinine clearance; electrolytes; needle biopsy of kidney.
stone: urine analysis; calcium; uric acid; urea; stone analysis.
infection of kidneys (pyelonephritis) or bladder (cystitis): urine analysis; urine microscopy and culture.
cancer: cystoscopic examination with biopsy.

Male reproductive system

urethritis: urethral fluid smear and culture.
prostatitis: prostatic fluid smear and culture.
prostate cancer: acid phosphatase; needle biopsy of prostate.
infertility and impotence: sperm examination; hormone studies.

Female reproductive system

pregnancy: chorionic gonadotrophin; hormone studies.
infertility: hormone studies; endometrial biopsy.
uterine cancer: dilatation and curettage (D and C), and cervical biopsy.
breast cancer: nipple discharge cytology; breast biopsy.

Endocrine glands and metabolism

diabetes mellitus: urine analysis; glucose (sugar); glucose tolerance; electrolytes.
thyroid diseases: thyroxine (T_4) and related hormone studies.
adrenal diseases: hormone studies; electrolytes.
parathyroid diseases: calcium; phosphate; alkaline phosphatase.
pituitary diseases: hormone studies; glucose tolerance.
acidosis and alkalosis: pH; CO_2; electrolytes.
water and salt disturbances: electrolytes; urea.
nutritional disorders: protein; haemoglobin; calcium; phosphate; iron; vitamin studies.
phenylketonuria: Guthrie test.

Blood

anaemia: blood film; red cell count; haemoglobin; haematocrit; iron; vitamin studies; occult blood; haemoglobin A_2 and F (Mediterranean immigrants); haemoglobin C and S (African immigrants); bone marrow examination; gastric analysis.
leukaemia: white cell count; differential count; bone marrow examination; platelet count.
bleeding and clotting disorders: coagulation time; platelet count; prothrombin time; partial thromboplastin time; bleeding time.
infectious mononucleosis (glandular fever): see *Lymph nodes and spleen*.

malaria : thick and thin smear.

erythroblastosis : Rh on baby and mother; bilirubin; Coombs' test.

infection : white cell count; differential count; sedimentation rate; blood culture.

Lymph nodes and spleen

infectious mononucleosis (glandular fever) : white cell count; differential count; Paul-Bunnell test.

Hodgkin's disease : white cell count; differential count; lymph node biopsy.

sarcoid : proteins; calcium; lymph node biopsy.

leukaemia : see *Blood.*

Nervous system

meningitis, poliomyelitis, encephalitis : cerebrospinal fluid analysis, culture, and microscopy.

multiple sclerosis : cerebrospinal fluid analysis.

stroke : cerebrospinal fluid analysis.

Bones and joints

fracture from minimal injury : calcium; phosphate; alkaline phosphatase; protein.

arthritis : sedimentation rate; LE cell preparation; rheumatoid factor; proteins; uric acid; synovial fluid examination.

cancer : calcium; phosphate; alkaline phosphatase.

rheumatic fever : see *Heart and blood vessels.*

Infectious diseases

malaria : see *Blood.*

typhoid fever : blood culture; stool culture; urine culture; agglutination tests (Widal).

brucellosis : agglutination tests; blood culture; skin tests.

diphtheria, streptococcal throat : throat swab culture.

whooping cough : nasal swab for culture.

rheumatic fever : see *Heart and blood vessels.*

meningitis and poliomyelitis : see *Nervous system.*

syphilis : dark field; VDRL; TPI; FTA-ABS; cerebrospinal fluid analysis.

virus : virus isolation; neutralization and complement fixation tests.

Tests to guide treatment

In one sense, all laboratory tests are used as a guide to treatment, since they promote accurate diagnosis. On the whole, however, they are probably more important for management of treatment than for diagnosis. In this section reference is made to the use of laboratory tests to select the type of treatment to be used, to determine how much treatment is required, to confirm that the desired effect is being obtained, and to avoid harmful side effects of treatment. The need for tests of this type is greatest in those chronic diseases where treatment must be continued for a long time, perhaps for life.

Tests of antibiotic efficacy In a dangerous infection such as meningitis, it is extremely important to obtain an optimum therapeutic effect without delay: therefore, treatment must be started immediately. Meanwhile, the sensitivity of the germs can be tested. Since meningitis may be due to different types of bacteria or viruses, and each of these may respond differently or not at all to the various antibiotic drugs, it is common practice to test the various antibiotic drugs directly against the bacteria that are present in the particular case. This can be done in the following way. Cerebrospinal fluid from the patient is spread over the surface of agar in a sterile dish. Tiny paper discs, each of which has been impregnated with a different antibiotic, are dropped onto the surface of the agar and the dish is set aside for several hours in an incubator. The bacteria that were present in the patient's cerebrospinal fluid begin to multiply and form colonies on the medium, except that where they are in contact with the paper discs their growth may be modified by the antibiotic. The test is a combination of cerebrospinal fluid culture and antibiotic sensitivity; from it the bacteriologist will have an indication of which drugs are most likely to be effective, and can so advise the physician.

Dosage regulation Probably the oldest use of laboratory tests is the regulation of drug dosage in the diabetic patient. Some diabetics have a different requirement of insulin from day to day, depending upon appetite, diet, exercise, infections, and the like. If the regular dose of insulin is sufficient, the urine test for glucose will be negative. If it is insufficient, the test will give a positive reaction of varying intensity, depending upon the amount of glucose present. The doctor teaches the patient how to test his own urine and to regulate the dose of insulin depending upon the result of the urine test. From time to time the diabetic patient must also have a glucose test on blood, so as to avoid incorrect insulin dosage.

The following are other examples of the many uses of laboratory tests to guide treatment. After an attack of coronary thrombosis or leg vein thrombosis, some patients are given drugs to reduce the clotting tendency of their blood. The effect must be precisely controlled by coagulation tests, since overdose of the drug could cause haemorrhage.

X-rays, radium, and drugs used in the treatment of

cancer sometimes destroy blood cells as well as cancer cells; occasional counts must be taken of white cells, red cells, and platelets to make sure that this harmful effect is avoided. Some drugs used in the treatment of high blood pressure produce in some patients a condition resembling a special form of sensitivity disease known as lupus erythematosus; blood examinations (LE preparation) can anticipate this effect.

Transfusions The use of blood transfusion is of life-saving importance in certain diseases. However, different people have different types of blood and it might be extremely dangerous to give a patient blood of a type different from his own. To detect these types and determine compatability between donor's and recipient's blood, ABO blood group and Rh tests must be carried out. Similar tests (ABO blood group and Rh) are of importance in determining whether the blood of an unborn baby is compatible with that of its mother. If incompatibility is present, it may be necessary to give the baby an exchange transfusion immediately after birth.

Frozen section The surgeon often calls upon the pathologist to help him to decide whether a lump in the breast should be simply removed or whether the whole breast and the nearby lymph nodes should also be removed. This provisional test, known as the frozen section, is performed while the patient is under anaesthesia and takes about 30 minutes; the normal definitive processing and examination of tissues removed at operation takes two or three days.

The surgeon removes the lump and passes it to the pathologist who freezes a portion of it in a jet of carbon dioxide gas. Once frozen, a very thin slice or section is cut, stained with a dye, mounted on a glass slide and examined under the microscope. If cancer is present, as determined by the pathologist, the surgeon will normally remove the entire breast and related tissue. If the pathologist determines that the lump is benign, the surgeon does not remove the remainder of the breast.

Definitions of certain laboratory tests and medical procedures

acid phosphatase: an enzyme test on blood, for diagnosis of prostatic cancer.

agglutination tests: antibody tests on blood, for the diagnosis of typhoid fever, brucellosis, and certain other infectious diseases.

alkaline phosphatase: an enzyme test on blood, used for the investigation of bone disease, and obstructive jaundice.

amniotic fluid: surrounds the unborn child in the womb; tested for alpha-fetoprotein for spina bifida (see page 225) and for fetal cells.

amylase: an enzyme test on blood, for diagnosis in acute pancreatitis.

antibiotic sensitivity: a bacteriological test, to determine which antibiotics are active against specific bacteria.

anti-streptolysin O: an antibody test on blood, used in cases of suspected rheumatic fever.

Australia antigen: see *HBAg.*

bicarbonate: see *electrolytes.*

bilirubin: a chemical test on blood, used for investigation of certain blood and liver diseases.

biopsy: a tissue test, usually used in cases of suspected cancer.

blood culture: a test to determine the presence of bacteria in the blood, for the diagnosis of fevers.

blood group (ABO and Rh): an antibody test on blood, used to select suitable blood for transfusions, and in pregnancy to evaluate the possibility of certain blood diseases in the baby.

bone marrow examination: a microscopic test on cellular material obtained by needle, used to diagnose leukaemia, anaemia, and certain other diseases of the blood.

breast biopsy: a tissue test, used in cases of suspected breast cancer.

bronchoscopic examination and biopsy: an investigative procedure combined with a tissue test, used in cases of suspected lung cancer.

BSP: bromsulphthalein, a chemical measurement of liver function; an injection is given, and some time later a blood specimen is taken for analysis.

calcium: a chemical test on blood, used for the investigation of bone diseases and certain parathyroid, kidney, intestinal, and pancreatic diseases.

cerebrospinal fluid examination: various chemical, microscopic, and bacteriological tests, used for investigation of infections and other diseases of the nervous system.

cervical biopsy: a tissue test, used in cases of suspected cancer of the uterine cervix.

cervical cytology: microscopic test of material obtained from the uterine cervix, smeared on a glass slide after the method of Papanicolaou; a screening test for cervical cancer.

chloride: see *electrolytes.*

cholesterol: a chemical test on blood, used in screening and investigation of arterial and heart disease, and also for the diagnosis of certain metabolic diseases.

chorionic gonadotrophin: an immunological test on urine, for the diagnosis of pregnancy.

coagulation time: a clotting test on blood, used for diagnosis in patients having a tendency to haemorrhage, and also as a guide to treatment in patients receiving anticoagulant drugs.

CO_2: a chemical test on blood, used as a guide to treatment in various conditions of acidosis and alkalosis.

complement fixation tests: antibody tests on blood, used for the diagnosis of certain viral and bacterial infections.

Coombs' test: an antibody test on blood, used in selecting blood suitable for transfusion, and in the diagnosis of certain anaemias.

creatinine: a chemical test on blood; a measure of kidney function.

creatinine clearance: a combined chemical test on blood and urine; a sensitive test of kidney function.

cystoscopic examination with biopsy: a surgical procedure combined with a tissue test, used in cases of suspected bladder cancer.

cytology: the study of cells; the term is often applied to the microscopic screening test for cancer first developed by Papanicolaou.

dark field: a microscopic test for the presence of certain bacteria.

differential count: a microscopic test done on a blood film, using for diagnosis of leukaemia and certain infections.

dilatation and curettage (D and C): a surgical procedure on the uterus; used to obtain a tissue specimen in cases of suspected uterine cancer.

duodenal drainage: an intestinal specimen is obtained by a swallowed tube and examined; for diagnosis of diseases of the pancreas.

electrolytes: chemical tests on blood or urine for sodium, potassium, chloride, and bicarbonate; used in the investigation of losses of body fluids, or of hormone disorders, and as a guide to treatment.

endometrial biopsy: a tissue test on the uterus, used in the study of infertility, and also for the diagnosis of cancer of the uterus.

enzyme: a broad group of tests, usually done on blood; mainly used in the diagnosis of heart, muscle, liver, and pancreatic diseases.

erythrocytes: see *red cell count.*

frozen section: a rapid tissue test, usually done during a surgical operation, for the diagnosis of suspected cancer.

FTA-ABS: fluorescent treponemal antibody absorption, a test on blood in suspected syphilis.

gastric analysis: a specimen of stomach juice is obtained by stomach tube, often after an injection of a stimulating drug, and examined chemically and microscopically in the investigation of ulcer, anaemia, and cancer.

gastric cytology: microscopic examination of stomach juice for cells in suspected stomach cancer.

glucose (sugar): a chemical test, either on blood or urine; used in the investigation of diabetes mellitus and other metabolic diseases, and as a guide to treatment.

glucose tolerance: a series of chemical tests for blood glucose after taking glucose by mouth; a test for early diabetes and other metabolic diseases.

Guthrie test: a combined chemical and bacteriological test on blood; used as a screening test for phenylketonuria.

haematocrit: a mechanical test on blood; used for the investigation of anaemia and also as a guide to treatment.

haemoglobin: a chemical test on blood; used for investigation and as a guide to treatment in anaemia.

haemoglobin C and S/A_2 and F: a physicochemical test on blood; for diagnosis of sickle-cell anaemia, thalassaemia, and related blood diseases.

HBAg (Australia antigen): a blood test for an infecting agent of hepatitis.

heterophile antibody test (Paul-Bunnell test): an antibody test on blood, used for diagnosis of infectious mononucleosis (glandular fever).

hormone studies: a broad group of tests, some chemical and some biological, usually done on blood, used in the diagnosis of endocrine and metabolic disorders.

iodine uptake: a radioisotope test for the diagnosis of thyroid diseases; done after taking a dose of radioactive iodine.

iron: a chemical test on blood, for investigation of anaemia.

LE preparation: lupus erythematosus preparation, a microscopic test of a blood preparation, for diagnosis of lupus erythematosus.

leucocytes: see *white blood count.*

lipase: an enzyme test on blood, for diagnosis of acute pancreatitis.

lymph node biopsy: a tissue test, used in cases of suspected cancer of the lymph nodes.

needle biopsy of kidney: a tissue test for diagnosis of kidney diseases, using as a specimen a small piece of kidney tissue obtained through a long needle.

needle biopsy of liver: a similar test for diagnosis of liver diseases, particularly cirrhosis.

557

Chapter 25 **Laboratory tests**

needle biopsy of prostate: a tissue test, used in cases of suspected cancer of the prostate.

neutralization test: a combined antibody and biological test for diagnosis of virus infections; blood is used.

nipple cytology: a microscopic test of nipple secretion in cases of suspected breast cancer.

occult blood: a chemical test on faeces, used to detect slight blood loss from the stomach or intestines.

partial thromboplastin time: a clotting test on blood; used as an investigation in patients having a tendency to haemorrhage.

pH: a test on blood used for diagnosis and as a guide to treatment in patients with acidosis or alkalosis.

phosphate: a chemical test on blood, used in the diagnosis of certain diseases of bone, kidney, and metabolism.

platelet count: a microscopic test on blood, used in the diagnosis of patients having a tendency to bleed.

potassium: see *electrolytes.*

proctoscopic examination and biopsy: a medical procedure combined with a tissue test, used in patients with suspected cancer of the rectum.

prostatic smear: a microscopic and culture test for diagnosis of infection of the prostate gland; the specimen is obtained by prostatic massage.

proteins: a chemical or physicochemical test on blood, used for diagnosis in diseases of nutrition, the liver, lymph nodes, and bone marrow.

prothrombin time: a clotting test on blood, used in patients having a tendency to haemorrhage, in liver diseases, and also as a guide to treatment in patients receiving certain anticoagulant drugs.

red cell count: a microscopic or electronic test for investigation of anaemia; blood is used.

Rh (Rhesus): an antibody test on blood, used in transfusion studies, and in pregnancy to evaluate the possibility of blood disease in the baby.

rheumatoid factor: an antibody test on blood used for the diagnosis of rheumatoid arthritis.

sedimentation rate: a mechanical test on blood; provides a nonspecific measure of inflammation, infection, and other conditions.

skin tests: sensitivity tests using the patient's skin; for identification of substances to which the patient is allergic, and to detect evidence of prior infection in tuberculosis and diphtheria.

sodium: see *electrolytes.*

sperm examination: a microscopic test of fertility in the male.

spinal fluid: see *cerebrospinal fluid.*

sputum cytology: a microscopic test of sputum in cases of suspected lung cancer.

sputum examination: various chemical, microscopic, bacteriological, and cytological tests on sputum, used for diagnosis of lung disease, especially tuberculosis, pneumonia, asthma, cancer, and abscess.

stool examination: a series of microscopic, bacteriological, and chemical tests on faeces, used for investigation of stomach and intestinal disease, including infections (for example dysentery), worms, amoebas, ulcer, and cancer.

sugar: see *glucose.*

sweat test: a chemical test on sweat, used for the diagnosis of fibrocystic disease of the pancreas.

synovial fluid examination: a series of microscopic and bacteriological tests for the diagnosis of gout and other forms of arthritis; joint fluid, removed by needle, is the specimen.

thick and thin smear: a microscopic test, using blood smears of different degrees of thickness, for diagnosis of malaria.

throat swab culture: a bacteriological test for diagnosis of such throat infections as diphtheria and streptococcal sore throat.

thyroxine: a test on blood, for the investigation of thyroid diseases.

TPI: treponema pallidum immobilization, an antibody test on blood, used in the diagnosis of syphilis.

transaminase: an enzyme test on blood, for the diagnosis of coronary thrombosis and liver diseases.

triglycerides: a chemical test on blood, used in screening and investigation of arterial and heart disease.

tubeless gastric analysis: a chemical test done on the urine after administration of a special preparation by mouth; serves as a test for gastric acid without passing a tube.

urea: a chemical test on blood; a measure of kidney function or tissue breakdown.

urethral smear: a bacteriological test used in cases of suspected gonorrhoea.

uric acid: a chemical test on blood, used in the diagnosis of gout.

urine analysis: a series of chemical and microscopic tests on urine, to investigate diseases of the kidney and bladder, and also many general diseases such as diabetes.

urine culture: a bacteriological test for diagnosis of infections of the urinary tract.

urine cytology: a microscopic test used in cases of suspected cancer of the kidneys or bladder.

uterine cytology: a microscopic test used as a screening procedure for uterine cancer.

VDRL: the Venereal Disease Research Laboratory

screening test for syphilis; blood is used.

virus isolation: biological tests for the diagnosis of virus infections; cerebrospinal fluid, bronchial washings, etc. may be used as specimens.

vitamin studies: tests on blood or urine for investigation of nutrition, intestinal function, and anaemia.

Wassermann: an antibody test that may be helpful for the diagnosis of syphilis; blood is used.

white cell count: microscopic or electronic test for the enumeration of leucocytes in blood; used for the diagnosis of infections and leukaemia.

Widal: an antibody test on blood, for diagnosis of typhoid fever.

Chapter 26
Medical genetics

Revised by Professor Paul E. Polani, MD FRCP FRCOG FRS

Parents are naturally concerned about their children. Before a baby is born they wonder whether he will be normal and most of the time all is well. But anxiety about a future baby can arise before conception, although very few prospective parents – or indeed couples contemplating marriage – have reason to undergo examination and investigation to assess the risk to their children. However, if a defective infant has already been born to a couple, or if some undesirable characteristic, a malformation, or a disease has occurred in the direct blood line and thus appears to be hereditary, there is reasonable cause for concern and for seeking advice and help.

In many such cases, or even when there are less firmly based, often hidden, anxieties, the family doctor, paediatrician, or obstetrician can often give reassuring answers. He can assure the non-haemophiliac brother of a haemophiliac that he cannot transmit the disease, or set a couple's minds at rest by telling them that cerebral palsy is usually not hereditary. Not only can he diagnose and treat, but also give counselling on the risks of occurrence or recurrence of the frequent forms of congenital disease. Additional advice may be needed for obscure disorders or conditions requiring special expertise. The doctor can refer the small number of patients who need this help to genetic counsellors. These are people who specialize in medical genetics, in the recognition and differentiation of the many clear-cut genetic diseases, and in the problems of transmission, the risk of a child being affected, and prenatal diagnosis. Medical geneticists also deal with the problems posed by those disorders in which a genetic element plays a relevant part but is by no means wholly responsible for the disease or malformation.

Genetic counsellors cannot give hard-and-fast answers to every problem. However, in general their answers are reassuring; the real facts concerning risks are much less ominous than the fears. Sometimes their answers must be tentative and qualified. Risks can be stated only in terms of odds or probabilities. More and more, however, they can give a firm opinion in a given pregnancy on whether the fetus is or is not affected by a specific disease or malformation for which he is at risk.

Congenital or hereditary?

Commonly a trait or a disease is considered *hereditary* if it is passed on from parent(s) to offspring by the mechanism of gene transmission. However, there are traits, diseases, or malformations which are the result of changes in the genetic material that have arisen anew, mostly in a given germ cell from either parent. These changes of the hereditary (or genetic) material may well be transmissible to future generations but the characteristics which they cause are *not strictly inherited*, in the sense that they are not present generally in the blood line. This is the case, for example, with most chromosome disorders, like Down's syndrome (mongolism), or with a proportion of persons with the form of short-limbed dwarfism known as achondroplasia, or in many male subjects with haemophilia, as well as in other genetic diseases.

A *congenital* abnormality is one that is present at birth. It is not necessarily hereditary. *Accidental* birth defects are not inherited and will almost certainly not be repeated in subsequent children. Among the causes of such accidents are infection of the mother with German measles or toxoplasmosis, or her exposure to drugs, toxins, or radiation, which may do harm by affecting the environment of the fetus in the womb at a critical stage of development. True *hereditary* birth defects are transmitted by parental germ cells, and follow rules which can be expressed in terms of mathematical odds or probabilities for or against repetition.

It is a platitude to say that the characteristics that we possess are the result of an interaction and mixed participation of heredity and environment. Reflection shows that this is why prevention and treatment of some genetic diseases is possible through manipulation of the environment, for example by diet to control abnormal metabolism. It is because of this interaction that many birth defects also result from an interplay of genes and environment in variable measure. The complexity can be great, for on the one hand an interaction of a number of different genes may create the predisposition, and on the other hand the interaction of genes interplays with different factors in the environment. This makes the genetics of many defects complex. In general the more complex the genetics of a particular anomaly (cleft palate, congenital heart disease) the less likely it is to be repeated in offspring. Parents of an infant with an isolated cleft palate may be told that the odds are 49 to one against repetition, or, to put matters the other way round, that there is a one in 50 chance of repetition, that is a two per cent risk of recurrence among subsequent children.

It is estimated that about three per cent of all live-born infants have a serious abnormality of development (congenital malformation), and it is against such a standard that individual family risks may well be measured in judging what constitutes an increased, or a greatly increased, risk. As is the case with many congenital malformations, some diseases are not directly inherited, but depend on a hereditary component, probably a subtle susceptibility which may be produced by multiple factors. Diabetes tends to recur in families, but a potential diabetic may never develop the disease if dietetic and other problems can be controlled. Women with close female relatives who have had breast cancer are three times more likely to develop the disease than the average woman. Pernicious anaemia patients inherit a predisposition to premature degeneration of the mucous lining of the stomach, and psoriasis patients a tendency to excessively rapid turnover of epidermal cells. But we do not yet know enough about the factors which underlie these diseases.

The impact of genetics on disease is substantial. Indeed, genetic causes account for between half and one and a half per cent of all congenital malformations. Major single gene abnormalities and disease affect about one in 300 newborn infants, chromosome abnormalities about one in 150, and complex conditions (such as schizophrenia, diabetes, and so on) can be taken to account for a genetic contribution of about two per cent. Altogether genetic disease and genetic contribution to disease of early life and adulthood is well over four per cent. In addition there is a smaller genetic contribution to common conditions such as cancer and heart disease which is by no means negligible. Medical genetics can play an important role in preventive medicine by informing susceptible people of their hereditary vulnerabilities so that suitable avoidance or other preventive action may be taken. Even when prevention is not possible, treatment may be started before symptoms appear.

Genetic blueprint

The body is made up of several million million cells of many different types and diverse functions, but they are all derived, by division, from a single original cell formed by the union of two germ cells, the egg from the mother fertilized by the sperm from the father. This cell, the zygote, carries within it in code form the information which is employed for making all the other cells and for directing their behaviour and function. We are, in fact, a collection of cells, and function in the way they dictate.

When the first cell divides into two, and in turn each of these two cells divides into two, and so on, the coded information, the blueprint for cell function and behaviour, is passed on from mother to daughter cells, having been faithfully duplicated first. So, each cell, with few exceptions, receives a copy of the original plan contained in the zygote. This information plan, in turn, is the result of two sets of partial information, one carried by each of the two germ cells; these are the hereditary directives derived from the mother and from the father. The blueprint of directives is written in a simple chemical code which uses basically four different "letters" to make coded "sentences" of different length and variable arrangement. The sentences convey the message of the hereditary or genetic language, and each sentence is a gene.

Within each cell the coded information of many sentences is interpreted and translated into the chemical language of cell function and structure. The chemicals made to the specification of the genetic blueprint are the enzymes, which promote the many types of chemical activities of the cells, and the other proteins which are used as building blocks for structure, or are employed for other specialized purposes. So all the directions for the structure and

561

Chapter 26 **Medical genetics**

functioning of our bodies are contained in our genes.

Genes are very long and very thin molecules of DNA (deoxyribonucleic acid). These molecules of DNA follow each other rather like a long thin tape, in an orderly fashion, separated by DNA spacers and by some other DNA stretches used for addressing, co-ordinating, or controlling (that is, turning on or off) the genes. These parts together form a chromosome. Thus each chromosome is a long stretch of DNA made up of genes and gene-regulating material – chromosomes are present in the nucleus of every cell, extremely thin and long, and invisible with ordinary microscopes. However there are times in the life of a cell, for example when it prepares to divide, that the chromosomes fold up regularly and become relatively compact and can, when suitably prepared and stained, be seen under a microscope. Human beings normally have 46 chromosomes, arranged in 23 pairs. One in each pair comes from the mother, one from the father.

Heredity is encoded in the DNA of the chromosome. The long DNA molecules consist of two intertwining chains coiled around a common axis, rather like spiral ladders, with thousands of connecting rungs or steps. The rungs are built of four simple chemical units, (the four letters of the gene code) repeated thousands upon thousands of times in different sequences along the length of the chain.

A gene is thus a relatively short stretch of the DNA. As an example it could be a specific sequence of 500 ladder steps. The relevant message of the gene is encoded only into one side of the DNA ladder; it represents in fact a half ladder. The other side is a chemical mirror image of the first part and represents an essential part of the vital mechanism used for copying genes (replicating DNA) before a cell divides and makes identical daughter cells which are therefore programmed to work like itself. Altogether, the thin DNA ladder within each cell nucleus could be well over a yard long if unravelled. It may contain several thousand, perhaps 50 thousand or so simple genes, and in addition a very large number of gene-coordinating, -correlating, and -steering DNA segments, as well as many additional features which make each chromosome a highly complex chemical structure.

The gene is a unit of heredity specifying some particular trait, primarily a simple chemical characteristic. For example it may determine a part of the haemoglobin molecule, the essential iron-containing substance of red blood cells. But genes often act together and, through the chemicals they programme, determine complex characteristics, such as the colour of the eyes. Here many genes act in a coordinated fashion to induce some cells to make one or other type of pigmented chemical, other cells to arrange themselves in a prescribed fashion within the eye at a certain stage in development, and yet other cells to undergo premature death. Gene action can thus be very complex – hence it needs to be coordinated – and genes may act *only at some times*, say in early development, or only after birth. Therefore there are vital cellular mechanisms for turning genes on or off, as the developmental blueprint of an organism demands. It is because of this complexity and versatility of cell function, and because of the extraordinarily difficult programme of development from conception to old age, that we need many genes, and yet many more switches, controls, and directives, all encoded in the DNA of our nuclei.

Ultimately a gene directs the assembly of an enzyme, or catalyst, essential for some bodily process. At times a gene may become chemically damaged because its DNA has been affected by radiation, by some chemical, or by some other obscure mechanism. The chemical change may produce a difference in only one letter within the sentence, but this can be sufficient to change the genetic message. Such a change of gene is known as a mutation and the changed gene as a mutant gene. As a result of the mutation, the mutant gene may produce an enzyme that is defective or even functionless. The effect may be harmless (as in pink coloration of the urine after eating beetroot, or the smell after eating asparagus) and unapparent; on the other hand, it may cause a major derangement of some physiological process. However, the effect of a mutant gene product generally depends on the environment in which persons with the mutant gene live. A mutant gene product which is harmful in one environment may not be so in a different setting. Indeed in some settings the products of the mutant gene can confer an advantage on those who carry it. In the end the advantage can have the result that those persons with the mutant gene are better able than those without it to pass on the gene in question to their children and so the gene is passed down through the generations. By this process the mutant gene, which arose by a single mutation, may eventually spread to many or even the majority of people within a population. It is often in this way that some hereditary differences between populations have arisen, spread, and become established.

Within the cell nucleus the DNA of the genes transcribes the genetic code upon a slightly different nucleic acid (RNA, ribonucleic acid). It is this RNA

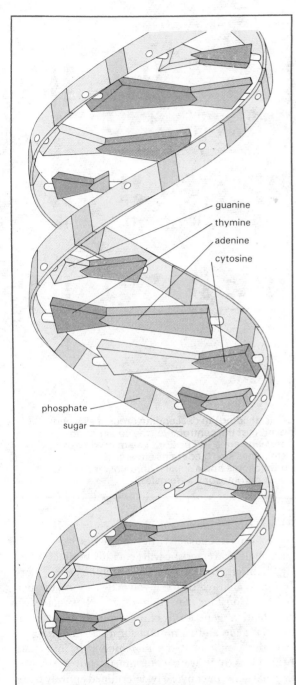

The double helix of DNA (deoxyribonucleic acid) which contains the encoded genetic information. The long molecule is shaped like a spiral staircase. The sides are chains of sugar (deoxyribose) and phosphate molecules; the steps or rungs are built of four bases (thymine and adenine; guanine and cytosine) taken two at a time, and repeated thousands of times in different sequences. It is the combination of sequences which carries the genetic information in code form.

which, in the cytoplasm that surrounds the cell nucleus, directs the cell to manufacture specific enzymes and other proteins by specifying the assembly of amino acids – of which some twenty are found in nature – in orderly sequences. Each sequence represents an individual protein, which therefore is the decoded and translated version of the message of each simple gene. As a result of a gene mutation a seemingly insignificant change – a different amino acid in a chain of perhaps a few hundred – may have far-reaching effects. Sickle-cell anaemia is a classic example of a molecular disease resulting from an amino acid change in a protein, haemoglobin. Owing to this change sickle-cell haemoglobin has different properties compared with other types of adult haemoglobins. Those persons who carry a single dose of the mutant gene may well be at a selective advantage in a malarial environment, while those with a double dose of the gene are affected by a severe and complicated anaemia. We have here an example of the influence of the environment, in this particular case malarial infection, on the effects of the mutant gene: in a malarial environment people who carry a *single dose* of the mutant gene are relatively protected from the effects of malaria. Naturally these people carry two different forms (alleles) of the gene, one from each parent: one form is that which determines the normal haemoglobin, and the other that which determines the sickle haemoglobin. From all this it can be seen that genes, like chromosomes, come in pairs, members of each pair being identical with each other or slightly different; for example, the normal form of a gene opposite the mutant form of the same gene. But in the male, the genes on the X and on the Y sex chromosomes have no matching partners.

Inheritance of traits

One of the 23 pairs of human chromosomes is a pair of sex chromosomes, designated XX in the female and XY in the male. The other 22 pairs are called autosomes. One of the pair of chromosomes is always of maternal derivation and the other paternal. The 50 thousand or so different simple genes that man is estimated to have are distributed between the X chromosomes and the autosomes more or less in relation to the size of each chromosome; the Y chromosome seems largely devoid of genes except for the important set responsible for the origin of maleness during early embryonic development.

Each individual gene has its special and constant position on a chromosome, whether it be an autosome

Chapter 26 Medical genetics

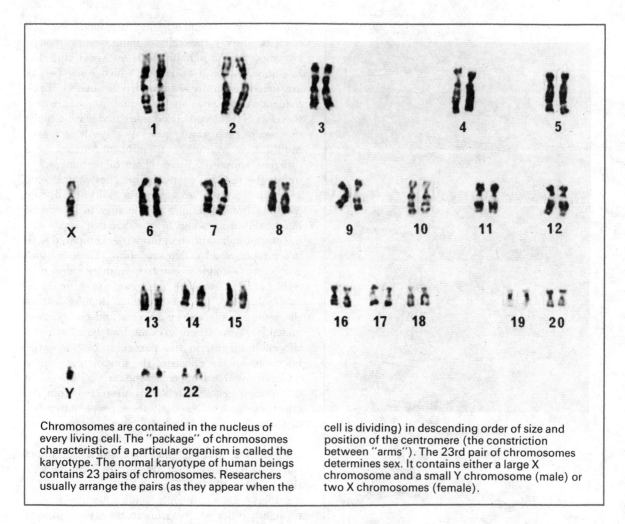

Chromosomes are contained in the nucleus of every living cell. The "package" of chromosomes characteristic of a particular organism is called the karyotype. The normal karyotype of human beings contains 23 pairs of chromosomes. Researchers usually arrange the pairs (as they appear when the cell is dividing) in descending order of size and position of the centromere (the constriction between "arms"). The 23rd pair of chromosomes determines sex. It contains either a large X chromosome and a small Y chromosome (male) or two X chromosomes (female).

or a sex chromosome; thus for each gene position on a given autosome there is a *corresponding position on the partner or matching chromosome*. For a matching pair of genes one comes from the mother and the other from the father. As we have seen, the two genes may be of identical form or their form may differ in various degrees, often in an important way. Sexual reproduction makes human variation possible by making new combinations of the genes in random ways. Sex determination, for instance, is a matter of chance: whether an X- or a Y-carrying sperm fertilizes an egg. If a paternal X unites with a maternal X the offspring will be female (the normal female chromosomes are always XX). If a paternal Y unites with a maternal X, the offspring (XY) will be male. So, quite clearly, the maleness-determining Y chromosome must always come from the father; which means that the single X chromosome that a normal male carries is always from his mother. Of the two Xs of the normal female one is from her mother and the other from her father.

These facts are important when we consider X-linked (or sex-linked) characteristics or diseases.

A single characteristic will generally be determined by the interaction of a pair of matching genes (more complex characteristics involve two or more such pairs). Consider the relationship between two nonidentical gene forms of a given pair (such as an original gene and its mutant form). It may happen that the trait which the matching pair influences behaves as if it were determined entirely by the original gene, or conversely determined entirely by its mutant form. In the first case the trait (and its gene) is called dominant and the mutant character (and the mutant gene) recessive, while in the second case things are the other way round. What is true of traits in general is equally true of disease determined by the action of single genes. One might think of a recessive gene as weak, unable to generate its specific enzyme, or producing too little of it, or making an enzyme whose function is inadequate. If it is paired with its standard, or normal, partner gene, the latter takes over the job and no abnormal symptoms appear. However, if two recessive genes – one coming from each parent – unite, the inadequacy can no longer be compensated for and the recessive character or disease appears in the offspring. Conversely, a dominant trait is transmitted by a gene from only one parent, which overrides the effects of the matching gene of different form from the other parent.

Most inherited metabolic diseases are transmitted recessively through recessive genes on the autosomes. If only one parent has a recessive gene, he or she is a carrier, but offspring will be normal. It is only when both partners are carriers that affected children will be produced, one in four on average. The most common examples of these disorders are cystic fibrosis and sickle-cell disease. Dominant hereditary disorders are quite rare (for instance, Huntington's chorea, and a form of dwarfism). X-linked traits and diseases are also nearly always recessive, so that a woman who carries a recessive gene on only one of her two X chromosomes does not usually manifest its presence since it has a matching partner. However, if she transmits this X chromosome to her XY son he will manifest the trait because in him the recessive gene has no dominant matching partner to take over the job. This is why X-linked recessive conditions like colour blindness are much more common in men than women and are usually transmitted through the mother, who is a carrier but does not have the condition herself.

In summary, in families with autosomal recessive disorders both parents of an affected child are almost invariably without symptoms, but both are carriers of the gene for the disease. In families with an X-linked recessive disease it is the male members who are affected and their sisters who may be carriers of the recessive gene. In a family with a history of a dominant hereditary disorder the affected members transmit the disease on average to half of their children. But in families in which a dominant disorder shows up irregularly, or appears only in later adulthood (as for example in Huntington's chorea), members who carry the gene, though not affected, have a 50–50 chance of transmitting it, and any child who receives this gene *may* manifest the disease. This obviously creates a difficult counselling problem.

What the odds mean

A statement of odds is a statement about chances or probabilities, not about certainties, but it gives a basis for decisions. If a child has a recessively transmitted disease, the chances that a subsequent child of the parents will have the disease are one in four, that is there is a 75 per cent chance that the next child will not be affected. If a disorder is dominantly transmitted there is a 50 per cent chance that offspring will be affected. Whatever the odds, it is quite possible that a given hereditary defect will appear in none of the children of a couple, or in all of them. Given the chances of one in four or one in two of producing an affected child, the birth of such an affected child does not alter the odds in the case of simply inherited conditions. For the next child the chance still remains one in four, or one in two. However, the birth of an affected child may make a difference in disorders in which the reasons for recurrence risk are complex. For example, if a couple has no affected children with neural tube defects (anencephaly, spina bifida) the risk in some regions may be about one in 200. Following the birth of an affected child the risk may rise to about one in 25; but following a second affected child the risk may be about one in eight.

Diagnosis and counselling

If presumptive hereditary diseases or birth defects are a cause for worry, the first step is accurate diagnosis. Rare and complex conditions may require careful investigation, detailed knowledge of genetics, and careful clinical and laboratory investigation. There are, for example, several forms of hereditary muscular dystrophy, and of deafness. Moreover, their manner of inheritance as well as their evolution with time can be quite different; and, further, some kinds of deafness may not be inherited though they may mimic inherited forms.

In the last few years great progress has been made towards the identification in early pregnancy of fetuses affected by serious genetic disease, or disease with a genetic component. When the risk is high tests may allow a precise or highly probable diagnosis of abnormality to be made. Usually the suspicion that such a high risk exists in a family derives from the birth of a child affected by the disease or malformation in question. By these new diagnostic procedures counselling can turn from a numerical estimate of odds to a precise statement about a given pregnancy. If tests reveal that a fetus is seriously defective, the parents have a choice, strictly their own, of seeking termination of pregnancy or of having an abnormal child.

At present four different sets of abnormalities of the fetus can be identified, but it must be stressed that the

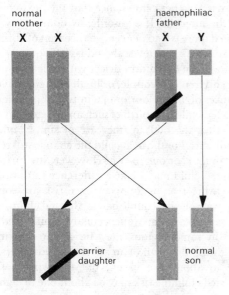

The inheritance of haemophilia

normal mother — X X

haemophiliac father — X Y

carrier daughter

normal son

The possible results of a marriage between a normal woman and a haemophiliac man. The black bar indicates the gene which carries the trait.

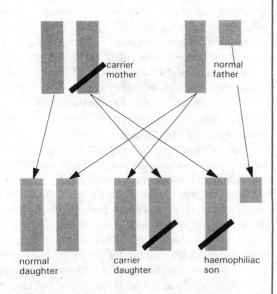

carrier mother

normal father

normal daughter

carrier daughter

haemophiliac son

The possible result of a marriage between a carrier woman and a normal man. The gene does not cause the disease in the carrier female because it is opposed by a normal gene on the other X chromosome. It causes the disease in the male because there is no corresponding normal gene to oppose its action.

tests are specific for one condition only; with one exception no multiple tests are carried out. So each test is capable only of answering a precise question, the one that is posed because of a high risk of a specific abnormality. The four sets of disorders are: a number of different specific inherited metabolic diseases; X-linked diseases (if the fetus is male he will almost always be affected); chromosome disorders, of which the main one is Down's syndrome (mongolism); neural tube malformations such as anencephaly or spina bifida. Diagnostic tests are carried out on the amniotic fluid, the fluid which surrounds the fetus in the womb and which can be obtained during pregnancy through an amniocentesis. This procedure consists in the withdrawal, through a hollow needle inserted into the mother's womb, of a sample of the fluid. The fluid contains fetal cells, which can be grown in culture, and other products mostly of fetal origin. The cells can be made to display their chromosomes, namely those of the fetus, or reveal their chemical functioning. Although considered to be safe in competent hands, amniocentesis is never to be resorted to lightly. It is invaluable if there is substantial risk of abnormality, as in a woman who has previously borne a child with a genetic disease, including Down's syndrome, or with anencephaly or spina bifida. In addition many specialists consider the test advisable if the mother is over 38 to 40 years old, because older women have a greater risk of giving birth to an infant with Down's syndrome or other chromosome disorders. The best time for amniocentesis is around the sixteenth week of pregnancy. Analysis takes about two to four weeks.

At present some 60 different inherited, grave, and incurable metabolic diseases can be diagnosed, each by a specific test, usually of a chemical nature.

The sex of the fetus can be determined by amniocentesis, and this is sometimes important for the purposes of genetic counselling. For example, the X-linked disease haemophilia cannot be recognised prenatally. However, if a high risk fetus is found to be female, the baby will not have haemophilia, although she may be a carrier like her mother; a male fetus, though, has a fifty per cent chance of being a haemophiliac, and the parents might consider termination of such a high risk pregnancy. In the near future, however, direct identification of haemophilia and other disorders of this type will become possible.

Chromosome studies

A number of birth defects can be diagnosed by finding abnormalities of structure in the number of chromosomes. Most such defects arise anew during the making of the germ cells. The most common chromosomal birth defect detectable by amniocentesis is Down's syndrome (mongolism) which affects about one in 600 newborn infants. There is a striking association between the frequency of Down's syndrome and the age of the mother. The affected child has a characteristic appearance, mental retardation, abnormalities of many systems of the body and is vulnerable to infections. These abnormalities are caused by an extra chromosome (No. 21), which is present because of a defect arising in the process of separation of chromosomes during the development of germ cells. The parents practically always have normal chromosomes. Chances that a subsequent child will be normal are quite good. Nevertheless the recurrence risk is generally increased regardless of the age of the mother.

A different, quite rare, form of Down's syndrome, seen proportionally more often among the affected infants born to younger women has a distinctive chromosome pattern: one chromosome (usually No. 14) carries a chromosome No. 21 attached to it. Thus, as in the standard chromosome type of Down's syndrome, there are *three* chromosomes No. 21, though *only two are free*. This form of Down's syndrome is often hereditary. One of the parents carries the attached chromosome No. 21 and *a single free No. 21* and thus, with two chromosomes No. 21, is not affected. If the mother is the carrier there is a ten per cent chance that her children will have Down's syndrome, but the risk is only two per cent when the father is the carrier. Differences in two seemingly identical disorders underline the importance of fine discrimination when undertaking genetic studies.

Conclusions

Although distressing symptoms of various disorders can often be relieved there is no useful treatment and at present no cure for most diseases in which the underlying defect is in the genes or chromosomes. Modifications of diet, if begun early, may prevent mental retardation in cases of galactosaemia and phenylketonuria. Cystic fibrosis of the pancreas may respond to pancreatic enzymes and mist inhalations. There is reason to hope that genetic disease may some day be more widely treatable and actually cured by other methods, for example, the implantation of normal cells into affected people – so that they may manufacture missing enzymes – or the actual administration, by suitable means, of purified enzymes to take over the functions of those that are defective. Research is exploring these and some other possibilities.

If the risk that some serious genetic condition will recur can be stated only in terms of odds, say one chance in four, the risks are real when viewed against the average background risk of about one in 30 (see above), but not so overwhelming as to be totally unacceptable to every couple. For some couples and some conditions termination of pregnancy may be the best course.

Genetic diseases vary in implication and handicap. Furthermore many developmental birth defects have no appreciable genetic basis. Not a few worries about alleged hereditary defects arise from misunderstanding. Genetic counselling can bring the facts to light and be of real help this way and in many other ways, as indicated.

Where to seek help The first source of help in matters of inherited disorders is the family doctor who, if necessary, can refer patients to reliable counselling centres. There are also assessment centres where a specialist can determine an infant's medical, social, and educational problems and recommend treatment and management in consultation with the family doctor and the parents. Another similar type of service is offered by handicapped children centres. Few communities are far away from laboratory and counselling services.

People or families who wish to know where genetic counselling is available can request a free list of such services. In the United Kingdom lists are published by the Department of Health and Social Security, Alexander Fleming House, Elephant and Castle, London SE1. There are also a number of societies and associations which will help sufferers from genetic diseases – such as:

Cystic Fibrosis Research Trust,
5 Blyth Road, Bromley, Kent BR1 3RS.

Down's Babies Association,
Quinborne Community Centre,
Ridgacre Road, Quinton, Birmingham B32 2TW.

Haemophilia Society, P.O. Box 9,
16 Trinity Street, London SE1 1DE.

National Society for Mentally Handicapped Children,
117 Golden Lane, London EC1.

Association for Spina Bifida and Hydrocephalus,
Tavistock House North, Tavistock Square,
London WC1H 9HT.

Chapter 27

Cancer

Revised by Sir Thomas Symington, MD

Throughout this book the authors have discussed cancer in relation to their medical specialties, since treatment is different according to the varying forms of cancer and in individual patients. The present chapter concerns general aspects of cancer and the current basis for research programmes which give hope that fundamental knowledge will lead to better measures of treatment, prevention, and control.

General features of cancer

Cancer is not inevitably fatal if it is promptly recognized and treated. More than one out of three cancer patients survives five years or longer and many are permanently cured. Prospects of successful treatment of some forms of cancer are excellent; for some other forms, the outlook is less heartening. Although cancer may exist for some time before it is detected or causes symptoms, authorities generally agree that early discovery and treatment enhance the prospects of cure. No little responsibility rests upon us as individuals to be aware of signals which may (or may not) warn of cancer, and not to procrastinate in going to a doctor. Any of the following symptoms, if it persists for two weeks or more, calls for prompt attention by the sufferer and investigation by a doctor:

Unusual bleeding or discharge
A lump or thickening in the breast, or elsewhere
A sore that does not heal
Change in bowel or bladder habits
Hoarseness or cough
Indigestion or difficulty in swallowing
Change in size or colour of a wart or mole
Apparently unexplained loss of weight, or pallor

Regular physical examinations are important in personal defence. For women, these include cervical smear tests and breast examination. If anything suspicious is discovered, a tissue specimen (biopsy) may be taken, and specific tests and X-rays may be ordered. Sometimes an exploratory operation is deemed necessary to determine the nature and extent of a patient's condition. Many tumours and abnormal growths are benign (noncancerous), though not necessarily harmless. Cancer is said to be malignant because of its life-threatening capacity to spread to distant parts of the body (metastasis), to press upon and invade nearby organs, and to drain vital resources of the body. We usually think of cancer as a localized solid tumour, but it can be manifested in nonsolid structures, as in leukaemia, which affects the blood-forming organs.

What is cancer?

Cancer is not a single disease but a group of several hundred diseases with a common characteristic – uncontrolled invasive growth at the expense of normal body systems. Something transforms a living cell into a cancer cell, reduces its control over orderly growth and function, and transmits this abnormality to succeeding cell generations. Many factors are associated with the occurrence of cancer, such as ageing, genetics, inhalation or ingestion of innumerable kinds of chemicals, radiation, sunlight, and chronic irritation, but the basic cause of cancer is unknown. Whatever the cause, it is now thought that we know where it acts. A cancer cell's heredity, its genetic control of orderly function, is drastically changed. This must involve a chemical change in the genes and nucleic acids of the cell (DNA), which control life processes. The main purpose of research is to find out what makes a living cell cancerous and then keeps it that way. Heredity-controlling molecules – nucleic acids – are now the prime targets of cancer research.

Carcinogenesis

Carcinogenesis is the name applied to the process by which a carcinogen, which may be a chemical substance, physical agent such as ultraviolet light or exposure to X-rays, or a virus, causes changes in the DNA of the cell nucleus which are faithfully replicated. Cell mutation occurs and, by some unknown means, malignancy results. This is the basis of the cell theory of carcinogenesis.

Chemical agents, inhaled or ingested, are believed to be the cause of 80 per cent of human cancer. The process by which cell mutation is believed to result can be followed below, where the carcinogen is a chemical substance (polycyclic hydrocarbon or aromatic amine) to which man may be exposed, particularly in occupational and industrial contact. The chemical makes its way (intercalates) between the bases which are important parts of the DNA of the cell nucleus. In this diagram the carcinogen is shown between the bases adenine (A) and guanine (G) of the upper strand of DNA. During DNA replication followed by cell division the lower strand of DNA, being normal, will faithfully reproduce normal daughter cells. Thus guanine (G) will form opposite cytosine (C), thymine (T) opposite adenine (A), and so on in accordance with the principles laid down by

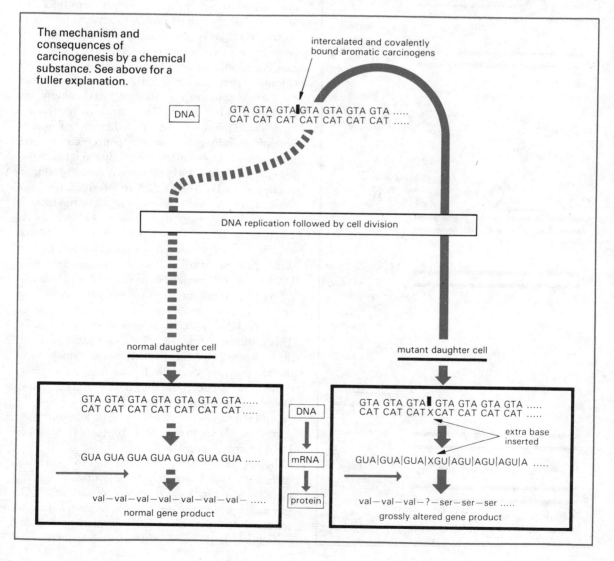

The mechanism and consequences of carcinogenesis by a chemical substance. See above for a fuller explanation.

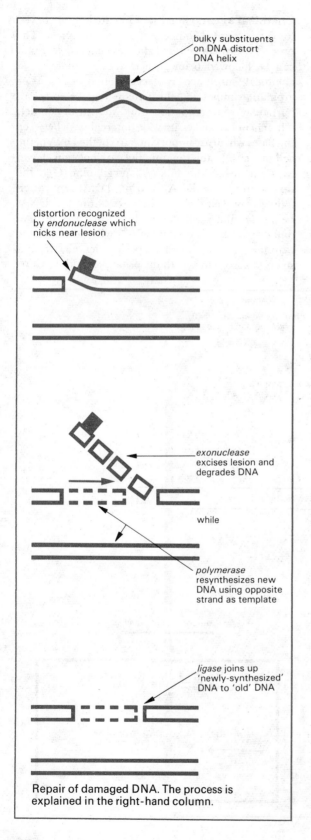

bulky substituents on DNA distort DNA helix

distortion recognized by *endonuclease* which nicks near lesion

exonuclease excises lesion and degrades DNA

while

polymerase resynthesizes new DNA using opposite strand as template

ligase joins up 'newly-synthesized' DNA to 'old' DNA

Repair of damaged DNA. The process is explained in the right-hand column.

Crick and Watson and illustrated by Watson in his book, *The Double Helix*. The DNA of this normal daughter cell will give rise to normal messenger RNA (mRNA) and normal gene products (proteins). However, during replication of the upper strand, the intercalated hydrocarbon is misread, an extra base is inserted at X, a mutant daughter cell results and faulty mRNA and proteins are formed. While such changes can explain cell mutation, it is still not clear how this process progresses to malignancy in the cell, and this is an area of active research.

Activation and inactivation of chemical carcinogens Since we are exposed to environmental chemical carcinogens every day of our lives it is surprising that cancer is not more common. To understand this, it is necessary to look at the existence of protective mechanisms in the cell cytoplasm and nucleus. Many chemical carcinogens are insoluble and accordingly inactive when taken into the body. However, the cell possesses in its cytoplasm a series of enzymes which can convert an inactive chemical carcinogen into an active one. Similarly, in the cell cytoplasm there is another enzyme which can render the active carcinogen inactive. Accordingly, in assessing the ability of a cell to activate or inactivate a chemical carcinogen and to predict the effect of a potential carcinogen, it would be necessary to take into account the balance of activating and inactivating enzymes in the cell cytoplasm. If a man or woman is a heavy smoker, their ability to inactivate the large amount of activated carcinogen in cigarette smoke is less than if they were light smokers or nonsmokers and so their chance of developing lung cancer is much greater. If the activated chemical carcinogen in sufficient concentration does reach and unite with DNA in the cell nucleus to produce bulky abnormal substances, there are mechanisms by which the affected cell can recognize and repair the chemically damaged DNA which has distorted the DNA helix. This is shown on the left. The abnormality is recognized by an enzyme, endonuclease, which nicks the abnormality near the lesion. Another enzyme, exonuclease, cuts out the lesion and degrades DNA while polymerase makes new DNA using the opposite strand as a template. A ligase joins up newly synthesized DNA to old DNA. In this way damaged DNA returns to normal.

In summary, when a cell is exposed to a chemical carcinogen, the latter may be activated in the cell cytoplasm and in this form can react with DNA. On the other hand, the activated carcinogen can be rendered inactive by other enzymes in the cell cytoplasm. If the activated carcinogen produces a bulky abnormality of the DNA, excision repair of the damaged DNA is carried out. It is perhaps only when the chemically damaged DNA is small in amount and is not recognized that defective replication occurs and leads to cell mutation.

Viruses There is no conclusive proof that viruses cause human cancers, but few scientists seriously doubt that they can. Numerous animal cancers are known to be caused by viruses, and there is no known biological reason why man alone should be immune. Viruses have their own genetic codes for transmitting hereditary traits. They contain the same classes of nucleic acids (DNA or RNA) as other forms of life. Their genetic machinery is enclosed in a protein coat which plays a part in causing familiar viral infections. Hypothetical ways in which viruses may cause cancer are mysteriously different from the ways in which we catch common viral diseases. One hypothesis is that a virus inserts some of its genetic material into the nucleic acids of a normal living cell. This changes the heredity of the cell, like a bad gene which gives distorted directions for some life processes. The viral material "sickens" the cell's nucleic acids so that daughter cells inherit a trait of wild proliferation at the expense of normal cells – a characteristic of cancer. Enormous difficulties confront investigators. The cancer-causing viral gene may lie latent for a long time until other factors, such as the chemical carcinogen mentioned or physical agents, trigger it into action. The viral part may be so broken up or so transformed that it is difficult for investigators to recognize it as having originated in a virus.

Immunity to cancer

If cells exposed to chemical or physical agents or to viruses undergo malignant transformation, the body recognizes them as abnormal and destroys them. This is the immunological theory of cancer defence. It seems likely that we all produce a few cancer cells every day but never know it. So-called immune systems defend the body against foreign agents by recognizing things that are not "self" and destroying them. We are most familiar with immunizing procedures such as vaccination, but defence systems are constantly alert to operate against anything foreign that gets into the body. Cancer cells are presumably different enough from normal cells to be recognized as foreign and rejected before they can gain a foothold.

There is, at least, considerable evidence that immunity is somehow involved in cancer. Patients who receive organ transplants are given drugs which suppress their immune systems, to improve the chances that the transplant will not be recognized and rejected as a foreign body. Such patients have an increased risk of developing cancer later. Many cancer patients have impairment of immune response, although whether this is a cause or a result of cancer is not known. Researchers are studying the surfaces of cells, where most immunological events are initiated, and looking into cancer cells for antigens which could be latent chemical fingerprints of long-vanished viruses.

Towards better therapies

Research pathways take unexpected turns and new directions. One can only make informed guesses about possible cancer cures and preventives that lie in the future. If specific chemical events that induce cells to become cancerous are discovered, chemicals to act against them and turn them off are conceivable. Little is known about constitutional differences of different kinds of cells, of the lung, uterus, bowel, and so on, which imply chemical differences in forms of cancer. If understood, the differences may lead to highly selective treatments which affect specific tissues rather than the whole body. If our genes worked incessantly to carry out every order they contain, the result would be chaos – mob rule instead of teamwork. Monstrous overgrowth, not unlike cancer, would ensue if our genes were not inactive most of the time. Fortunately cells have mysterious control units, probably chemical, which are sensitive to external conditions and give feedback orders that regulate gene activity. Repressor molecules that turn off gene activities have been identified in living cells. A repressor chemical that could stop the action of a malignant gene would be a cancer cure.

So-called "genetic engineering" has a futuristic sound. The concept is that human genes, and hence heredity, may be alterable by inserting correct genetic information into living cells, perhaps with the transport help of harmless viruses. Much speculation along this and related lines concerns management of genetic diseases, discussed in the preceding chapter, but ultimate discoveries would be just as relevant to cancer if, as many investigators believe, cancer is basically a disease of DNA.

Chapter 28
Drug use and abuse

Revised by Richard de Alarcon, MD FRCPsych

Many modern drugs have healing properties that would have been undreamt of a generation ago. Unfortunately the unquestioned benefits of properly used drugs can be endangered by the belief held by many people that medicines have the magic power to overcome the ordinary stresses of life and that there is a harmless pill for every problem. This is not true, and this way of thinking is not only unrealistic but also fraught with dangers, as it may lead to unwise self-medication and overmedication, and to the use of pills to feel carefree or "pepped-up", thus opening the doors to drug abuse and addiction. In a society where pill takers are prevalent it is important that we develop a healthy respect for all medical drugs and that we take our medicines exactly as directed. No drug is totally safe for all persons in all doses at all times. Over-the-counter drugs bought without a prescription are useful in many minor conditions, and their safety rests on the assumption that they will be taken exactly as specified on the instructions.

Drugs that can be obtained only on prescription differ from those bought over the counter in that they usually have a much smaller safety margin or can be harmful except when taken for a specific illness. They can be prescribed only by a doctor. The label of a prescription drug specifies the only person for whom the medicine is intended, and when and in what amounts it should be taken. It also states the name of the drug and the dosage. Unless for a chronic condition, expected to go on for months or years, prescription drugs should be discarded or returned to the pharmacist after recovery from the illness. Drugs can deteriorate and a stockpile of old drugs tempts one to take one or two tablets when not feeling well, or even to give them to others. This can be a dangerous thing, as it is difficult for the layman to know whether such and such a drug is indicated. Do not hoard drugs. Keep current drugs in a medicine cabinet, well apart from cosmetics and tooth brushes. Do not keep pills in handbags or on kitchen shelves where children can get at them. Teach children not to take medicines except those given to them, because other kinds of pretty pills might make them very sick. Remember that children tend to model their drug-taking behaviour on that of their parents. Set an example in the home. Bear in mind that it is not only the small child taking a pill accidentally who is at risk but also the adolescent who may be tempted to raid the medicine cupboard and try out some of the drugs "for kicks".

Dangerous drugs

Any drug is dangerous if taken to excess; some are dangerous when taken with other drugs – this is why a prescribed medicine should not be taken simultaneously with any other drug, however harmless the latter may seem, without consulting the prescribing doctor. In the present chapter the term dangerous drugs will refer to those which are taken by certain people not for a medical purpose, but mainly for their pleasurable or euphorizing effects. All these drugs affect the mind and mood even if only for a few hours and several of them lead to physical or psychological dependence. When taken regularly and in large amounts they affect not only mind and body but also the person's whole way of life. A vast illegal traffic spread over many countries has developed to supply these drugs to people who take them for nonmedical reasons.

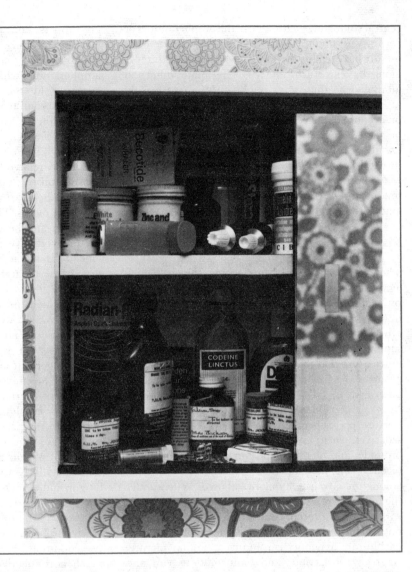

An example of the danger in many homes.

The main groups of drugs commonly open to abuse are the following:

Opiates

These include all the drugs obtained from the opium poppy such as opium, morphine, heroin, and codeine as well as a few synthetic drugs with morphine-like action, for example, pethidine. They are also known as narcotics. They are extremely valuable in medicine and surgery to relieve severe pain. Opiates quickly induce physical dependence. The body gets used to them, and then if they are stopped it cannot function properly and severe withdrawal symptoms develop. This makes opiates such dangerous drugs if taken for nonmedical reasons. Experimenters who think "I'll try it once or twice", "It cannot happen to me" easily become hooked and find they cannot do without the drug.

At present heroin is the opiate most commonly abused. It is a white powder that is much more powerful than morphine; heroin on the black market is often sold adulterated with quinine or other substances. It is usually injected into a vein but the powder can also be sniffed. On injection there is a marked reduction of tension and a small period of euphoria followed by drowsiness. Symptoms associated with heroin are blocked nose and sniffing, itchy skin, drowsiness, constipation, and contracted pupils. As the effects of the drug disappear the person, if strongly addicted, will become restless and increasingly anxious and after some hours severe withdrawal symptoms may appear if another dose is not injected. Often heroin is injected together with a central stimulant, such as one of the amphetamines or cocaine, to counteract the drowsiness. Chronic users usually have scars, abscesses, needle marks and tracks along the veins of arms and legs. The opiate addict and all those who abuse any drug by injection are greatly at risk of contracting serious illness and infections on account of the contaminated needles and syringes or the adulterants added to the drugs they take. Overdoses, frequently fatal, are also a constant threat. Life expectancy is reduced by fifteen to twenty years. Fortunately heroin and other opiate users are a small minority – though a severely affected one – among those who abuse drugs.

Hypnotics and sedatives

These include all types of sleeping tablets, which again are valuable medicines, but can be misused by respectable middle-aged people taking them quietly in private, by youngsters sharing them with others, or by the heavily involved addicts when opiate supplies are scarce or they wish to complement the other drugs that they are taking. The most powerful group is the barbiturates – their proprietary name often ends in "al", such as Seconal and Nembutal. Many household medicine cabinets contain barbiturates prescribed in the past. Nonbarbiturate sedatives, such as chloral hydrate, glutethimide, bromide, and many others, can also be misused. In recent years methaqualone (Mandrax) has been among the favourite hypnotics abused. When under the influence of a barbiturate, people act as if drunk, with slurred speech, uncoordinated movements, unsteady gait, and impaired judgement. The nonbarbiturate hypnotics can induce a similar picture. Aggressive behaviour and hallucinations can also occur. With the barbiturates particularly, a strong physical dependence develops among heavy regular users, and, if the drug is suddenly withdrawn, convulsions, twitching, agitation, and even death may occur. This is an acute medical emergency requiring hospitalization and intensive care. With any kind of sleeping pill there is also the risk of an accidental or intentional overdose. Alcohol and sleeping pills intensify each other's action, and relatively small doses of alcohol and certain sleeping pills if taken together can prove fatal. The same danger applies to sedatives and tranquillizers.

Stimulants

Whilst the slang terms for the hypnotics are downers and sleepers, the equivalent names for the stimulants are uppers and pep pills. These drugs increase alertness, produce a feeling of wellbeing, and reduce appetite. The most common stimulants are the amphetamines which are made as tablets, powder, or ampoules for injection. They have also been produced in combination with a barbiturate, such as the "purple hearts" which were much in vogue in Britain a few years back. There are other drugs such as methylphenidate hydrochloride (Ritalin) which are closely related to the amphetamines in action and can be abused in the same way. The amphetamines increase the heart rate, raise the blood pressure, and dilate the pupils. They cause palpitations, dry mouth, sweating, and headaches. Large amounts make the person overactive, unstable, talkative, and sometimes violent. If taken regularly in large amounts, they may cause mental symptoms in the form of hallucinations, ideas of persecution, and acute agitation. Sporadic users may occasionally take amphetamines to stay awake, drive long hours, or study for an examination. This type of use rarely leads to difficulties, but it can have a disorganizing effect upon judgement and if the person takes these drugs regularly he may come to rely on them whenever situations requiring some extra effort arise, or simply because he has developed a taste for their euphorizing action. In the past they were prescribed as appetite suppressants in cases of overweight or for the treatment of mild depression, but when the drug is taken regularly the person may come to fear the fatigue and depression that occur when it is stopped, and so become dependent on it. This was a common occurrence, mainly among middle-aged women, when amphetamines were prescribed for one of these two conditions. Fortunately in recent years safer and much more effective ways for treating both depressive illnesses and overweight have been discovered.

A more disturbing form of amphetamine abuse has been the widespread taking of the drug by the young since the early 1960's. For many it never went beyond the taking of amphetamines over the weekend with their friends in a setting of all-night dance halls, joy rides, and adolescent antisocial behaviour. For others, however, it led not only to the gradual taking of amphetamines during weekdays, but also to the injection of amphetamines as well as to a deeper involvement and experimentation with other drugs. The amphetamines can also be injected into a vein. Fortunately this is practised by a much smaller number of people than the adolescent and middle-aged users described above. Injection usually implies a heavier commitment to drug taking, and the majority of persons who inject amphetamines will also be injecting opiates or barbiturates and taking other drugs. The risks here are the same as those mentioned earlier for the opiates.

Cocaine Although this is a brain stimulant, some of its derivatives are useful in medicine as local anaesthetics. It is abused for the feeling of euphoria it produces. Heavy drug users take it by injection combined with heroin, but more commonly it is sniffed as a white powder. Strong dependence can develop and chronic use can, as with the amphetamines, lead to hallucinations, agitation, antisocial behaviour, and mental disturbances.

Hallucinogens

These drugs, also known as psychedelics, differ from the group described above in that they have practically no part in the treatment of disease. Apart from their occasional use by some psychiatrists in controlled clinical conditions, they are not used in the field of medicine, and are taken only for the experiences and sensations they produce. Many of these drugs have been used from time immemorial by North and Central American Indians in their religious ceremonies. Features common to this group of drugs are the extraordinary mental reactions they can produce, such as visions, hallucinations, and weird distortion of sensation, perception, thinking, self-awareness, and emotions. Often there is an illusion that one gains fantastic insights into the meaning of things or oneself. For a time they were fashionable among certain writers and poets who became self-appointed propagandists of the drugs.

The most widely used hallucinogen is LSD (lysergic acid diethylamide). Others are mescaline, psilocybin, and STP. LSD, often called "acid', is so potent that 30 gm (one oz) is enough for half a million doses. The drug can be taken in pill or capsule form but minute amounts are often dropped onto sugar cubes or other food. Immediate physical effects are enlarged pupils, flushed face, chilliness, and sometimes increased heart rate. The mental effects follow. The effects of LSD may be experienced as pleasant ("a good trip"), or take on a terrifying character with panic and horror ("a bad trip"). Although LSD and other hallucinogens do not produce dependence, their potential dangers should not be understated as not only can they unsettle the ordinary rhythm of life but also produce an acute panic state with wild behaviour and possible harm to the taker and others. In a few vulnerable persons mental illnesses lasting several months have been seen after LSD.

Cannabis

Another substance which at present has practically no medical use in Western medicine is cannabis, known also as marijuana or "pot". It is the dried material from the Indian hemp plant and resembles coarse tobacco. It is smoked rolled in cigarettes or in a pipe, and has a characteristic smell which has been compared with burning rope or leaves. Smokers sometimes try to mask this smell by burning joss sticks or incense. The plant produces a resin which contains the active principle. Poor quality stock is mild and contains a fair proportion of seeds, stalks, and leaves of low resin content. A much stronger variety is hashish which is the concentrated resin of the plant compressed into a mass from which portions are broken off to smoke.

The immediate physical effects of marijuana include reddening of the eyes, increased heart rate, and cough due to the irritating effects of the smoke. Mood effects vary. Time may seem extended, sounds and colours intensified. There may be a false feeling that one is thinking more keenly. Some experimenters get very little reaction, others find the effects unpleasant. The user may be relaxed, happy, silly, talkative, or may withdraw into himself. The smoking of cannabis has become widespread in the last decade. Its use covers the whole range from the experimenter or occasional smoker to the heavy regular user. In Britain the person who smokes cannabis daily or heavily is likely to be involved with other drugs and his work pattern and style of life often will be that of the heavy drug user. Cannabis does not produce physical dependence, but heavy chronic users may become psychologically dependent on it. There is no evidence that cannabis in itself leads to other and more dangerous drugs. Given the large numbers who have tried it, occasional use appears to be harmless from the medical point of view. More important than the drug itself is with whom it is taken. It is one thing to smoke it with one or more curious youngsters, another to do so in the company of people who are more committed to a drug-taking way of life and are likely to be taking other drugs also. The latter situation cannot be taken lightly as it is fraught with potential risk.

Sniffing

Some youngsters, even ten-year-olds, take to sniffing the vapours of volatile substances from plastic bags or directly from aerosol cans, expecting to get a feeling of exhilaration. They develop symptoms resembling drunkenness: slurred speech, double vision, unsteadiness, drowsiness. Substances favoured by sniffers include model glue, varnish, paint thinners, cleaning and lighter fluids, gasoline, spray-paint, refrigerants, spot removers, benzine, and any other vaporous substance they can experiment with. Some of these substances are immediately dangerous and some are cumulatively toxic when repeatedly used. They may cause temporary blindness and damage to bone marrow, kidneys, liver, brain, and lungs. Sudden death has resulted from paralysis of breathing following inhalation of freezing sprays, and from inhalation of some substances that act rapidly and irreversibly, so that there is no escape.

Alcohol

Last but not least is alcohol, which is the substance most widely abused. The effects of acute alcoholic intoxication and its consequences of impaired judgement and coordination are too well-known to require description. Occasional or social drinkers (the great majority) control their intake reasonably well even though their consumption may be quite impressive. Some problem drinkers go on several drinking sprees a year which may last for two days or more with intervening periods of sobriety. Another, often undiagnosed, form of problem drinking is that of the housewife who drinks secretly on her own during the day. If alcohol is consumed regularly and heavily over a number of years – usually about ten, though some people manage to shorten this period considerably – physical dependence on alcohol develops, and acute withdrawal symptoms may appear in the form of alcoholic hallucinations or delirium tremens if intake is suddenly stopped. This is an acute medical emergency requiring hospital care. Uncontrolled chronic heavy drinking disrupts work, family, and in fact the person's whole life, as well as physical health. Eventually the liver and the brain may be damaged permanently. The cure for alcoholism is abstention, which obviously requires great motivation on the part of the alcoholic. Chances of success are reasonably good if the alcoholic is not too old and has the emotional support of his family and friends; they are not so good if he has been drinking to excess for many years, is lonely most of the day and night, has nobody who depends on him (or her), and nobody who cares. Medical treatment is essential in the management of acute alcoholism and delirium tremens. Following withdrawal and the rebuilding of physical health, a long programme of rehabilitation lies ahead. The value of medical help at this stage is doubtful, except for some form of group therapy. A willing patient may benefit more from the active support of bodies like Alcoholics Anonymous, composed of ex-alcoholics who give aid, understanding, and fellowship to group members. In Britain advice and help may be obtained by telephoning the local branch of the National Council on Alcoholism or of Alcoholics Anonymous. A few psychiatrists specialize in the problems of alcoholism.

Treatment of drug misuse

From the description given above it should be clear that there are many different patterns of drug misuse, some more serious than others. At one end of the scale is the experimenter or occasional user whose drug taking is of little or no medical consequence. At the other are the alcoholic and the heavily committed drug taker who will use or have used a wide variety of drugs by mouth, inhalation, or injection. Life style and often health are likely to have been affected by drug taking. In the latter group the treatment is usually medical. Treatment and withdrawal are difficult to manage and are better carried out in hospital. As in the case of alcohol, it is in the subsequent rehabilitation where the success or failure of the treatment lies. This is easy to understand when one considers that the person has to learn to accept a life without drugs, make new friends among people with whom for many years perhaps he has had little in common, and develop new habits of perseverance. In many instances it will also require the person to achieve some changes in his set of values and in the way he regards himself, life, and the world at large. Here nonmedical bodies can often be of greater help than medically trained or orientated persons. With the occasional or less heavily involved drug taker it is in many cases a matter of adolescent curiosity, experimentation, or rebellion. In some cases, however, there may be a background of emotional problems or maladjustment, and drug taking, in the same way as delinquency, may be a way of acting out these inner conflicts. Expert help may be required here, but not necessarily from a Drug Addiction Unit which caters for a different type of drug taker, but from organizations experienced in helping adolescents.

The address of Alcoholics Anonymous is:

11 Redcliffe Gardens, London SW10 9BG.
There are branches in most large towns.

National Council on Alcoholism,
3 Grosvenor Crescent, London SW1X 3EE.
There are also regional councils.

Chapter 29

First aid

This chapter is based mainly on the *Digest of First Aid* published by the St. John Ambulance Association, with the permission and kind assistance of the Chief Medical Officer of the Association, P. A. B. Raffle, MD FRCP K.St.John.

Principles and practice of first aid

First aid is literally *first* aid, that is what to do before the doctor arrives. It is not a substitute for professional medical help.

First aid is based on the principles of practical medicine and surgery; a knowledge of the subject in case of accident or sudden illness enables trained persons to give such skilled assistance as will preserve life, promote recovery, and prevent the injury or illness from becoming worse until medical aid has been obtained. First aid consists of simple measures that anyone can learn, but if carried out correctly, quickly, gently, and as early as possible, they can be life-saving, and may prevent the necessity for more complicated treatment later which may be too late to save life. It includes the necessity of giving the casualty confidence by talking to him and by reassuring him.

The first-aider's responsibility ends when the casualty is handed over to the care of a doctor, nurse, or other responsible person, but not until they have taken over the whole responsibility for the case. The first-aider should not leave until he has made his report to the doctor or other responsible person, and has ascertained whether he could be of any further help. First aid, in general, is limited to the assistance rendered at the time of the emergency, with such material as is available, and often extensive improvisation will be necessary.

Remember at all times the importance of common sense in first aid as an addition to the actual knowledge of the subject. First aid manuals usually consider for treatment only one condition at a time. However, in real life it is found that serious accidents rarely produce only one single injury. Frequently, two injuries or more occur close together so that the correct treatment of one may interfere with the correct treatment of the other. One injury may require the casualty to be put on his back, but another that he should be in the recovery position. In such circumstances the first-aider must decide which injury is the most serious, or needs the most urgent treatment and treat that one in the correct way and then deal with the second injury as correctly as possible in the conflicting circumstances.

First aid consists of three parts:

1 Dealing with the situation, apart from the casualty.
2 Diagnosing what is the matter with the casualty and then giving the correct first aid treatment.
3 Disposing of the casualty, to doctor, hospital, or home and notifying those concerned about the accident.

In arriving at the diagnosis the first-aider is guided by:

1 The report given by persons present (which includes the conscious casualty) as to the cause of the injury or illness – HISTORY.
2 The account given by the casualty of his own sensations and feelings – SYMPTOMS.
3 His complete examination of the patient – SIGNS.

The situation Be calm and take charge. Ensure safety from traffic, fire, water, theft, the possibility of falling masonry, and so on. Ask those present to remain if they are able to help; otherwise they should be requested to stand clear. Give each one a specific job, for example:

Ring up and notify the Police.
Ask for an ambulance.

LIFE-SAVING MEASURES

Breathing stopped If the victim stops breathing, he will die unless breathing is restored at once. First tilt his head back to open the air passage from mouth to lungs, squeeze the nostrils together, then BLOW your own breath firmly through his mouth into his lungs. Repeat this at your own breathing rate until his is restored. See page 585.

Bleeding Bleeding from injuries must be controlled, as severe loss of blood may lead to death. The best way to stop bleeding is to squeeze the injured part together by direct PRESSURE of the fingers on the wound or squeeze the edges of the wound together. See page 588–9.

Unconsciousness The willing but untrained bystander is most helpless when confronted with the UNCONSCIOUS victim. The simple act of turning such a victim on his side, in the RECOVERY position so that he cannot drown in his own vomit, may save his life. See page 592.

Shock Shock is likely to be present in all cases of injury and many cases of sudden illness. Its effects, which may be extremely serious, can be made less severe by the comfort, confidence, and REASSURANCE supplied by the rescuer. See page 593.

Broken bones These are serious injuries. Stop any MOVEMENT of broken bones which may make the injury more severe. Injured limbs may be secured to the body or the other uninjured limb.

Burns and scalds These are common injuries and if a large part of the body is involved death may result. COOL the affected area with cold water, then cover with clean cloth or large dressing until it can be seen by a doctor.

Procedure for motor accidents See page 600.

Prevention of household accidents
See page 604.

In each case, state the place of the accident and describe what has happened.

Ask if anyone has any first aid knowledge. Ask for help in turning the casualty or in steadying a limb. In each case give exact instructions and, if necessary, show the bystander how your request should be carried out.

The casualty Depending on what has happened, the degree of severity of the injuries, and the circumstances, decide whether to treat the casualty where he is or whether to move him to a more suitable place. In a street accident note his exact position, as the Police may want to know this. If you decide to move him, carry out a quick preliminary examination of the head and neck, spine, and limbs. Then, decide on the most suitable method of removal in view of the injuries and the amount of skilled or unskilled help available. Then complete the examination of the casualty for injuries so that you can make a complete diagnosis and carry out the necessary treatment.

Stay with the casualty and reassure him until the ambulance or other aid arrives. Give your report and, if necessary, accompany the casualty to hospital and report there. Notify the nearest relative and any other person or organization that should be told. In serious outdoor accidents the Police should be sent for or notified.

The most urgent matters are:

1 To apply resuscitation if the casualty is not breathing.
2 To restart the heart if it has stopped beating.
3 To control bleeding.
4 To maintain a clear airway by correctly positioning the casualty.

If in doubt as to whether the casualty is alive or not, continue treatment until medical aid is available.

The most important procedures to prevent the condition becoming worse are:

1 To dress wounds.
2 To immobilize fractures and large wounds.
3 To place the casualty in the most comfortable position, consistent with the requirements of treatment.

Helpful measures in promoting recovery are:

1 To relieve the casualty of anxiety and promote his confidence.
2 To relieve him of pain and discomfort.
3 To protect him from the cold.
4 To handle him gently so as to do no harm.

579

Chapter 29 First aid

Priority in first aid

Do the things below quickly and methodically.

Reassure the casualty and those around, to lessen anxiety, while taking in the situation.

If breathing has stopped, start resuscitation.

Control visible bleeding.

Give priority to the most severe injuries.

Give priority where several are injured, to those who will benefit most by prompt treatment.

Guard against shock – and look for signs of internal bleeding.

Immobilize fractures and larger wounds before moving the casualty – handle gently.

Do not remove clothes unnecessarily, as this can be a painful or awkward procedure and the casualty may get cold.

Do not attempt too much – attend to essentials and prevent the condition from becoming worse.

Do not allow people to crowd round – they get in the way and may interfere with first aid procedures.

Arrange as soon as possible for careful conveyance of the casualty to hospital or to a doctor.

Breathing and resuscitation

Breathing is the mechanism of expansion and relaxation of the lungs by which, in normal circumstances, oxygen will pass from the air into the blood, while carbon dioxide, a waste product, is expelled from the blood by the lungs. The two lungs fill the greater part of the chest cavity, one on each side of the heart.

Respiration is carried out by the action of the diaphragm and the muscles between each pair of ribs. Air is drawn into the lungs (inspiration) and expelled from the lungs (expiration) at an average rate of eighteen times per minute in the adult. The more active the exercise, the faster will be the respiratory movement. Inspiration is produced by contraction of the diaphragm, whose dome-shaped centre becomes flattened and draws air in through the air passages. The ribs are raised by the action of the muscles between them and this also tends to increase the size of the chest and helps to suck air inwards. In expiration, air is forced out through the airway by the diaphragm and the ribs returning to their normal positions.

If an unconscious person is lying on his back there is the danger of the tongue falling back and blocking the airway. There is also the danger of secretions or regurgitated stomach contents entering the windpipe because of the epiglottis failing to function, which is why the recovery position must be used for the casualty.

The recovery position (see opposite) The casualty lies semi-prone, with his lower arm behind him and tucked in against his trunk – to prevent his rolling onto his back. The upper arm and leg are flexed as in the illustration – to prevent his rolling flat onto his face. The important thing is that his face should be inclined towards the ground. The object is to ensure that if vomit or other liquid comes up, it will pour out onto the ground and not down into the lungs.

Asphyxia Anything which interferes with the intake and absorption of oxygen (respiration) produces asphyxia. If the lungs do not receive a sufficient supply of fresh air, important organs, especially the brain, are deprived of oxygen. The result is loss of consciousness, and if the condition continues heart action will fail, causing death.

The commonest causes of asphyxia are:

1 *Those affecting the airway:*

Liquid in the air passages, as in drowning.

Foreign bodies in the air passages, such as portions of food or vomited matter getting into the windpipe.

Compression of the windpipe, as in throttling or hanging.

Smothering, as in overlaying of an infant.

Swelling of the tissues within the throat as a result of scalds or stings or infection.

2 *Those affecting the respiratory mechanism or control centres of the brain:*

Pressure or crushing of the chest.

Some acute infections of the nervous system such as tetanus and poliomyelitis.

Electric shock.

Harmful gases, such as coal gas, motor exhaust fumes, and after-damp in mines.

Poisons such as barbiturates, opium derivatives, and overdosage with some common household remedies, for example aspirin.

Rarefied atmosphere as experienced by mountain climbers, air travellers, and divers.

Symptoms and signs of asphyxia:

1 Breathing – rate and depth increase at first, later it can become noisy and frothing may occur from the mouth.

Recovery position

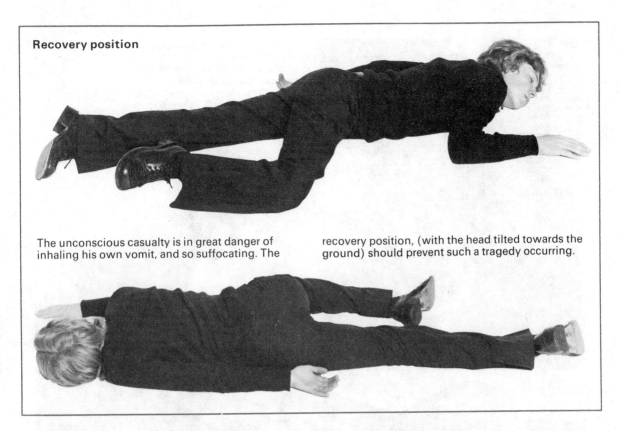

The unconscious casualty is in great danger of inhaling his own vomit, and so suffocating. The recovery position, (with the head tilted towards the ground) should prevent such a tragedy occurring.

2 Congestion of head and neck – resulting in swollen veins, lips, and face, and dizziness.
3 Face, lips, conjunctiva, and nail beds of fingers and toes are blue-grey (cyanosis).
4 Progressive loss of consciousness.
5 Fits may occur.

General treatment Depending on the cause and prevailing circumstances:

1 Remove the casualty from the cause, or the cause from the casualty.
2 Ensure an open airway and adequate air.
3 Start respiratory resuscitation at once. This must be continued until natural breathing is restored or until a doctor arrives.

Special treatments

Drowning While respiration is being restored, instruct bystanders to remove the casualty's wet clothing, rapidly dry him, and keep him wrapped in dry blankets.

Strangulation Cut and remove the constriction, while supporting the weight of the body in cases of hanging.

Choking A common incident at all ages. Although a foreign body may be present, the obstruction to breathing is largely due to spasm. The casualty has a fit of coughing. His face, neck, fingers, and toes are congested and may become blue. Violent and alarming attempts at inspiration are made. The object is to relieve the spasm, remove any foreign body and, if necessary, to get air into the lungs past the foreign body.

The method used is the same but its application differs somewhat depending on whether the casualty is an infant, a child, or an adult. First remove any obvious obstruction, such as false teeth or a lump of meat. If the obstruction is thought to be in the windpipe in the case of:

AN INFANT Hold infant by the legs. Smack him smartly three or four times between the shoulders.
A CHILD Lay the child prone with his head downwards over your knee. Give three or four sharp smacks between the shoulders.
AN ADULT Strike three or four sharp blows between the shoulders. After removing any debris from the throat, if necessary ventilate the lungs.

If the above method fails, stand behind the victim with your clasped fists over the upper abdomen. Then push upwards very strongly. Even if the obstructing material is successfully removed, it is wise for the patient to see a doctor.

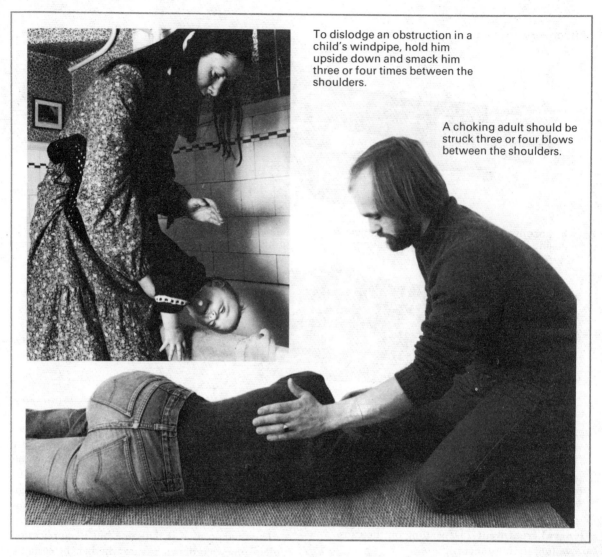

To dislodge an obstruction in a child's windpipe, hold him upside down and smack him three or four times between the shoulders.

A choking adult should be struck three or four blows between the shoulders.

Swelling of the tissues within the throat If the casualty is conscious, and can swallow, give ice or cold water by mouth.

Suffocation by smoke If no respirator is available and the casualty is easily accessible take a deep breath, pass quickly into the smoke-filled area and remove him to safety, both keeping as low as possible.

Suffocation by poisonous gases Take a deep breath and hold it. Pass quickly into the room, without breathing; remove casualty to safety. If possible, open doors and windows. The use of a lifeline by rescuers entering gas-filled chambers is of value in many cases.

Electrical injuries Even with domestic voltages, if an electric current passes through a person it may in some cases produce stoppage of breathing, burns, and cardiac arrest.

Treatment If possible, switch off the current or pull out the plug. Never attempt to cut the cable.

If it is not possible to switch off or break the current, the casualty must be removed from contact with it. Before doing so, ensure that you are properly insulated, otherwise you also may be affected.

With ordinary domestic voltages, sufficient insulation can be obtained by wearing rubber gloves or by standing on a rubber surface, or on partially insulating material, such as a thick carpet or thick layers of dry cloth or newspaper. Withdraw the casualty by grasping dry clothing or by pulling him away with a dry rope or walking stick. Avoid contact with anything damp or metallic. If breathing is absent, the heart will usually have stopped beating as well, so resuscitation of heartbeat and breathing must be started at once and continued until profes-

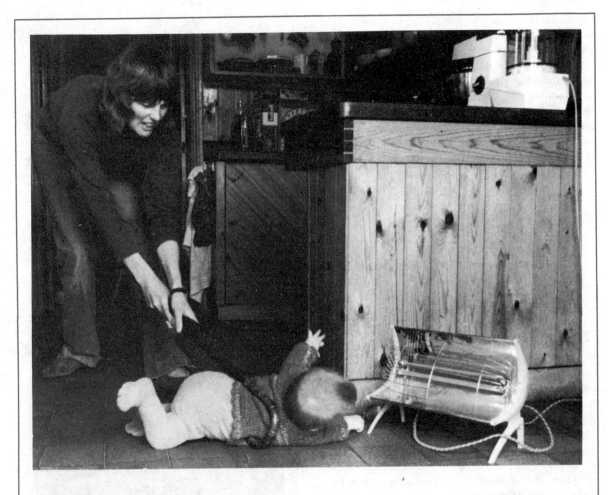

Be sure that you are insulated when attempting to rescue someone from contact with an electrical current.

sional help arrives, or natural breathing is restored.

With very high voltages, no rescue should be attempted unless specially clothed, equipped, and trained. It may even be dangerous to approach a casualty who has been thrown clear, but who is still in close proximity to the electric current.

Effect of oxygen deprivation If the brain is deprived of oxygen for four minutes, irreversible changes take place in it. The aim of respiratory resuscitation is the immediate oxygenation of the blood in order to forestall such changes.

Although the person performing this method passes on to the casualty some air that he has used himself, there is enough oxygen in it (fifteen per cent) compared with the 21 per cent in fresh air, to be effective.

The urgent need is for the lungs to be inflated.

Emergency resuscitation The mouth to mouth method of resuscitation is preferred. Its main advantage is that it can be more easily and effectively applied than other methods and used in some situations where they cannot; for example, in cases of drowning while the casualty is still in the water, or where he is trapped by a fall of earth and cannot be immediately released. Other advantages are:

It gives the greatest ventilation of the lungs and oxygenation of the blood.

The degree of inflation of the lungs can be assessed by watching the movement of the chest.

It is less tiring, does not require strength, and can be applied by a child.

Difficulty in employing this method, in cases of injury to the mouth or face and for other reasons, is recognized. There is an alternative method of

583

resuscitation, namely the Holger-Neilsen. This method, (described later) has the advantage that the rescuer can use it when there are facial injuries.

The aim of resuscitation is to prevent damage to the brain and other vital organs through lack of oxygen.

Prompt application can re-establish and maintain the casualty's oxygen requirements until breathing starts spontaneously, or is restored mechanically.

We breathe to live – the body's VITAL NEED IS AIR – seconds count.

The essential steps to be taken are:
Ensure an open airway. Ventilate the lungs.

If the casualty is not breathing:
1 Lay him on his back, on as firm a surface as possible. Remove false teeth.
2 Ensure a clear airway by pressing the top of the casualty's head backwards while supporting the nape of the neck so as to extend the head.
3 Improve his airway by pressing forward the angles of the jaw from behind, or by pressing the chin forward.

NOTE: These manoeuvres extend the head on the neck and lift the tongue clear of the airway, particularly necessary in an unconscious casualty on his back when the tongue falls back and blocks the airway.

If breathing does not start now, his condition is serious. Remember, permanent damage to the brain will occur after four minutes without breathing.

When the obstruction to the airway has been relieved, and if the casualty is capable of breathing:
He will gasp and start to breathe.
4 A few exhaled air inflations given in rhythm with his own breathing may then be of help.

During recovery there is often an outpouring of saliva and gastric secretions which may be followed by retching and vomiting.
5 Therefore, place him in the recovery position until fully conscious.
6 Keep close watch on the casualty, especially on his breathing.
7 Send him to hospital without delay, staying with him until hospital or ambulance staff have taken over responsibility.

IF NO RESPONSE. Keeping the head extended start expired air inflation of the lungs.

Opening and maintaining the airway

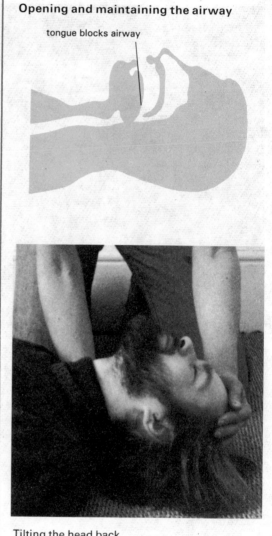

tongue blocks airway

Tilting the head back.

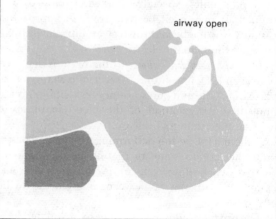

airway open

Method of ventilation

1 Open your mouth wide and take a deep breath.

2 Pinch the casualty's nostrils with the fingers, then seal your lips around his mouth.

3 Blow into the casualty's lungs until the chest rises, then remove your mouth and watch his chest deflate. The escape of air from his lungs will be clearly audible.

4 If the chest fails to rise remove any foreign body in the mouth or back of the throat.

5 Repeat, giving the *first four inflations as rapidly as possible* to saturate the blood with oxygen.

6 Lung inflation can also be carried out through the nose, when the casualty's mouth should be sealed with the thumb of the hand holding the lower jaw. This modification is used when the first-aider cannot seal the casualty's mouth with his own.

7 Continue to ventilate the lungs until breathing becomes spontaneous. Aim at a rate of one inflation every six seconds (ten per minute).

8 Do not leave the casualty but get someone to call an ambulance.

NOTE: In the case of an infant or young child, modify the technique above:

1 By sealing the casualty's nose as well as his mouth, with your lips.

2 By blowing *gently* into his lungs, until filled.

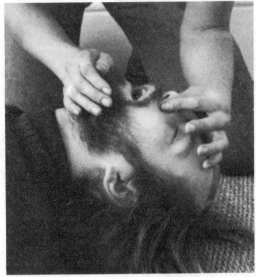

Mouth to mouth ventilation

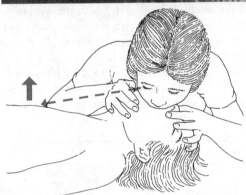

Blow in through the mouth, watching to make sure the chest rises.

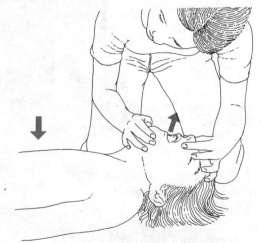

Remove your mouth and watch the chest deflate.

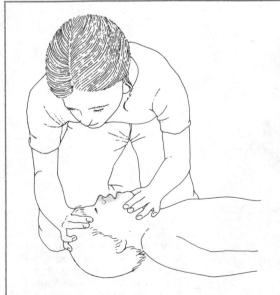

Modified technique for infant and young child. Cover the child's nose and mouth with your mouth.

Chapter 29 First aid

IF THE HEART HAS STOPPED BEATING (cardiac arrest) then no carotid pulse will be felt, the pupils are widely dilated, and the colour becomes, or remains, blue-grey:

1 Put the casualty on a firm surface (floor) on his back, if not already in that position.
2 Strike the chest smartly over the heart – this stimulus may restart it.
3 If a bystander is available, get him to raise the legs and keep them raised.

If still no response – start external cardiac compression while continuing to ventilate the lungs – in the ratio of one inflation of the lungs to about five compressions of the sternum.

1 Take up a position at the side of the casualty.
2 Find the lower half of the breast bone (sternum).
3 Place the heel of your hand on this part of the sternum – the palm and fingers being raised from the chest.
4 Cover the heel of this hand with the heel of your other hand and, with straight arms, rock forward and press down on the lower part of the sternum. The fingers should not be in contact with the chest wall. This rocking movement should be carried out evenly but not equally. The forward movement each time should be quicker and snappier than the recovery movement. The pressure in all cases should be firm and controlled – erratic or violent action can break ribs. (In an unconscious adult the sternum can be pressed towards the spine from 2·5 to four cm (one to $1\frac{1}{2}$ in).

5 In treating adults repeat the pressure once per second. With children the pressure of one hand will suffice and the rate is 60 to 100 times per minute. For small infants use fingertips only.

NOTE: If there are two persons present, one should undertake the external cardiac compression and the other should undertake the inflation of the lungs and feel for the pulsation of the carotid artery in the neck.

6 Check the effectiveness of the first aid by:
noting the size of the pupils, which should become smaller with effective treatment;
feeling for the carotid pulse, which will become apparent with each compression;
watching for improvement in the casualty's colour, which is sudden and striking when the heart resumes its functions.

7 This combined lung-heart resuscitation may have to be continued until the casualty reaches hospital. It is tiring, and responsible bystanders should be recruited to take turns in giving resuscitation under your supervision.

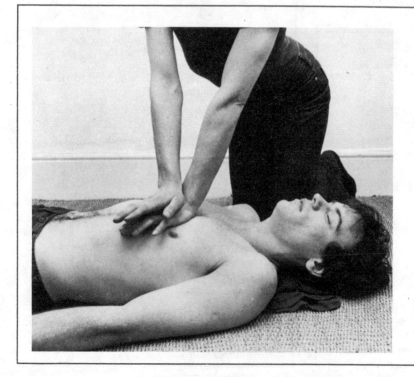

Cardiac compression should be performed only when you are sure that the heart has stopped beating. The hands should be placed on the casualty's chest as shown, and pressure applied with firmness and control. *Check the carotid pulse in the neck.*

Holger-Neilsen method (see illustrations) If ventilation of the lungs by the mouth-to-mouth or mouth-to-nose method cannot be undertaken because of severe facial injuries, or when the casualty is trapped in the face-downwards position, the Holger-Nielsen method is recommended. It is not practicable when there are gross injuries to the upper limbs, shoulder-girdle, or ribs.

Position of casualty The casualty should be placed face downwards on a flat surface. His hands, one over the other, should be placed level with his forehead, the casualty's head being turned to one side so that his cheek rests on the uppermost hand.

Position of the operator Kneel on one knee at casualty's head, and put the foot of the other leg near his elbow.

Place your hands on his back just below the shoulder blades.

Application Keeping the elbows straight, rock forwards until the arms are approximately vertical, exerting steady pressure on the casualty's chest.

Grasp the casualty's arms just above the elbow and rock backwards, raising his arms until resistance and tension are felt at the casualty's shoulders. The arms are then dropped.

The phases of expansion and compression should each last two and a half seconds, the complete cycle being repeated twelve times per minute.

Recovery On recovery at any stage, outpouring of saliva and fluid from the stomach and nose usually takes place: this may be followed by retching and vomiting. To prevent inhalation of this fluid or vomit, place the casualty carefully in the recovery position.

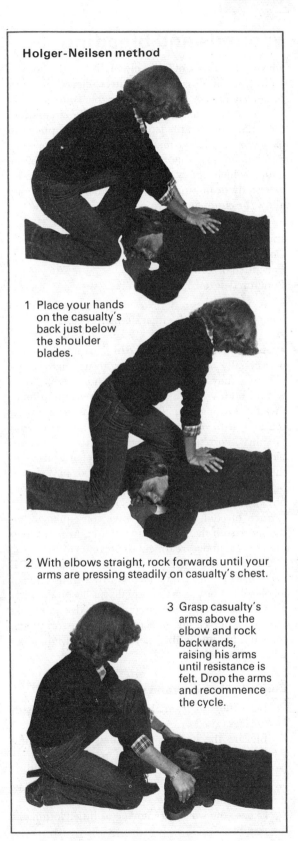

Holger-Neilsen method

1 Place your hands on the casualty's back just below the shoulder blades.

2 With elbows straight, rock forwards until your arms are pressing steadily on casualty's chest.

3 Grasp casualty's arms above the elbow and rock backwards, raising his arms until resistance is felt. Drop the arms and recommence the cycle.

Wounds and bleeding

The total quantity of blood circulating in the body of an average adult is about six litres (eleven pints) or roughly a litre per eleven kg (a pint per stone) of body weight. When much blood is lost from the circulation, the vital organs are deprived of fresh supplies of oxygen and nutritive matter, and shock develops.

A wound is an abnormal break in the tissues of the body, which may permit the escape of blood, externally or internally, and in either instance may allow the entrance of germs, causing infection.

There are four different types of wounds:

Incised or clean-cut
Contused or bruised
Lacerated or torn
Punctured or stab

As in the case of external bleeding, internal haemorrhage may be either slight or severe.

Wounds with severe bleeding   If an artery, or occasionally a vein, is cut or torn, such severe bleeding may occur that life is endangered. In a wound both vessels may be cut at the same time as they lie close together. Blood from an artery is bright red and, if the cut vessel is exposed, may come out in spurts, corresponding to the heartbeats. Venous blood is darker and flows continuously, or wells up in the wound. The colour of the blood may be in between these two, where bleeding is coming from both vessels at the same time.

Such bleeding may have grave consequences, all the more so if the casualty is suffering from a blood disease or is under treatment to prevent clotting.

The urgent need is to stop the bleeding and if necessary to replace the blood lost by a transfusion of whole blood or plasma (normally in hospital). First aid treatment should be directed towards controlling bleeding, preventing infection, and reassuring the casualty, because visible bleeding is very frightening when uncontrolled.

Control of bleeding and wound treatment

1 Place the casualty at absolute rest, preferably with the legs raised.
2 Elevate the injured part unless an underlying fracture is suspected.
3 Loosen all tight clothing.
4 Reassure him and explain the need to relax completely.
5 Expose the wound, removing as little clothing as possible.

6 Do not waste time washing your hands or cleaning the wound area in cases of severe haemorrhage.
7 Control haemorrhage by pressing sides of wound firmly together; if necessary, by direct digital pressure on the bleeding point or points, preferably over a clean dressing. Avoid disturbing blood clots.
8 Apply sufficient sterile dressing packed into the depth of the wound, until it projects above the wound, then cover with adequate padding and bandage firmly.
9 If bleeding continues, do not disturb the original dressing or bandage, but add more pads and again bandage firmly.
10 If foreign bodies are present in the wound and are visible and capable of removal, gently wipe off with a clean dressing, otherwise leave alone and proceed as in the next paragraph.

If a foreign body has to be left in the wound, or bone is projecting, cover the wound with a sterile dressing, and apply pads round the wound to a sufficient height to enable the bandage to be applied in a diagonal manner avoiding pressure on the projecting foreign body or bone.
11 All bandages should be applied just sufficiently firmly to stop bleeding.
12 Immobilize the injured part by a suitable method – e.g. a sling in the case of the upper limb, or by tying an injured lower limb to the uninjured one.
13 Keep the casualty comfortably warm with blankets.
14 Remove him to hospital as quickly as possible.
Dressings are used:
To assist in controlling bleeding.
To protect a wound from further injury.
To prevent or lessen the risk of infection.

An efficient dressing should be nonadhesive and have a high degree of porosity to allow for the effect of sweating and oozing.

Bandages   Bandages are made of flannel, domette (cotton and wool), calico, elastic net, or paper. They can be improvised from any of the above materials.

There are three different types:
Triangular bandage; roller bandage; elastic net.
Bandages are used:
To retain dressings and splints in position.
To maintain direct pressure over a dressing in order to control bleeding.
To reduce or prevent swelling.
To afford support in the form of a sling.
To assist in lifting or carrying casualties.
To act as padding.

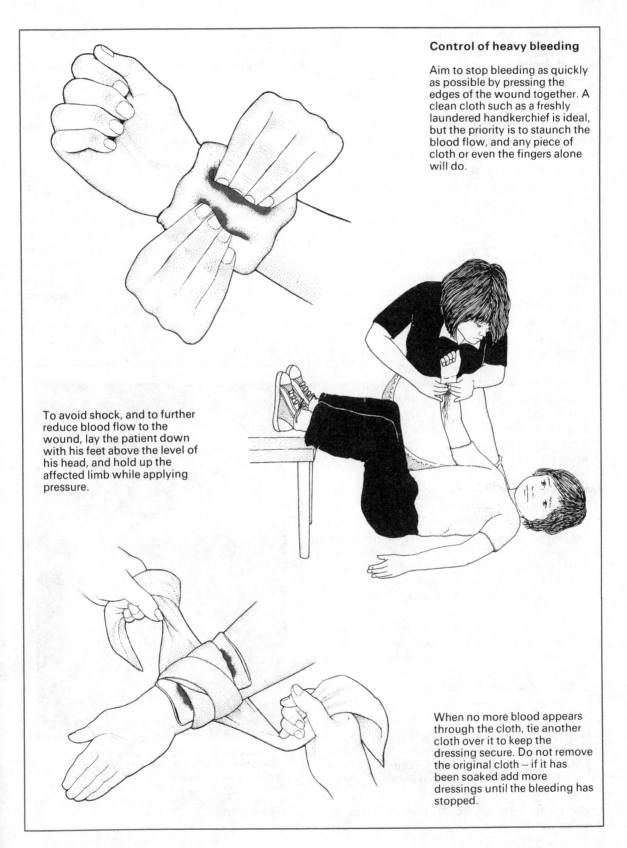

Control of heavy bleeding

Aim to stop bleeding as quickly as possible by pressing the edges of the wound together. A clean cloth such as a freshly laundered handkerchief is ideal, but the priority is to staunch the blood flow, and any piece of cloth or even the fingers alone will do.

To avoid shock, and to further reduce blood flow to the wound, lay the patient down with his feet above the level of his head, and hold up the affected limb while applying pressure.

When no more blood appears through the cloth, tie another cloth over it to keep the dressing secure. Do not remove the original cloth – if it has been soaked add more dressings until the bleeding has stopped.

589

Adhesive dressings The wound covering is of a nonadhesive film, which is supported by several layers of absorbent gauze or cellulose, held in place by a covering layer of adhesive material.

Sterilized adhesive dressings are sealed in a paper or plastic envelope.

Minor wounds with slight bleeding Slight bleeding comes from injured capillary vessels in or immediately under the skin, is red in colour, and may ooze from all parts of the wound. Such minor bleeding, although it may appear alarming, usually stops of its own accord, and is easily controlled by local pressure.

Treatment of minor wounds
1 Exert firm pressure to the bleeding points over a sterile dressing and bandage with pad if necessary. This can sometimes be done by the casualty himself. Adhesive dressing may be suitable.
2 Elevate the bleeding part – slings are rarely necessary.
3 If possible first scrub or wash your hands thoroughly in water, preferably hot and running.
4 If the wound area is dirty, wash the wound with running water. Protect with a sterile swab and gently clean the surrounding skin.
5 Dry the skin around with swabs of cotton wool, using each swab once only, wiping away from the wound.

Internal bleeding
This may occur into one of the body cavities (chest, abdomen, or skull), following a direct injury from a blow, crash, stab, or bullet, or from an indirect blow. It may also be due to certain medical or surgical conditions which include gastric ulcer, high blood pressure, and certain blood diseases, in each of which there is no external cause. Such concealed bleeding may also take place into muscles when crushed, or may be associated with a fracture. In the case of a complicated fracture of the femur, the large thigh muscles may swell considerably from the extra amount of blood in them which is lost to the circulation. Internal bleeding may be permanently concealed or subsequently visible.

Permanently concealed bleeding from an internal organ remains concealed in the following cases:
1 Fractured vault or base of skull, or in cerebral haemorrhage from high blood pressure.
2 Into muscles, associated with complicated fractures.
3 From the liver, spleen, or pancreas into the abdomen. This type of bleeding should be suspec-

ted where signs and symptoms of bleeding are present following a crash or blow to the abdomen.
4 Damage to the lungs when blood is not coughed up.

Subsequently visible bleeding may occur as the result of:
1 Fractured base of skull, when in some cases, blood may issue from the ear channel or nose, or cause bloodshot eyes.
2 Damage to the lungs (by rib fracture, bullet, or disease) when blood is coughed up which is bright red and frothy.
3 Ulceration of the stomach or adjacent bowel, when blood is vomited. It will be bright red if brought up immediately, but will resemble coffee grounds if it has remained in the stomach for some time.
4 Damage to upper bowel, when partly digested blood is mixed with the motions making them dark and tarry in appearance. If the lower bowel is injured, blood in the motions may be of normal colour.

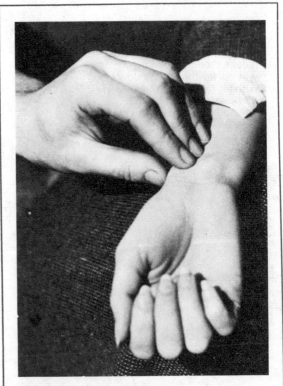

The usual pulse to be felt is at the radial artery. Lightly place the examining fingers (not the thumb) on the bone on the thumb side of the wrist and gently advance them until the bone can no longer be felt and is replaced by the pulsating artery.

5 Injury to the kidney, when a little blood escaping into the urine may make it look smoky, while more blood will make it look red. It is frequently accompanied by pain over the kidney area. If the bladder is bleeding, the urine will be bloodstained and passed with some pain and difficulty.

Treatment of internal bleeding (concealed or visible)

1 Lay the casualty in position of maximum comfort, except that if blood is vomited the recovery position should be used.
2 Loosen all tight clothing.
3 Give nothing by mouth.
4 Bear in mind possibility of other injuries; look for them.
5 Remove to hospital as soon as possible; avoid jolting casualty during transport.
6 Keep close watch on respiration.
7 Make a written note of pulse rate at ten to fifteen minute intervals, for information of hospital doctor.
8 Keep and report on any specimens passed or vomited.

Treatment for a wound of the abdominal wall
Place the casualty so that the wound does not gape, preferably on the back in the horizontal position, with head and shoulders slightly raised and a pillow under the knees. If no internal organs protrude, dress as for a wound, bandage sufficiently firmly, and give nothing by mouth.

If internal organs protrude through the wound cover lightly with a large clean soft towel or dressing, and fix in place, but avoid undue pressure.

In all cases of abdominal wounds remove casualty to hospital as quickly as possible. Do not use hot water bottles.

Bleeding from a fractured base of the skull Bleeding or discharge of blood and perhaps colourless or straw-coloured fluid from the ear and/or nose may occur as a result of a fractured base of skull, and the eyes may be bloodshot.

Treatment

1 Secure a sterile dressing or pad over the ear or nostril.
2 Place the casualty in the recovery position on the affected side.
3 Do not pack the nostril or ear channel, or allow him to blow his nose.
4 Remove to hospital immediately; keep close watch on breathing.

Unconsciousness

Unconsciousness is the result of injury or disturbed function of the brain, and is recognized by the fact that the casualty cannot be roused.

The first-aider may find it difficult to make a diagnosis of the cause of unconsciousness, although in some cases, such as head injuries producing concussion or compression, and diseases such as strokes, epileptic fits, and infantile convulsions, the diagnosis may be apparent.

General rules for treatment of an unconscious person

1 Provide and maintain a clear airway – remove dentures and clear mucus, saliva, or blood from the mouth and throat. Ensure a sufficient supply of fresh air by opening windows and keeping back crowds.
2 If breathing has stopped, commence respiratory resuscitation at once.
3 Search for and control any bleeding.
4 Check level of response, such as, can the casualty speak or answer questions? Does he respond in any other way if you try to rouse him?
5 Place the casualty in the recovery position; this will allow vomit to drain naturally without obstructing the air passage. Remain with him.
6 Loosen all tight clothing about the neck, chest, and waist.
7 Treat the cause of unconsciousness if known.
8 Do not apply heat. Wrap him in a blanket and place one underneath if possible.
9 Do not leave the casualty unattended.
10 Do not attempt to give food or fluids by mouth while the casualty is unconscious.
11 Make a full and thorough examination to see if there are any associated injuries, and, if found, treat these.
12 Remove him to hospital as a stretcher case.

Head injury Injuries to the head may cause wounds of the scalp and fracture of the skull bones, with or without damage to the underlying brain. If there has been damage or disturbance to the brain, consciousness may be clouded. Associated injuries to the spine, the chest, the abdomen, or fracture of the limb bones may be present, but masked.

Guiding principles Examine casualties with head injury very carefully to see whether or not there are associated injuries. Establish as soon as possible the casualty's level of response. Watch for any

The recovery position

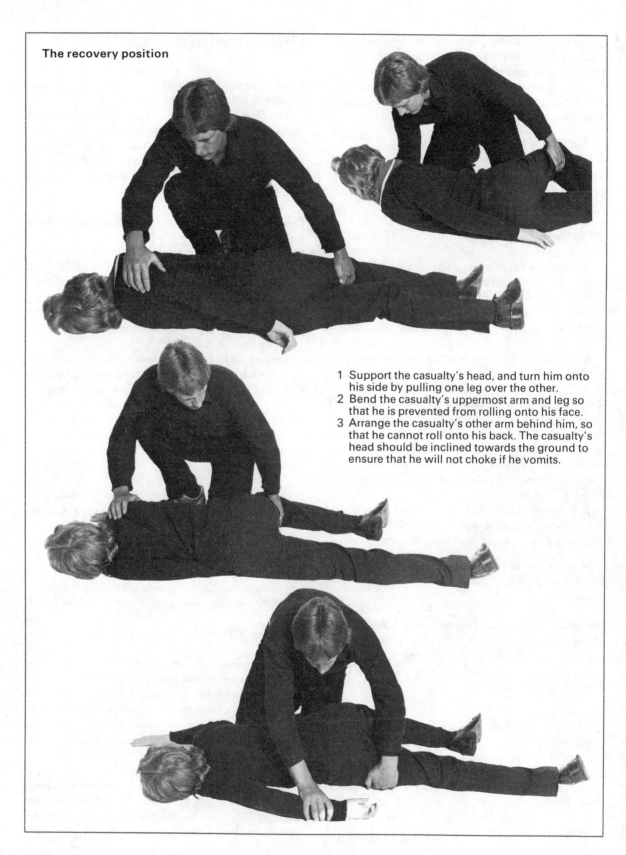

1 Support the casualty's head, and turn him onto his side by pulling one leg over the other.
2 Bend the casualty's uppermost arm and leg so that he is prevented from rolling onto his face.
3 Arrange the casualty's other arm behind him, so that he cannot roll onto his back. The casualty's head should be inclined towards the ground to ensure that he will not choke if he vomits.

deterioration in his condition as shown by alteration in his level of consciousness, and rates of pulse and respiration. If deterioration occurs, removal to hospital is urgent. A note giving the time and cause of the injury, his state of consciousness, rate of pulse and respiration should accompany him.

Examine carefully the casualty's pockets and belongings, if possible in the presence of a reliable witness, such as a police officer, for any treatment cards which may be helpful in deciding on the correct treatment. The person may be unconscious because of some condition such as diabetes (through an overdose of insulin) or may have excessive bleeding because of anticoagulant therapy.

A certain number of cards are issued for patients to carry about with them in case they are taken ill. Some of these cards are given out on a national scale, such as those carried by diabetics and epileptics while others, such as the steroid and anticoagulant cards, may be used only locally by a given hospital, or group of hospitals.

Guidance may also be found concerning the blood group of the patient. This may be of value in notifying hospitals and casualty departments when severe blood loss has taken place.

Shock

Shock is an abnormal condition of the body which can arise from a variety of causes. It can be slight or serious. It accompanies injuries, severe pain, or sudden illness, and may vary in severity from a feeling of faintness to collapse or even death. Shock may arise in one of two ways, from blood loss or from nerve reaction. The commonest and therefore most important cause of shock is loss of blood which may occur with injury or disease.

The brain may be deprived of blood in two ways:

From a haemorrhage – though this is more often external and visible, it can also be from concealed or internal bleeding. Loss of plasma from the blood vessels into the tissues, as in burns, or crush injuries, may produce a similar result. This loss, if severe, will have to be replaced by a blood or plasma transfusion (generally in hospital).

From nerve (neurogenic) shock, when much blood is pooled in internal blood vessels and is therefore not available for general circulation. If this condition is sufficiently severe or prolonged, consciousness is lost (fainting). As recovery takes place, circulation improves and gradually becomes normal.

Other common and contributory factors are pain, exhaustion, stimulation of the sensory nerves of smell, sight, and hearing, absorption of toxic substances from crushed muscles and burns, and from bacterial infection or inflammation. Other causes are acute medical and surgical conditions, such as a heart attack or perforated appendix.

Signs and symptoms of shock In nerve shock, these may vary from a slight feeling of faintness to a state of complete collapse. With slight degrees of shock there may be giddiness, pallor, nausea, cold clammy skin with a slow pulse at first, getting quicker before returning to normal. Where haemorrhage is the main cause, these signs and symptoms are aggravated, depending on the degree of bleeding. The severity of haemorrhagic shock will depend on the rate and extent of blood loss, how long the shocked condition has lasted, and the promptness of treatment.

Treatment of shock Nerve shock is almost always reversible with simple measures, used promptly. Haemorrhagic shock can be reversed by giving suitable blood in the necessary amount, if the bleeding has not been so severe as to cause irreversible damage.

The treatment of shock consists of two parts, preventive measures and general treatment.

Treatment of nerve shock (as in fainting) It has already been noted that before fainting, a person will go pale, perhaps have a cold sweat on the face, sway unsteadily, or complain of giddiness and sickness. If this occurs:

1 Take casualty away from a crowd, into the shade and fresh air.
2 Lay him on his back with head low and turned to one side, and legs raised. In certain cases, it may be more convenient and quicker to use the sitting position, with head placed between the knees.
3 Loosen tight clothing about neck, chest, and waist. It is rarely necessary to do more, as recovery is usually rapid.

General treatment of shock

1 Control the injury or cause.
2 Take casualty away from a crowd, into the shade and fresh air.
3 Lay him on his back with head low and turned to one side and legs raised; this may be done by tilting the stretcher. If he is unconscious, use the recovery position.
4 Loosen tight clothing about neck, chest, and waist.
5 Wrap casualty in a rug or blanket – protect, but do not overheat.

6 Reassure casualty and do not leave unattended. Let him smoke if he wishes.

7 Give nothing by mouth if the casualty is unconscious, or suffering from head injury, or internal or uncontrolled external bleeding, or when an operation may be necessary.

   When the cause of shock is purely emotional, a cup of tea or coffee (never alcohol) may be given during the recovery period.

8 Do not apply heat or friction to the limbs or use a hot-water bottle.

Where the condition of the casualty clearly indicates hospital or medical attention, valuable time should not be wasted by overelaborate first aid measures.

Treatment of shock (haemorrhagic) Blood or plasma transfusions and surgical operations are matters of grave urgency in cases of shock, so that the casualty must be removed to hospital as quickly as possible. The first-aider should prevent the casualty's condition deteriorating and only give treatment which is essential to maintain respiration, stop bleeding, for example by dressing a penetrating wound of the chest, or securing a badly broken limb.

Shock

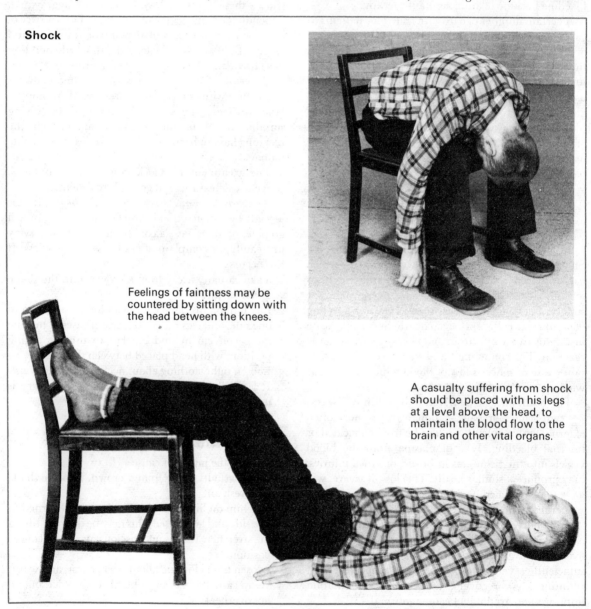

Feelings of faintness may be countered by sitting down with the head between the knees.

A casualty suffering from shock should be placed with his legs at a level above the head, to maintain the blood flow to the brain and other vital organs.

Injuries to bones and joints

A fracture is a broken or cracked bone. Where there is a history of force applied to a bone and the diagnosis is uncertain treat all such injuries as fractures.

Common causes of fractures

1 Direct force, such as a kick or blow.
2 Indirect force, which may break a bone at some distance from where the force is applied, such as a fall on the outstretched hand, which may cause a fracture of the collarbone.
3 Muscular contraction which may, for example, cause fracture of the kneecap.

Types of fracture

Closed or simple   When there is no wound leading down to the broken bone.

Open or compound   When there is a wound leading down to the broken bone, or when the fractured ends protrude through the skin thus allowing germs to gain access to the site of the fracture.

Complicated   When there is some other injury directly associated with the fracture, such as to an important blood vessel, the brain, nerves, or lungs, or when associated with a dislocation.

General signs and symptoms of fractures

(Comparison with the uninjured side will often help in diagnosis.)
Pain over the injured part.
Tenderness on gentle pressure.
Swelling and subsequent bruising.
Loss of control of the affected limb.
Deformity of the limb, such as shortening or angularity (bend appearing in unusual position). Irregularity of the bone may be felt.

General rules for the treatment of fractures

1 Severe wounds and bleeding must be dealt with before continuing with treatment of fractures.
2 Treat the fracture where the casualty lies. The injured part must be secured, even if only in a temporary way before the casualty is moved, unless life is immediately endangered.
3 Steady and support the injured part at once, and maintain this control until such time as the fracture is completely secured.
4 Immobilize the fracture either by securing the injured part to a sound part of the body by means of bandages or, where necessary, by the use of splints and bandages.

Bandages and splints   Bandages should be applied sufficiently firmly to prevent movement, but not so tightly as to prevent the circulation of the blood. If the casualty is lying down, use a splint or similar object to pass the bandage under the trunk or lower limbs in the natural hollows of the neck, waist, knees, and just above the heels. The bandages may then be worked gently into their correct position.

Splints must be well-padded and long enough to immobilise the joint above and below the fracture. They may be improvised by using such aids as firmly folded newspaper, an umbrella, a well-padded broom handle, or a piece of wood.

Slings are used when it is necessary to support and afford protection to the upper limb. The arm sling is effective only when the casualty is sitting or standing.

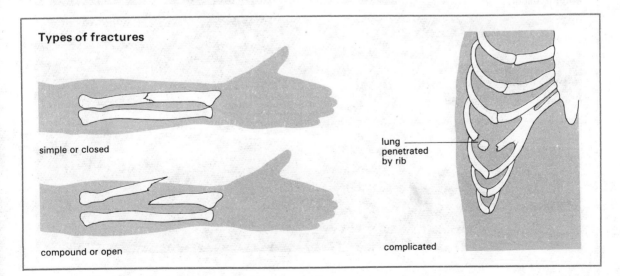

Types of fractures

simple or closed

compound or open

lung penetrated by rib

complicated

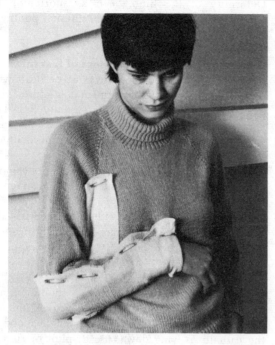

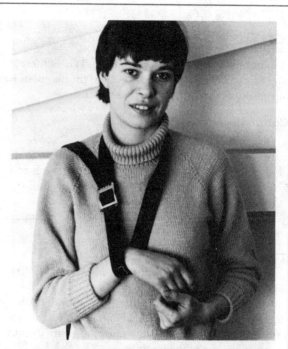

Arm slings can be improvised in various ways, see left and right above.

If the casualty is lying down, pass bandages underneath the natural hollows of the body, and then work them gently into the correct position.

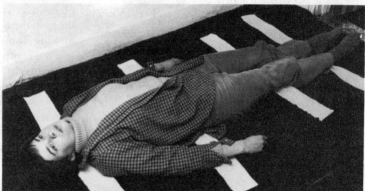

A broken leg can be splinted by bandaging it to the other, uninjured leg.

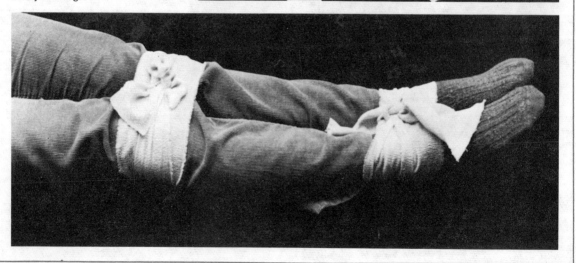

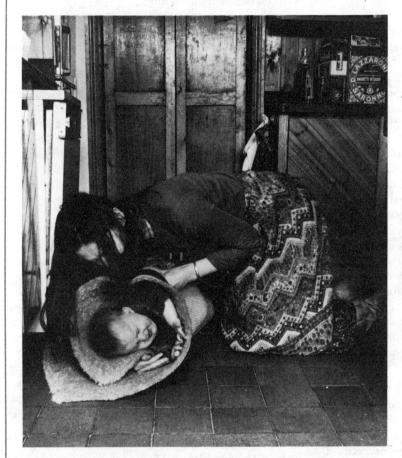

If clothes or hair are on fire, the flames may be smothered by a rug, blanket, or similar thick covering.

Burns and scalds

Minor burns and scalds should be immersed in cold water as quickly as possible.

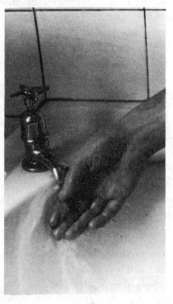

Burns and scalds

A burn is caused by:

dry heat – fire or hot objects;

contact with high tension electric current or by lightning;

friction from a revolving wheel or fast-moving rope;

strong acids and strong alkalis, such as sulphuric acid or caustic soda.

A scald is caused by:

moist heat – such as boiling water or steam, hot oil, or tar.

The injury to the skin is the same whether due to dry or moist heat, or due to corrosive chemicals. The contents of the cells solidify and they die. The injured area rapidly becomes red, swollen, blistered, and painful. The damage to the skin has been caused by heat. It is thus necessary to cool the part affected as soon as possible after it has been in contact with the heat source.

General rules for the treatment of burns and scalds

1 Place the part affected under cold running water, or immerse it in cold water.

2 Do not remove burnt clothing as it will have been rendered sterile by heat.

3 Do not break blisters but keep immersed in cold water if still painful.

4 Remove at once anything of a constricting nature – rings, bangles, belts, boots – before the part starts to swell.

5 Cover the area with a sterile dressing, clean lint, or freshly laundered linen.

6 If liable to get dirty, as in the case of a hand or foot, apply sterile or clean smooth dressing lightly.

Other conditions

Crush injuries   These may involve crushing of the trunk or limbs, occurring when casualties are trapped or crushed by some heavy weight. Injury may involve bones (fractures), soft parts (muscles and skin), or internal organs. On release the appearance of such casualties may be deceptive, and there may be little sign of injury except perhaps redness or swelling. Shock may well be severe and if not immediately apparent may be delayed in onset. There may be some bruising or blister formation and sometimes complaint is made of numbness and tingling.

When the pressure is relieved, two further complications may arise. The injured areas swell and become hard because plasma leaves the blood and enters the injured tissues. Blood pressure rapidly falls, partly from this fluid loss into the tissues, and partly because products from the injured muscle are absorbed into the bloodstream and make shock more severe. This condition is serious and liable to occur if the casualties are crushed for more than an hour by a heavy weight, such as masonry or machinery. The absorption of these toxic substances can lead to acute kidney failure and death.

Treatment

1 After release, keep casualty lying down with head low and legs raised.
2 Leave the injured part covered to prevent infection, with lightweight dressing if necessary.
3 Prevent increase in heart rate by warning the casualty not to move; keep him, and particularly the injured part, as cool as possible.
4 Remove casualty to hospital for further treatment with the least possible delay after removal of the pressure, as this is the danger period.

Blast injuries are caused by an explosion. The casualty may be apprehensive and tremulous, restless, and complaining of pain in the chest. Cyanosis (blue face, lips, and nail beds) is common, with frothy sputum coughed up, which may be bloodstained. This fluid in the lungs causes difficulty in assessing the severity of the injury. There may be no visible evidence of bruising or of fracture; and due to the shocked state, the casualty may not complain of pain or tenderness.

Treatment

1 Reassure the casualty and tell him that complete rest is essential.
2 Lay casualty down with head and shoulders raised and supported.

3 Loosen all tight clothing.
4 Keep sharp watch for any deterioration in breathing or pulse rate.
5 Remove to hospital quickly, avoiding long journeys if possible.

Poisons

A poison is any substance, solid, liquid, or gas, which when taken into the body in sufficient quantity is capable of destroying life or impairing health. Even a normally beneficial substance may be poisonous if taken to excess.

It may be taken:
through the lungs;
by the mouth;
by injection under the skin; or
by absorption through the skin.

Gas poisoning occurs mostly from breathing town gas or fumes from fires, stoves, or motor exhausts. Poisoning by industrial gases may also occur, from carbon tetrachloride (in fire extinguishers and dry cleaning solvents), trichloroethylene (for degreasing, dry cleaning, and as an anaesthetic), hydrogen sulphide (smells of rotten eggs), and cyanogen gas or cyanide fumes (heated fumes of cyanides which are rapidly fatal). Certain compounds used for agricultural purposes may be harmful if not used in accordance with the manufacturers' instructions.

Swallowed poisons   Some act directly on the food passages, causing sickness, pain, vomiting, and often diarrhoea. Common causes are poisonous fungi and berries or decomposing food.

Strong acids and strong alkalis (corrosives) will burn the lips, mouth, gullet, and stomach, causing intense pain.

Barbiturates and aspirin (noncorrosive) produce depression, drowsiness, and finally coma.

Food baits with rat poisons are often coloured and attract children.

General rules for the treatment of poisons

1 Send for ambulance aid giving any particulars available, and preserve for examination any remaining poison, any box or bottle which may have contained the poison, and any vomited matter.
2 If the casualty is unconscious, or appears to be likely to vomit, place him in the recovery position.
3 When poison has been swallowed and the casualty is conscious ask him quickly what happened as he may lose consciousness at any time.

4 If the casualty is not breathing (but his heart is still beating) start ventilating his lungs. If no response and the heart has stopped beating, commence external cardiac compression as well.

5 Get the casualty to hospital quickly. Do not leave him until a doctor or ambulance personnel have taken over responsibility for the case, because he may relapse.

Rules for treatment of special poisons

6 In the case of poisoning by an industrial gas, do not attempt rescue unless equipped with and practised in the use of a respirator and a life-line. Remove any contaminated clothing and wash contaminated skin thoroughly.

7 In the case of poisoning by pesticides the casualty must not be allowed to exert himself at all; if convulsions occur, treat as for a fit, remove all unnecessary clothing, sponge freely with cold water his head, back of neck, spine, and body. Place him in a current of air; if necessary, fan him. Give plenty of water or well-sweetened drink.

8 Food baits containing rat poison – send to hospital any children found eating these baits.

Notes on common poisons

Barbiturates There is depression, stupor, or collapse followed by coma, with failure of circulation and kidney function.

Alcohol The casualty smells of alcohol, is in a confused state, coordination poor, with dilated pupils, sleepiness, stupor, or coma. NOTE: Barbiturate plus alcohol is a dangerous combination of poisons. Send casualty immediately to hospital.

Aspirin The casualty is found with pain in the abdomen, nausea, depression, drowsiness, or coma, sweating profusely, sometimes with a flushed face, laboured breathing, and strong rapid pulse. In children the tablets are usually consumed by accident; in adults the consumption may be deliberate.

Ferrous sulphate (anaemia tablets) These attract a child because of their pretty colour (green) and the sweet sugar coating. Overdose causes retching and vomiting, often bloodstained. The child is cold, drowsy, and restless with a rapid pulse.

Belladonna (deadly nightshade) Children are attracted by the ripe coloured berries in the autumn. The skin is hot and flushed, temperature about 40°C (104°F), the mouth is dry, there is intense thirst, widley dilated pupils, and noisy breathing. The casualty may be excitable in the early stages and later becomes depressed. He may see nonexistent butterflies.

Household poisons

liquid bleach*
lavatory cleaner*
dishwashing liquid
window and mirror cleaner
general purpose liquid
fabric soaking and sterilizing fluid
scouring powder
scouring liquid
scouring cream
fabric rinse conditioner
carpet cleaner
lavatory blocks
detergent
toilet soaps
dishwashing machine powder
oven cleaning pads
oven cleaner aerosol
ammonia
garden sprays, weedkillers, flowers, seeds
cosmetics, perfume
batteries
glue
cigarettes

*can give off irritant gases in combination

All these substances, despite their common use around the home, should be kept away from young children. They are *all* causes of poisoning in children taken to hospital.

Some common poisonous plants

deadly nightshade

yew

laburnum

599

Motor accidents

If you are clear about the priorities in an accident (that is, the order in which things are done) you are well on the way to being a first-aider. The following are the priorities. If you do not deal with threatened danger you and your casualties may be killed.

Pile-ups and fire are the dangers in a road accident:
Get someone to flag down the traffic far enough away to secure compliance.
Switch off the engine.
Impose a "No Smoking" ban.
Send for an ambulance.

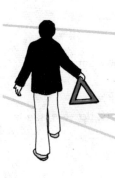

1

Warn other traffic by placing red warning triangle or similar 200 metres from accident in both directions. Switch on your 4 way hazard flashers and head lamps.

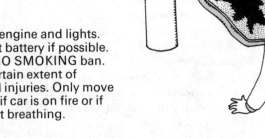

2

Switch off engine and lights. Disconnect battery if possible. Impose a NO SMOKING ban. Try to ascertain extent of injured and injuries. Only move occupants if car is on fire or if they are not breathing.

3

Sending for the ambulance
Dial 999 and ask for the
Police and ambulance
service, stating:
Where to come.
How many patients.
The nature of the injuries.
Whether specialist equipment
is required e.g. cutting gear.

First Aid procedures.
Examine casualties and look
for any who might have
been thown clear

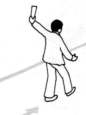

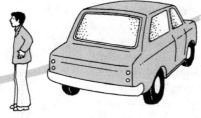

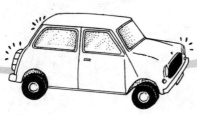

4

Breathing   A crash victim
is often unconscious and
cannot breathe because of a
kink in his airway.

Open the airway up by
extending the head
backwards.

Check for obstruction to
airway and relieve it.

If still not breathing pinch
nose, hold head back, and
inflate lungs by blowing.

Bleeding

Grasp sides of wound.

Elevate if possible.

Continue pressure on sides
of wound with pad and firm
bandage.

Unconsciousness   You
must try to keep the
unconscious patient alive
until the ambulance arrives.

Keep the airway open.

Turn into the recovery
position.
WATCH THE AIRWAY

Shock   In severe injuries
the patient will die in a few
hours unless he gets a blood
transfusion.

When sending for the
ambulance, mention the
probable need for
transfusion.

Fractures
Immobilize using common
sense measures, such as:

Upper limb: use arm sling or
pin sleeve to lapel

Lower limb tie to sound leg
after padding between
knees and ankles.

Wounds
Stop bleeding.

Cover with sterile or clean
dressing.

Immobilize.

Moving the casualty
DO NOT, unless you have to
(for example if the car
catches fire or you want to
treat one of the priority
conditions such as asphyxia
or severe bleeding).

First aid for motorists

First on the scene of an accident What do you do if you are first at the scene of an accident? The first instinct is to run to the car and start pulling people out. DON'T! It has been discovered that "A high percentage of the people hurt in cars and pulled out by frantic rescuers are made worse, even killed".

Every crash is so different that there are no set rules. But here is some basic advice gained from experience of accidents in several busy traffic areas.

What to do first Put out the authorized reflective warning triangles on both sides of the accident sufficiently far away to give adequate warning to oncoming traffic. If you have no triangles send people to flag down vehicles. At night use portable warning lamps. Stop for a second to think. What are the conditions at the scene? If the crashed vehicle is upside down, people may be trapped inside. How many people involved? Stop passing cars and send them in opposite directions to find telephones, dial 999, ask the operator for the Police, give all available information about the extent of crash, exact location, the number of injured, the number and types of vehicles involved, and the services required. It is wise to send one car and then another in each direction with this information. The Police will inform Fire Brigade, Ambulance Service, doctor, and break-down vehicle if necessary. What else can happen? More cars can crash into the crashed vehicle. It is often more important to protect the scene than go at once to the injured. Flag down the first cars, get the drivers to pull off the road, send them as flagmen with some white object to wave, *both ways*, and not fifteen to 30 m (50 to 100 ft) but 150 to 300 m (500 to 1,000 ft) where they can give adequate warning.

Dealing with victims As soon as you get to the crashed vehicles turn off the ignition and lights to prevent fire. If the victims of the crash are hurt but not bleeding profusely, leave them in the car(s) until trained help comes. DON'T TWIST, TURN, OR MOVE THEM. If they are lying on the road, cover them with a blanket or coat, leave them there, and take steps to guard them from the traffic. Monitor the breathing continually and move the casualties only when this appears to be failing.

If people are trapped Often accident victims otherwise unhurt appear to be trapped when they are merely held by a foot twisted under a seat. If so, crawl in and gently release the foot. Make sure the car will not roll while you do this.

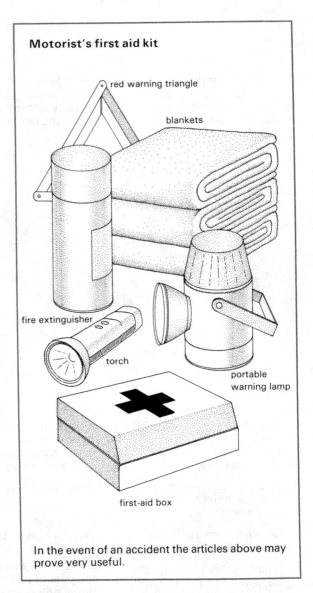

Motorist's first aid kit

red warning triangle

blankets

fire extinguisher

torch

portable warning lamp

first-aid box

In the event of an accident the articles above may prove very useful.

Lifting cars People sometimes get injured or further injuries are received because motorists try to lift cars, find they cannot, and let the car fall back. Four men can sometimes lift one side of a car, but if you try this, be sure you are not pushing the other side down onto someone.

Fire If a fire does not start right away, it rarely starts afterwards unless some thoughtless motorist lights a cigarette. Fire in the wiring usually begins as smouldering under the bonnet or dashboard. Do not let this panic you into immediately moving the injured. Do three things:

Disconnect the battery.

Locate the fire.

Attack it with a fire extinguisher, blanket, or earth.

Miscellaneous

Bee stings and wasp stings If the sting is visible, remove it gently with tweezers. Apply an alkali, such as washing soda. A single bee or wasp sting is unpleasant, but not likely to be dangerous. Multiple stings may require medical attention, as does the rare occurrence of a sting penetrating a vein (such as on the back of the hand) which may make the victim very ill.

Snake bite The only poisonous snake in the United Kingdom is the viper (or adder). It is a small snake, about 50 cm in length, with a brownish well-marked pattern and a "V" on its head. It will not directly attack a human being, but if molested (for example, by being accidently trodden on) it will strike. The first aid for a snake bite is to reassure the casualty and make him lie down. Physical exertion is harmful. The limb should be gently constricted above the bite to obstruct the veins, but NOT the arteries. This will encourage bleeding to wash out the venom. If possible wash the wound with soap and water. Keep the limb immobilized and seek medical advice. The appropriate antivenom serum is available at many hospitals.

Do not kill a large green snake (grass snake) or a small black one (slow worm or blind worm). Both are completely harmless, and do good by eating pests.

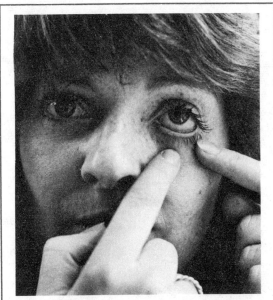

If a foreign body, such as glass, appears to be embedded in the eye, or cannot be reached easily, take the casualty to hospital immediately.

Foreign body in the eye Foreign bodies, such as small flies, can often be removed by repeated blinking. Do not rub the eye. If blinking fails, turn the affected eyelid outwards, and remove the object with the corner of a clean handkerchief. The lower lid is easily turned down simply by pulling down the skin just below the lid. The upper lid presents more difficulty, because it is less flexible, being larger and deeper. If a matchstick is laid against the upper part of the lid, it can be turned upwards by using the upper eyelashes as a handle and at the same time pressing downwards with the matchstick. The lid will appear to be completely inside out, but it is easily replaced.

If a chemical substance, whether acid or alkaline, gets into the eye, the first aid is free flushing with water.

Fish hooks If a fish hook catches in the ear, finger, or elsewhere, it cannot be pulled out because of the barb. However painful, it must be pushed on until the curve of the hook makes the point and barb come out through the skin. The barbed end can be cut off with pliers or a file and the rest of the hook withdrawn.

Frostbite Do not rub the affected part or expose it to great heat. Thaw by using the heat of another part of the sufferer's own body, or by contact with another person. Severe frostbite requires medical attention.

Snakes

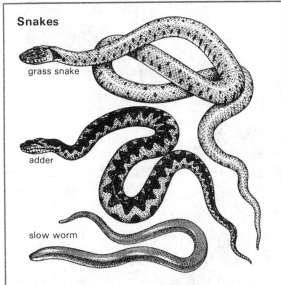

grass snake

adder

slow worm

Both the slow worm and grass snake are non-poisonous and harmless. The adder will not bite unless molested and its bite is seldom fatal, though painful.

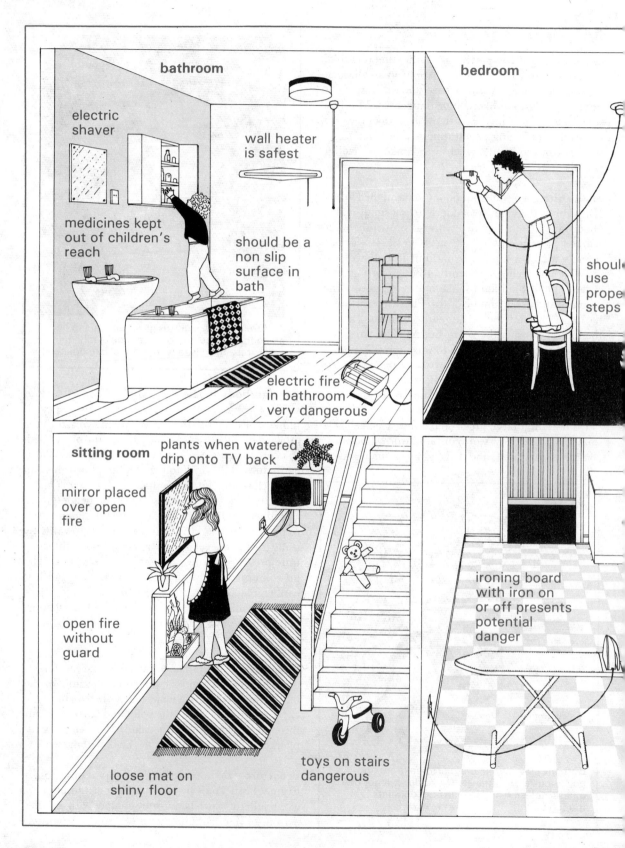

bathroom

electric shaver

medicines kept out of children's reach

wall heater is safest

should be a non slip surface in bath

electric fire in bathroom very dangerous

bedroom

shoul use prope steps

sitting room

plants when watered drip onto TV back

mirror placed over open fire

open fire without guard

loose mat on shiny floor

toys on stairs dangerous

ironing board with iron on or off presents potential danger

Prevention is better than cure

Some preventive DO's and DONT's for the home.

1 Keep medicines, especially coloured tablets, out of reach of young children, in a locked cupboard. Keep pesticides and other dangerous chemicals locked up.

2 Keep matches and cigarette lighters out of reach of young children.

3 Keep small objects, such as buttons, small coins, peanuts, orange pips, and pins out of reach of young children. Such objects may be placed up the nose or in the ear, or may lead to serious choking.

4 A young child's toys should be no smaller than his fist.

5 Don't leave a young child alone in the bath – he may turn on the hot tap and scald himself.

6 Teach your children never to run when carrying a knife, chisel, or other sharp object.

7 Teach them always to cut with the edge of the blade moving away from the body.

8 Remember that the most dangerous room in the house for children is the kitchen.

continued

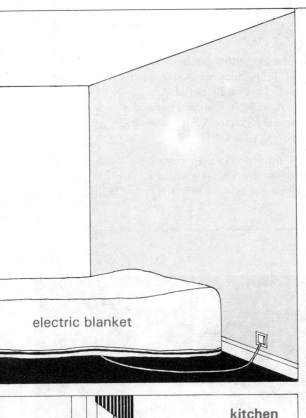

electric blanket

kitchen

cooker without guard

sharp knives

dangerous household chemicals in low cupboard

knife drawer within easy reach of toddler

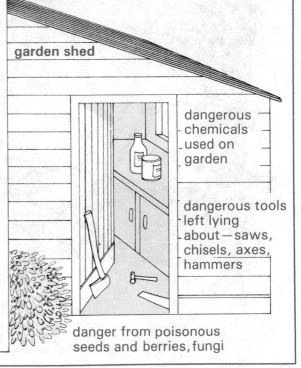

garden shed

dangerous chemicals used on garden

dangerous tools left lying about—saws, chisels, axes, hammers

danger from poisonous seeds and berries, fungi

9 Never have any electrical appliance or switch so placed that it can be reached by anyone in the bath.

10 Switch off the current at the mains before replacing a fuse or making any electrical repairs.

11 Replace frayed electric flex or any bare wire.

12 Do not leave objects lying about on the floor, especially in passages or on stairs, where people may trip over them in the dark.

13 Never use furniture as a step ladder.

14 If there are firearms in the house, keep them locked up and unloaded.

15 Metal wastepaper containers are safer than flammable ones.

16 Lift heavy objects by standing over them, not by leaning over them; act as a lift, not a crane.

17 Never run the engine of your car in the garage, especially if the door is closed.

First aid outfits can be obtained from: The Order of St. John (Supplies Dept.), St. John's Gate, Clerkenwell, London EC1M 4DA.

A suitable Family First Aid Box is No. 42 (code number F03200). The price in February 1979 was £13.55 plus VAT.

A trained first-aider can do so much more than an inexperienced well-wisher. Why not join the St. John Ambulance Brigade, or the British Red Cross?

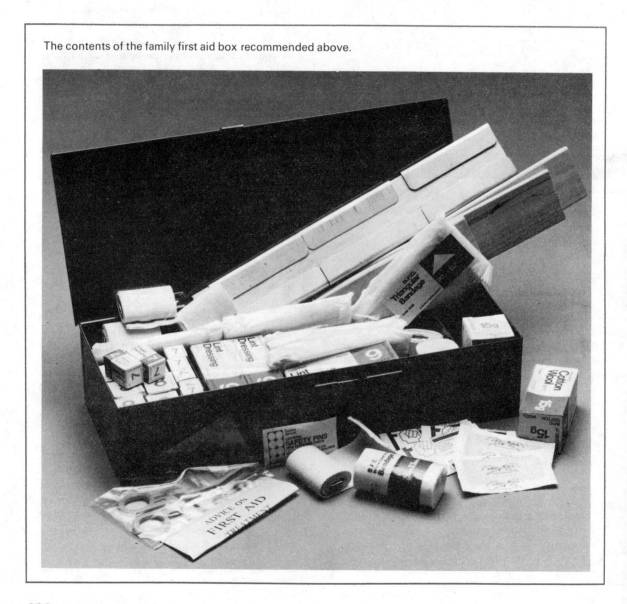

The contents of the family first aid box recommended above.

Chapter 30
Health and travel abroad

by Emeritus Professor Brian Maegraith, CMG TD MD DSc FRCP

During 1977 more than 400 million people moved from one country to another by air, usually without in-flight professional medical help. A much smaller number travelled by sea, mostly on cruises in large ships carrying their own medical staff. Some moved in a variety of ways, by air, sea, rail, sailing, canoeing, even walking, many of them on the expeditions mounted by universities or schools, which often present high health risks as they are usually without medical advice. There are also special groups of travellers such as servicemen and diplomats, who stay away for long periods, and people involved in travel itself, including the crews of planes and ships. These groups usually have their own medical services.

This chapter will deal with the ordinary traveller and look at some of his problems – firstly in the pre-travel period, secondly during travel, arrival, and adaptation to a new environment, and thirdly on the return home. The possible export and import of diseases spread by travellers will also be discussed, particularly in the case of travellers who have been in the developing world.

Pre-travel

In the period approaching departure many things have to be done. The golden rule is that, unless there is real urgency, you should proceed with your plans without fuss, and allow as long a time as possible, at least a month, to deal with preliminaries. The last few days before travel should be peaceful. Most of the planning problems of travel can be best solved by working through an established travel agency, which can help in dealing with things like checking the passport and getting visas, entry papers, and airport clearances.

Medical hazards of travel Travel anywhere has its health risks. These depend on three basic factors – present state of health, the possible hazards of travel itself, and the special health problems of the country to which the traveller is going. Health and age are major factors. The significance of existing illness depends to some extent on the mode of travel. Passengers are exposed to certain physiological stresses when travelling by air, which may affect particularly those suffering from chronic disease involving the heart and lungs, or those recently involved in major surgery. Older people often find long journeys tiring, but infants and young children are mostly little affected, provided the latter are kept under control, as they can be more trouble to other passengers than to themselves. There are certain conditions which are regarded as contraindications for air travel and, in some cases, for any form of travel. Considering the numbers of people who do travel without declaring their health state and with apparently little ill effect, it may be that some of these factors are overemphasized. Some, however, must be taken into consideration.

The recognizable infective stages of infectious diseases should prohibit travel, particularly in the confined space of aircraft. Airlines all have rules about travel by pregnant women. Consult a travel agency for details. In all medical problems, including the transport of critically ill patients, the medical authorities of the relevant airlines or shipping firms must be informed. The decision will rest entirely with them. If you are suffering from high blood pressure, some form of heart failure, recent myocardial infarction, from cerebral accidents – for example, a stroke – or from severe emphysema or chronic bronchitis, you must consult your doctor and accept his advice. If he does not think you should travel, do not go. If there is any doubt, ask him to contact the medical authorities of the proposed carrier direct. This applies particularly to air travel, since the pressurizing of the cabins means that you will be travelling at an atmospheric pressure equivalent to several thousand feet above sea level. This can have certain medical consequences. Metabolic disorders, if they are acute, should also be declared to the airline medical authorities, especially if the journey is long and crosses several time zones. Diabetes is a case in point, since large time changes and the associated effects on body rhythm may lead to mistiming of insulin injections.

Mental illness always causes difficulties. Psychotic conditions are often worsened in flight and the sufferer may require sedation. Full information must be given to the airline medical authorities, who will make the final decision about whether the patient may fly. Medical information can be given to the authorities confidentially in a sealed envelope, either by the travel agent or direct to the airline.

There are many other things which may worry the intending passenger but these are usually minor. Some people are afraid of flying but it is actually one of the safest forms of transport. A good travel agent can usually allay any fears by pointing out that sitting in the cabin is really just like travelling in an unusually large bus.

Protection against disease you may meet abroad   Going anywhere outside your own country (or even inside it) carries certain health risks, particularly if you are visiting the poorer unhygienic parts of the world. Most risks are trivial, some serious, and some even lethal. When you return, you may bring an infection back with you which does not normally occur in your country or occurs only rarely. It may involve you only, or both you and the community. There are various methods of protection available before you leave on your journey.

Vaccinations included in the International Health Regulations   Most countries (not including Australia) are signatories to these Regulations. Each country also has its own regulations about health and these vary from time to time according to disease outbreaks inside or outside its territory. It is essential to get up-to-date information and act on it. Otherwise there will be difficulties on arrival, or in countries passed through in transit. Information about vaccinations necessary for your particular visit will be given by the travel agent or the official agents

for the airline or shipping line with which you are concerned. If you wish to obtain the information yourself, apply to the Embassy or Consulate of the relevant countries. (The requirements will usually be printed on visa application forms.) A useful quarterly journal giving details of requirements of most major countries concerning visas, health, customs, and currency is the *ABC Guide to International Travel*, published by ABC Guides Ltd.

All vaccinations given under International Health Regulations must be recorded on the official yellow forms. Most vaccinations (other than for yellow fever) may be given by the general practitioner, but these will not be considered valid unless the entry on the form is stamped by the local Health Authority. It is probably easiest to get your vaccinations done by the latter. In the United Kingdom this can be done under the National Health Service. Carry your vaccination and any other health documents in your passport.

Smallpox   The recent campaigns are believed to have eradicated this infection from most former endemic areas. Nevertheless, many countries still require the traveller to have a valid vaccination certificate. This does not apply to the United Kingdom, Western Europe, United States of America, and Canada, unless the traveller comes from an area where the disease is active. There are a few contraindications for giving smallpox vaccine, which is live attenuated virus. These include diseases such as eczema, and certain genetic deficiencies of white blood cells. Your doctor will know about these and should write a letter explaining why you ought not to be vaccinated. A copy should be given to the medical authorities of the carrier concerned and you should keep one available for inspection by the health authorities on arrival at your destination. Your doctor may also give you a note merely stating that for medical reasons (not detailed) you should not be vaccinated. This may be required by the travel agent. Most countries exempt children under twelve months old from smallpox vaccination. A few have no age limits. Avoid vaccination of infants if possible. Vaccination is inadvisable during pregnancy. Vaccine is given intradermally, that is, it is dropped onto the skin and rubbed in with a special needle. A first (primary) vaccination or a vaccination a long time after a previous one, may cause a severe local reaction which may last a week or more with some mild fever over the first few days. If the vaccination is successful, it is regarded as protective after eight days, and is valid for three years. Revaccination, to which there is usually little local and no general response, is valid from the time of vaccination for three years.

609

Yellow fever Yellow fever vaccination certificates are required in areas where the disease exists (mostly in Africa, and Central and South America), and (if the traveller has recently been in or through such an area) in "receptive" areas, where the mosquito that carries the disease exists but the disease has not yet appeared (mostly in Asia). Infants are usually exempt from vaccination. Only a few countries still have no age limits. Avoid vaccination of infants unless demanded. Vaccination is inadvisable during pregnancy. Vaccination is given subcutaneously and reaction is slight. There may be some pain, redness, and tenderness in the site for a few days. Vaccination can be regarded as protective after ten days and is valid for ten years. Yellow fever vaccine is also a living attenuated virus and the contraindications for its use are similar to those for smallpox.

Vaccination with both smallpox and yellow fever vaccine If you are going to an area where both vaccines may be required, for example West Africa or Brazil, allow three weeks between the vaccinations. If you are having a primary smallpox vaccination, have it first and do not be vaccinated against yellow fever until the reactions have subsided. Many regular travellers prefer to have the yellow fever vaccination first, followed by smallpox revaccination three weeks later. If circumstances demand, both vaccines may be given at the same time (with a very small risk of encephalitis) but not in the same part of the body.

Cholera If you are going to, or passing through, a country where the disease is permanently present (an endemic area) or where there is a temporary outbreak, you will require vaccination. If not vaccinated, you will not be admitted at your destination, or will have to undergo vaccination on the spot, followed by surveillance. Cholera vaccine is not highly effective. It may be given as two subcutaneous injections a week apart; often one injection is accepted as adequate. There is occasionally some very mild swelling and soreness at the site of injection lasting one to two days, but no general reaction. The vaccine gives some protection lasting for up to six months, starting six days after injection. On a long stay in an endemic area, vaccinations must be repeated at six monthly intervals.

Other vaccinations not included in the International Health Regulations

Typhoid, paratyphoid, tetanus Vaccination against typhoid and paratyphoid A and B is advisable and it is usual to add tetanus toxoid. The multiple vaccine (TABT) is injected into the skin. Local reaction is minimal and there is usually no general

reaction. Maximum protection requires several injections at intervals, but a single injection gives good protection within ten days, and is thus worthwhile if you are visiting unhygienic areas. For those frequently exposed, a booster dose is needed every three years. No matter what protective vaccination you have had, a heavy intake of organisms – even at a single meal – can lead to infection. If you are going abroad to do dirty engineering or agricultural work, you should be more thoroughly protected against tetanus by a course of injections of tetanus toxoid. Children should be covered by routine vaccination in infancy, followed by a booster dose three to four years later.

Poliomyelitis Normally, children in developed countries are protected by vaccination (three drops of vaccine once every three weeks for three doses). The adult traveller should be given a booster dose of vaccine if he has not received one within the previous five years. This is particularly important if he is likely to be going to developing countries with bad sanitation or if, for example as a teacher, he is to be associated with children while abroad. The Sabin vaccine (a live attenuated virus) is given orally on sugar and there are no reactions.

Diphtheria, whooping cough, and tetanus The triple vaccine is commonly given in infancy. There is some controversy over the occasional brain damage caused by the whooping cough vaccine. This may be omitted on request and a diphtheria-tetanus vaccine substituted. Dosage for either is one dose injected each month for three successive months, with a booster dose three to four years later.

Tuberculosis Under normal conditions in the developed world, protection where necessary should have been provided from infancy with BCG vaccination.

Infective hepatitis This disease occurs occasionally in most countries but is highly endemic in some, particularly in West, Central, East, and North Africa, and the Far East. Travellers going to these areas should obtain medical advice about protection by injection and gamma globulin.

Plague and typhus Vaccination is not recommended except in certain circumstances for people going to the few endemic areas.

Malaria protection by chemical substances (chemosuppression, chemoprophylaxis) This is of practical importance to the ordinary traveller only if going into malaria endemic areas, most of which lie in Africa, the Middle East, India and Southeast Asia, certain Pacific Islands, or South or

Central America. You should be advised about possible malaria risks by the travel agent or the airline. Details of methods of chemosuppression can now be obtained from the medical authorities of the latter, and the possibility of contracting malaria is pointed out in a pamphlet issued by the United Kingdom government to all travel agents (who are, unfortunately, not obliged to pass the information on to customers). Warnings are in future to be issued by cabin staff in British Airways. The most effective antimalarial drug is proguanil. For the adult, one tablet (100 mg) should be taken every day by mouth during exposure, starting on the day of arrival in the infected area and continuing for a month after permanently leaving the area. Children may be given pyrimethamine (which is practically tasteless) by mouth twice weekly. Drugs and details of how they should be taken can be obtained from the airline health authorities or your doctor. On return, after the taking of the drug has been stopped, it is unlikely that malignant tertian malaria (a highly dangerous disease) will occur, as the drugs taken for suppression usually cure the infection. This is not the case with the other three forms of malaria, which are not lethal but may relapse after periods of weeks or months. They can be safely and successfully treated.

Travel by sea

The liner that carried passengers on regular services to distant parts has largely disappeared and its place has been taken by the aeroplane. There are still relatively small numbers of people who travel by sea, mainly on highly organized cruises in large vessels which carry their own medical personnel and have provision for looking after the sick. A few also go on smaller cargo ships taking a limited number of passengers to the Caribbean Islands, the Far East, South America, even to Australia. Most of these do not have a doctor on board and medical services are limited. It is essential, therefore, if such a trip is contemplated, to have a medical check before you complete your plans and to carry with you whatever drugs or appliances you may require. Your doctor should supply an account of your medical record, treatment, and so on. Keep one copy for yourself – another (sealed, but for opening if necessary) can be handed to the Purser. The medical authorities of the shipping line should also be informed.

It is unwise to travel on long sea voyages if you are chronically sick or seriously incapacitated, or in the late stages of pregnancy. Many cruises include in their schedules stays in ports and excursions to places of interest, which may take you into unhealthy insanitary environments or areas in which serious diseases such as malaria are endemic. You should, therefore, be adequately advised and protected by vaccinations and possibly chemosuppression. Such advice is usually provided in the brochure issued by the shipping agents concerned and by the travel agent. At a later stage, after return, should you become ill, you must remember to include these special visits in your description of your travels given to the doctor. Seasickness is the main hazard of the short voyage, such as in a Channel ferry. Larger ships have stabilizers which provide much steadier progress. Seasickness is not specific to sea travel. It is merely a form of motion sickness, arising from disturbances of the inner ear. There are a number of satisfactory preventive tablets. Ask your doctor.

Travel by air

People without much experience of flying are often afraid of it, or are troubled by the confined space of the plane and sometimes by the endless rows of seats separated by narrow corridors. If the traveller really finds the environment unbearably claustrophobic, for everyone's sake he should not travel by air. Fortunately, most people quickly adapt. Fear is at its maximum at takeoff and landing, but it is usually well-contained and no sedative is needed.

The major disadvantages of long journeys in tourist class, which carries by far the greatest numbers, are the cramped conditions, the very restricted leg space, the constant movement, noise, and slight vibration, and the smells. Of the last, the smell of tobacco smoke is probably the most objectionable, especially from pipes (usually forbidden) and cigars (permitted on some airlines). The growing limitation of smoking to certain areas of the cabin has reduced this inconvenience. In any case, you should reduce your own smoking levels. The smells are minimized by the remarkable ventilation of the modern aeroplane. The air is completely changed about every ten minutes. This is a great source of comfort, and is probably also of some hygienic value in keeping down the atmospheric carbon monoxide concentration which is raised by excessive smoking, and also in lowering the transmission rate of droplet infection.

Sitting closely packed, sometimes for several hours, is physically bad, especially if you have varicose veins or other vascular disturbances, or are physically disabled. Venous congestion of the legs inevitably results. This can be kept to a minimum by frequent movement of the limbs and by occasional standing

Chapter 30 Health and travel abroad

and walking about. The sensible traveller will wear light, loose shoes or bring slippers with him. Avoid tight boots and undo shoe laces. Even so, some swelling of the ankles may appear. This is usually of no significance. Clothes should be loose and comfortable, and chosen with a view to the climatic conditions likely to be met at fuelling stops – when you should get off, if permitted, and walk about – and at your destination. If you are flying from cold Europe to hot Southeast Asia or the reverse, it is wise to carry a change of clothing with you in your overnight bag.

The cabin is pressurized during the journey to an atmosphere equivalent to that at 1,500 to 1,800 m (5,000 to 6,000 ft) above sea level. This occurs rapidly during the climb and the reverse during descent. There is often some slight temporary disturbance of the ears which may upset young children whose loud protests are commonest at these times. The disturbance can be overcome by swallowing, aided by sucking sweets, which were once routinely issued to passengers, a practice which is no longer often seen. Despite pressurization there is a slight rarefaction of the atmosphere which may exacerbate heart or lung disorders and will increase the volume of any gas contained in the body by some twenty per cent. This applies to the gases in the abdomen, and leads to distension and often intestinal discomfort – relieved by loosening the clothing. On long journeys it may lead to flatus and diarrhoea.

The air in many aircraft is not always adequately moistened, and the dryness may lead to some dehydration. You should, therefore, take a reasonable amount of fluid. Do not drink to excess and avoid overintake of either alcohol or food, both common practices in aircraft.

Motion sickness See also under *Travel by sea* (seasickness). This was common in air travel in the days of relatively low altitude flight in propeller-driven planes which were unable to fly above the turbulences of storms, as do the modern jets, in which airsickness has become rare. It should be added that there is a psychological element in some cases, possibly partly due to the prominence of the paper vomit bag in the rack in the back of the seat. Vomiting may even occur before the plane has taken off. It is also catching and may induce trouble in adjacent passengers. If you are inclined to motion sickness, choose an aisle seat in the middle section of the plane, where movement is least, and avoid the back of the plane where movement is greatest.

Circadian (diurnal) rhythm The rhythms of everyday life, sleeping, waking, working, eating, passing urine, defaecation, may be temporarily upset on long flights from West to East or East to West. They are not affected by flying North or South along roughly the same meridian. These disturbances are often known as "jet lag". Every 15° meridian of longitude represents a change of one hour, either way. Thus flying west from London to Washington means passing through a time zone of five hours, and flying east from London to Bangkok a time zone of about eight hours. The effects of flying through these time zones are usually noticed after three hours and are distinct by five hours. They appear to be more pronounced when flying west to east than east to west.

The change in rhythms is subjectively indicated by a sense of fatigue on arrival, and is usually more obvious in chronically ill and older people. There is some associated loss of efficiency and ability to make decisions, often not appreciated by the traveller. These features are sometimes more pronounced in people who have been abroad for some time, especially in a different kind of environment, to which they have become acclimatized. The loss of standards of performance is a significant factor which should be allowed for in any traveller, particularly those concerned with politics or business. Do not go direct from the plane to an important meeting or a party. If you do, your major decisions may be thoroughly bad.

It may take some days for the physiological functions to adjust completely to the new situation. The accustomed time for defaecation, for instance, may come at an inconvenient moment and lead to enforced constipation. Carry a mild laxative with you. The desire to urinate may also have to be withstood. The major troubles usually come from interference with the normal sleep rhythm. On the first day, at least, try to go to bed at the local time which is equivalent to the time you would normally go to bed at home. With the overlay of excitement, a mild sedative may be needed, depending on advice from your doctor at home or locally. The most sensible solution is to accept that these changes occur and put aside at least a whole day for adjustment on arrival. An alternative is to break the flight into relatively short journeys and pause for a day or two in each place to adjust.

Troubles with disturbed rhythms have worsened in the jet age, probably because people can now travel so far so quickly, as compared with flying in propeller craft, when it took days, not hours, to go halfway around the world. On the other hand, travelling even faster may reduce the impact of the time zones and jet lag over relatively short distances, say London to New York.

Adaptation at journey's end

Arrival after a long flight usually means fatigue, frustration, interminable airport corridors, delays in customs, and worry about baggage and its transport. These are probably inevitable, but the irritation can be eased for the elderly and handicapped, since the airline, if notified in advance, can provide wheelchairs at both ends of the journey.

Exposure to disease   Travellers should note that they are going to be exposed to unfamiliar conditions and diseases in any environment. Some of the latter may not occur in one's native country, or may occur only rarely; others are common to both. In particular, the traveller is likely to be exposed to local infections, such as malaria, which may be acquired and taken back home. The chances of getting such diseases depend, of course, on destination, but they also depend on common sense and self-discipline and often on the kind of work to be undertaken. Thus, the engineer who goes up-country in Africa to build a dam is more likely to get malaria or some other tropical disease than a tourist or businessman, based in an air-conditioned hotel.

It must be appreciated that you can acquire a disease and show no signs of it until after your return, since modern travel is so fast that you can come back during the incubation period. You can also become infected and be temporarily protected from the clinical effects while abroad, only to become ill some time after your return. It is therefore essential that, should you become ill after returning home, you must seek medical help at once and tell the doctor exactly where you have been and when. All details are important, even the refuelling stops. It needs only one mosquito bite to give you malaria, and you may be flying from one clean place to another but come down in transit in an infected area.

Food and drink   Be careful, not frightened. Infection with typhoid and bacillary dysentery can come from any food or drink (rarely from manufactured bottled drinks or hot drinks made from boiling water). Eating cooked food bought in open market places or warmed-up meats, puddings, and so on is very risky; so is drinking milk, unless you can be sure of the source. It is said, not without truth, that the only really sterile drink in the tropics is breast milk; gastrointestinal troubles abound in bottled milk prepared for infants. Avoid eating fresh salads in areas where human compost is used, as in the East.

Vegetables may be heavily laden with cysts which cause amoebic dysentery and possibly later amoebic liver abscess. Where infection is likely, all drinking water should be boiled. Alcoholic drinks are usually safe, unless the diluent is infected. The amount of alcohol consumed is up to the traveller. In moderation it has no ill effects, and ordinary table wines are often safer than water. No special health virtues lie in expensive chateau-bottled wines. Antimalarial drugs can be taken with alcoholic drinks.

Traveller's diarrhoea   Short-term diarrhoeas are common in travellers. Many are unimportant. Some result from unusual additives. Food containing hot peppers or curries may cause diarrhoea, anal pain, and discomfort. This sort of disturbance lasts for only a day or two, but it may become advisable to avoid chillies and other hot foods altogether. Travellers accustomed to bland English food may sometimes suffer temporarily from the rich sauces, oils, and seasoning of French, Spanish, or Italian cooking. Diarrhoea and vomiting soon after eating indicate food that is off rather than infection. If accompanied by nettle rashes the disturbance may be caused by sensitivity to some food, commonly shellfish. In hot countries, ice is a great temptation, but it should never be taken in drinks served in markets, small shops, and so on, where it is usually dirty and served by hand, and nearly always infected. Unopened drinks from a refrigerator are usually safe, and so is ice made in a refrigerator, provided the water has been boiled before freezing.

Salt and water balance   In a hot country you need roughly 28 gm of salt daily (about one oz). The normal European diet contains about fifteen gm. There may be enough in the local food, but if you need more, add table salt to your food or drink water with salt well diluted. Salt tablets should be avoided, as they may not dissolve in the gut and are thus not absorbed. Drink plenty of water or other fluids. Alcohol is damaging only in excess. Beer is probably the best way to take fluid, but the cleanest alcoholic drink is usually regarded as whisky, well diluted with clean water or soda water. One way of avoiding excess alcohol is to start the evening with a glass of soda water to allay your thirst.

Effects of heat   Heat in itself – unless excessive – is harmless. Most people can quickly adjust to it. The early effects of exposure to heat can be alarming, but are seldom serious.

Syncope   Unacclimatized persons exposed to

heat may develop heat syncope or collapse after exercise or prolonged standing, often the result of exhausting sightseeing. The patient becomes restless, pale, dizzy, and may faint. He feels cold and clammy and the pulse is fast; the blood pressure is low. This condition has nothing whatever to do with salt: water imbalance. Rest in a cool place will adjust everything.

Heat exhaustion This arises in people who have been working in a hot environment, for example, in mines underground or in closed vehicles, such as military tanks. It results from great loss of salt and water in sweat and can be serious, leading to shock. Occasionally the cause is primarily excessive loss of water, as in people caught in the desert. The two situations produce different clinical pictures. The ordinary traveller, taking adequate quantities of salt and water and not too much strenuous exercise, will not be likely to suffer from heat exhaustion.

Heat stroke This is a serious condition caused by inability to lose heat, due to overcrowding, over-clothing, febrile illness, or similar conditions. Very high fever usually over 41°C (106°F), dry skin, and central nervous symptoms are the usual features. A very similar condition may develop in malignant tertian malaria.

Neurosis This is common in those who have been exposed to hot conditions for some time, and is exacerbated by alcohol. It is unlikely to be seen in the short-term visitor.

Effects of light These may be very unpleasant. Even a few days in bright light may result in glare effects – headache, dizziness, and eye discomfort, sometimes with blurring and distortion of vision. Keeping well in the shade and using tinted glasses can usually deal with this. Tinted glasses should be adjusted to your vision. Long and continued exposure to sunlight in fair-skinned individuals can give rise to various forms of skin reactions which may lead to serious rodent ulcers or even cancer.

Sunburn Direct exposure to sunlight or to light reflected from sand, sea, or snow may cause severe burns on the skin, due to ultraviolet light. These may be very serious and occasionally fatal. Most sunburn results from too rapid and prolonged exposure to sunlight, often deliberate. It can be avoided by gradual exposure, increasing by a few minutes each day. Salt water and wind exacerbate the effects. There are protective lotions and creams which contain chemical filters which withhold the ultra-violet light. Some let through the longer infrared waves, which mobilize the protective skin pigment and lead to the much desired tanning effect (craved

by European women and shunned by their Eastern sisters). Sunburn from gross overexposure can also occur in persons with a dark skin.

Care of the skin In hot countries, care of the skin is essential. Cleanliness, frequent washing with bland soaps (shaving soap is excellent), showers rather than baths, careful drying, and subsequent powdering are most important. Prickly heat can usually be controlled by such measures, though it may occasionally become serious in infants and young children and require their return to a cooler climate. Control of skin fungus infections occurring between the toes or in the groin and between the legs is important. These infections are easily picked up in public baths and changing places, and from using communal towels. There are many quite successful proprietary preparations for these infections, but if they are serious, get medical help.

Coming home – imported diseases

Many travellers may return suffering from a disease acquired abroad which is unusual in their own country. Thus, uncommon diseases are being exported from countries abroad and brought into the United Kingdom by the returning holidaymaker, businessman, or by the visitor from abroad, and the immigrant.

As pointed out above, most of these diseases are trivial, but some are dangerous to the individual and may threaten the community as well. It is essential, therefore, that these diseases are detected and dealt with quickly. Two elements are involved in this. One is the awareness and knowledge of the medical profession. The other is the awareness of the travelling public. Public appreciation of the risk of acquiring infection abroad is essential to the control of such diseases. For this reason every traveller, should he become ill after return, must see his doctor and must tell him in complete detail, where he has been and when. The problem in regard to the present-day traveller is that he is still not yet properly informed of his responsibility in this respect.

Every travel agent in the United Kingdom is issued by the Department of Health and Social Security with copies of a pamphlet "Notice to Travellers: Health Protection" which covers the broad details of the subject and advises the returned traveller, should he become ill, to see his doctor and tell him where he has been and when. The agent is not legally required to give the potential passenger a copy of the pamphlet or tell him about its contents. However, if you are not offered a copy, it is advisable to ask for one. Warnings should also be issued by all concerned in travel, including the port or airport authorities on departure, those in the countries visited, and on return.

When the traveller returns, the main responsibility regarding imported infection rests with the United Kingdom health authorities, beginning at the seaport or airport. In the latter, but for some curious reason not the former, by arrangement with the Council of Europe, a yellow card is given to each passenger returning from anywhere overseas except Europe. This tells him to see a doctor if he becomes ill, and show him the card, which states that the holder has been in an area where he may have acquired an infectious disease unusual in this country, including malaria. After this, it is up to the medical profession, which must be equally aware that unusual disease can enter in this way and must be on the look-out for it.

As a layman, the thing to remember is that you may have been exposed to such infections. Before you go abroad, you should see that you are well advised and protected. When abroad, take reasonable precautions and use antimalarial drugs where they are required. In your own interest, and that of others, be scrupulous with hygiene. Above all, *if you become ill on return at any time, see your doctor and tell him exactly where you have been and when.*

Encyclopedia of medical terms

Numbers in brackets refer to pages where a topic is
discussed more fully or illustrations are given.
SMALL CAPITALS in the text below indicate that the topic
can be looked up under its own heading. Also consult the
INDEX.

A

Abduction   The moving of a part away from its midline
or from the axis of the body; for example, moving the arm
away from the body. The opposite of ADDUCTION.

ABO   Blood groups are based on the presence or absence
of factors in red blood cells, determined by heredity. Type A
blood contains factor A; type B blood contains factor B;
type AB contains both factors; type O contains neither.
These types are further subdivided by the presence or
absence of anti-A or anti-B factors in red cells or serum, and
by even more complicated factors (103).

Abortion   Expulsion of an embryo or fetus from the
uterus before it is capable of independent life. *Spontaneous*
abortion is not uncommon; the lay term is miscarriage.
Some expulsions of an embryo too malformed to live occur
so early in pregnancy that they may not be recognized.
Induced abortions, performed under safe and sterile
conditions in a hospital, are permissible if doctors agree that
the mother's life or health is endangered. *Criminal* abortions
(illegal operations) are performed under conditions of
furtiveness, crudity, and haste which can lead to infection,
sterility, and even death (222).

Abrasion   A scraped skin surface, such as a grazed knee
which oozes blood.

Abscess   A collection of pus within a well-defined space
in any part of the body. Treatment is by drainage and
overcoming the infection.

Accommodation   Change in curvature of the lens of the
eye to bring objects into sharp focus (397).

Accouchement   The French word for childbirth.

Acetabulum   The cup-shaped cavity in the pelvis in
which the upper end of the femur rests (462).

Achalasia   Inability to relax a hollow muscular organ;
especially, the lower portion of the oesophagus (*cardiospasm*), producing a feeling that swallowed food has lodged
itself at the entrance to the stomach (342).

Achilles tendon   The thickest and strongest tendon of the
body, extending upwards about 15 cm from the back of the
heel. It binds the muscles of the calf of the leg to the bone in
the heel.

Achlorhydria   Absence of free hydrochloric acid in the
stomach. The condition is a feature of pernicious anaemia,
sometimes of stomach cancer or other diseases, but it may
occur in elderly people who are quite healthy.

Acholic   Without bile. Clay-coloured *acholic stools* indicate some obstructive disorder of the liver or bile ducts.

Achondroplasia   A form of dwarfism; the head and torso
are of normal size but arms and legs are very short. The
condition results from a congenital defect· in the formation
of cartilage at the growing ends of long bones which
prevents normal lengthening (560).

Acid and alkaline foods   There is no reason for a normal
person to be in the least concerned about the acidity or
alkalinity of foods. Doctors sometimes put patients who
have acid kidney stones on a high alkaline ash diet, and
patients who have alkaline kidney stones on a high acid ash
diet. Persons with peptic ulcer should not drink large
amounts of citrus or other acid juices on an empty stomach,
because the immediate effect is to increase acidity and
irritate the ulcer. But the ultimate effect of most acid juices
and of foods which contain organic acids and taste sour is to
leave an alkaline ash – that is, their ultimate reactions in the
body are alkaline. Almost all fruits and vegetables,
although they may taste acid, are alkaline-producing foods.
The major acid-producing foods are cereals, meats, eggs,
and cheese, which do not taste acid at all. An ordinary
mixed diet provides perfectly adequate acid-alkaline ash
balance, and even if it does not, the body has remarkably
efficient buffering systems to maintain a balance.

Foods with alkaline ash
All fruits except cranberries, plums, prunes, and rhubarb
All vegetables except maize and dried lentils
Milk
Almonds
Brazil nuts
Chestnuts
Coconut
Treacle

Foods with acid ash
Bread
Cereals
Cranberries, plums, prunes, rhubarb
Bacon
Beef

Cheese
Chicken
Eggs
Fish
Ham
Lamb
Liver
Pork
Veal
Peanut butter
Peanuts
Walnuts
Maize
Lentils

Neutral foods
Butter
Cornflour
Cream
Lard
Oils
Sugar
Tapioca
Coffee
Tea

Acid-base balance   Blood is slightly alkaline; it is never acid during life. Mechanisms which maintain this delicate balance are remarkably efficient and do not require attention except in presence of disease which a doctor can recognize. Acid-base balance is kept constant by elimination of carbon dioxide from the lungs, excretion of acid by the kidneys (urine is normally acid), and buffer systems of the blood. The chief acid-maker is carbon dioxide, which forms carbonic acid when dissolved in water. Sodium bicarbonate constitutes a large alkaline reserve in the blood. Interplay between carbonic acid and bicarbonate keeps the blood balanced. *Acidosis* (reduced alkalinity of the blood, but not to the extent that it becomes acid) can result from disturbance of the balancing system by kidney insufficiency, diabetes (216), prolonged diarrhoea with loss of bicarbonate, and other conditions. Significant acidosis practically never occurs except in diseases which are or should be under treatment. Strenuous exercise can also produce mild and harmless acidosis because breathing cannot quite keep pace with carbon dioxide accumulation. Excessive intake of antacids or bicarbonate may produce the opposite condition, *alkalosis*, slightly increased alkalinity of the blood. Alkalosis may be induced by hyperventilation; overbreathing washes out carbon dioxide. The same type of alkalosis occurs in MOUNTAIN SICKNESS when overbreathing results from thinness of the air at high altitudes. Alkalosis can also result from prolonged vomiting which removes a large amount of acid from the system.

Acidosis   Decreased alkalinity of the blood and other body fluids. See ACID-BASE BALANCE.

Acid stomach   Burning, gnawing pain in the upper abdomen is often attributed by the layman to acid stomach, especially if distress is not continuous. The stomach is naturally acid. Stomach discomfort may be due to hunger, or inflation by gas-producing foods, or irritants, or too much smoking, or food allergy, or overeating, or a dozen causes other than acid. If distress persists, see a doctor; it is unwise to take antacids continuously over long periods to subdue symptoms when some possibly serious condition is involved.

Acne rosacea   A chronic disease, entirely unrelated to common acne, resulting from dilatation of superficial blood vessels, giving an appearance of constant redness to the area of the middle part of the face (132).

Acne vulgaris   Common acne; a skin disorder, most conspicuously affecting the face, with pimples and blackheads as the most obvious lesions. Acne has nothing to do with "bad blood"; it is due to overactivity of oil-secreting glands and hair follicles. It is associated with the increase of sex hormones at puberty, and is in large degree a physiological condition that most young people pass through on their way to sexual maturity. Acne usually subsides in the twenties, but in the meantime various treatments are beneficial (122). Severe cases should have good medical care in order to prevent scarring and pitting.

Acromegaly   A disorder of adults due to overproduction of growth hormone by the pituitary gland (202). The word means "large extremities." There is enlargement of the bones and soft parts of the face, hands, and feet. The face with its thickened tissues, enlarged jaw, nose, and bony ridges over the eyes, has a characteristic appearance. Height is not increased. However, if the same hormone overproduction occurs in a young person before the growing ends of the bones have closed, he becomes a giant up to eight feet tall (gigantism).

ACTH   Abbreviation of *adrenocorticotrophic hormone*; a hormone of the pituitary gland which stimulates the adrenal gland to produce cortisone (208).

Actinomycosis   (called by farmers "wooden tongue") An infectious disease caused by fungi which produce unsightly lumpy pus-draining abscesses, especially common on the face and jaw.

Acuity   The degree of sharpness of sight or hearing.

Acupuncture   An ancient Oriental (especially Chinese) system of folk medicine in which needles are inserted into parts of the body and twisted, to treat disease or induce anaesthesia. Traditional acupuncture recognizes about 300 regions of the body arranged on lines associated with major organs. Theoretically, needles inserted into appropriate sites on appropriate lines restore the ebb and flow of opposing forces (*yin* and *yang*; male and female) to natural rhythms, thus benefiting affected organs. Interest of Western physicians in the theories and mysteries of acupuncture was stimulated by doctors who visited China and watched major operations in which acupuncture was apparently used successfully as the only form of anaesthesia. A few experiments with acupuncture (modified, in some instances, by attaching a source of electric current to needles instead of twisting them) suggest that the procedure might have limited value for anaesthesia in some circumstances. Whether acupuncture is a temporary fad, how many of its anaesthetizing effects are attributable to autohypnosis, and whether it is really practical, are undetermined. Hypnosis itself can produce anaesthesia, but few doctors use it because of time required for preparation and induction, and alternatives are always at hand, as with acupuncture. A disadvantage of acupuncture in major surgery is that, while it may ease pain, it does not – unlike conventional anaesthetics – produce muscle relaxation, which is important in surgical procedures.

Addison's disease   A chronic disease characterized by weakness, easy fatigability, skin pigmentation, low blood pressure, and other symptoms (208). The underlying cause is atrophy or disease of the outer layer of the adrenal gland.

Adduction   The moving of a part towards another or towards the axis of the body: for example, moving the thumb towards the index finger. The opposite of ABDUCTION.

Adenoviruses A group of viruses responsible for respiratory infections like the common cold (38), viral conjunctivitis, intestinal infections, and latent infections which may cause swelling of tonsils, adenoids, and other glandular tissue, especially in children. There are more than 30 different types of adenoviruses. They are widespread and sometimes give rise to epidemics. Most people have been infected by them. Except in small infants, adenovirus infections are rarely serious. They generally run their course in a week or less. Vaccines have been developed but their use is largely limited to military establishments where conditions are favourable for epidemics among young people.

Adhesions Abnormal sticking together of tissues which should slip or slide freely over each other. Diseases may produce adhesions: in the chest cavity as a result of pleurisy, in injured joints restricted in movement, and in other areas of inflammation. Adhesions in the abdominal and pelvic cavities may occur after surgical operations, particularly if pus has spilled from a ruptured abscess. It is not usually desirable to perform further surgery to free the adhesions unless they threaten to obstruct the bowel.

Adipose tissue Fatty connective tissue; commonly, the part of the body where fat is stored. Usually, adiposity is a way of saying "too fat".

Adiposis dolorosa See DERCUM'S DISEASE.

Adolescence The years between the beginning of puberty, when the reproductive organs become functionally active, and maturity.

Adolescent bent hip A condition of older children resulting from disconnection of the upper end of the thighbone from its normal hip joint attachments, producing a wobbly painful hip, and limping (463).

Adrenalin The hormone produced by the medulla of the adrenal gland (208). It stimulates heart action, constricts blood vessels, relaxes small bronchial tubes and other smooth muscle, and has many medical uses in allergic and other disorders. Also known as epinephrine.

Aerobic Usually describes bacteria which live or function in air or free oxygen.

Aetiology The study of causes of disease or disorder. Aetiology is not a word which means causes, but rather the study of causes.

African sleeping sickness A disease with a high fatality rate caused by organisms that get into the blood through the bites of tsetse flies indigenous to parts of Africa. It is not the same as sleepiness associated with some forms of encephalitis.

Afterbirth The placenta and membranes discharged from the uterus a few minutes after the birth of a baby.

After-image A visual image which remains for a few seconds after the eyes are closed or light has ceased to stimulate. An after-image can be produced by looking at a bright light or bright objects for a few seconds, then closing the eyes, or turning them on a dark surface, or fixing the gaze on a bright sheet of white paper. An image of the object will slowly float into view, become more distinct, and gradually fade away. After-images are either positive or negative. A positive after-image shows the object in its correct shade of black or white or colour. A negative after-image reverses dark and light parts and, if the object was coloured, shows the complementary instead of the original colour; for instance, a red object produces a green after-image.

NEVER LOOK DIRECTLY AT THE SUN.

Agammaglobulinaemia Blood deficiency of GAMMA GLOBULIN, protein molecules which produce protective antibodies against infections. The deficiency leaves the patient extremely susceptible to infections.

Agranulocytosis An acute, rare, and sometimes fatal illness associated with extreme reduction or complete absence of granular white blood cells (98) from the bone marrow and blood. Absence of cells which protect against infection results in weakness, rapid onset of fever, sore throat, prostration, ulceration of the mouth and mucous membranes. The disease may arise from unknown causes, but usually it can be traced to some chemical or drug which injures the bone marrow; the agent may be a widely used valuable drug which is harmless to most people but to which the patient is peculiarly sensitive (116). Treatment aims to combat infection while the bone marrow becomes normal.

Air embolism Plugging of blood vessels by air bubbles carried in the bloodstream, fatal if large numbers of bubbles reach the heart. Air can enter the bloodstream by accidental injection or through wounds of the neck. Air embolism is also a hazard of scuba diving; holding the breath while ascending from even relatively shallow depths may cause rupture of a part of the lung, forcing air bubbles into the pulmonary veins and thence to arteries of the brain.

Air-swallowing (*aerophagy*) The habit, usually unconscious, of swallowing excessive amounts of air. The gas may escape by a belch, or lead to FLATULENCE, or may cause distension of the gut. A small amount of air is naturally swallowed with food or drink or conversation, but excessive intake may be promoted by gulping, chewing with the lips parted, drinking fluids from a narrow-necked bottle, talking while eating, chewing gum, smoking, and nervous swallowing. More often than not the air-swallower has no idea that he is doing it, and is usually able to overcome the habit if it is called to his attention.

Albumin One of the proteins in blood plasma.

Albuminuria Presence in the urine of albumin, a protein like egg white (190). The kidneys do not normally excrete albumin, which is a useful substance, and albuminuria suggests damage to the filtering apparatus, but this is not always the case.

Aldosteronism (primary) A remediable form of high blood pressure with weakness, headaches, and other symptoms (86), due to excessive production of aldosterone, a hormone produced by the cortex of the adrenal gland. The hormone is a powerful regulator of salt and water balance. Excess causes retention of sodium and loss of potassium. If the excess is caused by an adrenal gland tumour, its removal is indicated. All the manifestations of primary aldosteronism can be reversed in a few weeks by oral doses of an antagonistic drug, spironolactone.

Alkaline ash diet A diet consisting mainly of fruits and vegetables, with only small amounts of meat and cereals, sometimes prescribed for patients who have kidney disease or kidney stones of the uric acid type. Alkaline environment has been found to deter the formation of acid stones.

Alkalosis Increased alkalinity of the blood. See ACID-BASE BALANCE.

Alkaptonuria A rare hereditary disorder in which the body is unable to produce enzymes for the proper utilization of certain AMINO ACIDS of protein foods. By-products of incomplete metabolism cause the urine to turn dark brown on long standing. The disorder does not affect life expectancy but in later life leads to discoloration of cartilage and possibly to a severe form of arthritis.

Allergen A substance that produces ALLERGY.

Allergy A capacity to react abnormally to specific substances which cause no symptoms in most people (486);

a general term for all kinds of hypersensitivities. Atopy is a synonym for allergy.

Allopurinol A drug which reduces the body's production of uric acid; used in treatment of GOUT.

Alopecia Baldness; loss of head hair. Some types of hair loss are temporary, some are irreversible (132). Neither hair tonics nor any other medical measure can overcome male pattern baldness. This type affects men who have a genetic predisposition, who produce adequate amounts of male hormone, and who have attained puberty. New surgical techniques for transplanting hairs from an area of growth to the bare scalp have had some success but are not widely popular. The technique consists of punching plugs of skin containing four or five hairs out of the back of the neck and inserting them into the scalp in hope that they will take root and spread. In time, after transplants of scores of tufts, the plugs may grow together to cover the scalp.

Alveolus A sac or chamber; a saclike dilatation at the end of a passage; especially, an air cell of the lung (140), the bony socket of a tooth, or certain cells of the stomach.

Amblyopia Dimness of vision without any organic lesion of the eye. Amblyopia may result from various toxins, or an eye, such as a squinting eye, may lose its vision from long disuse (407).

Amenorrhoea The abnormal absence of menstruation (214).

Amino acids Building blocks of PROTEIN. There are about twenty important amino acids. An amino acid molecule has an acid group of atoms at one end and an amino (nitrogen-containing) group at the other. In between are carbon units with different side chains which give each amino acid its individuality. The acid end of an amino acid links with the amino end of another, a sort of chemical hook-and-eye arrangement. In this way amino acids form short chains (peptides) or large complex molecules containing many hundreds of different amino acids in exact sequences (protein). Eight amino acids are called essential because the body cannot synthesize them and they must be obtained ready-made from protein foods (356). The amino acids of protein foods are separated by digestion and go into a general pool from which the body takes the ones it needs to synthesize its own proteins; thus an amino acid which we may have obtained from a pork chop may become a part of a fingernail, skin, hair, of a hormone such as insulin, or of an enzyme that activates some vital chemical process.

Amnion The innermost of the fetal membranes, forming the BAG OF WATERS which surrounds and protects the developing child.

Amoebiasis Amoebic dysentery (48).

Amyloidosis Abnormal masses of protein infiltrating various organs; primary or secondary to chronic diseases; treatment depends on the underlying disease. Diagnosed by biopsy.

Amyotonia Lack of muscle tone; a congenital form in infants is characterized by small undeveloped muscles and weakness of the limbs and trunk.

Amyotrophic lateral sclerosis A disease of the spinal cord which produces progressive paralysis and wasting of muscles on both sides of the body (166).

Anabolic steroids Drugs related to male hormones, sometimes given for anabolic (building-up) action, to stimulate growth, weight gain, strength, and appetite. The drugs are more accurately called androgenic-anabolic steroids, since they are related to testosterone and retain some of the male hormone's masculinizing action. Although the masculinizing action has been minimized in some anabolic steroids, the separation is not complete and prolonged use in women or children will cause virilization.

Anabolism The building-up part of metabolism; constructive processes of body cells which build complex substances from simpler ones. The opposite of CATABOLISM.

Anaerobic Usually describes bacteria which live or function in the absence of free air or free oxygen. TETANUS and GAS GANGRENE organisms are anaerobic.

Such organisms thrive best where there is no oxygen, as in deep puncture wounds, and cannot survive if oxygen is present.

Anaesthesia Loss of feeling. This can occur from natural processes or accidents; for example, nerve injury, frostbite, hysteria, blood vessel spasms, etc. Ordinarily the word refers to obliteration of pain by anaesthetic drugs, with or without loss of consciousness. There are many kinds of anaesthetic drugs and gases, administered by inhalation, infusion, or injection (537). Each anaesthetic has specific properties, advantages, and disadvantages; selection of the best agent or combination for a particular patient requires special knowledge. The safety and relative comfort of modern surgery, and the ability to perform complex prolonged operations without haste, depend upon the anaesthesia team.

Anaphylaxis Anaphylaxis is an ANTIGEN-ANTIBODY reaction which occurs in seconds or minutes after a foreign substance has entered the body. The immediate, severe, and sometimes fatal reaction is manifested by nettle rash (urticaria), rhinitis, wheezing, shock, ANGIONEUROTIC OEDEMA, and difficult breathing, in varying combinations and degrees of severity. The most frequent causes of anaphylactic reactions are sera, drugs, and vaccines; next most common are insect stings (495). Skin tests may detect hypersensitivity to a substance, but sometimes even the minute amount used in a test may provoke a reaction. If a doctor asks you to wait for fifteen minutes or so after giving an injection, it is not a waste of time; he has emergency measures at hand if a dangerous reaction occurs. Because accident victims are often given routine injections of tetanus antitoxin or penicillin, persons who know they are sensitive to these substances should carry a warning card in their wallet or handbag where a doctor who is a stranger is sure to see it.

Anasarca Generalized OEDEMA.

Androgen A substance which has masculinizing effects (215).

Aneurysm A blood-filled sac formed by dilatation of artery walls; it is susceptible to rupture and haemorrhage (82).

Angiitis Inflammation of a blood or lymph vessel.

Angina pectoris A crushing or gripping pain in the chest, often related to exertion or excitement, caused by insufficient blood passing through the coronary arteries of the heart.

Angiogram An X-ray of blood vessels, usually performed by injecting a substance which is opaque to X-rays into the bloodstream. X-ray films taken in rapid succession may give important information about blood vessels in some types of heart trouble (547).

Angioma A tumour composed of blood vessels; one kind of birthmark.

Angioneurotic oedema Acute local swelling, like giant nettle rash under the skin, frequently a result of food allergy (489). The swelling is serious if it occurs around the tongue and larynx, threatening suffocation.

Anhidrosis Abnormal deficiency of sweat production.

Ankylosis Stiffening or growing together of a joint; the fusion may be part of a disease process (483), or it may be a deliberate surgical immobilization.

Anomaly Deviation from normal of an organ or part; abnormality of structure or location.

Anorexia Loss of appetite.

Anorexia nervosa A nervous disorder manifested by profound aversion from food, leading to extreme emaciation. The typical patient is a young single woman. Usually she is not particularly concerned about her extreme thinness and may even insist that she eats a lot. Management of the condition requires explanation, encouragement of eating, possibly hospitalization and psychiatric help.

Anoxaemia Deficiency of oxygen in the blood.

Anoxia Oxygen deficiency in organs and tissues and the disturbance resulting therefrom.

Antacid A substance that counteracts or neutralizes acidity. Most commonly, a substance taken to reduce the acidity of gastric juice.

Anthrax (*wool-sorters' disease*) A bacterial disease of herbivorous animals. The causative organism sometimes infects persons who have close contact with raw wool, bristles, or hides (53).

Antibiotics Chemical substances produced by certain living cells, such as bacteria, yeasts, and moulds, that are antagonistic or damaging to certain other living cells, such as disease-producing bacteria. Different antibiotics may kill disease germs or prevent them from growing and multiplying.

Antibody A protein in the blood, modified by contact with a foreign substance (*antigen*) so that it exerts an antagonizing or neutralizing action against that specific substance. Antibodies are chiefly associated with GAMMA GLOBULIN in the blood and are key elements of IMMUNITY mechanisms of the body. Usually the antibody-antigen reaction is protective. Measles virus is an antigen which stimulates the body to produce measles antibodies, so measles seldom occurs twice. But antibody-antigen reactions may also be distressing or harmful, as in allergies; see chapter 21. So-called AUTO-IMMUNE DISEASES presumably result, at least in part, from harmful reactions of antibodies against normal proteins of the patient's own body.

Anticoagulants Drugs which slow down the clotting process of the blood. Clots forming in blood vessels are potentially dangerous (see THROMBOSIS, EMBOLISM). Anticoagulants are useful in reducing the clotting tendency. The doctor's problem is knowing when and when not to use them; administration requires frequent checks of the patient's blood since overdosage can induce haemorrhage. Anticoagulants are sometimes given to patients for a few weeks after a heart attack caused by a blood clot in coronary arteries. There is wide difference of medical opinion as to whether the drugs should be continued for preventive purposes for many months or years or the remainder of a lifetime.

Anticonvulsants Drugs which are used to reduce the number and severity of chronic epileptic seizures. The doctor's choice of drugs depends upon the type of seizure (171). Since the drugs must be used for a prolonged period, it is important that the patient be told of possible adverse effects and be instructed to report unusual symptoms to his doctor.

Antidiuretic hormone A hormone produced in brain areas linked with the pituitary gland; it checks the secretion of urine (200).

Antiemetic A drug or treatment which stops or prevents nausea or vomiting.

Antigen Any substance which stimulates the production of ANTIBODIES.

Antihistamines A large family of drugs which block some of the effects of histamine, a normal substance in body cells which plays a part in allergic reactions. Histamine, triggered by an allergen, may escape from local groups of cells and cause symptoms of hay fever. Deliberate injection of histamine causes the walls of capillaries to become so permeable that fluids leak into nearby tissues. This leakage is characteristic of allergies. The effect may be superficial, as in weepy eyes or running nose or nettle rash, or more deep-set, as in dangerous swelling and constriction of the breathing passages.

Antihistamine drugs are most effective in the treatment of acute nettle rash and seasonal hay fever, and generally give good results in subduing allergic tissue swellings (angioneurotic oedema). They may often give symptomatic relief of allergic skin disorders and of itching which is not of allergic origin. The most widely prescribed preventives for motion sickness belong to the antihistamine family; they are effective against symptoms of dizziness, nausea, and vomiting, and have some sedative action. Although many attacks of asthma are allergic in origin, antihistamines have only limited value in this disease.

The drugs differ one from another in potency, effects, and duration of action; facts weighed by the doctor in prescribing a specific drug. Some antihistamines have a pronounced tendency to cause drowsiness; others have very little sedative action. A person taking an antihistamine with sedative action should be aware of its effects on driving ability. Some sleeping pills and insomnia remedies contain small amounts of an antihistamine compound. These may cause drowsiness but the effect is not uniform. Most persons will acquire tolerance to the drug, and antihistamines cannot be considered reliable remedies against insomnia. Because of the depressant action of antihistamines, patients should not drink alcoholic beverages or take barbiturates which in combination may magnify depressant effects.

Anti-Rh serum Prevention of ERYTHROBLASTOSIS (Rh disease) is now possible. Pregnant women lacking a substance in their red blood cells (Rh factor) may develop ANTIBODIES against their own babies whose blood does possess the factor. These antibodies can cause severe anaemia and damage to the unborn child. The risk increases with each pregnancy after the first, which usually is normal because the mother has not yet become sensitized. A preventive measure is treatment of the Rh-negative mother with a specially prepared anti-Rh serum after the birth of each Rh-positive baby, to destroy quickly any Rh-positive blood cells of the baby which might have entered her circulation, thus greatly reducing the chance of her sensitization. Wide use of the serum may in the future eliminate this important cause of stillbirth and serious birth defects.

Antitoxin A substance which neutralizes a specific bacterial, animal, or plant toxin. Most of the antitoxins injected by doctors for treatment or prevention of disease are prepared from serum obtained from a horse which has been immunized by gradually increased doses of a particular toxin. Harmful reactions may follow injection if a patient is sensitive to the serum component.

Antivenin An antitoxin to venom, especially snake venom.

Antrum See MAXILLARY SINUS.

Anuria Total suppression of urine secretion; suggestive of but not confined to kidney damage.

Aorta The great blood vessel which arches from the top of the heart and passes down through the chest and abdomen (65). It is the main trunk of the arterial system.

Aphakia Absence of the lens of the eye, as after cataract surgery (412).

Aplastic anaemia A grave form of anaemia due to progressive failure of the bone marrow to develop new blood cells; it may be caused by chemicals which poison the cell-producing mechanisms of the marrow (116).

Apnoea Temporary cessation of breathing because of absence of stimulation of the breathing centre, as by too little carbon dioxide or too much oxygen.

Apoplexy A stroke; cerebrovascular accident; rupture or haemorrhage of blood vessels in the brain.

Appendicitis Acute inflammation of the appendix (349). It occurs in all age groups but is most common in children and young persons. Typically, pain is felt in the region of the navel before it moves down to the appendix area in the lower right quarter of the abdomen, but not all cases are typical. The early pain may be mistaken for colic. If a child's severe stomachache persists for more than an hour or two, a doctor should be called to diagnose the trouble, which most often is not appendicitis, but if it is, prompt action is important because an inflamed appendix can reach bursting point in a few hours.

Appetite depressants (*anorectic drugs*) These are drugs used to allay hunger and to make the early phases of adjusting to a diet easier. The drugs should be used only for a short time as adjuncts to a low-calorie diet for overcoming obesity, because long-continued use is habit-forming and dangerous.

Aqueous humour Watery fluid which fills the chamber of the eye in front of the lens (395). Obstruction of drainage causes pressures that lead to glaucoma (412).

Arcus senilis A white ring around the outer edge of the cornea of the eye, especially in the aged.

Areola A pigmented ring surrounding a central point; for example, the pigmented area encircling the nipple.

Argyll Robertson pupil A pupil of the eye which does not react to light but does react to accommodation; a feature of syphilis (58) of the central nervous system.

Arrhythmia Any departure from normal rhythm of the heartbeat (78).

Arteriosclerosis A thickening and hardening of the walls of arteries, leading to loss of their elasticity.

Artificial insemination Mechanical introduction of semen into the vagina or uterus to induce pregnancy. If successful, conception, pregnancy, and childbirth occur in a normal way. The first recorded attempt at human artificial insemination was performed by the famous surgeon, John Hunter, in 1799. Artificial insemination is widely employed in animal husbandry, but its availability to couples troubled by *infertility* has largely come about in the past twenty-five years. Technically, there are two forms of artificial insemination: AIH, in which semen is provided by the husband, and AID, in which semen is provided by a donor. Because the husband's infertility is usually the dominant factor, AID is the most frequently used method. There are no exact figures on the number of children conceived by artificial insemination, but the number runs into the thousands and some of these children have themselves become parents.

Artificial kidney A device, of which there are several types, which passes a patient's blood over a membrane outside the body, to extract waste materials and return cleaned blood to the circulation (190).

Artificial pneumothorax Surgical collapse of a lung for therapeutic purposes (139). Not much used now.

Asbestosis Slowly progressing inflammation of the lungs, resulting from inhalation of fine asbestos fibres (151). It occurs in miners and workers in construction trades exposed to asbestos-containing materials. The lungs cannot eliminate asbestos dusts, and normal tissue is replaced by fibrous tissue; the incidence of a particular kind of cancer in persons with asbestosis is high.

Ascariasis Infestation with a species of round-worms which inhabit the small bowel (59).

Ascites Painless accumulation of yellowish fluid in the abdominal cavity, indicative of impaired circulation often related to heart failure, cirrhosis of the liver, malignancy, or kidney disease. Diuretic drugs or sodium and fluid restriction may control this, depending on the underlying disease.

Aspiration Removal of fluids or gases from a body cavity by suction. Also, inhalation of foreign material, as in aspiration pneumonia.

Aspiration pneumonia A form of pneumonia caused by foreign matter in the lungs. The foreign substance may be inhaled, it may trickle into the windpipe, or it may be forced into the windpipe by choking or difficulties of swallowing. Lipoid or oil pneumonia can occur in infants and elderly persons (41). It is important to avoid putting oils into an infant's nose. Give oily substances such as cod liver oil only when the child is in an upright position and can swallow properly.

Asthma A condition of paroxysmal, difficult, laboured, wheezy breathing.

Astigmatism Distortion of vision resulting from imperfect curvature of the cornea or lens of the eye (403). The defect may be so slight that nothing need be done about it, or severe enough to cause eye strain. The condition is corrected by using a lens that bends light in only one direction.

Astragalus The anklebone.

Ataxia Loss of muscular coordination. There are many causes.

Atelectasis A retracted or collapsed state of the lung which leaves all or part of the organ airless. The condition may arise from obstruction of bronchial tubes; gases in the affected part of the lung are gradually absorbed and the area collapses. *Fetal atelectasis* is a condition in which the lungs of an infant do not expand adequately immediately after birth, as they normally should (137).

Athetosis A condition usually occurring in children as the result of a brain lesion, characterized by rhythmical movements of fingers, toes, or other parts.

Atopy See ALLERGY.

Atresia Closure or failure to develop of a normal opening or channel in the body.

Atrial Of or relating to the atria of the heart (64).

Atrophy Wasting away or shrinking in size of organ, tissue, or part.

Atypical pneumonia See PNEUMONIA.

Audiometer An electrical instrument which emits pure tones that can be made louder or fainter (424). It is used in measuring acuity of hearing for sounds of different frequencies.

Aura A premonitory sensation preceding an epileptic seizure.

Auscultation Determination of the condition of organs, particularly the heart and lungs, by study of sounds arising from them.

Autoclave An apparatus for sterilizing instruments by steam under pressure.

Autograft A piece of tissue taken from one part of a

patient's body and transplanted to another part, as in skin grafts to cover raw areas, burns, and so on.

Auto-immune diseases Several diseases of unknown cause may reflect a strange inability of the body to "recognize" itself, so that mechanisms which normally create immunity to foreign invaders establish a specific sensitivity to certain of the body's own tissues, with harmful consequences. The concept is complex, relatively new, and the mechanisms are not fully understood.

Avascular Without blood or lymphatic vessels; the nails, the cornea, and some types of cartilage are avascular.

Avulsion The forcible tearing away of a part.

Axilla The armpit.

Axon A single long fine fibre which conducts impulses away from the body of a nerve cell (154). Most axons are covered with a sheath of material called *myelin*; abnormalities of this covering occur in demyelinating diseases such as multiple sclerosis (166).

Azoospermia Absence of active spermatozoa in semen.

B

Bacillary dysentry (*shigellosis*) Acute diarrhoea, acquired by person-to-person contact, eating contaminated food or handling contaminated objects, or through spread of contamination by flies (48). The causative germs are present in the excretions of infected persons. Infection is caused by rod-shaped bacteria called shigella, of which there are several types of variable virulence. Good sanitary and hygienic practices prevent infection. In infants and small children, bacillary dysentery can cause serious loss of fluids and ELECTROLYTES in a short time; the onset of severe diarrhoea is cause for calling a doctor promptly.

Bacteraemia The presence of living bacteria in circulating blood.

Bacteria Tiny single-celled organisms (32). Bacteria can be seen with a microscope. They are shaped like spheres, rods, spirals, or commas. Most bacteria are harmless and even useful to man. Those which cause diseases are called *pathogenic* bacteria.

Bagassosis Chronic inflammation of the lungs caused by inhalation of bagasse, the material left from crushed sugar cane after its juices have been extracted.

Bag of waters The fluid-filled sac which protects the fetus during pregnancy. During labour the bag of waters helps to dilate the outlet of the uterus for passage of the baby through the birth canal. Usually the bag of waters ruptures at the height of a strong contraction and the fluid escapes with a gush, but rupture may occur even before labour pains begin (dry labour).

Baldness See ALOPECIA.

Ballistocardiograph An instrument for measuring the jerk given by the heartbeat to the body (66). It is useful in some aspects of diagnosis.

Bamboo spine A spine deformed by ankylosing spondylitis, having the jointed appearance of bamboo.

Banti's syndrome Enlarged spleen and anaemia, associated with cirrhosis of the liver and ASCITES.

Barber's itch (*tinea sycosis*) A fungus infection of bearded parts of the face, producing reddish patches covered with dry hairs and scales. A more severe condition, *sycosis barbae*, is caused by bacterial infection of follicles of the beard, producing crusts, pimples, and numerous pustules perforated by hairs.

Barbiturates Drugs now used mainly for the control of epilepsy. They have been superseded by safer drugs as sleeping pills.

In the United Kingdom barbiturates have become much less popular with doctors in recent years, because they are habit-forming, they have bad long-term effects, they are liable to serious abuse by drug-takers, and used often to be taken for attempted suicide.

A number of nonbarbiturate sleeping pills with a greater margin of safety than the barbiturates have been developed.

All these drugs are sold only on medical prescription.

Barium meal and barium enema A suspension of insoluble barium sulphate in water, swallowed in preparation for a stomach X-ray. The barium has greater density to X-rays than surrounding tissues and thus defines structures. To outline the large intestine the barium is given by enema.

Barrel chest A rounded, bulging, barrel-shaped chest which moves poorly with the intake and output of air and is more or less fixed in a position of deep inhalation; characteristic of advanced emphysema (153).

Bartholin glands Small glands on the floor and sides of the vaginal opening which secrete lubricating material. The glands are subject to infection and cyst formation.

Basal ganglia Aggregations of nerve cells in the region of the base of the brain; Parkinson's disease is associated with abnormalities in this area (163).

Basal metabolic rate (BMR) A baseline of the minimal rate of energy expenditure for maintaining basal activities such as heart action, breathing, and heat production when the body is at rest; useful in diagnosis of certain diseases, especially those involving the thyroid gland (204).

BCG Bacillus of Calmette and Guérin; a vaccine which gives immunity to tuberculosis for a variable time. The vaccine contains strains of live tubercle bacilli grown on ox bile for a long period to reduce their virulence. It is a safe vaccine, extensively used, mostly in persons with special hazards of exposure to tuberculosis, such as doctors, nurses, and members of families of tuberculosis patients. BCG vaccination interferes with the interpretation of tuberculin tests (144), but proponents point out that there are other ways of detecting tuberculous infection.

BDS Twice a day.

Bearing down pains Pains which occur in the second stage of labour when the mother, feeling that something must be expelled, makes powerful contractions of her abdominal muscles in coordination with the contractions of the uterus.

Bed cradle A frame to prevent the weight of bedclothing from pressing on a patient's body.

Bedsores PRESSURE SORES.

Bed-wetting Nocturnal enuresis (265).

Bejel A nonvenereal form of syphilis, transmitted by such means as contaminated eating and drinking utensils. Occurs chiefly in the Middle East.

Bell's palsy Paralysis of the facial nerve, usually temporary; the patient is unable to move muscles of the mouth, eye, and forehead on one side (166).

Bence Jones protein An abnormal protein in the urine, occurring most often in association with *multiple myeloma* (115). The substance is readily deposited in kidney tubules and leads to impaired kidney function.

Bends See CAISSON DISEASE.

Benign Mild; usually the word means that a tumour is not cancerous. Benign tumours are not necessarily harmless; they can cause a wide range of symptoms related to pressure, obstruction, twisting, and excessive production of potent substances such as hormones.

Beriberi A deficiency disease, rare in this country, chiefly the result of a deficiency of thiamine (vitamin B_1) in the diet (363). *Dry* beriberi chiefly affects the nerves of the extremities; *wet* beriberi is characterized by oedema and congestive heart failure.

Bezoar A solid mass of compacted indigestible material in the stomach or intestines, found occasionally in mentally disturbed persons who swallow rags, rubber, hair, rope, and other inedible materials. A hair ball is called a *trichobezoar*.

Bile A yellowish or greenish fluid continuously manufactured in the liver; it is stored and concentrated in the gallbladder and released as required into the duodenum (351). Bile helps to emulsify and absorb fats and to alkalinize the intestine. It is a complex, bitter-tasting fluid (gall) containing pigments, salts, fatty acids, cholesterol, and other materials. Bile salts are sometimes used in medicine to stimulate the secretory activity of the liver.

Bilharziasis See SCHISTOSOMIASIS.

Biliousness A nondescript word for vague symptoms attributed, usually wrongly, to the liver. Probably the word survives from ancient times when a "choleric" person was said to have an excess of yellow bile and a "melancholy" person an excess of black bile. Many symptoms, including jaundice, can indeed arise from abnormalities of bile, but only a doctor can diagnose them.

Bilirubin The principal pigment of bile; a substance derived from the breakdown of HAEMOGLOBIN. Bilirubin tests are useful in determining the nature of certain blood and liver diseases, in distinguishing different types of jaundice, and in evaluating excessive destruction of blood cells.

Biological clocks Some people can set a mental clock to awaken them before an alarm clock goes off. A few are confident enough to dispense with alarm clocks entirely. Many familiar physiological rhythms recur approximately every 24 hours – sleep, waking, ups and downs of body temperature and heart rate. These are called *circadian rhythms*. There are also many shorter rhythms, such as brain wave patterns, superimposed upon longer ones. All of these are rather like biological clocks distributed through the body.

Biopsy Removal of tissue from the living body for purposes of diagnosis, as in cases of suspected cancer. The specimen may be subjected to biochemical tests; more often, it is set in a paraffin block, cut into very thin slices, stained, and studied under a microscope. If necessary, the procedure can be completed in a few minutes by quick-freezing the tissue. This is frequently done while the patient remains under anaesthesia on the operating table and surgeons await the pathologist's verdict as to whether a tumour of the breast or other organ is or is not malignant.

Birth control See CONTRACEPTION.

Birth defects Some live newborn infants have abnormalities recognizable at birth. Some defects such as a slightly twisted toe or a cleft lip are obvious *congenital malformations* (present at birth). Others have abnormalities which are not recognizable at birth, but which become apparent as they grow older. Many abnormalities are relatively minor, and about 80 per cent of birth defects, including the most serious forms such as congenital malformations of the heart, can be corrected and treated.

Causes, if not the total mechanisms, of some birth defects are known. Some are hereditary, determined by parental CHROMOSOMES, and genetic counselling is helpful to prospective parents concerned about some real or imagined abnormality that runs in the family (see MEDICAL GENETICS). Some defects are *environmental*, quite unrelated to heredity.

A disturbance of the environment of the fetus may distort its growth. The best-known example of environment-caused abnormalities is infection of the mother with German measles at a critical time of pregnancy. Some abnormalities are believed to be caused by a combination of hereditary and environmental factors, or by an accident at the time of delivery, as in cases of brain damage due to interruption of the oxygen supply to the newborn during delivery.

Time of vulnerability. It is now well established that certain birth defects originate at a critical time of pregnancy; in general, during the first three months, at the time when the cells of the embryo are developing into arms and legs and vital organs. At this time the embryo is peculiarly vulnerable to harmful agents. Before then it is too young; afterwards, too old to be seriously affected. It has also been established that in early pregnancy, excessive amounts of alcohol and tobacco have similar harmful effects on the embryo. See page 229.

Blackwater fever An acute complication of MALARIA, especially in persons who have been treated with quinine. An attack is marked by high fever, shivering, and profound anaemia; the urine is very dark, hence the name (56).

Black widow spider (*Latrodectus mactans*) A small black spider with a globe-shaped abdomen marked by a reddish design like an hourglass or dumbbell. Its bite is very painful and can be serious if treatment is neglected. This spider is not native to Britain, but is occasionally imported in crates of fruit.

Blastomycosis A group of diseases caused by yeastlike fungi, variously affecting the skin, lungs, or body as a whole.

Bleb A small blister usually filled with blood or fluid.

Blepharitis Inflammation of the eyelids, usually due to bacterial infection; sometimes associated with allergies or seborrhoea of the face and scalp.

Blind spot A small spot on the retina, where the optic nerve enters, which is insensitive to light (398).

Blood-brain barrier Some natural body substances, drugs, and chemicals circulating in the blood are unable to reach active brain cells. The apparent blood-brain barrier permits some substances to enter and prevents others. It is thought by some authorities to consist of a layer of cells around small capillaries in the brain. The barrier is presumably a natural protective mechanism.

Blood poisoning A general term for the presence of germs or their toxins in circulating blood. See BACTERAEMIA, SEPTICAEMIA, TOXAEMIA.

Blood tests Laboratory tests of blood can yield a vast amount of information. The extent of testing depends on what is being looked for. There are many special tests for special purposes. A routine blood test does not include unusual procedures, but does include standard studies, for which the following are normal physiological values:

pH (acid-alkaline ratios; pH 7 is neutral, above 7 is alkaline) 7.35–7.45

Red blood cells (erythrocytes)
    4,500,000–5,000,000 per cu. mm.

White blood cells (leucocytes)
    5,000–10,000 per cu. mm.
    Polymorphonuclear neutrophils 60–70%
    Lymphocytes 25–33%
    Monocytes 2–6%
    Eosinophils 1–3%
    Basophils 0.25–0.5%

Platelets 200,000–400,000 per cu. mm.

Haemoglobin 14–16 gm per 100 ml.

Bleeding time 1–3 minutes

Coagulation time 6–12 minutes

Serum cholesterol 150 to 250 mg per 100 ml.
Glucose 80–120 mg per 100 ml.
Albumin 3.5–5.5 gm per 100 ml.
Nonprotein nitrogen 25–38 mg per 100 ml.

Blue baby An infant with a congenital heart defect which allows venous and arterial blood to mix, resulting in insufficient oxygen in the blood, producing blue skin and mucous membranes (72).

Body build See SOMATOTYPE.

Boeck's sarcoid See SARCOIDOSIS.

Bone age An index of physiological maturity, based on the fairly definite schedule of development of bone from birth to maturity, independent of chronological age. Bone age is commonly estimated by taking X-rays of a child's hands and wrists and comparing the centres of ossification with standards appropriate to his age. There are normal variations; bone age may be advanced or retarded a year or so without necessarily being abnormal. Advanced bone age may be associated with overactivity of the adrenal or thyroid glands, retarded bone age with deficient thyroid activity or malnutrition. Tall children who reach sexual maturity at an early age usually have advanced bone age; those who have retarded bone age are probably late maturers.

Bone banks Stored collections of pieces of human bone. When transplanted, the dead sterile bone somehow stimulates the growth of new bone around it, eventually is incorporated into that new bone, and is slowly replaced. In the meantime the graft is a barrier which prevents soft fibrous tissue from filling the hole or defect in the patient's own bone. Bone grafts are used most frequently to correct curvature of the spine in children, and after fractures, if the bone ends fail to unite properly.

Bone conduction Bones of the head are natural channels for conduction of sounds to the ears. This can be demonstrated by stopping the ears and touching a vibrating tuning fork to the skull or teeth. Some types of hearing aids, in contact with bone behind the ear, make use of this phenomenon. Bone conduction explains why our own voices do not sound the same to us as they do to others.

Bone marrow examination Microscopic study of bone marrow tissue obtained by needle, used in diagnosing certain diseases of the blood.

Booster dose Injection of a vaccine or immunizing agent given some time after an original vaccination, to enhance its effectiveness. Immunizations tend to wear off in the course of time; a booster rejuvenates them. Some primary immunizations are given in two or three spaced injections, several days or weeks apart, to produce maximal immunizing action.

Bornholm disease (*Devil's grip, epidemic pleurodynia*) An infectious disease of sudden onset, produced by COXSACKIE VIRUSES, marked by knifelike pains in the chest or abdomen.

Botulism A dangerous form of food poisoning caused by toxins of botulinus organisms in improperly preserved foods. This disease is now seldom seen from food poisoning, but has recently arisen spontaneously in infants (50).

Bougie A slender cylindrical instrument introduced into a body orifice to explore or dilate a passage or act as a guide for other instruments.

Boutonnière deformity Bending of the middle joint of a finger with extension of the other joints, resulting from the cutting or rupture of a tendon (460).

Bowlegs (*genu varum*) Outward bowing of the knee joints; common in young children just beginning to walk, usually requiring no treatment unless bowing persists after five or six years of age (464).

Bowman's capsule The cup-shaped capsule of a *nephron*, the minute filtering unit of the kidney (182).

Bradycardia Abnormal slowness of the heartbeat, with a pulse rate of less than 60 per minute.

Brain waves Minute electric currents of brain cells which, when amplified and transcribed, have the form of spiked or wavy lines. See ELECTROENCEPHALOGRAPH.

Breast support A common source of breast pain, especially if the breasts are unusually large, is a poorly fitted brassiere which supports most of the weight from above by shoulder straps. Correct breast support sustains most of the weight of the breasts from *below*, by the portion of the brassiere which encircles the chest under the breasts; the main function of shoulder straps is to hold the garment in position.

Breath-holding Crying of infants and small children so furious that they hold their breath until they turn blue or even lose consciousness for a moment. A breath-holding spell can be frightening the first time a parent is confronted with it, but the episode is just a bout of temper, and nature has arranged that we cannot hold our breath long enough to do serious harm.

Breech delivery Presentation of an infant's buttocks instead of the head at the outlet of the birth canal.

Bright's disease An old term for several diseases which fall under the general category of *glomerulonephritis* (189).

Bromhidrosis Foul-smelling perspiration, caused by decomposition of sweat and debris by bacteria.

Bromism Chronic poisoning from long continued use of bromides; these drugs are now seldom used.

Bronchial tree The breathing passages which extend from the windpipe in finer and finer ramifications (139).

Bronchiectasis Dilatation of bronchial tubes, usually a result of pus-producing infections or obstruction by foreign bodies.

Bronchitis Inflammation of the linings of bronchial tubes (146).

Bronchography The taking of an X-ray film of the lungs after injection of a radiopaque substance.

Bronchoscope A tubelike instrument, inserted into the windpipe for purposes of inspecting tissues, withdrawing secretions or tissue samples, administering medicines, or extracting foreign bodies.

Bronzed diabetes See HAEMOCHROMATOSIS.

Brucellosis (*Malta fever, undulant fever*) An infectious disease transmitted from animals to man, most commonly by contact with cattle or consumption of raw milk products (51). Called *undulant fever*, from the type of fever. Recovery from acute brucellosis is usually spontaneous but convalescence may be prolonged. Chronic brucellosis may be unrecognized and hard to diagnose; varied symptoms – obscure fever of long duration, weakness, fatigability, excessive sweating – may puzzlingly resemble those of infectious mononucleosis, tuberculosis, malaria, or rheumatic fever. Positive diagnosis is made by recovery of brucella organisms from body excretions.

Bruxism The habit of grinding the teeth.

BSP A test for liver function.

Bubo An inflamed, swollen lymph node, usually in the groin or armpit, caused by absorption of infective materials.

Buccal Of or relating to the cheek or mouth.

Buerger's disease Inflammation of the inner walls of blood vessels with clot formation and interruption of blood supply. The legs, feet, and toes are especially affected. Shutting off the blood supply can lead to GANGRENE and amputation. The cause of the disease is unknown but it chiefly affects young men and is almost never seen in nonsmokers. Absolute prohibition of smoking for the rest of the patient's life is an essential part of treatment; resumption of smoking can provoke renewed attacks and gangrene.

Bulimia Insatiable appetite, requiring enormous meals for satisfaction.

Bulla A large blister.

Bunion (*hallux valgus*) Enlargement and thickening of the big joint of the big toe, bending the big toe towards the little toe (469). The deformity becomes progressively worse if untreated. Surgical correction is not so simple as it seems, but is indicated for young persons. In older persons, a special shoe made to fit the deformity comfortably may be the most practical solution.

Buphthalmos Enlargement of the eye.

Burkitt's lymphoma A form of malignant tumour, especially affecting the jaw and facial bones, most frequent in children of central Africa, but also occurring elsewhere. The tumour responds well to therapy. The disease is thought to be caused by a virus (Epstein-Barr).

Bursa A sac between opposing surfaces that slide past each other. It is filled with lubricating fluid, which permits free motion. Inflammation of a bursa causes painful *bursitis* (456), as of the shoulder, elbow, knee, or ankle.

Butterfly suture A strip of plastic or adhesive tape with a relatively thin bridge between wider ends, used to draw together the opposing edges of a minor laceration on a smooth skin surface.

Byssinosis An occupational disease of textile workers caused by inhalation of dusts produced during certain processing stages in cotton, flax, and hemp mills. Initial symptoms are chest tightness, cough, wheezing, and shortness of breath, which occur predominantly on the first working days after absence from work, as over a weekend. The cause is thought to be a chemical substance in textile dusts which constricts the bronchi and causes asthma-like symptoms.

C

Cachexia Profound weakness, emaciation, general ill health, resulting from serious disease such as cancer.

Caecum The blind pouch in which the large bowel begins; the appendix projects from it (336).

Caesarean section Delivery of a baby through an incision in the abdomen and uterus. Legend has it that Julius Caesar was born in this way.

Cafe au lait spots Multiple pigmented patches in the skin, the colour of coffee with milk, associated with NEUROFIBROMATOSIS.

Caffeine A chemical substance contained in tea, coffee, and cola beverages. Caffeine is a powerful stimulant of the central nervous system and tends to increase both mental and physical performance. A great variety of drug preparations contain caffeine, often in combination with other drugs.

Caisson disease Divers' paralysis; cramping pain in the abdomen, legs, and other parts, called "the bends" by divers. Symptoms are caused by nitrogen bubbles in the blood. The nitrogen gets into the blood from air inhaled under pressure, as under water or in caissons or wherever surrounding pressure greatly exceeds that of the atmosphere. Attacks can be prevented by gradual ascent from a deep dive, or treated by putting the patient into a decompression chamber where high pressure is gradually reduced while nitrogen slowly dissipates from body fluids.

The bends can affect scuba divers who stay too long under water at depths of 100 feet or so and ascend too rapidly.

Calcaneus The heel bone.

Calcification The process by which tissues become hardened by deposits of calcium salts.

Calcium A mineral element that is an essential constituent of bone and is essential for blood clotting, muscle tone, and nerve function.

Calculus A stone formed in a duct, cyst, or hollow organ of the body, especially in the gallbladder (351) and kidney (193). Most calculi are composed of mineral salts, often with a mixture of organic matter. The composition of a stone may sometimes give the doctor information of value in preventing future stone formation. Stones range in size from specks of sand to stones which fill the entire interior of the organ. The material that stones are made of is somehow extracted and condensed from fluids of the body. Infection and stagnation of fluids play a part in stone formation, but exactly why some people form stones and others do not, is not known. Drinking hard water is not a causative factor. Stones may cause few symptoms if they stay where they are, but severe pain ensues if a stone tries to squeeze through a passage too small for it. *Dental calculus* is tartar that accumulates on teeth (379).

Callus A patch of hard, thickened skin, usually on the hands or feet; a protective reaction to pressure or friction. A callus is like a corn except that it is more diffuse and has no core, and it tends to disappear spontaneously when the cause is removed. Persons who stand a great deal often develop thick calluses of the heel or ball of the foot. The hard skin may be removed by rubbing with pumice stone, emery board, or a coarse Turkish towel after soaking the foot in hot water. Persistent calluses which cause a great deal of discomfort should have the attention of a chiropodist. Callus is also a word for the bony material which exudes from and surrounds broken bony ends and plays a part in the healing of a fracture.

Calorie A unit of heat. The unit used in measuring body metabolism and the fattening propensities of foods is the large Calorie, the amount of heat necessary to raise the temperature of one kilogram of water one degree Centigrade. Nowadays the unit joule is preferred (354).

Calyx One of the several small cuplike chambers which receive urine from the kidney tubules and channel it into the funnel-shaped cavity of the kidney which merges with the ureter (184).

Candidiasis Infection caused by *Candida albicans*, which has a predilection for mucous membranes. Common sites of infection are the skin, nails, mouth, vagina, gastrointestinal tract. See vaginal yeast infections (310), in pregnancy (227), thrush (126).

Cannula A hollow tube for insertion into a body passage or cavity; within the cannula there is usually a *trocar*, a sliding rod with a pointed tip, designed to puncture a cavity and release fluid, after which the trocar is withdrawn and fluid drains through the cannula.

Canthus The angle formed where the eyelids meet at the outer or inner side.

Capillary The smallest size of blood vessel.

Carbohydrate The primary fuel of muscular activity, the major source of energy we need for moving, working, acting, living. Carbohydrates occur as sugars and starches, in many complex forms; the starches are converted to sugar by the digestive processes (359). Cereals, vegetables, and fruits are inexpensive carbohydrate foods which are major sources of food for much of the world's population. Carbohydrate is necessary to burn fats efficiently, and it spares protein, which can be burned for energy if necessary but is more valuable for other purposes. Cellulose, the indigestible matter in many carbohydrate foods, supplies useful bulk in the intestines. Most of the carbohydrate in the body is stored in the liver and muscles in the form of glycogen (animal starch), but not much more than a day's needs are held in storage. As the supplies become depleted, hunger pangs remind us that it is time to replenish our energy reserves.

Carbon dioxide snow Extremely cold snowlike particles about $-73°C$ $(-100°F)$ formed by rapid evaporation of liquid carbon dioxide. Application of the snow freezes the skin instantly. It is used in treatment of various skin lesions, such as birthmarks (120).

Carbon monoxide A colourless, odourless gas which can cause fatal poisoning. Immediate first aid is imperative (580). Carbon monoxide kills by depriving tissues of oxygen; it combines 200 times more readily than oxygen with HAEMOGLOBIN of the red blood cells. The gas is produced by any incompletely burned fuel. A common belief that a fire in a closed space is dangerous because it burns up all the oxygen is erroneous; it is dangerous because it emits carbon monoxide. It is dangerous to let a car run in a closed garage even for seconds. Gas can also seep into a car from a leaky silencer or exhaust pipe. Relatively small amounts of the gas in a car driven with windows closed can dull a driver's senses or cause him to fall asleep at the wheel. It is wise to drive with one window at least partly open and to have the exhaust system checked for leaks during routine inspections.

Carbuncle A deep-seated infection of the skin, like several boils joined together; pus is discharged from a number of points on the tight, reddened skin surface (124).

Carcinogen Any agent which tends to produce cancer.

Carcinoma Cancer comprised of epithelial cells, the type that cover the skin and mucous membranes and form the linings of organs. Carcinomas may arise in almost any structure of the body; many forms are curable if proper treatment is begun early.

Cardiac Of or relating to the heart.

Cardiac asthma (an undesirable term) Paroxysms of difficult breathing, often occurring at night, characteristic of congestive heart failure (75). It is a quite different condition from bronchial asthma.

Cardiac catheter A slender tube which is threaded into a vessel of the arm and on into the heart to obtain several kinds of important diagnostic information (73).

Cardiac pacemaker A device which electrically stimulates the heart, triggering the beat and producing contractions at or near the normal rate when the organ itself cannot do so reliably (80).

Cardiac sphincter The valve of ringlike muscle at the junction of oesophagus and stomach (330).

Cardiospasm See ACHALASIA.

Cardiovascular Of or relating to the heart and blood vessels.

Caries Decay of bone; the dentist's word for tooth decay (dental caries).

Carotene A yellow pigment occurring in carrots, leaves, yellow vegetables, egg yolk, and other foodstuffs. The body converts it into vitamin A. Excessive intake over a long period of time of carrots or other carotene-rich foods may raise the blood's content of carotene to such an exaggerated level that the skin takes on a yellowish hue, sometimes mistaken for jaundice. This condition, known as *carotenaemia*, is harmless.

Carotid The principal artery that runs up each side of the neck. At approximately the middle of the neck it divides in a Y shape; one branch continues as the external carotid artery which goes to the face and scalp, and the other as the internal carotid artery which goes directly to the brain. Some strokes are caused by obstruction of the artery at the Y; the structure is close to the surface, readily accessible to a surgeon, and an operation may result in great improvement of the patient's symptoms (177). Overstimulation or compression of nerves at the point where the artery divides can cause dizziness and loss of consciousness.

Carpal Of or relating to the wrist. The *carpal tunnel* through which a large nerve passes from the wrist to the hand may become constricted and cause tingling and numbness of the fingers (460).

Car sickness See MOTION SICKNESS.

Cartilage Gristle; white, elastic, connective tissue. It is the substance of soft parts of infants which later become bone. It forms part of the skeleton. Pads of cartilage cushion the opposing surfaces of joints; thinning or wearing away of cartilage is associated with some forms of arthritis (476). The stiff but flexible substance of the external ear is cartilage. Cartilage does not have a blood supply and if injured cannot heal. Tearing or other injury of cartilage is quite common among athletes. This often requires surgical removal of the cartilage, for example from the knee (465).

Caruncle A small, nonmalignant, fleshy growth; a type which causes pain and bleeding (urethral caruncle) occurs at the urinary outlet of women, most frequently at the menopause.

Castration Removal of the testicles or ovaries. Functional powers of both can be destroyed by radiation. Sometimes necessary in treatment of disease; this is called nonsurgical castration.

Casts *renal* Shed material in sediments of urine, sometimes indicative of latent forms of kidney disease (188). There are four forms of casts, *hyaline* (glassy), *red cell*, *granular*, and *epithelial*, from which inferences concerning the nature of kidney lesions may be drawn.

Catabolism The breaking-down aspect of METABOLISM; the breaking-down of complex substances by cells is often accompanied by release of energy. The opposite of ANABOLISM.

Cataract An opacity of the lens of the eye. A cataract is not a foreign substance, but a biochemical change in structure. Babies may be born with cataracts and some of these cases are hereditary. Increasing age, physical injury, chemical injury from certain drugs and industrial chemicals, diabetes and other endocrine diseases, are associated with cataract formation, but the great majority of cataracts seem to be a part of the ageing process. The only way to restore useful vision is to remove the lens surgically (412); this permits light to enter the eye once again. Of course the light-bending powers and power of ACCOMMODATION of the absent lens are lost. The patient has to wear spectacles to replace the missing lens. He can see quite well again – a wonderful reprieve from partial or total blindness – but it takes some adjustment and re-education. Many improvements have been and are being made in cataract glasses but they do not restore normal ease of seeing completely. Contact lenses have been improved and come closer to restoring normal visual function but they are not suitable for everyone. Replacement of the opaque lens with a plastic substitute is becoming increasingly successful.

Catarrh A flowing down; an old-fashioned term for inflammation of mucous membranes, especially of the nose and throat, with free-flowing discharge, as in a cold.

Catatonia A phase of schizophrenia in which the patient stands or sits in some fixed position for hours on end and resists all attempts to get him to speak or move.

Cat cry syndrome A peculiar condition of infants who give a cry like that of a cat, because of defective development of the larynx. It is an inherited abnormality, resulting from lack of a short arm on one of the infant's CHROMOSOMES.

Cathartic A purgative medicine; a substance that increases evacuation of the bowels. Regular use of cathartics is unwise; they can be habit-forming, and do not correct an underlying condition. Cathartics or laxatives should not be used if abdominal pain is present, and powerful cathartics such as castor oil or epsom salts should be used only as the doctor directs.

Catheter A hollow tube for insertion through a canal into a cavity to discharge fluids, especially of the urinary bladder (186). The heart may also be catheterized for diagnostic purposes (73).

Cat scratch disease An infection characterized by painless swelling of lymph nodes, acquired from a scratch by a cat.

Caul The head of a baby born with a caul is covered with a fetal membrane, the AMNION, which has become detached.

Causalgia Burning pain caused by injury to sensory nerves, especially of the palms and soles; often associated with poor circulation to the part and discoloration, clamminess, and coldness of the skin. Blocking the affected nerves with procaine may give relief.

Cautery Application of heat or a chemical to destroy tissue. In ancient times, a red hot iron was applied to wounds to stop bleeding and infection. Today the most common form is *electrocautery*, in which a wire loop heated by electric current is used to seal bleeding vessels or destroy tissue.

Cellulitis Diffuse septic inflammation of soft, loose connective tissue beneath the skin.

Cementum The bonelike substance which covers the roots of teeth (377).

Centigrade (C) A thermometer scale, in which water freezes at o degrees C and boils at 100 degrees C. To convert to Fahrenheit degrees, multiply degrees Centigrade by nine fifths and add 32. Average body temperature is 37° Centigrade (98.6° Fahrenheit).

Central nervous system (*CNS*) The brain and nerves of the spinal cord (159). The system is central because it is the functional headquarters of the whole nervous system, and all the nerves of the body enter or leave the brain or spinal cord.

Cephalic Of or relating to the head. Turning the fetus so that the head presents at the cervix is called *cephalic version*.

Cerebellum A specialized part of the brain, underneath the CEREBRUM at the back of the head (155). It is concerned with equilibrium and coordination of movements.

Cerebral palsy A form of paralysis manifested by jerky, writhing, spastic movements, resulting from damage to brain centre controls of muscles (169). Cerebral palsy is not a single disease but a group of syndromes with a common factor, some form of injury to motor control centres in the brain. It is not always possible to determine the cause of brain damage. It may result from birth injury, from infections of the mother or fetus, from errors of development, and other causes.

Cerebrospinal fluid Clear colourless fluid that surrounds the spinal cord and is continuous with the same fluid in the ventricles of the brain. Examination of the fluid assists in the diagnosis of various diseases (such as meningitis, polio, brain tumour) which cause changes in the fluid. The fluid may contain blood, pus, and other abnormal constituents; it may be given chemical, microscopic, and bacteriological tests and may be cultured to determine the presence and identity of germs.

Cerebrovascular accident A stroke, resulting from interruption of blood supply to the brain (176). The cause may be obstruction by a clot of a vessel supplying the brain, or rupture of a vessel with bleeding into brain tissue.

Cerebrum The main part of the brain; the great mass of nerve tissue that occupies the entire upper part of the skull. *Cerebral* refers to phenomena that occur in the cerebrum; for example, cerebral haemorrhage.

Cerumen Ear wax (428).

Cervical erosion A rough spot in the membrane lining the opening of the cervix.

Cervical rib An extra rib in the cervical or neck region, in addition to the usual twelve on each side. It can sometimes be felt as a bony projection at the root of the neck. The rib may cause no trouble, but if pressure or other disturbing symptoms develop, it may require operation.

Cervicitis Inflammation of the neck of the uterus.

Cervix A neck; the word applies to any necklike or constricted part of the body; especially, the tapering neck of the uterus (304). Also, the neck of the urinary bladder. The seven cervical vertebrae (442) constitute the topmost part of the spine; cervical lymph nodes occur in the neck region.

Chadwick's sign A blue discoloration around the entrance to the vagina and on the neck of the uterus; an early indication of pregnancy.

Chafing See INTERTRIGO.

Chalazion A painless small tumour or cyst of the eyelid due to an obstructed drainage duct; dammed-up secretions cause the swelling. Hot compresses can be applied, together with an antibacterial medicine if the doctor so directs. If the tumour does not disappear spontaneously incision may be necessary.

Chancre The primary lesion of syphilis; a hard sore or ulcer at the site where syphilis germs gained entrance to the body.

Chancroid (*soft chancre*) A nonsyphilitic venereal disease caused by a specific bacillus, *Haemophilus ducreyi*. Initially a soft sore appears, usually on the genitals. In a few days it breaks down into a painful pus-discharging ulcer.

Chemotherapy Treatment with chemicals which favourably alter the course of a disease.

Cheyne-Stokes respiration An abnormal form of breathing in some patients with heart, kidney, or vascular disease. Intensity of breathing gradually decreases until no breath at all is taken for a few seconds or longer. This is followed by increase in breathing and shortage of breath. The pattern occurs in repeated cycles. One of the causes is thought to be a decrease in blood supply to the brain.

Chilblain (*erythema pernio*) An acute or chronic form of cold injury, less severe than frostbite, characterized by inflammation of the skin, itching and swelling, frequently followed by blisters. The immediate cause is exposure to cold, to which some persons have an exaggerated sensitivity; it is advisable for them to stay indoors or wear heavy garments and fleece-lined gloves and overshoes during cold weather. Such persons should begin to wear protective clothing early in the winter when the environmental temperature drops below 15°C (60°F).

Chloasma Discoloration of the skin with yellow-brown spots and patches. The condition is often associated with some endocrine disturbance. Chloasma frequently occurs in pregnancy as a result of increased secretion of a pituitary hormone, MSH, which stimulates pigment-producing cells.

Encyclopedia of medical terms

Hormone production returns to a normal level soon after delivery and the pigmented areas fade, though not always completely.

Chocolate cysts Cysts of the ovary filled with chocolate-coloured material, characteristic of *endometriosis* (313).

Cholangitis Inflammation of the bile ducts.

Cholecystitis Inflammation of the gallbladder. It may occur in acute or chronic forms (351).

Cholelithiasis Stones in the gallbladder or its ducts (351).

Cholera A serious epidemic infectious disease caused by comma-shaped germs transmitted in bowel discharges of carriers to food and water. It is characterized by profuse watery diarrhoea, cramps, vomiting, prostration, and suppression of urine. The principal mechanism by which cholera weakens and kills is through extreme losses of body fluids and ELECTROLYTES. Travellers going to regions where cholera outbreaks occur (India, Pakistan, South East Asia) should be vaccinated with a cholera vaccine which gives some immunity for about six months.

Cholesteatoma A mass that forms in the middle of the middle ear. The first sign may be a scanty discharge from the ear when the mass liquefies and perforates the drum. This also causes erosion of bone, which may extend dangerously into neighbouring structures. In most cases, surgical removal of the cholesteatoma is the best treatment (427).

Cholesterol A waxy substance resembling fat in its properties, closely related to the sex hormones and vitamin D. It is present in all animal tissues. It regulates the passage of substances through cell walls, keeps us from becoming waterlogged when we bathe, and prevents us from losing too much water from evaporation. It is so important to the body that it is manufactured by the liver and other tissues whether we get cholesterol in our diets or not. Despite these virtues, cholesterol has become something of a scare word, blamed for degenerating the walls of arteries and setting the stage for heart attacks. However, most specialists are reluctant to indict cholesterol as the predominant factor in heart and blood vessel diseases (69). One reason for cholesterol's bad publicity is that it is easier for doctors to measure than other fatty components of blood serum. Clinically, such measurement is useful as an index of the overall pattern of fatty substances in the blood. The normal range of serum cholesterol is about 125 to 265 mg per 100 ml. It tends to rise in later years, and changes can be caused by variations in thyroid activity, diabetes, kidney insufficiency, and stress. Moderation of fat intake, reduction of weight if obese, and substitution of polyunsaturated fats for some of the hard fats in the diet are prudent measures in the present state of knowledge.

Chondroma A tumour with the structure of CARTILAGE, usually benign, but with a tendency to recur after removal.

Chorea A disease of the nervous system manifested by involuntary, irregular, rapid, jerky movements of muscles of the face, legs, and arms. Its common form (also called *St. Vitus' dance* and *Sydenham's chorea*) is a disease of childhood, often a manifestation of rheumatic fever (76). The jerky movements and facial grimaces subside in a few weeks. Signs of rheumatic disease may never appear, but about half the patients with chorea develop or have rheumatic fever. HUNTINGTON'S CHOREA is an entirely different hereditary disease.

Chorion The outermost of the fetal membranes. The fetal part of the placenta develops from it.

Choroid The middle coat of the eye, continuous with the iris in front; a thin, pigmented layer composed largely of interlaced blood vessels, vital to the eye's nutrition (394).

Christmas disease A hereditary bleeding disease, having the same symptoms as classic haemophilia but resulting from deficiency of a different blood-clotting factor (111). Named after the family in whom it was discovered.

Chromosomes Threadlike bodies in the nucleus of a cell; they contain the GENES and DNA (see chapter 26).

Chronic Long continued ill health as opposed to *acute* illness.

Cilia Minute hairlike processes of specialized cells which beat rhythmically and keep debris-laden fluids flowing in one direction; for example, out of the lungs. The word also means eyelashes.

Ciliary body The part of the eye which suspends the lens and secretes aqueous humour (395).

Circadian rhythms. Cycles and rhythms of body processes that recur approximately every 24 hours. See BIOLOGICAL CLOCKS.

Circumcision Removal of the foreskin or prepuce of the penis.

Cirrhosis of the liver Chronic, progressive inflammation of the liver, with increase of nonfunctioning fibrous tissue, distortion of liver cells, enlargement or shrivelling of the organ, and various eventual complications such as oedema, digestive complaints, weight loss, jaundice, bleeding veins of the oesophagus (35).

Cisternal puncture Puncture at a point beneath the skull in the back of the neck to withdraw CEREBROSPINAL FLUID, when the more usual method of lumbar puncture is not possible.

Claudication Lameness, limping. *Intermittent claudication*, characterized by cramplike pain in the legs which comes on when walking, is usually a symptom of obliterative arterial disease (81).

Clavicle The collarbone (445).

Cleft lip, -palate Congenital malformation of structures of the lip, palate, or both, which fail to fuse properly during fetal development (441). The bilateral parts of the lips and palate normally fuse at about the eighth week of pregnancy.

Climacteric The change of life. See MENOPAUSE and MALE CLIMACTERIC.

Clinical Of or relating to the bedside; by extension, observation and treatment of patients, results and experience thus gained, as opposed to theoretical, laboratory, or experimental medicine.

Clitoris The small erectile sex organ of the female, situated above the vagina (302); homologue of the penis.

Clofibrate A drug that lowers fat levels in the blood, prescribed in the hope that such lowering may reduce the incidence of heart attacks.

Clonic Spasmodic muscular contractions and relaxations which succeed each other alternately and jerkily. It may be combined with *tonic* contractions which are continuous.

Clonorchis A chronic Asiatic disease caused by liver flukes transmitted by raw, smoked, or pickled fish.

Clubbed fingers Short, broad, bulbous finger ends with overhanging nails. The condition results from local deficiency of oxygenated blood and is usually associated with abnormalities of the heart and respiratory system such as congenital heart malformation, emphysema, bronchiectasis, chronic disease of the heart and chest.

Clubfoot (*talipes*) A foot twisted out of shape so that the sole does not rest flat on the floor when standing; there are several types (468). Heredity has little if anything to do with the condition. The principal causative factor is thought to be a fixed position of the fetus in the uterus, maintained for a long period of fetal life; scantiness of amniotic fluid possibly inhibits free movement of the fetus. Pressures of long-maintained fixed posture tend to modify the development of body parts in a mechanical way.

Coagulation time The time it takes a sample of blood to form a clot, determined by laboratory procedures. This information is useful in treating patients with a tendency to haemorrhage, and as a guide to treatment of patients receiving anticoagulants.

Coarctation of the aorta Congenital constriction of the great vessel which carries arterial blood from the heart (72).

Cobalt bomb In medicine, not really a bomb but a device employing radioisotopes of cobalt for powerful irradiation of patients, usually suffering from cancer.

Coccus A small round bacterium. Some types, such as those which cause gonorrhoea and pneumonia, occur in pairs; other types form chains and others cluster in irregular masses like bunches of grapes.

Coccyx The fused vertebrae at the tip of the spine; the tailbone (443).

Cochlea A bony pea-sized structure of the inner ear, shaped like a snail shell, lined with fine hairs and nerve endings which are the essential organs of the sense of hearing (420).

Coeliac disease A disorder, believed to have a hereditary basis, in which the small intestine is unable to absorb fat from foods. See MALABSORPTION SYNDROME.

Coenzyme A partner needed by some enzymes to accomplish a biochemical change. Many vitamins are coenzymes.

Coffee-ground vomit Dark brown or blackish granular vomited material, somewhat resembling coffee grounds; the colour comes from changed blood and indicates slow bleeding in the upper digestive tract (344).

Coitus Sexual intercourse.

Colchicine A drug prepared from roots of the meadow saffron which is specific in relieving acute attacks of GOUT (477).

Collagen Fibres in the connective tissue which supports the body; it constitutes 40 per cent of the body's protein. In ways not fully understood, it is associated with rheumatic and other diseases, collectively called collagen or connective tissue diseases (483). Collagen fibres vary greatly in structure and function. Some, as in the cornea of the eye, are transparent. Collagen is the cushioning material of cartilage in the joints, the matrix on which minerals are laid down to form bones, the inelastic material of tendons which transfer muscle movements over joints, the elastic part of skin, a part of webs and struts which hold the body together, a substance which when boiled yields glue or gelatine. Once laid down in the body, collagen is not renewed or replaced. Old collagen is less elastic than young collagen. It is related to stiffness of joints and laxity of skin with increasing age, and may be a good index of a person's biological rather than chronological age.

Collapsed lung Pneumothorax or atelectasis (521).

Colles' fracture A common fracture of one of the forearm bones (*radius*) near the wrist joint on the thumb side. It is usually a consequence of falling with an arm thrust out and hand bent backward to break the fall.

Colloid goitre Soft, smooth, symmetrical enlargement of the thyroid gland, usually as a result of iodine deficiency; simple goitre.

Colon The large bowel (336).

Colostomy A surgically created opening of the colon (artificial anus) in the wall of the abdomen (519). A colostomy may be temporary, to divert intestinal contents while a portion of the colon is healing, or it may be permanent, as is usually the case if a large section of the bowel must be removed because of disease. A *colostomy bag* is a container which covers the artificial opening and receives excretions.

Colostrum The first milk secreted by the mother's breasts shortly after the birth of a child. Colostrum is not true milk but a clear or slightly cloudy fluid containing fats and sugars which have a slight laxative effect on the newborn baby. Colostrum also contains IMMUNOGLOBULINS which pass on to the baby some of the immunities acquired by the mother; this immunity is not long lasting.

Colour blindness Inability to distinguish colours. There are many types and degrees of colour blindness, some so slight that an affected person may never be aware of it. Colour blindness does not affect keenness of vision and is no great handicap except in occupations where safety or fine colour discrimination is important. A colour blind man may choose a shirt, tie, jacket, socks, and trousers of violently clashing hues. Total colour blindness in which everything is seen as shades of grey is rare. The most common type is red-green colour blindness, which may range from ability to see only the brightest hues of red and green to inability to see the two colours as other than shades of grey. Injury to the retina or ocular disease may produce colour blindness, but this is very rare. Colour blindness is almost always inherited; a few women are partially colour blind but the condition predominantly affects the male sex. Common red-green colour blindness is a sex-linked trait, transmitted to her sons but not her daughters by a mother who herself is not colour blind. The inherited defect is in the structure of the CONES, the colour-sensitive nerve cells of the retina (398). Nothing can be done to change the defect, although some improvement in discrimination of shades may be attained by training.

Colpotomy Any surgical cutting of the vagina.

Coma Unconsciousness so deep that it is impossible or extremely difficult to rouse the patient. Many different conditions cause coma; advanced liver and kidney disease, diabetes, poisoning, head blows, tumours, strokes, to mention a few.

Comedo Blackhead.

Comminuted fracture One in which the bone is broken into pieces (471).

Compound fracture One in which the broken bone breaks through the skin or into an open wound.

Concussion Violent jarring, shocking, shaking, or the resulting condition. *Concussion of the brain* (165) may result from a fall or violent blow on the head. The injured person may not be knocked out, but may be dizzy, sleepy, nauseated, or he may lose consciousness and have a feeble pulse, cold skin, and pallor. Medical help should be sought immediately, even though the person seems to have recovered or to be only slightly dazed. A doctor treating concussion may wish to keep the patient under observation, or to make tests, to be sure that the skull has not been fractured, or the brain damaged.

Conduction deafness Failure of airborne sound waves to be conducted efficiently through and over the external and middle ear structures, so that adequate messages do not reach the nerves of the inner ear (424).

Condyloma A warty growth on the skin around the anus and external sex organs.

Cones Specialized cells of the central part of the retina which distinguish colours and are responsible for finely detailed vision (398).

Congenital malformations Abnormalities that are present at birth. See BIRTH DEFECTS.

Conization Reaming out of a cone-shaped piece of tissue by high-frequency current; usually a gynaecological procedure performed on a diseased cervix.

Conjunctiva The thin mucous membrane which covers the insides of the eyelids and is reflected over the front of the eye (407). *Conjunctivitis* is an inflammation of this tissue resulting from infection, allergies, irritation, or inflammation from within the eye itself.

Consanguinity Blood relationship.

Contact dermatitis Skin eruption, redness, or inflammation, resulting from contact with any of hundreds of substances (124).

Contact lenses Plastic or glass lenses worn over the cornea of the eye (404). Meticulous fitting to the eye contours is essential. The lenses must have proper hygienic care. Serious complications are rare, minor ones not uncommon. The most painful complication appears to result from wearing the lenses too long. They should not be worn while sleeping, or when the eye is infected, or when there are cold sores on the face (the cold sore virus can infect the eyes dangerously). Flush-fitting contact lenses which cover the white of the eye permit a thin layer of tears to circulate beneath them and have special medical uses as healing aids. Such lenses improve the healing of chemical burns of the cornea, ulcerations, corneal transplants, and other conditions. Plastic lenses which absorb moisture have become available; see SOFT CONTACT LENSES.

Contraception Prevention of conception or impregnation.

Contraindication A medical term meaning that something is undesirable, or should not be done; for example alcohol is contraindicated in extreme cold.

Contrast medium A substance which has greater density to X-rays than tissues which are objects of study. Contrast media are given by injection or other means to obtain clearly outlined X-ray images of structures being examined.

Contusion A bruise.

Coombs' test An antibody test on blood, used in determining the compatibility of bloods for transfusion and in diagnosis of certain anaemias.

Cornea The curved transparent tissue covering the iris and pupil on the outside of the eye; the window of the eye (395).

Corneal transplant The cornea may become scarred or clouded, obstructing vision. If the rest of the eye is in good condition, sight may be restored by transplanting a disc taken from the cornea of a recently deceased person. It is like replacing an opaque pane of glass with a transparent one. The procedure requires a supply of donor eyes, and eye banks have been established in many cities to receive and preserve donated eyes, which must be removed promptly after death of the donor. It is useless to donate one's eyes in a will, because of legal delays. Anyone wishing to donate his eyes after death should do so through his doctor or an eye bank.

Corns Rough skin thickenings about the size of peas which occur principally on or between the toes. Soft corns between the toes are softened by sweat. The common hard corn has a cone-shaped core which presses on nerves to cause dull discomfort or sharp pain. Corns are caused by continued pressure and friction, as from too tight or ill-fitting shoes and stockings. Pressure can be relieved by wearing softer shoes with ample toe-room and by foam rubber pads and inserts. The hard tissue of a corn usually must be removed as required for comfort's sake. Soaking the feet in hot water and paring the surface of the corn with a razor blade often relieves friction and pressure, but there is a risk of cuts and infection. Superficial hard tissue may be removed with an emery board, nail file, or pumice stone. The core may be sufficiently loosened by soaking to be lifted out by sterilized tweezers. Corn plasters and medicines usually contain salicylic acid which softens the hard growth. Diabetics should be especially careful in care of the feet because of the risk of ulcers (220).

Coronary thrombosis Commonly called a heart attack; a blood clot in a coronary artery of the heart (71).

Cor pulmonale A form of heart disease secondary to chronic disease of the lungs.

Corpuscle Any small round body; the word used to be a synonym for cell. Technically, a cell has a nucleus; the mature red blood cell does not, and is sometimes called a corpuscle.

Corpus luteum The yellow body which develops from a follicle of the ovary after a ripened egg has been discharged. The yellow body produces progesterone, a hormone which prepares the lining of the uterus to receive a fertilized egg (212). If fertilization occurs, the corpus luteum enlarges and continues to produce pregnancy-sustaining hormone for several months. If conception does not occur, the corpus luteum shrinks and degenerates.

Cortex The surface layer of an organ such as the brain, kidney, adrenal gland. The cortex of an organ has different functions from its inner part (medulla); for example, the adrenal cortex produces hormones entirely different from those of its inner part. The thin surface layer of the brain (*cortex cerebri*) consists of grey matter, largely composed of small-bodied nerve cells with rich interconnections, interspersed with larger neurons which send AXONS into underlying white matter.

Corticosteroids Substances having the properties of hormones secreted by the cortex of the adrenal glands (208). Cortisone, hydrocortisone, prednisone, and many other corticosteroids have important medical uses.

Coryza An old word for the common cold.

Cosmetic dermatitis Inflammation of the skin, usually allergic, produced by contact with cosmetic creams, dyes, lotions, perfumes, and the like (124).

Cowper's glands Two small glands of the male which secrete lubricating fluids into the urethra (185).

Cowpox A disease of cattle, so closely related to smallpox, and so mild in man, that inoculation with vaccine containing cowpox virus has long been the standard method of immunizing against smallpox.

Coxsackie viruses A family of viruses named after a community in New York from whom the viruses were first isolated and identified. A score or more of different Coxsackie viruses cause diseases such as HERPANGINA, BORNHOLM DISEASE, and forms of *meningitis*.

Crabs Infestation by pubic lice (128).

Cradle cap Patchy areas of greasy crusts on an infant's scalp, arising from secretions of oil glands (271).

Cranial nerve A nerve attached directly to the brain, leaving it through a perforation in the skull. There are twelve pairs of cranial nerves, with names that suggest their function or location: transmission of the sense of smell (*olfactory*), sight (*optic*), hearing (*acoustic*); control of movement – of the eyeball (*trochlear*), a muscle of the eyeball (*abducens*), the pupil (*oculomotor*), muscles of the upper throat and taste sensations from the back of the tongue (*glosso-pharyngeal*), sense of taste, salivary glands and muscles of the face (*facial*), muscles of the larynx and throat (*accessory*), the tongue (*hypoglossal*); sensory nerve of the face and front part of the scalp (*trigeminal*); sensory and motor nerve branching to the heart, stomach, and oesophagus (*vagus*).

Craniotomy   Surgical opening of the skull cavity.

Cranium   The skull.

Creeping eruption   (*larva migrans*)   A parasitic infection of the skin: thin, red, tortuous lines creep ahead at one end an inch or more a day while fading at the other end. The moving lines mark the progress of larvae burrowing under the skin. The burrowers, often immature forms of cat or dog hookworm, get into people who go barefoot on beaches, children in sandpits, gardeners, and repairmen who work under porches or houses. Freezing the larvae in the skin with an ethyl chloride spray usually stops their migrations.

Creeping ulcer   One which creeps slowly outward from its centre.

Cremaster   The muscle which retracts the testicle.

Cretin   A child born with an underactive thyroid gland (206).

Crohn's disease   See REGIONAL ILEITIS.

Crossed eyes   Eyes that do not work as a pair in holding the gaze straight on an object, because of imbalance of muscles that control movements of the eyeballs (407). An eye that turns in or out in young children may lose its vision completely unless the condition is corrected before it is too late.

Croup   Difficult laborious breathing and coughing of a child. *Spasmodic croup* is more frightening than serious; another type, *laryngotracheobronchitis*, is one of the most serious conditions of infancy and is a medical emergency (272).

Crowning   The stage in childbirth when the crown or top of the infant's head first becomes visible in the dilated outlet of the vagina.

Cryosurgery   Use of extreme cold to destroy or to freeze and later revive tissues. Pioneering cryosurgical work was done in the field of brain surgery, especially in surgical management of *Parkinson's disease*. Complete destruction of tissue by super-freezing has been used to relieve benign or malignant obstruction of the *prostate* gland. The freeze treatment for *gastric ulcer* does not permanently destroy stomach tissue, but tends to decrease acid production; long-term benefits are considered disappointing by many. A newer application of cryosurgery (more exactly, cryotherapy, since tissue is not destroyed) is in the treatment of *glaucoma* (410). The purpose is to decrease production of fluid in the eye. Cryotherapy is a reserve method if drugs or surgery fail to stop the advance of glaucoma.

Crypt   A cavity, pit, or follicle; such as the natural depressions in the tonsils.

Cryptorchidism   Failure of the testicles to descend into the scrotum during fetal development; the undescended organs remain in the abdominal cavity or groin (212).

Curettage   Scraping out of a body cavity with a spoon-shaped instrument called a *curette*.

Curling's ulcer   An ulcer of the stomach or duodenum, associated with severe skin burns.

Cushing's syndrome   Disorders resulting from excessive output of certain adrenal hormones.

Cuticle   The dead outer layer of skin; the crescent of skin at the base of nails.

Cyanosis   A bluish tinge of the skin and mucous membranes resulting from insufficient oxygen in the blood. There are many different causes; for example, congenital heart defects (72), congestive heart failure, emphysema, mountain sickness, respiratory and blood disorders. The lips or the beds of the nails may sometimes take on a bluish discoloration without a deficiency of oxygen in the general circulation, simply from slow circulation due to cold.

Cyesis   Pregnancy.

Cyst   A normal or abnormal sac with a definite wall, containing liquid or semisolid material. Frequent sites of cysts that may require surgery or other measures are the ovaries, kidneys, skin, the coccygeal area (pilonidal cyst), and breast.

Cysticercosis   Infestation of the body with tapeworm larvae, sometimes present in raw beef. Beef should be cooked at least to the rare stage (60°C, 140°F) to avoid danger.

Cystic fibrosis   An inherited disease of the *exocrine* glands which pour secretions into or out of the body rather than into the blood; for example, the pancreas and bilary, intestinal, and sweat glands. Thick viscid secretions obstruct or depress the functioning of many different organs and tissues and produce a variety of symptoms; respiratory distress is prominent (272). Cystic fibrosis was discovered in 1938, at which time it was thought to be a disease of the pancreas; it is now known that nearly all the exocrine glands are affected to some degree. The earliest sign of cystic fibrosis in a newborn infant is MECONIUM ILEUS. Prompt recognition and treatment of cystic fibrosis, with aerosol aids for breathing, postural drainage, digestive enzymes, and antibiotics to combat infection, have carried affected infants through critical periods of childhood. The disease is being increasingly recognized in adults who have had it from infancy, without realizing it. Doctors think it likely that many patients treated for bronchial asthma or various chronic lung conditions actually have cystic fibrosis. The disease is transmitted as a recessive trait (the mother and father are carriers but do not have the disease themselves). An abnormal protein in the blood serum of cystic fibrosis patients and of blood-related persons is the possible basis for a test to detect carriers of the trait; if two carriers marry, the chance that each of their children will have cystic fibrosis is one in four.

Cystinuria   An inherited disease in which cystine, a sulphur-containing amino acid, is excreted in large quantities in the urine. The poorly soluble cystine tends to form recurrent kidney stones (193); alkalinizing the urine and drinking large amounts of water may help to reduce the likelihood of cystine stone formation.

Cystocele   Sagging of the base of the bladder into the vaginal canal (315).

Cystoscope   An instrument for examining the interior of the urinary bladder (187).

Cytological diagnosis   Microscopic study of cells shed by body tissues to detect abnormalities, especially the presence of cancer cells. The PAPANICOLAOU SMEAR test for detection of cancer of the cervix is the most widely used cytological screening test, but the technique is applicable to smears obtained from the lungs, stomach, bladder, and a number of other organs.

Cytology   Scientific study of the structure, elements, and functions of cells.

Cytoplasm   The substance of a cell outside its nucleus.

Cytotoxic drugs   Drugs that are poisonous to body cells. Cancer cells are often more vulnerable to such drugs than normal tissues, and so these drugs have a valuable part to play in the treatment of some kinds of cancer.

D

D & C   Dilatation and curettage, a common minor operation on women; the canal of the uterus is dilated and the lining of the uterus scraped with a spoon-shaped instrument called a curette (321).

Dandruff Fine, whitish, somewhat greasy scales formed upon the scalp (133); the condition is controllable but rarely curable.

Deaf-mutism Inability to hear and speak. The two disabilities are interrelated. A totally deaf child cannot learn to speak in the normal way because he cannot hear sounds to imitate. Various signs may arouse suspicion of deafness in an infant as young as six months (424). While the child is still young, he can be taught to speak by training techniques used in special schools for the deaf.

Débridement Surgical cleaning of a wound; removal of foreign material and dead tissue.

Decalcification The withdrawal of calcium from the bones where it has been deposited. It may be caused by an inadequate supply of calcium in the diet so that calcium has to be taken from the bones, or by hormonal imbalances.

Decibel The unit of measurement of the loudness of sound, used in tests of hearing (424). A whisper is about twenty decibels loud.

Decidua That part of the lining of the uterus which is modified during pregnancy and cast off after delivery.

Decubitus ulcer See PRESSURE SORES.

Defaecation Passage of faeces; evacuation of the bowels.

Deficiency diseases Those caused by insufficiency of some constituent of the diet, such as vitamins, minerals, protein, fatty acids (359).

Deglutition The act of swallowing.

Dehiscence A splitting open, as of a sutured wound.

Dehydration Drying out of the body; loss of more water than is taken in. Dehydration may be induced for medical reasons, but often it is an aspect of disease or injury, characterized by dry mucous membranes, fever, scanty urine, soft or even wrinkled skin, possible shock. Treatment, which may present an emergency, requires recognition of underlying circumstances, calculation of water and ELECTROLYTE deficits, and usually replacement of water and salts (sometimes of plasma or blood) by infusion into a vein.

Déjà vu Already seen; an illusion that a present experience has occurred at some previous time.

Delirium A state of mental confusion, excitement, incoherent talk, restlessness, hallucinations. Delirium may be associated with high fever, poisoning, drug intoxication, infections, and metabolic disturbances. Treatment is directed to the underlying condition while the patient is kept in a quiet room, and closely watched to prevent injury. Tranquillizers may be prescribed. Reassurance by a close member of the family may help significantly to allay fears.

Delirium tremens (D.T.'s) A serious, sometimes fatal form of delirium, most often occurring in persons with a long history of alcoholism, but occasionally associated with other poisoning of the brain cells, senile brain changes, and psychoses. The patient has vivid visual hallucinations, often of moving coloured animals, large or small; he may feel as well as see them crawling over his skin. Anxiety, fear, coarse trembling of the hands, mental confusion, and sleeplessness are other manifestations. Physical restraints may be necessary but skilful attendants can often avoid this. The delirium lasts for a couple of days to a week or more and usually terminates in deep sleep. The patient is often malnourished and run down physically. Appropriate tranquillizers and large doses of B vitamins are commonly a part of treatment. KORSAKOFF'S PSYCHOSIS may begin as delirium tremens.

Deltoid Triangular in shape, like the Greek letter *delta*; specifically, the muscle which covers the shoulder joint and extends the arm out from the side.

Dementia A general term for mental deterioration, usually implying serious impairment of intellect, irrationality, confusion, stupor, insane behaviour. Dementia may result from poisons, physical changes in the brain, toxins produced by disease, or psychoses of which the basic cause is unknown.

Dendrites Fine, branched fibres, which accept and convey incoming impulses to the central body of a nerve cell (154).

Dengue Sudden high fever, called breakbone for the severe pain it causes in muscles, bones, and joints. It is not a dangerous disease.

Dental implants Replacement of lost teeth, as by reimplantation of a knocked-out tooth (381).

Dental plaque A thin, transparent film that builds up on the teeth. It is made up of material from saliva. The plaque contains bacteria which are thought to be a factor in tooth decay.

Dentine The ivory-like material, harder and denser than bone, which underlies the enamel of the teeth (377).

Denture The set of natural teeth; also, a set of artificial teeth; "false teeth" (390).

Denture stomatitis Sore mouth due to ill-fitting dentures or allergy to substances in the plates (382).

Depilation Removal of hair. Permanent removal of unwanted hair is best accomplished by ELECTROLYSIS, which destroys the hair follicle.

Depot desensitization A single injection technique for desensitization to allergens, using oily emulsions (497).

DeQuervain's disease (*stenosing tenovaginitis*) Thickening of the sheaths covering the tendons of the thumb, resulting in pain at the base of the thumb, and radiating to the nail and into the forearm (459). Surgery corrects the condition, or it may cure itself if the wrist is immobilized.

Dercum's disease (*adiposis dolorosa*) A rare disease of middle-aged and older women. Firm fat nodules, slightly sensitive or very painful, are distributed over various parts of the body except the face, lower arms, and lower legs; the overlying skin is red and shiny. There is pronounced muscular weakness and degree of psychological disturbance. The cause is not known. Nonspecific methods of treatment include measures to relieve pain, reduce weight, and combat the mental disturbances that may be associated.

Dermabrasion A method of removing layers of skin with an abrasive instrument, usually a rapidly rotating wire brush, for cosmetic improvement of scars or blemishes.

Dermatitis Inflammation of the skin. Its causes are manifold, its symptoms varied. Chemicals, plants, common household agents, cosmetics, drugs, X-rays, and many other things can produce dermatitis; allergies to various substances are often involved.

Dermatoglyphics The study of the ridges, whorls, lines, and creases which form highly individual patterns of the skin of the hands and feet. Skin patterns determined by GENES begin to form in the fetus at about the fourth month of pregnancy. Several abnormal patterns, such as a single crease instead of the usual two which run across the top of the palm, are characteristic of infants with congenital diseases. Some disorders such as MONGOLISM and KLINEFELTER'S SYNDROME result from abnormal CHROMOSOMES. Others, such as malformations associated with the mother's infection by German measles, result from unfavourable environment of the fetus at the time when skin patterns as well as organ systems are developing. It is not yet possible to identify specific diseases by abnormal palmprints, but they usually indicate some congenital abnormality. Palmprint studies may give early warning of a congenital disorder, or confirm some suspected condition, such as mongolism, without the need for analyzing chromosomes.

Dermatome An instrument for cutting thin layers of skin for grafts.

Dermatomyositis An ill-defined disease of unknown cause, affecting connective tissue, manifested principally in the skin and voluntary muscles; characterized by pain and swelling in muscles, weakness, inflammation and swelling of skin of the face, upper trunk, and extremities.

Dermatophytes Fungi which produce blistery, scaly, crusty lesions of the skin; most notoriously those responsible for *dermatophytosis* or athlete's foot.

Dermis The true skin, as opposed to the epidermis; the *corium*; a dense elastic layer of fibrous tissue underlying the topmost epithelial layers.

Dermographia Skin writing; a condition in which a tracing made on the skin by a fingernail or blunt instrument produces a pale streak bordered on each side by a reddened line. The marks disappear after a few minutes. The condition may be associated with NETTLE RASH but in itself is not injurious to health. Dermographia occurs in persons whose mechanisms for expanding and constricting blood vessels are sensitive to any irritation.

Dermoid cyst A congenital cyst (often of the ovary) which contains fragments of skin appendages such as strands of hair, sweat and oil glands, and sometimes cartilage, bone, and teeth, remnants of development.

Desensitization Reduction of a person's allergic reaction to a specific substance such as pollen or house dust. Sensitivity is reduced by spaced injections of small amounts of extracts of specific allergens; hay fever injections are a familiar example (497).

Desquamation Shedding of the skin in scales or sheets, as after scarlet fever or severe sunburn.

Detached retina Separation of the light-receiving layer of the back of the eye from its underlying layer (413). In the majority of cases, the detached filmy structure can be welded back into place by surgical procedures.

Deviated septum Diversion from a straight line of the bony wall that divides the nose into two equal parts, usually a result of injury but sometimes congenital (434). The deformity may not be obvious from the outside. Depending on its nature, a deviated septum may partially obstruct air passages, deflect air currents, and lead to mouth-breathing and profuse, annoying postnasal drip.

Dextrocardia Congenital transposition of the axis of the heart towards the right side of the chest.

Dextrose (*glucose*) A sugar which is a source of energy, and necessary for combustion of fats. The liver converts dextrose into *glycogen* (animal starch) and stores it. This reservoir is drawn upon for dextrose, reconverted from glycogen, as energy needs of the body require. Dextrose solutions are often infused into the veins of patients.

Dhobi itch See TINEA CRURIS.

Diabetes The word comes from a Greek term for syphon, or to flow through, referring to the excessive flow of urine and excessive thirst. Used alone, diabetes means *diabetes mellitus* or sugar diabetes (216). There are other forms of diabetes, such as *diabetes insipidus* (204), a hormone imbalance causing enormous thirst and compensating urinary outflow, and *bronzed diabetes*, associated with HAEMOCHROMATOSIS.

Diagnosis The art and science of identifying a patient's disease, a prerequisite to treatment. Some diagnostic techniques date back to the time of Hippocrates: the patient's history, symptoms, and physical signs; tapping and listening, feeling, inspecting, applying all the senses. Modern tools project the perceptions of physicians into chemical and electrical processes of the body. Instruments amplify and transcribe minute currents of the heart and brain and muscles; instruments of many kinds carry trained eyes into caverns of the body; a film of tissue yields secrets to a pathologist; X-rays probe hidden structures.

Dialysis Separation of substances in solution by passing them through a porous membrane; this is done naturally by the kidney and mechanically by an ARTIFICIAL KIDNEY (190).

Diaphragm The transverse, dome-shaped muscle which separates the chest from the abdomen; the chief muscle of breathing (140). Contraction of the diaphragm expands the rib cage and lungs so that air flows in; relaxation allows the rib cage and lungs to collapse partially, and air is exhaled. A *vaginal diaphragm* is a ringed latex cup which covers the cervix for contraceptive purposes.

Diaphragmatic hernia See HIATUS HERNIA.

Diarrhoea Abnormal frequency and liquidity of stools (348). In young infants, profuse diarrhoea (and vomiting) can cause serious loss of fluids and ELECTROLYTES, and the baby should be under the care of a doctor.

Diastole The resting stage of the heart during which relaxed chambers are filling with blood (64). Diastolic pressure is the lower of the two figures (such as 120/80) by which doctors express blood pressure readings (see SYSTOLE). Diastolic pressure gives the doctor significant information about the condition of blood vessels and the harmful effects of sustained hypertension (86).

Diathermy Generation of heat in body tissues by passing high-frequency electric currents through them. Resistance of the tissues produces the heat, which is very penetrating and can build up to dangerous levels unless treatment is supervised by an experienced operator. In surgical diathermy, heat is sufficient to destroy tissues or to cut tissues with little or no bleeding.

Diathesis Inborn constitutional susceptibility or predisposition to a certain disease or condition.

Digitalis A drug derived from the foxglove which is a powerful stimulant of heart muscle contractions. Whole digitalis contains a number of active agents called *glucosides*; some of these, such as *digitoxin*, are prepared pharmaceutically in pure form. *Digitalization* is the procedure of administering digitalis until a desired concentration of the drug is built up in the patient's body, after which maintenance doses suffice. The toxic effect of digitalis is close to the therapeutic effect and medical supervision of dosage is necessary.

Diopter The unit of measurement of the refractive (light-bending) power of a lens, including the lens of the human eye, which has a power of about 10 diopters. Abbreviated as D in prescriptions for glasses; +D (plus D) indicates a convex lens for correcting a farsighted person, −D (minus D) a concave lens for correcting a short-sighted person (404).

Diphtheria An acute contagious disease, once responsible for many deaths of children, but no longer a threat to the child who is properly immunized (282).

Diplegia Paralysis of like parts on both sides of the body.

Diplopia Seeing double; one object is seen as two. The condition may be temporary or persistent and can be caused by a number of diseases and disorders, including head injuries, alcoholism, and poisoning. The double vision effect is the result of paralysis or improper functioning of muscles that control the eyeball movements, or paralysis of one of the nerves controlling action of the eye muscles. Persistent double vision may be the result of a nervous system ailment such as multiple sclerosis, myasthenia gravis, meningitis, tabes dorsalis, or a brain tumour affecting the nerves running between the brain and eye muscles. Treatment of persistent diplopia may require surgery, the use of special corrective lenses, or both.

Dipsomania Compulsion to drink alcoholic beverages to excess.

Dislocation Displacement of a bone from its normal position in a joint, usually the result of a severe blow, fall, or twisting force; often there is an accompanying sprain (471).

Diuretic An agent which increases the output of urine; a drug prescribed for this purpose. Along with other treatment, physicians prescribe diuretics for a variety of conditions associated with excessive retention of water; for example, congestive heart failure (75); hypertension (86); premenstrual tension (214); cirrhosis of the liver (351).

Diverticula Small thin-walled pouches opening from a hollow organ. They can occur anywhere along the digestive tract from the oesophagus to the colon, but the most common site is the colon (348). A person with these little pockets has *diverticulosis* but may never know it as they may not cause symptoms. It is estimated that ten per cent of people over 40 years of age have diverticulosis. Chances that existing pockets may become infected, inflamed, or ruptured, resulting in *diverticulitis*, increase with advancing age. Diverticulitis is sometimes called left-sided appendicitis because the patient's symptoms are similar to those of appendicitis except for reversal of position. Many patients with diverticulitis are well controlled with medical measures. Sometimes surgery is necessary to remove a diseased portion of the bowel (517).

Dizygotic Developed at the same time from two fertilized eggs; (of twins) fraternal.

Dizziness A feeling of unsteadiness and of the world revolving about one (429). The disturbance may be primarily in the inner ear (423), in nerves serving this area, in reduced blood supply to the brain, in nervous messages from the heart, eyes, or stomach, or in association with many other conditions. An ordinary mild bout of dizziness can usually be cured by sitting or lying down. Dizziness is not usually a symptom of serious disease but recurrent attacks should be investigated to determine the cause.

Dominant eye The eye unconsciously preferred in visual tasks, such as aiming a rifle (394).

Dorsum The back; any part of the body corresponding to the back, as the back of the hand.

Double-blind study A technique often used in studying the effects of drugs. Neither the doctor nor the patient knows whether a given medicine contains an active drug or totally inert ingredients. This eliminates unconscious bias in knowing that a drug should or should not have some effect.

Double vision See DIPLOPIA.

Douche A stream of water directed against or into a part of the body; used alone, the word usually refers to a *vaginal douche* (308).

Down's syndrome See MONGOLISM.

Dreams See SLEEP.

Dropsy An old term for OEDEMA.

Drug addiction Certain drugs (including alcohol) have an effect on body cells, particularly those of the nervous system, called *tissue tolerance*. Body chemistry is upset and the cells adjust their metabolism to accommodate the drug. The tissues become physically dependent upon the drug to maintain their normal functions.

Over a period of time, increasingly large doses of the drug are necessary to obtain the same original effect and the body, in turn, constantly alters its chemistry to accommodate the larger doses. Eventually the addict is able to tolerate doses of drugs which would be fatal to a non-addict. When an addict suddenly stops using drugs, he experiences severe WITHDRAWAL SYMPTOMS because of physical dependency; he also has psychological dependency. Because addiction and habituation are often used interchangeably, the World Health Organization to banish confusion has adopted a more general term, drug dependence. Dependence is defined as "a state arising from repeated administration of a drug on a periodic or continuous basis." This is subdivided into dependence of the morphine type, cocaine type, barbiturate type, marijuana type, amphetamine type, and alcohol type, applying to all types of drug abuse. (See chapter 28.)

Dry labour See BAG OF WATERS.

Dry socket Failure of a protective blood clot to develop in the socket left after extraction of a tooth, or premature loss of a clot, causing pain and delay in healing (392).

Ductus arteriosus In the fetus, a tube which bypasses blood from the pulmonary artery to the aorta; normally it closes and ceases to function at birth (72). In certain cases the channel fails to close. Usually the condition can be corrected by surgery.

Dumping syndrome Symptoms of abdominal distension, diarrhoea, vomiting, and distress, occurring soon after eating in persons whose stomachs have been partially removed (345).

Duodenum The first part of the small intestine (333). Here, just beyond the acid stomach, the intestinal environment begins to become alkaline. Alkaline bile and digestive juices of the pancreas flow into the duodenum. *Duodenal ulcer* is the most common type of peptic ulcer (343).

Dupuytren's contracture Thickening of connective tissue (FASCIA) of the palm of the hand, pulling one or more fingers down into the palm (460).

Dura mater The outermost membrane of tough connective tissue which covers the brain and spinal cord (162).

Dyscrasia Abnormal state, especially of the blood.

Dysentery Inflammation of the colon with severe diarrhoea, abdominal cramps, painful and ineffectual rectal straining; the stools may contain blood and mucus. Chemical poisons and various irritants of the bowel can cause dysentery, but there are two major forms of the disorder: BACILLARY DYSENTERY produced by certain bacteria and amoebic dysentery produced by protozoa (48).

Dysfunction Abnormality or impairment of the normal activities of an organ or bodily process.

Dyslexia Literally and in its widest sense the word means difficulty in reading. This may be due to many causes, for example defective vision, mental backwardness, psychological causes, or the effects of physical disease. The word is also used to describe a particular disorder; a congenital defect of brain function, in an otherwise normal and intelligent person, which impairs or prevents his learning to read. In children, special teaching can often improve the condition.

Dyslogia Impairment of speech.

Dysmenorrhoea Difficult, painful menstruation (305).

Dyspareunia Painful or difficult sexual intercourse; the cause may be physical, mental, or both.

Dyspepsia Disturbed digestion; indigestion. There are

several disorders (see MALABSORPTION SYNDROME) in which foods are inadequately digested or assimilated. But the terms dyspepsia and indigestion are often rather casually applied to symptoms which do not arise primarily from incomplete digestion of food but which originate in the digestive canal or adjacent organs. Inaccurate use of the word does no harm if it sends one to a doctor to find out what the trouble is.

Dyspnoea   Difficult breathing, distress, often but not invariably associated with heart or lung disease.

Dystocia   Painful or difficult labour, delivery, childbirth.

Dystrophy   Degeneration, wasting, abnormal development.

Dysuria   Difficult or painful urination.

E

Ecchymosis   Bleeding into the skin and the discoloration of skin so produced. It may be from a bruise, or from disease of blood vessels or the blood itself.

ECG   An electrocardiogram. See ELECTROCARDIOGRAPH.

Echinococcus cysts   Multiple fluid-filled cysts, particularly in the liver or lungs, produced by tapeworm larvae; *hydatid disease*.

ECHO viruses   The initials mean Enteric Cytopathic Human Orphan, the orphan indicating that the viruses are not associated with known diseases. The designation has become less appropriate since some of the viruses have been identified as the causative agents of certain diseases.

Eclampsia   Convulsions. A serious form which can occur in late pregnancy or even during or after delivery; it is an extreme manifestation of *toxaemia of pregnancy*, often associated with kidney disorders. Early signs of impending eclampsia are practically always evident to the doctor, in time to institute effective preventive measures. Eclampsia is rare in women who receive proper prenatal care.

Ectomorph   See SOMATOTYPE.

Ectopic   In the wrong position, out of place; for example, *ectopic pregnancy* in which the embryo is implanted in a fallopian tube or elsewhere outside the uterus.

Ectropion   Outward-turning of an eyelid, drooping away from the eyeball.

Eczema   Is not a disease, but a general term for inflammation of the skin (121).

Edentulous   Toothless.

EEG   An electroencephalogram; a brain wave tracing or record. See ELECTROENCEPHALOGRAPH.

Effleurage   A stroking movement used in massage.

Effusion   Outpouring of fluid into a body part or tissue.

Ejaculation   Ejection of semen.

Elective treatment   Treatment which is not immediately urgent. *Elective surgery* can be put off until a more convenient or desirable time.

Electric knife   A surgical instrument employing electric current to cut and seal vessels bloodlessly.

Electrocardiograph   An instrument which amplifies tiny electric currents in contracting heart muscle and records these on paper. The written record is an *electrocardiogram* (ECG). Electric impulses are conveyed to the machine from surfaces over several areas of the heart. Interpretation of electrical events within the heart muscle, recorded in an ECG, gives valuable information in the diagnosis of heart disease and in following the progress of a patient during his recovery from a coronary attack (66).

Electroconvulsive therapy   (ECT)   A treatment for some forms of mental illness; an electric current is passed from temple to temple through the patient's brain, producing unconsciousness (506). The patient has no memory of the shock.

Electroencephalograph   An instrument which amplifies minute electric currents from brain cells and transcribes them to a moving strip of paper. This record, called an *electroencephalogram* (EEG), shows aspects of brain activity, popularly called brain waves, in the form of spiked or wavy lines (165). Electrodes taped to the subject's scalp pick up tiny currents from brain cells near the surface of the skull. The brain has several characteristic rhythms. Modern electroencephalographs have a number of channels, each recording changes in electric potential between two electrodes taped to different areas of the scalp. The instrument is useful in diagnosing various disturbances of brain function, such as epilepsy, and is a research tool for investigating the workings of the brain. Recent advances in studies of SLEEP and dreams have been greatly aided by the electroencephalograph's ability to identify rhythms characteristic of different and changing levels of consciousness.

Electrolysis   Permanent removal of superfluous hair by means of an electric needle which renders the hair follicle incapable of further growth. The word also means decomposition of a salt or chemical compound by means of an electric current.

Electrolytes   Electrolytes are dissolved salts or ions in body fluids, analogous to electrolytes in a car battery. Our electrolytes conduct electric currents, they participate in countless chemical processes of life, they are bearers of electrical energy within our cells, they are in constant motion and exert outward pressure, and they are vital regulators of acid-base balance. The principal regulator of water and electrolyte balance is the kidney (182). The major electrolytes are ions of sodium, chlorine, and potassium. Numerous conditions affect the composition of the body fluids: vomiting, diarrhoea, kidney or liver disease, congestive heart failure, dehydration, severe burns, diabetes, drug treatments, surgery, or oedema. There may be excessive loss or excessive retention of electrolytes. Sodium chloride (salt) locks considerable amounts of water in the body. This is the reason for *low-sodium diets* (372), designed to ease waterlogged tissues of their burden. But a gross deficiency of sodium may produce leg cramps and other symptoms. Correction of electrolyte deficits or excesses is an important part of the management of many illnesses.

Electromyography   Tracings of electric currents produced by muscle action.

Elephantiasis   Gross enlargement of a body part (legs, scrotum) due to fluids in tissue spaces under the skin, dammed back by obstruction of lymphatic drainage channels. See LYMPHOEDEMA. The most extreme forms of elephantiasis are seen in persons in tropical countries who suffer from FILARIASIS.

Elimination diets   Menus which start with a few foods that rarely cause allergic reactions, and then add one new food at a time to determine to which one a patient reacts (491).

Embolism   Obstruction of a blood vessel by an EMBOLUS. Consequences vary according to the size of the blocked vessel and the part of the body deprived of blood. The lungs, brain, and heart are frequent sites of embolism. *Pulmonary embolism* which can cause sudden death results from blockage of the pulmonary artery or its large branches. *Fat embolism* results from a severe injury of bone or fatty tissue which disperses fat into the bloodstream, whence it is disseminated to many organs. Fat embolism may be fatal.

Encyclopedia of medical terms

Embolus Any abnormal substance – a blood clot, fat globule, air bubble, clump of cells – which is swept along in the bloodstream until it lodges in a vessel and blocks the flow of blood.

Embryo A term given to the developing human being in the uterus up to the third month of pregnancy, after which it is known as a fetus.

Emetic Productive of vomiting.

Emphysema Too much air in the lung, either from distension or, more usually, from destruction by disease of the divisions between the air sacs.

Empyema Accumulation of pus in a body cavity, especially in the pleural cavity.

Encephalitis Inflammation of the brain. Some forms of encephalitis are caused by viruses (166), others are complications of other diseases or conditions.

Encephalogram An X-ray of the brain.

Endarterectomy Surgical removal of a clot or plaque from the inner wall of an artery (524).

Endarteritis Inflammation of the innermost layer of an artery.

Endemic Of or relating to diseases which occur constantly or repeatedly in the same locality.

Endocarditis Inflammation of the lining of the heart, especially attacking the heart valves.

Endocrine glands Ductless glands which secrete hormones directly into the circulation (198).

Endodontics A branch of dentistry concerned with disease and treatment of inner structures of the teeth.

Endogenous Originating within or inside the cells or tissues.

Endometriosis Presence in abnormal locations of fragments of the membrane which lines the cavity of the uterus (313). The displaced tissue menstruates wherever situated, and so produces cystic collections of blood.

Endomorph See SOMATOTYPE.

Endoscopy Visual examination of hollow parts of the body by insertion of a lighted instrument through a natural outlet. There are many types (sigmoidoscope, bronchoscope, cystoscope, and others) named after the inspected organs. Some have systems of lenses, and auxiliary devices for removing foreign objects or pieces of tissue for examination.

Endotoxin A toxin produced by internal processes of a germ, liberated when the cell of the germ is destroyed.

Enteric coating A coating of drug tablets which permits them to pass through the acid stomach without dissolving and to liberate their dose in the alkaline intestine.

Enteritis Inflammation of the intestine, particularly of the small intestine (346).

Enterobiasis Threadworm infection (59).

Enteroviruses Viruses, such as polio and ECHO viruses, whose preferred habitat is the intestinal tract.

Enucleation Removal of the tonsil or eyeball.

Enuresis Bedwetting; involuntary discharge of urine (192).

Eosinophils Certain white blood cells which take up a pink stain called eosin. Large numbers of eosinophils are present in nasal and other secretions during allergic attacks. They are also increased in parasitic infestation.

Epidemic Rapid spread of disease attacking large numbers of people in the same locality at the same time.

Epidemic pleurodynia See BORNHOLM DISEASE.

Epidemiology The study of epidemic diseases.

Epidermis Popularly, the skin; technically, the outermost part of the skin consisting of four layers without blood vessels (118).

Epididymitis Inflammation of that part of the semen-conducting duct which lies upon and behind the testicle.

Epigastrium The upper middle abdomen. A hand stretched across the lower end of the breastbone covers the episgastrium.

Epiglottis A structure like a hinged lid above the voice box (larynx); it opens to admit air and shuts like a trapdoor during swallowing to prevent food from going down the windpipe (440).

Epilation Removal of hair, including the roots. The same as DEPILATION. See ELECTROLYSIS.

Epilepsy A nervous disorder of varying severity, marked by recurring explosive discharge of electrical activity of brain cells, producing convulsions, loss of consciousness, or brief clouding of consciousness (171).

Epiphysis The end part of a long bone which in children is separated from the shaft of the bone by a layer of cartilage. It is the site of growth in long bones. As growth progresses, the cartilage layer disappears, the epiphysis is said to have closed, and the bone does not grow longer. Therefore growth in height ceases.

Episiotomy An incision in the margin of the vulva to enlarge the area through which the baby's head passes in childbirth; the purpose is to prevent or minimize tearing in less desirable sites.

Epispadias A malformation of the penis in which the urinary canal remains open on the upper side of the organ (188). The problem is to restore urinary control and then to form a new tube by plastic surgery.

Epithelial Refers to those cells that form the outer layer of the skin, those that line all the portions of the body that have contact with external air (such as the eyes, ears, nose, throat, lungs), and the liver, kidneys, digestive, urinary and reproductive tracts.

Epitheliomas Skin tumours of varying malignancy.

Epithelium Specialized tissue which covers all free surfaces of the body, forms the EPIDERMIS, lines hollow organs, glands, and respiratory passages; it does not possess blood vessels.

Epizootic Epidemic disease in animals.

Eponym The name of a person applied to a disease, syndrome, or theory which it is presumed he was the first to discover or describe; for example, *Bright's disease, Addison's disease*. This form of commemoration has become less common since more precise and specific descriptions of disease have been made possible by scientific advances.

Equinovarus A form of clubfoot (468).

Ergotism Poisoning with *ergot*, a substance contained in a fungus that grows on rye and other grains. Ergot has a powerful constrictive action on small blood vessels; chronic poisoning may produce closure of blood vessels, resulting in gangrene of the extremities. Various ergot drugs and combinations have medical uses, as in obstetrics and prevention of migraine headaches.

Eructation A belch.

Erysipelas An acute bacterial infection of the skin and underlying tissue (124).

Erythema Abnormal redness of the skin. The pattern, intensity, distribution, duration, and appearance of the reddened areas give clues to disease, which may be trifling, or a disease of childhood manifested by a rash, or an allergy or systemic disorder.

Erythroblastosis (*Rh disease*) A disease of newborn infants associated with incompatible Rh blood factors of mother and child (103).

Erythrocytes Red blood cells; minute elastic discs containing HAEMOGLOBIN (96).

Erythrocytosis A condition of too many red blood cells in the circulation; *polycythaemia* (106).

Erythropoiesis The process of red blood cell formation.

Eschar Sloughed-off tissue produced by a burn or corrosive substance.

Ethmoid A bone of the upper nose behind the frontal sinus; nerve fibres of the sense of smell pass through perforations in it (436).

Eunuch A castrated male; a boy or man whose testicles have been removed. Eunuchs cannot produce SPERMATOZOA or father children, but if only the testes are removed, and this operation is done after sexual maturity, some eunuchs retain a degree of sexual potency. *Eunuchoidism* is a natural condition in which the sex organs are malformed or physiologically inactive (211).

Euphoria Feeling of wellbeing; often implies exaggerated elation.

Eustachian tube A tubular passage about an inch and a half long which leads from the middle ear to the throat (418). Air passing through it equalizes pressure on both sides of the eardrum, enabling the drum to vibrate freely. Infectious material can enter the middle ear through the tube.

Exanthem A skin eruption or the disease which causes it. *Exanthem subitum* (also called *roseola infantum*) is a disease of childhood; fever comes on suddenly, persists for three or four days, then drops, a skin rash appears, and the child is well. The rash of scarlet fever or measles is an exanthem.

Exchange transfusion Replacement of a baby's blood with suitable whole blood of a donor; resorted to in some instances to save the life of a baby with severe blood-destroying anaemia resulting from incompatibility of the mother's and baby's Rh blood factors.

Excision The act of cutting out.

Excoriation A scratch mark of the skin, usually deep enough to bleed or become crust-covered, produced by scraping or scratching.

Exfoliation Peeling or shedding of surface skin in scales or sheets.

Exocrine Outpouring; glands which do not deliver their secretions to the bloodstream but through ducts and channels to organs and surfaces; for example, sweat glands, sebaceous glands, digestive glands. Inherited disabilities of the exocrine glands are the fundamental defects in CYSTIC FIBROSIS.

Exogenous Originating from outside the cells or tissues.

Exophthalmos Bulging eyes, a condition characteristic of some kinds of thyroid disease (205).

Exostosis Projection of a bony growth from the surface of a bone; a bony spur.

Expectorant A substance that softens or increases bronchial secretions and helps to bring up phlegm from the chest.

Exstrophy of the bladder A congenital malformation in which the bladder has no abdominal covering and urine comes out onto the surface of the body.

Extensor A muscle which straightens or extends a body part.

External cardiac massage A first-aid measure to make a stopped heart start to beat, used in conjunction with mouth-to-mouth resuscitation (586); the latter supplies fresh oxygen. With the victim on his back, place the heel of one hand on the lower part of his breastbone (over the heart), and the other hand on top of the first one. Press down with your weight on the breastbone to force blood out of the heart into vessels. Relax the pressure; blood flows into the heart chambers. Repeat at intervals of about one second. Too much pressure can hurt the heart or break ribs; if the patient is a child, pressure of one hand may be sufficient. Ideally, one person gives mouth-to-mouth resuscitation while the other applies external heart massage. If one person must do it all, he can give external massage for half a minute, then mouth-to-mouth breathing for ten seconds or so, and repeat.

Extrasystole A premature beat of the heart; a contraction that is triggered too soon and is followed by a compensating delay in the next beat (78). The pause between the premature beat and the succeeding one, which is likely to come with a thump, gives a feeling that the heart has skipped a beat. The phenomenon is quite common and usually not serious.

Extravasation Escape of fluids from a vessel, especially a blood vessel, into surrounding tissues. A black eye is a good example.

Extrinsic asthma A form of asthma in which the provoking substance enters the body from outside (148). *Intrinsic asthma*, which has its source within the body, can coexist with extrinsic asthma.

Extrinsic factor Literally, a constituent from outside; medically, the term commonly refers to vitamin B_{12} which prevents pernicious anaemia (105). The vitamin is assimilated from food in conjunction with a substance secreted by the stomach called INTRINSIC FACTOR.

Exudate Anything that is exuded, oozed, trickled, pushed out. One exudes sweat, for example. Although many exudates are entirely normal, in medical usage the word often refers to pus or other materials of pathological importance.

Eye bank See CORNEAL TRANSPLANT.

Eye tooth A canine tooth.

Eye wash A simple and effective eye wash can be made by adding a level teaspoon of salt to a pint of boiled water.

F

Face lift An operation to remove wrinkling caused by loose skin and to tighten fatty tissues which tend to sag in the face and neck with advancing years.

Face presentation Appearance of the face of the fetus at the outlet of the uterus during delivery, instead of the top of the head, as is normal.

Faeces Contents of a bowel movement; the stool. Faeces are not simply unabsorbed food residues. The greatest part of the solid matter is made up of materials excreted from blood, and cells shed by lining membranes of the intestines; about ten per cent is bacteria (see INTESTINAL FLORA). Practically all the protein, fat, and carbohydrate that is eaten is absorbed. Unabsorbed food residues consist largely of indigestible vegetable cellulose, the amount of which varies with the diet. This indigestible roughage stimulates activity and secretions of the bowel. Large amounts of undigested food elements in faeces are associated with diseases which impair assimilation.

Fahrenheit (F) The thermometer scale formerly generally used. It marks the freezing point of water at 32 degrees F and the boiling point at 212 degrees F. See CENTIGRADE.

Fainting (*syncope*) Brief loss of consciousness due to diminished blood supply to the brain. Usually self-corrected; the fainting person drops to the floor and blood flows more easily to the brain. Blood vessels in the abdominal area have immense capacity to hold blood when fully dilated. Shock or strong emotion may cause these vessels to dilate and fill with so much blood that blood pressure drops and fainting results. Rarely is fainting due to heart trouble. A soldier standing at attention for some time may faint, because of lack of muscular movement to aid the return flow of blood through the veins. Feelings of faintness may be cured by lying down, or placing the head between the knees.

Fallen womb Prolapse of the uterus; sagging of the organ into the lower vagina or occasionally protrusion, due to weakness, stretching, or tearing of supporting structures (314).

Fallopian tubes The tubes through which the egg cell is transported to the uterus, and in which fertilization usually occurs.

Fallout RADIOISOTOPES from nuclear explosions which settle out of the atmosphere.

False pregnancy (*pseudocyesis*) Signs and symptoms of pregnancy occurring without conception. The woman herself is usually deceived, and even an obstetrician may be deceived for a while. The patient is usually a woman with an overpowering, obsessive desire to have a child, who through autosuggestion is somehow able to mimic the signs of pregnancy – cessation of menstruation, breast changes, morning sickness, enlargement of the abdomen at the rate of normal pregnancy. Careful examination and tests can determine that no pregnancy exists, but in some instances it is difficult to convince the woman until the expected date of delivery passes.

Fanconi's syndrome Multiple inherited abnormalities which impair kidney function and progressively depress blood cell formation in the bone marrow.

Farmer's lung An inflammatory disease of the lungs which principally affects agricultural workers exposed to mouldy hay, grain, fodder, or silage. The disease resembles pneumonia but does not respond to antibiotics as bacterial pneumonias do. Symptoms of chills, fever, cough, headache, and chest tightness are thought to be caused by allergy-like sensitivity to inhaled mould dusts, and may appear a few hours after heavy exposure. Total avoidance of mouldy vegetable matter is most important during the illness and after recovery.

Fascia Tough sheets of connective tissue which give support under the skin, between and around muscles, blood vessels, nerves, and internal organs.

Fat embolism Plugging of a blood vessel by fat droplets carried in the bloodstream; this can occur from crushing injuries of fatty tissue or bone, or injection of oily solutions.

Fatty acid A compound of carbon, hydrogen, and oxygen which combines with glycerol to make a fat.

Favism Acute anaemia with red blood cell destruction, caused by eating fava beans. The condition occurs only in genetically susceptible persons who do not possess an enzyme that is important in red blood cell metabolism. Certain drugs, such as aspirin and sulphonamides, may produce the same symptoms in susceptible persons.

Febrile Feverish.

Felty's syndrome Chronic arthritis of rheumatoid type with enlargement of the spleen and decreased numbers of certain white blood cells.

Female urethral glands Two glands with ducts just inside the opening of the female urethra. Inflammation of the glands may involve the bladder and cause urgency of urination; the most common cause is gonorrhoeal infection.

Femur The thighbone.

Fenestration An opening in a part of the body, or the act of making one. The *fenestration operation* for improving the hearing of persons with OTOSCLEROSIS creates a bony window for passage of sound waves to the inner ear (527).

Fertile period The period of about one week around the midpoint of the menstrual cycle when conception can occur. The fertile period cannot be pinpointed precisely, but occurs approximately from days eleven to eighteen counting from the onset of menstruation (213).

Festination The taking of hurried short steps to prevent falling forwards, characteristic of *Parkinson's disease* (169).

Fetus The unborn child after the third month of pregnancy; before that it is called an embryo.

Fever Abnormally high body temperature. Normally, body temperature varies slightly through the day, is higher in the evening than in the morning, higher internally than at the skin surface, and is increased by eating and exercise. The most common fevers accompany infections, but disturbances of heat-regulating centres of the brain, as in heatstroke, and other noninfectious conditions can produce fever. Experienced people can often recognize fever by the feel and appearance of the patient's hot, dry, flushed skin. Accurate fever reading, however, requires the use of a thermometer (26). Temperature charts are kept in hospital, and may be desired by the doctor for patients under home nursing care.

Fever increases the body's rate of metabolism about seven per cent for each degree Fahrenheit of temperature elevation. The heart's ability to contract decreases and it beats more rapidly in an attempt to move more blood to the skin to increase heat loss. Excessively high (*hyperthermic*) fever of 40.5°C (105°F) and more cannot be endured for a long period; the very high fever of HEATSTROKE is so quickly lethal that immediate efforts to bring it down must be made by immersing the patient in an ice bath or applying a stream of cold water to the body. Young children react to the slightest infection with fever, sometimes as high as 40°C (104°F); the height of the fever does not necessarily indicate the seriousness of the infection. If a doctor cannot be reached promptly, a very high fever can be reduced by a cool sponge or cool enema (276).

Whether or not fever is part of nature's treatment to cure infection is an unsettled question. In tissue cultures, temperatures of feverish degree inhibit the multiplication of some viruses. There is some evidence that fever increases the production of INTERFERON. But fever-producing organisms in patients survive the temperatures they produce and many authorities doubt that fever has any direct effect on the patient's resistance to infection. All agree, however, that fever is an important guide to the progress of an illness; sometimes it is the only important diagnostic clue.

Fibrillation Fine twitching of muscle fibres, especially of the heart muscle. Individual muscle fibres act independently, uncoordinated, out of rhythm, causing rapid, irregular, ineffective heartbeats. The condition may affect the *atria* or *ventricles* (79) of the heart. Defibrillating devices that administer an electric shock are used to restore normal rhythm.

Fibrinogen A protein manufactured in the liver and distributed into the bloodstream where it acts as a clotting agent when a blood vessel is cut or injured. Fibrinogen combines with another substance, *thrombin*, to yield long threads of *fibrin* which form a mesh to trap blood corpuscles in a clot.

Fibroid A muscle and connective tissue tumour of the uterus (311).

Fibrositis Inflammation of connective tissue (475); often, combined inflammation of muscle and connective tissue (*fibromyositis*), producing pain, tenderness, and stiffness.

Fibula The slender bone on the outer side of the lower leg.

Filariasis A chronic disease caused by the presence of threadlike worms (*filaria*) in the body. The organisms get into the blood through the bites of mosquitoes. The adult worms live in the lymphatic system and cause overgrowth of fibrous tissue which obstructs drainage. Obstructed fluids accumulate in tissue spaces and cause the affected part to swell (LYMPHOEDEMA). The result is some degree of ELEPHANTIASIS. The most extreme forms of the disease occur in residents of tropical countries who are frequently reinfected from mosquito bites.

Fimbria A fringelike structure; especially, fimbriae of the opening of the FALLOPIAN TUBES, close to the ovary. The fringelike projections are covered with *cilia*, minute hairlike processes which wave back and forth and set up rhythmic currents in surrounding peritoneal fluid. Their function is to sweep a mature egg cell released by the ovary into the tube where fertilization usually occurs.

Fish skin disease See ICHTHYOSIS.

Fissure A break or crack in the skin or in a membrane, most frequent in the rectal area (349).

Fistula An abnormal channel between body parts, or leading from a hollow organ to a free surface, which usually discharges fluids or material from an organ. A fistula may be caused by disease, injury, or an abscess which makes an abnormal drainage channel for itself. Many fistulas are named after the body parts they connect; for example, *vesicovaginal* fistula (bladder and vagina). Some fistulas never heal by themselves because of continual infection, and surgical correction is necessary to close the abnormal channels.

Flank The fleshy outer part of the body between the ribs and hip.

Flat foot Ordinarily, if a print of a bare foot on a piece of paper shows that the sole has made flat contact all over, without an open space under the middle inside part of the foot, it is construed as a sign of flat feet caused by fallen arches. This is not always true. Babies' feet are always flat. Some people have naturally flat feet which are perfectly efficient and comfortable. When feet become *flattened*, and hurt, troubles arise and treatment is necessary (466).

Flatulence Excessive gas in the stomach or intestines. A normal bowel always contains some gas; balance is maintained by unostentatious gas exchange mechanisms. Excessive gassiness, vented by belching or passing wind, may result from indiscretions of diet or some disorder of the digestive tract which requires the attention of a doctor. Sometimes, excessive belching is a consequence of unconscious AIR SWALLOWING.

Flexor A muscle which bends a limb or part, as in flexing the biceps.

Floaters Cells or strands of tissue which float in the VITREOUS HUMOUR and move with movements of the eyeball, casting shadows on the retina (415). The floaters, particularly when seen against a bright background such as open sky, look like moving spots and threads of diverse shapes. Floaters are most prevalent in nearsighted and older persons. Usually they are more annoying than serious, but if they become worrying or excessive, an eye examination is indicated.

Floating kidney A kidney which is abnormally movable from its normal location because of slack attachments and inadequate support from surrounding fat.

Flora (intestinal) Bacteria and other small organisms found in the intestinal contents.

Flukes Parasitic flatworms, rarely encountered, which cause infestations of the intestines, liver, or lungs.

Fluorides Salts of fluorine, a gaseous element. The role of fluorides in helping to lessen tooth decay is well known (384). Recent studies have furnished evidence that fluorides contribute importantly to normal bones as well as teeth and may play a part in the treatment and prevention of *osteoporosis* (470), a condition of abnormal porousness, thinning, and easy fracturing of bone, common in women after the menopause and in old people. One study of more than a thousand persons over 45 years of age has shown osteoporosis to be much less frequent in those who lived most of their lives in areas of relatively high fluoride content of drinking water than in those who lived in low-fluoride areas. There was also much less hardening of the AORTA in those who lived in high-fluoride areas. It appears that fluoride helps to keep calcium deposited in hard tissues of the body and not in soft tissues. If such action is confirmed, fluorides may assume an important preventive role in osteoporosis and hardening of the arteries.

Fluoroscope A device for viewing X-ray images on a fluorescent screen. The patient stands behind the screen, and X-rays passing through the body make structures visible to the radiologist. The digestive tract, heart, lungs, and other organs can be viewed in action, and the progress of a BARIUM MEAL can be followed through the digestive tract. Closed circuit television is now used, which exposes the patient to less radiation.

Flutter Rapid, fluttery, but rhythmic beats of the heart atria.

Foley catheter A tube inserted through the urethra into the bladder for drainage of urine; it has a small balloon at the bladder end which is inflated after insertion and serves to hold the catheter in place.

Folic acid A vitamin of the B complex. Also known as *pteroylglutamic acid*. It is a bright yellow compound needed in very small amounts in the diet of animals and man. A deficiency results in poor growth, anaemia, and other blood-related disorders.

Folie à deux A form of mental disorder, usually occurring in close friends, where both have the same delusions.

Follicle A small sac or cavity which produces secretions or excretions. Hair grows from a follicle linked with sebaceous glands which produce skin oil (119).

Fontanelle The soft spot on the top of a baby's head. The area, which is covered by a very tough membrane that is by no means so fragile as some mothers fear, will be filled with bone as the skull grows. It takes anywhere from one to two years for the spot to close.

Food diary A complete record of everything that is eaten for a period of time, a guide to detection of food allergies (491).

Food poisoning Intestinal infection caused by bacteria or their toxins in foods. Many attacks of food poisoning are not recognized for what they are. Even severe attacks with nausea, vomiting, violent diarrhoea, perhaps abdominal cramps, fever, and dizziness, may be blamed on influenza or a 24-hour virus unless several people who attended the same banquet or picnic are simultaneously stricken. The most common causes of food poisoning are strains of *salmonella* bacteria (48) which are widespread in the animal kingdom, and *staphylococci*, readily spread by human carriers. An originally small population of salmonella in pies, eclairs, egg dishes, cakes, custards, and salads can multiply enormously if such foods are left to incubate for a short time at room temperatures. Violence of food poisoning symptoms varies with the dose of bacteria and with individual susceptibility. Attacks two or three hours after eating suggest that the poisoning was caused by bacterial toxins rather than by live bacteria. Thorough cooking destroys bacteria and some toxins (see BOTULISM) but heat must be sufficiently high, penetrating, and long continued. A large turkey may not be thoroughly cooked because the stuffing acts as a sort of internal insulation. Proper refrigeration and sanitation guard against food poisoning (373).

Foot drop Drooping of the foot, due to paralysis or injury of muscles or tendons that extend or lift it.

Foot supports Simple arrangements of bedding or accessories to keep the weight of blankets off a bedridden patient's upturned feet (15).

Foramen A perforation or opening in a body part. There are many such perforations, especially in bones, to permit passage of blood vessels and nerves. Some are abnormal, such as openings in congenitally malformed hearts.

Forceps An instrument with two opposing blades and handles, for grasping, compressing, or holding body parts or surgical materials. *Forceps delivery* is extraction of the fetus from the birth canal with the mechanical aid of OBSTETRIC FORCEPS of special design (200).

Foreskin The fold of skin covering the head of the penis; the part removed in circumcision.

Formication Sensation that ants are crawling over the skin.

Fortify To add one or more nutrients to a food so that it contains more of the nutrients than were present originally before processing. Milk is often fortified with vitamin D, margarine with vitamin A, beverages with vitamin C, various cereal products with thiamine and riboflavin. Foods with vitamins added to replace lost values are said to be restored.

Fossa A pit or trenchlike depression in a body part.

Fovea A pit, cup, or depression in a body structure; especially, the *fovea centralis*, a small depression near the centre of the retina which is the area of sharpest, most detailed vision (398).

Fraternal twins Twins of either sex originating from two separate eggs; they are no more closely related genetically than other brothers and sisters.

Free grafting Transplantation of a completely detached piece of skin from one part of a patient's body to another (532).

Frenum A fold of tissue which partially limits the movement of an organ. A small frenum can be seen as a band of tissue connecting the underside of the tongue with the floor of the mouth.

Frigidity Sexual coldness in women. There may be some physical cause, but more often the aversion has a psychological origin which may be difficult to recognize and overcome. Frigidity which occurs after the menopause, in women who have previously had normal sex drive, may respond to hormone treatments (321).

Froelich's syndrome Excessive fat deposits in the pelvic area and lack of genital development in young men, often with retardation of growth, somnolence, and other symptoms. The condition results from impairment, as by a tumour of the pituitary gland, of the functions of the *pituitary* and *hypothalamus* (200). Careful diagnosis is necessary because most obese, genitally underdeveloped adolescent boys do not have this specific disorder.

Frozen section A piece of tissue removed from the body, and quickly frozen by carbon dioxide spray, sliced, and examined immediately under a microscope. This is most often done when cancer is suspected and the patient is on the operating table, while surgeons await the verdict which will determine the extent of the operation.

Frozen shoulder Pain, stiffness, and limitation of movement in the shoulder and upper arm (457).

Frozen sperm SPERMATOZOA frozen at very low temperatures, with a small amount of glycerol added, come alive when thawed and are capable of fertilization. See ARTIFICIAL INSEMINATION.

FSH Follicle-stimulating hormone (202).

Fulguration Destruction of tissue by DIATHERMY.

Fulminating Sudden in onset, explosive, severe, rapid in course.

Functional disease Disease without any discoverable organic basis.

Fundus The part of a hollow organ farthest from its opening: for example, the back part of the eye; the top part of the uterus farthest from its cervical outlet.

Fungi Forms of plant life, including moulds and yeasts, some of which are capable of causing infection. For example, *mycoses; ringworm; otitis externa; thrush; yeast infections.*

Funnel chest (*pectus excavatum*) A congenital deformity in which the breastbone is depressed towards the spine, forming a more or less funnel-shaped cavity. The deformity rarely affects the heart and lungs adversely unless unrelated diseases are present.

Funny bone The upper end of the ulna at the elbow, so-called because a blow there causes the fingers to tingle.

Furuncle A boil.

Fusiform Spindle-shaped.

Fusion Union, cohesion, merging together; for example, *spinal fusion*, the uniting of two vertebrae by disease or by surgical procedures to improve some painful condition of the back. Also, the fusion of images from the two eyes for efficient binocular vision.

G

Galactagogue An agent that promotes the flow of milk.

Galactosaemia A hereditary condition of infants who cannot digest milk sugars (*lactose, galactose*) because their bodies lack a necessary enzyme (368). Milk feedings lead to toxic accumulations of galactose in the blood, injuring the lens of the eye, the brain, and kidneys, with formation of cataracts and mental retardation unless all milk and milk products are immediately and stringently removed from the diet. The outlook with strict dietary control is good, and children who survive early infancy are often normal. Galactosaemia is inherited as a recessive trait (see chapter 26). If a galactosaemic infant is born into a family, the doctor should test later offspring of the same parents and institute a galactose-free diet immediately after birth if necessary.

Gallbladder The saclike organ attached to the liver in which bile is stored, concentrated, and delivered to the digestive tract as needed (336).

Gallop rhythm Sounds of the heart resembling the gallop of a horse, indicative of failing heart muscle.

Gallstones Stones in the gallbladder; they may or may nor cause symptoms (351).

Gamete A germ cell; an egg or sperm.

Gamma globulin An IMMUNOGLOBULIN; a protein in the blood which gives immunity to certain diseases through ANTIBODY production. Gamma globulin injections containing specific antibodies are sometimes given in the hope of preventing an infection in a person who has been exposed to it, or making it milder. Antibodies which protect against bacterial and viral infections are mostly in gamma globulin circulating in the blood; other closely related immunoglobulins occur in internal and external secretions outside the blood, as in saliva, tears, nasal, bronchial, and intestinal fluids.

Ganglion (usually of the wrist) A cyst of a tendon sheath on the back of the wrist. If troublesome, it can be removed surgically (459). A *ganglion* is also a cluster of nerve cells which serves as a centre of nervous activity.

Ganglionic blockage agents Drugs, prescribed for some patients with high blood pressure, which reduce the actions of ganglia that transmit impulses which constrict blood vessels and increase pressures. Ganglionic blockers produce the greatest fall in blood pressure when the patient is standing, relatively little change when the patient is lying down. Sometimes a patient who has been lying down may feel faint when he suddenly rises to a sitting position.

Gangrene Death of tissue due to failure of blood supply to the area. There are many precipitating causes – vascular disease, frostbite, burns, crush injury, pressure, obstruction of blood vessels, too tight a tourniquet. *Wet gangrene* has an offensive watery discharge and becomes infected so that complications of infection are superimposed upon the gangrene. Amputation of the part may be necessary to save the patient's life. *Dry gangrene* does not become infected but the part becomes dry and mummified. Small areas of dry gangrene may sometimes be saved by appropriate treatment, but amputation may be necessary. Diabetics are especially prone to gangrene of the feet and legs and preventive measures are very important (220).

Gargoylism A hereditary condition in children characterized by opacities of the cornea, protruding abdomen, large head, short arms and legs, mental deficiency.

Gas gangrene A serious infection of injured tissues with bacilli which produce bubbles of foul-smelling gas.

Gastrectomy Surgical removal of all or part of the stomach.

Gastric analysis Analysis of stomach juices for acidity, presence of cells, and other elements. The juice, obtained after the patient has fasted twelve hours, is withdrawn with a syringe connected to a tube passed through the nose into the stomach.

Gastric flu A term more current among patients than doctors. Usually the complaint is of nausea, vomiting, and diarrhoea, which run their course in a couple of days or even 24 hours and have nothing to do with influenza. Gastrointestinal viruses may cause such upsets but it is practically never possible to identify the viruses. Many cases of self-diagnosed gastric flu may actually be instances of unsuspected FOOD POISONING.

Gastric freezing A treatment sometimes used for peptic ulcer; the patient swallows a balloon which is cooled by passing freezing agents through it.

Gastritis Inflammation of the stomach (343).

Gastrocnemius The long muscle of the inner side of the lower leg which bends the leg and extends the foot.

Gastroenteritis Inflammation of the stomach and intestines, producing such symptoms as diarrhoea, abdominal pain, nausea, vomiting, fever. There are many causes: infections, food poisoning, parasites, allergies, bacteria, viruses, and toxins.

Gastroenterostomy Joining the stomach to a loop of intestine to bypass the duodenum (516).

Gastrointestinal Of or relating to the stomach and intestines.

Gastrostomy A surgically created outlet of the stomach onto the skin surface of the abdomen.

Gaucher's disease A disorder of LIPID metabolism, transmitted as a recessive trait (see chapter 26). It is characterized by enlarged spleen and liver, bone and joint pains, and brown pigmentation of the skin, due to accumulation of abnormal fatlike substances.

Gavage Feeding of liquid nutrients into the stomach by a tube.

Genes The units involved in transmission of hereditary characteristics, contained in the CHROMOSOMES.

Genitalia The reproductive organs.

Genitourinary Of or relating to genital and urinary organs – kidneys, ureters, bladder, urethra, prostate, testes – which are interrelated; see chapter 8.

Geographic tongue Fancied resemblance of the surface of the tongue to a relief map gives this disorder its name. Thickened patches occur on the tongue and shift positions from day to day. This odd appearance is the only symptom. The cause is not known. The disorder usually occurs in children and adolescents; debilitated persons appear to be more susceptible.

Geophagia Dirt-eating. See PICA.

Geotrichosis An infection caused by species of fungi, affecting mucous membranes of the mouth, lungs, or intestinal tract. Chronic cough is a common symptom. The condition responds well to proper treatment.

Geriatrics The medical specialty concerned with care of old people.

German measles (*rubella*) A mild viral infection producing a pink rash which spreads all over the body, sometimes with symptoms of headache and slight fever, sometimes with symptoms so slight that the infection passes unnoticed (45, 282). On the other hand rubella in a woman in the first three months of pregnancy may cause serious damage to the embryo.

Gestation Pregnancy.

G.I. Gastrointestinal.

Gigantism Abnormal tallness, most often a result of excessive secretion of GROWTH HORMONE by the pituitary gland before the growing ends of the bones have closed, but other factors may produce excessive height (202). Boys up to six feet six inches tall and girls up to six feet are not considered to be giants; they fall at one extreme of a normal bell-shaped distribution curve of height in the population, with unusually short people who are not dwarfs at the other extreme.

Gingiva The gum. *Gingivitis*, inflammation of the gums, is the most common form of *periodontal disease*.

Gland A cell or organ which makes and releases hormones or other substances used in the body. *Endocrine* glands secrete their products into the bloodstream; *exocrine* glands, to body surfaces or elsewhere, by ducts or channels (for example, sweat glands).

Glandular fever INFECTIOUS MONONUCLEOSIS.

Glaucoma A common cause of blindness in adults, produced by destructive pressure of fluid inside the eye (410). An acute form may come on suddenly and cause intense pain; a chronic form may cause no symptoms that the patient is aware of, although his vision is being insidiously impaired. Measurement of internal pressures of the eye with a *tonometer* (411) is an important part of an eye examination. The condition is treated either by instillation of eye-drops, or by operation.

Gleet Chronic gonorrhoeal discharge.

Glia Supporting cells and fibres of nervous tissue. *Glioma* is a tumour of glial tissue, occurring principally in the brain and spinal cord.

Globulin One type of protein in the blood plasma.

Encyclopedia of medical terms

Globus A "lump in the throat" which does not disappear on swallowing; also called *globus sensation* when no disease or organic cause can be discovered (342). The condition, most common in women, is associated with anxiety, and tightness or spasms of throat muscles. The feeling may also be caused by a foreign object in the throat, or swelling of lymphoid tissues such as tonsils or adenoids. The complaint, if persistent, calls for medical examination to rule out possible physical causes.

Glomeruli Tufted networks of capillaries which bring blood to chambers of the kidney for filtration of waste materials (182).

Glomerulonephritis Acute or chronic inflammation of fine blood vessels of the glomeruli, usually preceded by a streptococcal infection (189).

Glossitis Inflammation of the tongue.

Glottis The aperture between the vocal cords, including parts of the voice box concerned with sound production.

Glucagon A hormone produced by cells of the pancreas, comparable to insulin but opposite in action. Glucagon's function is to correct LOW BLOOD SUGAR levels by stimulating the liver to convert more of its reserves of GLYCOGEN into sugar.

Glucocorticoids Cortisone-like hormones of the adrenal gland which influence carbohydrate, protein, and fat metabolism (208).

Glucose tolerance test A test for early diabetes and other metabolic disorders. It measures the patient's ability to reduce blood sugar levels at a normal rate. After fasting, a blood sugar level is taken as a baseline and the subject is given a measured amount of dissolved sugar to drink. Blood sugar levels are taken at half-hourly intervals. Abnormal rise or persistence of blood sugar is indicative of diabetes. The test is used in borderline cases.

Glue-sniffing The dangerous and foolish practice of inhaling volatile intoxicating fumes of airplane glues and similar cements, indulged in by some teenagers. See chapter 28.

Gluteal Of or relating to the *gluteus* muscles of the buttocks.

Gluten-free diet A regimen which excludes wheat, rye, oats, and their products from the diet of patients with *coeliac disease*. See MALABSORPTION SYNDROME.

Glycerol Glycerine.

Glycogen Animal starch, similar to vegetable starch; the form in which carbohydrate is stored in the liver and released as energy needs demand. The liver manufactures glycogen from DEXTROSE (glucose), a sugar, and reconverts glycogen to sugar as needed.

Glycogen storage disease A group of hereditary disorders of infants. The infant lacks certain enzymes necessary for glucose metabolism. This leads to abnormal deposits of glycogen in various tissues of the body, with progressive slowing down of body processes.

Glycosuria Sugar in the urine.

Goitre Enlargement of the thyroid gland. There are several types (207).

Goitrogens Substances such as are contained in plants of the cabbage family and some other vegetables, which in excessive amounts induce goitre.

Gold salts Compounds of gold, used in progressive, crippling *rheumatoid arthritis* (479) in the hope of suppressing the active inflammatory disease and decreasing bone and cartilage destruction.

Gonads The primary sex glands, ovaries or testes.

Gonioscope An instrument for studying angles of the eye where fluids drain.

Gonorrhoea The most common venereal disease, an infection produced by kidney-shaped bacteria (59). Recovery from gonorrhoea does not give significant future immunity; reinfection is frequent. Incidence of the disease has increased in recent years.

Gonorrhoeal arthritis A specific form of arthritis associated with gonorrhoea, responsive to penicillin.

Gonorrhoeal ophthalmia A serious eye disease of newborn infants, acquired in passage through the birth canal of a mother who has gonorrhoea. Obstetricians sometimes put drops into the baby's eyes at birth to prevent the infection.

Gooseflesh Little skin bumps induced by cold or shock. The bumps arise around hair follicles in response to minute muscles which attempt to raise the hair.

Gout A hereditary disorder of body chemistry, resulting in too much uric acid in the blood, with chalklike deposits of urate crystals (derived from uric acid) in cartilage of the joints and sometimes elsewhere (477).

GP General practitioner.

Graafian follicles Tiny, round, transparent cysts embedded in the ovary. Each follicle contains an immature egg cell. Under the influence of the follicle-stimulating hormone of the pituitary gland, one of the blisters is stimulated to grow, and its egg matures in preparation for fertilization. The follicle bursts at about the fourteenth day of the menstrual cycle and releases the ripened egg; this is called *ovulation*.

Gram-positive, -negative Classification of bacteria according to whether they do or do not accept a stain, named after Hans Gram, a Danish bacteriologist. Different life processes and vulnerabilities of germs are reflected by their Gram-positive or Gram-negative characteristics. For instance, an antimicrobial drug effective against certain Gram-positive germs may be ineffective against Gram-negative ones, or vice versa.

Grand mal Severe epileptic seizure; convulsions, loss of consciousness, jerking and stiffening of the body (171).

Granulation tissue Tiny red, rounded, fleshy masses having a soft granular appearance; the type of tissue that forms in early stages of wound healing. Each granule has new blood vessels and reparative cells. Proud flesh is an excessive overgrowth of granulation tissue.

Granulocytes White blood cells containing granules that become conspicuous when dyed (98). They are manufactured in the red marrow of the bones. One of their functions is to digest and destroy invading bacteria.

Granuloma A tumour, new growth, or chronically inflamed area in which GRANULATION TISSUE is prominent.

Granuloma inguinale A mildly contagious venereal disease produced by rod-shaped bacteria. It is named after the *inguinal* region (groin) where lesions appear.

Gravel Fine, sandlike particles of the same substance as kidney stones, often eliminated in the urine without anything being noticed.

Graves's disease Hyperthyroidism, toxic goitre.

Gravid Pregnant. In obstetrician's language, a *gravida* is a pregnant woman; a *primigravida*, one who is pregnant for the first time; a *multigravida*, one who has had several pregnancies.

Greenstick fracture An incomplete fracture of a long bone, usually in children whose bones are still pliable (471). The break does not go all the way through the bone, which is splintered on one side only, in much the same way that a green stick splinters on the outside if you hold an end in each hand and bend it until it breaks.

Gristle CARTILAGE.

Groin The lowest part of the abdomen where it joins the legs; the groove at this junction. Also called the *inguinal* area, a common site of hernia (521).

Ground substance Semi-fluid material which fills spaces between connective tissue fibres and cements them together.

Growing pains Pain in a child's legs or arms may be associated with subacute rheumatic fever and the complaint should be investigated by a doctor, but there are other quite harmless causes of what are called growing pains. Non-rheumatic muscle pains at night are quite common in normal children. These pains are most probably an after-effect of vigorous playtime activities. They usually occur in muscles of the legs and thighs at the end of the day or soon after the child goes to sleep; there is no pain on motion and the child does not limp; he is vague in pointing out where it hurts and is free of pain in the morning. In fact, except for cutting the teeth, growth is painless. So-called growing pains should always be investigated in case they are due to disease.

Growth hormone A hormone of the anterior pituitary gland which stimulates growth (202).

G.U. Genitourinary.

Guaiac test A dye test, usually of urine or a stool specimen, for the presence of blood.

Gullet The oesophagus; the muscular tube through which food passes from mouth to stomach (330).

Gumboil A swelling of the gum produced by an abscess at the root of a tooth, usually painful.

Gumma A firm, rubbery mass of tissue resembling GRANULATION TISSUE, occurring almost anywhere in the body but most frequently in the skin, heart, liver, or bones. It is a characteristic lesion of late syphilis (58).

Guthrie test A blood test for *phenylketonuria*.

Gynaecoid Resembling a woman; female-like; as, a gynaecoid pelvis.

Gynaecologist A physician who specializes in diseases of women.

Gynaecomastia Abnormal enlargement of either or both male breasts. It may result from therapeutic use or unintentional absorption of female hormones, from glandular abnormalities, from drugs such as digitalis, amphetamine, or reserpine, or it may be associated with conditions which have little in common, such as thyroid disease, adrenal or testicular tumours, cirrhosis of the liver. Gynaecomastia frequently occurs in perfectly healthy adolescent boys and usually disappears in a few weeks; this form is a transient phase of the body's coming into mature hormonal balance.

H

Haemangioma A red, often elevated birthmark; strawberry mark. It may or may not be present at birth. Only superficial blood vessels are involved. The mark often disappears spontaneously after some months, but in some cases treatment may be required (120).

Haematemesis Vomiting of blood.

Haematocele A swelling produced by effusion of blood into a cavity.

Haematocrit The percentage by volume of red blood cells in whole blood; a reading is obtained by spinning whole blood in a centrifuge to pack the cells.

Haematoma A swelling filled with blood which clots to form a solid mass. The blood accumulates from vessels injured by a blow or disease. A *subdural haematoma* is one that

occurs under the skull. The cauliflower ear of boxers results from a neglected haematoma.

Haematuria Blood in the urine. *Occult* blood in the urine is not visible but can be detected by tests. Haematuria may occur from relatively harmless causes (for example, prolonged marching, and severe stress of physical contact sports), but it may portend serious disease and always requires medical investigation (190).

Haemochromatosis (*bronzed diabetes*) A progressive disease characterized by abnormal deposits of iron in many organs of the body, associated with bronzing of the skin, diabetes, and impaired functioning of the liver and pancreas. Mild forms of the disease with few if any clinical symptoms may require liver biopsy to make the diagnosis. It is thought that the patient has an abnormal capacity to absorb iron, rather than lessened ability to excrete it, and that the trait is genetically determined. A key treatment of severe haemochromatosis is frequent bloodletting (PHLEBOTOMY) as often as once a week, to deplete the stores of iron that harm the patient.

Haemocytometer A device for counting blood cells.

Haemodialysis Separation of waste materials from blood by passage over a semipermeable membrane, especially as performed by an artificial kidney (190).

Haemoglobin The colouring matter of red blood cells. The molecule contains a protein part (*globin*) joined with an iron-containing pigment, *haem* (from which comes the prefix *haem-* for many medical words denoting some relationship to the blood). *Haem* is the oxygen-carrying portion of haemoglobin. Haemoglobin picks up oxygen in the lungs, holds it loosely, carries it in arterial blood, and delivers it as a fuel to cells. In exchange, the blood plasma picks up carbon dioxide which cells must get rid of and carries it to the lungs where it is exhaled, while a fresh load of oxygen is taken on. Iron is the key element of this remarkable gas-transporting molecule but the protein part is vital too; not all kinds of anaemias are benefited by merely taking iron.

Haemolysis Dissolution, breakdown of red cells with release of HAEMOGLOBIN. Old worn-out red cells are constantly being broken down and replaced; the process balances out in healthy persons. Excessive haemolysis may result from chemicals, incompatible transfusions, snake venom, and congenital or acquired conditions leading to haemolytic jaundice and anaemia (107).

Haemophilia A bleeding disease (110). Hope that haemophilia may be conquered received great impetus in 1967 with development of concentrated antihaemophilic globulin for preventing bleeding episodes.

Haemoptysis Coughing up blood.

Haemorrhage Bleeding. The only normal form of bleeding is menstruation. Otherwise, bleeding is a sign of something wrong, often the major symptom to be dealt with immediately in giving first aid (588). *Arterial bleeding* comes in spurts of bright red blood with each beat of the heart, unless blood wells up into a wound from a deep artery. *Venous bleeding* is indicated by a continuous flow of dark blood. *Capillary bleeding* is a general oozing from a raw surface such as a grazed knee. *Internal bleeding* is to be suspected if the patient has suffered severe blows, crushing, falls, or penetrating injuries which may lacerate internal organs. Disease, such as erosion of a peptic ulcer, may cause haemorrhage into closed body cavities, with signs of shock (590).

Haemorrhoids (*piles*) Dilated varicose veins in and around the rectal opening. The condition is common, is often tolerated quite well for years, sometimes is temporary, as in pregnancy, and frequently responds to medical treatment and improvement of bowel habits (349). Haemorrhoids may shrink by themselves, or get worse. Some are best removed by surgical operation, *haemorrhoidectomy* (531).

Haemostat An instrument which stops bleeding by clamping a blood vessel, or an agent which stops bleeding.

Hair transplants See ALOPECIA.

Hairy tongue A rare condition which may occur after use of antibiotics, or from unknown causes; intertwining hairlike filaments form black or brownish patches on the tongue. The disease, if it may be called such, is harmless. The hairy patches may disappear quickly or persist for months.

Hallucinogenic drugs Chemical agents which produce distortions of the mind. See chapter 28.

Hallux The big toe.

Hallux valgus See BUNION.

Hammer toe A toe which is bent upwards like an inverted V and cannot flatten out, usually caused by cramping the toes into too small a shoe (470).

Hamstrings Tendons above the back of the knee.

Hand-Schuller-Christian disease An insidiously developing disease in the first decade of life, manifested by bulging eyes, excessive thirst, deposits of CHOLESTEROL in bones and tissue under the skin.

Hansen's disease See LEPROSY.

Hashimoto's disease A form of chronic thyroiditis occurring most frequently in middle-aged women (207). It is thought to be an AUTO-IMMUNE DISEASE.

Hay fever Pollinosis; an allergic reaction to inhaled pollens, characterized by reddened weepy eyes, running nose, and sneezing (487).

Hearing aids Choice of the right hearing aid requires hearing tests by an ear specialist, since there are many kinds of hearing impairment, improved by different types of instruments (430). The ear specialist will suggest which type of hearing aid is suitable. The decision depends upon the type of hearing loss, its severity, and other factors. The specialist may suggest a National Health Service instrument or a brand-name of hearing aid.

In selecting a hearing aid:

Compare for clarity and quality of sound. Listen to familiar voices with different aids.

Compare how well you understand speech with each of the aids. Listen in noisy places as well as in quiet. Try the aids outdoors as well as indoors.

Compare for comfort and convenience. Controls should be easy to operate. Batteries, parts, and minor repairs should be available locally.

Compare costs. A low-priced aid may be just as satisfactory as a high-priced aid, depending on your needs. Does the price include the ear mould, the cord and the receiver, and the battery? Ask about the costs of batteries.

Compare extra services. Does the dealer give you a convenient repair and replacement service? Will the dealer help you to learn to use your aid?

Heart attack Common term for *coronary thrombosis* (71).

Heart block Heart block, of various degrees, occurs when the transmission of impulses from the atria to the ventricles is interfered with.

Heartburn Mild to severe burning sensations in the upper abdomen or beneath the breastbone, usually resulting from regurgitation of stomach contents into the oesophagus. Heartburn typically occurs after a heavy meal containing fatty foods, often occurs when the patient is lying down, or sitting with feet slightly elevated, and is relieved by sitting up. Occasional heartburn associated with dietary excess is not uncommon and does not necessarily require treatment. Weight reduction, antacids, diet regulation, and sleeping with the head of the bed elevated are helpful measures. Persistent or severe heartburn, or pain thought to be heartburn, may be associated with disease requiring medical diagnosis. Heartburn is the most common symptom of *hiatus hernia* (340). It is frequent in the middle and later months of pregnancy.

Heart-lung machine A device which infuses oxygen into a patient's venous blood (a lung function) and pumps the freshened blood to the circulation (a heart function). Several types of such devices make open heart surgery feasible (522).

Heart murmurs Various sorts of blowing, soft, or swishing sounds made by the heart. The mere presence of murmurs does not necessarily indicate serious disease. Some murmurs are congenital, some are acquired (as from rheumatic fever), some are functional and of no great significance. Murmurs are heard in many healthy children and adults. The meaning of murmurs, as of all signs, must be interpreted by a physician.

Heat cramps Painful muscle spasms of legs and abdomen, resulting from loss of salt through profuse prolonged sweating (614).

Heatstroke A very serious reaction to exposure to extreme heat. The heat-regulating centres in the brain are paralyzed; the victim's extremely high temperature must be reduced immediately with ice packs or streams of cold water (614).

Heberden's nodes Small swellings at the end joints of the fingers in older people (476). The condition is a form of osteoarthritis which does not progress to severe crippling. The classic description by William Heberden is as valid today as when he published his account in 1802: "... little hard knobs, about the size of a small pea, which are frequently seen upon the fingers, particularly a little below the top, near the joint. They have no connection with the gout, being found in persons who never had it; they continue for life; and being hardly ever attended by pain, or disposed to become sores, are rather unsightly than inconvenient, though they must be of some little hindrance to the free use of the fingers."

Helminthiasis Infestation with *helminths*, parasitic worms.

Hemianopsia Half vision; blindness of one half of the field of vision. One or both eyes may be affected.

Hemiplegia Paralysis of one side of the body, due to a clot or rupture of a brain artery (stroke, 176). It may be temporary or permanent, and associated with hemianaesthesia.

Henoch-Schönlein purpura An allergic form of haemorrhage into the skin, beginning with pain in the abdomen and joints. Recovery is usually spontaneous unless the kidneys are affected. The condition may be associated with streptococcal infection, rheumatic fever, or food allergy (493).

Hepatitis Usually virus-caused inflammation of the liver (52). There are also nonviral forms, such as amoebic, alcoholic, toxic, and syphilitic.

Hepatolenticular degeneration See WILSON'S DISEASE.

Hepatoma A tumour of the liver.

Heredity See chapter 26.

Hermaphrodite A person with the sex organs of both sexes. True hermaphrodites are rare. More common are *pseudohermaphrodites*, examples of *intersex*. Such persons, assigned to the wrong sex at birth, may in later life be candidates for sex reversal operations, which do not actually change the basic sex, but give it better expression. Assignment of true sex at birth can be very difficult because of great variation in external and internal structures. Males with HYPOSPADIAS and CRYPTORCHIDISM may be assigned a female role; females may be mistaken for males with these abnormalities. Surgical exploration is often necessary in doubtful cases, and it may be possible for surgery to correct the condition, if not completely, at least to a degree of satisfactory adjustment. But the varieties of hermaphroditism are far too numerous and complex for any single rule of sex assignment. Even the genetic sex may be wrong. Girls with testicular feminization have internal testes and are genetically male, but they have a body of normal female appearance, with a vagina but without a uterus or menstruation; their hormones at puberty are exclusively feminizing and their entire psychological outlook is feminine. Cases of doubtful sex require individual study and technical knowledge. If the sex of an infant is in doubt, appropriate steps, surgical or otherwise, should be taken at an early age, not only that the child may identify with its appropriate sex, but because in some cases an endocrine disturbance detrimental to health may underlie the condition.

Hernia (*rupture*)   Protrusion of an organ or part of an organ through a weak spot in tissues which normally contain it. There can be herniations of the brain, lung, or other organs, but the most common herniations are of organs contained by the abdominal wall. A natural weak spot in the groin area, especially in men, who have an opening through which the spermatic cord passes, is the site of *inguinal* hernia, the most common type in both men and women. It is curable by surgical operation, as indeed are other forms of hernia (521).

Herniorraphy   Any operation for repair of hernia which includes suturing.

Herpangina   A COXSACKIE VIRUS infection, usually of infants and children, producing fever, sore throat, loss of appetite, sometimes nausea and vomiting.

Herpes simplex   The cold sore or fever blister (52).

Herpes zoster   See SHINGLES.

Hiatus hernia   Protrusion of part of the stomach into the chest cavity through a weak spot in the DIAPHRAGM (340).

Hiccups (hiccough)   The annoyance is known to all; its medical definition is spasmodic contraction of the DIAPHRAGM and sudden closure of the glottis. Irritation of nerves that control the diaphragm (140) causes spasm, and the glottis, the chink between the vocal cords, snaps shut, causing a peculiar sound. The hiccup trigger may be an overloaded stomach, trapped gas, something that went down the wrong way, swallowing hot foods or irritants, gulping, or unknown trifling provocations. Virtually all the popular cures for hiccups (re-breathing from a paper bag, holding the breath as long as possible, taking a dozen sips of water without stopping to breathe) increase the carbon dioxide content of the lungs and thus help to stabilize the breathing centre. Severe hiccups which continue for hours or days may be associated with liver, abdominal, or intestinal disease, or lesions of the breathing centre; temporary surgical interruption of the phrenic nerve may be necessary to stop incessant spasms.

Hip dislocation (congenital)   Spontaneous dislocation of the hip before or shortly after birth (462).

Hippocratic oath   A statement of ethics traditionally demanded of the young physician on entering practice. It contains some anachronisms – mention of freemen and slaves, and apparent ruling out of operations for bladder stone (*lithotomy*) as beneath the dignity of reputable men of medicine. But the ethical precepts of the Oath endure. The Oath bears the name of Hippocrates, the famous Greek physician, born about 460 B.C., who is called the Father of Medicine for his sound and close observations of patients and diseases which began to give the medical arts a scientific foundation, but whether or not Hippocrates himself wrote the Oath is not known; it is probably a collective expression of his followers. There are several English translations of the Oath; the wording that follows is best known:

"I swear by Apollo the physician, by Aesculapius, Hygeia, and Panacea, and I take to witness all the gods, all the goddesses, to keep according to my ability and my judgment the following Oath:

"To consider dear to me as my parents him who taught me this art, to live in common with him and if necessary to share my goods with him, to look upon his children as my own brothers, to teach them this art if they so desire without fee or written promise, to impart to my sons and the sons of the master who taught me and the disciples who have enrolled themselves and have agreed to the rules of the profession, but to these alone, the precepts and instruction.

"I will prescribe regimen for the good of my patients according to my ability and my judgment and never do harm to anyone. To please no one will I give a deadly drug, nor give advice which may cause his death. Nor will I give a woman a pessary to procure abortion. But I will preserve the purity of my life and my art. I will not cut for stone, even for patients in whom the disease is manifest. I will leave this operation to be performed by specialists in this art.

"In every house where I come I will enter only for the good of my patients, keeping myself far from all intentional ill-doing and all seduction, and especially from the pleasures of love with women or with men, be they free or slaves. All that may come to my knowledge in the exercise of my profession or outside of my profession or in daily commerce with men, which ought not to be spread abroad, I will keep secret and will never reveal.

"If I keep this oath faithfully, may I enjoy my life and practise my art, respected by all men and in all times, but if I swerve from it or violate it, may the reverse be my lot."

Hirschsprung's disease   See MEGACOLON.

Hirsutism   Abnormal hairiness.

Histamine   A normal chemical of body cells which plays a part in allergic reactions (486).

Histoplasmosis   Systemic infection due to inhalation of dusts containing spores of a species of fungus.

Hoarseness   Generally a trivial symptom resulting from using the voice too much; if it persists for more than a couple of weeks, a doctor should be consulted to determine the cause.

Hobnail liver   A liver studded with small nodules, the most common form of CIRRHOSIS OF THE LIVER.

Hodgkin's disease   A form of malignancy of the lymph nodes (114).

Hookworm   Infestation of the small intestine by a parasitic worm.

Hordeolum   A stye, or abscess of the eyelid (407).

Horseshoe kidney   Kidneys linked at their lower ends by a band of tissue instead of being separate; their shape somewhat resembles a horseshoe (187).

Hot flushes   See MENOPAUSE.

Household pets   The family dog, cat, or other pet is a pleasure-giving member of the household – if the animal is healthy and well cared for. Puppies and kittens should be wormed by a vet to prevent contamination of soil and materials with worm eggs in their excretions. Ingested eggs of the common dog roundworm can enter the bloodstream and larvae can reach many parts of the body. Mysterious cases of SCABIES, the itch, have occurred in persons who never dreamed that the family dog carried the mites. Animals with fur or feathers (even stuffed toy ones) are suspect if someone in the family has allergies, even though skin tests may not show sensitivity to a particular animal. Allergic persons have a tendency to become sensitized to scurf. Pets should have veterinary attention if they show any of the following symptoms: abnormal discharges; abnormal lumps or difficulty in getting up or lying down; loss of appetite, marked weight loss or gain, or excessive water consumption; excessive head shaking, scratching, and biting any part of the body.

Housemaid's knee Inflammation of the knee bursa.

Housewife's eczema A dermatitis associated with soaps, detergents, and water.

Humour Any fluid or semi-fluid of the body; for example, aqueous and vitreous humours of the eye (395). There is no connection with the ancient humoral theory of disease, which held that sickness results from disproportions of four body humours – blood, phlegm, yellow bile, and black bile – respectively associated with sanguine, phlegmatic, choleric, and melancholic temperaments. The word melancholy literally means black bile.

Hunner's ulcer An ulcer of the lining of the urinary bladder, associated with chronic interstitial cystitis (shrinkage of the bladder wall, splitting, decreased capacity).

Huntington's chorea A rare hereditary disease, appearing in middle life or later; there is progressive deterioration of the nervous system, manifested in jerky involuntary movements of the arms, legs, and face; personality changes, speech defects, difficulties of walking and swallowing. Profound nervous degeneration ultimately leads to idiocy and death. The disease is transmitted as a dominant trait (see chapter 26). Members of families in which the disease has appeared should have the benefit of genetic counselling; if they are carriers of the defective genes, half their children, statistically, will have the disease, and for that reason they may choose to forgo parenthood.

Hutchinson's teeth Widely spaced, narrow-edged upper central incisors with notching at the biting edge; a sign of congenital syphilis, though not always of that origin.

Hyaline membrane disease A condition of pronounced respiratory distress which affects newborn infants, especially premature infants, at birth, and may be fatal in a day or two. It is the most common cause of death of liveborn premature infants. The affected infant cannot get enough oxygen because ducts leading to tiny air sacs in the lungs are lined with hyaline (glassy) material, probably derived from the baby's own secretions. Breath is rapid and laboured almost from the moment of birth; CYANOSIS appears; the heart works desperately to push enough blood through the lungs. Absence of a substance, surfactant, which reduces surface tension and normally lines the air sacs seems to be the most important abnormality. Treatment consists of measures to avoid premature delivery if possible, rapid resuscitation at birth of premature infants, care in an incubator and, recently, the forcing of moist oxygen-rich air under pressure into the infant's lungs.

Hydatid disease Infestation with animal tapeworms which produce clusters of fluid-filled cysts in the lungs and other organs.

Hydatidiform mole A rare complication of early pregnancy, resulting from degeneration of membranes which would normally become a part of the placenta. The mass resembles a bunch of grapes of irregular size.

Hydramnios An excess of fluid produced by the innermost of the fetal membranes (*amnion*) which forms the BAG OF WATERS that surrounds the fetus. *Acute hydramnios* is rare; it begins during mid-pregnancy and rapidly expands the uterus to enormous size. The condition terminates in spontaneous abortion or abortion induced to save the mother's life. *Chronic hydramnios* is a more common and less threatening form, does not often terminate in miscarriage, but frequently provokes premature labour.

Hydrocele Swelling of the scrotum from accumulation of fluid in the sac of the membrane that covers the testicles (280). It is painless but weight of the fluid causes a dragging sensation. Usually only one side is involved. The condition may be related to some injury but in most cases the cause is obscure and the testicles function normally. Chronic hydrocele, most frequent in middle-aged men, is relieved by withdrawal of fluid (TAPPING) but the swelling tends to recur. The sac can be removed surgically.

Hydrocephalus Water on the brain; actually water *in* the brain – abnormal amounts of CEREBROSPINAL FLUID in brain cavities, exerting destructive pressure on brain substance (170).

Hydronephrosis Swelling of the cavity of the kidney because of obstruction to outflow of urine, as from a stone, stricture, or tumour, in the kidney itself, in a ureter, or within the bladder (194).

Hydrophobia See RABIES.

Hydrotherapy Treatment by means of water.

Hymen A membranous partition which partially blocks the external orifice of the virginal vagina.

Hyperbaric therapy Treatment by inhalation of oxygen at greater than atmospheric pressure; an auxiliary to other appropriate treatment. The patient, doctors, and nurses occupy a large chamber in which the atmospheric pressure is increased to about three times the sea level pressure. The patient breathes pure oxygen to increase the amount delivered to body cells. The technique has been employed experimentally in treatment of carbon monoxide poisoning, tetanus, and infections caused by bacteria which do not thrive in the presence of oxygen.

Hyperchlorhydria Excessive hydrochloric acid in gastric juice.

Hypercholesterolaemia Excessive amount of CHOLESTEROL in the blood.

Hyperemesis gravidarum Vomiting of pregnancy, more severe than simple MORNING SICKNESS which clears up by itself; may require hospital treatment.

Hyperhidrosis Excessive sweating.

Hyperinsulism A condition of abnormally low blood sugar resulting from an excess of insulin or deficiency of sugar; similar to insulin shock.

Hypermetropia Longsightedness.

Hypernephroma A malignant tumour of the kidney which occurs in persons over 40 years of age (195).

Hyperplasia Overgrowth of an organ or tissue from an increase in the number of its cells which are, however, in normal arrangement.

Hypertension Abnormally high arterial blood pressure (86).

Hypertensive heart disease A form of heart disease associated with high blood pressure which forces the heart to work harder to pump blood against resistance.

Hyperthyroidism (*thyrotoxicosis, toxic goitre*) Overactivity of the thyroid gland (204).

Hypertrophy Increase in size of an organ, without an increase in the number of cells. It is usually a response to increased activity or functional demands; voluntary, as when a much exercised muscle increases in size, or involuntary, as when the body enlarges one kidney to compensate for a deficiency of the other.

Hypnosis Hypnosis is not a curative treatment, but at times can be helpful. Medical hypnosis first of all requires that the practitioner be trained as a doctor. The hypnotic trance itself is harmless but it can be misused by the medically untrained; a headache which can be temporarily hypnotized away may result from a brain tumour. The major medical uses of hypnosis are for relief of pain and anxiety; for example, in childbirth, dentistry, psychological preparation for anaesthesia and surgery. Hypnosis may reduce the amount of an anaesthetic that is needed, and is especially useful when anaesthetics and sedatives are for some reason undesirable. Unreasonably high hopes for medical hypnotic miracles are not justified.

Hypnotic Inducing sleep; a sleeping pill.

Hypodermic Under the skin; commonly refers to hypodermic injection, or the needle which effects it.

Hypoglycaemia Deficiency of sugar in the blood. *Hypoglycaemic shock* due to an overdose of insulin is the same as *insulin shock*.

Hypo-ovarianism Inadequate functioning of the ovaries.

Hypophysis The pituitary gland (200).

Hypospadias A congenital malformation in which the urethra, the urinary outlet, fails to fuse completely, but takes the form of an open troughlike channel on the underside of the penis (188). A similar malformation in the female permits urine to escape into the vagina.

Hypotension Low blood pressure; sometimes significant, but usually harmless, not warranting treatment or concern, and indeed a factor in longevity (89).

Hypothalamus A part of the brain concerned with primitive functions such as appetite, procreation, sleep, body temperature; closely associated with the pituitary gland.

Hypothyroidism Deficiency of thyroid hormone, leading to a slowing down of mental and physical processes. If the deficiency occurs in an infant before birth, it is known as *cretinism*; if it occurs in an adult, it is known as *myxoedema* (206).

Hysterectomy Surgical removal of the uterus (321), either through an abdominal incision or through the vagina, which leaves no abdominal scar.

I

Iatrogenic diseases Those unintentionally induced by words or actions of a doctor. A patient may misconstrue a doctor's remark or ominous look and be convinced that he has a grave disease which does not exist or is not nearly so grave as he fears. Iatrogenic heart disease is not uncommon; a doctor's casual mention of a murmur or premature beat may send a nervous patient into iatrogenic invalidism, although he would be much better off if he remained active. Some iatrogenic disease is unavoidable, the side effect of drugs which are necessary for the patient's welfare.

Ichthyosis (*fish skin disease*) Dry, fishlike scaliness of the skin, a congenital abnormality (122). There are two forms of ichthyosis, both of which are hereditary. The commoner form is transmitted as a dominant trait; the other is determined by a sex-linked recessive gene. The latter type affects males only but is transmitted by apparently normal females. It is not a danger to life or limb.

Icterus Same as JAUNDICE.

Identical twins Twins, always of the same sex and having the same heredity, developing from a single fertilized egg.

Idiopathic Originating spontaneously from unknown causes, not the result of any other disease; it is peculiar to the individual.

Idiosyncrasy Peculiar personal capacity to react differently from most people to drugs, foods, or treatment.

Ileitis Inflammation of the ILEUM.

Ileum The lower portion of the small intestine, a tube several feet long in which major processes of digestion and assimilation take place (335). It is continuous with the *jejunum*, a section of the small intestine which lies above it, and joins the colon at the *caecum*, a pouch to which the appendix is attached. The *ileocaecal valve* at this junction controls the admission of its contents into the colon.

Ilium The broad upper part of the pelvis.

Immediate dentures Artificial dentures worn immediately after extraction of the front teeth, the other teeth having been removed previously. While the gums are healing, the denture is prepared and is worn as soon as the front teeth are removed. This saves the patient the embarrassment of being conspicuously toothless for a while, and helps to prevent the gums from shrinking.

Immunity Complex body mechanisms which create immunities to disease germs and foreign substances are not well understood, but research in this area has produced exciting knowledge which may ultimately be relevant to cancer, arthritis, and other diseases which many authorities think may be related to the inability of immunity mechanisms to cast out abnormal cells and substances. The role of the thymus in producing protective ANTIBODIES has only recently been clarified (see THYMUS GLAND). Immunity is partly humoral (that is, chemical) and partly cellular. There are two kinds of humoral immunity. *Passive immunity* is the kind borrowed from someone else, when a doctor injects GAMMA GLOBULIN or some other substance containing preformed antibodies made by another person or animal, or when a mother's antibodies are transferred to her unborn child. *Active immunity* is the kind produced by vaccination or exposure to disease germs; the body is stimulated to produce its own antibodies, continues to do so for a long time, and steps up antibody production when renewed by a booster dose or another contact with the same germs.

Immunization Procedures by which immunities to diseases are produced in a person; especially, by vaccines and toxoids. See IMMUNITY, *active* and *passive*.

Immunoglobulins Substances in the blood and in other body fluids which build immunities to various diseases; loosely synonymous with ANTIBODIES.

Impacted Firmly lodged, wedged in place; as, an impacted wisdom tooth, embedded in the jawbone (382).

Imperforate hymen Complete closure of the membrane at the opening of the vagina (300).

Impotence Incapacity of the male to have a penile erection and perform the sexual act. Impotence is an impediment of delivery rather than of production of SPERMATOZOA; it is not the same as infertility, which may affect perfectly potent males. Anatomical defects, injuries, or disorders of the nervous or endocrine systems, and systemic diseases may cause impotence, and the possibility should first be investigated. But the majority of cases have a psychological basis; the affected male may be impotent with one sexual partner but not with another; emotional factors are varied and complex, and counselling or psychiatric help may be required.

Encyclopedia of medical terms

Incisors   The four cutting teeth at the front of the upper and lower jaws.

Incontinence   Inability to retain urine or faeces.

Incubation period   The time between infection with disease organisms and the first appearance of symptoms. The period varies for different diseases, as short as a day or two for influenza and as long as 100 days for serum hepatitis.

Incus   A tiny anvil-shaped bone, the middle bone in the chain of *ossicles* of the middle ear which conduct sounds to the inner ear (419).

Indigestion   A general lay term for abdominal distress with such symptoms as heartburn, distension, gas, cramps, and fullness (343).

Induction of labour   Artificial stimulation of labour before it starts naturally; accomplished by rupturing the BAG OF WATERS, use of drugs such as *oxytocin*, or mechanical means.

Infantile eczema   An eruptive skin disorder of infancy, frequently due to food sensitivities (280).

Infant sleep patterns   Newborn infants do not sleep most of the time. They sleep about 16 hours out of 24, and can sleep only about four hours at a stretch. One study of newborn infants showed only a gradual decrease in amount of sleep per day over a 16-week period. By the time they were four months of age they slept about $14\frac{1}{2}$ hours a day, while increasing the length of a single sleep period to a little more than eight hours. Waking periods of newborn infants are more frequent from 5 p.m. to 3 a.m. than during the day. Long intervals between feedings may account for night-time wakefulness. At two to three weeks of age, CIRCADIAN RHYTHMS (24-hour cycles) of sleep and wakefulness begin to develop. At three years of age a child has generally consolidated his sleep time and sleeps about ten hours a night. Difficulties in sleeping may be aggravated about the fifth year when daytime naps are given up. There is no arbitrary time for giving up afternoon naps, but generally they should be tapered off when a nap delays the onset of sleep in the evening and keeps the child awake after going to bed.

Infarct   An area of dead tissue resulting from complete blockage of its blood supply. This frequently occurs in *coronary thrombosis* when a clot in a coronary artery stops the supply of blood to a portion of the heart muscle, producing *myocardial infarction* (71).

Infectious jaundice   See LEPTOSPIROSIS.

Infectious mononucleosis   An infection thought to be caused by the Epstein-Barr (EB) virus. It generally lasts about two weeks; patients with the most acute symptoms require on the average only four days of bed rest, the majority require no bed rest, but there may be relapses.

Inflammation   Inflammation is a defensive reaction to all sorts of tissue injury. The names of inflammatory processes are designated by the suffix "-*itis*," preceded by the name of the affected tissue – for example, *appendicitis*, *arthritis*. The four characteristics of inflammation are reddening, swelling, pain, and heat. Reddening results from increased blood supply to the affected part; white blood cells whose job it is to trap and destroy germs are also increased. Concentration of fluids causes swelling. Increase of blood supply and local metabolism produces heat. Pain is a warning not to abuse the part and to get something done about it. A doctor is needed if inflammation is at all serious, to find out what is wrong and what to do about it.

Influenza (*grippe, flu*)   An acute highly infectious viral disease tending to occur in epidemics, see chapter 2.

Infusion   Introduction of fluid into a vein.

Ingrown hairs   Curled, corkscrew-like hairs that burrow into the skin, particularly affecting the bearded area. Shaving may cut such hairs more or less longitudinally, leaving a sharp point which turns in upon its owner. The ingrown hair may cause inflammation of the follicle, and the usual treatment is to pull it out with antiseptic precautions.

Inguinal   Of or relating to the GROIN. A frequent site of hernia.

Inoculation   Introduction of a disease agent into the body to produce a mild form of the disease, giving immunity; for example, cowpox vaccination for smallpox.

Insemination   Introduction of semen into the vagina, by natural means or by artifical insemination.

In situ   In a normal place.

Inspiration   Inhaling, breathing in.

Inspissated   Thickened, from absorption or evaporation of fluid.

Insufflation   Blowing gas or powder into a body cavity, as the lungs or vagina.

Insulin   A hormone produced by the islet cells of the pancreas, essential for metabolism. Insulin in treatment of *diabetes* (216) must be given by injection, since it is a protein molecule broken down by digestion. Pharmaceutical companies prepare insulin in a number of different forms from animal sources. The structure of insulin was worked out by Frederick Sanger, a British biochemist. Insulin is a rather small protein molecule composed of 51 amino acids in two chains held together by sulphur links. Human and animal insulins have the same properties but differ in a sequence of three amino acids in one of the chains.

Intention tremor   Involuntary movements caused or intensified by voluntary movement.

Intercostal   Between the ribs.

Interferon   Infection caused by one virus may prevent concurrent infection by another virus. This phenomenon is called viral interference. An apparent mechanism which gives this protection has recently come under study. It is now known that body cells invaded by a virus produce a substance called *interferon* which diffuses out of the cells and into neighbouring cells. The cells then become resistant to infection by viruses. Interferon is a complex protein. Its production by the body is a generalized phenomenon occurring when cells are exposed to viruses. Its unique properties suggest that it might be developed into an agent for treatment of viral diseases, but great practical difficulties stand in the way. Interferon is too complex for synthetic manufacture and difficulties of producing large amounts of the pure substance are formidable. Even if interferon becomes available, its medical uses would be limited. Interferon must be absorbed into cells to block the multiplication of viruses, and means must be found to get interferon into cells in time to produce a curative or beneficial response.

Intermenstrual pain   A usually brief attack of moderate to severe pain which some women experience about midway between menstrual periods, coincidental with OVULATION, rupture of an egg-sac of the ovary and release of a mature ovum (212). Primary DYSMENORRHOEA never occurs in the absence of ovulation; intermenstrual pain of this nature is a rough guide to the time of ovulation and the fertile period. Discovery in 1940 that ovulation is essential for menstrual cramps, and that administration of oestrogen early in the cycle could eliminate the cramps, later led to the development of oral contraceptive pills. The right ovary lies near the appendix and midmenstrual pain in that region may be mistaken for a symptom of appendicitis. A doctor can distinguish between intermenstrual pain and appendicitis on the basis of laboratory tests and dates of the menstrual cycle.

Intermittent claudication   Pain in the calf muscles and limping on exercise, due to inadequate blood supply (81).

Intersex   See HERMAPHRODITE.

Intertrigo (*chafing*)   Redness, abrasion, and maceration of opposing skin surfaces that rub together. Common sites are the armpit, groin, anal region, and beneath the breasts. Moisture and warmth with friction of adjacent skin set the stage for chafing, which may be complicated by bacterial or fungus infection. Cleanliness, regular use of a dusting powder, and reduction in weight if obese are helpful preventives. Diabetes increases the susceptibility to intertrigo.

Intervertebral discs   Cartilaginous cushions between vertebrae (442).

Intestinal flora   Bacteria which normally inhabit the intestine, do no harm, and in fact are helpful. Varieties of intestinal bacteria vary somewhat with diet. Diseases or antibiotics or other circumstances sometimes incapacitate one or more floral species, permitting others to thrive disproportionately from lack of competition; this may cause disturbing symptoms. A few kinds of bacteria may get through the stomach, but most kinds do not survive the antiseptic acid gastric juices. The floral population flourishes increasingly from the stomach downwards. Some intestinal bacteria synthesize all the vitamin K we need, some synthesize other B vitamins, but not all these products are well absorbed.

Intestinal juices   Digestive juices secreted by the intestinal walls, in contrast to gastric juices secreted by the stomach, and pancreatic juices secreted by the pancreas. Intestinal juices contain enzymes which complete the final stages in digestion of protein, fat, and carbohydrate.

Intestine   The digestive tube from the outlet of the stomach to the outlet of the rectum. Although it is a continuous structure, each of the different sections has a different function. See DUODENUM, JEJUNUM, ILEUM, CAECUM, COLON, RECTUM.

Intima   The inner lining of an artery; the innermost of its three coats or layers.

Intracutaneous test   Introduction of allergens into the skin; a positive reaction indicating sensitivity to a test substance will manifest itself in a few minutes in the form of an itching skin eruption.

Intradermal   Into or within the skin.

Intramuscular   Into or within a muscle. Some drugs are injected into muscles, usually the buttocks.

Intrauterine contraceptive devices (IUD, IUCD)   Flexible devices of stainless steel, silk-worm gut, or plastic, inserted by a doctor into the uterus and retained there indefinitely for prevention of conception. Various devices are shaped like a bow, spiral, ring, or loop.

Intravenous (*I.V.*)   Into or within a vein; as, *intravenous feeding* (514).

Intrinsic factor   A substance produced by the stomach for the transport of vitamin B_{12} across membranes into the blood. The fundamental defect in *pernicious anaemia* (105) is absence or deficiency of intrinsic factor so that vitamin B_{12}, necessary for normal development of red blood cells, cannot be absorbed from foods.

Intubation   Introduction of a tube into a hollow organ such as the larynx, to keep it open.

Intussusception   Sliding of a part of the intestine into its hollow interior; telescoping, like the pushed-in finger of a glove (286).

In vitro   Literally, in glass; of or relating to studies done in test tubes or by laboratory methods, outside the living body. *In vivo* studies are done with living persons or organisms.

Ionizing radiation   The effect of radiation (X-rays, radium, radioisotopes, and so on) is to drive electrons out of atoms; the electrons become attached to other atoms or molecules, forming chemical units called *ions*. Such alteration of the electron patterns of components of living cells, changing their functional capacities, is the basis for the therapeutic use of X-rays (550).

Iridectomy   Excision of a piece of the iris to open drainage channels for relief of *glaucoma* (535).

Iris   The circular, pigmented structure of the eye, perforated by the pupil (395). The iris controls the amount of light entering the eye and gives the eyes their colour. *Iritis* is an inflammation of the iris (409).

Iron   The essential mineral of HAEMOGLOBIN. The body preserves its iron stores, and constantly reuses iron salvaged from broken-down red blood cells. The small amount lost each day is replaced from the diet, but if reserves are severely depleted, food alone will not restore them. Infants and children particularly need good sources of iron; milk, which may constitute a large proportion of their diet, is relatively low in iron and a paediatrician's advice about addition of solid foods or possible supplements should be followed. Pregnancy increases a woman's requirements for iron; supplements are usually given.

Chronic blood loss, dietary deficiencies, or disorders of absorption may result in iron-deficiency anaemia (104). It is easy for a doctor to determine if iron-deficiency anaemia exists in a patient. Unless it does, iron will do nothing to correct fatigue or a possibly serious underlying disease of which fatigue is a symptom. In men, iron-deficiency anaemia leads the doctor to look for some cause of chronic blood loss, such as bleeding ulcer or haemorrhoids. Women of childbearing age are more susceptible to iron-deficiency anaemia because of monthly blood losses, but the loss normally is very small in terms of iron.

Good food sources of iron
Whole grain and enriched cereals
Dried beans and peas
Greens
Eggs
Apricots
Meat and poultry
Liver and kidney
Prunes and raisins
Molasses
Dried figs and peaches
Bouillon cubes
Brewer's yeast
Wheat germ
Nuts

Iron lung   Popular name for a machine which expands and contracts the chest, so that a person with paralysed respiratory muscles can breathe; a respirator.

Iron poisoning   Common iron pills or tablets, prescribed for iron-deficiency anaemia and commonly for pregnant women, are dangerous and even deadly to small children who get hold of a bottle and swallow the pills which sometimes look like sweets. Children have died from swallowing such tablets, usually five-grain tablets of ferrous sulphate. Symptoms of poisoning develop in an hour or so, with signs of shock, coma, vomiting, diarrhoea. Iron poisoning is an acute emergency requiring immediate medical treatment. So keep all medicines locked away from children.

Irradiation, *medical* Treatment or diagnosis of disease with X-rays, RADIOISOTOPES, or other sources of IONIZING RADIATION. The body normally contains a certain amount of radioactive potassium and is subject to radiation from rocks and other unavoidable background sources.

Irreducible Incapable of being put back into the normal position; said of a hernia.

Irrigation Washing out of a cavity.

Irritable bowel syndrome Overreaction of the colon to emotions or other stimuli, without discoverable organic cause (348). Symptoms include pain in the lower abdomen, distension, and abdominal aching.

Ischaemia Local deficiency of blood supply, due to spasm or obstruction of an artery. A frequent concomitant of *coronary artery disease* (68).

Ischium One of the bones of the pelvis. The bone we sit on (448).

Islet cells The cells of the pancreas which produce INSULIN (216). Also called *islets of Langerhans.*

Isometric exercise A form of exercise in which a muscle group exerts utmost force without moving a part. No special equipment is needed. Muscles of the abdomen or other parts of the body can be held at maximum tension while sitting or standing; arms can push against the sides of a doorway while standing in the opening; the palms of the hands can strain upward under the kneehold space of a desk while one sits in front of it. Isometric exercise builds strength up to a plateau. After the plateau is reached, increasing frequency of exercise does not increase strength further. Mild effort is useless. Strength increases only if maximum effort is maintained for at least six seconds.

I.V. Intravenous.

J

Jacksonian seizure A *focal* epileptic seizure, so called because the spasm or convulsion originates in a local part of the brain and its effects are limited to one part of the body; for example, a twitching arm or leg (172).

Japanese encephalitis A virus-caused infection, occurring in eastern Asia, transmitted by the bites of mosquitoes.

Jaundice Yellow discoloration of the skin and tissues by bile pigments in the blood (351). The skin may itch. The urine is dark yellow or brown. The whites of the eyes have a yellowish tinge; in skin discolorations which might be mistaken for jaundice, the whites of the eyes remain clear. The symptom indicates that something has happened to cause bile pigments to mount up in the blood. The underlying abnormality may be in the liver, in the bile passages outside the liver, or in the blood itself. *Haemolytic jaundice* is due to increased destruction of red blood cells; the stools are dark. A harmless form of haemolytic jaundice occurs in newborn babies and lasts for three or four days; the baby has an excess of red cells which are destroyed during the first few days after birth. *Toxic* or *infective jaundice* reflects injury to liver cells by some agent which interferes with their ability to eliminate bile pigment. *Obstructive jaundice* results when bile ducts are blocked by disease, inflammation, gallstones, infection, or tumours. In this type of jaundice the discoloration of skin and mucous membranes is intense, the stools clay-coloured, and the urine deeply coloured. Underlying causes of jaundice are numerous. Various laboratory tests help to detect what is wrong.

Jejunal ulcer A peptic ulcer occurring near the opening between the stomach and jejunum, after a surgical operation to establish a direct connection between the organs (*gastrojejunostomy*).

Jejunum A portion of the small intestine, several feet long, continuous from the DUODENUM to the ILEUM (335). Absorption of food is practically limited to the small intestine. Digestion is accelerated in the jejunum which is the recipient of gruel-like materials from the stomach after thorough mixing with bile and pancreatic juices in the duodenum.

Jellyfish stings See PORTUGUESE MAN-OF-WAR.

Jet injection A technique for vaccinating without a needle. A volume of liquid is suddenly compressed and forced through a very fine orifice at such speed that it penetrates the skin painlessly and delivers a cone-shaped spray of material into the tissues under the skin. Various types of jet injectors have been developed; some have reservoirs holding enough material for several hundred doses. The devices have been used principally for mass vaccination of large numbers of people.

Jiggers Sand fleas; pregnant females of the species bore into the skin, causing intense itching and inflammation.

Joint mice Small loose fragments of bone that have become separated within a joint, often the knee.

Joule The unit of energy. Has largely replaced the Calorie in dietetics.

Jugular veins Veins of the side of the neck which drain blood from the head and neck towards the heart. The internal jugular veins are deep-lying; the external ones are near the surface.

K

Kahn test A blood test for syphilis.

Kala-azar An infection transmitted by the bites of sandflies, occurring in Mediterranean, tropical, and oriental regions. It is characterized by fever, anaemia, enlarged spleen, emaciation, and has a high fatality rate if left untreated, but responds well to medical treatment.

Kaposi's disease See XERODERMA PIGMENTOSUM.

Keloids Irregular ridges, nodules, and cordlike bands of skin like raised scars, at first rubbery and later very dense and hard. They tend to occur on the site of previous scars. The cause of such excessive growth is not known. Keloids can be removed by surgery or shrunk by radiation, but have a tendency to recur.

Keratin The hard, horny protein which is the chief structural material of the outermost layer of the skin, of hair and nails, and in animals lower than man, of claws, horns, hooves, and feathers.

Keratitis Inflammation of the cornea.

Keratoconjunctivitis Acute inflammation of the cornea and conjunctiva, tending to occur in epidemics, caused by a specific virus.

Keratoconus Cone-shaped projection of the cornea; vision impaired by the bending of light waves in distorted ways. Good vision may be restored by contact lenses.

Keratoplasty Surgical procedures on the cornea, such as CORNEAL TRANSPLANT.

Keratosis Overgrowth of the horny layer of the skin; for example, a wart or callus.

Kerion Fungus infection of the beard or scalp, producing pustules.

Kernicterus A severe form of JAUNDICE characterized by

deposits of bile pigments in parts of the brain and degeneration of nerve cells, occurring in infants with ERYTHROBLASTOSIS.

Ketosis A condition produced when more fat is eaten than can be burned completely by the body. The unburned fats produce acid chemical substances called *ketone bodies*. An excess of ketones produces a form of ACIDOSIS to which some diabetics are especially susceptible; acetone derived from incomplete combustion of fats can produce a characteristic odour to the breath of diabetics with *ketoacidosis*.

Kidneys Paired organs in the small of the back behind the abdominal cavity. The kidneys regulate the volumes and composition of body fluids, filter out impurities, keep ELECTROLYTES and blood composition in balance, and secrete substances which modify blood pressure. The kidneys are subject to infections, stone formation, tumours, malformations, circulatory and other diseases.

Kimmelsteil-Wilson disease (*diabetic nephropathy*) A specific form of kidney disease (sclerosis of the GLOMERULI) associated with diabetes of long duration.

Kinaesthesia The sense by which we perceive weight, position, movement, resistance, and rapidly integrate countless muscle-registered stimuli – from a grasped steering wheel, tennis racket, bicycle handlebars, or from muscles that tell us an arm is outstretched or bent without our looking at it.

Kinins Miniature proteins associated with rheumatism and allergic reactions(486).

Kiss ulcer One that appears to result from parts that press upon or are in contact with each other.

Klebsiella pneumonia A type of pneumonia caused by a type of bacteria other than the common pneumococci (41). It tends to produce chronic lung abscesses.

Klinefelter's syndrome Undeveloped testes and female characteristics such as breast enlargement in males, due to an abnormality of the sex-determining pair of CHROMOSOMES. A normal female has two X chromosomes (XX), a normal male, an X and a Y (XY). A person with Klinefelter's syndrome has an extra and harmful X chromosome (XXY).

Kline test A blood test for syphilis.

Knee jerk The patellar reflex; sudden jerking forward of the lower leg when tapped below the kneecap. A test of the integrity of nerves.

Knock-knees (*genu valgum*) Inward bending of the knees at the joint; in young children it usually corrects itself spontaneously (464).

Koplik's spots Small bluish-white spots on mucous membranes of the cheeks, present shortly before the rash of MEASLES appears.

Korsakoff's psychosis This severe mental disturbance usually, but not always, follows a bout of DELIRIUM TREMENS which blends into it. The outstanding manifestation is loss of memory for recent events, and falsifications of memory, such as remembering things that never happened. The psychosis is associated with chronic alcoholism and chronic malnutrition; treatment is much the same as for delirium tremens. Some patients recover their memories after weeks or months, but others never do.

Kraurosis Progressive drying and shrivelling of the skin, due to atrophy of glands, often accompanied by severe itching; especially, kraurosis of the vulva in elderly women (321).

Kwashiorkor A PROTEIN deficiency disease occurring most often in children in tropical countries who are raised on cereal diets after weaning. Affected children have pot bellies, apathy, muscular wasting, oedema, and fail to grow. It is an extreme form of disease which may occur in lesser degree in persons whose diets are very low in protein. The basic deficiency is lack of AMINO ACIDS for synthesis of proteins.

Kyphosis Humpback curvature of the spine. A mild form is round shoulders. Kyphosis may result from poor posture or from diseases such as rickets, tuberculosis, and osteoarthritis, which affect the spine.

L

Labia Lips or liplike organs. *Labia majora*, folds of skin on either side of the entrance of the vulva; *labia minora*, folds of tissue covered with mucous membrane within the labia majora (302).

Labour Childbirth. There are three stages: dilatation of the cervix; expulsion of the child; expulsion of the placenta.

Labyrinth Intricate passageways, intercommunicating canals; especially, structures of the inner ear (420).

Laceration A wound caused by tearing of tissue; for example, laceration of the perineum in childbirth.

Lacrimal Of or relating to tears, produced by the *lacrimal gland* in the upper outer region of the orbit (400).

Lactation Secretion of milk (203). Interacting hormones initiate and sustain this complicated process. The milk-duct system of the breast enlarges during pregnancy under the influence of *oestrogen*, an ovarian hormone. Milk-secreting lobules also proliferate under the influence of a different hormone, *progesterone* (214). During labour, OXYTOCIN, another hormone, takes effect. Shortly after the baby is born the breasts secrete COLOSTRUM, which is not true milk but a secretion containing protective antibodies of the mother. True milk appears when *prolactin*, a pituitary gland hormone, acts upon breasts already prepared by oestrogen and progesterone. Lactation can be suppressed by giving suitable hormones.

Lactose The sugar of milk.

Lactovegetarian A person who lives on a diet of vegetables, cereals, fruits, and dairy products.

Laennec's cirrhosis The most common form of cirrhosis of the liver; portal cirrhosis (351).

Laminectomy Surgical opening of the wall of the spinal canal to expose underlying structures (529).

Lancet A short, pointed, double-edged surgical knife, used for *lancing* – that is, cutting open.

Lancinating A description of sharply cutting, shooting pain.

Lanugo Fine downy hair on the body of the fetus and on the adult body, except the palms and soles.

Laparotomy Opening of the abdomen by an incision; a variety of surgical procedures may be used subsequent to the opening.

Larva migrans See CREEPING ERUPTION.

Laryngectomy Surgical removal of all or part of the voice box, usually because of cancer. There is a high rate of cure if the cancer is discovered early. The patient is left without vocal cords, but with persistence and encouragement can learn to speak again by swallowing and belching air and manipulating it with muscles of the tongue and mouth.

Laryngitis Inflammation of the LARYNX (voice box). Acute laryngitis is often associated with a common cold, infection, or overuse of the voice. The throat is dry, swallowing may be affected, it is not possible to speak above a hoarse whisper, if at all. Absolute rest of the voice is an essential part of treatment (440).

Encyclopedia of medical terms

Laryngoscope A hollow metal tube with a light, inserted into the throat for examining the LARYNX.

Laryngotracheobronchitis An acute, serious condition of children, rapid in onset, requiring immediate medical care. The outstanding symptom is extreme difficulty in breathing, due to thick mucus and fluid which can plug the breathing passages.

Larynx The vocal apparatus, located between the base of the tongue and the windpipe (439). It includes the vocal cords and muscles which modify the vibrations of air passing through them, to produce controlled sounds.

Laser A device which gets its name from the initial letters of Light Amplification by Stimulated Emission of Radiation. Essentially, a laser multiplies the energy of a light source, such as the flash of a photographic bulb, into a very powerful emission of parallel light waves of the same wavelength, all in step. The original laser employed a ruby crystal about the size of a cigarette, impregnated with chromium atoms, with a reflective mirror at one end and a semitransparent mirror at the other. Setting off a high-powered flash bulb excites atoms in the crystal to higher energy levels; they drop to normal levels and in doing so excite other atoms, trapped between mirrored ends of the tube, rebounding, intensifying, until an extremely intense burst of coherent (nondiffuse) light is emitted from the semitransparent end of the tube. For a very brief time, hundredths of thousands of a second, a laser beam is more brilliant than the sun and its parallel rays can be focused on a spot no wider than a millionth of a millimetre. Medical uses of a laser are still experimental and many problems remain to be solved. Laser beams have successfully destroyed pigmented skin cancers in human patients, have been used to remove portwine stains and tattoos, and have been employed to secure *detached retinas* (534) into position.

Laurence-Moon-Biedl syndrome A rare genetic disorder of the pituitary gland, producing obesity, mental retardation, degeneration of the retina, webbed fingers or toes, and underdevelopment of the genitals.

Lavage Washing out of a hollow organ such as the stomach or a sinus.

Lead poisoning Intoxication from absorption of lead or its salts into the body; *plumbism*. Mild lead poisoning may produce no apparent symptoms but the metal can accumulate in the body over a period of time and produce chronic poisoning. Some of the signs of lead poisoning are abdominal pain, constipation, muscle weakness, pallor, drowsiness, mental confusion, and a blue line on the gums. Lead poisoning occasionally occurs in young children who chew objects containing paints with a lead base. Insidious lead poisoning is not rare in children who live in old, poorly maintained houses with flaking paint and plaster. Fortunately, lead paint is little used now. Infants explore the world by putting all sorts of things into their mouths. About the time when they begin to walk and have a few teeth, they may develop an abnormal appetite for non-food substances (see PICA). It is a dangerous habit which should be corrected by teaching the child as early as possible what should and should not go into his mouth.

L E cell A white blood cell which has undergone changes characteristic of *lupus erythematosus* and related diseases (483).

Left-handedness When a left-handed child appears in a right-handed family there may be some worry. The left-handed may suffer unjustly in a right-handed world. Perhaps it is such considerations that lead some parents to force a naturally left-handed child to favour his right hand. The consensus of medical opinion is that if a child wants to use his left hand, let him. Some things we learn to do with either the right or left hand because it is more convenient. A left-handed person shakes hands with his right hand because that is the way the world shakes hands. A right-handed person holds a telephone receiver with his left hand and uses his left ear to leave his right hand free for writing. We are left- or right-eyed as well as handed; it is easy to determine one's dominant eye (394). Teachers and parents never make any effort to change eye dominance. If handedness is to some extend hereditary, the mode of transmission has not been elucidated.

Leishmaniasis A parasitic disease transmitted by sandflies; it has several forms.

Leprosy (*Hansen's disease*) A chronic disease which inflicts deformities and mutilations, caused by bacteria closely related to those that cause tuberculosis. About twelve million people suffer from leprosy today. Most of them live in tropical or subtropical countries. The disease affects the skin and nerves of all patients, but is usually classified according to which tissue is predominantly involved. Patients with nerve leprosy develop discoloured skin areas, devoid of feeling because nerves are deadened. Ultimately, fingers, toes, or other parts may shrivel. Patients with skin leprosy develop thick swellings which grossly distort the features. Drugs known as sulphones seem to prolong the lives of some patients but others appear to get worse after chemotherapy is begun. Close skin contact with a patient who has leprosy seems a likely route of entry of organisms into the body. Leprosy is generally thought not to be very catching. Husbands and wives of patients with leprosy may remain apparently uninfected after living many years together. Some investigators feel that leprosy is a highly contagious disease but only to a few people who are highly susceptible.

Leptospirosis (*infectious jaundice; spirochaetal jaundice*) An infectious disease caused by certain spirochaetes (*leptospira*). The germs are spread in the urine of infected animals – rats, mice, dogs, cows, pigs – and most people who acquire the infection have had contact with animals or with water or moist soil to which animals have access. Several local outbreaks have been traced to swimming or wading in ponds or slow-moving streams in rural areas where waste disposal is not properly screened. The germs enter the body through mucous membranes or minute breaks in the skin. Typically, the infection produces sudden fever, chills, headache, and muscle pains. In some cases there may be few if any symptoms; in others, jaundice may develop. Usually leptospirosis is a brief self-limited illness, but *Weil's disease* (54) is a severe form in which jaundice, kidney failure, haemorrhage, anaemia, and heart damage may become threatening complications. Leptospirosis responds well to antibiotics.

Lesion Alteration of tissue or function due to injury or disease. A pimple, fracture, abscess, scratch, wart, or ingrowing toenail may be called a lesion.

Leucocytes White blood cells (98).

Leucocytosis Abnormal increase in numbers of white blood cells. The cell count normally increases slightly after eating and in pregnancy, but the word implies an abnormal increase, often associated with bodily defences against infection and inflammation. For instance, a high count may help to confirm a diagnosis of appendicitis. Disorders of the blood-forming organs may also induce leucocytosis.

Leucopenia Diminished number of white blood cells. The condition may result from allergies, drug reactions, irradiation, certain kinds of infections, or anaemias.

Leucorrhoea Whitish discharge from the vagina.

Increased flow of mucus about midway between menstrual periods often accompanies OVULATION. The discharge is sometimes called the whites. It may also result from yeast or protozoal infection. See TRICHOMONIASIS and CANDIDIASIS.

Leukaemia Malignant disease of the blood-forming organs. The characteristic abnormality is gross overproduction of white blood cells. There are several acute and chronic forms of leukaemia, so diverse that the word does not refer to a single specific disease but to a variety of leukaemic states (112).

Leukoderma See VITILIGO.

Leukoplakia Whitish, leathery patches on mucous membranes of the mouth (382) or vulva (310). No specific cause is known, but continued irritation is considered to be a factor. Patients with oral leukoplakia are forbidden to smoke and the white patches may regress if this and other irritations are removed. Leukoplakia by no means progresses inevitably to cancer, but it is considered to be a precancerous lesion and requires medical care and supervision.

Leydig cells Interstitial cells of the testes which produce testosterone, the male hormone (and small amounts of female hormone). The cells are separate structures from those that produce SPERMATOZOA. Thus, infertile males whose production of spermatozoa is impaired may produce adequate amounts of male hormone and be normally potent.

LH Luteinizing hormone of the pituitary gland. It causes a GRAAFIAN FOLLICLE which has released an egg to become a yellow body which produces *progesterone*, a hormone which helps to prepare the lining of the uterus for implantation of a fertilized egg (212).

Libido Commonly means sexual desire.

Lichenification Leathery thickening and hardening of the skin, usually the result of long-continued irritation from scratching and rubbing.

Lichen planus An itching eruption of unknown cause; dull purplish-red spots appear on thin-skinned areas of the body (128).

Ligament A band of tough, flexible fibrous tissue which connects bones or supports organs.

Ligate To tie up; for example, a bleeding blood vessel. In surgery, a *ligature* is a thread of silk, catgut, wire, or other material used for tying vessels.

Lightening The time around the middle of the last month of pregnancy when the baby's head settles more deeply into the pelvis preparatory to birth. This slightly decreases the mother's feeling of abdominal distension.

Limbus A border; the edge of the cornea where it joins the white of the eye.

Lipids A broad term for fats and fatlike substances. Lipids contain one or more fatty acids. Lipids include fats, cholesterol, phospholipids, and similar substances which do not mix readily with water.

Lipoid pneumonia See ASPIRATION PNEUMONIA.

Lipoma A tumour composed of fat tissue, occurring chiefly on the trunk, back of the neck, forearms, or armpits. Lipomas must be distinguished from other tumours. Lipomas usually stop growing after they reach a certain size and remain at that size indefinitely. True lipomas are painless, harmless, never become malignant, and are best left untreated unless they are so large and cosmetically objectionable as to justify surgical removal.

Lithiasis Stone formation (gallstones, kidney stones); the condition of having stones.

Lithotomy Cutting into the bladder to remove a stone (193). Structures are close to the surface, and because of this accessibility the operation has an ancient history. Mortality was high in the centuries before antiseptic surgery, but some patients did recover.

Little's disease Cerebral palsy of children, affecting both sides of the body.

Liver fluke A disease acquired by ingesting food or water contaminated with cysts of sheep liver flukes, a species of flatworm.

Lobotomy Cutting into a lobe of an organ, especially a lobe of the brain.

Lochia The discharge from the vagina which continues for a week or two after childbirth. It is a normal aftermath of childbirth and ceases when the uterus returns to its pre-pregnancy state.

Locked knee A painfully swollen knee joint which cannot be extended fully, due to a torn CARTILAGE. Surgical removal of the injured cartilage is usually necessary (465).

Lockjaw See TETANUS.

Locomotor ataxia See ATAXIA.

Longsightedness (*hypermetropia*) A condition in which light from near objects is focused behind rather than upon the retina, usually because the eyeball is too short (403). Close objects are blurred but distant ones are distinct. Longsighted persons may read and do close work with some success through ACCOMMODATION, but this effort of ciliary muscles can give rise to complaints of eye strain, tired eyes, and distaste for tasks of close seeing. With increasing age, the lens of the eye loses flexibility and longsighted people tend to hold their newspapers at arm's length to read them. Glasses for reading, or a reading segment in bifocal glasses, can do much to give comfort.

Lordosis Exaggeration of the normal forward curve of the spine at the small of the back. The general aspect is that of an abdomen thrust forward and shoulders thrust back. The characteristic posture of late pregnancy is a lordosis. Abnormalities of the hip joint sometimes cause lordosis.

Low blood sugar (HYPOGLYCAEMIA) Less than normal amounts of glucose (sugar) in circulating blood. Blood sugar naturally drops if there is a long interval between meals. Mild transient symptoms of hunger, weakness, faintness, are perfectly normal and no surprise to anyone who omits food long enough to deplete his reserves; a meal restores the balance. *Chronic* hypoglycaemia may be associated with various endocrine and other disorders. Insulin, which reduces abnormally high blood sugar levels, is only one agent in nature's complicated balancing scheme. Another hormone, *glucagon*, also produced by the pancreas, but by different cells from those which produce insulin, stimulates the liver to convert GLYCOGEN to blood sugar and raise low blood sugar levels.

LSD Lysergic acid diethylamide. See chapter 28.

Lues Syphilis.

Lumbago A general term for pain in the lumbar region (453). Lumbago is not a specific disease but a symptom to be investigated.

Lumbar puncture Withdrawal of CEREBROSPINAL FLUID through a hollow needle inserted between lumbar vertebrae of the small of the back (165). Withdrawal may be done for purposes of diagnosis, to relieve pressure, or the puncture may be made to introduce medication, such as an anaesthetic.

Lumen The open space inside a tubular structure such as an intestine or blood vessel.

Luxation Dislocation.

Lymphangitis Inflammation of lymphatic vessels due to spread of an infection. Red lines mark the paths of inflamed vessels. There is a danger of bacteria getting into the blood. Treatment is directed to overcoming the original infection.

Lymphoedema Swelling of a part of the body, especially the legs or arms, from accumulation of fluids because of obstruction or inadequacy of the lymphatic drainage system. The condition may cause huge enlargement of a part (ELEPHANTIASIS). Lymphoedema of the arm sometimes occurs after breast removal surgery. Obstructive lymphoedema is secondary to other conditions such as tumours or FILARIASIS. A less frequent, sometimes congenital form results from primary defects in the functioning of lymphatic channels in the skin and its deep layers. This type of lymphoedema manifests itself as a grossly swollen leg in the teens or middle life. The unsightly swelling may be controlled to some degree by rest in bed, elevation of the limb to promote drainage, and wearing a firm rubber bandage over a stocking when up and about. However, this does not cure a chronic condition which tends to worsen with time, and surgery to remove the diseased tissue before extensive changes occur may be advisable.

Lymphogranuloma venereum - A disease produced by viruses transmitted by sexual contact.

Lymphosarcoma A malignant tumour of lymphatic tissue. *Lymphogranulomatosis* is sometimes a synonym for HODGKIN'S DISEASE.

Lysozyme A natural antibacterial substance contained in some bodily secretions, such as tears (400).

M

Maceration Softening and deterioration of tissue in constant confined contact with fluids.

Macula lutea A small, round, yellowish spot near the centre of the retina; the area of colour perception and most distinct vision (398).

Macule A flat discoloured spot on the surface of the skin. The rash of measles is macular.

Madura foot (*mycetoma*) A chronic fungus infection of the foot, occurring in tropical regions. The swollen foot becomes filled with connecting cystlike areas from which fungus-containing pus drains. In time the disease destroys the tissues, and amputation may be necessary.

Maidenhead The HYMEN.

Malabsorption syndrome A descriptive term for several disorders resulting from defective absorption of foodstuffs in the small intestine (347). Certain diseases or surgical procedures may disturb previously normal assimilative processes, but the most common forms of the syndrome (variously called *coeliac disease, sprue, idiopathic steatorrhoea*) seem to involve hereditary defects in the absorptive surface of the small intestine, and deficient activity of intestinal enzymes. Large amounts of unabsorbed fat produce frequent, pale, loose stools (steatorrhoea). *Coeliac disease* in children is the same as *nontropical sprue* in adults. Symptoms in adults – diarrhoea, weakness, loss of weight, anaemia deceptively like pernicious anaemia – are insidious and require careful diagnosis. Young children with coeliac disease commonly have poor appetite, various signs of malnutrition, stunted growth, bulging abdomen, and frequent frothy stools containing excessive amounts of fat. Gluten, a wheat protein, has a toxic effect on the small bowel of many patients with malabsorption syndromes. Strict elimination of gluten from the diet often restores bowel function to normal and maintains it even though there is no structural improvement in the bowel. A gluten-free diet prohibits wheat, rye, oats, and their products such as bread, buns, cakes, and biscuits, as well as foods such as gravies and soups which have wheat flour added to them.

Malacia Softening of part of an organ.

Malaise Listlessness, tiredness, irritability, depression, distress, and general feeling of illness; often a forerunner of some feverish infection.

Malar Of or relating to the cheek; the cheekbone, the *zygoma*.

Malaria An infection characterized by chills and intermittent or remitting fever, caused by parasites transmitted to man by the bites of mosquitoes (55).

Mal de mer Seasickness; a form of MOTION SICKNESS.

Male climacteric An indefinite state in elderly men, analogous to the menopause in women but without a clearcut sign comparable to cessation of menstruation which marks the female climacteric. Some physical changes occur with age as the hormone output of the sex glands diminishes; it may be difficult to separate physical factors from psychological reactions to fears, worries, boring environment, retirement, decreased sexual function and opportunity, unrecognized illness, depression, apprehensive brooding on the passage of time. Vague symptoms self-attributed to the male climacteric call for a visit to the doctor, who may decide that hormone treatment is worth a trial, or may find some condition that requires quite different treatment. Symptoms associated with diminished male hormone production (restorable to normal maintenance levels by replacement therapy) are decreased sexual potential, irritability, depression, lack of concentration, and diminished growth of beard and body hair.

Malignant Life-threatening; the usual medical meaning is cancerous.

Malingering The feigning of illness. The motive may be to avoid work, collect damages, or gain sympathy. The deception can usually be exposed by tests and observations not recognized or understood by the malingerer.

Mallet finger A dislocation of the end joint of a finger, which cannot be lifted, due to rupture or tearing of a tendon by a direct blow from a cricket ball or other object upon the end or back of the finger (460).

Malleus One of the three tiny bones (*ossicles*) of the middle ear which amplify vibrations of the eardrum and conduct them to the inner ear (419). Malleus means "hammer"; the handle of the hammer, attached to the eardrum, amplifies vibrations which are transmitted to the adjacent anvil-bone.

Malocclusion Inharmonious meeting of the upper and lower teeth; poor bite; bad alignment of teeth and jaws.

Malpresentation Any position of the fetus in the birth outlet other than the normal head-down position at childbirth; for example, breech, forehead, or foot presentation.

Malta fever See BRUCELLOSIS.

Mammography X-rays of the breast; several views are taken, to improve accuracy in detecting very small lesions (547).

Mammoplasty Plastic surgery of the breast; especially an operation to correct sagging breasts. It is performed by excising tissue and fixing the glands in their normal position.

Mandible The lower jawbone.

Manic-depressive psychosis A form of mental illness (505). It is characterized by swings from intense elation and hyperactivity to deep depression; between swings the patient may act quite normally. In the manic phase, the patient is enormously optimistic, overtalkative, physically busy, always on the go; his thoughts skip wildly from one subject to another; he is excited by grandiose projects. In the depressive phase, he may be hopelessly discouraged, have feelings of utter worthlessness, hear voices which nag him, and may have difficulty in performing the simplest mental and physical tasks.

Manubrium   The uppermost part of the breastbone.

Marasmus   Wasting and emaciation of infants; causes are various.

March fracture   Painful swelling and fracture of bones of the foot, not produced by acute injury but by excessive strain, as in marching.

Marfan's syndrome   A rare hereditary disorder, characterized by unusual flexibility of joints, disproportionately long legs, flabby tissues, funnel chest or pigeon breast, spider fingers, flat foot, displacement of the lens of the eye, and heart defects. The fundamental defect appears to be in connective tissue which breaks down or fails to produce normal amounts of fibres to support body structures.

Marginal ulcer   A peptic ulcer occurring at the junction where the stomach and jejunum have been surgically united.

Marie-Strumpell disease (*ankylosing spondylitis*)   A progressive disease of joints of the spine, different from rheumatoid arthritis (483).

Marrow   Soft material which fills the cavities of bones. Formation of blood cells takes place in the *red marrow* of certain bones of adults and of all bones in early life. *Yellow marrow* is fatty material which does not perform any blood-making function.

Masseter   A muscle that moves the lower jaw in chewing.

Mastectomy   Surgical removal of the breast, usually because of cancer (528).

Mastitis   Inflammation of the breasts, from bacterial infection or other causes. The most common disease of the female breast is *chronic mastitis*; the breasts contain nodules and small cysts of rubbery consistency, usually painful. A lump in the breast is not necessarily cancer, but it is imperative to consult a doctor to determine its nature.

Mastodynia   Pain in the breast.

Mastoid   Refers to mastoid air cells which surround the middle ear. Infection reaching these cells from the middle ear may require *mastoidectomy*, surgical removal of affected cells (527).

Materia medica   Substances used in medicine, and the science concerned with the origin, preparation, dosage and administration, and actions of such substances.

Maxilla   The upper jawbone.

Maxillary sinus   A pyramid-shaped cavity, largest of the nasal sinuses, located in the front of the upper jaw on each side of the nose (435). Also called the *antrum*. The floor of the cavity is close to the root of the eye-tooth.

Measles (*rubeola*)   An infectious disease caused by a virus (44, 282). Although most children recover from a natural attack of measles without suffering serious after-effects, the disease can be treacherous. It can lead to ENCEPHALITIS and mental retardation. Immunizing vaccines make it unnecessary for any child to be exposed to such risk. One injection of live-virus measles vaccine gives long-lasting, probably lifetime immunity.

Meatus   An opening or passage, such as the external opening of the urethra.

Meckel's diverticulum   A pouch opening from the small intestine, a blind tube two to five inches long (345). It is normally obliterated in the course of fetal development, but in some people it remains as a vestigial remnant. It may become inflamed and cause symptoms resembling appendicitis.

Meconium   Pasty, greenish material which fills the intestines of the fetus before birth and forms the first bowel movement of the newborn. *Meconium ileus*, obstruction of the intestines by viscid meconium, is the earliest manifestation of *cystic fibrosis* (272).

Mediastinum   The space in the middle of the chest between the lungs, breastbone, and spine, containing the heart, great blood vessels, oesophagus, windpipe, and associated structures.

Medical genetics   The science concerned with associations of heredity with defects and disease. See chapter 26.

Medulla   The inside parts of certain organs, such as glands and bones, as distinguished from the cortex or surface layer of the organ. The word also means marrow-like.

Medulla oblongata   The lowest part of the brain, where it merges with the spinal cord. It resembles a bulb at the end of the spinal cord. It contains vital nerve centres which control such functions as heart action, breathing, and swallowing.

Megacolon   Gigantic colon. In a congenital form known as *Hirschsprung's disease*, the colon lacks nerve cells necessary for its emptying (347). The symptoms are a greatly enlarged abdomen and intractable constipation; days may go by without a bowel movement. An acquired type of megacolon usually has a psychological basis; the child refuses to have a bowel movement and the rectum and colon become greatly distended from the mass of retained faeces.

Megakaryocyte   A giant cell of the bone marrow. Fragments of this cell are blood PLATELETS, essential for normal coagulation of blood (100).

Meibomian glands   Sebaceous glands of the eye-lid, subject to infection (*stye*) and obstruction (CHALAZION).

Melaena   Black, tarry stools discoloured by the presence of blood altered in the intestinal tract, as in bleeding from the stomach or intestines. Melaena of the newborn occasionally occurs from seepage of blood into the alimentary tract and is rarely a symptom of disease. Otherwise, passage of tarry stools calls for medical investigation.

Melanin   A brown to black pigment which is a factor in skin colour. It is derived from an AMINO ACID, tyrosine, through the action of an enzyme; if the enzyme is missing the person is an albino. Its production is stimulated by a hormone of the pituitary gland. Suntan, freckles, and flat brown spots on the skin of elderly people are examples of melanin deposits.

Melanoma   A dark mole coloured by melanin granules. The word often means *malignant melanoma*, a dangerous form of cancer, arising from pigment-producing cells. Blue or black moles may be removed as a preventive measure. Moles that darken or increase in size or appear after the age of 30 can be dangerous and should be removed (130).

Membrane   A thin layer of tissue which lines a part, separates cavities, or connects adjacent structures.

Menarche   The time of first occurrence of menstruation (303). The periods may be irregular while the menstrual cycle (213) is becoming established. The average age at onset of menses is eleven to thirteen years; variations of a year on either side of the average are not unusual. If menstruation is not established before or shortly after the sixteenth year, the cause should be investigated.

Meninges   Membranes which cover the brain and spinal cord (162).

Meningitis   Inflammation of the MENINGES.

Menopause   Cessation of menses; the milestone which marks the end of a woman's reproductive years (320). The average age at menopause is 48 years, but it is not unusual for women to continue to menstruate up to or beyond 50 years of age. At menopause, menstruation may cease abruptly, or there may be a gradual increase in the number of days between menstrual periods over a year or two. The final menstrual cycles are usually *anovulatory* – that is, no egg cells are produced by the ovaries. Many cycles which occur long before the menopause are probably anovulatory, but this cannot be relied on as assurance against conception. The average menstrual life span is about 33 years, during which a mature egg cell is released from the ovaries every month. Over the years, fewer and fewer cells which develop into ova remain in the ovaries. Along with the dwindling numbers of such cells there is a progressive decrease in production of ovarian hormones. Hot flushes and other symptoms of the menopause reflect this decline. Most women adjust to the menopause with little difficulty. A few have to seek medical attention for symptoms which are likely to be more annoying than incapacitating. However, symptoms occurring at this time may be wrongly blamed on the change of life and should be investigated to determine the cause, which may be quite unrelated to the menopause.

Menorrhagia Excessive menstrual bleeding.

Mental subnormality Mental subnormality is categorized in three main groups; broadly speaking, a child with an IQ between 70 and 50 is classed as *educationally subnormal*, and a child with an IQ of 50 or below may be classed as *mentally retarded* or *severely mentally retarded*. Children in the last two categories can never live without constant supervision, but the educationally subnormal may be expected to undertake some protected occupation and might live semi-independently, for example in supervised lodgings with meals provided.

Mescaline See chapter 28.

Mesentery The flat, fan-shaped sheet of tissue which carries nerves and blood vessels and supports the intestine, from the handle of the fan attached to the back wall of the abdomen (335). The arrangement allows considerable freedom of intestinal movement within the abdomen.

Mesomorph See SOMATOTYPE.

Metabolism The sum total of all the chemical activities by which life processes are organized and maintained; the breakdown and build-up of complex substances by body cells, assimilation of nutrients, and transformations which make energy available to the living organism. *Basal metabolism* is the minimal amount of heat (energy) needed to sustain activities when the body is in a state of complete rest.

Metaplasia Alteration of a cell to an abnormal type.

Metastasis Spread of disease from one part of the body to an unconnected part, by transfer of cells or organisms by blood and lymph channels. Ability to metastasize is characteristic of invasive cancer.

Metatarsalgia Foot pain in the instep area (468), usually due to weakness of muscles and ill-fitting shoes.

Metatarsals The five long bones of the foot, overlying the longitudinal arch, between toe joints and heel (467).

Meteorism Distension of stomach or intestines with gases.

Metritis Inflammation of the uterus.

Metrorrhagia Abnormal bleeding from the uterus at times other than the menstrual period.

Microtome An instrument which cuts extremely thin slices of tissue which are placed on slides, stained, and studied by pathologists.

Micturition The act of passing urine.

Middle ear The air-filled cavity between the eardrum and the inner ear. It contains the chain of three tiny bones over which sound vibrations are conducted (418).

Miliaria Prickly heat, heat rash. Obstruction of sweat glands traps sweat under the skin, producing small blisters. The condition disappears when the stimulus to sweating is removed, as by a cool environment.

Milk leg A form of THROMBOPHLEBITIS which occasionally occurs a week or two after childbirth. The affected leg swells and the tense skin has a white appearance, hence the name. Getting out of bed and moving around soon after delivery helps to prevent clot formation in veins. There is very little risk of EMBOLISM in this condition.

Milk line Extra breasts or nipples are congenital anomalies that occur occasionally in men and women. Supernumerary nipples with little or no underlying breast tissue are more common than miniature out-of-place breasts. In some instances, superfluous breasts of women may attain considerable size and even produce milk. The most frequent site of accessory breasts is about three inches below the normal pair, but they may occur anywhere along an imaginary line running from the armpit to the groin on either side. This is called the milk line, and marks the course of structures which permit the development of multiple breasts in mammals other than man. Development of accessory breasts along this line is determined early in fetal life.

Milk teeth Baby teeth; the twenty teeth which are shed when the permanent teeth erupt.

Miller-Abbott tube A double-channelled tube for insertion through the nose into the stomach to relieve distension of the small bowel. One channel has a small balloon at the end which is inflated in the stomach; peristaltic movements carry the tube farther down. Intestinal contents are withdrawn through the other channel.

Mineralocorticoids Hormones of the cortex of the adrenal gland which regulate salt and water balance (208).

Miscarriage Expulsion of the fetus before it is capable of independent life. See ABORTION.

Mitochondria Minute sausage-shaped particles in body cells, which contain the chemical machinery for generating energy. A typical mitochondrion has an outside membrane and numerous connecting interfolds. The outer membrane extracts energy from molecules derived from food and moves it to inner membranes which make ATP (*adenosine triphosphate*), the form of energy that keeps life processes going.

Mitral valve The valve on the left side of the heart which admits oxygenated blood to the main pumping chamber, the left ventricle (64). The valve has two peaked flaps shaped somewhat like a bishop's mitre. The valve may be damaged by rheumatic fever so that it leaks, or is scarred and thickened and cannot open widely enough (76).

Mittelschmerz A sign of OVULATION; lower abdominal pain produced by escape of blood into the peritoneal cavity as a result of ovulation, about midway in the menstrual cycle. The nature of the pain is usually identified by absence of any signs of pelvic disease and onset of menses about fourteen days later.

Molar pregnancy See HYDATIDIFORM MOLE.

Molluscum contagiosum A contagious viral infection of the skin, producing yellowish pimples containing cheesy material.

Mongolian spot A bluish spot or spots in the region of the lower back, seen in some newborn infants. The congenital spots usually disappear by the fourth or fifth year. Not related to MONGOLISM.

Mongolism (*Down's syndrome*) A congenital abnormality. Mongol babies tend to have upward slanting eyes, broad face, flattened skull, short hands, feet, and trunk, stubby nose, and lax limbs. The average mongol seldom achieves a mental capacity beyond that of a three to seven-year-old child, but is often lively and lovable. Life expectancy is not great. Placement in an institution is often recommended, especially if there are other children in the family. Mongolism results from a specific defect in CHROMOSOMES, called *trisomy*. One set of chromosomes (No. 21) is not a normal pair, but a triplet. The extra mongolism chromosome causes defects of physical and mental development. The mongoloid child has 47 instead of the normal complement of 46 chromosomes. The parents are in no way responsible for this accident, which occurs sporadically. The older the mother, the greater the risk. See chapter 26.

Monocyte A type of large white blood cell with a single central mass or nucleus (99). *Infectious mononucleosis* gets its name from an excess of such cells, arising from infection.

Monosodium glutamate A substance used to enhance the flavours of foods. It is a concentrated source of sodium and would not be permitted in diets in which sodium intake must be kept low.

Monozygotic Developed from a single fertilized egg, as identical twins.

Mons veneris The rounded prominence of fatty tissue above the external female sex organs.

Morning sickness The nausea or vomiting of pregnancy. Nausea and vomiting usually occur around breakfast time, then subside, only to recur the next morning. The symptom usually persists for two or three weeks and clears up without treatment. About 50 per cent of pregnant women experience morning sickness. A more serious form of vomiting of pregnancy (*hyperemesis gravidarum*) may go on for weeks, produce serious weight loss, and require medical treatment or a period in hospital.

Morphinism Addiction to morphine.

Motion sickness Nausea and vomiting induced by forms of motion which rotate the head simultaneously in more than one plane (sea sickness, car sickness, train sickness, air sickness). The trouble originates in the labyrinth of the ear where the organs of equilibrium are located (423). Confusing impulses reach the vomiting centre in the brain. Motion sickness may sometimes be prevented or minimized by not overeating or overdrinking; by lying down; by taking a position where motion is least exaggerated; by not reading or looking out of a car window or watching a rolling horizon from a boat. A number of drugs help to prevent or lessen motion sickness.

Mountain sickness A temporary condition brought on by diminished amounts of oxygen in the air at high altitudes. Persons who live at high altitudes adapt to the thin air; their red corpuscles increase in number. Acute mountain sickness is most likely to affect persons who are suddenly transported to high altitudes and do strenuous work. The symptoms usually abate in a few days to a week.

Mouth breathing The habit of breathing through the mouth instead of the nose has a drying action on the mouth tissues, which become inflamed, sometimes swollen and painful. Mouth breathers usually have a high incidence of colds and upper respiratory infections because they do not have the normal protection of the filtering, warming, air-conditioning functions of the nose. Physical factors may encourage mouth breathing. Children with narrow nasal passages, easily stuffed up by a minor cold, tend to breathe through the mouth. Enlarged adenoid or tonsil tissue, which normally grows in excess up to about ten years of age and then diminishes, may obstruct the airway and force the child to breathe through the mouth, which can easily become a habit. A doctor or dentist can diagnose mouth breathing easily, determine if there is a physical cause, and help a child to overcome a harmful habit with unpleasant consequences.

Mouth ulcers (*aphthous ulcers*) Little blisters on membranes of the mouth and cheeks which break and leave open sores. The painful ulcers usually heal spontaneously in a week or so, but attacks may be recurrent. It is no longer thought that mouth ulcers are caused by viruses (the sores may appear at the same time as cold sores or fever blisters which are caused by herpes simplex virus). A bacterial cause is suspected. Persons who have repeated or continuous crops of mouth ulcers may be allergic to some substance in the bacterium's make-up. The organism is sensitive to tetracycline, an antibiotic; oral suspensions of the drug held in the mouth for two minutes and then swallowed (four times daily) shorten the healing time but do not prevent recurrences.

Mucous colitis Not an organic disease, but the over-reaction of an easily irritated colon to various stimuli such as emotions or foods. Passage of mucus with bowel movements is harmless.

Mucous membrane Mucus-secreting tissue lining the inner walls of body cavities and passages which contain or may contain a certain amount of air and hence could dry out if not moistened. Mucous membranes are similar in general design but perform somewhat different functions in various parts of the body. Mucous membranes of the nose warm and moisten air before it reaches the lungs. Membranes of the windpipe are equipped with fine hairlike processes which sweep a thin film of mucus containing trapped particles of dust and dirt outwards from the lungs. Membranes of the stomach have special glands concerned with digestion; the membrane of the uterus undergoes periodic changes of engorgement and recession linked with the menstrual cycle.

Mucus Watery material secreted by mucous membranes, normally thin and unobtrusive, profuse in the presence of head colds, and subject to thickening and stickiness if its water content becomes greatly reduced.

Multipara A woman who has previously given birth to several children.

Multiple births The statistical chance of a mother's giving birth to twins is about one in 90 and the odds against triplets, quadruplets, or quintuplets are very much greater. Twins are more frequent in countries with high birth rates and more frequent among coloured than white people. There is some tendency for fraternal (two-egg) twins to run in families. Women under the age of 20 have the lowest incidence of twins and women between 35 and 39 have the highest. Likelihood of having twins is greater if a woman has already borne children, and greater yet if any of those children were twins. Treatment with gonadotrophin hormones to stimulate fertility seems to increase the likelihood of multiple births.

Mummification Drying and shrivelling of tissue to a mummy-like mass, a result of dry GANGRENE.

Mumps vaccine It is of the attenuated live virus type (see VACCINE) which gives lasting immunity.

Muscae volitantes Spots and threads before the eyes; floating specks (415). This common condition increases with age, and is not of serious significance.

Muscle About half the body's weight is muscle, a remarkable tissue which has the ability to contract and shorten its length. It is about 80 per cent water and most of the rest is protein. We have three types of muscle, different in function and visibly different under a microscope. Muscles we are most aware of are the ones that move our bones and make it possible to chew, walk, and execute all manner of movements. This type is called *striped, voluntary*, or *skeletal* muscle. It has dark and light crossbands giving a striped appearance. Voluntary muscles move when we will them to; their ends are connected to the parts they move. (The only voluntary muscle that is not attached at both ends is the tongue.)

Another type of muscle is called *smooth, visceral*, or *involuntary*. It has no cross-striping. It is present in the walls of the digestive tract, blood vessels, bladder, uterus, lungs, and other tissues, where it works without our conscious command. The pupil of the eye changes its size involuntarily; we are propelled into the world by the involuntary contractions of smooth uterine muscles.

A third type of muscle is unique. It constitutes the heart muscle (*myocardium*). It is a firm network of fibres connected to one another to function as a unit. Muscle contraction requires energy, produces heat, and is responsible for most of the body temperature. Even when resting, muscles are in a constant state of mild contraction (*tonus*). *Muscle cramps* result from continuous nerve impulses which keep a muscle in a painful state of contraction. A pulled muscle results from tearing or stretching by some massive effort. Exercise increases the size of muscles by enlarging individual cells, not by adding more cells. (Muscle table 446.)

Muscular dystrophies See chapter 19.

Mutation A change in the hereditary material of an organism, producing a change in some characteristic of the organism; especially, alteration of the character of a GENE. Mutations may occur spontaneously or they may be induced by some external stimulus, such as irradiation.

Myasthenia gravis A chronic disease characterized by rapid fatigue of certain muscles, with prolonged time of recovery of function. The muscles of the eyes and throat are most often affected, producing such symptoms as inability to raise the eyelids, difficulties of swallowing and talking, loss of chewing power, impairment of breathing. The muscles do not waste away. It is thought that the patient lacks some chemical concerned with nerve transmission. A drug called *neostigmine* acts at nerve and muscle fibre junctions to restore considerable muscle power quite rapidly. Many myasthenia gravis patients have an enlarged *thymus gland* or tumours of the thymus. X-ray treatment or surgical removal of the gland has produced some remissions, but results of these treatments for individual patients are not predictable.

Mycetoma See MADURA FOOT.

Mycoses Infections caused by fungi.

Myelin White fatty material which covers most nerve AXONS, in the manner of insulation around an electric wire; it is essential to proper transmission of nerve impulses. Degeneration or disappearance of the myelin sheath is the characteristic lesion of *demyelinating disease* (165).

Myelitis Inflammation of the spinal cord or bone marrow. *Poliomyelitis* is inflammation of grey matter of the cord.

Myelogram An X-ray film of the spinal canal made after injecting a contrast medium opaque to X-rays.

Myeloma, *multiple* Malignant tumours of the bone marrow (115).

Myiasis Infestation with larvae of flies which may develop in the skin, eyes, ear, or nose, and in wounds.

Myocarditis Inflammation of the heart muscle.

Myocardium The heart muscle; a highly specialized, cross-layered, very powerful involuntary muscle (65). Shutting off the blood supply to a portion of the muscle, as in coronary thrombosis, results in local death of tissue (*infarction*), a common sequel to heart attack.

Myocyte A muscle cell.

Myoglobin A form of HAEMOGLOBIN, slightly different from that of the blood, which is present in muscles and serves as a short-term source of oxygen to tide muscle fibres from one contraction to another.

Myoma A tumour composed of muscle elements; it is a common benign tumour of the uterus (311).

Myometrium The muscle of the uterus.

Myopathy Any disease of muscle.

Myopia Shortsightedness (403).

Myositis Inflammation of muscle.

Myringitis Inflammation of the eardrum.

Myringoplasty Surgical repair of a damaged eardrum.

Myringotomy Incision of the eardrum to relieve pressure of pus behind it (427).

Myxoedema Thyroid deficiency, *hypothyroidism* in adults (206). Congenital thyroid deficiency in children is known as *cretinism*. The patient with untreated myxoedema has dry, thick, puffy skin, thinning hair, low metabolism, is sensitive to cold, thick of speech, and mentally sluggish.

Myxoma A tumour derived from connective tissue.

N

Naevus A local area of pigmentation or elevation of the skin; a mole, a birthmark.

Nappy rash An ammonia burn resulting from breakdown of urine (288).

Narcissism Self-love, undue admiration of one's own body; a psychological term indicating self-admiration fixed at a level appropriate to infants but not to adults.

Narcolepsy Irresistible attacks of sleep, often with transient muscular weakness. Attacks occur during normal waking hours, not only under conditions conducive to drowsiness – after a heavy meal, during a dull lecture, in a train – but in inappropriate and even hazardous circumstances, as in driving a car. The affected person usually sleeps a few minutes, wakes refreshed, but may fall asleep again in a short time. The sleep does not differ from normal sleep except in its untimeliness; there are no signs of disease or physical abnormality. Treatment with drugs is usually successful in warding off attacks of sleepiness during the day.

Narcosis A state of deep sleep, unconsciousness, and insensibility to pain. *Narcotics* are drugs that produce such effects. Such drugs are very important in medicine, but if misused can lead to drug addition.

Nasopharynx The top part of the throat, behind the nasal cavity (432).

Nausea of pregnancy See MORNING SICKNESS.

Near point The point closest to the eye where an object, such as small print, is seen distinctly, normally 25 cm (10 in).

Necropsy Autopsy; a postmortem examination.

Necrosis Death of a localized portion of tissue surrounded by living tissue.

Negri bodies Round or oval particles in certain cells of animals dead of *rabies* (54). Their presence is proof that the animal had rabies.

Neisserian infection Usually means infection with gonorrhoea germs, *Neisseria gonorrhoeae* (59).

Neonatal Newborn: the first two or three days of life.

Neoplasm Any abnormal new growth; a tumour which may be malignant or benign. Neoplastic disease is a common term for cancer.

Nephrectomy Surgical removal of a kidney.

Nephritis Inflammation of the kidney (189).

Nephrolith Kidney stone.

Nephroma Malignant tumour of the cortex of the kidney.

Nephron The urine-forming unit of the kidney (182). It consists of a double-walled cup-shaped structure (*Bowman's capsule*) within which a tuft of tiny blood vessels (the *glomerulus*) exudes blood constituents which pass as a dilute filtrate into the tubule of the capsule. Most of the water and some essential materials in the filtrate are reabsorbed and the remainder is concentrated as urine.

Nephrosclerosis Nephritis due to hardening of kidney blood vessels (189).

Nephrosis Degeneration of the kidney without signs of inflammation; usually refers to nephrotic disease of children (190).

Nephrotoxic Poisonous to the kidneys.

Nerve Any of the cordlike bundles of fibres, composed of microscopic neurons, along which nerve impulses travel. See chapter 7.

Nerve deafness Impairment of hearing from partial or complete failure of the auditory nerves to transmit impulses to the brain (429).

Nettle rash (*urticaria*) Whitish, intensely itching elevations of the skin; weals, resembling mosquito bites and usually larger, sometimes covering patches as large as the palm (493). An attack may be a solitary event, never again experienced, subsiding in a few days, but in some instances nettle rash is repeated and persistent. Frequently the condition is an allergic reaction to certain foods (strawberries, shellfish, etc.), to drugs (495), to cold (496), to heat, or to sunlight (497).

Neuralgia Severe pain in a nerve or along its course, without demonstrable change in the structure of the nerve (167). The pain is typically sharp, stabbing, and severe, though short-lasting.

Neurasthenia A somewhat unfashionable term for a state of great fatigability, listlessness, aches and pains, once attributed to depletion or exhaustion of nerve centres, but without any demonstrable abnormality of the nervous system. Neurasthenic symptoms may have some organic cause and medical examination may disclose some treatable condition quite unrelated to nerves. If not, the label neurasthenia indicates a functional disorder with a psychological basis.

Neuritis Inflammation of a nerve, due to infection, toxins, compression, or other causes.

Neurodermatitis A chronic skin condition of unknown cause, not related to infection or allergy. It occurs most frequently in nervous women and may have a neurotic basis. Itchy patches of thickened skin (see LICHENIFICATION) occur especially on the neck, the inner surfaces of the elbows, and the backs of the knees. Treatment to relieve itching and discourage rubbing of the skin helps to alleviate the condition.

Neurofibromatosis A condition of multiple tumours in the skin along nerve pathways. The tumours, mainly composed of fibrous material, tend to increase in size and number. The growths are not cancerous, but very rarely may undergo malignant transformation. Sometimes the tumours can be removed surgically, often permanently, although in some cases they have a tendency to recur. The disorder is thought to be hereditary.

Neurogenic Of nervous origin.

Neuron The complete nerve cell, including the cell body, *dendrites* which bring incoming impulses to the body, and the *axon* which carries impulses away from it (154).

Neuropsychiatry The medical specialty concerned with both nervous and mental disorders and their overlap.

Neurosis See PSYCHONEUROSIS.

Neurosurgery The surgery of the central nervous system.

Neurosyphilis A late stage of syphilis affecting the central nervous system.

Neutrophil A type of white blood cell stainable by neutral dyes (98). *Neutropenia* is scarcity of such cells in the blood (111).

Nictitation Blinking.

Nidation Implantation of a fertilized egg in the uterus.

Nidus A nest; a point of origin or focus.

Nieman-Pick disease A rare hereditary condition occurring almost exclusively in children of Jewish families. It is a disorder of LIPID metabolism (inability to handle fatlike substances) which progresses to anaemia, emaciation, mental retardation, blindness, and deafness. Affected children rarely survive their second year. There is no treatment. The disease is inherited as a recessive trait.

Night blindness (*nyctalopia*) Imperfect vision at night or in dim light; reduced dark adaptation. The symptom may result from deficiency of vitamin A, which is necessary for regeneration of nerve cells of the retina (rods). These do most of the seeing when light is poor (398). Certain diseases of the retina can also cause night blindness.

Nitrogen balance An expression of the body's PROTEIN balance, determined by measurements of its nitrogen constituents. If nitrogen intake exceeds excretion, the balance is positive. Excessive retention of nitrogen may indicate kidney disease or other conditions. Negative nitrogen balance may indicate inadequate dietary protein, excessive loss of protein due to toxic goitre, burns, draining wounds, and so on, impaired absorption of protein, or defective metabolism of protein as in some liver diseases.

Nitrogen mustard A drug, derived from mustard gas, used to destroy malignant cells in lymphomatous diseases.

Nitrous oxide Laughing gas; an inhalant for producing brief anaesthesia, as for tooth extraction.

Nocturia Excessive urination at night.

Node A small protuberance, swelling, rounded knob, knot of cells. A *nodule* is a small node.

Nodular goitre Enlargement of the thyroid gland, characterized by lumpy masses in the gland (207).

Nonviable Incapable of living.

Normotension Normal blood pressure.

Nosocomial Of or relating to a hospital.

Nuchal Of or relating to, or in the region of, the nape of the neck.

Nuclear medicine Radioisotopes of an element decay spontaneously, ultimately reverting to a stable atom, and in the process give off energy in the form of radiation which is detectable by sensitive devices. Thus, substances marked or labelled with radioisotopes (for example, radioactive iodine, phosphorus, chromium) can be followed in their course through the body, giving information about the chemical processes of life. Drugs can be marked in this way to gain new knowledge of how they work. Recently developed *scintillation cameras* translate isotope emissions into dots on film, giving a pattern of radiation within a

659

patient's body. Certain tissues are selective for certain elements; the thyroid gland, for instance, takes up iodine, Radioisotopes which tend to concentrate in such tissues may be given in larger doses with the object of destroying or reducing the functioning of cells. Diagnostically, radioisotopes help to measure the functional abilities of certain tissues, are useful in evaluating some blood disorders, and in locating and marking the boundaries of tumours.

Nucleus The rounded central body of a cell, surrounded by cytoplasm. It contains the CHROMOSOMES and mechanisms of cell division and heredity.

Nullipara A woman who has never born a child.

Nummular eczema Dry skin with coin-shaped plaques on the back of the hands and outer surfaces of the arms, legs, and thighs.

Nyctalopia See NIGHT BLINDNESS.

Nymphomania Excessive sexual desire in a woman.

Nystagmus Involuntary, rhythmic oscillation of the eyeballs, horizontal, vertical, or rotatory. Most people experience nystagmus if the body is whirled to produce dizziness and an attempt is made to fix the gaze on a stationary object. Simple forms of nystagmus can result from eye strain or refractive errors. Nystagmus may be a symptom of inner ear disturbance or disorder of the nervous system.

O

Obstetric forceps Two curved flat blades (right and left) which are separately placed with great care around the head of the fetus in the birth passage; the handles are then interlocked. Used to assist extraction of the baby in difficult deliveries.

Obstetrician A doctor specializing in the care of pregnant women.

Occiput The back part of the head.

Occlusion Closure or shutting off, as of a blood vessel; also, the meeting position of upper and lower teeth when closed.

Occult Hidden, not evident to the naked eye; as, occult blood in faeces.

Ocular Of or relating to the eye.

Ocular muscle imbalance Disharmony of muscles which move the eyeball. Associated with such conditions as squint, poor fusion of images, amblyopia (407).

Oculist Same as OPHTHALMOLOGIST.

Oedema Excessive accumulation of fluid in body cavities and spaces around cells. The fluid produces swelling of waterlogged tissues. Oedema is not a disease but a symptom of varying importance. The waterlogging may be mild and localized, such as the puffiness around a bruise or a slight swelling of the ankles after standing all day, or it may distend almost all the body like a balloon. The underlying cause may be trivial, as in PREMENSTRUAL TENSION, or serious. Pitting oedema, the kind which leaves a little pit or depression when pressed, is often associated with heart or kidney disorders. Oedema results from some disturbance of the mechanisms of fluid exchange in the body, of which there are many causes; salt and water retention by the kidneys (see ELECTROLYTES), congestive heart failure, allergy, protein deficiency, obstruction of lymphatic drainage (see LYMPHOEDEMA), inflammation, injury, liver and kidney disease, tumours. Modern diuretic drugs which increase the output of urine and dispose of excess fluid are helpful in the management of oedema while the underlying disease is treated.

Oesophagitis Inflammation of the lining of the oesophagus (341).

Oesophagus The gullet; the muscular tube through which swallowed food passes into the stomach by muscular action (330).

Oestrogen A general term for female sex hormones (212).

Oil pneumonia See ASPIRATION PNEUMONIA.

Olecranon A curved part of one of the forearm bones (*ulna*) at the elbow end. It is what we lean on when we rest an elbow on a table.

Olfactory bulb A structure just above the thin bone which separates the top of the nasal cavity from the brain. It receives nerve fibres that pass upwards through small holes in the bone from the nose (436).

Oligomenorrhoea Scanty menstrual flow, or abnormally long time between menstrual periods.

Oligophrenia Mental deficiency, feeblemindedness.

Oligospermia Abnormally few SPERMATOZOA in the semen.

Oliguria Scanty secretion of urine; abnormal infrequency of urination.

Omentum A layer of tissue, a fold of the peritoneum, that hangs from the stomach and transverse colon and covers the underlying organs like an apron. It forms a fat pad on the front of the abdomen, sometimes conspicuously thick.

Onchocerciasis A form of FILARIASIS occurring in tropical areas. Infection with threadlike worms produces tumours in the skin and sometimes blinding disease of the eyes.

Oncology The science of tumours, new growths.

Onychia Inflammation of the bed of a nail, often resulting in loss of the nail.

Ophthalmia Inflammation of the eye, especially with involvement of the conjunctiva.

Ophthalmologist A doctor who specializes in medical and surgical care of the eyes (400).

Ophthalmoscope An instrument which gives a view of structures inside the eye (400).

Opiates Narcotics derived from or related to opium; for example, morphine, heroin, codeine, paregoric, laudanum. In a broad sense the word applies to any sense-dulling, stupor-inducing drug.

Opisthotonos A position of the body in which the head and lower legs are bent backwards and the trunk arched forwards, due to convulsive spasm of muscles of the back, such as in strychnine poisoning.

Optic atrophy Irreversible degeneration of optic nerve fibres.

Optic chiasma An arrangement of nerve fibres in which the optic nerves of both eyes cross at a junction near the pituitary gland (398).

Optic disc The area at the back of the eye where all the nerve fibres of the retina merge with the optic nerve. Because light is not perceived at the point where the optic nerve enters the eye, the area is a normal BLIND SPOT. When using both eyes together, one is unaware of a blind spot.

Optician A technician who carries out the prescription of an ophthalmologist for glasses or contact lenses; a manufacturer or designer of optical equipment.

Optic nerve A bundle of a million or so nerve fibres which transmits impulses from the RETINA to the occipital lobe at the back of the brain where they are transformed into vision.

Oral Of or relating to the mouth; in the case of medicines, administered by the mouth. (Not to be confused with *aural* – of or relating to the ear.)

Oral contraceptives STEROID compounds taken by mouth by women to prevent conception; the pill. The tablets contain combinations of oestrogen-progestogen or they may be sequential, furnishing oestrogen alone on certain days of the cycle, followed by combined oestrogen-progestogen. Regularity of dosage is very important.

Orbit The bony socket that contains the eyeball (394).

Orchidectomy Castration; surgical removal of the testicles.

Orchitis Inflammation of the testicles. It may be a complication of mumps.

Organ of Corti The centre of the sense of hearing in the inner ear. It contains hairlike cells which oscillate in response to pulsating fluids, stimulating nerve endings which merge into the nerve of hearing that carries impulses to receiving centres in the brain.

Organic disease Disease that has a physical cause, a lesion, disorder of an organ, as opposed to FUNCTIONAL DISEASE.

Orgasm The climax of the sexual act, terminating in ejaculation of semen by the male and release of tension in the female.

Oriental sore (*cutaneous leishmaniasis*) Single or multiple skin ulcers produced by infection with organisms transmitted by sandflies.

Orifice The opening or outlet of a body cavity or passage.

Ornithosis (*parrot fever, psittacosis*) A pneumonia-like disease produced by viruses from infected birds.

Orthodontics Tooth straightening; the branch of dental science concerned with prevention and correction of irregularities of the teeth and jaws (391).

Orthopaedics The surgical and medical speciality concerned with correction of deformities, diseases, accidents, and disorders of body parts that move us about – limbs, bones, joints, muscles, tendons, and so on.

Orthopnoea The need to sit upright in order to breathe comfortably, manifested by persons with congestive heart failure (75).

Orthoptics Teaching, training, and exercises for improving the fusion of images from both eyes (as in squint), putting a lazy eye back to work, and generally making visual mechanisms more efficient.

Orthostatic Induced or intensified by standing upright; for example, *orthostatic hypotension*, a lowering of blood pressure brought on by changing from a lying-down to an upright position.

Osgood-Schlatter disease Degeneration of the protuberance on the knee-end of the TIBIA, the long bone of the lower leg. A form of OSTEOCHONDRITIS, occurring most frequently in young persons.

Osmosis The phenomenon of transfer of materials through a semipermeable membrane that separates two solutions, or between a solvent and a solution, tending to equalize their concentrations. *Osmotic pressure* is that exerted by the movement of a solvent through a semipermeable membrane into a more concentrated solution on the other side. This pressure is the driving force that causes diffusion of particles in solution to move from one place to another. Walls of living cells are semipermeable membranes and much of the activity of the cells depends upon osmosis.

Osseous Composed of bone or resembling bone.

Ossicle One of the three tiny bones of the middle ear (*malleus, incus, stapes*) which conduct sound vibrations to the inner ear (419).

Ossification The process of forming bone. CARTILAGE is made into bone by the process of ossification. Calcium phosphate is deposited in the cartilage, changing it into bone.

Osteitis Inflammation of bone.

Osteitis deformans PAGET'S DISEASE. A chronic process of bone overgrowth, destruction, and new bone formation, ultimately producing deformities (471). The skull, spine, and weight-bearing bones are most commonly affected.

Osteochondritis Inflammation of both bone and CARTILAGE. *Osteochondritis dissecans* is a fairly common condition of late adolescence in which there is local death of a section of the joint surface of a bone (usually of the knee) and its overlying cartilage (465). *Osteochondritis deformans juvenilis* (Perthé's disease) is a degenerative condition of the upper end of the thigh bone in children three to eight years of age, which eventually heals but may leave some permanent deformity of the hip joint.

Osteogenesis imperfecta A rare hereditary condition of defective formation of bony tissues, resulting in brittle bones which fracture easily.

Osteomalacia Adult RICKETS; softening of bone, abnormal flexibility, brittleness, loss of calcium salts. Usually due to vitamin D deficiency or impaired absorption of nutrients (470).

Osteomyelitis Infection of bone and marrow due to growth of germs within the bone. Infection may reach the bone through the bloodstream or direct injury (450).

Osteoporosis Enlargement of canals or spaces in bone, giving a porous thinned appearance. The weakened bone is fragile and may be broken by some minor injury, or may fracture spontaneously. The condition is common in women after the menopause and occurs to some degree in old men.

Osteotome A surgical instrument used for cutting through bone.

Otalgia Earache.

Otitis Inflammation of the ear. *Otitis externa* is a bacterial or fungal infection of the ear canal (425). *Otitis media* is an acute or chronic infection of the middle ear (426).

Otoplasty Plastic surgery for correction of malformed ears. See PROTRUDING EARS.

Otorhinolaryngologist A specialist in diseases of the ear, nose, and throat. An *otologist* confines himself to the ear.

Otorrhoea Chronic discharge from the ear (427).

Otosclerosis Overgrowth in parts of the middle ear of spongy bone which dampens vibrations, and impairs hearing (428). This type of hearing loss is often correctible by surgery (527).

Outpatient A patient who comes to a hospital for treatment but does not reside there.

Oval window A membrane-covered opening to the inner ear, to which the footplate of the STAPES is attached (420). Sounds conducted by the chain of bones in the middle ear are hammered against the oval window and transmitted to fluids behind it and thence to the inner ear.

Ovarian cyst A sac containing fluid or mucoid material arising in the ovary (312). A cyst with a stem may become twisted and produce sudden severe pain in the lower abdomen.

Ovariectomy Surgical removal of one or both ovaries. Also called *oophorectomy*.

Ovulation Release of a mature egg cell from the follicle in the ovary in which it develops (212). This is the time during the menstrual cycle when conception can occur. There are no infallible signs of ovulation that a woman can recognize, but there are suggestive signs. Ovulation usually occurs about midway between menstrual periods in a normal menstrual cycle of approximately 28 days. Body temperature tends to rise, though to a small degree, at the time of ovulation. Abdominal pain and a pinkish discharge from the vagina may also occur at the time of ovulation; see INTERMENSTRUAL PAIN, and MITTELSCHMERZ.

Ovum   The female reproductive cell; an egg. The ovum is the largest human cell but it is barely discernible by the naked eye. It is about half of the size of the full stop at the end of this sentence. It is a round cell with a clear capsule, and with the consistency of stiff jelly. Like the sperm, the ovum contains only 23 CHROMOSOMES, which at conception pair off with those of the sperm to give the embryo a normal complement of 46 chromosomes. Although the ovum is about 85,000 times larger than the sperm, both contain the same number of GENES. The relatively huge size of the ovum is partly accounted for by its content of nutrient yolk. Only about 400 ova ripen to maturity and are released by ovulation during a woman's reproductive lifetime; of these, only a very few are fertilized.

Oxyhaemoglobin   HAEMOGLOBIN carrying a full load of oxygen; the haemoglobin in bright red arterial blood.

Oxytocin   A hormone of the pituitary gland which stimulates the uterus to contract. It is frequently administered into a vein in order to stimulate labour and ensure effective contractions (200).

Oxyuriasis   Threadworm or pinworm infection.

Ozaena   A chronic disease of mucous membranes of the nose, giving off a foul-smelling odour or discharge.

P

Pacemaker   A small knot of tissue in the right atrium of the heart which triggers the heartbeat (65). In certain heart disorders, battery-powered devices connected to the heart can take over the pacemaking function. See CARDIAC PACEMAKER.

Pachydermatous   Thick-skinned.

Paediatrician   A doctor specializing in the care of children.

Paget's disease   Two diseases bear this name. *Paget's disease of the breast* is manifested by thickened, eczema-like scaliness of the area around the nipple, with fissuring, oozing, and destruction of the nipple as the underlying disease (cancer of the central ducts of the breast) advances. The other Paget's disease, also known as *osteitis deformans*, is a chronic disease of bone metabolism. The skull, pelvis, spine, and long bones are especially affected. Calcium and phosphorus are lost from the bones, which become soft and bend easily. Irregular replacement of the minerals causes thickening and deformity. Bone pain, impaired hearing, and muscle cramps are frequent symptoms. The disease progresses slowly and after many years may lead to chronic invalidism (471).

Painful menstruation   Primary dysmenorrhoea (305) is characterized by pain, cramps, or mild to severe discomfort occurring at the onset of menstrual periods, in the absence of any organic disorder. Physical exercises may help to banish distress. Any exercise which involves systematic twisting, bending, and extending of the trunk is helpful.

Painful shoulder syndrome   Limitation of motion and pain about the shoulder may arise from injury, calcium deposits, bursitis, osteoarthritis, diseases of the chest, coronary heart disease. The predominant symptom is severe pain in the shoulder area and inability to raise the arm because of pain and weakness.

Painter's colic   LEAD POISONING.

Palliative   Relieving pain, suffering, or distressing symptoms of disease but without any curative action.

Palpation   A method of obtaining information about a patient's condition by manipulating or feeling a part of the body with the hand.

Palpebral   Of or relating to the eyelid.

Palpitation   Throbbing, pounding, rapid, or fluttering heartbeat, sufficiently out of the ordinary to make the patient aware of it. More often than not the condition is temporary and not of serious importance, but there are many causes and if the symptom is repeated or alarming it should be investigated.

Palsy   Paralysis.

Pancreatitis   Inflammation of the pancreas. It occurs in acute and chronic form (353).

Pandemic   A super-epidemic, one that occurs on a large scale over a very wide area of a country or of the world.

Panhypopituitarism   Severe loss of function of the anterior pituitary gland (203).

Panniculus   A layer of fat beneath the skin; the layer on the front of the abdomen sometimes expands the waistline noticeably.

Panophthalmitis   Pus-producing inflammation of all the tissues of the eye, threatening total and permanent blindness.

Papanicolaou smear   (*Pap test*)   A screening test for cancer of the cervix and the uterus. Cell scrapings obtained painlessly from the surface of the cervix are spread on glass slides, stained, and examined under a microscope. Detection of cancer cells in the specimen, and confirmation of cancer of the cervix by other diagnostic measures, leads to prompt treatment of a form of cancer which in its early stages is almost invariably curable (307).

Papilla   A small conical or nipple-shaped elevation, like a pimple. Papillae give the front of the tongue its slightly rough appearance, and orderly lines of papillae projecting into the upper skin layer give us fingerprints.

Papilloedema   (*choked disc*)   Noninflammatory swelling of the optic nerve where it enters the eye, due to increased pressure within the skull or interference with flow of blood from the veins of the eye. It occurs most frequently in patients with brain tumour, brain abscess, or meningitis; concussion, haemorrhage, or severe hypertension may also be responsible. Vision is good in the early stages, but gradually deteriorates. Treatment depends on detection of the underlying cause.

Papilloma   A tumour of lining tissues – skin, mucous membranes, glandular ducts – composed of epithelial cells covering supporting papillae. It is usually benign.

Papule   A small solid elevation on the skin; a solid pimple containing no pus or fluid.

Paracentesis   Surgical puncture of a body cavity to withdraw fluid.

Paraesthesia   Abnormal sensations of crawling, burning, and tingling of the skin, due to neuritis or lesions of the nervous system.

Paraffin wax packs   A way of heating body parts, especially painful arthritic hands. The hands are dipped into melted paraffin until a thick heat-retaining layer is built up.

Paralytic ileus   Intestinal obstruction resulting from decreased peristaltic activity of the bowel (345).

Paranoia   A form of mental illness characterized by suspiciousness, delusions, feelings of being persecuted, spied upon, or endangered. The patient's delusions are so systematized and seemingly logical that they can be quite convincing to others, especially since the paranoid patient often seems quite sane and reasonable except on one or a few subjects. Mild paranoid trends are not uncommon in suspicious people who think others have it in for them, put obstacles in their way, and are responsible for their failures, but the extreme paranoid, who may do violence to his supposed persecutors, has a severe mental illness.

Paraplegia Paralysis of both legs, usually due to injury or disease of the spinal cord. The bladder and bowels may be paralysed as well as the legs, depending on the controlling part of the nervous system that is injured. Rehabilitation training may restore a good measure of function to the paraplegic patient.

Parathyroid glands Four pea-size glands embedded superficially on the back and side surfaces of both lobes of the thyroid gland. The glands secrete hormones which maintain a stable concentration of calcium in the blood. Either an excess or deficiency produces mild to serious bodily disturbances (207).

Paratyphoid An acute infectious disease which resembles typhoid fever but is less severe. It is caused by Salmonella bacteria transmitted directly or indirectly from the faeces and urine of infected persons.

Parenchyma The functioning, specialized part of an organ, as distinguished from connective tissue that supports it.

Parenteral Outside the digestive tract. The word commonly refers to substances given by injection or infusion instead of by mouth.

Paresis Slight or incomplete paralysis. Also, a term for general paralysis of the insane, resulting from syphilis.

Parietal Of or relating to the wall of a cavity; especially, the bones of the skull at the top and sides of the head behind the frontal bones.

Parkinson's disease (*parkinsonism*) A chronic progressive disease of which the chief symptoms are tremor, stiffness, and slowness of movement, resulting from disturbance of a small centre at the base of the brain (169).

Paronychia Pus-producing infection of tissues around the nails, caused by yeasts (134) or bacteria. Acute bacterial paronychia is usually treated with antibiotics. Surgical drainage may be necessary. Chronic bacterial paronychia may require prolonged treatment with hot soaking, drainage, and local application of an antibiotic ointment. During treatment the involved finger or fingers should be kept as dry as possible.

Parotid gland One of the saliva-producing glands, located in the angle of the jaw in front of and below the ear (330).

Parotitis Inflammation of the parotid gland. Epidemic parotitis is another name for mumps.

Paroxysmal tachycardia Periodic attacks of extremely rapid beating of the heart, 200 or more beats per minute. Attacks may last only a few seconds or as long as several hours (79).

Parrot fever See PSITTACOSIS.

Parturition Childbirth.

Passive transfer An indirect method of testing for skin allergies. Serum of the patient is introduced into areas of the skin of another person, and a couple of days later these sites are tested for reactions to suspected allergens (496). The other person acts as a guinea pig, demonstrating skin reactions to substances to which he himself is not allergic.

Patch test A method of identifying allergic sensitivities by applying suspected material to the skin (490).

Patella The kneecap.

Paternity tests Blood groups (103) are determined by unvarying laws of heredity. This is the basis of tests for excluding paternity. If a child's red blood cells contain substances which are incompatible with the blood groups of its presumed parents, one of the couple cannot be the father or the other cannot be the mother. A person with AB blood cannot have a child of group O; a person of group O cannot have a child of group AB; a person of group M cannot have a child of group N. Presence or absence of a number of other factors follows the same hereditary rules. The blood factors of the mother, child, and putative father are determined by tests using antiserums and red blood cells known to contain A, B, O, M, or N factors. If the factor tested for is present, the red cells clump together; if it is absent they do not. Tests cannot prove that a man *is* the father of a certain child. They prove only that he cannot be, and they cannot always do that because by coincidence his blood may contain the same factors as the actual father. The chance that nonpaternity can be proved is a little better than 50 per cent. Only three blood groups (ABO, MN, Rh) are used for medicolegal purposes, but several other factors are known and it is theoretically possible to distinguish 50,000 different blood group combinations. Indeed, it is believed that blood is as individual as fingerprints, and when its chemical markers are more fully revealed it may become possible to determine that a child is the offspring of a particular couple.

Pathogen An agent causing disease.

Pathogenic Having the capacity to produce disease. Many bacteria are harmless and even beneficial to man, but the types that cause disease are pathogenic organisms.

Pathology The science and study of the nature of disease: its processes, effects, causes, manifestations; changes from normal in structure and function. Pathology does not mean disease, but its study. *Pathologists* examine stained cells and tissues, do autopsies, and employ chemical and laboratory methods to assist in diagnosis of disease, identify normal and abnormal structures, and to add to scientific knowledge of disease processes in general.

Pectoral Of or relating to the chest.

Pedicle graft A flap of a patient's own skin attached to the body by a stalk or pedicle containing blood vessels that supply nourishment while the flap is taking hold in an area to which it is grafted (533).

Pediculosis Infestation with body lice (128).

Pellagra A DEFICIENCY DISEASE manifested by rough skin, diarrhoea, sore mouth and tongue, and sometimes mental disturbance (363).

Pelvimetry Measurement of the dimensions of the bony pelvis, usually done to determine whether the outlet of the birth canal is of sufficient size to permit the fetus to be born naturally.

Pelvis A basin-shaped cavity, especially that formed by the bones in the hip region. The bony pelvis supports the spinal column, rests on the legs, and contains structures of the lower end of the trunk (448). The female bony pelvis is slightly different from that of the male. The *kidney pelvis* is a cavity which collects urine from the organ's filtration units and carries it to the ureter and thence to the bladder (181).

Pemphigus An uncommon but serious skin disease manifested by crops of large blisters which rupture and leave raw surfaces.

Penicillin reactions The major single cause of systemic reactions to drugs is penicillin. Reactions occur in persons previously sensitized to the drug by therapeutic doses, or sometimes by indirect contact, as in milk products. The most serious and fortunately the most rare reaction is

ANAPHYLAXIS; its most common pattern is acute breathing difficulty, swelling of the larynx threatening suffocation, and profound shock. This reaction occurs within seconds or minutes after administration of penicillin to sensitized patients. Far more common and less serious, but distressing, are skin reactions such as nettle rash and itching. SCRATCH TESTS on persons with no previous history of penicillin sensitization may be performed before administering the drug, but if patients with past histories of penicillin sensitivity are to be tested, emergency treatment facilities should be immediately available.

Penis The male sex organ.

Pepsin A protein-digesting enzyme in the gastric juice. It is active only in an acid environment, which the stomach provides (333).

Peptic ulcer An ulcer associated with the digestive action of acid juices; it may be located in the stomach or duodenum, or at the site of surgical joining of the stomach and jejunum. The most frequent form is duodenal ulcer (343).

Percussion A method of physical diagnosis. Short firm blows are tapped upon a body surface by a finger or small hammer to produce sounds or vibrations. Solid, fluid-filled, tense, empty, or congested organs have different resonances. Percussion is most often applied in examination of the lungs and abdomen.

Perennial allergic rhinitis A condition similar to hay fever but running a more or less continuous course without seasonal variations (492).

Perforated eardrum The eardrum may be punctured by direct injury (never stick hairpins or toothpicks into the ear canal!) or by infections of the middle ear which break through the drum. A punctured eardrum may heal itself, but if not, a route of invasion for infectious material from the outside world is open. A person with a punctured eardrum should not dive or swim or put the head under water because of the danger that infectious material may be forced into internal ear parts. Ear plugs do not give dependable protection. A perforated eardrum can be closed by an operation known as *tympanoplasty* (527).

Perianal Situated around the anus.

Pericarditis Inflammation of the PERICARDIUM from causes such as rheumatic fever or extension of infection from neighbouring parts (65).

Pericardium The sac or membrane that encloses the heart (65). It secretes lubricating fluid that permits free movements of the heart.

Perineum The area between the anus and scrotum in men, and the anus and the vulva in women.

Periodontal disease Inflammation of the membranes that cover the roots of the teeth (380); laymen commonly call it PYORRHOEA.

Periosteum The membranous covering of nearly all bone surfaces (449).

Peripheral At or near an outer surface; for example, peripheral blood vessels, near skin surfaces.

Peristalsis Wavelike movements of constriction and relaxation which propel materials along the digestive tube. Encircling muscle contracts to squeeze material forward while muscles in front of the material relax; the latter muscles constrict in their turn, and so on.

Peritoneum The strong smooth membrane which lines the abdominal cavity and covers the abdominal organs.

Peritonitis Inflammation of the PERITONEUM; the most frequent cause is a ruptured appendix, but infection can occur from other routes (347).

Perlèche Cracks at the side of the mouth, thickened, covered with whitish material. The condition is classically associated with deficiency of a vitamin, riboflavin. Usually the patient has excessive folding of the skin at the corners of the mouth – perhaps congenital, or the result of missing teeth or poorly fitting dentures – and the moist opposing surfaces rub together, resulting in maceration, inflammation, possible infection. The patient licks the cracks, fostering further maceration; spicy or acid foods may be irritating. An ointment may be prescribed, together with appropriate measures to keep the area dry – correction of malocclusion or poorly fitting dentures, abstention from smoking, chewing gum, and chewing tobacco.

Perthé's disease Degeneration of the upper end of the thighbone in young children (463).

Pertussis Whooping cough (43).

Pessary One of many devices of metal, rubber, or plastic, of different shapes and sizes, placed in the vagina or the uterus or parts of it to support displaced pelvic structures. Also used of medicated preparations for vaginal insertion.

Petechiae Tiny pinpoint haemorrhages in the skin (110).

Petit mal A form of epileptic attack, consisting of sudden loss of consciousness lasting for only a few seconds (172).

Pets See HOUSEHOLD PETS.

pH Technically, a symbol expressing hydrogen ion concentration; practically, a scale of the acidity or alkalinity of substances. The neutral point is pH 7. Below 7, acidity increases. Above 7, alkalinity increases.

Phaeochromocytoma A tumour, usually arising in the inner part of the adrenal gland, which secretes excessive amounts of hormones, producing such symptoms as tremor, cramps, palpitations, headache, nausea, and high blood pressure. Treatment is surgical removal (210).

Phalanx One of the bones of the fingers or toes. The plural is *phalanges*.

Phantom limb The illusion that a limb which has been amputated is still attached to the body and feels pain and other sensations.

Pharmacopoeia An authoritative collection of formulas and methods of preparing and using drugs, which sets standards of purity, safety, and potency.

Pharyngeal tonsils Lymphoid tissue better known as *adenoids* (439).

Pharyngitis Sore throat.

Pharynx The membrane-lined cavity at the back of the nose, mouth, and throat; the place where a sore throat hurts.

Phenylalanine An essential AMINO ACID, present in protein foods.

Phenylketonuria Hereditary inability to metabolize phenylalanine, an essential amino acid, because of a genetically determined lack of a necessary enzyme; an inherited error of metabolism. Breakdown products of incompletely metabolized phenylalanine accumulate in the infant's body and impair brain function. The *Guthrie* test of an infant's blood gives evidence of the condition soon after birth. A diet of special foods, very low in phenylalanine, lessens the threat of damage to the developing nervous system.

Phimosis Tightness of the foreskin of the penis, preventing retraction over the tip of the organ.

Phlebitis Inflammation of the walls of a vein, which may lead to formation of a clot, *thrombophlebitis* (94).

Phlebothrombosis Formation of a clot in a vein. Not due to local inflammation.

Phlebotomy Bloodletting, by cutting into a vein;

venesection. Irrational bloodletting for almost any state of ill health was practised wholesale in the seventeenth and eighteenth centuries. The practice undoubtedly weakened and even caused the death of patients. It fell into deserved disrepute as a panacea. But there are some conditions for which bloodletting is recognized as a part of modern treatment; see HAEMOCHROMATOSIS and POLYCYTHAEMIA (106).

Phobia An abnormal, excessive dread or fear. There are scores of specific phobias, each with its own medical name. Some of the more common are:

phobia	fear of
acrophobia	heights
agoraphobia	open places
aichmophobia	sharp objects
ailurophobia	cats
algophobia	pain
androphobia	men
bacteriophobia	germs
ballistophobia	missiles
belonephobia	needles, pins
claustrophobia	confined spaces
cynophobia	dogs
dipsophobia	drink
erythrophobia	blushing
genophobia	sex
gymnophobia	nakedness
haemophobia	blood
hypnophobia	falling asleep
lalophobia	talking
lyssophobia	becoming insane
melissophobia	bees
mysophobia	dirt, contamination
ochlophobia	crowds
osmophobia	odours
paedophobia	children
photophobia	light
pyrophobia	fire
siderodromophobia	railways
sitophobia	eating
tocophobia	childbirth
triskaidekaphobia	number 13
xenophobia	strangers

Photoscanner An instrument which measures the concentration of radioisotopes (measured doses of radiation) in a patient's body. See NUCLEAR MEDICINE.

Photosensitivity A number of disorders are caused or made worse by exposure to sunlight. Photosensitive reactions may result from certain drugs taken internally, from materials in cosmetics or substances applied to the skin, from contact with certain plants (parsnips, celery, carrots, dill, parsley), or from underlying disease which increases the sensitivity of the skin to sunlight. A clue to photosensitive reactions is the presence of lesions on exposed areas of the forehead, nose, edges of the ears, and backs of the hands, while areas under the jaw not exposed to sunlight are not affected. Patients with *lupus erythematosus* (483) are sensitive to sunlight.

Phototherapy Treatment with light rays, including invisible ultraviolet and infrared wavelengths.

Phrenic nerve The principal nerve of breathing which activates the muscle of respiration, the *diaphragm*. The nerve also serves the PERICARDIUM and PLEURA.

Phthisis An old term for pulmonary tuberculosis.

Physical allergy Allergic reactions induced by purely physical factors such as heat, cold, or light (496).

Phytobezoar A compact ball of vegetable matter in the stomach.

Pia mater The innermost of the three membranes that cover the brain and spinal cord (162).

Pica A craving to eat strange foods or unnatural substances – wood, clay, coal, dirt, chalk, starch, and so on. Pica is more common in children.

Pigeon-breeder's lung A recently recognized respiratory disease occurring in pigeon breeders or others in close contact with pigeons. Chills, fever, cough, and shortness of breath develop a few hours after inhaling dusts in an environment of pigeons. The disease is not a bacterial or viral infection, but appears to be a hypersensitivity reaction to ANTIGENS in pigeon feathers and droppings, a disease similar to FARMER'S LUNG.

Pigeon toe Inward turning of the feet and toes when walking. Children in the early stages of walking are often pigeon-toed but usually outgrow the condition (468).

Piles See HAEMORRHOIDS.

Pill rolling Involuntary movement of thumb and fingers, as if a pill were being rolled, a feature of Parkinson's disease (169).

Pilonidal cyst A congenital hair-containing sac under the skin overlying the coccyx at the top of the cleft of the buttock. There may be only a dimpling of the skin or a hairy overlying tuft to mark the presence of the cyst until it becomes infected, swollen, and painful, and perhaps develops a FISTULA through which fluids are excreted. Surgical removal of the cyst is usually necessary to accomplish a permanent cure.

Pimple The term for what doctors call a *pustule*.

Pineal gland A structure about a quarter of an inch long which lies very nearly in the centre of the brain. For centuries physiologists were unable to ascribe any function to it. Now there is evidence that the pineal is a sort of biological clock which influences the activities of hormones. Experiments with animals indicate that in some way the pineal regulates the sex glands.

Pink eye One variety of acute *conjunctivitis*, a highly contagious infection of the eye (407). Discharges contain the infective organisms.

Pinna The external ear; the protruding part of the hearing mechanism, mainly a sound collector.

Pinworm infection Threadworms, oxyuriasis.

Pityriasis rosea A noninfectious, noncontagious skin disease of young adults, characterized by scaly patches (128).

Placebo An inert substance such as a sugar pill, without drug effect, given to please the patient or as a comparison with a drug being tested. Oddly, seeming therapeutic benefits and even side effects from placebos are not uncommon. The phenomenon, called the placebo effect, has to be taken account of in the evaluation of drug effects.

Placenta The organ on the wall of the uterus through which the fetus receives nourishment and eliminates wastes. Structures of the implanted embryo grow into the uterine wall and the placenta develops until it occupies about half the area of the uterus at the fourth month of pregnancy. The fetus and placenta are connected by the UMBILICAL CORD. The placenta has a definite life span and is a senile organ by the time labour pains begin. It is expelled as the AFTERBIRTH shortly after the baby is born. It is flat, about an inch thick and six or seven inches in diameter.

Encyclopedia of medical terms

Complications of pregnancy may be caused by a mislocated placenta (*placenta praevia*) or by premature detachment.

Plague An acute feverish disease caused by bacilli (*Pasteurella pestis*). It is primarily a disease of rats and other rodents, which tend to be inhabited by fleas, which can transmit plague to man (57). *Bubonic plague* is characterized by swellings (*buboes*) under the arms and in the groins. *Pneumonic plague* affects the lungs and has a high fatality rate. The plague, or black death, which ravaged Europe in the fourteenth century, was a form of bubonic plague with an exceptionally high incidence of haemorrhage.

Plantar Of or relating to the soles of the feet. The most frequent affliction of this area is *plantar warts* which usually form at points of pressure on the ball of the foot (125).

Plantar reflex (*Babinski sign*) Upward movement of the big toe and downward movement of the other toes when the sole of the foot is stroked; an indication of certain nervous system disorders.

Plaque Patches or unnatural formations on tissues such as on tooth surfaces and on inner arterial walls. *Atheroma*, plaques that are found in walls of arteries, contain some LIPIDS and some connective or scar tissue. They contribute to stiffening of blood vessel walls, narrowing of arteries, choking of circulation, and ruptured arteries, associated with heart attacks.

Plasma The fluid part of the blood, minus the blood cells (96).

Plasma cell A type of white blood cell closely related to *lymphocytes* (100). Multiple MYELOMA and a form of leukaemia are associated with plasma cell abnormalities.

Plasmodium The genus of parasites that cause malaria, transmitted by the bites of mosquitoes (55).

Platelets (*thrombocytes*) Tiny, colourless structures in the blood, about a quarter of the size of a red blood cell, which help to initiate blood clotting (100). They are formed in the bone marrow. Platelets are fragile and short-lived outside the circulation, and there are various methods of salvaging and transfusing them. *Platelet transfusions* may be necessary in some bleeding disorders such as *purpura* (110). Platelet transfusions may be of fresh whole blood, or of recently stored blood collected in specially treated glass containers or plastic bags. Since it is the platelets themselves rather than whole blood which the patient usually requires, a recently developed procedure promises to be less wasteful of hospital blood bank supplies. Platelets for transfusion are separated from blood given by a donor, and the donor's blood, minus the platelets, is returned to his circulation. The donor soon makes new platelets.

Pleura The thin, glistening membrane attached to the outer surface of the lungs and the inner surface of the chest wall (136). The opposed fluid-lubricated surfaces glide over each other as the lung contracts and expands, so that breathing is painless.

Pleurisy Inflammation of the pleura, causing knifelike pains aggravated by a deep breath or coughing. There are wet and dry forms of pleurisy (147).

Pleurodynia Sharp pain in the muscles between the ribs. It is characteristic of *Bornholm disease*, an acute virus-caused epidemic disease.

Plumbism LEAD POISONING.

Pneumoconiosis Chronic inflammation of the lungs, due to long-continued inhalation of various kinds of mineral dusts (152).

Pneumonectomy Removal of an entire lung (522).

Pneumonia Inflammation of the lungs caused by various organisms (41). In the past it was customary to classify pneumonias according to the part of the lung affected – *lobar pneumonia* if a lobe or lobes were involved, *bronchopneumonia* if infection was localized to air sacs connecting with bronchi. Now the trend is to classify pneumonia according to the organism that causes it. A common causative organism is the pneumococcus. The terms *viral pneumonia* and *primary atypical pneumonia* came into vogue after World War II to describe pneumonias not caused by recognized bacteria. Viruses may be implicated, but it is now known that most cases of atypical pneumonia are caused by *mycoplasma*. These are strange organisms like bacteria, but they lack the stiff outer covering that holds conventional bacteria in shape and are enveloped only in a flexible membrane. During the progress of research the organisms have been called *Eaton's agent* and *pleuropneumonia-like organisms* (PPLO), the latter because they resemble organisms which cause a respiratory disease of cattle called pleuropneumonia. They have recently been given a category of their own, the genus *mycoplasma*. Respiratory infection caused by these germs comes on gradually, producing fever, chills, and cough. The patient does not appear to be very ill, and often does not consult a doctor, although he may stay at home from work for a few days with a "bad cold." The organisms are sensitive to tetracycline, an antibiotic. Another form of pneumonia, of which the cause may not be immediately suspected, is parrot fever (*ornithosis, psittacosis*), an infection transmitted by parrots and other birds. Other unusual pneumonias may result from foreign material that gets into the lungs; see ASPIRATION PNEUMONIA.

Pneumothorax Collapse of a lung due to air in the pleural cavity.

Podagra Gout.

Poisonous plants Any plant that is not a familiar food plant is poisonous if parts of it are eaten. That is the safest rule to follow, even though parts of some strange or common plants may be harmless. Children are particularly attracted by berries which look good to eat but may be highly poisonous. They should be taught never to chew or eat unknown berries, leaves, roots, or barks. Many highly toxic plants are cultivated in gardens; others, some of them quite attractive, grow wild.

A partial list of toxic plants includes many cultivated for their beauty: foxglove leaves and seeds, poinsettia leaves, oleander leaves and branches, iris roots, larkspur, delphinium, lily of the valley, monkshood, yew, daphne, Christmas rose, bittersweet. Bulbs of hyacinth, narcissus, and daffodil are toxic; as purchased, plant bulbs may be treated with toxic chemicals. Rhubarb leaves (the stalks are edible), wisteria seeds, any part of laurels, rhododendrons, and azaleas can produce serious poisoning. Play safe by never putting any part of a growing plant into the mouth. Immediate treatment of plant poisoning is emptying of the stomach by inducing vomiting, unless the victim is unconscious or having a fit, and calling a doctor.

Pollen counts Measurements of the number of pollen particles in the air at a given time, made by counting the number of particles adhering to a glass slide covered with sticky material and exposed to the atmosphere.

Pollinosis A state of allergic reaction to inhaled plant pollens; for example, hay fever, asthma (487).

Polyarteritis A rare disease characterized by inflammation and nodular swellings of artery walls, sometimes leading to local death of tissues. Also called *periarteritis nodosa* and *polyarteritis nodosa*. The cause is not known.

Polycystic kidney A congenital developmental defect in which the kidneys are filled with bubble-like cysts (187).

Polycythaemia   Too many red cells in the blood (106).

Polydactyly   More than the normal number of fingers or toes.

Polydipsia   Enormous thirst, characteristic of *diabetes insipidus* (204), and sometimes of *diabetes mellitus*.

Polyps   Smooth outgrowths or tumours of mucous membranes which line body cavities. Usually the polyp hangs from a stem or stalk. Polyps occur most commonly in mucous tissues of the nose (434), uterus (311), and colon (349). They rarely cause symptoms, but nasal polyps may be associated with allergies, and some polyps, as of the colon, may be precancerous and are best removed when discovered. Surgical removal is relatively simple.

Polyunsaturated fats   Much interest has been aroused by well-publicized knowledge that high levels of CHOLESTEROL in the blood may be reduced by increasing the proportion of polyunsaturated fats in the diet. The hope is that reduction of blood cholesterol may slow the process of *arteriosclerosis* (68) which leads to heart attacks. It is not possible to speak with complete assurance about prevention of an extremely complex and incompletely understood process, but most authorities agree that it is unwise to flood the body with large amounts of unsaturated fats (69). Saturated is a technical word referring to bonds between the carbon atoms of fatty acids which combine with glycerol to form fats and oils. These bonds in *saturated fats* contain all the hydrogen atoms they can hold. *Unsaturated* and *polyunsaturated* fatty acids have additional bonds between carbon atoms and can take on additional atoms; thus they are more chemically active. Most of the animal fats and some of the vegetable oils (for example, coconut oil) are formed from fatty acids which are highly saturated. Fish oils, corn oil, sunflower oil, cottonseed oil, and some other vegetable oils are highly unsaturated. The polyunsaturated fatty acid of principal nutritional importance is *linoleic acid*. Most of the fat stored in the adult human body is relatively unsaturated.

Polyuria   Excessive output of urine.

Popliteal   Of or relating to the hind part of the knee joint.

Portuguese man-of-war   Creatures that people call jellyfish sometimes empty beaches in a hurry. The most formidable, not exactly a jellyfish, is the Portuguese man-of-war, a creature – actually composed of many separate organisms – which floats on the surface and drapes scores of tentacles into the depths. The tentacles, as long as 50 feet, contain venom-injecting surfaces for killing prey. The stingers feel like a hot iron to the bather who comes in contact with them. There is immediate pain, burning, feeling of tightness in the chest, and nausea after a minute or so. The muscles cramp and it feels as if every muscle of the body is contracting. The stung areas should be flushed with water while medical help is on the way. The skin may be rubbed with a cloth, or better still, lathered and shaved with a safety razor to remove venomous particles. Antihistamine drugs seem to give the most rapid relief of pain, cramping, and spasm. Persons with weak hearts may be dangerously affected by the man-of-war toxin and should have prompt medical care.

Postpartum   After childbirth.

Postprandial   After a meal. *Postcibal* has the same meaning.

Postural drainage   Use of gravity to assist in draining secretions from the lungs and chest. The patient lies face down over the edge of a bed or table, his head, shoulders, and chest hanging down lower than the waist. In this position, gravity helps to drain secretions. Coughing, and thumping the back encourage drainage.

Precordial   Of or relating to the area of the chest overlying the heart. Precordial pain may or may not come from the heart; there are many structures in this area.

Precursor   Forerunner; something that precedes. In biology, a compound that can be used by the body to form another compound. For example, the body converts vegetable *carotene* into vitamin A.

Premenstrual tension   Cyclic occurrence of emotional symptoms associated with body changes about a week before onset of a menstrual period. Most women are aware of some change in disposition during the premenstrual week and learn to live with it, but some have sufficient distress to seek medical attention. Nervous symptoms such as irascibility, tension, fatigue, moodiness, weepiness, severe enough to upset domestic tranquillity, are not all in the mind but reflect bodily changes. Physical symptoms such as abdominal swelling, weight gain, swelling of the hands, and swelling and tenderness of the breasts, indicate that the fundamental disturbance which provokes emotional irritability is cyclic OEDEMA – transitory retention of fluids, which exert pressure on internal organs and have far-reaching effects. The tension state ends at the onset of menstruation. A doctor may prescribe diuretics, sedatives, stimulants, or other measures according to individual need. Explanation that premenstrual tension is not abnormal is reassuring.

Prenatal   Before birth.

Prepuce   A fold of skin covering the head (glans) of the PENIS or CLITORIS; the foreskin; the part that is removed in circumcision.

Presbycusis   Normal diminution of acuteness of hearing that comes with increasing age (423). Mainly, sensitivity to the highest sound frequencies is reduced while sensitivity to lower frequencies – those most important in conversation and daily affairs – remains good.

Presbyopia   The change in eyesight caused by ageing. It begins to come on in middle life when the lens of the eye loses some of its elasticity and power of ACCOMMODATION. Near objects have to be held farther away to see them distinctly. In a culture that depends on reading, close vision, and paperwork, corrective glasses are a necessity and an aid to efficiency.

Pressure sores   Sores or ulcers resulting from pressure on parts of the body in persons confined to bed for long periods; good nursing care can do much to relieve and prevent them (25).

Priapism   Abnormal, painful, sustained erection of the PENIS, unrelated to sexual stimuli. It may result from obstruction of vessels that drain the organ, from injury to nerve centres, or from stimuli such as bladder stones or PROSTATITIS.

Prickly heat   See MILIARIA.

Primary irritants   Caustic, acid, corrosive, or otherwise irritating substances which are harmful to anyone's skin on first exposure in sufficient concentration; no allergic reaction is involved (124).

Prodromal   Premonitory; early warning signs of an oncoming condition before overt symptoms appear.

Prognosis   A doctor's forecast of the course and duration of an illness based on the best information available to make a judgment.

Projectile vomiting   Forceful ejection of stomach contents (292).

Prolactin   A hormone of the pituitary gland which stimulates milk production (202).

Prolapse   A falling downward of a part from its normal position; for example, *prolapse of the uterus* (314).

Prophylaxis   Prevention of the spread or development of disease, for example by public health measures, vaccination, or inoculation against infections.

Prostaglandins A group of hormone-like substances which occur in minute amounts in virtually all body tissues. The name, something of a misnomer, originated with discovery of the substances in semen, to which the prostate gland contributes. Different prostaglandins (at least sixteen natural forms are known) have different and even opposite effects. Prostaglandins are so versatile that many investigators expect them to become major therapeutic agents if experimental and clinical trials prove their safety and effectiveness in a wide range of conditions. Prostaglandins stimulate or relax smooth muscle, appear to regulate cell behaviour, and inhibit and potentiate hormones. On the evidence of clinical and experimental studies, specific prostaglandins may become valuable drugs for: induction of labour at term; contraception; induced abortion; prevention and treatment of peptic ulcer (by shutting off gastric secretions); induction of delayed menstruation; control of high blood pressure; treatment of bronchial asthma, emphysema, even the common cold (by opening closed airways). Aspirin tends to halt production of prostaglandins, which sheds some light on the way aspirin works. Various prostaglandins can cause fever, inflammation, and headache, symptoms commonly relieved by aspirin.

Prostatectomy Removal of all or part of the *prostate gland* by surgical operation (524).

Prostatitis Acute or chronic inflammation of the *prostate gland* (190).

Prosthesis A substitute for a missing part of the body; for example, artificial eye, limb, or denture.

Prosthodontics The branch of dentistry that relates to the replacement of missing teeth and oral structures by artificial devices.

Proteins Large complex molecules built up of long chains of simpler AMINO ACIDS. Skin, hair, nails, muscles are largely protein. It is the characteristic matter of life. Enzymes which carry out multitudes of living chemical processes of the body are proteins. About one half of the dry weight of the body is protein. Protein constituents of foods are broken down into their constituent amino acids by digestion, assimilated, and the separated parts are reassembled by body cells into specific and unique personal proteins (see GENES, HEREDITY). Bodily synthesis of proteins is essential not only for growth and repair of tissues but for the continuance of the multitudes of chemical processes we live by. Protein elements of foods can be burned for energy if necessary, but carbohydrates and fats are superior energy providers.

Prothrombin A plasma PROTEIN, one of many elements necessary in the complicated processes of blood coagulation. Tests of prothrombin time are used in patients having a tendency to haemorrhage and as a guide to treatment of patients receiving anticoagulant drugs.

Protoplasm Living matter; the material which is the essential matter of living cells, never found in the inanimate world. The word was meaningful years ago when the best that scientists could do was to analyse the cell constituents – carbohydrates, proteins, fats, salts, water, and so on – of what they considered to be one substance. Today, many of the structures and activities of specific elements of protoplasm are known – mechanisms of heredity, protein synthesis, energy transformations, chemical directives of life – and the word is outliving its usefulness except as a very general term for living matter.

Protozoa Single-celled organisms. Most protozoa do not cause disease, but those that do are responsible for malaria, amoebic dysentery, and a number of other diseases (32).

Protruding ears Plastic surgery to correct protruding, flattened, or deformed ears is usually performed on children, but is just as suitable for adults. The operation (*otoplasty*) is performed by means of incisions behind the ears. The procedure takes from an hour to an hour and a half. The patient may be discharged from the hospital as soon as 24 hours after surgery. A bandage is worn over the ears for about one week after surgery, and the ear is further protected during sleeping for another two weeks.

Proud flesh An excess of GRANULATION TISSUE.

Prurigo A chronic skin ailment characterized by small, deep-seated, solid pimples that itch intensely.

Pruritus Severe itching.

Psilocybin A hallucinogenic drug; see chapter 28.

Psittacosis (*ornithosis, parrot fever*) A pneumonia-like disease transmitted by infected birds (42). The disease affects not only birds of the parrot family, but pigeons, chickens, ducks, turkeys, and other birds.

Psoriasis A chronic disease of the skin, of unknown cause, usually persisting for years with periods of remission and recurrence (122). It is characterized by elevated lesions in various parts of the body – elbows, knees, scalp, nails, lower back – covered with dry silvery scales that drop off. General health is rarely affected, although *psoriatic arthritis*, a form of arthritis in the fingers and toes, may develop in some patients.

Psychedelic The word means mind-manifesting, and is applied to drugs which affect the mood and the mind.

Psychoanalysis A system of mental therapy created by Sigmund Freud, originally as a research method to gain insight into mental processes. Essentially, the patient speaks to the psychoanalyst about whatever comes to mind, during a long series of sessions which usually total several hundred hours for a complete analysis. Unconscious conflicts expressed through dreams, slips of the tongue, symbolism, and so on, are interpreted by the psychoanalyst with the object of giving the patient insight into his conflicts and thus lessening their injurious effects. The therapeutic value of psychoanalysis is controversial (509).

Psychomotor seizure A relatively mild form of epileptic attack which the patient never remembers (172). He does not fall but may stagger, make restless movements and strange sounds, and lose contact with his environment for a minute or two.

Psychoneurosis An emotionally based disturbance of the personality, often severe enough to be handicapping, generally a defensive reaction to psychological conflicts.

Psychosis Serious mental illness, disabling, usually requiring treatment in a hospital. Some psychoses have organic causes and others primarily psychological causes or possibly metabolic disturbances too subtle to be identifiable.

Psychosomatic disease A disease, sometimes but not always without accompanying physical causes, in which disturbing emotions of the patient play an important part in inciting, worsening, or continuing the disability (504).

Psychosurgery Operations on parts of the brain to alter a personality. *Prefrontal lobotomy*, an operation in which the frontal lobes of the brain are cut into, at one time had many advocates. Unmanageable, violent, manic patients subjected to this procedure usually become tractable and even amiable, but too often with gross deterioration of personality to a vegetative level. Psychosurgery is a drastic procedure that is resorted to only when other measures have failed.

Psychotherapy Treatment of emotional and mental disorders by psychological methods as opposed to physical or medical methods (509).

Ptomaines Putrid substances produced by decay of dead animal matter. Food poisoning is not caused by ptomaines, which are too malodorous for anyone to ingest. Food poisoning is commonly caused by salmonella or staphylococcus organisms.

Ptyalin An enzyme in saliva which initiates the digestion of starch (330). *Ptyalism* is the condition of excess of saliva; salivation.

Puberty The age at which the reproductive organs become functionally active. It occurs when a person is between twelve and seventeen years old and is indicated in the girl by the beginning of menstruation and in the boy by development of semen and deepening of the voice.

Pudenda The external sex organs.

Puerperium The time of childbirth and return of the uterus to its pre-pregnancy size.

Purpura A disorder of blood coagulation; tiny blood vessels bleed into the skin and mucous membranes, and cause purplish patches to pinpoint haemorrhages (110). There are many causes.

Purulent Containing, exuding, or producing pus.

Pus A fluid derived from the blood, containing many white cells, the response to certain infections.

Pustule A small elevation of the skin containing pus.

Pyaemia Pus in the blood.

Pyelogram An X-ray film showing the pelvis of the kidney and ureter.

Pyelonephritis Infection of the kidney and its urine-collecting pelvis.

Pyloric stenosis In babies, obstruction of the outlet of the stomach due to abnormal thickening of the pyloric muscle that encircles it. The condition is completely relieved by an operation which cuts some of the muscle fibres. In adults, it usually arises from scarring or a growth (292).

Pylorospasm Spasm of the circular muscle at the outlet of the stomach, manifested by PROJECTILE VOMITING of an infant shortly after birth (292). Usually the condition can be corrected by medication which relaxes the muscle and permits normal passage of food to the intestines.

Pyogenic Pus-producing.

Pyorrhoea Literally, flow of pus; a common term for *periodontoclasia*, inflammation and gradual destruction of supporting tissues of the teeth. Pockets form and enlarge between the gum surface and tooth, bacteria and debris fill the pockets, pus forms, and bone is absorbed. Eventually the tooth becomes loose in its socket and is lost from lack of support. The condition can be arrested but lost tissue cannot be restored (380).

Pyrexia Fever.

Pyridoxine One of the B vitamins, commonly designated as vitamin B_6.

Pyrosis Heartburn.

Pyuria Pus in the urine (188).

Q

Q fever A self-limiting disease caused by RICKETTSIAE, resembling pneumonia, often mild and unrecognized (42).

Q.i.d. Four times a day.

Quadriceps The large muscle which extends the thigh.

Quadriplegia Paralysis of both arms and both legs.

Quick A tender, vital part, such as the bed of a fingernail.

Quickening The time about the middle of pregnancy when kicks and flutters within the uterus give unmistakable evidence that life is present.

Quinsy An abscess in and around a tonsil, causing a very sore throat.

Quotidian Occurring every day – usually referring to fever.

R

Rabies (*hydrophobia*) A lethal disease caused by viruses which have an affinity for brain and nervous tissue (54). The virus is transmitted to man by the bite of an infected (rabid) animal. Mere contact of an infected animal with abraded or scratched skin can transmit the disease. Mad dogs are not the only sources of rabies. A considerable reservoir exists in wildlife in certain areas. Bats, foxes, squirrels, and other rabid animals can transmit the disease directly by biting people or indirectly by infecting domestic animals which in turn can transmit the disease by their bites or saliva. The disease is invariably fatal but has an incubation period of a month to a year or more. The incubation period is shortest if bites are inflicted on the head, face, neck, or arms, and are severe and numerous. Prompt Pasteur treatment – daily injection of rabies vaccine for two weeks – usually prevents rabies from taking hold. The treatments are painful and the type of vaccine cultivated in animal nerve tissue sometimes has bad side effects. A newer type of duck-embryo rabies vaccine greatly reduces the serious problem of nervous system reactions. Immediate preventive injections may not be necessary if the biting animal can be caught and kept under observation. If killed, the animal's body and particularly the head should be kept for laboratory studies which can determine whether or not the animal was rabid. If injections have been started, and the animal proves not to be rabid, they can be discontinued. The problem of what to do about the bite of a possibly rabid animal should be turned over immediately to the doctor and local health department.

Radiation sickness Illness resulting from intense or cumulative exposure to sources of radiation. Exposure to massive doses of radiation, as in the neighbourhood of a nuclear explosion, is very rare. An overwhelming dose of radiation is extremely serious if not fatal. Necessary therapeutic use of X-rays may sometimes be followed by mild radiation sickness – lassitude, nausea, vomiting – which usually disappears quickly and can be coped with effectively by the physician or radiologist. There is virtually no threat of radiation sickness from the use of diagnostic X-rays (550).

Radiculitis Inflammation of a spinal nerve root.

Radiograph An X-ray photograph.

Radioisotopes See NUCLEAR MEDICINE.

Radiologist A physician who specializes in the making and interpretation of X-ray studies and applications of radiation (540).

Radiopaque Not transparent to X-rays. Radiopaque substances (for example, BARIUM MEAL) are introduced into parts of the body to give clear delineation of structures which otherwise would not show up distinctly on an X-ray film or fluoroscopic screen.

Radiosensitivity The capacity of tissues to react with different degrees of intensity to radiation. This quality is used in the treatment of some kinds of cancer.

Radiotherapy Treatment of disease by X-rays, radium, radioisotopes, and other forms of ionizing radiation (550).

Radon A radioactive gas given off by the decay of radium. *Radon seeds* are tiny radon-containing tubes of gold or glass for implantation into tumours (551). The gas decays at a steady rate and after a week or so loses all its radioactive power, so no harm is done if radon seeds remain in or are lost in tissues.

Rales Abnormal sounds from the lungs or air passageways, heard over the chest. The sounds, described as coarse, medium, fine, wet, dry, and so on, are not specific but help the doctor to judge the condition of the patient.

Raynaud's disease Intermittent blanching and reddening of the skin, especially of the fingers, brought on by exposure to cold. Blood vessels first constrict, causing pallor and numbness, the affected area becomes blue and then red as large amounts of blood return. An attack may last for minutes or hours. The condition may be secondary to other diseases, but more often the peculiar blood vessel spasms occur without apparent cause; 90 per cent of patients are women. There is some evidence that affected persons may be unusually susceptible to collagen diseases such as SCLERODERMA in later life, but in itself Raynaud's disease is more a nuisance than a serious condition. Patients are usually instructed to protect themselves well against cold, by wearing warm clothes, lined gloves, and overshoes, because a certain amount of exposure to cold is necessary to trigger attacks. Smoking, which tends to constrict superficial vessels, is forbidden. In its most extreme form, Raynaud's disease may lead to dry GANGRENE of the fingers. Surgical severing of nerves which serve blood vessels of affected areas may be resorted to in patients with severe symptoms.

Rectocele A bulging of the rectum through the rear wall of the vagina (315).

Rectum The terminal part of the bowel, about six inches long, ending in the narrow muscular anal canal and anus (336).

Red palms (palmar erythema) The palms often become deep pink or reddish, like a sustained blush, during pregnancy. The reddening, caused by a high level of circulating hormones, fades after delivery and needs no treatment. A similar phenomenon occurs in some patients with cirrhosis of the liver.

Reed-Sternberg cell A type of cell characteristic of HODGKIN'S DISEASE.

Referred pain Pain that does not originate where it hurts. For instance, pain which originates in an inflamed gallbladder may be felt in the back under the right shoulder blade.

Reflex An action in response to a stimulus, occurring without conscious effort or thinking about it (158); for example, dilatation or contraction of the pupil in response to different intensities of light. Some 300 different reflexes have been catalogued. They are useful in helping to diagnose or locate the sites of disorders, infections, or injuries that may involve the nervous system.

Refraction Bending of light waves from a straight line in passing through lenses or transparent structures of different densities. In ophthalmology, the measurement and correction by lenses of defects of the eye (*shortsightedness, longsightedness, astigmatism*) which prevent light waves from being brought to a sharp focus exactly on the retina.

Regional ileitis (*Crohn's disease*) Inflammatory disease of the lower portion of the small bowel (346). The disease may be principally inflammatory, obstructive, or diffuse, with varied symptoms. Total recovery may be made after a single attack and there may be no symptoms for many years although abnormalities of the small bowel still persist.

Medical treatment usually is effective but complications may require surgery.

Regurgitation Effortless bringing up of food from the stomach soon after eating; spitting up of food. Babies are adept at it (297). Not to be mistaken for vomiting. The word also means backflow of blood through a leaky heart valve (76).

Reiter's syndrome A form of arthritis with inflammation of the mucous membrane of the eyes and of the urethra. It resembles rheumatoid arthritis but in many respects is less crippling and is self-limiting.

Relapsing fever Episodes of fever which subside spontaneously, then recur. Specifically, an acute infectious disease caused by organisms spread by lice and ticks.

Renal insufficiency Incapacity of the kidneys to filter toxins adequately from the blood (190).

Renin A kidney protein capable of raising blood pressure by activating *angiotensin*, a powerful pressure-elevating agent.

Resect To cut out a part of an organ or tissue; a term used by surgeons.

Residual urine Significant amount of urine left in the bladder after urination. This symptom in men may be associated with prostate trouble; in women, with CYSTOCELE or pressure of tumours of the uterus.

Respirator A mechanical breathing device for patients whose breathing muscles are paralysed by disease or injury.

Respiratory distress syndrome See HYALINE MEMBRANE DISEASE.

Resuscitation Artificial respiration applied to a person suffering from asphyxia.

Reticuloendothelial system A pervasive mechanism like a network throughout the body, which defends against foreign invaders (102).

Retina The thin light-receiving structure at the back of the eye, composed of ten layers (397). Hundreds of thousands of nerve endings in the retina merge into the optic nerve which conveys impulses to the seeing part of the brain at the back of the head.

Retinitis pigmentosa Hereditary degeneration and atrophy of the retina.

Retinoblastoma A malignant tumour of the retina; a congenital form of cancer occurring in infants and young children. An early sign is a white pupil; this sign in an infant or young child has serious import and immediate medical diagnosis is imperative. Retinoblastoma is life-threatening, but improved methods of treatment, given as soon as the tumour is discovered, usually save life though sometimes at the cost of partial or total blindness. If only one eye is affected, it is usually removed. If both eyes are involved the more seriously affected one is usually removed and the other is treated in the hope of destroying the tumour and preserving as much vision as possible. X-rays, radioactive applicators, photocoagulation, and other measures may be used in an effort to save the eye. The disease is thought to be inherited as a dominant trait.

Retinopathy Any abnormal condition of the retina.

Retractors Instruments designed to hold or pull back the edges of an incision or wound.

Retrobulbar Behind the eyeball.

Retroflexion Condition of being bent backwards.

Retroversion A backward-tilted position of an organ, as a retroverted uterus (313).

Rh disease See ERYTHROBLASTOSIS.

Rheumatism A general term for painful, disabling conditions affecting the joints, muscles, and surrounding structures (474).

Rheumatoid factor An abnormal PROTEIN in the blood of about 70 per cent of patients with *rheumatoid arthritis* (480). The rheumatoid factor acts like an ANTIBODY against one of the patient's own normal body proteins, with resulting inflammation and damage to tissue. This is much like an acquired allergy to a part of one's self. Mechanisms which produce the rheumatoid factor have not been proved to be a cause of rheumatoid arthritis, but better knowledge about the factor may throw light on the fundamental nature of the disease. Tests for the factor are commonly given in diagnosing a suspected case of rheumatoid arthritis.

Rhinitis Inflammation of the mucous membranes of the nose. It may arise from something as common as a cold, or from infections or allergies (491).

Rhinophyma Overgrowth of blood vessels, sebaceous glands, connective tissue, and skin of the nose, giving the enlarged organ a knobbly, reddish, bulbous appearance. The condition is sometimes associated with overindulgence in spirits. Correction is surgical.

Rhinoplasty Plastic surgery of the nose, for cosmetic purposes or correction of deformities (438).

Rhinorrhoea Running nose.

Rhinoviruses A family of 30 or more viruses which are major causes of the common cold.

Rhodopsin A purple pigment in the retina. It is bleached on exposure to light and requires vitamin A for regeneration.

Rhythm method (*calendar method*) A method of contraception which relies on abstinence from sexual intercourse during the fertile phase of the menstrual cycle. OVULATION occurs around the midpoint of the menstrual cycle (213); the fertile period of about one week is assumed to span this midpoint, during which abstinence is practised. If the menstrual cycle is regularly 28 days in length, the fertile period can be counted as beginning eleven days after onset of menstruation and continuing through the eighteenth day (or for extra assurance, beginning on day ten and continuing to day twenty). Menstrual cycles are rarely of exactly the same duration month after month. Calendar records may give a reasonably good average over several months, but if swings are great the accuracy of calculations is lessened. Some subjective signs suggest, but do not positively prove, that an egg has been released and that conception is possible; see OVULATION. In general, for couples who adopt the rhythm method, the safest period when conception is unlikely is the few days just before and just after menstruation.

Rice diet A diet providing about ten ounces of boiled rice a day, with fruit juices and sugar, introduced in 1949 as an adjunct to the treatment of patients with severe high blood pressure. Benefits of the diet have been attributed largely to its very low sodium (salt) content. Since the introduction of antihypertensive and diuretic drugs, it is usually no longer necessary to restrict salt intake drastically.

Rickets A vitamin DEFICIENCY DISEASE of infants, resulting from insufficient dietary vitamin D or insufficient exposure to sunshine, which creates vitamin D from substances in the skin (362). Infantile rickets is manifested by distortion, softening, and bending of incompletely mineralized bones, and sometimes by nodules strung like beads over the ribs. *Renal rickets* is not a deficiency disease but a congenital incapacity of the kidneys to reabsorb the phosphate necessary for normal bone structure.

Rickettsiae Disease-causing microbes smaller than bacteria but larger than viruses. They are transmitted to man by the bites of fleas, ticks, and lice. Among the diseases they cause are *typhus, trench fever*, and *Q fever*.

Rifampicin A recent addition to the antituberculosis drugs; a synthetic antibiotic which, in combination with at least one other well-known drug (isoniazid, streptomycin, ethambutol) is effective in eliminating tubercle bacilli from the sputum of most patients in about twenty weeks.

Ringworm Infection by various fungi of the skin, hair, nails, and scalp (127). The troubles they cause have a general medical name, *dermatophytosis*, and a general word, *tinea*, linked with a name for the affected area, as *tinea capitis, tinea barbae, tinea pedis* (the last is better known as athlete's foot).

Rodent ulcer A form of skin cancer (*basal cell epithelioma*, 130) which does not spread to other areas of the body but which, if long neglected, tends to penetrate deeply and erode soft tissues and bones. The ulcers usually occur on sun-exposed areas of the face, especially at margins of the eyes, lips, nose, and ears. The edges of the ulcer have a rolled appearance. The lesion usually begins as a single pinhead to pea-sized nodule, waxy or pearly, which slowly enlarges by development of other waxy nodules near it and coalescence with them. In early stages before undermining of skin and bones begins, surgical removal or X-ray treatment is effective and leaves little scarring.

Rods Cylindrical structures in the retina, about 100,000,000 to each eye (397). The rods see only shades of grey but are extremely sensitive to faint light and are responsible for most of what we see in dim surroundings. Rods cover most of the cup-shaped RETINA and discern movements which we do not look at directly but perceive at the corner of the eye. There are no rods in the small round spot near the centre of the retina (*fovea*) where all colour vision and fine discriminating seeing takes place. The fovea is composed of different, close-packed nerve structures called CONES.

Roentgen A quantitative unit of X-radiation, used in measuring intensity of exposure.

Root canal A small channel in the root of a tooth, continuous with the pulp chamber above it. A tooth dead or dying from injury to its pulp may sometimes be saved by root filling or root resection (388).

Rosacea See ACNE ROSACEA.

Roseola Any rose-coloured eruption of the skin. *Roseola infantum* is a viral infection of young children producing a fever which lasts three or four days, after which the temperature falls to normal, a skin rash appears, and the child is well (284).

Roughage Indigestible food residues in the intestinal tract, mostly composed of cellulose. A reasonable amount of bulky material is a mechanical aid to intestinal function.

Roundworms Several varieties of worms that invade the human body, gaining entrance by their eggs or larvae in contaminated soil or by hand-to-mouth transmission. The largest of the species is *Ascaris lumbricoides* (59); roundworms of lesser size are HOOKWORMS, WHIPWORMS, THREADWORMS. Good hygiene and cooking are preventive measures.

Royal jelly A substance from the salivary glands of bees, fed by the worker bees to the queen bee. No important nutrient has been reported to be present in royal jelly that cannot be obtained readily from ordinary foods. It has no therapeutic value.

Rubefacient Any agent that makes the skin red.

Rubella See GERMAN MEASLES.

Rubeola Measles.

Rubin test A test of female fertility; also called *tubal insufflation*. It determines whether the FALLOPIAN TUBES through which egg cells are transported to the uterus are open or obstructed. A gas, usually carbon dioxide, is introduced through the cervix under pressure. An instrument records significant changes in pressure as the gas flows through. If the fallopian tubes are open, bubbles of gas pass into the abdominal cavity.

Rugae Wrinkles, folds, elevations, ridges of tissue, as of the linings of the stomach and vagina.

Running ear Chronic discharge from an ear, a warning that serious infection may erupt at any time (427).

Rupture See HERNIA.

Ruptured disc Protrusion of the pulpy, cushioning pad between vertebrae through a tear in the surrounding ligament (454).

S

Sabin vaccine Oral poliovirus vaccine for immunization against polio. It contains weakened live polio viruses which produce an inapparent infection that establishes long-lasting immunity.

Sac A pouch or baglike covering of an organ or tissue; for example, the pericardial sac of the heart, the sac of a cyst, hernia, or tumour.

Saccular Sac-shaped.

Sacroiliac strain Backache in the region of the sacroiliac joints. The sciatic nerve traverses this area and ligaments and muscles are subject to injury. Many mechanisms can produce low back pain; treatment depends upon determination of the cause (453).

Sacrum A large, triangular, curved bone of the lower back, just above the coccyx, composed of five vertebrae fused together. The sacrum forms the back wall of the bony pelvis. On each side of the sacrum is the hipbone, the *ilium*, and their junction with the sacrum forms the *sacroiliac joint*.

Safe period The days during the menstrual cycle when conception is not likely to occur. See RHYTHM METHOD.

St. Anthony's fire Erysipelas (124).

St. Vitus' dance See CHOREA.

Salicylism A condition produced by overdosage with drugs of the aspirin family (salicylates), causing ringing in the ears, rapid breathing, nausea, visual disturbances, dizziness.

Salivary glands The three saliva-producing glands on each side of the face: the *parotid* gland in front of and below the ear (the one that is affected in mumps); the *sublingual* gland under the tongue; and the nearby *submaxillary* or *submandibular* gland (332).

Salivation Excessive secretion of saliva. Ordinary MOTION SICKNESS, irritation of the nervous system, poisoning, local inflammations, certain infectious diseases, and disturbances of the stomach or liver can produce it.

Salk vaccine A killed-virus vaccine for establishing immunity to polio. It is given in spaced injections; booster doses are recommended every two years. Oral polio vaccine (see SABIN VACCINE) is considered to have superiority.

Salmonella A family of bacteria which cause gastrointestinal infections (48). They are the most common causes of FOOD POISONING. There are some 400 varieties of salmonella, one of which produces typhoid fever. Most cases of salmonella food poisoning are not definitely identified. The most frequent symptom is gastroenteritis, ranging from a few cramps to fulminating diarrhoea. A small percentage of recovered patients become carriers of the infection. The organisms are widely distributed in eggs, poultry, and other animal products. Thorough heating, above 74°C (165°F) destroys the organisms.

Salpingitis Inflammation of one or both FALLOPIAN

TUBES (*oviducts*). Symptoms are pain in the lower abdomen, tenderness, discharge from the cervix.

Saphenous veins Two large veins of the leg near the skin surface which sometimes become varicose (90).

Sarcoidosis A disease of unknown cause, somewhat resembling tuberculosis. Small tumours arise in almost any tissue, but particularly in the lungs, skin, bones, eyes, lymphatic system, liver, and muscle (149). The nodules may persist more or less unchanged for years or they may heal and recur. Symptoms vary with the organs affected. There is no specific treatment, but steroids help.

Sarcoma A form of cancer arising mainly from connective tissue. *Osteogenic* sarcoma is a bone tumour, usually requiring amputation of the part. *Ewing's* sarcoma of children and young adults affects the shafts of long bones; the outlook is poor. A somewhat similar tumour, *reticulum cell* sarcoma, is sensitive to X-rays, and treatment by irradiation or amputation offers a good chance of survival.

Saturated fat See POLYUNSATURATED FATS.

Satyriasis Excessive sexual desire in the male.

Scabies The itch; infestation with female mites that burrow tiny tunnels in the skin and lay eggs in them (127).

Scaphoid A small boat-shaped bone of the wrist and of the ankle.

Scapula The shoulder blade.

Scheuermann's disease Wedge-shaped deformation of parts of certain vertebrae; a relatively common cause of backache in adolescents (455).

Schistosomiasis (*bilharzia*) A parasitic disease of the tropics acquired by wading in fresh water where free-swimming forms of a blood fluke penetrate the skin and migrate to various organs by the bloodstream. Snails, in which eggs of the parasite develop into free-swimming larvae, are reservoirs of the disease.

Schlemm, canal of A small channel at the junction of the white of the eye and the cornea through which fluids drain from the chamber of the eye in front of the lens. Narrowing or blocking of the drainage channel builds up pressures within the eye (*glaucoma*, 410). Damage caused by glaucoma cannot be repaired. Glaucoma may be kept from progressing by eye drops, or surgery may be necessary to reopen channels.

Sciatica Not a disease, but a symptom: pain in the back of the thigh and leg along the course of the sciatic nerve. Sciatica may be a form of neuritis (167) or severe forms may result from disc trouble (454).

Scirrhous Hard.

Sclera The strong, elastic outer coat of the eye, visible in front as the white of the eye (394).

Scleroderma A connective tissue disease of unknown cause. The first signs usually appear in the skin of the hands and feet, in patchy areas which gradually involve more and more of the body. The skin slowly becomes hard, thickened, stiff, smooth, and shiny. The face may become mask-like because of loss of flexibility. Internal organs – lungs, heart, digestive tract, kidneys – are progressively affected. There is no specific treatment.

Sclerosing agents Substances injected to harden and close up blood vessels, as in varicose veins and haemorrhoids.

Sclerosis Hardening of tissue, especially by overgrowth of fibrous tissue. The sclerosing process affects many kinds of tissues; for example, nerve tissue (*multiple sclerosis*) and linings of the arteries (*arteriosclerosis*). What initiates and perpetuates the process is not understood.

Scoliosis Sideways curvature of the spine (455).

Scorbutus SCURVY.

Scotoma A blind or partially blind area in the field of vision, indicating some change in the optic nerve or retina requiring examination by an ophthalmologist. *Scintillating scotomas*, frequently coloured, which have saw-toothed shimmering edges and spread out from a small spot to a large area then disappear in a few minutes, are often migraine-like phenomena.

Scratch test A skin test for allergic sensitivity, especially to inhaled and contacted substances, done by scratching test materials lightly into the skin without drawing blood (490). If the patient is sensitive to the substance, a positive reaction appears within a few minutes.

Scrofula Tuberculosis of lymph nodes of the neck. The affliction was once common but has almost vanished since the advent of modern methods of treating tuberculosis.

Scrotum The pouch containing the testicles (185).

Scrub typhus (*tsutsugamushi fever*) A feverish disease from eastern Asia, transmitted by mites.

Scurf Minute skin particles shed by animals. Inhalation of scurf is a frequent cause of allergic reactions.

Scurvy A DEFICIENCY DISEASE due to lack of vitamin C (362), easily preventable and curable by taking the vitamin. Advanced scurvy with its classic symptoms of spongy, bleeding gums, loose teeth, and haemorrhages under the skin is now rare, but mild scurvy due to monotonous diets, food aversion, or inadequate supplementation of infant foods is still encountered occasionally.

Seasickness See MOTION SICKNESS.

Sebaceous cyst A wen; a localized skin swelling produced by obstruction of the outlet of an oil-secreting gland (122).

Sebaceous glands Glands of the skin which secrete *sebum* or skin oil; usually associated with hair follicles. Their function is to waterproof the skin (118).

Seborrhoea Overproduction or change in quality of skin oil secreted by sebaceous glands, producing oily skin, crusts, or scales.

Sedimentation rate The rate at which red blood cells settle out of a prepared specimen of blood under laboratory conditions; useful in diagnosis of certain diseases.

Self-limiting A disease that comes to an end all by itself in a limited time, such as an uncomplicated cold.

Semen The whitish secretion containing SPERMATOZOA which is ejaculated by the male during orgasm. It is a mixture of secretions of the testes and prostate gland, which contributes most of its bulk.

Semicircular canals Three interconnecting fluid-filled canals of the inner ear which lie in planes at right angles to each other (423). Our sense of balance is located here. Fluid in the canals responds to movements and sends information over nerve pathways to the brain.

Semilunar Shaped like a half moon, as the *semilunar valves* of the heart (64).

Seminal vesicles Accessory part of the male reproductive system (185). The two pouchlike vesicles lie behind the bladder. Each consists of a single tube coiled upon itself. The vesicles store spermatozoa and secrete a fluid which is added to secretions of the testes. Infection of the vesicles is rare.

Seminoma A tumour of the testicle.

S.E.N. State-enrolled nurse.

Septal defects Abnormal openings between chambers of the heart which permit blood to leak from one side of the heart to the other (72).

Septicaemia Blood poisoning; fever, prostration, the reaction to growing bacteria in the blood. Since the advent of antibiotics, septicaemia is less common and more controllable.

Septum A partition or wall between two compartments or cavities; for instance, the nasal septum which divides the nostrils.

Sequestrum A small piece of dead bone which has become detached from its normal position.

Serum The amber-coloured fluid of blood that remains after the blood has coagulated and the clot has shrunk. It contains ANTIBODIES to bacteria and toxins. This is the basis of serums and antitoxins for treatment of disease. Animals, commonly horses, are inoculated with gradually increasing doses of bacteria or toxins until they build up large amounts of corresponding antibodies. The animal's serum is withdrawn, purified, and injected to increase the person's resistance to a particular disease.

Serum sickness A reaction to injected animal sera (496). The most common symptom is nettle rash. Some patients have a skin rash; some have fever, pain in the joints, enlarged lymph nodes. Serum sickness is closely related to ANAPHYLAXIS, but much milder, and symptoms do not appear until several days after contact with the offending serum.

Sessile Broad-based; as in a tumour that does not have a stem or stalk.

Sex determination Although sex is almost always evident at birth, there are borderline cases where anomalies of development make the true sex difficult to determine (see HERMAPHRODITE). A guide to determination of genetic sex has been found to be the presence or absence in the subject's body cells of minute particles called *chromatin bodies*, which are visible under a microscope. Female cells contain chromatin bodies. Male cells do not, although the chromatin may be undetectable rather than absent. The sex chromatin method has been used to predict the sex of an infant before birth by study of cells obtained from the fluid which surrounds the fetus.

Sex-linked heredity Certain traits such as COLOUR BLINDNESS and HAEMOPHILIA show a form of inheritance called *sex-linkage*. For example, mothers who do not themselves exhibit a trait may transmit it to their sons, who do exhibit it, but not to their daughters. However, the daughters may carry the trait, which is in turn manifested in their sons. There are many technical and complex differences in sex-linked transmission lines, but the general principle is fairly simple: sex-linked traits occur because the GENES for expressing them are located in the pair of sex CHROMOSOMES which all normal persons possess. A female has two X chromosomes, one from her mother and one from her father, in her pair (XX). A male has an X chromosome from his mother and a Y chromosome from his father (XY). The Y chromosome is smaller and contains fewer genes. Many genes in the X chromosome have no counterpart in the Y. If there is a defective gene in one X chromosome of a woman, she has another X which is likely to be normal and to suppress the defective gene trait (although she still carries it). But the same defective gene in a man's X chromosome is paired with a Y which has no complementary gene to neutralize the trait, which therefore is fully expressed.

Sheehan's disease See PANHYPOPITUITARISM.

Shigellosis See BACILLARY DYSENTERY.

Shingles (*herpes zoster*) A virus infection of nerve endings, manifested in the skin by crops of small blisters (167). The face and trunk are most often affected. Red patches appear and develop into fluid-filled blisters which become dry and scabbed in four or five days and eventually heal. The skin should be kept clean and dry and a doctor can prescribe measures to relieve distress. Infection of one nerve may reach the eye and threaten to leave scars on the *cornea*; competent care is important. In older people, shingles is sometimes followed by painful long-lasting *neuralgia* that is difficult to treat. Viruses that cause shingles and chickenpox are thought to be identical. Some adults exposed to chickenpox have developed shingles.

Shoe dermatitis   Not all cases of dermatitis of the feet are due to athlete's foot. Some, which may be mistaken for common fungus infection of the feet, are instances of shoe dermatitis – sensitization and reaction to rubber, leather, dyes, adhesives, and innumerable substances used in the manufacture of shoes. The skin may be dry and scaly, or red and itchy, and crops of small blisters may develop. Sweating and maceration of the skin promote sensitization by irritant substances from the shoes. Shoe dermatitis may first be suspected when treatments for supposed athlete's foot do not give any benefit. Unlike fungus infection of the feet, shoe dermatitis does not affect the webs of the toes or cause crumbling of the nails. Shoe dermatitis may be suspected if both feet are affected in the same symmetrical pattern, which may correspond with the design of the shoes. If the irritation subsides when a particular pair of shoes is not worn, and flares up when they are worn again, some irritant in that pair of shoes may be suspected. Shoes are made of dozens of different materials, and scores of different chemicals are used in processing these materials. Identification of a specific irritant depends upon a PATCH TEST done with samples taken from the patient's shoes. The only remedy is to stop wearing a pair of shoes that gives trouble.

Show   A small amount of red or pink discharge from the vagina indicating the onset of labour.

Sickle cell anaemia   A hereditary abnormality of haemoglobin. Crises marked by fever and attacks of pain occur (108).

Siderosis   A form of *pneumoconiosis*; chronic lung inflammation due to prolonged inhalation of dusts containing minute particles of iron.

Sigmoid   S-shaped; especially, the *sigmoid flexure*, in the part of the colon above the rectum.

Silicosis   Lung inflammation caused by inhalation of high concentrations of very fine particles of silicon over a period of time (150).

Simmonds's disease   See PANHYPOPITUITARISM.

Singer's nodes   Nodules like calluses on the vocal cords of singers, orators, and others who use the voice to excess.

Singultus   HICCUPS.

Sinus   A hollow space, cavity, recess, pocket, dilated channel, suppurating tract. Of the scores of medically designated sinuses, the *paranasal sinuses* – membrane-lined cavities in bones around the nose – are most familiar to laymen (434). *Sinusitis* (inflammation of the sinuses) is experienced to some degree by everyone who has a head cold, and more severely if drainage channels become blocked and congested and infection sets in.

Situs inversus   Transposition of all the organs of the chest and abdomen from the normal side of the body to the opposite side. For example, the liver is on the left side instead of the right. Total transposition does not necessarily impair general health.

Sitz bath   Application of wet heat to relieve pain, congestion, or spasm in the pelvic area, by sitting in a tub of warm water, 48°C (110°F) or more, which covers only the hips and buttocks.

Skin writing   See DERMOGRAPHIA.

Sleep   New insight into sleep has come from studies with the ELECTROENCEPHALOGRAPH, but no one can yet say precisely what sleep is. Brain waves of experimental subjects show that we fall asleep in four stages, from Stage 1 (light sleep) to Stage 4 (deepest sleep), and awaken in reverse order. It takes about an hour and a half to go from light sleep to deep sleep and back again. There are about five such cycles in an average uninterrupted night's sleep of approximately eight hours. At the top, or light sleep phase of each cycle, we are close to waking, and may even wake and go back to sleep without remembering it. Perhaps this is the most critical time for insomniacs who fall asleep easily enough but wake in a little while and cannot get to sleep again. The discovery that dreaming is accompanied by a peculiar but characteristic kind of rapid eye movement has given some new information about dreams. Studies confirm that we generally have the first dream of the night after we ascend to light sleep from the first deep sleep. The average sleeper spends about two hours a night in dreams which occur in four or five cycles corresponding to light sleep. Experimenters believe that everybody dreams repeatedly every night but that dreams are almost immediately forgotten, remembered only if we awaken while a dream is in progress, and then not usually remembered for long.

Sleeping sickness   (*African trypanosomiasis*)   A disease with high fatality caused by organisms that get into the blood through the bites of tsetse flies indigenous to parts of Africa. It is not the same as sleepiness associated with some forms of encephalitis, which used to be called sleepy sickness.

Sleepwalking   (*somnambulism*)   Parents are often concerned about sleepwalking in children; the condition is less common in adults. Sleepwalkers may perform dangerous feats, but they may also injure themselves by falling out of windows or crashing against objects. Anxiety and tension are often strong components of sleepwalking, and investigation of such factors is desirable if sleepwalking persists. The belief that it is dangerous to wake a sleepwalker has no basis in fact. It is better to wake him, to prevent injury to himself or others.

Slipped disc   See RUPTURED DISC.

Slough   A mass of dead tissue cast off from or contained in living tissue.

Smallpox vaccination   See VACCINIA.

Smears   Secretions or blood spread on a glass slide for examination under a microscope. Smears are often stained with various dyes to bring out the details of structure.

Smegma   Thick whitish material that sometimes accumulates under the PREPUCE in men and around the CLITORIS in women.

Snoring   The sounds of snoring are produced by vibrations of air passing in and out over the soft palate and other soft structures. Variations of sound are modified by the force of air flow, frequency of vibration, and the size, density, and elasticity of affected tissues. Sleeping on the back is conducive to snoring, but some people can snore while sleeping on their sides. A few causes of snoring may be correctable; it is worth consulting a doctor to find out. Most cases of snoring in children are associated with enlarged tonsils and adenoids. Snoring is often associated with mouthbreathing, and if blocked nasal passages or predisposing conditions are treatable, the condition can be relieved. Nasal polyps are readily removed, a deviated septum can be corrected, blockages associated with infections and allergies are treatable. However, many snorers cannot be cured and often the best that can be done is to keep them from sleeping on their backs by sewing a rubber ball or something else uncomfortable, into the back of their pyjamas. The most practical remedy, useless to the snorer but of great value to his auditors, is ear plugs.

Soft contact lenses Conventional contact lenses are made of optical glass or hard plastic. Soft lenses are made of water-absorbing plastic which stays soft and supple by absorbing moisture from the eye. Advantages claimed for soft lenses are: easier to fit (the lens moulds to the shape of the cornea); greater comfort; less chance of falling out (soft lenses cover about twice as much eye surface as hard ones). Disadvantages are: greater routine care (daily sterilization); inadequate correction of astigmatism; greater susceptibility to wear and damage; sometimes, alternate clearing and blurring of vision; higher cost. Progress in this field is rapid; improvement of materials and resolution of problems of sterilization are to be expected, as well as probable use of soft contacts as bandages for the eyes in certain conditions, and as carriers of medicines in conditions requiring frequent applications.

Solar urticaria Nettle rash produced by exposure to sunlight.

Solitary kidney A rare congenital condition; only one kidney is present.

Somatic Of or relating to the body.

Somatotype Body build, constitutional type. Somatotyping procedures most widely used today were developed by Dr. William H. Sheldon whose terms, *endomorph, mesomorph,* and *ectomorph* have entered the common medical language. Constitution-classifying is based on the three primitive cell layers of the embryo from which particular organs and systems develop. Skin and nervous system derive from the outside layer, the *ectoderm*. Bones, muscles and vascular system derive from the middle layer, the *mesoderm*. The lining of the gut derives from the inner layer, the *endoderm*. Everyone has all three components, but in varying proportions. The circus weight lifter, fat man, and living skeleton are extreme constitutional types. An extreme mesomorph has a predominance of muscle and bone and a hard, square build. An extreme endomorph has a good digestive tract, soft roundness of body, and great facility for getting fat. An extreme ectomorph with a preponderance of skin and nervous tissue has a slender build and great alertness to what is going on around him. Accurate somatotyping requires accurate measurements and photographing of the nude body.

Somniferous Producing sleep.

Somniloquy (talking in sleep) It is quite common for children to talk in their sleep. Even some adults worry that they may babble secrets when sleeping. Words spoken in sleep are usually fragmentary, mumbled, even ludicrous, and probably indicate participation in dreams or remembered events of the previous day. Talking during sleep probably reflects decreased depth of sleep and is nothing to be alarmed about. See SLEEP.

Spasm Sudden, severe, involuntary contraction of muscles, interfering with function and often causing pain. If tightening of muscle is steady and persistent, as in leg cramps, it is called *tonic* spasm. If contractions alternate with relaxations, causing jerky movements, the spasms are called *clonic*. Both voluntary and involuntary muscles can be affected, causing a variety of *spastic* conditions. Spasms of involuntary muscle may involve the bronchial tubes (ASTHMA), intestines, blood vessels (RAYNAUD'S DISEASE), and sphincters of the gallbladder and urethra. Antispasmodic drugs such as belladonna may be prescribed to ease spastic conditions of involuntary muscle.

Speculum A tubular instrument for viewing the interior of a passage or body cavity; for instance, the vagina, rectum, nose, ear.

Spermatocele A swelling of the SCROTUM caused by cystic dilatation (fluid-filled sac) of the sperm-conducting tubules of the testicle (197). Surgical removal of the painless cyst is usually desirable if it is persistent.

Spermatocide An agent that kills SPERMATOZOA.

Spermatozoa Male germ cells; sperm (185). The sperm is the smallest human cell, and the only one capable of independent locomotion, by virtue of its tail. Sperms are produced in enormous numbers in the seminiferous tubules of the testicle. Primitive cells in the lining of the tubules develop into maturing sperms which fall off and are carried into a coiled tube, the *epididymis*, and thence into a straighter tube, the *vas deferens* (185). The journey takes about two weeks, during which the sperms continue to mature. They do not move under their own power until they are suspended in SEMEN at the time of ejaculation. Sperm production is a continuous process from puberty to old age. The average man produces a vast number of sperms in his lifetime. The average ejaculate contains from 200 to 250 million sperms. An individual sperm has a head, neck, midpiece, and a tail. The head carries the nucleus which contains 23 CHROMOSOMES, one of which is a sex chromosome – either an X (female-determining) or a Y (male-determining) chromosome. The sex chromosome of the human egg is always an X. Hence, it is the sperm that determines the sex of offspring. If the sperm contains a Y chromosome to pair with the X chromosome of the egg, the XY combination produces a boy. If the sperm contains an X chromosome to pair with the X of the egg, the combination produces a girl.

Sperm count A laboratory procedure for estimating the number of SPERMATOZOA in a specimen of semen, useful in assessing male fertility. Although a count of 40,000,000 sperms per cubic centimetre of ejaculate is generally considered normal (counts two to three times greater are not unusual), conception can occur with a relatively low sperm population. Vigorous activity of sperms, and relative lack of abnormal forms, may be more significant to fertility than a relatively low sperm count. If sperms are vigorous and well-shaped, a sperm count of 20,000,000 per cubic centimetre is generally considered adequate for fertility. The volume of ejaculated semen ranges from two to six cubic centimetres.

Sphenoid Wedge-shaped; especially, the bone which lies behind the upper part of the nasal cavity.

Sphincter A muscle which surrounds and controls opening and closing of a natural orifice; for example, the anal sphincter.

Sphygmomanometer The instrument used for measuring arterial blood pressure.

Spider (arterial) Dilatation of small blood vessels in the skin, branching somewhat like the legs of a spider. Spider naevi may be associated with liver disease, pregnancy, varicose veins, and other conditions but may also occur in normal persons.

Spider bite The BLACK WIDOW SPIDER, a common American spider, sometimes reaches the United Kingdom in fruit. Its bite is dangerous.

Spina bifida A congenital malformation of the spine in which some of the vertebrae fail to fuse, so that a sac containing the covers of the spinal cord and even the spinal cord itself may protrude under the skin (170).

Spinal cord The soft column of nerve tissue enclosed in the vertebral column (159). *Spinal nerves* (all the nerves of the body except the twelve pairs of cranial nerves) enter or leave the spinal cord through openings in the vertebrae.

Spirochaete   A microbe shaped like a corkscrew. Many kinds of spirochaetes are harmless, but some cause syphilis, yaws, relapsing fever, tropical ulcer, ratbite fever, and other infections.

Splenomegaly   Enlargement of the spleen.

Split graft   A flap of skin from which the deeper layers have been cut away, leaving the outer layers for grafting (533).

Spondylitis   Inflammation of vertebrae.

Spondylolisthesis   Deformation of the lower spine, due to the slipping forward of a lumbar vertebra, usually on the sacrum (455).

Spoon nail   A nail with a concave outer surface instead of the normal convexity, slightly resembling a spoon; often found in iron-deficiency anaemia.

Spore   An inactive form of a microorganism that is resistant to destruction and capable of becoming active again. For example, TETANUS spores.

Sporotrichosis   Infection by a kind of fungus that is parasitic on plants. The disease produces nodules along the course of lymphatic vessels which enlarge, ulcerate, and discharge pus. Nurserymen, farmers, and persons in contact with plants and woods are most susceptible. The infection is stubborn and may persist for months but usually responds to treatment.

Spotting   A slight show of blood in the vaginal discharge at times other than menstruation. Slight spotting is not uncommon at the approximate time of OVULATION between menstrual periods. Spotting in pregnancy or after the menopause should be reported promptly to a doctor.

Sprain   Tearing or laceration of ligaments that hold bones together at a joint, a result of severe wrenching. Sprains are sometimes difficult to distinguish from fractures; both may result from the same injury (471). Diagnosis should be left to the doctor.

Sprue   See MALABSORPTION SYNDROME.

Sputum   Matter which is coughed up from the lungs – that is, mucus and the substances entrapped in it.

Squint (*strabismus*)   Failure of the two eyes to direct their gaze simultaneously at the same object because of muscle imbalance (407).

S.R.N.   State-registered nurse.

Staghorn calculus   A large stone which more or less fills the pelvis of the kidney and has irregular projecting surfaces resembling antlers (193).

Stamp grafts   Small pieces of skin about the size of a postage stamp, used for grafting (533).

Stapes   A tiny stirrup-shaped bone of the middle ear (419). Fixation of the footplate of the stapes by bone growing around it (*otosclerosis*) prevents free conduction of sound to the inner ear. Several types of operations aim to correct this form of hearing loss (527). *Stapes mobilization* is a procedure to unfreeze the stirrup bone from its surroundings and restore free vibratory movements. In *stapedectomy*, the stirrup bone is replaced by a plastic substitute.

Staphylococci   Spherical bacteria which tend to grow in clumps like a bunch of grapes. They are common inhabitants of the skin and nasal passages.

Stasis   Stagnation; slowing of normal flow of body fluids, blood, intestinal contents.

Status   A severe, refractory condition. *Status asthmaticus*: intractable asthma, extreme difficulty in breathing, cyanosis, exhaustion, lasting a few days to a week or longer (149). *Status epilepticus*: epileptic attacks coming in rapid succession, during which the patient does not regain consciousness.

Steatorrhoea   Stools containing large amounts of undigested fats.

Stein-Leventhal syndrome   A rare condition of sterility, absence of menstruation, and hairiness, in women having enlarged ovaries with many cysts. Treatment is surgical removal of a wedge-shaped section of tissue from each ovary.

Stenosis   Narrowing or constriction of a duct or aperture of the body.

Sterilization   Any procedure which leaves a man or woman incapable of having children; usually, a surgical procedure. See TUBAL LIGATION and VASECTOMY.

Sternum   The breastbone.

Sternutation   Sneezing.

Steroids   Natural hormones or synthetic drugs whose molecules share a common basis of four rings of carbon atoms (the steroid nucleus) but which have different actions according to the attachment of other atoms. Natural steroids include the male and female sex hormones and cortisone-like hormones of the cortex of the adrenal glands (208). Oral contraceptives (the pill) are steroids. Many synthetic steroids increase activity, enhance desired effects, minimize side effects, or otherwise improve the actions of a molecule by shifting, attaching, or detaching a few atoms.

Stethoscope   An instrument which conducts bodily sounds, especially those of the heart, but of other organs as well, to the ears of the examiner. A piece of paper rolled into a cylinder, one end of which is placed on the chest of the patient and the other at the ear of the listener, demonstrates the principle. The stethoscope was invented by René Laennec, a French physician, in 1819.

Still's disease   A disease of children, like rheumatoid arthritis, affecting many different joints.

Stokes-Adams syndrome   Loss of consciousness, and sometimes convulsions, resulting from temporary cessation of the heartbeat in heart block. Nowadays the condition is often alleviated by the use of an electrical pacemaker.

Stomatitis   Inflammation of the mouth. The inflammation may be limited to the mouth or it may be a symptom of some systemic disease. Viruses, bacteria, or fungi may infect the mouth tissues, membranes may be sensitized to certain materials, some drugs may produce oral inflammation. Stomatitis may be an aspect of blood disorders, vitamin deficiencies, mechanical injuries from jagged teeth or ill-fitting dentures, and skin diseases. Treatment is as varied as the causes.

Stool   The bowel evacuation; faeces.

Strabismus   Squint (407).

Stratum corneum   The topmost horny layer of the outer skin or epidermis, composed of dead cells that are shed and replaced from below (118).

Strawberry mark   A birthmark comprised of superficial blood vessels, present at birth or developing shortly after, which has a tendency to disappear spontaneously (120).

Strawberry tongue   A bright red tongue seen especially in scarlet fever; the blood-engorged papillae are enlarged and prominent.

Streptococci   Bacteria which tend to grow like chains of little balls. They are responsible for scarlet fever, sore throat, and many other infections.

Stria (pl. *striae*)   A streak, line, stripe, narrow band. Whitish striations of the abdomen may appear as the skin is stretched during pregnancy and in the breast after milk production ceases. Obesity or an excess of cortisone-like hormones (210) may produce such marks on the abdomen. Striations may appear temporarily in adolescent girls as the sexual hormone balance is established.

Stricture Narrowing or tightening of the passageway of a duct or hollow organ; may result from inflammation, contraction, injury, or scarring.

Stroke Apoplexy, cerebrovascular accident (176).

Stroma The supporting tissue of an organ, as opposed to its active, specific tissue.

Stupe A cloth wrung out of hot water and applied to the skin; turpentine is sometimes sprinkled in the water as a counterirritant.

Subacute An almost acute condition; intermediate between chronic and acute illness.

Subclinical disease A disease, usually mild, that has no definite symptoms or signs which can be recognized by the usual visual or clinical means.

Subcutaneous Beneath the skin, as a hypodermic injection.

Subluxation Partial or incomplete dislocation, sprain.

Substernal Underneath the breastbone.

Sudorific Sweat-inducing.

Sunburn, suntan Prolonged unaccustomed exposure to intense sunlight will, as practically everyone has learned, cause sunburn, which is in every sense a burn. What most people want to acquire is a suntan, not a burn. The amount of sun that individuals can stand varies with thickness, pigmentation, and personal structure of the skin. The sun usually is intense enough to affect the skin between 9.30 a.m. and 4.30 p.m. from April to August. Of the ultraviolet rays: 5% are reflected off the skin surface, 65% absorbed by the horny layers of skin, 27% absorbed by the rest of the epidermis, 3% reach the dermis ("true skin"). To develop a tan without a burn, the skin should be exposed gradually, starting with an exposure of no more than twenty minutes on the first day, increasing exposure by about one third each successive day. After a week the skin should have been conditioned sufficiently to permit a moderate amount of sunbathing through the summer. Suntan is produced by the darkening and moving towards the surface of melanin granules made by cells in deeper skin layers. Exposure to sun not only darkens the skin, but thickens it. The extra thickness gives much of the protection against sunlight, but this thickness lasts only six weeks or so after exposure has ceased. Unlimited exposure to burning rays of the sun has undesirable long-term effects. Continued exposure ages the skin prematurely, thickening and wrinkling it.

Superfluous hair Hirsutism; especially, excessive hairiness of the lips, cheek, chin, or legs of women, more obvious in brunettes. There may be an underlying endocrine disorder (215), a family tendency to hairiness, or hair may be unduly conspicuous in an area where it is not normally present. Electrolysis performed by a skilled operator employs electric current to destroy the hair root permanently, but its application is tedious. Chemical depilatories remove hair satisfactorily but directions must be followed carefully to avoid skin irritation. A bleach may mask the condition if hair growth is fine.

Supernumerary More than the normal number, as a sixth finger or toe.

Suppuration Formation of pus.

Suprarenal glands Adrenal glands (208).

Supraspinatus syndrome A term for disorders of the shoulder region which make it painful or impossible to lift the arm completely (456).

Suture To sew up a wound, or the threadlike materials used for this purpose; catgut, linen, silk, wire, cotton, and so on. *Absorbable* sutures such as catgut are often used to close wounds in deep tissues. Sutures used to sew surface tissues are usually nonabsorbable and removable.

Swimmer's ear Athlete's foot of the ear canal; water incompletely drained from the ear sets up moist conditions favourable to fungus infection.

Sycosis Inflammatory disease of the hair follicles, especially of the beard. Usually a STAPHYLOCOCCAL infection, characterized by pus-filled pimples around hairs.

Sydenham's chorea See CHOREA.

Sympathectomy Surgical removal of fibres of the sympathetic nervous system.

Sympathetic ophthalmia Inflammation of one eye due to injury of the other eye. Prompt treatment of an injured eye is important to prevent involvement of the other eye and possible blindness.

Symphysis The junction of originally distinct bones which have grown together; for example, the lines of fusion of the sacrum and the coccyx, and of the pubic bones.

Symptoms and signs Symptoms are subjective, that is, things of which the patient is aware, such as pain, stiffness, giddiness. Signs are objective, that is, things of which the patient is not aware, but the doctor finds, such as a heart murmur, a lump in the abdomen, or an absent reflex.

Synapse A point of communication between the processes of nerve cells which come close together but do not actually touch.

Syncope Fainting.

Syndactyly Webbed or fused fingers or toes.

Syndrome A set of symptoms which occur together and collectively characterize a disease.

Synovial fluid The clear fluid which lubricates the movements of tendons and joints.

Systemic disease One which affects the body as a whole, not limited to a particular part; for example, an infection spread through the bloodstream.

Systole The period of contraction of the heart. Systolic pressure is the higher of the two figures (such as 120/80) by which doctors express blood pressure readings. See DIASTOLE.

T

Tabes dorsalis See ATAXIA.

Tachycardia Rapid heartbeat (79).

Taenia TAPEWORM.

Talipes Foot deformity; clubfoot (468).

Tampon A plug of absorbent material inserted into a body cavity, such as a pack for nosebleed or a vaginal tampon to absorb menstrual flow.

Tapeworm A ribbonlike flatworm which may invade the intestines of consumers of undercooked beef, fish, or pork (59).

Tapping Emptying fluids from a body cavity by surgical puncture; resorted to when accumulated fluids affect the functioning of the heart, lungs, abdomen, or other organs.

Tarsus The instep of the foot (467).

Tartar (*dental calculus*) Hard, mineralized deposits on the surface of teeth, irritating to the gums and underlying bone (379). Toothbrushing helps to prevent the deposits when they are in a soft state, but they solidify quickly. Periodic removal by a dentist is good insurance against disease of supporting tissues of the teeth, popularly called pyorrhoea.

Tattooing Insertion of permanent colours into the skin through punctures, as by a needle. Unsterilized tattoo needles can transmit viral HEPATITIS and other diseases. In competent medical hands, tattooing has recognized but limited value, primarily for minimizing skin discolorations.

Encyclopedia of medical terms

Portwine stain, a bluish-red birthmark (120), may be made less conspicuous by tattooing opaque skin-coloured pigments into the affected area.

Tay-Sachs disease A hereditary disease occurring mostly in Jewish children, manifested early in infancy, characterized by muscle weakness and blindness. With an ophthalmoscope a characteristic bright cherry spot can be seen at the back of the infant's eye. No known treatment can reverse the condition and life expectancy is short. Certain related diseases which occur later in life do not have a racial incidence.

Telangiectasis Dilatation of groups of small blood vessels, appearing as fine red or blue lines on the skin, sometimes associated with diseases of the skin, cirrhosis of the liver, and other disorders. The dilatations may form hard, red, wartlike spots the size of a pinhead or pea. In *hereditary haemorrhagic telangiectasis*, a rare form, the dilated vessels become thin and fragile, rupture spontaneously, and bleed into the skin, intestines, or other parts of the body. It is inherited as a dominant trait; see chapter 26.

Temporomandibular joint The joint in front of the ear in which the hinge of the lower jaw fits into a socket in the base of the skull. Its close relationship to the teeth may bring about changes not common in other joints. Uneven bite, tooth-clenching habits, poorly fitting dentures, or tooth restorations may limit sideways motion, limit the opening of the mouth, cause pain, soreness, clicking noises, and even headaches.

Tendinitis Inflammation of tendons and their attachments.

Tendon A band or cord of tough white fibrous tissue that connects a muscle to a bone. Muscle fibres merge into one end of a tendon, the other end of which is attached to a bone. Sometimes a tendon conveys muscle action over a considerable distance, as in the back of the leg, where a long tendon inserted into the rear of the ankle transmits the pull of calf muscles above it. This makes it unnecessary to have a huge mass of muscle around the ankle itself. Most tendons are covered by sheaths which secrete lubricating fluid for easy sliding. Tendons and their sheaths are subject to injury by tearing, stretching, twisting stresses (pulled tendon is a common athletic injury) and to inflammations, for which there are technical names such as *tenosynovitis* and *tenovaginitis*.

Tenesmus Painful straining to empty the bowel, without success.

Tennis elbow This painful condition of the outer side of the elbow joint can affect anyone who overvigorously uses a screwdriver as well as a tennis racket. It is a form of BURSITIS produced by violent extension of the wrist with the palm downward or vigorous rotary movement of the forearm against resistance, putting severe stress on the elbow joint.

Teratology The branch of science concerned with the study of malformations. A *teratoma* is a tumour containing hair, teeth, bones, or other material not normal to the part in which it grows.

Term (at term) The end of the normal period of gestation or pregnancy when birth occurs.

Testicles, testes The primary male sex glands or gonads; paired organs, enclosed in the SCROTUM, together with accessory structures (185).

Testosterone The male sex hormone, a STEROID hormone produced by cells of the testicle independent from cells which produce SPERMATOZOA.

Tetanus (*lockjaw*) A serious infection caused by toxins of tetanus organisms which get into the body through perforating, penetrating, or deep wounds and thrive in the absence of oxygen (53). The main features are violent spasms of muscles. The disease is easily prevented by *tetanus toxoid* injections. These are routinely given to infants and should be just as routine for adults.

Tetany Painful muscle spasms, especially of wrists and feet; sometimes convulsions. Insufficient calcium in the blood causes the muscular irritability and consequent symptoms. Insufficiency of circulating calcium may result from vitamin D deficiency or underactivity of the parathyroid glands (207). Treatment is with calcium salts, orally or by infusion if the condition is severe. Not to be confused with TETANUS.

Tetralogy of Fallot Congenital malformation of the heart, exhibiting four defects: aorta turned to the right, ventricular septal defect, constriction of the pulmonary artery or valve, hypertrophy of the right ventricle.

Thalassaemia A congenital form of anaemia which occurs primarily in people native to Mediterranean countries or their descendants (109).

Therapy Treatment of disease. Anything that is therapeutic is designed to help or heal.

Thermography Body surfaces emit slightly different amounts of heat because of local differences in underlying blood supply. This is the principle of thermography, which employs sensitive instruments to scan body areas and record slight heat differentials. Thermography has been used to detect and localize very small breast tumours, to investigate blood vessel obstructions, and to localize the site of the placenta.

Thoracentesis Puncture of the chest wall with a hollow needle for withdrawal of fluid.

Thorax The chest.

Threadworms Small roundworms which may infest the intestines, usually in children.

Thrombin An enzyme present in blood oozing from a wound, but not in circulating blood. It acts upon a blood protein to produce *fibrin*, which is the essential portion of a blood clot.

Thromboangiitis obliterans See BUERGER'S DISEASE.

Thrombocytes Blood PLATELETS, which help to initiate blood clotting.

Thrombocytopenia Deficiency of platelets necessary for blood coagulation, resulting in bleeding from tiny blood vessels into the skin and mucous membranes, known as PURPURA (110).

Thrombophlebitis Presence of a blood clot (THROMBUS) in a vein, with inflammation; *venous thrombosis* (94). Veins of the leg are most commonly affected. If superficial, the affected vein may be felt as a tender cord. Thrombosis of deep veins is serious because blood clots may break off and be carried in the bloodstream until they plug vital vessels. A large piece (EMBOLUS) may reach the lungs and cause death. The tendency of clots to form in slightly injured veins is greatly increased by physical inactivity such as prolonged bed rest. Getting the patient out of bed soon after surgery or childbirth, and encouraging bedridden patients to carry out frequent movements of the legs, are preventive measures. Treatment of active deep venous thrombosis includes such measures as elevation of the foot of the bed, warmth, and anticoagulant drugs which retard blood clotting.

Thrombosis Formation of a clot in a blood vessel, and the partial or complete plugging of the vessel that ensues. The most familiar example is *coronary thrombosis* (71), but the process can occur in many vessels besides those which supply the heart.

Thrombus A clot which forms in a blood vessel and

remains at the site of attachment. If a fragment or the entire clot breaks off and is carried through the bloodstream, it is called an EMBOLUS.

Thrush   See CANDIDIASIS.

Thymus gland   An organ in the chest which for years puzzled anatomists who could find no function for it. Recent research has shown that immediately after birth, the thymus begins to activate the body's defences against infections. The thymus produces and sends out millions of *lymphocytes* (100) to the spleen and lymph nodes, where they synthesize ANTIBODIES. Once these seedbeds are established with the aid of a hormone from the thymus, production of lymphocytes in lymphoid tissues continues throughout life. The thymus then shrinks. In infants the thymus is a large organ, relative to body size. It continues to grow for eight to ten years. By that time the body's immunity systems are running smoothly and the thymus is no longer necessary. The gland begins to shrink and in adults is very small. At one time it was thought that an enlarged thymus was a cause of sudden unexplained deaths of infants, because the thymus of infants dead from infections was much smaller than the thymus of infants who died suddenly from unknown causes. It is now realized that the thymus of infants who die from infections is abnormally small because the gland shrinks rapidly in the presence of infections and stresses, and that a relatively large thymus is normal in infancy.

Thyroglobulin   An iodine-protein substance, the form in which thyroid hormone is stored in the gland (204).

Thyroid   The shield-shaped gland in the neck, covering the front and sides of the windpipe (204). It is a regulator of metabolism, the rate at which the body burns its fuel.

Thyroidectomy   Surgical removal of part of the thyroid gland (525).

Thyroiditis   Acute or chronic inflammation of the thyroid gland (207).

Thyrotoxicosis   Hyperthyroidism; a toxic condition due to excessive activity of the thyroid gland, or to a tumour of the gland (204).

Thyroxine   The hormone released from the thyroid gland (204).

Tibia   The larger and more prominent of the two bones in the lower leg.

Tic douloureux (*trigeminal neuralgia*)   Stabbing, excruciating pain in one side of the face along the course of the fifth cranial nerve, set off by touching a trigger area (167).

Tics   Habit spasms; quick, repetitive movements of certain muscle groups, always in the same manner: pouting the lips, blinking the eyelids, wrinkling the nose, making faces, shaking the head, shrugging a shoulder, tilting the neck, and so on. These nervous habits develop most commonly in children and often disappear in the course of time if the child is not nagged about them. Usually the child is tense to begin with; he may be a target of excessive demands, expectations, and pressures. A little loosening of the reins by those who hold them may help to relax a child who, after all, does not consciously decide to indulge in tics. Nervous habits should be distinguished from purposeless movements associated with some physical disorder. Genuine tics never appear during sleep.

T.i.d.   Three times a day.

Tinea   Ringworm; fungus infection of the skin (126).

Tinea cruris (*Dhobi itch*)   Ringworm of the groin; a fungus infection of the skin of the upper thighs near the genital organs (126). It is caused by the same group of organisms responsible for athlete's foot. Because the symptoms are similar to those of psoriasis and other skin diseases, a doctor should be consulted. It is easily cured.

Tine test   A form of TUBERCULIN TEST. A small disposable stainless steel disc with four prongs covered with dried *tuberculin* is pressed into the skin. The unit is used on only one patient, never reused. The technique is advantageous in screening large population groups of school children and susceptible young adults for tuberculosis.

Tinnitus   Head noises; ringing, roaring, clicking, or hissing sounds in the ears (429).

Tipped uterus   Forward, backward, or other displacement of the uterus from its normal position (313).

Tissue culture   A method of growing cells in a suitable nutrient in flasks or test tubes outside the body, and of propagating viruses in the cells. Polio viruses and some others are grown in tissue culture for manufacture of vaccines. Viruses can be identified by tissue-culture reactions under laboratory conditions. More than 100 new viruses have been isolated and identified by tissue culture techniques in the past decade and some have been associated with diseases.

Tolerance   Ability to withstand abnormally large doses of a drug, induced by its continual use.

Tomograms   X-ray films of layers or planes of the body. A tomogram shows a plane of the body about a half inch thick. The layer shows fine detail but structures above and below it are blurred (548).

Tonometer   An instrument for measuring the pressure in the eyeball, used in screening for *glaucoma* (411).

Tophi   Urate deposits in the external ear, joints, and other structures composed largely of CARTILAGE; characteristic of *gout* (477).

Torticollis (*wryneck*)   A condition in which the muscles of one side of the neck are in a state of more or less continuous spasm, pulling the head into an unnatural position (455).

Toxaemia   A poisoned condition due to absorption into the blood of toxic substances produced by bacteria or body cells, but without the presence of bacteria in the blood. *Toxaemia of pregnancy* is a disturbance of metabolism which in severe form (rare if the patient has good prenatal care) is attended by fever, headache, convulsions, and a rapid rise in blood pressure.

Toxic goitre   THYROTOXICOSIS, hyperthyroidism.

Toxin   A poisonous substance originating in microbes, animals, or plants. Injection of a specific toxin into an animal stimulates the production of specific ANTIBODIES. This is the basis for pharmaceutical preparation of an antitoxin that neutralizes a particular toxin, for example: *botulinus, tetanus, diphtheria, snake venom*.

Toxoid   Resembling a toxin; a substance prepared by treating a toxin with agents which produce a *toxoid* that has the same immunity-stimulating ability as the toxin but is itself harmless and nontoxic. Tetanus and diphtheria toxoids are widely used in routine immunization.

Toxoplasmosis   A disease caused by infection with protozoan organisms. Inapparent infection of a pregnant woman may cause severe abnormalities in her baby.

Tracer elements   See RADIOISOTOPES.

Trachea   The windpipe.

Tracheobronchitis   Inflammation of the windpipe and bronchial tubes.

Tracheotomy   Cutting a hole in the windpipe to bypass an obstruction and permit air to flow into the lungs (526).

Trachoma   A contagious disease of the eyes, caused by viruses which attack the lining membranes of the lids and eyes (408), leading to ulcers and blindness.

Tranquillizers   A popular, nonmedical term for a variety of drugs which more or less selectively depress the central nervous system to produce calming, sedative effects but which, in proper doses, do not dull consciousness or induce sleep. Tranquillizer is a broad term that includes many drugs of somewhat different individual actions. The drugs are often categorized as *major* and *minor* tranquillizers.

The major tranquillizers, most of which belong to chemical families known as *phenothiazines* and *piperazines*, have their greatest use in treating severely disturbed psychotic patients. They tend to reduce agitation, excitement, panic, and hostility, and to quiet the wild destructive behaviour associated with those emotional states, and there may be a reduction of psychotic symptoms such as hallucinations and delusions. This often makes the calmed patient more receptive of and amenable to other forms of therapy. Many patients must continue on the drugs for varying lengths of time, but this often can be supervised by the doctor, and recovery tends to be assisted by a comfortable home and family environment.

The major tranquillizers are sometimes used in non-psychiatric patients for their secondary actions in preventing or arresting nausea and vomiting, and for intensifying the actions of anaesthetics and pain-relievers so that smaller doses of the latter can be given.

The minor tranquillizers (sometimes called *ataractics*) are mainly used to suppress mild to moderate manifestations of anxiety and tension in psychoneurotic patients as well as in normal persons who react tensely to stresses of their environment. Their action is similar to, and probably not superior to, that of the hypnotics in easing anxiety-tension states. However, the classic sedatives cause some drowsiness and loss of alertness; in correct doses, the minor tranquillizers produce mild sedation without dulling consciousness or impairing performance. Some of them have moderate muscle-relaxing action. The minor tranquillizers have a considerably greater margin of safety than potent sedatives, and massive overdosage is less likely to be serious or fatal, although huge overdoses, taken with suicidal intent, can lead to coma, collapse, and even death. Patients who take excessive amounts of the drugs for long periods may become dependent upon them and suffer withdrawal reactions when they are discontinued.

Transillumination Examination of a cavity or structure by means of light passing through it; for example, examination of nasal sinuses with a light in the patient's mouth.

Transplantation Surgical techniques for transplanting an organ from one person to another are well advanced. The best known procedure is kidney transplantation (535), but the heart, lung, liver, and spleen have occasionally been transplanted, demonstrating that surgical techniques of transplantation have been mastered. The major obstacle to permanent transplantation is the body's ultimate rejection of a donated organ as foreign tissue by the patient's immune mechanisms.

Transvestism Desire to wear the clothes of the opposite sex; a person who does so is a *transvestite*.

Trauma Injury, wound.

Traveller's diarrhoea See chapter 30.

Tremor Involuntary quivering and trembling of muscle groups, other than from obvious causes such as shivering from cold. Tremor is a symptom which may give information about a constitutional disease. A doctor may ask a patient to hold out the arms at shoulder level with palms down and fingers stretched; fine, rapid tremor of the fingers may suggest hyperthyroidism. There are fine, coarse, slow, and rapid tremors; harmless hereditary tremors; tremors that appear when at rest; and intention tremor that appears when voluntary movement of a part is attempted. Tremors may or may not indicate a disorder of the nervous system; there are hysterical tremors that have no organic basis.

Trench fever A louse-borne, typhus-like RICKETTSIAL INFECTION. Many cases occurred in World Wars I and II but the disease has since disappeared.

Trench mouth (*Vincent's infection*) Painful, swollen, malodorous inflammation of the mouth and gums (380). The disease is not considered to be contagious. Susceptibility is increased by malnutrition, poor mouth hygiene, and heavy smoking.

Trepanning Cutting a circular section of bone out of the skull with a *trephine*, an instrument with sawlike edges.

Treponema A kind of corkscrew-shaped microbe responsible for a number of infectious diseases, including syphilis (58).

Triceps The muscle that extends the forearm.

Trichinosis (*trichiniasis*) A parasitic disease due to ingestion of encysted larvae of worms present in raw or undercooked pork.

Trichobezoar A ball of hair formed in the stomach.

Trichomoniasis A common infestation of the vagina with minute pearshaped protozoa (310). Their presence produces vaginal irritation and a thin, white, watery, offensive discharge. Men may also be infected but often have no symptoms. Local methods of treatment by insufflation of powders, medicated douches, and so on give relief but the organisms are hard to eradicate. Infection may be retransmitted by marital partners and for total eradication, both partners may be treated. A new oral drug, *metronidazole*, is highly effective in eradicating the infection.

Trichophytosis Ringworm of the scalp (127). The causative fungi fluoresce when exposed to ultraviolet light. The condition, which is contagious, occurs in children before puberty.

Tricuspid valve A valve with three triangular-shaped leaflets through which blood moves from atrium to ventricle in the right side of the heart (64).

Trigeminal neuralgia See TIC DOULOUREUX.

Trigger finger A condition in which efforts to unbend a finger are at first unsuccessful, but it soon straightens with a snap or a jerk, like the release of a trigger. It is caused by a constriction which prevents free movement of a tendon in its sheath.

Trimester Three months, or one third of the nine months of pregnancy. The nine months of pregnancy are traditionally divided into the first, second, and third trimesters.

Triple vaccine Vaccine combining immunizing agents against *diphtheria, pertussis* (whooping cough), and *tetanus*, administered in a single injection instead of separate injections for each disease.

Trismus Spasmodic tightening of muscles of the jaw, as in lockjaw (tetanus).

Trocar A perforating instrument for puncturing a cavity to release fluid; it fits inside a *cannula*.

Tropical ulcer Chronic, tissue-destroying ulceration of the lower leg or foot, caused by a spirochaete.

Truss A device, usually a pad attached to a belt, designed to hold in place a HERNIA or internal organ which tends to protrude.

Trypanosomiasis African sleeping sickness, produced by organisms transmitted to the blood by the bite of an infected insect.

Tryptophane One of the essential AMINO ACIDS. It is frequently inadequate in food protein of plant origin.

TSH Thyroid-stimulating hormone (201).

Tsutsugamushi disease See SCRUB TYPHUS.

Tubal ligation (*salpingectomy*) An operation for sterilization of women. The surgeon makes a small incision in the abdomen and cuts and ties the FALLOPIAN TUBES. This prevents the meeting of sperm and egg and makes conception impossible. The procedure is comparable in severity to an appendix operation and is always performed in hospital. It is frequently performed a few hours after delivery of a baby but can be done at any time for a nonpregnant woman. Tubal ligation does not interfere with menstruation or sexual capacity; the ovaries continue to produce hormones. It is important to regard the sterilization as permanent, but restoration of fertility can sometimes by achieved by a further operation. A recent development entails nipping the tubes with a plastic clip or ring, instead of severing them. This procedure damages the tube less, so that if fertility is desired there is a better chance of this being achieved. It must always be understood that no surgeon, however skilful, can guarantee to re-establish fertility.

The operation is often done with a laparoscope – that is, a special telescope which is passed through the abdominal wall.

Tubal pregnancy Implantation of a fertilized egg in the walls of the Fallopian tube instead of in the uterus; the most common form of ECTOPIC PREGNANCY.

Tubercle A small nodule or prominence; especially, a mass of small spherical cells produced by tubercle bacilli that is characteristic of tuberculosis. The word also means a small rounded prominence on a bone.

Tuberculin test A skin test for tuberculosis (144). Tuberculin in various forms is a sterile fluid containing substances extracted from dead tuberculosis germs. Tissues of a person with tuberculous infection are sensitive to products of tubercle bacilli. Injection of a small amount of tuberculin under the skin gives a positive or negative reaction. A positive reaction, indicated by redness and swelling of the injected area within a few hours, indicates the presence of tuberculous infection but does not tell whether the infection is old or new, active or inactive. It merely indicates that tuberculous infection was acquired at some time.

Tubule A little tube; any minute tubular structure, such as the kidney tubules or the seminiferous tubules of the testes.

Tumefaction Swelling.

Turbinates Scroll-shaped bones of the outer walls of the nasal cavity, covered by spongy tissue which warms, moistens, and filters inhaled air (431).

Turner's syndrome A congenital condition in which the ovaries neither mature nor produce egg cells (214). The affected girl develops along female lines but breast enlargement and menstruation do not occur at puberty, unless the condition is recognized early and treated with female hormones; however, the patient is permanently sterile. A woman with Turner's syndrome has only 45 instead of the normal 46 CHROMOSOMES. One sex chromosome is missing. A normal woman has two XX (female) chromosomes; in Turner's syndrome, one X chromosome is lacking. Its absence results in ovaries lacking egg-producing follicles, and there is retardation of body growth; ultimate adult height is usually less than five feet.

Tussis Cough.

Twins See MULTIPLE BIRTHS.

Tympanoplasty Plastic surgery of the middle ear to clean out and reconstruct the cavity (527).

Tympanum The eardrum, the *tympanic membrane*.

Typhoid fever Acute feverish illness caused by germs of the salmonella family, contained in the faeces of infected patients and unknowing carriers; usually transmitted by contaminated water or food or poor personal hygiene (47). Modern sanitation, alert health departments, and medical progress have made typhoid fever a rare disease where it was once common, feared, disabling, and often deadly. An antibiotic, chloramphenicol, is effective in treating typhoid fever. Vaccination against the disease (three inoculations a week or more apart, and an annual booster dose if one remains in an infected area) is recommended for travellers to regions where typhoid fever is endemic (610).

Typhus A RICKETTSIAL DISEASE transmitted to man by infected lice and fleas, with rats and mice as intermediaries. There are several varieties of typhus (57). The disease is endemic in parts of Asia, the near East, India, and other areas. Vaccination is recommended for travellers to such areas (610).

U

Ulcer An open sore with an inflamed base; local disintegration of tissues of the skin or mucous membranes, leaving a raw, sometimes running surface. The cause may be infection, pressure (as in PRESSURE SORES), erosive irritation (PEPTIC ULCER), varicosities, systemic disease, impaired circulation.

Ulcerative colitis Inflammation of the colon and rectum, characterized by ulcers inside the tube and blood-streaked diarrhoea. The disease may be mild and responsive to medical treatment or so severe as to require surgical removal of the affected part of the colon (349).

Ulna The bone on the side of the forearm opposite to the thumb; its companion bone is the radius.

Ultrasound Sound waves of high frequencies above the range of human hearing. Ultrasonic devices have several medical uses. Instruments which register the echoes of ultrasound have been used to locate and define brain tumours, to locate the position of the placenta and fetus, and to identify the site and severity of arterial obstruction by registering the rate of blood flow in deep vessels. Therapeutically, ultrasonic equipment is used to clean tartar from teeth, to treat bursitis, and an ultrasound probe has had some success in destroying nerve endings in the inner ear, without damage to hearing and the sense of equilibrium, in patients with Menière's disease who have not responded to medical treatment.

Ultraviolet rays Wavelengths of radiation too short to be seen as visible light. They lie between the wavelengths of visible light and X-rays. The spectrum of visible light runs from short violet rays to long red rays. The sequence of colours in a rainbow or sunlight scattered by a prism is violet, indigo, blue, green, yellow, orange, red. Beyond red lie the long invisible *infrared rays*, sometimes used to deliver dry heat to parts of the body. Ultraviolet rays contained in sunshine or produced by ultraviolet lamps (sunlamps) act upon substances in the skin to make vitamin D. They also produce a skin tan (see SUNBURN). These are the only known benefits of ultraviolet rays in moderation. Excessive exposure to natural or artificial ultraviolet radiation can produce burns, and age the skin prematurely. It is wise to ask for and follow a doctor's advice on the use of sunlamps.

Umbilical cord The long flexible cord which is attached to the PLACENTA at one end and to the abdomen of the fetus at the other. It is the lifeline of the fetus. Through vessels of the cord the fetus receives nutrients and disposes of wastes. The cord allows considerable freedom of movement in the womb. The cord continues to function until it is tied and severed at birth.

Umbilical hernia   A protrusion of the intestines through a weakness in the abdominal wall in the region of the navel, not uncommon in infants (279).

Umbilicated   Depressed like a navel.

Umbilicus   The navel, belly-button; a depressed round scar in the middle of the abdomen, a reminder of the umbilical vessels that once nourished the fetus by the placenta.

Uncinaria   HOOKWORMS.

Underweight   Body weight ten per cent less than desirable weight is usually considered to be underweight. However, healthy people vary in bone and muscle proportions and rates of energy expenditure. Underweight may be a symptom of some disease process and should be evaluated by a doctor; sudden unexplained loss of weight requires medical investigation.

Undescended testicles   See CRYPTORCHIDISM.

Undulant fever   See BRUCELLOSIS.

Uniovular   Of or relating to or originating from a single egg, as identical twins.

Universal donor   A person with Type O blood does not have factors which would antagonize the blood of Types A, B, or AB, and hence is presumably compatible with all blood types. However, there are many blood factors besides the ABO group (Rh, M, N, Lewis, Kell, Duffy, Lutheran, and others) which may make the blood of a Type O donor antagonistic to a recipient. A universal donor's blood may be given in an emergency, but cross-matching of blood is necessary for greatest safety in transfusions (103).

Unsaturated fats   See POLYUNSATURATED FATS.

Upper respiratory infection   Infection of nasal passages or throat above the lungs. An infection may extend from the original site of symptoms.

Uraemia   Presence in the blood of toxic substances due to incapacity of the kidney to filter and excrete them in urine; *uraemic poisoning* (189). Symptoms may develop in a few hours or over a period of weeks: headache, dimness of vision, drowsiness, restlessness; later, diarrhoea and vomiting, difficult breathing during the night, convulsions, coma, death. It is the way in which serious kidney disease usually terminates.

Urea   A nitrogen-containing substance in blood and urine, formed mainly from nitrogen groups removed in the liver from the AMINO ACIDS of protein foods. Some is formed from nitrogen released by the wear and tear of body tissues. Increasing the protein portion of the diet increases the output of urea in the urine. The *urea clearance test* of blood is a test of kidney function.

Ureter   The narrow tube through which urine from the kidneys passes into the bladder (184). Urine is not drawn down the tube by gravity, nor does it descend in a steady flow. The ureter has walls of smooth muscle which contract in waves (PERISTALSIS) to move urine into the bladder in jets which occur a few times a minute.

Urethra   The canal from the neck of the bladder to the outside, through which urine is passed. The female urethra is about 4 cm (1½ in) long; the male urethra, 20 to 23 cm (8 to 9 in). Voiding of urine is regulated by circularly arranged sphincter muscles which in the adult are largely under voluntary control.

Urethritis   Inflammation of the URETHRA.

Uric acid   A nitrogen-containing compound present in normal blood and urine. It is derived from substances in the nuclei of cells called *purines*, in which liver, sweetbreads, kidney, and other glandular meats are rich. An excess of uric acid products is characteristic of GOUT (477), a disorder in which tiny urate crystals tend to be deposited in cartilage and cause pain.

Uricaemia   Excessive amounts of URIC ACID in the blood.

Urinalysis   Inspection and chemical analysis of urine. The extent of analysis depends on what the doctor wants to find out. At the minimum, observations of colour, clarity, specific gravity, acidity, sugar, and ALBUMIN content are usually made. More extensive microscopic or chemical analysis of possible constituents – pus, bile, blood cells, crystals, casts – may be necessary to throw light on what is going on in the body (558)

Urine   The amber-coloured, slightly acid fluid secreted by the kidneys. It is mostly water but normally contains about four per cent of dissolved materials such as salt, ammonia, urea, uric acid, hormones or their breakdown products, and pigments. Excessive or deficient amounts of normal constituents may indicate disease, and abnormal constituents – fat, blood, pus, bacteria, spermatozoa, bile – almost always do. Acidity of the urine varies with the diet. Most fruits reduce the acidity of the diet; starvation or a high protein diet increases it. Acidity of the urine indicates that the kidneys are doing their job of maintaining the slight alkalinity of the blood (see ACID-BASE BALANCE). The average adult forms about 1.5 l (2½ pints) of urine a day. The volume of urine is reduced in hot weather, by strenuous muscular exercise or scanty fluid intake, and is greater on a high than a low protein diet. The most concentrated urine is passed after getting up in the morning. Doctors have good reason for specifying that a sample of urine should be taken at a certain time. Formation of urine is decreased during sleep; decided and persistent increase of volume of night urine may be a sign of chronic kidney or other disease. The yellow pigment that gives urine its colour is called *urochrome*.

Urogenital   See GENITOURINARY.

Urologist   A medical specialist in diseases of the urinary tract in females and of the genitourinary tract in male patients.

Uterine tubes   FALLOPIAN TUBES.

Uterosalpingography   X-rays of the uterus and tubes, after injection of iodized oil to determine whether or not the tubes are open.

Uterus   The womb; the pear-shaped, muscular, hollow, distensible home of the fetus in pregnancy. In the adult nonpregnant woman the uterus is about 7.5 cm (3 in) long, 6 cm (2½ in) wide near the top, tapering to a neck (*cervix*) about 2.5 cm (1 in) wide, which occupies the upper part of the vagina. The uterus has walls of smooth muscle with a lining of mucous membrane (endometrium). Its triangular cavity is continuous with a narrow canal through its neck which affords an entrance for SPERMATOZOA and an exit for menstrual discharges. The uterus lies between the bladder and the rectum, tilted forward, its upper part resting on the bladder. It is loosely supported by eight LIGAMENTS which allow freedom of motion and position in adjusting to pressures of surrounding organs and enlargement in pregnancy. The organ enlarges slightly during menstruation, enormously during pregnancy, and after childbirth returns almost to its previous size, but its cavity is larger than before.

Uvea   Pigmentary layers of the eye: the IRIS, CILIARY BODY, and CHOROID coat, composed largely of interlaced blood vessels vital to the eye's nutrition.

Uveitis   Inflammation of the UVEA, and associated eye structures. It is a serious condition that can cause blindness.

It may be associated with systemic diseases (TOXOPLASMOSIS, HISTOPLASMOSIS, LEPTOSPIROSIS), but there are many types of uveal inflammation for which no specific cause can be found. One form is thought to be an AUTO-IMMUNE DISEASE resulting from a patient's sensitization to tissues of the lens of his own eyes.

Uvula The blob of tissue hanging from the soft palate at the back of the mouth. It can be seen with a mirror by opening the mouth wide and depressing the tongue. It rarely causes any trouble, except that it may be implicated in snoring.

V

Vaccine The word derives from the Latin word for cow, the source of cowpox virus used to vaccinate against smallpox. It has come to mean any bacterial or viral material for inoculation against a specific disease. Virus vaccines are of two types, *live virus* or *killed virus* vaccines. Live virus vaccines contain living viruses, so weakened that they cannot cause significant disease, but can still stimulate the body powerfully to make protective ANTIBODIES against a particular disease. Killed virus vaccines contain viruses treated by physical or chemical means to kill or inactivate them so they cannot cause disease but nevertheless can stimulate immunity-producing mechanisms of the body. In general, live virus vaccines are more potent and create longer lasting immunity than killed virus vaccines.

Vaccinia Cowpox; a disease of cattle caused by a virus which, inoculated into man, creates immunity to smallpox. Babies used to be vaccinated against smallpox before they were a year old but routine vaccination is no longer recommended (infants with eczema, impetigo, or skin rashes should not be vaccinated until the condition clears up, nor should they be in close contact with others who have just been vaccinated). About three days after smallpox vaccination a red pimple appears at the site of inoculation, enlarges, becomes a blister, and is surrounded by a reddened area. The lesion begins to dry in a week to ten days. It forms a scab which falls off by the end of the third week or sooner, leaving a flat whitish mark. Reaction to one's first smallpox vaccination is known as a primary take. Reactions in persons who have been vaccinated previously are milder, but if there is no reaction at all it does not necessarily mean that one is naturally immune, but that the vaccine was weak or did not get through the skin. Smallpox is now a very rare disease.

Vacuole A clear space in tissue.

Vacuum extractor (ventouse) A cuplike device within which a partial vacuum is created when it is placed over the presenting part of a baby's head during childbirth. The adherent cup with its handle facilitates extraction of the baby and the device is sometimes used in delivery as a substitute for obstetric forceps.

Vagina A sheath; the female organ of copulation, a muscular canal lined with mucous membrane which opens at the surface of the body and extends inward to the cervix of the uterus.

Vaginal diaphragm A contraceptive device consisting of a spring-rimmed rubber dome inserted into the vagina to cover the cervix.

Vaginal hysterectomy Surgical removal of the uterus through the vagina (322).

Vaginismus Painful spasm of the female pelvic muscles, making sexual intercourse difficult or impossible (309).

Vaginitis Inflammation of the vagina, characterized by discharge and discomfort; see CANDIDIASIS and TRICHOMONIASIS. A form occurring after the menopause is called *atrophic* or *senile vaginitis*.

Vagotomy Cutting of certain branches of the VAGUS nerve. The object is to diminish the flow of nerve impulses, such as those which stimulate the stomach to produce acid (516).

Vagus The tenth cranial nerve which arises in the brain and extends its fibres to the pacemaker of the heart, to the bronchi, oesophagus, gallbladder, pancreas, small intestine, and secretory glands of the stomach.

Valsalva manoeuvre Originally a technique devised by an Italian anatomist for pushing air into the middle ear by exhaling forcibly while keeping the glottis closed. A similar condition is produced by coughing or straining when passing a stool. The manoeuvre is used by cardiologists as a diagnostic test of congestive heart failure. Increase of pressure in the chest and abdomen prevents the return flow of blood from the head, hands, and feet. Heart output decreases and venous blood pressure increases. When the effort is ended, a surge of venous blood into the right side of the heart causes temporary overloading of the heart chambers. The mechanism explains why some persons feel light-headed or dizzy during bowel movements or while coughing.

Valve A structure that prevents backflow of fluids. There are valves in the heart (64), in many veins, at the stomach outlet, and at junctions along many tubes, to keep blood or fluid moving in the right direction.

van den Bergh test A qualitative test of blood serum, useful in determining the origin of different types of JAUNDICE and measurements of liver function.

Varicella Chickenpox (43, 282).

Varices VARICOSE VEINS.

Varicocele Varicose, twisted veins of the spermatic cord; a soft mass in the SCROTUM that feels like a bag of worms. The condition occurs most frequently in adolescence and tends to disappear with maturity. Usually it is a minor affliction, often undetected, causing no discomfort, or sometimes a slight dragging feeling, relieved by wearing a suspensory bandage. Varicocele does not significantly affect the health of the testes or lead to impotence or sterility. Only a few cases warrant surgery.

Varicose veins Swollen, dilated, tortuous veins (90). The site most frequently affected is the legs. Varicose veins frequently develop during, or are aggravated by, pregnancy.

Variola Smallpox.

Vas A tube or vessel, usually applied to the vas deferens.

Vascular Of or relating to or abundant in vessels, especially blood vessels. Well-vascularized tissues have abundant blood supply; *avascular* tissues such as the CORNEA have none.

Vas deferens The duct through which SPERMATOZOA are transported from the testicle to the seminal vesicles and urethra (185).

Vasectomy A simple surgical procedure for sterilization of a man. The excretory duct of the testis (VAS DEFERENS) is severed or a portion cut out of it to prevent SPERMATOZOA from entering the SEMEN. The structures are close to the surface and the operation can be done under local anaesthesia. There is no interference with sexual capacity since the hormone-producing tissues of the testicle are not affected. It is prudent to regard the sterilization as permanent, although in a few cases the severed ends of the ducts have been rejoined, with restoration of fertility. It should be remembered that the sterilizing effect of vasectomy is not immediate. There are still spermatozoa in the seminal vesicles.

Vasoconstrictor A drug or natural substance or mechanism that narrows the calibre of small blood vessels and reduces the volume of blood flowing through.

Vasodilator An agent that dilates small blood vessels so that more blood flows through them; blood pressure is usually lowered. The opposite of VASOCONSTRICTOR.

Vasomotor Of or relating to mechanisms that control dilatation or constriction of walls of blood vessels, and thus the volume of blood flowing through them. Impulses from centres in the brain go to muscle fibres in walls of blood vessels causing constriction or dilatation. Feedback mechanisms of the vasomotor system are exceedingly intricate. In haemorrhage, for instance, the fall in blood-pressure caused by loss of blood makes the vasomotor machinery constrict blood vessels and speed the heart, which tends to restore blood pressure to normal.

Vector A carrier, spreader of disease; especially, an insect or animal host that carries disease germs and transmits them to human beings.

Veins Thin-walled, strong blood vessels that collect dark used blood from tissues and carry it to the heart at low pressure to be pumped through the lungs, where the blood leaves carbon dioxide and takes up oxygen. Blood from capillaries is collected into *venules* (tiny veins) which enter into larger veins and finally into the *vena cava* which opens into the right atrium of the heart. When a vein is cut the blood wells out in a steady flow with no evident pressure.

Venereal warts CONDYLOMA ACUMINATA.

Venesection Bloodletting; same as PHLEBOTOMY.

Ventricle A small cavity or chamber; especially, the ventricles of the heart and brain. The lower part of the heart has a right ventricle which receives venous blood and pumps it to the lungs, and a left ventricle which receives oxygenated blood from the lungs and pumps it to the body (64). The brain has several ventricles filled with CEREBROSPINAL FLUID. Increased volume and pressure of fluid in brain ventricles, due to impaired drainage, results in HYDROCEPHALUS.

Ventriculogram An X-ray of the brain taken after introducing air or a contrast medium into the ventricles.

Venules The smallest veins, communicating with capillaries.

Vermiform Wormshaped.

Vernix caseosa A greasy substance that covers and waterproofs the skin of the fetus.

Verruca A wart.

Version Turning, manipulation of the fetus in the uterus to attain a better position for delivery, such as turning the feet in podalic version.

Vertebra (pl., *vertebrae*) One of the 33 bones which constitute the spine (442). Vertebrae are roughly circular bones with knobs for muscle attachments and a hole in the middle for passage of the spinal cord. Individual vertebrae, except those which are fused to form the SACRUM and COCCYX, are separated by pads of elastic cartilage (*intervertebral discs*) which absorb shocks and give a certain amount of flexibility.

Vertex The highest point of the skull, the topmost part of the head.

Vertigo See DIZZINESS.

Vesicant An agent that produces blisters, such as mustard gas.

Vesicle A small sac containing fluid, like a skin blister.

Viable Capable of living.

Vibrissae Hairs in the nose. Also, a cat's whiskers.

Villi Minute finger-like projections from the surface of a mucous membrane. The small intestine contains millions of villi which increase the surface area in contact with foods (334).

Vincent's infection TRENCH MOUTH.

Virilism Development in a female of masculine characteristics (beard growth, deep voice, and so on), usually due to a masculinizing tumour of the ovary, overactivity of the cortex of the adrenal glands, or administration of androgenic hormones (210).

Viruses Very small agents that may cause disease (32).

Visceroptosis Sagging of abdominal organs from their normal position.

Viscid Sticky, adhesive.

Viscus (pl., *viscera*) An internal organ, such as the intestines, stomach, heart, lungs, and kidneys.

Visual field The area of space seen when the gaze is fixed straight ahead (402).

Visual purple A pigment produced by RODS of the RETINA, essential for good vision in dim light. The purplish pigment bleaches to yellow when exposed to light. A product of its breakdown is vitamin A, which is also needed for its regeneration. Severe deficiency of vitamin A causes night blindness because of the inability of visual purple to regenerate adequately.

Vitiligo (*leukoderma*) Irregular white patches of skin, sometimes streaks of white or grey hair, due to lack of pigment. Often there is a family tendency to develop the condition. The white patches are most conspicuous when surrounded by deeply tanned skin. No infallible way of inducing repigmentation of the spotty patches is known, but in some instances the taking of an oral drug, *methoxypsoralen*, followed by controlled exposure to sunlight, may produce some deposit of pigment. However, results are uncertain and the treatment may cause some irritation of affected areas and excessive pigmentation of surrounding skin. Vitiligo is not a systemic disease but a purely cosmetic defect which, if distressing, can usually be covered satisfactorily with a tinted preparation.

Vitreous humour Transparent colourless material which fills the eyeball behind the lens (395).

Volvulus Twisting or knotting of the bowel, leading to intestinal obstruction and possibly GANGRENE of the part (346).

Vomiting Forcible ejection of stomach contents. A protective mechanism for getting rid of toxic or irritating materials. Ordinarily, vomiting is a transient event of no great significance in itself, provoked by gastric indiscretion, motion sickness, or some infectious illness accompanied by other symptoms. Vomiting from minor intestinal upsets can be managed simply. Either PROJECTILE VOMITING or COFFEE-GROUND VOMIT is a symptom requiring immediate investigation. Intractable, prolonged vomiting (or diarrhoea) can seriously deplete body fluids and ELECTROLYTES, especially in infants who have small reserves. Common causes of ordinary infant vomiting are stomach dilatation from *overfeeding* (too-frequent feeds or too much at a time) or *underfeeding*, leading to hunger, crying, air-swallowing and distension. Too-hot feeds may induce vomiting. Vomiting may be controlled by ice-cold feeds.

von Gierke's disease GLYCOGEN STORAGE DISEASE with involvement of the heart, liver, and kidneys.

von Recklinghausen's disease See NEURO-FIBROMATOSIS.

Vulva The external female sex parts.

Vulvovaginitis Inflammation of both the VULVA and VAGINA. A severe gonorrhoeal form occasionally is transmitted to female infants and children by careless hygiene. See TRICHOMONIASIS and CANDIDIASIS.

W

Wall-eye Outward turning of an eye; divergent squint, a condition of ocular muscle imbalance (407).

Warts Harmless but unsightly small growths from the skin (125). Common warts of the hands, face, and feet, most frequent in children, are caused by viruses, are contagious, and the sufferer may reinoculate himself over and over again. Common warts can be removed by a great variety of methods, including magic, and they tend to disappear in time with no treatment at all. An isolated wart is probably best left alone, unless it is very disfiguring or painful, or is enlarging or changing its appearance, or is in a part of the body subject to constant irritation.

Warts at the edges of fingernails or underneath them are hard to treat; applications of cold – dry ice or liquid nitrogen – are commonly used. Warts in the scalp or beard area are especially troublesome because shaving and combing the hair tend to spread them. A man with warts in the beard area should use an electric shaver.

Wassermann test The original blood test for syphilis. It is not specific for syphilis; false positive reactions may be produced by malaria, hepatitis, mononucleosis, and other unrelated diseases.

Water on the brain HYDROCEPHALUS.

Wax epilation A method of removing superfluous hair, usually of the legs or lips. A waxy compound is warmed to make it fluid and a layer is applied in the direction in which the hair lies. After the layer has hardened, the sheet is pulled sharply against the direction of hair growth. Embedded hairs are pulled out by the roots. The hair follicle is not permanently destroyed, as it is in ELECTROLYSIS. Fine hair tips reappear in two or three weeks, but wax epilation does not leave a stubble as shaving does. Repeated wax epilation tends to damage some follicles and in time to reduce the number of hairs. Slight irritation lasts for a few hours after wax epilation. The treatment is considered to be safe in competent hands, but the skin of some women will not tolerate it.

W.B.C. White blood cell count.

Weals Temporary skin swellings resembling mosquito bites, but often much larger (486). Weals may result from allergy, drugs, irritants, or injection of substances in skin tests of sensitivities.

Webbed fingers Connection of adjacent fingers by a thin fold of skin between them. A similar condition may affect the toes.

Weber test A hearing test to determine which ear hears better by bone conduction. It is performed by touching a vibrating tuning fork to various parts of the head.

Weil's disease An acute feverish illness caused by spirochaetes (54). A severe form of LEPTOSPIROSIS.

Wen A sebaceous cyst, a skin tumour ranging up to the size of a marble or larger, filled with cheesy material; movable, firm, rarely painful. Wens usually occur on the scalp, face, or back, and result from obstruction of an oil-secreting gland. They are harmless, and easily removed.

Whiplash injury A popular term for injury sustained when the head is suddenly thrown forwards and jerked backwards, as in cracking a whip (456). This may occur in car accidents. The injury is something like a sprained neck; muscles and ligaments may be strained and torn but bones and nerves are rarely damaged.

Whipple's disease A rare progressive disease of unknown cause characterized by multiple arthritis, fever, fatty stools, lymph node enlargement, diarrhoea, loss of weight and strength, and abnormalities of the small intestine. Antibiotic treatment continued for many months may reverse the course of the disease, which may possibly be of bacterial origin.

Whipworms Slender worms which inhabit the CAECUM of dogs, pigs, sheep, and goats. Their eggs can be transmitted to man by contact with contaminated soil. The infection may be symptomless or it may produce diarrhoea or acute appendicitis.

Whites Vaginal discharge; see LEUCORRHOEA.

Whitlow See PARONYCHIA.

Whooping cough (*pertussis*) A serious but preventable disease of childhood, especially dangerous and sometimes fatal in young infants whom it readily attacks (43, 286). It can be prevented by immunization, which is often combined with the toxoids of diphtheria and tetanus.

Widal test An ANTIBODY test of blood for the diagnosis of typhoid fever.

Wilms tumour A malignant tumour of the kidney occurring in children (195). The tumour may first be noticed as an abdominal mass by mothers in caring for their babies. Early discovery and immediate treatment (surgery and radiation) give the best hope of permanent cure. Simultaneous administration of an antibiotic which causes the tumour to regress has recently been shown to improve the chances of cure.

Wilson's disease (*hepatolenticular degeneration*) A disease inherited as a recessive trait, see chapter 26. Abnormal deposits of copper in many tissues, especially the brain, eyes, kidneys, and liver, cause damage producing various symptoms as the disease progresses: tremor, clumsiness, psychological disturbances, weakness, emaciation, blue half-moons of the nails, retraction of the upper lip exposing the upper teeth. Treatment is directed to decreasing the intake of copper-rich foods (chocolate, molasses, shellfish, kale, liver, peas, nuts, corn, whole-grain cereals, dried beans, mushrooms, lamb, pork, dark meat of chicken), and use of drugs to prevent absorption of copper and speed its excretion.

Witch's milk A milklike secretion, resembling COLOSTRUM, exuded from the breast of newborn infants of either sex. If left alone, the secretion dwindles and disappears in a few days.

Withdrawal symptoms Physical reactions to withdrawal of certain drugs (narcotics, barbiturates) from persons addicted to them, who have established physical dependence on the drug. The patient has nausea, diarrhoea, a runny nose, watery eyes, chills, waves of gooseflesh. His arms and legs ache, muscles twitch, he perspires and even in hot weather may cover himself with a heavy blanket. Usually the worst is over within a week.

Womb The UTERUS.

Wood's light A device used in diagnosing ringworm of the scalp. Light passed through a special glass filter has no visible rays left but the ultraviolet rays are still present, and cause certain fungi to fluoresce.

Wool-sorters' disease So named because of its occurrence in persons who handle raw animal hides and hairs; *anthrax* (53).

Wrist drop Drooping of the hand at the wrist, inability to lift or extend it, due to paralysis or injury of muscles or tendons which extend the fingers and hands.

Encyclopedia of medical terms

X

Xanthelasma A form of XANTHOMA occurring as soft yellow-coloured plaques on the eyelids.

Xanthoma Yellow tumour; a yellowish nodule or slightly raised yellow-coloured patch in the skin.

Xanthomatosis A generalized condition attended by many deposits of yellowish fatty material in tissues, due to some disturbance of CHOLESTEROL and LIPID metabolism. A hereditary form characterized by yellowish deposits around tendons, especially in the elbows, wrists, and ankles, may appear early in life. It is transmitted as a dominant trait (see chapter 26). In this condition (*familial hypercholesterolaemia*) blood levels of cholesterol are very high and patients have a tendency to develop premature hardening of the arteries. The inborn trait cannot be corrected but blood cholesterol levels may be lowered by stringent dietary restriction of saturated fats.

Xanthopsia Yellow vision, a condition in which objects look yellow. It sometimes accompanies JAUNDICE.

Xanthosis Yellow discoloration of the skin, due to eating excessive amounts of carrots and other vegetables which contain pigments (*carotenoids*) that are deposited in the skin. The condition clears up when yellow vegetable intake is restrained. The condition is harmless.

X chromosome The female sex-determining chromosome: females have two of them, males only one. See CHROMOSOMES. The X chromosome is larger than the Y chromosome and contains some GENES for which there are no complements on the Y chromosome.

X disease An epidemic form of encephalitis, first recognized in Australia, now called *Murray Valley encephalitis*.

Xeroderma Dry skin; a mild form of *ichthyosis* (122). A rare form, *xeroderma pigmentosum*, begins in childhood. Pigmented spots, made worse by sunlight, appear in the skin, and there are scattered TELANGIECTASES.

Xerophthalmia Extreme dryness of membranes which line the eyelids and front of the eye. Lack of tears may cause infection and ulceration of the CORNEA. The condition is associated with NIGHT BLINDNESS and severe deficiency of vitamin A. Specific treatment consists of prescribed daily doses of the vitamin. There are also other causes of xerophthalmia.

Xerostomia Dryness of the mouth, due to deficient salivary secretion, drugs, dehydration, or secondary to fevers or other diseases.

Xiphoid Shaped like a sword; applies to the structure at the lower tip of the breastbone.

X-rays (*roentgen rays*) Electromagnetic radiation of shorter wavelength than visible light. X-rays can penetrate solid substances, produce shadows of structures of different densities on film, and destroy living tissues (540). Some living cells, said to be RADIOSENSITIVE, are more easily destroyed by X-rays than others; this is the basis for the use of X-rays in the treatment of cancer.

Y

Yaws A tropical disease caused by spirochaetes resembling syphilis organisms. It is non-venereal, and possibly transmitted by insect bites. It is characterized by fever, rheumatic pains, red skin eruptions, and destruction of skin and bones of the nose if not treated.

Y chromosome The male sex-determining chromosome. See CHROMOSOME.

Yellow fever An acute, infectious, feverish disease caused by viruses transmitted by the bites of mosquitoes. The disease exists in tropical America where yellow fever is endemic. Travellers should be protected by a vaccine which is highly effective (610).

Yellow spot The *macula lutea*, the small spot near the centre of the RETINA which is the focus of finely detailed vision, and coloured vision.

Yoghurt A milk product formed by the action of acid-producing bacteria. It has the same food value as the milk from which it is made. When made from partially skimmed milk, as it often is, yoghurt is lower in fat, vitamin A, and calories than when it is made from whole milk. Yoghurt is a good source of the other nutrients obtained from milk, especially calcium, riboflavin, and protein.

Z

Zoonoses Diseases of animals transmissible to man.

Zoster, zona SHINGLES.

Zygoma The cheekbone.

Zygote The fertilized egg cell before it starts to divide.

Glossary

It is a convenience for doctors to have their own language. *Tonsillectomy* has exactly half the number of syllables of *surgical removal of the tonsils*. Compound words, although apt to be long, convey a great deal of information. Most importantly, as the majority of medical terms are derived from Greek or Latin they form a common language for doctors in different countries. Words such as patella (kneecap), encephalitis (inflammation of the brain), tracheostomy (an artificial opening made into the windpipe), tomography (a special X-ray technique) and countless others would be understood by any doctor speaking a European language, and many speaking other languages. From the building blocks of these basic roots, words can be built up in all sorts of combinations.

a-, an- Absent, lacking, deficient, without. An*aemia*, deficient in blood.

aden- A gland. Aden*oma* is a tumour of glandlike tissue.

alg-, algia Pain. A prefix such as *neur-* tells where the pain is (*neur*algia).

ambi- Both.

andro- Man, male. An andro*gen* is an agent which produces masculinizing effects.

angi, angio- Blood or lymph vessel. An angi*oma* is a tumour consisting of blood vessels.

anti- Against. An anti*biotic* is "against life" – in the case of a drug, against the life of disease-causing microbes.

arthro- Joint. Arthro*pathy* is disease affecting a joint.

bleph- Of or relating to the eyelid.

bronch-, broncho- The large air passages.

cardi-, cardio- Of or relating to the heart.

carp- The wrist.

-cele Swelling of herniation of a part, as *hydro*cele, *recto*cele.

-cephal- Of or relating to the head. *En*cephal-, "within the head", pertains to the brain.

cervi- A neck.

chol-, chole- Relating to bile. Chole*sterol* is a substance found in bile.

chon-, chondro- Cartilage.

costo-, costal Of or relating to the ribs.

cranio- Skull. As in cranio*tomy*, incision through a skull bone.

cry-, cryo- Cold.

cyan- Blue.

-cyst Of or relating to a bladder or sac, normal or abnormal, filled with gas, liquid, or semi-solid material. The root appears in many words concerning the urinary bladder (cyst*ocele*, cyst*itis*).

-cyte, cyto- Cell. *Leuco*cytes are white blood cells.

dent-, dento- Of or relating to a tooth or teeth.

-derm, derma- Skin.

dia- Through.

-dynia Condition of pain, usually with a prefix identifying the affected part.

dys- Difficult, bad. This prefix occurs in large numbers of medical words, since it is attachable to any organ or process that is not functioning well.

-ectomy A cutting out; surgical removal. Denotes any operation in which all or part of a named organ is cut out of the body.

endo- Within, inside, internal. The endo*metrium* is the lining membrane of the uterus.

-enter-, entero- Of or relating to the intestines. *Gastro*enter*itis* is an inflammation of the intestines as well as the stomach.

eryth-, erythro- Redness. An erythro*cyte* is a red blood cell.

eu- Good. A eu*thyroid* person has a thyroid gland that is normal. A eu*phoric* one has a sense of wellbeing.

gastr-, gastro- Of or relating to the stomach.

-gen- Producing, *gen*erating.

glosso- Of or relating to the tongue.

-gogue Eliciting a flow. A *chole*gogue stimulates the flow of bile.

-gram, -graph These roots refer to writing, inscribing. They appear in the names of instruments which record bodily functions on graphs or charts. The *-graph* is the instrument that does the recording; the *-gram* is the record itself, as *electrocardio*graph and *electrocardio*gram.

gyn-, gynae- Woman, female. Gynae*cology* literally means the study and knowledge of woman, but its common meaning is the medical specialty concerned with diseases of women.

haem-, haemato-, -aem- Pertaining to blood. Haemat*uria* means blood in the urine. When the roots occur internally in a word, the "h" is often dropped for the sake of pronunciation, leaving -*aem-* to denote blood, as in anox*aemia* (deficiency of oxygen in the blood).

hemi- Half. The prefix is plain enough in hemi*plegia*, half paralysis, affecting one side of the body. It is not so plain in *migraine* (one-sided headache), a word which shows how language changes through the centuries. The original word was hemi*crania*.

hepar-, hepat- The liver.

hyal- Glassy, transparent.

hyper- Over, above, increased. The usual implication is overactivity or excessive production, as in hyper*thyroidism*.

hypo- Under, below; less, decreased. The two different meanings of this common prefix can be confusing. Hypo*dermic* might mean that a patient has too little skin. The actual meaning is *under* or *beneath* the skin, the proper site for an injection. The majority of "hypo" words, however, denote an insufficiency, lessening, reduction from the norm, as in hypo*glycaemia*, too little sugar in the blood.

hyster-, hystero- Of or relating to the womb.

ia A suffix indicating 'condition", preceded by the name of the affected organ or system, as *pneumon*ia. A doctor wishing to be more specific might call it *pneumon*itis.

-iasis Indicates a condition, as *trichin*iasis.

-iatro- Of or relating to a doctor. A related root, -*iatrist*, denotes a specialist – *psych*iatrist.

idio- One's own, personal, distinct. As in idio*syncrasy*.

inter- Between.

intra- Within.

-itis Inflammation.

labio- Lips or lip-shaped structures.

leuc-, leuco- White.

lig- Binding. A lig*ament* holds two or more bones together.

lipo- Fat, fatty.

-lith Stone, calcification. Lith*iasis* is a condition of stone formation.

mamma-, mast- Of or relating to the breast. The first root derives from Latin, the second from Greek. *Mamma-* is obvious in *mammal* and *mammary* gland. The *mast-* root is usually limited to terms for diseases, disorders or procedures, as mas*tectomy* (excision of the breast) and mast*oidectomy* (hollowing out of bony processes behind the ear).

mega-, megalo- Large. The prefix *macro-* has the same meaning.

melan- Black. The root usually refers in some way to cells that produce *melanin*, the pigment that produces suntan. But it also endures in melan*choly*, "black bile", a gloomy humour once supposed to be the cause of depression.

men, meno- Of or relating to menstruation, from the Greek word for "month".

metr-, metro- Of or relating to the womb. *Endometrium* is the lining membrane of the womb.

myelo- Of or relating to marrow, and also to the spinal cord.

my-, myo- Of or relating to muscle. *Myocardium* is heart muscle.

necro- Of or relating to death (of a tissue).

nephr-, nephro- From the Greek for kidney. See *ren-*.

neur-, neuro- Of or relating to the nerves.

ocul-, oculo- (Latin) and *ophthalmo-* (Greek) Both roots refer to the eye, "ophth" words more often to diseases.

odont-, odonto- Of or relating to a tooth or teeth.

-oid Like, resembling. *Typhoid* fever resembles typhus fever, or was supposed to when the name was given, but the two diseases are quite different.

olig-, oligo- Scanty, few, little. Olig*uria* means scanty urine.

-oma A tumour, not necessarily a malignant one.

onych-, onycho- Of or relating to the nails of fingers or toes.

oo- Denotes an egg. Pronounced oh-oh, not ooh. The combining form *oophor-* denotes an ovary.

orchi- Of or relating to the testicles. Orchi*dectomy* means the removal of a testicle.

ortho- Straight, correct, normal. Ortho*paedics* literally means straightening out children.

oro, os- Mouth, opening, entrance. From the Latin, which also gives *os* another meaning, to complicate matters. See below.

os-, oste-, osteo- Pertaining to bone. The Latin *os-* is most often associated with anatomical structures, the Greek *osteo-* with conditions involving bone. Osteo*genesis* means formation of bone.

-osis Indicates a condition of production or increase (*leucocyto*sis, abnormal increase in numbers of white blood cells) or a condition of having parasites or pathogenic agents in the body (*pedicul*osis).

-ostomy Indicates the surgical creation of a mouth, opening, or entrance. The opening may be external, as in *colo*stomy, the creation of an artificial outlet of the colon as a substitute for the anus, or internal, as in *gastroenter*-ostomy, establishment of an artificial opening between stomach and intestine. Compare with *-otomy*.

ot-, oto- Of or relating to the ear. Oto*rrhoea* means a discharge from the ear.

otomy Indicates a cutting, a surgical incision (but not the removal of an organ; compare with *-ectomy*). *Myring*otomy means incision of the eardrum.

pachy- Thick. A pachy*derm* is thick-skinned.

paed- Child, hence paed*iatrics*.

para- (Greek) Alongside, near, abnormal. As in para*proctitis*, inflammation of tissues near the rectum. A Latin suffix with the same spelling, *-para*, denotes bearing, giving birth, as *multi*para, a woman who has given birth to two or more children.

path-, patho-, -pathy Feeling, suffering, disease. Patho*genic*, producing disease; *entero*pathy, disease of the intestines; patho*logy*, the medical specialty concerned with all aspects of disease. The root appears in the everyday word *sym*pathy (to feel with).

ped- Of or relating to the foot, as in ped*al*.

-penia Scarcity, deficiency, poverty.

peri Denoting around, about, surrounding Peri*odontium* is a word for tissues which surround and support the teeth.

phag-, -phagy Of or relating to eating, ingesting. As in *geo*phagy, dirt eating; *oeso*phagus, the gullet; phago*cyte*, a cell capable of engulfing and ingesting foreign particles.

phleb- Of or relating to a vein. As in phleb*otomy*, cutting into a vein to let blood; phlebo*thrombosis*, a condition of clotting in a vein.

plast-, -plasia, -plasty Indicates moulding, formation. An objective of *plastic* surgery, as in *mammo*-plasty, an operation for the correction of sagging breasts.

-plegia From a Greek word for stroke; paralysis. *Quadri*plegia means paralysis of all four limbs.

pneumo- (Greek) and **pulmo-** (Latin) Both terms relate to the lungs.

-pnoea Of or relating to breathing. *Dys*pnoea is difficult breathing.

-poiesis Production, formation. *Haemato*poiesis means formation of blood.

poly- Many.

presby- Old. As in presby*opia*, eye changes associated with ageing.

psych-, psycho- Of or relating to the mind, from the Greek word for "soul".

pur-, pus- (Latin) and **pyo-** (Greek) Indicates pus, as in pur*ulent*, *sup*pur*ative*, pus*tule*, and pyo*derma*, suppurative disease of the skin.

pyel-, pyelo- Of or relating to the urine-collecting chamber (pelvis) of the kidney.

pyr-, pyret- Indicates fever.

-raphy A suffix indicating a seam, suture, sewing together; usually describes a surgical operation, such as *hernior*raphy, a stuture operation for hernia.

ren- Latin for kidney; this root form is usually found in anatomical terms, such as ren*al* and *supra*ren*al*. The Greek-derived root, *nephr-*, usually occurs in words describing diseases, for example, nephr*itis*.

retro- Backward or behind.

rhag-, rhagia- Indicates a bursting, breaking forth, discharge from a burst vessel; usually denotes bleeding, as in *haemor*rhage, with an aspect of suddenness.

rhin-, rhino- Of or relating to the nose.

-rhoea Indicates a flowing, a discharge, as in *otor*rhoea, discharge from the ear.

scler- Indicating hard, hardness. *Arterio*sclerosis is a condition of hardening of the arteries.

somat-, somato- Of or relating to the body.

stom-, stomato- The mouth or a similar opening.

supra- Above, upon.

tachy- Indicates fast, as in tachy*cardia*, abnormally rapid heartbeat.

thromb- Blood clot.

-ur-, ure-, ureo- Of or relating to urine.

urethr-, urethro- Relating to the urethra, the tube leading from the bladder for discharge of urine.

veni-, veno- Relating to the veins.

xanth- Yellow.

xero- Indicates dryness, as xero*stomia*, dryness of the mouth.

Index

Main references to a subject are in **bold** type, whereas illustrations or their captions are indicated by page number in *italic*. Where repeated references are made to a subject over several consecutive pages the first page number is given with the letters ff (for "and following pages"). Sub-headings: further detail may often be found where the sub-heading appears elsewhere as a main entry. Extra information, and definitions of some terms, may be found in the **Glossary** and **Encyclopedia** sections on the preceding pages.

Index

nervous disorders 166
noise, excessive 423
"noises in ear" *see*
TINNITUS
otosclerosis 428–9
Paget's disease 470
pressure-change 418–19
speech delay 294–5
stroke 176
tinnitus *see* TINNITUS
wax-blockage 418, 425,
428
see also HEARING;
HEARING AID
decibel 424
defaecation
anal fissure 270–1, 349
haemorrhoids 349
irritability 318, **348**
see also BOWEL; FAECES
deficiency
mental 46, 174 *see also*
RETARDATION
nutritional 359, **362–3**,
470
dehydration 363
child 538
cholera 50
dysentery 48
"hangover" 204
pyloric stenosis 292
salt depletion 182
travel 612, 613
see also PLASMA LOSS
delirium 507–8
delirium tremens 576
delivery of baby
breech **245**
Caesarean section 231,
246, 247
breech presentation
245, 246
diabetics 220, 244
"disproportion" 246
elective/emergency
246
fetal distress 246
haemorrhage 239, 246
placenta praevia 239
subsequent
pregnancies 246
toxaemia 246
date (E.D.D.) 241
forceps 231, **245**
induced **244–5**
accidental
haemorrhage 239
diabetics 220
Rhesus factor 240
toxaemia 240
premature *see*
MISCARRIAGE
vacuum extraction **245**
see also BIRTH; LABOUR
delusion, schizophrenic
507
see also HALLUCINATION
dementia 508

dentine 374ff, **377–8**, 379,
383–5
dentist 374ff
dentures 11, 374, **382**,
390–1
allergy 492
appearance 390–1
care 382, 390
children 374
handicapped people 392
sore mouth 382
ulcers 381–2
deodorant 310
**Dept of Health and
Social Security**
abortion 234
child employment 291
contraception 303
maternity benefits 231
travel 614–15
depression 500, **505–6**
amphetamines 574
in elderly 508
hypothyroidism 206
manic *see* MANIC
neurosis 503–4
postmenopausal 320
postnatal 248, **505**, 508
postoperative 508
situational reaction
501–2
suicide 501–2
see also ANXIETY; TENSION
dermatitis 121, **124**, 131,
489–90ff
dermis 118–19ff
desensitization 148,
497–8
hay-fever 492
see also SENSITIZATION
detergent
allergy 124, 490
development of child
254–60, 273–4
see also BEHAVIOUR;
GROWTH
dhobi itch *see* TINEA CRURIS
diabetes insipidus 204,
221
**diabetes mellitus/
diabetic** 10, **216–21**,
353, 561
boils 124
British Diabetic
Association 221, 298
coma 219–20
complications 218, 220
constipation 348
contraception 220–1, 252
diet 218, 219
eyes 412, 414
feet, care of 220
gangrene 530
heart/artery disease 68,
76, 81, 88
hypoglycaemia 219
insulin 218–20
itching 131, 310

neuritis 166–7
obesity 217
pregnancy 217, 220–1,
244
symptoms 217–18
thrush 126
travel 609
ulcers 93
diagnosis 552–9
dialysis
renal *see* RENAL
diaphragm 136–7, **140**
contraceptive *see*
CONTRACEPTION
hiatus hernia 332, 340–1
diarrhoea 47ff, **274**, **348**
allergy 274, 487, 493
bloodstained *see* FAECES
bottle-feeding 274
coeliac disease 268
cholera 50
with constipation 348,
350
dehydration 50, 363
drugs, cause of 218
dysentery 48
enteritis 346
intestinal disorders **345ff**
pregnancy 226
severe 9
travel 612
"travellers" **59**, 333,
346–7
diet 29–30, 354ff, **370–3**,
561
allergies 489
bland 30
bulk-forming 30
coeliac disease 269, 347
constipation 240, **270**,
348
convalescent 29–30
diabetes 216, **218–19**
diarrhoea 348, 372
elimination 481, 489
fat, low 82, 352, 372
fibrocystic disease 146
galactosaemia 369
gluten-free 269, 347
and heart disease 69, 76,
82
high-residue 30
kidney stone 193
light 29–30
meat-free 340
milk-free 269, 369
normal recommended
356–7
obesity *see* slimming
below
osteoporosis 470
peptic ulcer 344
phenylketonuria 368
piles 349
polyunsaturated fat *in*
372
pregnancy 223, **226**, 370
toxaemia 239, 370–1

reducing *see* slimming
below
salt/sodium, low/poor
30, 76, 189, 239, 370,
372–3
Ménière's syndrome 430
slimming 10, 354, **364–5**,
370
anorexia nervosa
504–5
teeth 385, **386**
therapeutic **370–3**
underweight 368
Wilson's disease 368
digestion 330ff, *355*, 515
digestive juice 330ff, *355*
digestive system/tract
330–53
see also GASTRO-
INTESTINAL
dilatation
and curettage ("D&C")
224, **321**, 557
see also CURETTAGE
dioptre 404
diphtheria 33, **45**, **282–3**
immunization 34, 40, 45,
274, 281
disabled persons
epilepsy 174–5
stroke 179
travel 608ff, 611–12
disc, intervertebral 167,
442, *452*, **454–5**, 528–9
discharge 568
ear 426–7
eye 405, 407
mole 131
nipple (breast cancer)
325–6
vaginal *see* VAGINA
see also BLOOD; MUCUS
discipline 291–2
dislocation 471
**disseminated lupus
erythematosus (SLE)**
483–4
diuresis 200
anti-diuretic hormone *see*
ADH
diuretic drug *see* DRUG
diverticulum
intestinal **518–19**, 545
Meckel's 345, 519
diverticulitis 349, **518–19**
diverticulosis 348–9
divorce 307
children 289
sexual problems 309
dizziness 79, **168**, **429–30**
see also VERTIGO
**DNA (deoxyribonucleic
acid)** 562–3
cancer 569–71
repair 570–1
**doctor, family (general
practitioner, GP)** 9ff,
12–13, 179, 254ff

Index

Index

Index

Index

Index

nicotine 204, 429
 see also SMOKING
nicotinic acid 357, **358**,
 360–1
night blindness 362, 398
nipple 246–7, *324–7*
 pregnancy 223, **228**
 see also BREAST
nits 128
node
 heart 65, 78–9
 Heberden's 462, 476–7
 lymph *see* LYMPH NODE
noise
 excessive 423, 429
 "in ear" *see* TINNITUS
noradrenalin 87, 88, 211
nose **431–9, 491–2**
 allergy 486ff, **491–2**
 congestion 487
 discharge (*see also* MUCUS)
 590–1
 infection 38ff, **433**
 and ears 425ff
 "picking" 292–3
 respiration 139
 rhinophyma 132
 "runny" 435
 sinuses *see* SINUS
 smell, sense of 436–7
 surgery, plastic 438–9
nosebleed 77, 110, 590–1
nucleic acid *see* DNA;
 RNA
numbness
 crush injuries 598
 feet 81
 fingers 460
 nervous diseases 166–7
 diabetic neuropathy
 220
 stroke 177
 pernicious anaemia 106
nurse
 home (district) 13
nursing at home 12–31
nutrient/nutrition
 354–9ff
 see also FOOD
nystagmus 295

O

obesity 10, 363–5
 arthritis 465–6
 breathlessness 142
 contraceptive pill 252
 diabetes 217, 218
 heart disease 69
 hernia 340
 hypertension 89
 incidence 69
 osteoarthrosis 477
 pregnancy 226
 rheumatoid arthritis 483
 see also DIET, SLIMMING; FAT

obsession, neurotic
 503–4, 509
obstetrics/obstetrician
 222ff, 300
 congenital disorders 270,
 560
 ultrasound 549
occlusion
 arterial *see* THROMBOSIS
occupational
 disease/hazard 150
 allergy 486ff, **489**
 anthrax 32–3, 36, 53
 back trouble 453, 455
 brucellosis 52
 cancer 569ff
 deafness 423
 dust, organic 149–50,
 486ff, **489**
 eye injury 405
 leptospirosis(Weil's
 disease) 54
 see also INDUSTRY
occupational therapy
 482
 autism 265
 stroke 178–9
oedema (dropsy) 75,
 93–4
 angioneurotic 129, 493
 baby 240, 247
 beriberi 363
 child 190
 eye 409
 face 189, 190
 nephritis 189
 nephrosis 190
 pregnancy 226, 239, 247
 premenstrual 364
 sodium excess 182
 toxaemia 239
 weight-increase 363–4
 see also FLUID; SWELLING
oesophagitis 341–2
oesophagus/oesophageal
 139, **330–2**, 431, 439–40
 bleeding 342, 343, 351
 disorders **340–3**
 rupture 343
 stricture 340ff, **342**
oestrogen 211, **212–15**
 contraceptive pill 214,
 250
 deficiency 215, 321
 menopause 215, 309,
 320–1
 ovarian tumour 301,
 318–19
 protection against
 infection 307
 therapy 215, 309, 321
 adverse effects 318,
 321
 after ovary-removal
 322
operation *see* SURGERY
ophthalmoscope 401,
 411, 413

opiate/narcotic 573–4,
 580
opium 573–4
 see also DRUG
optician, ophthalmic
 401ff
optic nerve 159, 166,
 394ff, **398–9**
oral contraception *see*
 CONTRACEPTIVE, PILL
oral hygiene 385–6
 dentures 390
 gingivitis 391
 handicapped people 392–3
orbit of eye 394
orchitis 45, 59
orgasm 185, 309–10
orthodontics 391–2
orthopaedics/
 orthopaedic surgeon
 469, **529–30**
osteitis deformans *see*
 PAGET'S DISEASE
osteoarthrosis/osteo-
 arthritis 474, 476–7
 see also ARTHRITIS,
 DEGENERATIVE
osteochondritis
 dissecans 458, 465
osteomalacia 470
osteomyelitis 450–3
osteoporosis 470, 471
otitis
 externa **425–6**
 media **426–7**
 deafness 296
otosclerosis 428–9, 527–8
ovary 212–15, 300ff, *304*
 location 198–9, *213*
 virilism *see* VIRILISM
 see also MENSTRUATION;
 OVULATION
overactivity
 brain 171ff
 manic-depressive illness
 505
overweight *see* OBESITY
ovulation 212–14
 adolescence 304
 contraception 250
 menopause 215
ovum 212ff

P

pacemaker
 artificial 65, 79–80
 natural (sinus node) 65,
 78–9
paediatrics/paediatrician
 coeliac disease 347
 congenital disorders 270,
 273, 279, 560
 cot-death 271
 examination of newborn
 300

Paget's disease 471
pain 9, 119
 anaesthesia 537–8
 childbirth *see* LABOUR
 felt away from injury
 142, 156, 475
 surgery 512ff
 see also DRUG
palate *297, 436*, **439**
 artificial 384
 cleft **384, 441**
 mucous membrane 378
 soft *436, 439*
 see also MOUTH
pallor/paleness 9, 568
 anaemia 105ff, 307
 child
 head injury 268
 stomach ache 295
 heat syncope 614
 hypoglycaemia 219
 leukaemia 287
 shock 593
palpitations
 adrenalin excess 211
 hyperthyroidism 205
 neurosis 503
 pregnancy 227
 see also HEARTBEAT
palsy
 Bell's 166–7
 cerebral 169
pancreas 216ff, 330, *331*,
 334–5, **336–8**, 353
 cancer 343, **353**
 disorders **353**
 enzymes 216–17, 334–5,
 353
 excess 353
 failure 347
 fibrocystic disease 146,
 272–3
 hormone production
 198–9, 353
 laboratory tests 340, 554
 tumours 353
 X-ray 548
panhypopituitarism
 203, 206
Papanicolaou/"Pap"
 test *see* TEST
paracetamol
 child **276**
 convulsions 271
 fever 271, 276
 headache 168
 pregnancy 228
 rheumatoid arthritis
 481
 teething 296, 376
paralysis/paralytic 159
 agitans *see* PARKINSON'S
 DISEASE
 breathing-muscles 51
 diplegia 169
 facial 166–7
 flaccid 164
 general, of the insane 58

Index

Index

712

Index

Index

Index

Acknowledgments

Senior designer
Arthur Lockwood

Designers
Ray Carpenter: Chap 12, 15
Brian Lee: Chap 7, 8, 9, 14, 17, 18
Robert Wheeler: Chap 2, 23, 26, 27, 29

Illustrators
Corinne and Ray Burrows: Chap 1, 2, 4, 5, 11, 12, 14,
    15, 16, 21, 24, 26, 27, 29
Brian Delf: Chap 7, 9, 13
Eleanor Fein: Chap 6, 18, 20, 23
Vanessa Luft: Chap 29 (p. 599, 603)
Gillian Newing: symbols
Michael Woods: Chap 3, 8, 19

Photographers
Geoffrey Drury: Chap 28 (p. 573), 29 (p. 581, 587,
    592, 606)
Daisy Hayes: p. 247
Carolyn Johns: Chap 1, 13 (p. 327–329), 24, 29
    (p. 582, 583, 584, 585, 586, 589, 590, 594, 596,
    597, 603)

Photograph acknowledgments
Abbot Laboratories Ltd (p. 41)
American Hospital Supply (UK Ltd) (p. 80)
Bencard (p. 488)
Camera Press Ltd (p. 39)
Bruce Coleman Ltd (p. 127)
KeyMed Ltd (p. 146)
Mr. James Webb (p. 211)
Churchill Hospital
Guy's Medical School
Nuffield Orthopaedic Centre, Oxford
Radcliffe Infirmary, Oxford

Special thanks to
Dr. Peter Elmes
Dr. Keith Thompson
Professor Gerald Winter and M. Jeremy Shaw

Cover acknowledgment
© Howard Sochurek, from the John Hillelson Agency

Indexer
Judy Batchelor

In-house editor
Ruth Swan